NEET

National Eligibility cum Entrance Test

AF646230

Objective Chemistry

Part–II

NEET

National Eligibility cum Entrance Test

Objective Chemistry

Part–II

Dr. Manu Kaushal

G K Publications (P) Ltd

Title : NEET 2022 : Objective Chemistry Part II - Guide

Language : English

Author's Name : Dr. Manu Kaushal

Typeset & Published by :

Career Launcher Infrastructure (P) Ltd.

A-45, Mohan Cooperative Industrial Area, Near Mohan Estate Metro Station, New Delhi - 110044

Marketed by :

G.K. Publications (P) Ltd.

Plot No. 9A, Sector-27A, Mathura Road, Faridabad, Haryana-121003

ISBN : **978-93-89310-04-7**

Printer's Details : Printed in India, New Delhi.

ABOUT THE AUTHOR

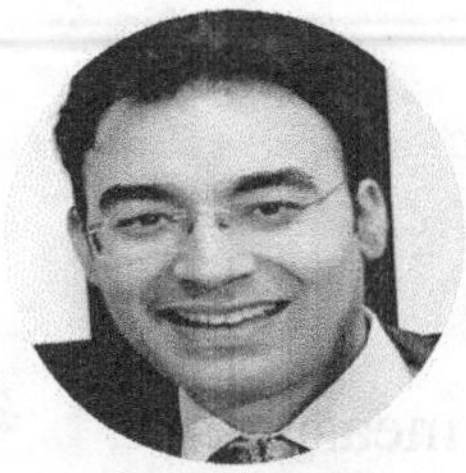

Dr. Manu Kaushal is a renowned faculty of Chemistry and has teaching experience of more than 15 years. He has worked as a senior faculty with institutes like Aakash Institute (New Delhi) and Helix Institute (Chandigarh). Through this book, he wants to share his vast experience with each and every student in India and help them prepare the best for their most important exam.

PREFACE

Students appearing for NEET cannot rely on conventional books and measures to crack the entrance examination. Keeping in mind the cut-throat competition, it becomes mandatory for all the aspirants to have a thorough exposure of all types of problems, especially in Chemistry (Part II).

The objective of this book is to help students get rid of any phobia about Chemistry. Through this book I have made every possible effort to include variety of questions in every chapter.

The questions have skillfully been set along with solutions to help students develop an all round problem solving methodology.

I am thankful to the almighty, my parents, son 'Yuvraj', daughter 'Neyhal' and my wife for their immense support.

I am also thankful to Mr. Nishant Pathak and Mr. Nitin Sharma for their help in writing this book.

Finally, I would like to thank GK Publications (P) Ltd. for giving me an opportunity to write this book. For any queries, you can connect me at 8968706718 (Whats app only)

Regards

Dr. MANU KAUSHAL

CONTENTS

CHAPTER 1

Solid States

Types of Solid, Space Lattice & Its Types

1. Which one of the following is anisotropic & covalent solid?

(a) NaCl (b) Diamond

(c) Copper (d) Tin

2. Identify the mismatch:

(a) Molecular solid → Solid CO_2

(b) Ionic solid → sugar crystals

(c) Covalent solid → Solid silicon

(d) Metallic solid → tungsten

3. The nature of intermolecular forces in silicon carbide are:

(a) London forces (b) Electrostatic forces

(c) Metallic forces (d) Covalent forces

4. A match box exhibits :

(a) Cubic geometry

(b) rectangular geometry

(c) Orthorhombic geometry

(d) monoclinic geometry

5. A metal has primitive cubic lattice with unit cell edge length of 5 Å. Then, the volume of the unit cell (in cm^3) is:

(a) 5×10^{-23} (b) 12.5×10^{-23}

(c) 1.25×10^{-24} (d) 2.5×10^{-24}

6. Which of the following crystal structures has the parameters as: $a = b \neq c$ & $\alpha = \beta = \gamma = 90^\circ$

(a) hexagonal (b) monoclinic

(c) tetragonal (d) orthorhombic

7. The crystal system of a compound with unit cell dimensions, a = 0.387 nm, b = 0.387 nm, c = 0.504 nm & $\alpha = \beta = 90^\circ$, $\gamma = 120^\circ$ is :

(a) Cubic

(b) Hexagonal

(c) Orthorhombic

(d) Rhombohedral

8. Glass is considered a super cooled liquid because it:

(a) Can be moulded into various shapes

(b) becomes crystalline on heating

(c) has a tendency to flow, though very slowly

(d) has a sharp melting point.

9. SO_2 molecules are held in the crystal lattice by:

(a) Covalent bonds

(b) dipole-dipole interactions

(c) Metallic bonding

(d) dispersion forces

10. Match the crystal system in Column-I with their possible variations in column-II.

Column-I	Column-II
(a) Cubic	p. Face centred
(b) Tetragonal	q. End centred
(c) Orthorhombic	r. Body centred

(a) a – p, r; b – q, r; c – p, q

(b) a – p, r; b – r; c – p, q, r

(c) a – q, r; b – r; c – p, q, r

(d) a – r; b – p, r; c – q, r

11. In a bcc lattice, a unit cell is shared equally by:

(a) 8 unit cells (b) 4 unit cells

(c) 2 unit cell (d) 6 unit cells

12. Metals X, Y & Z crystallise in simple cubic, fcc & bcc unit cells respectively. What would be the correct order of metallic radii if volume of each unit cell is same?

(a) $r_x > r_y > r_z$ (b) $r_z > r_x > r_y$

(c) $r_x > r_z > r_y$ (d) $r_y > r_x > r_z$

13. Packing fraction in two dimensional primitive square unit cell is:

(a) $\frac{\pi}{4}$ (b) $\frac{2\pi}{a}$

(c) $\frac{\pi a^2}{4}$ (d) 4π

14. Which of the following is a characteristic of ionic solid?

(a) They have low melting & boiling points.

(b) They are always electrical insulators

(c) Ionic solids when dissolved in water or in molten state, they conduct electricity.

(d) Both (a) & (b).

15. Match the compounds in column–I with their types in column-II

Column-I	Column-II
(i) H_2, Cl_2 & I_2	p. Hydrogen bonded molecular solids
(ii) HCl, SO_2	q. Non polar molecular solid
(iii) H_2O (ice)	r. Polar molecular solid

(a) i – q; ii – r; iii – p

(b) i – r; ii – q; iii – p

(c) i – q; ii – p; iii – r

(d) i – p; ii – q; iii – r

16. In two dimensional square close packing, the co-ordination number is:

(a) 2 (b) 4

(c) 6 (d) 8

17. Which of the following statement is not true about amorphous solids?

(a) On heating they may become crystalline at a certain temperature.

(b) They may become crystalline on keeping for long time.

(c) Amorphous solids can be moulded by heating.

(d) They are anisotropic in nature

18. Which of the following features are not shown by quartz glass?

(a) It is a pseudo solid

(b) Refractive index is same in all directions

(c) It has a definite heat of fusion

(d) It is also called super cooled liquid

19. Match the type of packing given in column-I with the items in column-II.

Column-I	Column-II
(i) square close packing in 2-D	A. Triangular voids
(ii) Hexagonal close packing in 2-D.	B. pattern of spheres is repeated in every fourth layer (ABCABC)
(iii) Hexagonal close packing in 3-D	C. Co-ordination no. = 4
(iv) Cubic close packing in 3-D.	D. Pattern of sphere is repeated in alternate layers (ABABA...)

(a) i – D, ii – A, iii – C, iv – B

(b) i – A, ii – D, iii – C, iv – B

(c) i – B, ii – C, iii – A, iv – D

(d) i – C, ii – A, iii – D, iv – B

20. The axial angles in triclinic crystal system are:

(a) $\alpha = \beta = \gamma = 90°$ (b) $\alpha = \beta = \gamma;\ \beta \neq 90°$

(c) $\alpha \neq \beta \neq \gamma \neq 90°$ (d) $\alpha = \beta = \gamma \neq 90°$

21. In tetragonal crystal system, axial distances or edge lengths are:

(a) $a = b = c$

(b) $a = b \neq c$

(c) $a \neq b \neq c$

(d) $a \neq b = c$

22. Match the unit cell in column-I with their number of lattice points in column-II

Column-I	Column-II
(i) End-centred cubic	p. 9
(ii) Face centred tetragonal	q. 10
(iii) Body-centred cubic	r. 14

(a) i – p, ii – q, iii – r

(b) i – r, ii – q, iii – p

(c) i – q, ii – p, iii – r

(d) i – q, ii – r, iii – p

Formula Making

23. A compound is formed by element X & Y. Atoms of X are in simple cubic lattice while atoms Y are at centre of each face. If atom of X from one corner is missing then the formula is:
(a) X_7Y_{24} (b) XY
(c) X_7Y_3 (d) XY_3

24. In a binary compound having cubic unit cells, the anions B are located at the corners of the cube & face centres whereas cations A occupy all the tetrahedral voids. What is the formula of the compound?
(a) A_2B (b) AB
(c) AB_3 (d) A_2B_3

25. A compound of A and B crystallizes in a cubic lattice in which 'A' atom occupy the lattice points at the corners of a cube and two atoms of B occupy the centres of each of the cube faces. Then, the formula of compound is:
(a) AB_3 (b) AB_4
(c) AB_2 (d) AB_6

26. If the anions (A) form hexagonal closest packing & cations (C) occupy only $\frac{2}{3}$ Octahedral voids in it, then general formula of compound is:
(a) CA (b) CA_2
(c) C_2A_3 (d) C_3A_2

27. The formula of compound made of P, Q, R and S with P occupying all the corners of a cube, two Q on each face diagnol, two R on each body diagnol and S present at the body centre and at all edge centres, is :
(a) $PQ_{11}R_4S_8$ (b) $PQ_{12}R_8S_4$
(c) $PQ_8R_{12}S_3$ (d) $PQ_4R_4S_{12}$

28. A solid has a structure in which X atoms are located at all corners of the cube, Y atoms at all edge centres and Z atom at cube centre, then formula of the compound is:
(a) ZXY_3 (b) XYZ
(c) XYZ_3 (d) ZYX_3

29. In a solid with ccp arrangement of O^{2-} ions, atoms X are present at body centre and atoms Y at alternate face centres of a unit cell. Then, the formula of the solid is:
(a) XYO_4 (b) XYO_2
(c) XY_2O_4 (d) XYO

30. In a ccp lattice of X & Y, the X atoms are present at corners while Y at all the face centres. If one of the X atoms from a corner is replaced by Z atom, then the formula of the compound is:
(a) $X_7Y_{24}Z_2$ (b) $X_7Y_{24}Z$
(c) $X_{24}Y_7Z$ (d) $XY_{24}Z$

31. In a crystalline solid, anions Y^- are arranged in ccp. Cations X^+ are equally distributed b/w octahedral & Tetrahedral voids. If all the octahedral voids are occupied, then the chemical formula of the compound is:
(a) XY_2 (b) X_2Y
(c) XY_3 (d) X_3Y

32. A compound of iron & oxygen crystallises in a hexagonal close packed array of oxide ions with two out of every three octahedral voids occupied by Fe^{X+} ions. Then the formula of compound is:
(a) FeO (b) Fe_3O_4
(c) Fe_2O_3 (d) $Fe_{1.94}O$

Radius Ratio, Voids & Structures of Ionic Compounds

33. A compound AB has NaCl type structure. The face diagnol of the unit cell is $120\sqrt{2}$ pm. The nearest interionic distance between Na^+ & Cl^- in pm is :
(a) 30 (b) 120
(c) 60 (d) 45

34. What is true about NaCl structure with edge length of X pm?
A. Minimum distance between two Na^+ is $\frac{X}{\sqrt{2}}$
B. Minimum distance between Cl^- is $\frac{X}{\sqrt{2}}$
C. Co-ordination number of each Cl^- is 6.
D. Each Cl^- at corner is surrounded by 8 Tetrahedral voids.
(a) A, C, D only (b) A & C only
(c) B, C & D only (d) All are correct

35. In NaCl unit cell, if all the ions along one axis joining opposite face centres are removed, then the mass of one unit cell is:
(a) 175.5 amu
(b) 234g
(c) 234 amu
(d) 175.5g

36. The radius ratio of Cs^+ to Cl^- is 0.90.

If the radius of Cl^- is 1.80, the false statement regarding CsCl structure is:

(a) the distance between the centres of two Cl^- is greater than 3.6

(b) the distance between the centres of two Cl^- ions is exactly 3.6

(c) the distance between Cs^+ and Cl^- is 3.42

(d) both (b) & (c) are correct

37. The number of Na^+ ions present at edge centres of unit cell in 58.5g of NaCl is (N_A is Avogadros Number):

(a) 1.33 N_A (b) 0.75 N_A

(c) 0.25 N_A (d) 6N_A

38. A solid AB has rock salt structure. If spheres from a face in a unit cell are removed, then the number of octahedral voids destroyed (i.e., the voids which can no more be regarded as octahedral voids) in an unit cell is/are:

(a) 9 (b) 8

(c) 12 (d) 1

39. Consider the radii:

0.095 nm (Na^+), 0.181 nm (Cl^-), 0.074 nm (Zn^{2+})

0.2 nm (S^{2-}), 0.169 nm (Cs^+)

Choose the correct statement (s).

(a) Na^+ ions are packed in octahedral voids between the planes of close packed Cl^- ions.

(b) Zn^{2+} are packed in tetrahedral voids in ZnS

(c) Cs^+ ions are placed in cubic void in CsCl

(d) All are Correct

40. The number of next nearest neighbours of Cs^+ ion in Cs^+Cl^- crystal is:

(a) 12 (b) 8

(c) 6 (d) 4

41. If the volume occupied by a unit cell of NaCl is 4.7×10^{-23} ml, the volume of a crystal of NaCl weighing 1 gm is:

(a) 2.73×10^{22} ml (b) 8.93×10^{-25} ml

(c) 10.88 ml (d) 0.12 ml

42. In CaF_2 (fluorite type structure),

(a) Ca^{2+} forms fcc and F^- occupy all tetrahedral voids.

(b) Ca^{2+} forms fcc & F^- occupy all octahedral voids.

(c) Ca^{2+} form bcc & F^- occupy all Tetrahedral voids.

(d) None of these

43. Two ions P^+ & Q^- have radii 88 pm & 200 pm respectively. In the close - packed crystal of compond PQ, the Co-ordination number of P^+ is:

(a) 4 (b) 6

(c) 8 (d) None of thses

44. In diamond structure, the packing fraction of unit cell is:

(a) 0.66 (b) 0.69

(c) 0.34 (d) 0.12

45. An octahedral void at body centre (in FCC) is formed by:

(a) 3 face centred atoms + 3 corner atoms

(b) 6 face centred atoms + 8 corners atoms

(c) 6 face centred atoms only

(d) 4 face centred atom + 2 corners atoms

46. An octahedral void at edge centre (in FCC) is formed by:

(a) 6 corner atoms

(b) 2 corner atoms + 4 face centred atoms

(c) 8 corners atoms

(d) 4 corner atoms + 2 face centred atoms

47. A Tetrahedral void (in FCC) is formed by:

(a) 4 face centred atoms

(b) 2 face centred atoms + 2 corner atoms

(c) 3 face centred atoms + 1 corner atom

(d) 6 face centred atoms + 1 corner atom

48. What angle is made by the lines connecting any Zn^{2+} to any two of its nearest neighbours?

(a) 120° (b) 90°

(c) 109° 28′ (d) 60°

49. In fcc crystal lattice, edge length is 400 pm. Then, the diameter of the greatest sphere which can be fitted into the interstitial void without distortion of the lattice is:

(a) 152.5 pm (b) 121.3 pm

(c) 148.6 pm (d) 117.1pm

50. A cation 'X' fits exactly in trigonal void formed by anions 'Y'. Then the radius ratio must be:

(a) 0.225 (b) 0.155

(c) 0.732 (d) 1

51. In ionic solids AB & CD, radius ratios are x & y respectively. If x + y = 0.75 & x–y = 0.25, then cations in AB & CD are respectively, in:

(a) T-voids, O-voids (b) O-voids, T-voids

(c) T-voids, T-voids (d) O-voids, O-voids

52. A metal crystallises as in fcc structure with edge lengh of 300 pm. The radius of smallest atom that can fit into the octahedral void of its lattice (without distorting the lattice) is nearly :

(a) 44 pm (b) 88 pm

(c) 50 pm (d) 125 pm

53. In an ionic crystal, the radius of cation A^+ & the radius of anion B^- is 1.00 & 3.3 pm respectively then the approximate edge length of unit cell of AB is:

(a) 10 pm (b) 3.46 pm

(c) 0.5 pm (d) 4.3 pm

54. In a normal spinal type structure, the oxide ions are arranged in ccp whereas $\frac{1}{8}$ tetrahedral voids are occupied by Zn^{2+} ions & 50% of octahedral voids are occupied by Fe^{3+} ions. Then, the formula of the compound is:

(a) $Zn_2\ Fe_2\ O_4$ (b) $Zn_2\ Fe_2\ O_3$

(c) $Zn\ Fe_2\ O_4$ (d) $Zn\ Fe_2\ O_2$

55. r_{Na^+} & r_{Cl^-} represents radius of Na^+ & Cl^- ions respectively. If 'n' represents the number of NaCl units per unit cell, then the equation to obtain molar volume is:

(a) $\frac{8(r_{Na^+}+r_{Cl^-})^3}{n}\times N_A$

(b) $\frac{3\sqrt{3}(r_{Na^+}+r_{Cl^-})^3}{2n}\times N_A$

(c) $\frac{2\sqrt{2}(r_{Na^+}+r_{Cl^-})^3}{n}\times N_A$

(d) $\frac{2\sqrt{3}(r_{Na^+}+r_{Cl^-})^3}{4n}\times N_A$

56. Select the correct statement (s) among the following:

(a) In ZnS structure, Zn^{2+} occupy alternate tetrahedral voids.

(b) In NaCl structure, the Co. No of Na^+ & Cl^- are same.

(c) In NaCl, the next nearest neighbour of Na^+ are 12 Na^+.

(d) All are correct.

57. The distance between tetrahedral voids in fcc is:

(a) $\frac{\sqrt{3}a}{2}$ (b) $\frac{a}{\sqrt{2}}$

(c) $\frac{a}{2}$ (d) All of these

58. In the crystal of CsCl, the nearest neighbours of each Cs^+ ion are:

(a) 6 Chloride ions (b) 8 Chloride ions

(c) 6 Cesium ions (d) 8 Cesium ions

59. The edge length of unit cell of diamond is 356.7 pm. The distance b/w C atoms is

(a) 154.45 pm (b) 318 pm

(c) 297 pm (d) Name of these

Density

60. A metal crystallizes in two cubic lattices, fcc & bcc, whose edge lengths are 3.5 & 3.0 A° respectively. The ratio of densities of fcc & bcc unit cells is:

(a) 1.295 (b) 1.259

(c) 2.915 (d) None of these

61. Sodium (Na = 23) crystallizes in bcc arrangement with the interfacial seperation between the atoms at edge 53.6 pm. The density of sodium crystal is:

(a) 3.5 g/cc (b) 2.66 g/cc

(c) 1.19 g/cc (d) None of these

62. An element crystallizes as body centred cubic lattice. Its density is 7.12g/cm^3 and the length of side of unit cell is 2.88 A°. Then the number of atoms present in 288g of the element are:

(a) 1.693×10^{23} (b) 1.693×10^{24}

(c) 3.386×10^{23} (d) 3.386×10^{24}

63. A solid contains A & B atoms in a cubic arrangement in which 'A' atoms occupies corners & B the face centres of the unit cell. If the edge length is 5 A°, the density of unit cell is (Given atomic weights of A & B as 60 & 90, respectively)

(a) 7.2 g/cm^3 (b) 4.38 g/ cm^3

(c) 6.6 g/cm^3 (d) 1.8 g/cm^3

64. Sodium has a bcc structure with nearest neighbour distance of 365.9 pm. Density of its unit cell is:

(a) 1.5g/ cm^3 (b) 3g/cm^3

(c) 4g/cm^3 (d) 5g/cm^3

65. The density of a pure substance 'A' whose atoms pack in cubic close pack arrangement is 1g/cc. If 'B' atoms can occupy all tetrahedral voids, What is the density of resulting solid in g/cm^3?

(At mass of A = 30g/mol & at mass of B = 50 g/mol)

(a) 3.33 (b) 4.33

(c) 6.33 (d) 1.33

66. Copper has fcc crystal structure. Assuming an atomic radius of 130 pm for copper atom, what is the volume of the unit cell?

(At mass of Cu = 63.54 g/mol)

(a) 4.94×10^{-23} cm^2 (b) 6.63×10^{-25} cm^3

(c) 7×10^{-30} cm^3 (d) None of these

67. An atomic solid crystallizes in a body centred cubic lattice & the inner surface of the atoms at adjacent corner are seperated by 60.3 pm. If the atomic weight of 'A' is 48, the density of solid is nearly:

(a) 1.75 g/cc (b) 2.8 g/cc

(c) 3.2g/cc (d) 7.1 g/cc

68. A metal crystallises into two cubic faced fcc & bcc whose edge lengths are 3.5 & 3.0 A° respectively. The ratio of densities of fcc & bcc unit is cell

(a) 1.26 (b) 3.2

(c) 4.1 (d) 0.23

69. Iron crystallizes in several modifications. At about 910k, 'bcc' form (called α form) undergoes transition to γ-form with fcc lattice. Assume that the distance between the nearest neighbours is the same in two forms at the transition temperature. Then, the ratio of density of γ-iron to that of α-iron at the transition temperature is:

(a) 1.08 (b) 0.74

(c) 0.83 (d) 0.108

70. Calculate mass of a unit cell of an element which crystallises in ccp arrangement if its atomic mass is 56 amu.

(a) 3.72×10^{-22}g (b) 1.86×10^{-22}g

(c) 9.3×10^{-23}g (d) insufficient data

71. A compound AB has NaCl type structure. The density of AB is 6.25 g/cm^3 & its molecular mass is 60 g. If the radius of cation A^+ is 60 pm, then radius of anion B^- is ($N_A = 6 \times 10^{23}$)

(a) 60 pm (b) 140 pm

(c) 120 pm (d) 10 pm

Defects in Crystals

72. Which one of the following is not observed when Na Cl is heated in the atmosphere of Na vapour?

(a) electrons are trapped in anion vacanceis

(b) Non-stoichiometric defect results

(c) Extra Na^+ ions occupy interstitial positions

(d) Both (a) and (b)

73. At Curie temperature,

(a) diamagnetic solid changes to paramagnetic

(b) Ferromagnetic solid changes to paramagnetic

(c) Anti ferromagnetic solid changes to paramagnetic

(d) Ferrimagnetic solid changes to paramagnetic

74. The density of crystal always increases in which of the following defects:

(a) Schottky defect (b) Vacancy defect

(c) Frenkel defect (d) Interstitial defect

75. Which of the following intrinsic defect is shown in the figure below?

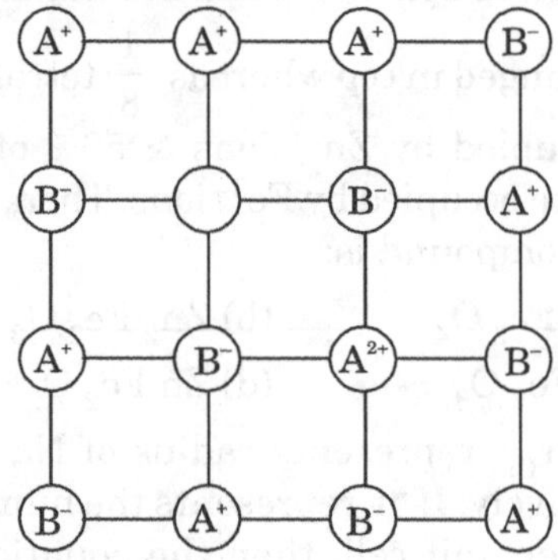

(a) Schottky defect

(b) Frenkel defect

(c) Metal deficiency defect

(d) Metal excess defect

76. Which of the following statement is WRONG about schottky defect?

(a) Density of the crystal decreases

(b) It is due to occupation of an interstitial site by cation

(c) Stability of crystal decreases

(d) All of these are WRONG.

77. If 'Y' is the ratio of the observed to the theoretical densities of a solid, then the value of 'Y' for schottky defect, interstitial defect & Frenkel defects present in the solid, respectively, are:

(a) <1, > 1, = 1 (b) > 1, < 1, = 1

(c) < 1, = 1, = 1 (d) < 1, > 1, < 1

78. Carbon (diamond), silicon and copper are crystalline solids. These are characterised by conduction band and valence band separated by energy gaps respectively, equal to $(E_g)_C$, $(E_g)_{Si}$ and $(E_g)_{Cu}$ Then

(a) $(E_g)_C = (E_g)_{Si} = (E_g)_{Cu}$

(b) $(E_g)_C > (E_g)_{Si} > (E_g)_{Cu}$

(c) $(E_g)_C < (E_g)_{Si} < (E_g)_{Cu}$

(d) $(E_g)_C < (E_g)_{Si} > (E_g)_{Cu}$

79. Which of the following crystals show Frenkel defect?

(i) AgBr (ii) AgCl

(iii) KBr (iv) ZnS

(a) (i), (ii) & (iv) (b) (i), (ii) & (iii)

(c) (ii), (iii) & (iv) (d) both (iii) & (iv)

80. Which of the following statement regarding electrical conductivity is/are true?

(a) The electrical conductivity of semi-conductors increases with rise in temperature

(b) Conductivity of silicon crystal increases on doping with gallium

(c) Metals behave like super conductor at very low temperature

(d) All are correct

81. Which one of the following is a combination of both vacancy & interstitial defect?

(a) Frenkel defect (b) Schottky defect

(c) Impurity defect (d) None of these

82. Which of the following are stoichiometric defects?

1. Schottky defect 2. Frenkel defect

3. Interstitial defect 4. Vacancy defect

(a) (2) & (4) only (b) (2) & (3) only

(c) (1), (2) & (4) only (d) All of these

83. Zinc oxide on heating changes to yellow. This is because:

(a) Zinc oxide becomes a stoichiometric compound

(b) Zinc oxide is a covalent compound

(c) Zinc oxide shows metal excess defect

(d) It has F-centres

84. The alignment of magnetic dipoles is shown below:

↑ ↓ ↓ ↑ ↓ ↓

Which of the following property is represented by these dipoles?

(a) Diamagnetism (b) Ferrimagnetism

(c) Ferromagnetism (d) Anti-ferromagnetism

85. Match the types of defects given in column-I with the statement given in column-II.

Column-I	Column-II
(i) Impurity defect	A. NaCl with anion vacancies having e^- trapped in them (F-centres)
(ii) Metal excess defect	B. FeO with Fe^{3+}
(iii) Metal deficiency defect	C. Na Cl with Sr^{2+} & some cationic sites are vacant.

(a) (i – A), (ii – C), (iii – B)

(b) (i – C), (ii – B), (iii – A)

(c) (i – C) (ii – A) (iii – B)

(d) (i – B), (ii – A), (iii – C)

86. Select the incorrect match.

(a) Ferromagnetic substances → Fe, Ni, Co

(b) Antiferromagnetic substances → FeO, MnO

(c) Ferrimagnetic substance → Fe_3O_4

(d) None of these is incorrect

Brain Teasers

87. How many unit cells are present in a ccp arrangement of NaCl of mass 1g?

(a) 5.14×10^{21} (b) 1.28×10^{21}

(c) 1.71×10^{21} (d) 2.57×10^{21}

88. If the radius of the anion in an ionic solid is 200 pm, what would be the radius of the cation that fits exactly into the cubic void?

(a) 146.4 pm (b) 82.8 pm

(c) 45 pm (d) 90 pm

89. If the ratio of co-ordination number of A to that of B is X:Y, then the ratio of number of atoms of A to that of number of atoms of B in unit cell is:

(a) X : Y (b) Y : X

(c) $X^2 : Y$ (d) $Y^2 : X$

90. Which statement is correct regarding the voids?

(a) Cubic void & octahedral void, both are formed at the centre of cube

(b) Cubic void is located at face centre where as octahedral void is located at body centre

(c) Octahedral void is located at corner where as cubic void is located at edge centre

(d) Cubic void & octahedral voids are same

91. In XY_3, Y^- ions have ccp arrangement & X^{3+} ions are present in octahedral voids. The fraction of total number of voids occupied is:

(a) $\frac{1}{3}$ (b) $\frac{1}{6}$

(c) $\frac{1}{9}$ (d) $\frac{1}{12}$

92. The total volume occupied in a face centred cubic unit cell of a metal is (r is the atomic radius):

(a) $\frac{12}{3}\pi r^3$ (b) $\frac{16}{3}\pi r^3$

(c) $\frac{20}{3}\pi r^3$ (d) $\frac{24}{3}\pi r^3$

93. In a sample of FeO when 12% Fe^{2+} ions get replaced by Fe^{3+}, the composition of this Wustite sample is:

(a) $Fe_{0.98}O$ (b) $Fe_{0.93}O$

(c) $Fe_{0.96}O$ (d) $Fe_{0.94}O$

94. An alkali metal (at weight = 40) has a bcc structure with nearest neighbour distance = $\sqrt{3}$ A°. Its density in kg m^{-3} is d × 10^4. The value of 'd' is

(a) 3.32 (b) 1.66

(c) 2.55 (d) 0.83

95. A transition metal M can exist in two oxidation states + 2 & + 3. It forms an oxide whose experimental formula is M_XO (where X < 1).

The ratio of number of metal ions in + 3 Oxidation state to those in + 2 oxidation state is:

(a) $\frac{1-x}{1+x}$ (b) 1 + 2x

(c) $\frac{2+x}{2(3x-2)}$ (d) $\frac{2(1-x)}{3x-2}$

96. If carbon atoms from one of the body diagnol plane of a diamond unit cell are removed, then the reduction in densities is:

(a) 43.75% (b) 50%

(c) 33.3% (d) 62.4%

97. The edge length of diamond unit cell was measured as 0.4 nm. Then the density of the unit cell is:

(a) 0.250 g/cm^3 (b) 2.50 g/cm^3

(c) 2.50 kg/cm^3 (d) 2.50 g/m^3

98. Packing fraction in 2-D hexagonal arrangement is:

(a) 0.6 (b) 0.74

(c) 0.524 (d) 0.906

99. In a non-stoichiometric sample of ferrous oxide with NaCl structure, the ratio of no. of Fe^{3+} ions to Fe^{2+} ions was found to be 0.15. Calculate the fraction of octahedral sites occupied by vacancies?

(a) 0.9384 (b) 0.0612

(c) 0.75 (d) 0.025

100. In ccp structure of mixed oxides, the oxide ions occupy all the corners & all the face centres. Cations 'A' occupy 25% Octahedral voids & 12.5% tetrahedral voids are occupied by B. The nearest neighbour distance wrt oxide ion is:

(a) $\frac{\sqrt{3}a}{4}$ (b) $\frac{a}{\sqrt{2}}$

(c) $\frac{a}{4}$ (d) $\frac{\sqrt{3}a}{8}$

101. Pervoskite crystallizes with Ca^{2+} ions at corners of a cubic unit cell, Ti^{4+} in its body centre & O^{2-} ions at all the face centres. The co-ordination numbr of Ti^{4+} ion is:

(a) 6 (b) 8

(c) 14 (d) 7

102. Next nearest neighbour of S^{2-} ion in zinc blende structure is/are:

(a) 6 (b) 8

(c) 12 (d) 10

103. CsCl unit cell has an edge length equal to 4.3 nm. Then, the shortest distance between two Cs^+ ions is:

(a) 4.3 nm (b) 8.6 nm

(c) 2.15 nm (d) None of these

104. Three lines are drawn from a single corner of a fcc unit cell to meet the other corner such that they are found to pass through; exactly only octahedral void (line one), onvoid of any types (line two) and exactly two tetrahedral void with one octahedral void (line three). The lines in same order are:

(a) Edge, face diagonal, body diagonal

(b) Face diagonal, edge, body diagonal

(c) Body diagonal, face diagonal, edge

(d) Edge, body diagonal, face diagonal

105. For a unit cell of edge length 10 Å and having density equal to 1g/cm^3, the atomic radius is (given at mass = 150 amu)

(a) 3.53 Å (b) 6.77Å

(c) 12.52 Å (d) 13.10Å

106. The arrangement of spheres in a hexagonal unit cell is shown below. If the labelled atoms are missing then the number of effective atoms in unit cell left after removing the labelled atoms are:

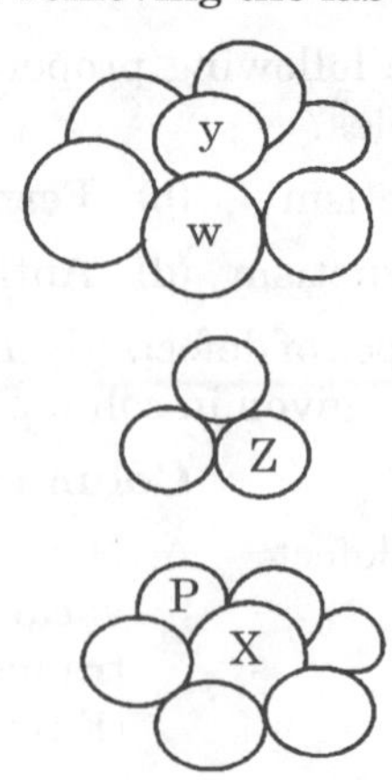

(a) $\frac{21}{8}$ (b) $\frac{11}{3}$

(c) 6 (d) 4

107. An ionic compound consists of X^+, Y^{2+} & Z^{3-} ions. Which of the following option (s) is/are Correct wrt their possible structure?

(a) X^+ ions occupy alternate corners of a simple cube. Y^{2+} occupy the body centre & Z^{3-} occupy a single tetrahedral void.

(b) Z^{3-} ions form ccp, X^+ ions occupy all the octahedral voids & Y^{2+} ions occupy half of the tetrahedral voids.

(c) Y^{2+} ions form hcp, X^+ occupy all the octahedral voids & Z^{3-} ions occupy half of the tetrahedral voids.

(d) Both b & c are correct

108. A monoatomic solid element exists in a cubic crystal. If its atomic radius is 1 Å & the ratio of packing fraction & density is 0.1 cm^3/gm, then the atomic mass of the element is:

(a) 8π

(b) 7.5π

(c) 64π

(d) 32π

109. Ratio of effective No. of atoms (Z) for a 2D hexagonal close packed unit cell (I) to 3D hexagonal centred unit cell (II) is :

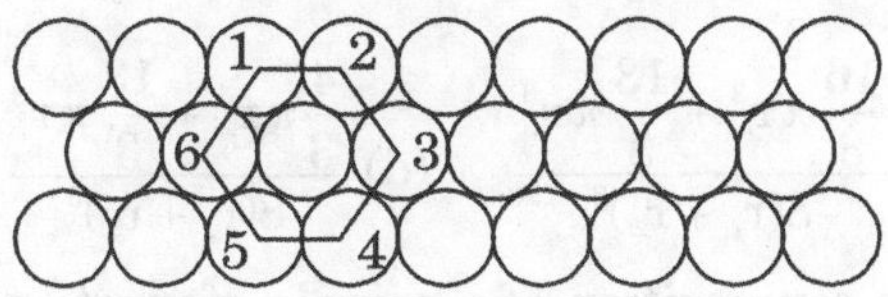

(I)

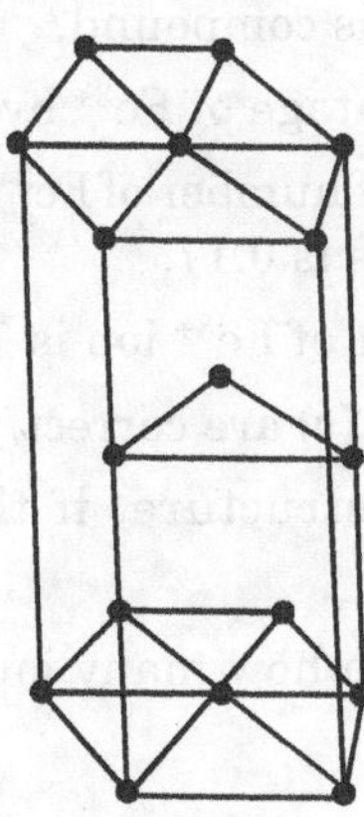

(II)

(a) $\frac{2}{3}$ (b) 1

(c) $\frac{1}{2}$ (d) $\frac{1}{3}$

110. XY_2 has ideal fluorite structure. The incorrect statement is/are:

1. each X^{2+} at corner is sorrounded by 18 Tetrahedral voids
2. each X^{2+} is sorrounded by 6 octahedral voids
3. shortest distance between two Y^- ions is half of edge length
4. shortest distance between X^{2+} & Y^- is half of edge length

(a) only 3 (b) 1, 3 & 4 only

(c) 1 & 4 only (d) 1, 2 & 4 only

111. In a face centred cubic lattice, atoms A are at the corners & atoms B at the face centres. If atom B is missing from one of the face centred points, the formula of the ionic compound is:

(a) AB_2 (b) A_5B_2

(c) A_2B_3 (d) A_2B_5

112. In a monoclinic unit cell, the relation of sides and angles, are respectively:

(a) $a = b \neq c$ and $\alpha = \beta = \gamma = 90^\circ$

(b) $a \neq b \neq c$ and $\alpha = \beta = \gamma = 90^\circ$

(c) $a \neq b \neq c$ and $\beta = \gamma = 90^\circ \neq \alpha$

(d) $a \neq b \neq c$ and $\alpha \neq \beta \neq \gamma \neq 90^\circ$

113. Ice crystallises in a hexagonal lattice having volume of the unit cell as 132×10^{-24} cm^3. If density is $0.92 g\ cm^{-3}$ at a given temperature, then number of H_2O molecules per unit cell are:

(a) 2 (b) 3

(c) 4 (d) 6

114. An oxide has a ccp structure in which oxide ions are present at all lattice points (face centres & corners) whereas Na ions are located at all the edge centres and W ion at the body centre. Then, the oxidation state of 'W' is:

(a) + 2 (b) + 3

(c) + 4 (d) + 5

115. The packing fraction in zinc blende (sphalerite) structure unit cell is (assuming ideal crystal)

(a) 0.749 (b) 0.385

(c) 0.575 (d) 0.912

116. A crystalline solid AB has NaCl type structure with radius of B^- ion as 250 pm. Which of the following cation can be made to slip into the tetrahedral site of crystal of A^+B^-?

(a) C^+ (ionic radius = 180 pm)

(b) D^+ (ionic radius = 90 pm)

(c) E^+ (ionic radius = 200 pm)

(d) G^+ (ionic radius = 150 pm)

117. In FCC unit cell, if on one of the face, unoccupied space between the atoms is 20 pm, what will be the edge length of this unit cell?

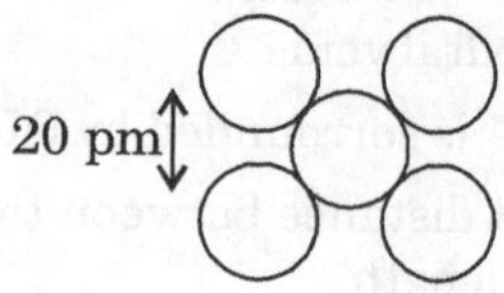

(a) 68.25 pm (b) 100 pm
(c) 143.88 pm (d) 190 pm

118. If NaCl is doped with $10^{-3}\%$ $AlCl_3$, what is the concentration of cation vacancies?

(a) 6.02×10^{18} (b) 12.04×10^{18}
(c) 2 (d) 12.04×10^{20}

119. Three layers of bcc are shown as:

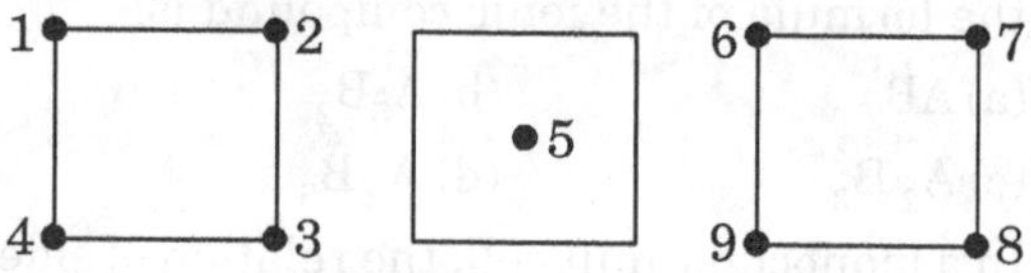

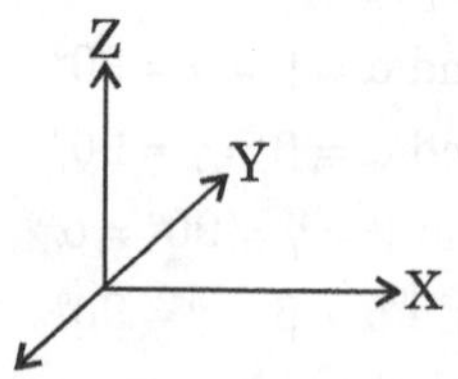

Which one of the following is correct?

(a) Distance between atoms labelled 6 & 7 = 2R
(b) Distance between atoms labelled 5 & 3 = 4R
(c) Ratio of distance between 7 & 9 and that between 7 & 5 = $\sqrt{\frac{8}{3}}$
(d) Ratio of distance between 4 and 5 & that between 8 and 5 = $\sqrt{\frac{3}{8}}$

120. If NaCl is doped with $AlCl_3$ and has 5 mole% vacancies. Then the formula of the compound is:

(a) $Na_{0.925}\,Al_{0.025}Cl$ (b) $Na_{0.075}\,Al_{0.025}Cl$
(c) $Na_{0.975}\,Al_{0.05}Cl$ (d) $Na_{0.045}\,Al_{0.05}Cl$

121. The packing efficiency of the two dimensional square unit cell shown below is:

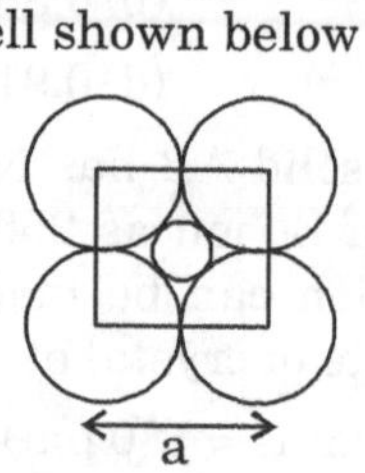

(a = 2r)

(a) 78.5% (b) 66.2%
(c) 20% (d) 52.4%

122. If a solid A^+B^- having ZnS structure is heated so that the ions along two of the axis passing through the face centre, particles are lost & bivalent ion (Z) enters here to maintain electrical neutrality so that the new formula becomes $A_X\,B_Y\,Z_C$. Then value of X + Y + C is:

(a) 7 (b) 9
(c) 5 (d) 6

123. In a fcc unit cell, atoms are numbered as shown below.

The atoms not touching each other are (Atom numbered 3 is face centre of front face)

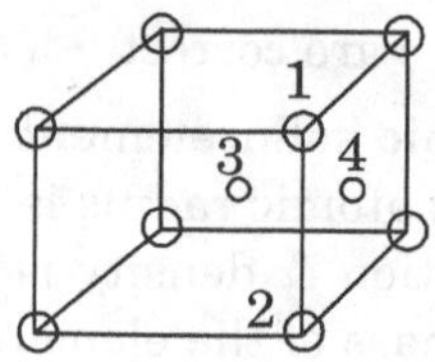

(a) 3 & 4 (b) 1 & 3
(c) 1 & 2 (d) 2 & 4

124. Which of the following expression is correct for packing fraction of NaCl if all the ions along the face are diagonally removed?

(a) $\dfrac{\frac{13}{3}\pi r_-^3 + \frac{16}{3}\pi r_+^3}{8(r_+ + r_-)^3}$ (b) $\dfrac{\frac{13}{3}\pi r_-^3 + \frac{4}{3}\pi r_+^3}{8(r_+ + r_-)^3}$

(c) $\dfrac{\frac{16}{3}\pi r_-^3 + \frac{13}{3}\pi r_+^3}{8(r_+ + r_-)^3}$ (d) $\dfrac{\frac{4}{3}\pi r_-^3 + \frac{13}{3}\pi r_+^3}{8(r_+ + r_-)^3}$

125. The composition of a sample of wustite is $Fe_{0.93}O_{1.00}$. Which of the following statement(s) is/are correct wrt this compound?

(a) The percentage of Fe^{3+} by mass is 11.5%
(b) The ratio of number of Fe^{3+} ions to the number of Fe^{2+} ions is 0.17.
(c) The weight of Fe^{3+} ion is 7.84g.
(d) Both (b) & (c) are correct.

126. In the CaF_2 structure, if the radius ratio is $\left(\frac{\sqrt{3}}{\sqrt{2}} - 1\right)$, then how many ions does each cation touch?

(a) 4 anions (b) 12 cations
(c) 8 anions (d) both (b) and (c)

127. The packing fraction for spinel structure (ideal) is :

(a) 0.768 (b) 0.56
(c) 0.356 (d) 0.16

128. Certain metal crystallizes in bcc lattice. The distance between the nearest neighbours is 433 pm. Then, the distance between the next nearest neighbours is:

(a) 400 pm

(b) 500 pm

(c) 600 pm

(d) 650 pm

129. The carbon-carbon bond length in diamond is 173.2 pm. If diamond's structure were considered to be ZnS type & having radii equal to half the bond length, then what would be its expected density?

(a) 2.49 g/cm^3

(b) 1.76 g/cm^3

(c) 7.65 g/cm^3

(d) 8.8 g/cm^3

130. If NaCl is doped with 10^{-3} mol% of $AlCl_3$, the concentration of cation vacancies is:

(a) 12.04×10^{18}

(b) 6.02×10^{16}

(c) 6.02×10^{20}

(d) 3.01×10^{18}

131. The figure given below shows the location of atoms in a crystallographic plane in fcc lattice, which of the following plane will show this arrangement?

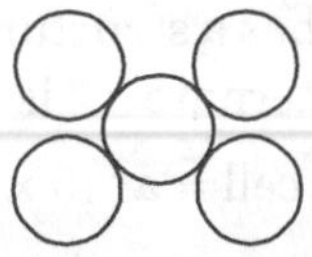

(a) Face plane (b) Body diagonal plane

(c) Rectangular plane (d) Any imaginary plane

132. Which of the following statement is NOT true about hexagonal close packing in 3D?

(a) The co-ordination No. is 12.

(b) It has 74% packing efficiency

(c) Tetrahedral voids of the 2nd layer are covered by the spheres of the 3rd layer.

(d) In this arrangement, spheres of the fourth layer are exactly aligned with those of the first layer.

133. The tetrahedral voids formed by ccp arrangement of Cl^- ions in rock salt structure are –

(a) Occupied by Na^+ ion

(b) Occupied by Cl^- ion

(c) Occupied by either Na^+ or Cl^- ion

(d) Vacant.

Answers

1. (b)	**2.**(b)	**3.** (d)	**4.** (c)	**5.** (b)	**6.** (c)	**7.** (b)	**8.** (c)	**9.** (b)	**10.** (b)
11. (d)	**12.** (c)	**13.** (a)	**14.** (c)	**15.** (a)	**16.** (b)	**17.** (d)	**18.** (c)	**19.** (d)	**20.** (c)
21. (b)	**22.** (d)	**23.** (a)	**24.** (a)	**25.** (d)	**26.** (c)	**27.** (b)	**28.** (a)	**29.** (a)	**30.** (b)
31. (b)	**32.** (c)	**33.** (b)	**34.** (d)	**35.** (a)	**36.** (b)	**37.** (b)	**38.** (a)	**39.** (d)	**40.** (c)
41. (d)	**42.** (a)	**43.** (b)	**44.** (c)	**45.** (c)	**46.** (b)	**47.** (c)	**48.** (c)	**49.** (d)	**50.** (b)
51. (b)	**52.** (a)	**53.** (a)	**54.** (c)	**55.** (a)	**56.** (d)	**57.** (d)	**58.** (b)	**59.** (a)	**60.** (b)
61. (c)	**62.** (d)	**63.** (b)	**64.** (a)	**65.** (b)	**66.** (a)	**67.** (a)	**68.** (a)	**69.** (a)	**70.** (a)
71. (b)	**72.** (c)	**73.** (b)	**74.** (d)	**75.** (c)	**76.** (b)	**77.** (a)	**78.** (b)	**79.** (a)	**80.** (d)
81. (a)	**82.** (d)	**83.** (c)	**84.** (b)	**85.** (a)	**86.** (d)	**87.** (c)	**88.** (a)	**89.** (b)	**90.** (a)
91. (c)	**92.** (b)	**93.** (c)	**94.** (b)	**95.** (d)	**96.** (a)	**97.** (b)	**98.** (d)	**99.** (b)	**100.** (a)
101. (a)	**102.** (c)	**103.** (a)	**104.** (a)	**102.** (a)	**106.** (b)	**107.** (d)	**108.** (a)	**109.** (c)	**110.** (c)
111. (d)	**112.** (c)	**113.** (c)	**114.** (d)	**115.** (a)	**116.** (b)	**117.** (a)	**118.** (b)	**119.** (c)	**120.** (a)
121. (a)	**122.** (a)	**123.** (c)	**124.** (a)	**125.** (d)	**126.** (d)	**127.** (a)	**128.** (b)	**129.** (a)	**130.** (a)
131. (a)	**132.** (d)	**133.** (d)							

Explanations

3. Silicon carbide has a structure similar to diamond where every alternate 'C' is replaced by silicon.

5. Volume of unit cell = a^3 $(5 \times 10^{-8}\ cm)^3$

$125 \times 10^{-24}\ cm^3$

9. SO_2 has a net dipole moment & is hence polar.

So, SO_2 molecules are held in lattice by dipole-dipole interactions.

11. In any lattice, a unit cell is shared equally by 6 unit cells.

12. Volume of unit cell = a^3

Same volume of each unit cell means that edge length of each unit cell is same.

For simple cubic,

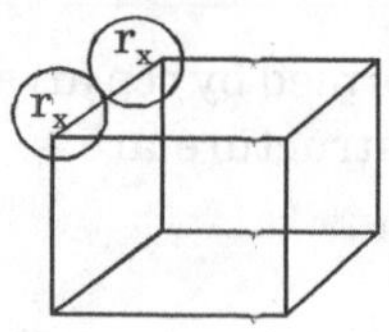

$2r_x = a$

$\boxed{r_x = \frac{a}{2}}$

For fcc,

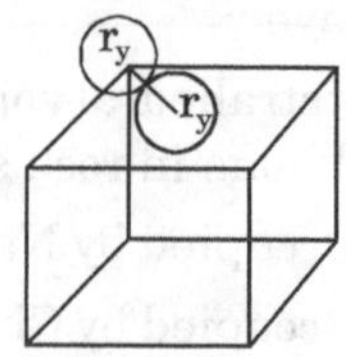

$2r_y = \frac{\sqrt{2}a}{2}$

$r_y = \frac{\sqrt{2}a}{2 \times 2}$

$\boxed{r_y = \frac{a}{2\sqrt{2}}}$

$\boxed{r_y = 0.353a}$

For bcc,

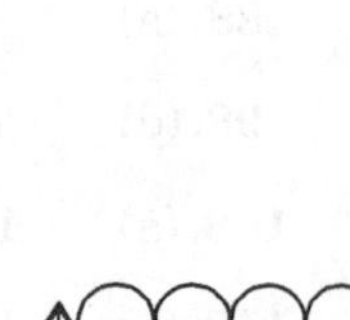

$2r_z = \frac{\sqrt{3}a}{2}$

$\boxed{r_z = \frac{\sqrt{3}a}{4}}$

$\boxed{r_z = 0.433a}$

13.

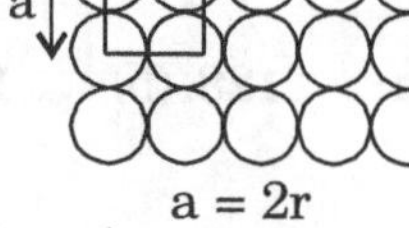

a = 2r

$$P.F = \frac{\text{Area covered by atoms}}{\text{Total area}}$$

$$= \frac{1 \times \pi r^2}{a^2} = \frac{\pi r^2}{(2r)^2} = \frac{\pi r^2}{4r^2} = \frac{\pi}{4}$$

16.

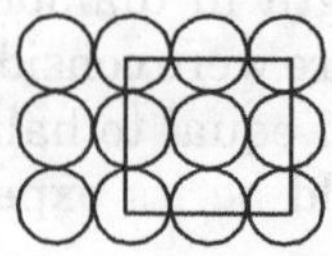

22.

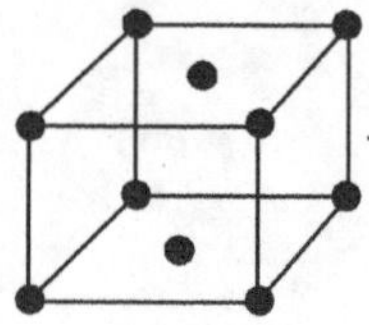

→ End - Centred Cubic

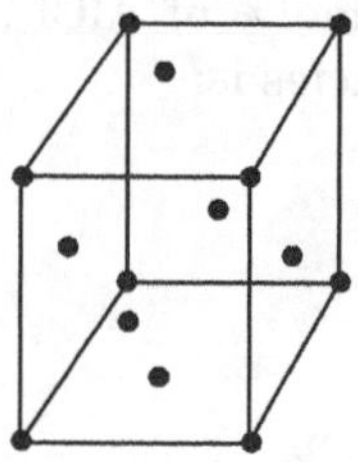

→ Face Centred tetragonal

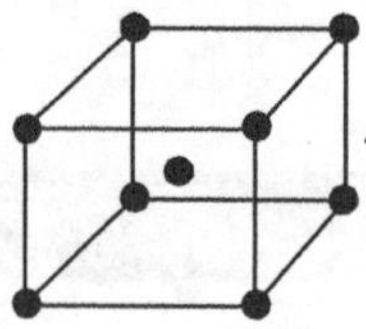

→ Body Centred Cubic

23.

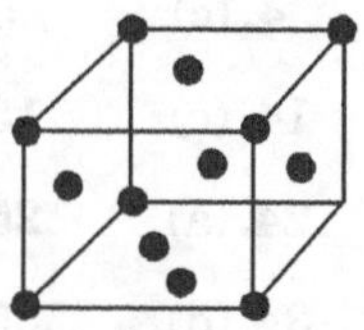

Locations occupied by X atoms = 7 corners (1 corner atom is missing)

Effective No. of X atoms = $7 \times \frac{1}{8}$

Y atoms are at locations = 6 (6 face centres)

Effective No. of Y atoms = $6 \times \frac{1}{2} = 3$

$X_{\frac{7}{8}}\ Y_3$

$\boxed{X_7\ Y_{24}}$

24. B-located at → Corners → $8 \times \frac{1}{8} = 1$

→ Face Centers → $6 \times \frac{1}{2} = 3$

So, effective 4 B^- ions are present per unit cell.

Tetrahedral voids formed = 8

So, effective A^+ cations = 8

Formula is $A_8 B_4 = A_2B$

25. A → Corners $\left(8 \times \frac{1}{8} = 1\right)$

B → 2 atoms a each face centre $\left(12 \times \frac{1}{2} = 6\right)$

Formula is AB_6.

26. Effective No. of atoms in hcp (3D) = 6

So, A^- = 6

Effective No. of Octahedral voids = 6

No. of octahedral voids occupied by $C^+ = \frac{2}{3} \times 6$

So, formula is $C_4 A_6 = C_2A_3$

27. P → at all corners $\left(8 \times \frac{1}{8} = 1\right)$

Q → 2 on each face diagnol $\left(24 \times \frac{1}{2} = 12\right)$

R → 2 on each body diagnol (2 × 4 = 8)

S → one at body centre + at all edge centres

Effective no. of S atoms = $1 + 12 \times \frac{1}{4} = 4$

So, formula is $P_1 Q_{12} R_8 S_4$

28. X atoms → at all corners $\left(8 \times \frac{1}{8} = 1\right)$

Y atoms → at all edge centres $\left(12 \times \frac{1}{4} = 3\right)$

Z atom → 1 (at cube centre)

So, formula is $X_1 Y_3 Z_1$.

29. O^{2-} in ccp → Effective atoms = 4

(fcc) (Corners = $8 \times \frac{1}{8}$ + face centres

$= 6 \times \frac{1}{2} = 4$)

X (at body centre) = 1

Y (at alternate face centres) = $2 \times \frac{1}{2} = 1$

So, formula is $X_1 Y_1 O_4$

30. Effective no. of X atoms = $7 \times \frac{1}{8}$

(one corner is removed)

Effective no. of Z atom = $1 \times \frac{1}{8}$

Effective no. of Y atoms = $6 \times \frac{1}{2} = 3$

$X_{7/8}\ Y_3\ Z_{1/8} = X_7\ Y_{24}\ Z_1$

31. Effective Y^- in ccp (or fcc) = 4

$\left(8 \times \frac{1}{8}\text{(from corners)} + 6 \times \frac{1}{2}\text{(form face centres)}\right)$

No. of Octahedral Voids formed = 4

No. of Octahedral Voids occupied by X^+ = 4 (given)

No. of T. Voids (Tetrahedral) formed = 8

No. of T. Voids occupied by X^+ = 4

(∵ Cations equally distributed)

So, formula is $X_8 Y_4 = X_2 Y$

32. No. of effective O^{2-} ions = 6

No. of effective O. Voids = 6

No. of O. voids occupied = 4

by Fe^{x+}

Total Anionic charge = – 12

Total Cationic charge = + 12

Wrt Fe^{x+} = 4

4x = 12

$\boxed{x = +3}$

$Fe^{3+} \times O^{2-} = Fe_2O_3$

33.

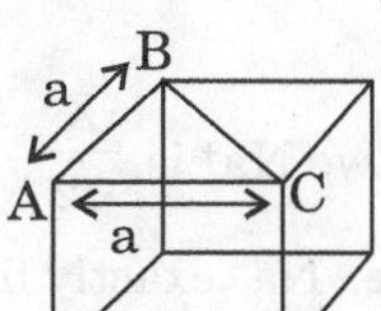

Apply pythagoras theorem

For Δ ABC

$BC^2 = AB^2 + AC^2$

$BC^2 = a^2 + a^2$

$\boxed{BC = \sqrt{2}\,a}$

So, face diagnol (BC) = $\sqrt{2}a$

$\therefore \sqrt{2}a = 120\sqrt{2}$

$\boxed{a = 120 \text{ pm}}$

For NaCl, Na^+ are at O. voids & Cl^- occupy fcc locations.

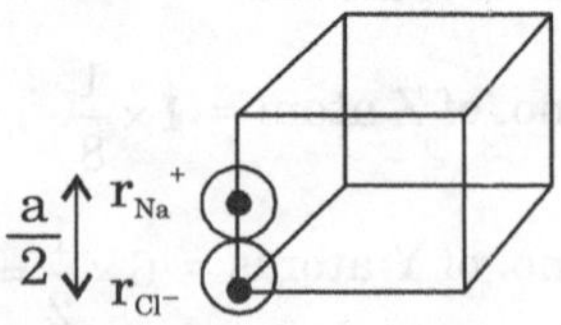

$$r_{Na^+} + r_{Cl^-} = \frac{a}{2}$$

$$r_{Na^+} + r_{Cl^-} = \frac{120}{2} = 60$$

So, nearest interionic distance between Na^+ & Cl^- = 60 pm.

34. Na^+ occupy Octahedral Voids & Cl^- occupy fcc lattice points.

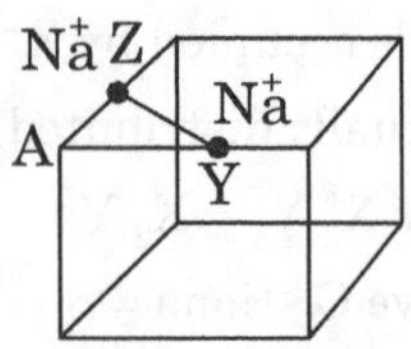

Apply Pythagoras Theorem for Δ ZAY –

$$ZY^2 = AZ^2 + AY^2$$

$$ZY^2 = \left(\frac{X}{2}\right)^2 + \left(\frac{X}{2}\right)^2$$

$$ZY^2 = \frac{X^2}{4} + \frac{X^2}{4}$$

$$ZY^2 = \frac{2X^2}{4}$$

$$ZY = \frac{X}{\sqrt{2}}$$

So, min. distance between two Na^+ is $\frac{X}{\sqrt{2}}$.

For ideal NaCl structure (i.e., Na^+ exactly fitting in Octahedral void), Anion-anion contact is maintained.

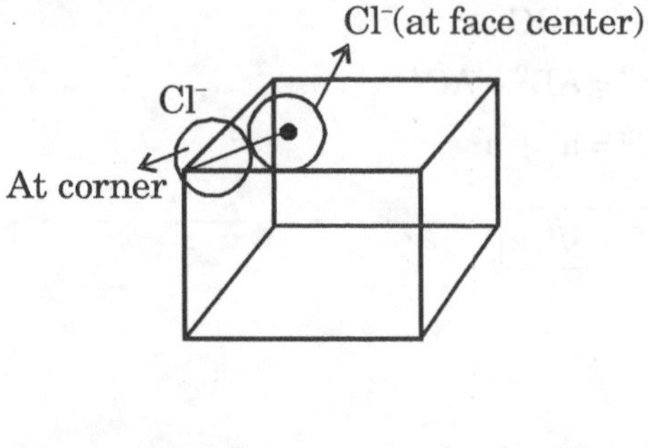

$$2r^- = \frac{\sqrt{2}\,X}{2} = \frac{X}{\sqrt{2}}$$

So, minimum distance between Cl^- = $\frac{X}{\sqrt{2}}$

Wrt 'C' statement

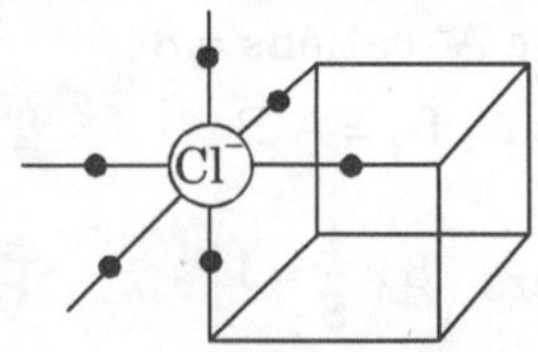

Cl^-, sorrounded by 6 Na^+ ions

Co-ordination No. wrt Cl^- = 6

Wrt 'd' statement

Each Cl^- at corner is sorrounded by 8 T.V. at 8 Body diagnols which emerge from corner.

35.

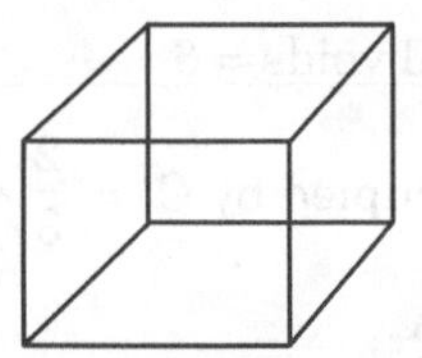

In NaCl structure

Na^+ occupy all O.V.

Cl^- occupy fcc locations

Cl^- → Corners → $8 \times \frac{1}{8} = 1$

Cl^- → Face Centers → $6 \times \frac{1}{2} = 3$

Effective Cl^- ions per unit cell = 4

So, Octahedral voids present (Effective) = 4

Effective Na^+ ions per unit cell = 4

Hence, formula units of NaCl

Per unit cell = 4

After removal of ions

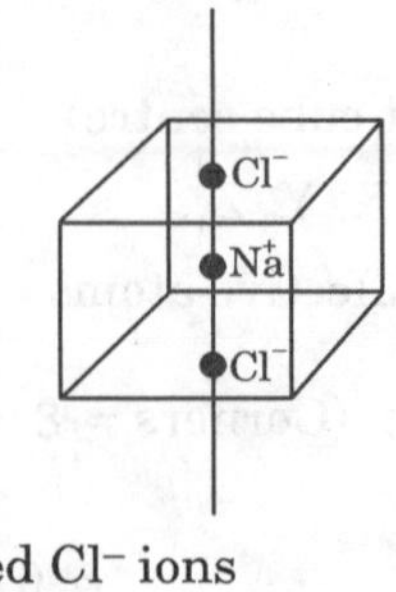

2 face centred Cl^- ions

and one Na^+ at body centre (O. V.) is lost.

Now, effective Cl^- ions

→ Face center $4 \times \frac{1}{2} = 2$

Corners $8 \times \frac{1}{8} = 1$

So, effective total Cl^- ions = 3

Effective Na^+ ions = $12 \times \frac{1}{4} = 3$

So, formula = $Na_3\,Cl_3$

Mass of unit cell = 3 × 23 + 3 × 35.5

= 69 + 106.5

= 175.5 amu

36. For CsCl,

$$\frac{r_{Cs^+}}{r_{Cl^-}} = 0.90$$

$$\frac{r_{Cs^+}}{1.80} = 0.90$$

$$\boxed{r_{Cs^+} = 0.90 \times 1.80 = 1.62}$$

wrt Cs^+Cl^-, Cl^- is at corners & Cs^+ at body centre (in cubic void)

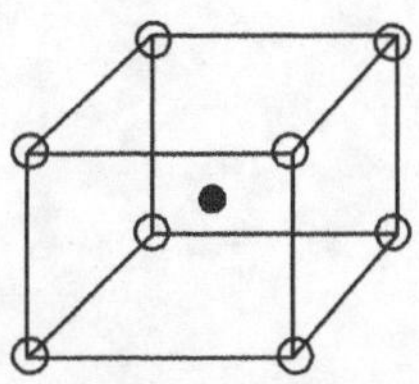

O → Cl^-

● → Cs^+

Since, radius ratio is > 0.732. So, Cs^+ is not exactly fitting & hence ANION-ANION Contact is not maintained.

Wrt the present structure,

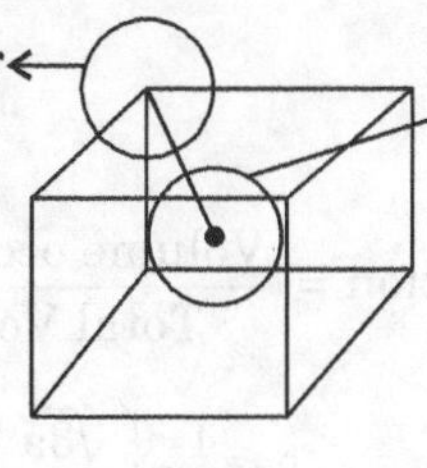

$$r^- + r^+ = \frac{\sqrt{3}a}{2}$$

$$1.80 + 1.62 = \frac{\sqrt{3}}{2} \times a$$

$$\frac{3.42 \times 2}{1.732} = a$$

$$\boxed{3.94 = a}$$

Also,

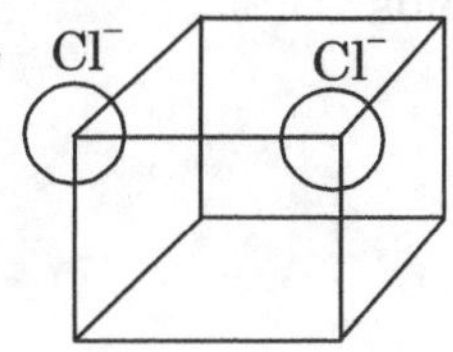

So, distance between 2 Cl^- ions = 3.94

Also, distance between Cl^- & Cs^+ = 1.80 + 1.62

= 3.42

37. Wrt NaCl structure, Na^+ occupy all O. Voids.

Effective Na^+ at edge centres = $12 \times \frac{1}{4} = 3\,Na^+$

3 Effective Na^+ are present at edge centres per unit cell & 4 formula units of NaCl are present per unit cell.

4 formula units of NaCl $\xrightarrow[\text{to}]{\text{Correspond}}$ 3 Effective Na^+ at edge centres

$\frac{58.5}{N_A} \times 4\,gm \xrightarrow[\text{to}]{\text{Correspond}}$ 3 Effective Na^+ at edge centres

$$58.5\text{ gm} \xrightarrow[\text{to}]{\text{Correspond}} \frac{3}{58.5 \times \frac{4}{N_A}} \times 58.5$$

$$= \frac{3}{58.5 \times 4} \times N_A \times 58.5$$

$$= \frac{3}{4} N_A = 0.75\ N_A$$

38. Na^+ occupy all O.Voids.

O.Voids are present at all edge centres & body centre in fcc.

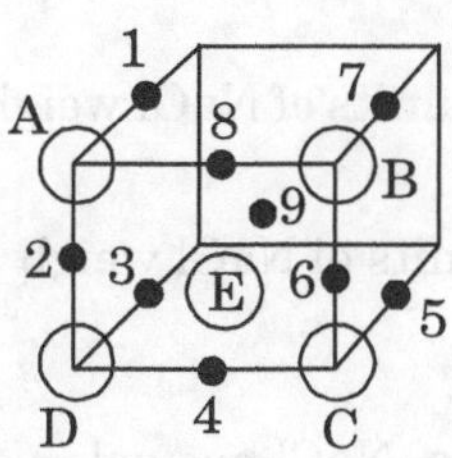

If Cl^- at A, B, C, D & E locations are destroyed, then O.Voids at edge centres 1, 2, 3, 4, 5, 6, 7 & 8 are destroyed. Also, O.void labelled 9 (at body centre) is also destroyed.

39. Radius ratio

$$\text{(for NaCl)} = \frac{r_{Na^+}}{r_{Cl^-}} = \frac{0.095}{0.181} = 0.524$$

For, Octahedral void, $\frac{r^+}{r^-} = 0.414 - 0.732$

& 0.524 lies between the range.

So, Na^+ are in O. voids.

For ZnS,

$$\frac{r_{Zn^{2+}}}{r_{s^{2-}}} = \frac{0.074}{0.2} = 0.37$$

Now, for tetrahedral void, $\frac{r^+}{r^-} = 0.225 - 0.414$ & 0.37 lies in the range. So, Zn^{2+} ions occupy tetrahedral voids.

For Cs^+Cl^-,

$$\frac{r_{Cs^+}}{r_{Cl^-}} = \frac{0.169}{0.181} = 0.933$$

For cubic void, $\frac{r^+}{r^-} = 0.732 - 1.00$ & 0.933 lies within this range. So, Cs^+ is present in cubic void.

Hence, all the three statements are true.

40. Nearest neighbour of Cs^+ are Cl^- ions. Next nearest neighbour of Cs^+ will be 6 Cs^+ ions at a distance 'a'.

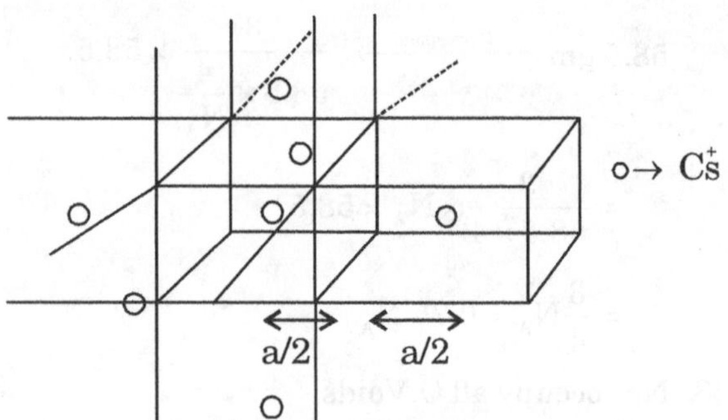

41. One unit cell of NaCl has 4 formula units of NaCl and

N_A formula units of NaCl weigh = 58.5g

4 formula units of NaCl weigh $= \frac{58.5}{N_A} \times 4g$

So, $\frac{58.5}{N_A} \times 4g$ NaCl has vol. $= 4.7 \times 10^{-23}$ ml

$$1 \text{ gm NaCl has vol.} = \frac{4.7 \times 10^{-23}}{58.5 \times \frac{4}{N_A}}$$

$$= \frac{4.7 \times 10^{-23}}{58.5 \times 4} \times 6.02 \times 10^{23}$$

$$= \frac{28.294}{234} = 0.12 \text{ ml}$$

43. Calculating the radius ratio, we get:

$$\frac{r^+}{r^-} = \frac{88}{200} = 0.44$$

It lies in the range, 0.414 – 0.732.

So, Co-ordination No. is 6.

44. Diamond has ZnS type structure where all S^{2-} ions & Zn^{2+} ions are replaced by C atoms.

Location of C atoms → at alternate tetrahedral voids (4); at corners; at face centers

at corners: $8 \times \frac{1}{8} = 1$ at face centers: $6 \times \frac{1}{2} = 3$

So, there are effective (1 + 3 + 4) 8 C atoms per unit cell.

Hence, volume occupied by 8C atoms

$$= 8 \times \frac{4}{3}\pi r^3 \quad \text{...(1)}$$

Total volume of the cube = a^3

Also,

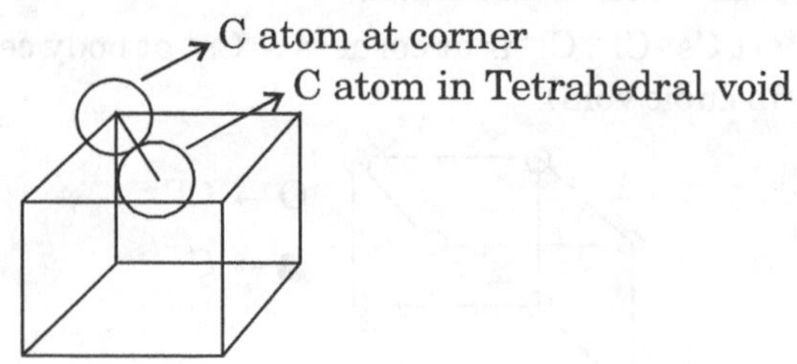

$$r + r = \frac{\sqrt{3}a}{4}$$

$$\boxed{2r = \frac{\sqrt{3}a}{4}}$$

$$\boxed{r = \frac{\sqrt{3}a}{8}}$$

$$\text{Packing fraction} = \frac{\text{Volume occupied by atoms}}{\text{Total Volume of cube}}$$

$$P.F = \frac{8 \times \frac{4}{3}\pi r^3}{a^3} = \frac{8 \times \frac{4}{3}\pi\left(\frac{\sqrt{3}a}{8}\right)^3}{a^3} = 0.34$$

45.

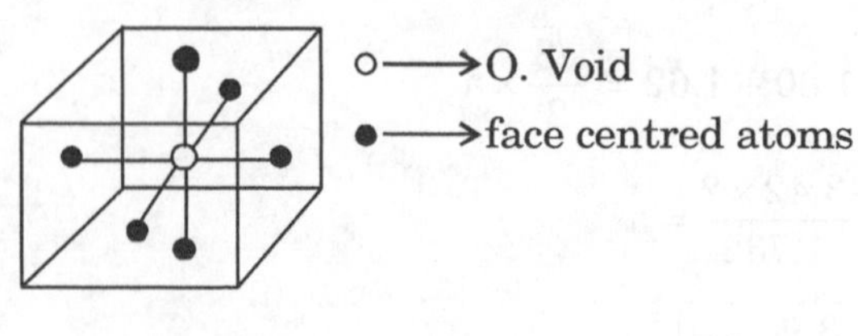

48. Zn^{2+} is in Tetrahedral void.

49. FCC has 2 voids, tetrahedral & octahedral. Greatest sphere can be accomodated only in greatest void (octahedral). To fit in O.Void without distortion,

$$\frac{r_{void}}{r_{(atom\ packed\ in\ fcc)}} = 0.414 \quad ...(1)$$

For fcc $2r = \frac{\sqrt{2}a}{2}$

$$2r = \frac{\sqrt{2}}{2} \times 400$$

$$r = \frac{\sqrt{2}}{4} \times 400$$

r(radius of atom in fcc) = $100\sqrt{2}$

Now, placing the value in equation 1, we get

$$\frac{r_{void}}{100\sqrt{2}} = 0.414$$

$$r_{void} = 0.414 \times 100\sqrt{2}$$

$$r_{void} = 0.414 \times 100 \times 1.414 = 58.53 \text{ pm}$$

diameter of greatest sphere that can fit

$= 2 \times 58.53 = 117$ pm

50.

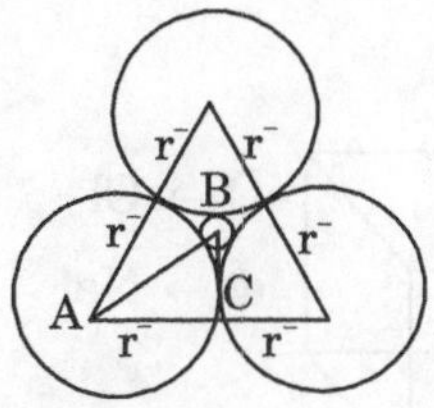

In ΔABC,

$$\cos 30° = \frac{r^-}{r^- + r^+}$$

$$\frac{\sqrt{3}}{2} = \frac{r^-}{r^- + r^+}$$

Reciprocating both sides

$$\frac{2}{\sqrt{3}} = \frac{r^- + r^+}{r^-}$$

$$\frac{2}{\sqrt{3}} = \frac{r^-}{r^-} + \frac{r^+}{r^-}$$

$$\frac{2}{\sqrt{3}} - 1 = \frac{r^+}{r^-}$$

$$\frac{2-\sqrt{3}}{\sqrt{3}} = \frac{r^+}{r^-}$$

$$\boxed{0.155 = \frac{r+}{r^-}}$$

51. Given

$$x + y = 0.75 \quad ...(1)$$

$$x - y = 0.25 \quad ...(2)$$

Add (1) and (2)

$$2x = 1$$

$$x = \frac{1}{2} = 0.5$$

Place volume of x in (1)

$0.5 + y = 0.75$

$\boxed{y = 0.25}$

So, $\boxed{x = 0.5}$

$$\frac{r_{A^+}}{r_{B^-}} = 0.5 \quad ...(3)$$

$$\frac{r_{C^+}}{r_{D^-}} = 0.25 \quad ...(4)$$

From equation 3, radius ratio = 0.5 which lies between 0.414 – 0.732.

So, cation is in octahedral void.

From eqn. 4, radius ratio = 0.25 which lies b/w 0.225 – 0.414, So, cation is in Tetrahedral void.

52. For exactly fitting in octahedral void,

$$\frac{r_{void}}{r_{metal\ atom}} = 0.414 \quad ...(1)$$

Also, in fcc

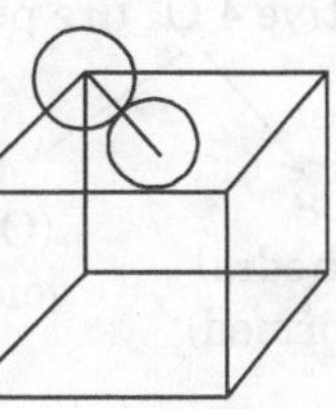

$$2r = \frac{\sqrt{2}a}{2}$$

(where r is radius of metal atoms packed in fcc)

$$2r = \frac{a}{\sqrt{2}}$$

$$r = \frac{300}{2\sqrt{2}} \text{ (a = 300 pm (given))}$$

$$r = \boxed{\frac{150}{\sqrt{2}} = 106.08 \text{ PM}}$$

Placing the value of radius of metal atom in equation 1.

$$\frac{r_{void}}{106.08} = 0.414$$

$$r_{void} = 0.414 \times 106.08 = 43.91 \approx 44\text{pm}$$

53. We can identify the kind of crystal (or ionic compound) by calculating the radius ratio.

$$\frac{r^+}{r^-} = \frac{1}{3.3} = 0.303$$

So, the cation is placed in tetrahedral void. Let us assume it to be ZnS type structure.

Hence,

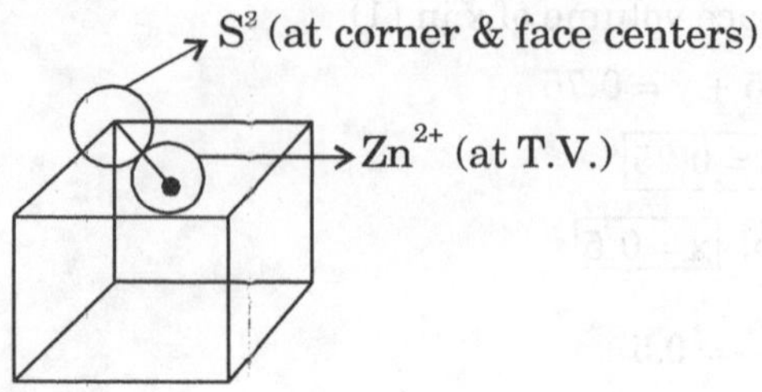

Now, $r^+ + r^- = \frac{\sqrt{3}a}{4}$

$$1 + 3.3 = \frac{\sqrt{3}}{4} \times a$$

$$\frac{4.3 \times 4}{1.732} = a = 10 \text{ pm}$$

54. O^{2-} are in ccp (fcc)

Corners: $8 \times \frac{1}{8} = 1$

Face centers: $6 \times \frac{1}{2} = 3$

So, total effective 4 O^{2-} are present per unit cell

8 (Tetrahedral voids formed)

4 (Octahedral voids formed)

Tetrahedral voids occupied $= \frac{1}{8} \times 8 = 1$ by Zn^{2+}

Octahedral voids occupied by $Fe^{3+} = \frac{50}{100} \times 4 = 2$

So, formula is $Zn\ Fe_2\ O_4$.

55. In NaCl structure, Na^+ occupy all the octahedral voids & Cl^- are placed in fcc locations. 4 formula units of NaCl are present per unit cell (= n (given))

4 formula units (= n), have volume = a^3

N_A formula units (1 mole) have volume

$$= \frac{a^3}{n} \times N_A$$

So, molar volume $= \frac{a^3}{n} \times N_A$ ...(1)

Also,

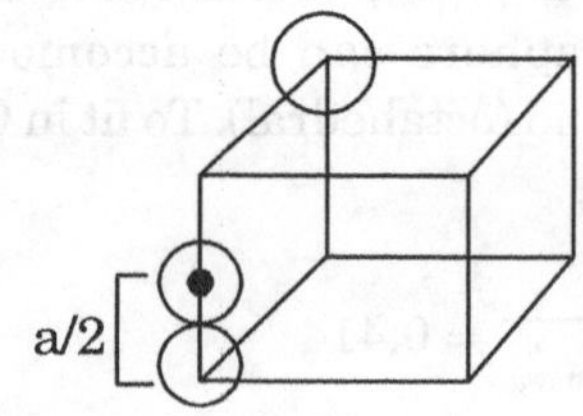

$$r_{Na^+} + r_{Cl^-} = \frac{a}{2}$$

$$\boxed{a = 2(r_{Na^+} + r_{Cl^-})}$$

Place the value of a in equation (1)

$$\text{Molar volume} = a^3 \times \frac{N_A}{n}$$

$$= \left[2(r_{Na^+} + r_{Cl^-})\right]^3 \times \frac{N_A}{n}$$

$$\boxed{\text{Molar volume} = 8\,(r_{Na^+} + r_{Cl^-})^3 \times \frac{N_A}{n}}$$

56. wrt option a, in Zns structure, Zn^{2+} occupy alternate tetrahedral voids.

Wrt option b, in NaCl structure, Cl^- occupy fcc locations whereas Na^+ occupy all octahedral voids.

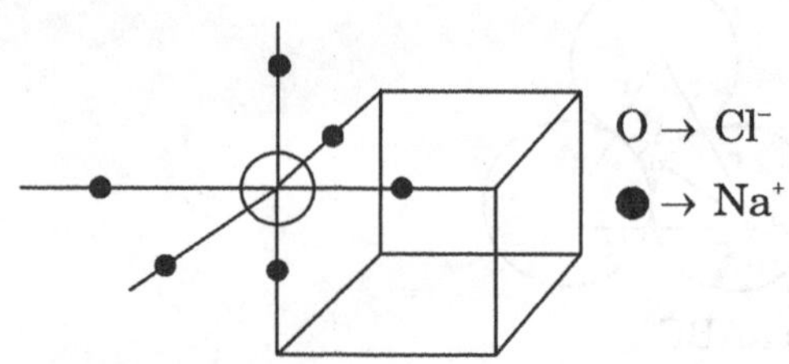

Co. No. wrt $Cl^- = 6$

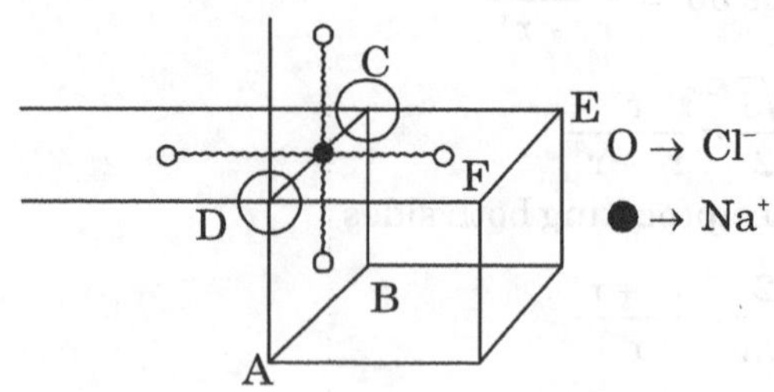

Co. No. wrt $Na^+ = 6$

wrt option c,

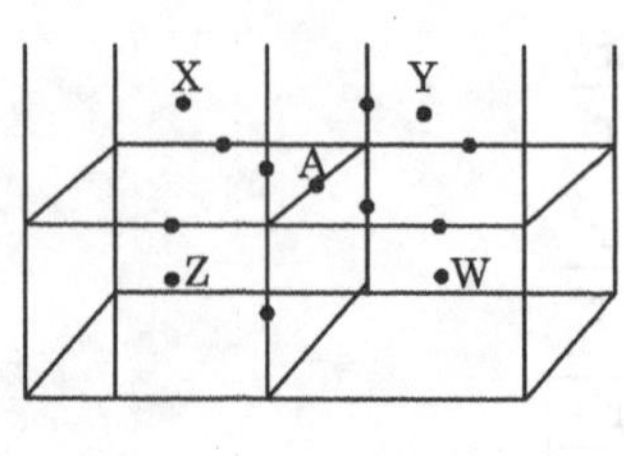

wrt Na^+ labelled 'A', the next nearest neighbours will be 12 Na^+ (8 Na^+ placed at edge centre & 4 Na^+ at body centres, all in octahedral voids) all at a distance of $\frac{a}{\sqrt{2}}$.

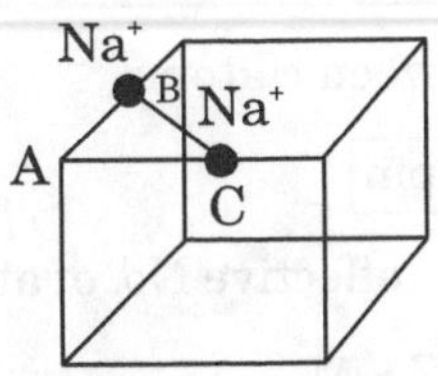

distance between 2 Na^+ions

For ΔABC

$$BC^2 = AB^2 + AC^2$$

$$BC^2 = \left(\frac{a}{2}\right)^2 + \left(\frac{a}{2}\right)^2$$

$$BC^2 = 2 \times \frac{a^2}{4}$$

$$BC^2 = \frac{a^2}{2}$$

$$\boxed{BC = \frac{a}{\sqrt{2}}}$$

57. Consider a big cube (FCC) & divide it into 8 equal cubes.

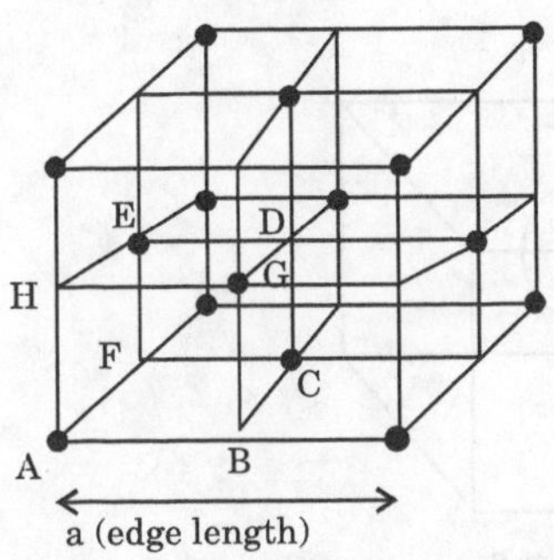

...(1)

Consider the cube ABCDEFGH

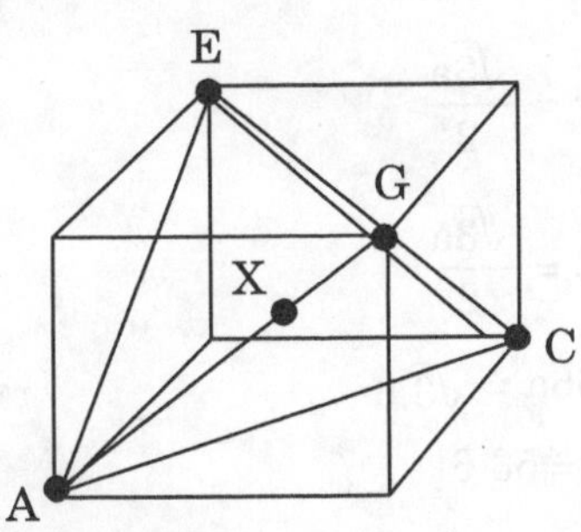

A tetrahedral void 'X' is formed at the centre of each small cube.

Similarly, a tetrahedral void each is formed at centre of each small cube, there by generating a small cube inside a big cube.

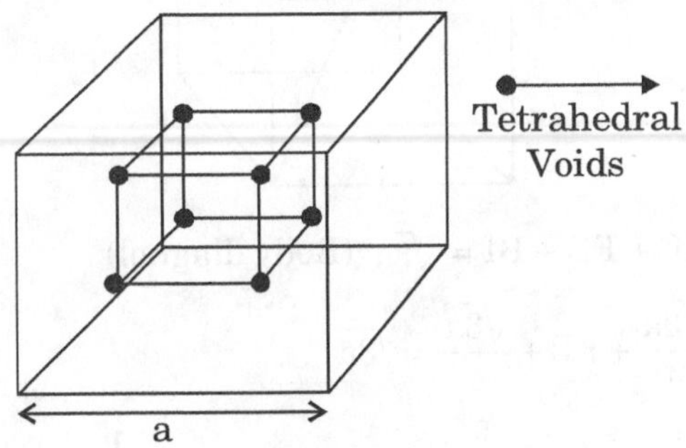

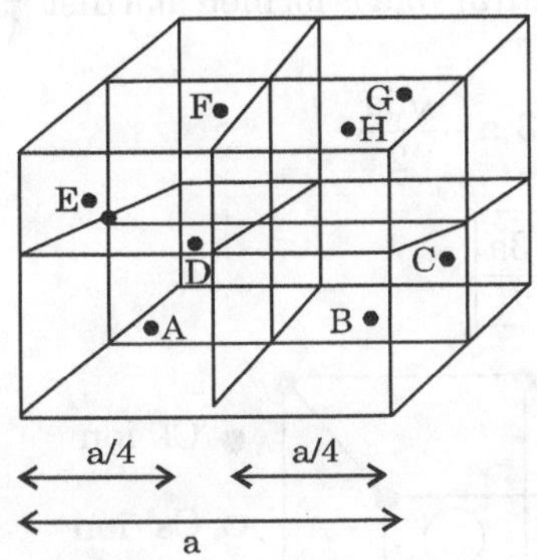

Distance between tetrahedral voids A & B = $\frac{a}{2}$

Joining these points & forming $\left(\frac{a}{4} + \frac{a}{4}\right)$ Cube,

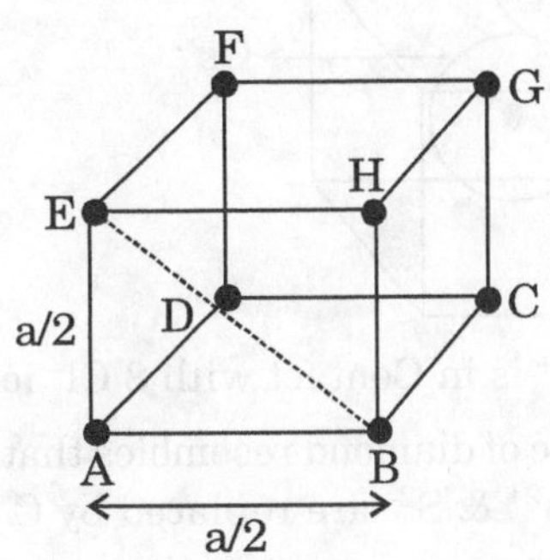

Distance between E & B (tetrahedral voids)

$$EB^2 = \left(\frac{a}{2}\right)^2 + \left(\frac{a}{2}\right)^2$$

$$EB^2 = \frac{2a^2}{4}$$

$$\boxed{EB = \frac{a}{\sqrt{2}}}$$

Also, distance between F & B Tetrahedral voids (these are present along body diagnol of big cube (fcc))

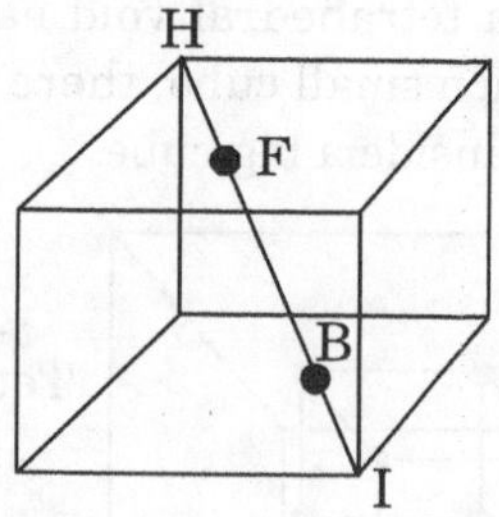

$$HF + FB + BI = \sqrt{3}a \text{ (Body diagnol)}$$

$$\frac{\sqrt{3}a}{4} + FB + \frac{\sqrt{3}a}{4} = \sqrt{3}a$$

Tetrahedral void is formed at a dist $\frac{1}{4}$ from corner

$$FB = \sqrt{3}\,a - \frac{\sqrt{3}a}{2}$$

$$\boxed{FB = \frac{\sqrt{3}a}{2}}$$

58.

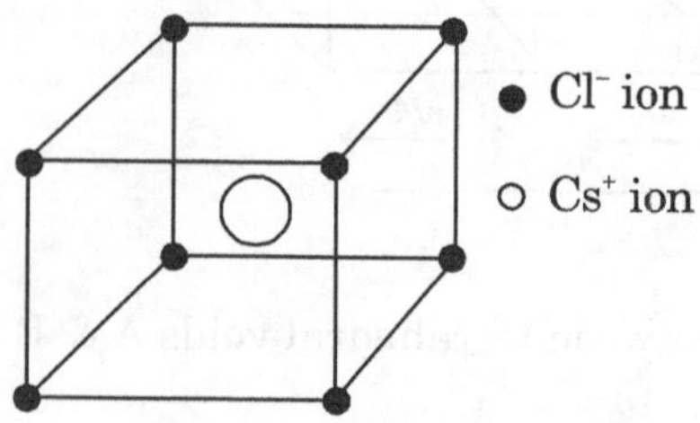

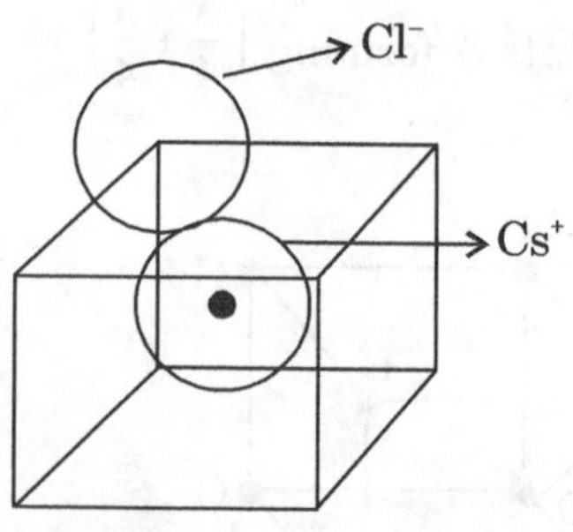

Here Cs^+ is in Contact with 8 Cl^- ions.

59. Structure of diamond resembles that of ZnS where every Zn^{2+} & S^{2-} are replaced by C atoms.

So, C atoms are at fcc locations (substituting S^{2-} ions) & also at alternate tetrahedral voids (substituting Zn^{2+} ions)

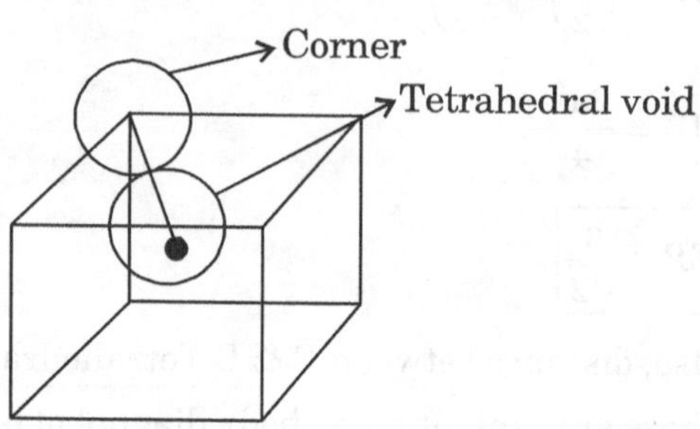

$$2r = \frac{\sqrt{3}a}{4}$$

(where r = radius of c)

$$2r = \frac{\sqrt{3}}{4} \times 356.7$$

distance between c atoms

$$\boxed{2r = 154.45\,\text{pm}}$$

60. For fcc, Z = 4 (effective No. of atoms per unit cell)

$$\text{Apply, } \rho = \frac{Z \times M}{a^3 \times N_A}$$

$$\rho_{fcc} = \frac{4 \times M}{(3.5)^3 \times N_A} \quad \text{...(1)}$$

For bcc, Z = 2

$$\rho_{BCC} = \frac{Z \times M}{a^3 \times N_A}$$

$$\rho_{BCC} = \frac{2 \times M}{(3)^3 \times N_A} \quad \text{...(2)}$$

$$\frac{\rho_{fcc}}{\rho_{BCC}} = \frac{4 \times N}{(3.5)^3 \times N_A} \times \frac{3^3 \times N_A}{2 \times M}$$

$$\frac{\rho_{fcc}}{\rho_{Bcc}} = \frac{2 \times 27}{3.5 \times 3.5 \times 3.5} = \frac{54}{42.875} = 1.259$$

61.

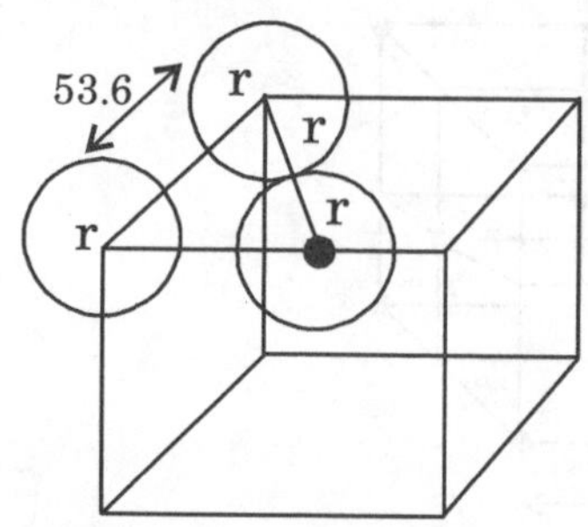

Given: 53.6 + 2r = a

$$2r = a - 53.6 \quad \text{...(1)}$$

$$\text{Also, } 2r = \frac{\sqrt{3}a}{2} \quad \text{...(2)}$$

$$a - 53.6 = \frac{\sqrt{3}a}{2}$$

$$a - 0.866a = \sqrt{3.6}$$

$$0.134\,a = 53.6$$

$$\boxed{a = \frac{53.6}{0.134} = 400 \text{ pm}}$$

Apply,

$$\rho = \frac{Z \times m}{a^3 \times N_A} = \frac{2 \times 23}{(400 \times 10^{-10}\text{cm})^3 \times 6.02 \times 10^{23}}$$

$$\rho = \frac{46}{64 \times 10^6 \times 10^{-30} \times 6.02 \times 10^{23}}$$

$$\rho = \frac{46}{64 \times 6.02} \times 10 = \frac{460}{64 \times 6.02}\ \text{g/cm}^3$$

$$\rho = \frac{460}{385.28}\ \text{g/cm}^3 = 1.19\ \text{g/cm}^3$$

62. Apply, $\rho = \dfrac{Z \times M}{a^3 \times N_A}$

$$7.12 = \frac{2 \times M}{(2.88 \times 10^{-8}\text{cm})^3 \times 6.02 \times 10^{23}}$$

$$M = \frac{7.12 \times 2.88 \times 2.88 \times 2.88 \times 10^{-24} \times 3.01 \times 10^{23}}{2}$$

M = 51.19g

So, 51.19g element has atoms = N_A

$$288 \text{ g element has atoms} = \frac{N_A}{51.19} \times 288$$

$$= \frac{6.02 \times 10^{23}}{51.19} \times 288$$

$$= 33.86 \times 10^{23}$$

or 3.386×10^{24}

63. 'A' at corners

Effective No. of 'A' atoms = $8 \times \dfrac{1}{8} = 1$

'B' at face centres

Effective no. of 'B' atoms = $6 \times \dfrac{1}{2} = 3$

So, formula of the compound is AB_3

M. Mass of AB_3 = 60 + 90 × 3 = 60 + 270

= 330 g

Apply, $\rho_{(\text{density})}$

$$= \frac{Z \times M}{a^3 \times N_A} = \frac{1 \times 330}{(5 \times 10^{-8}\text{cm})^3 \times 6.02 \times 10^{23}}$$

$$\rho = \frac{330}{125 \times 6.02 \times 10^{-1}}$$

$$\rho = \frac{3300}{125 \times 6.02}\ \text{g/cm}^3$$

$$\rho = \frac{3300}{752.5}\ \text{g/cm}^3$$

$$\boxed{\rho = 4.38\ \text{g/cm}^3}$$

64.

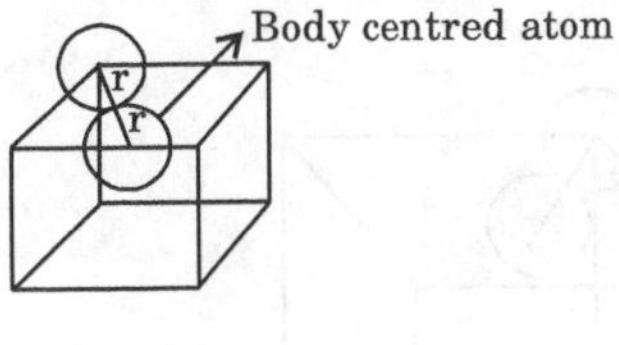

$$2r = \frac{\sqrt{3}a}{2}$$

$$365.9 = \frac{\sqrt{3}}{2} \times a$$

$$\frac{365.9 \times 2}{1.732} = a = 422.51 \text{ pm}$$

$$\rho = \frac{Z \times M}{a^3 \times N_A} = \frac{2 \times 23}{(422.5 \times 10^{-10}\text{cm})^3 \times 6.02 \times 10^{23}}$$

$\rho = 1.5\text{g/cm}^3$

65. 'A' atoms in fcc

Corners: $8 \times \dfrac{1}{8} = 1$

Face Centers: $6 \times \dfrac{1}{2} = 3$

Total, effective 'A' atoms = 4

So, Tetrahedral voids = 8

∴ B atoms = 8

Hence, formula is $A_4 B_8 = A B_2$

So, 4 formula units of AB_2 are present per unit cell. Initial density when 'A' above was packed in fcc,

$$\rho_A = \frac{Z \times M}{a^3 \times N_A} = \frac{4 \times 30}{a^3 \times N_A}$$

$$1 = \frac{4 \times 30}{a^3 \times N_A} \text{ (given } \rho = 1 \text{ g/cc)} \quad ...(1)$$

Now, density when 'AB_2' is packed

M. Mass of AB_2 = 30 + 2 × 50 = 130 g/mol

$$\rho_{AB_2} = \frac{4 \times 130}{a^3 \times N_A} \quad ...(2)$$

Divide $\dfrac{(1)}{(2)}$

$$\frac{1}{\rho_{AB_2}} = \frac{4 \times 30}{a^3 \times N_A} \times \frac{a^3 \times N_A}{4 \times 130}$$

$$\frac{1}{\rho_{AB_2}} = \frac{30}{130}$$

$$\rho_{AB_2} = \frac{130}{30} = 4.33 \text{ g/cc}$$

66. For fcc,

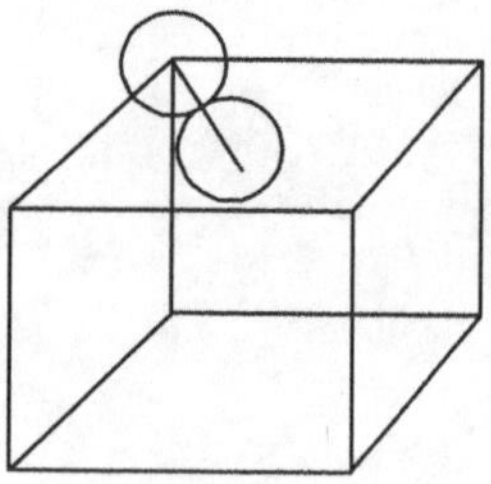

$$2r = \frac{\sqrt{2}a}{2}$$

$$2 \times 130 = \frac{\sqrt{2}}{2} \times a$$

$$\frac{260 \times 2}{\sqrt{2}} = a$$

$$\boxed{260\sqrt{2} = a}$$

Volume of the unit cell $= a^3 = \left(260\sqrt{2}\right)^3$

$$= (260)^3 \times 2\sqrt{2} \text{ pm}^3$$

$$= (260)^3 \times 2\sqrt{2} \times (10^{-10} \text{cm})^3$$

$$= (260)^3 \times 2\sqrt{2} \times 10^{-30} \text{cm}^3$$

Volume of unit cell $= 4.94 \times 10^{-23}$ cm^3

67.

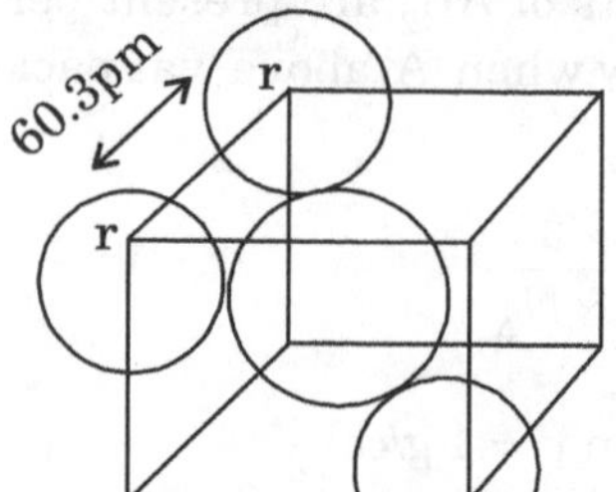

$$2r + 60.3 = a \qquad \text{...(1)}$$

Alos, $4r = \sqrt{3}a$

$$r = \frac{\sqrt{3}a}{4} \qquad \text{...(2)}$$

Place the value of 'r' in equation (1)

$$2 \times \frac{\sqrt{3}a}{4} + 60.3 = a$$

$$\frac{\sqrt{3}a}{2} + 60.3 = a$$

$$60.3 = a - \frac{\sqrt{3}a}{2}$$

$$60.3 = a - \frac{1.732a}{2}$$

$$60.3 = a - 0.866a$$

$$60.3 = 0.134a$$

$$\boxed{\frac{60.3}{0.134} = a} = 450 \text{ pm}$$

Apply

$$\rho = \frac{Z \times M}{a^3 \times N_A} = \frac{2 \times 48}{(450 \times 10^{-10} \text{cm})^3 \times 6.02 \times 10^{23}}$$

(For bcc, Z = 2)

$$\boxed{\rho = 1.75 \text{ g/cc}}$$

68. For fcc

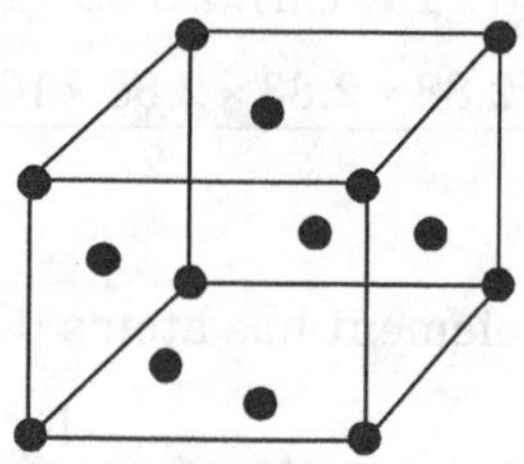

Apply, $\rho_{fcc} = \dfrac{Z \times M}{a^3 \times N_A}$

$$\rho_{fcc} = \frac{4 \times M}{(3.5)^3 \times N_A} \qquad \text{...(1)}$$

Z = 4

(Corners $= 8 \times \frac{1}{8} = 1$, Face centre $= 6 \times \frac{1}{2} = 3$)

For bcc, apply $\rho_{BCC} = \dfrac{Z \times M}{a^3 \times N_A}$

$$\rho_{BCC} = \frac{2 \times M}{(3)^3 \times N_A} \qquad \text{...(2)}$$

From (1) & (2)

$$\frac{\rho_{fcc}}{\rho_{BCC}} = \frac{4 \times M}{(3.5)^3 \times N_A} \times \frac{(3)^3 \times N_A}{2 \times M}$$

$$= \frac{2 \times (3)^3}{(3.5)^3} = \frac{54}{42.875} = 1.26$$

69. For bcc, (α-form)

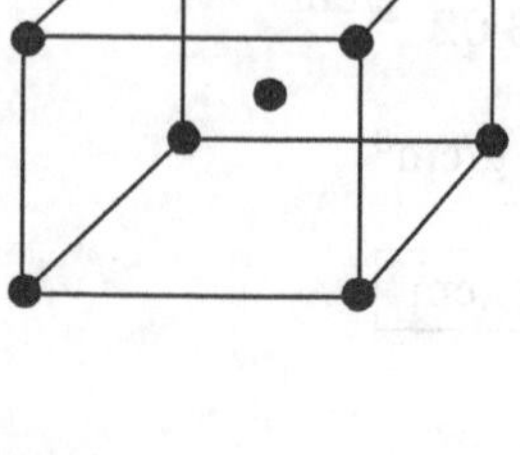

$$Z = 8 \times \frac{1}{8} \text{ (from corners)} + 1 \text{ (at body centre)} = 2$$

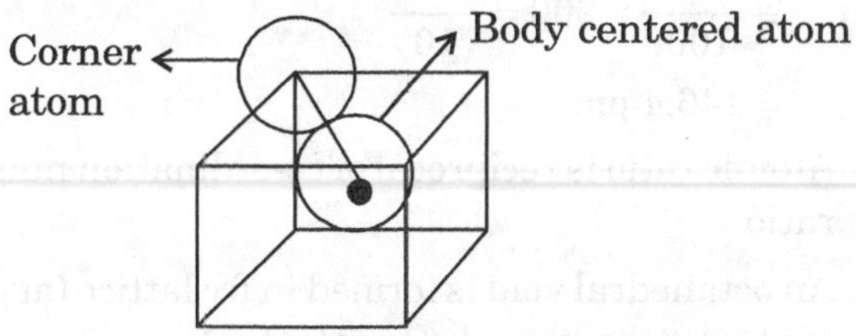

$$2r = \frac{\sqrt{3}a_1}{2} \text{ (nearest neighbour distance)} \quad ...(1)$$

For fcc (γ – form)

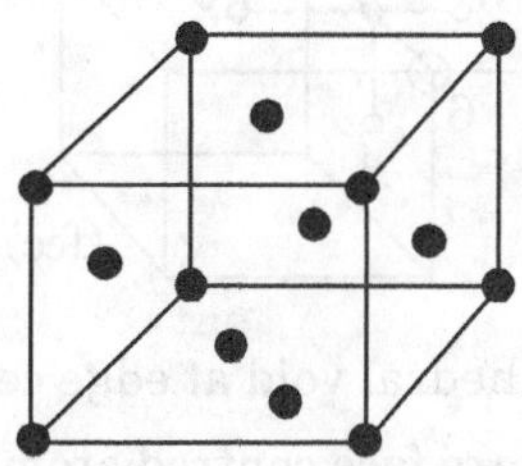

$$Z = 8 \times \frac{1}{8} + 6 \times \frac{1}{2} = 4$$

(from corner) (from face centre)

In fcc, nearest neighbour distance is

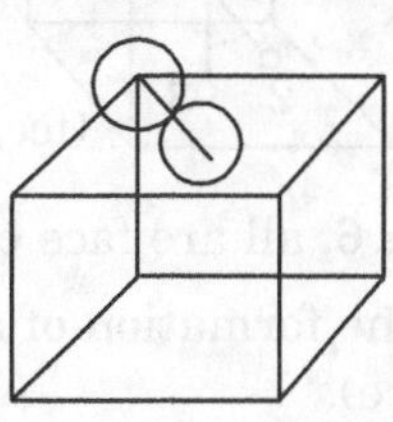

$$2r = \frac{\sqrt{2}a_2}{2} \quad ...(2)$$

Now, nearest neighbour distance in bcc & fcc are equal,

$\therefore$ from (1) & (2)

$$\frac{\sqrt{3}}{2}a_1 = \frac{\sqrt{2}}{2}a_2$$

$$\boxed{\frac{a_1}{a_2} = \frac{\sqrt{2}}{\sqrt{3}}}$$

or $\boxed{\frac{a_{bcc}}{a_{fcc}} = \sqrt{\frac{2}{3}}}$ ...(3)

$$\frac{\rho_{\gamma-\text{iron}}(\text{fcc})}{\rho_{\alpha-\text{iron}}(\text{bcc})} = \frac{\dfrac{2_{fcc} \times M}{(a)^3_{fcc} \times N_A}}{\dfrac{2_{BCC} \times M}{(a)^3_{BCC} \times N_A}}$$

$$\frac{\rho_{\gamma-\text{iron}}}{\rho_{\alpha-\text{iron}}} = \frac{4 \times M}{(a_{fcc})^3 \times N_A} \times \frac{(a_{BCC})^3 \times N_A}{2 \times M}$$

$$\left(\frac{a_{Bcc}}{a_{fcc}}\right)^3 = 2 \quad ...(4)$$

From eqn. (3), $\frac{a_{BCC}}{a_{fcc}} = \sqrt{\frac{2}{3}}$

So, placing value in (4)

$$\frac{\rho_{\gamma-\text{iron}}}{\rho_{\alpha-\text{iron}}} = 2 \times \left(\sqrt{\frac{2}{3}}\right)^3 = \frac{2 \times 2\sqrt{2}}{3\sqrt{3}}$$

$$= \frac{4 \times 1.414}{3 \times 1.732} = \frac{5.656}{5.196} = 1.08$$

70. Mass of unit cell is because of atoms occupying the unit cell.

Effective No. of atoms per unit cell = 4

$$\left(8 \times \frac{1}{8} + 6 \times \frac{1}{2} = 4\right)$$
(Corners) (face centre)

So, mass of 4 atoms = 56 × 4 = mass of unit cell

224 amu = mass of unit cell

$$\boxed{\text{Now, } 1\text{amu} = \frac{1}{N_A}\text{gms}}$$

So, mass of unit cell (in gms)

$$= 224 \text{ amu}$$

$$= 224 \times \frac{1}{N_A} \text{gms}$$

$$= 224 \times \frac{1}{6.02 \times 10^{23}} \text{ gms}$$

$$= 37.20 \times 10^{-23} \text{ gms}$$

$$= 3.72 \times 10^{-22} \text{ gms}$$

71. Apply, $\rho = \frac{Z \times M}{a^3 \times N_A}$

$$6.25 = \frac{4 \times 60}{a^3 \times 6.02 \times 10^{23}}$$

$$a^3 = \frac{4 \times 10}{6.25 \times 6 \times 10^{23}}$$

$$a^3 = \frac{40}{6.25} \times 10^{-23}$$

$$a^3 = 6.4 \times 10^{-23}$$

$$a^3 = 64 \times 10^{-24}$$

$$\boxed{a = 4 \times 10^{-8} \text{ cm}}$$

$$\boxed{1 cm = 10^{10} pm}$$

$$\boxed{a = 4 \times 10^{-8} \times 10^{10} pm = 400 pm}$$

If AB is NaCl type, then

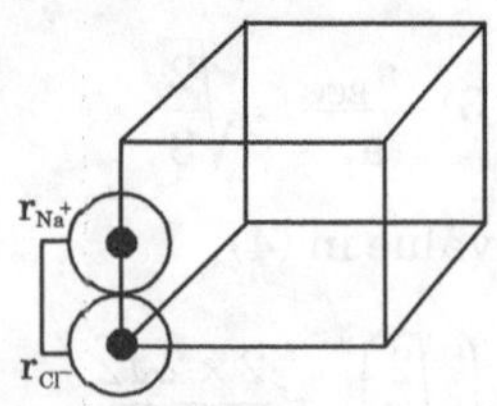

$$\boxed{r^+ + r^- = \frac{a}{2}}$$

$$\therefore r^+ + r^- = \frac{400}{2} = 200$$

60 + r⁻ = 200

$$\boxed{r^- = 200 - 60 = 140 \text{ pm}}$$

77. Density of a crystal is decreased in schottky defect, increased in interstitial defect & remains same in Frenkel defect.

78. Copper is a metal (least energy gap) silicon is a semi-conductor (moderate energy gap) C(diamond) is a non-metal (biggest energy gap)

79. Small size of cation in an ionic compound favors Frenkel defect

87. 4 formula units $\xrightarrow{\text{Correspond to}}$ 1 unit cell of NaCl

(Mass of 4 formula units of NaCl = $\frac{58.5}{N_A} \times 4$ gms)

$$\therefore \frac{58.5}{N_A} \times 4 \text{ gm} \xrightarrow[\text{to}]{\text{Corresponds}} 1 \text{ unit cell}$$

$$1 \text{ gm} \xrightarrow[\text{to}]{\text{Corresponds}} \frac{1}{58.5} \times \frac{4}{N_A} \text{ unit cell}$$

$$= \frac{1}{58.5 \times 4} \times 6.02 \times 10^{23} \text{ unit cells}$$

$$= \frac{6.02}{234.0} \times 10^{23}$$

$$\boxed{= 1.71 \times 10^{21} \text{ unit cells}}$$

88. For exactly fitting in cubic void,

$$\frac{r^+}{r^-} = 0.732$$

$$\frac{r^+}{200} = 0.732$$

$$r^+ = 0.732 \times 200$$

$$= \frac{732}{1000} \times 200 = \frac{1464}{10}$$

$$= 146.4 \text{ pm}$$

89. Atomic ratio is reciprocal of co-ordination number ratio.

90. An octahedral void is formed in fcc lattice (at edge centres & body centre) with Co. No. = 6

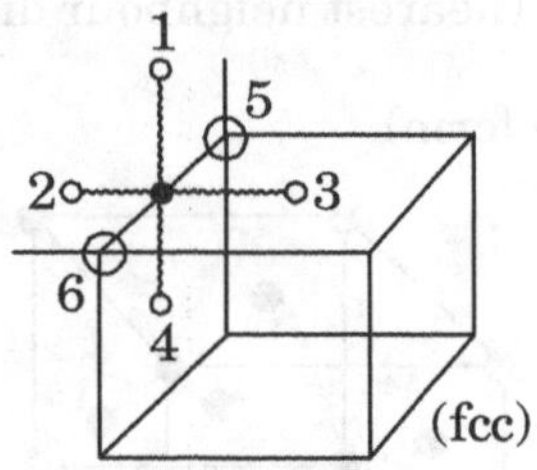

Octahedral void at edge centre

1, 2, 3, & 4 are face centred atoms whereas 5 & 6 are corner atoms

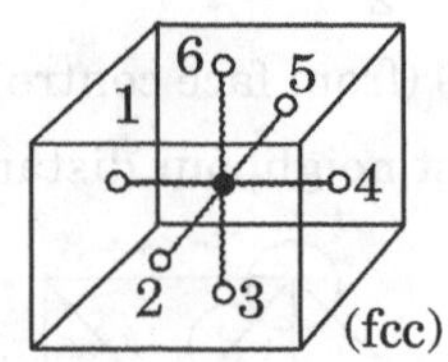

1, 2, 3, 4, 5, & 6, all are face centred atoms resulting in the formation of an octahedral void (at body centre).

→ Cubic void is formed at body centre in simple cubic arrangement & has Co. No. = 8.

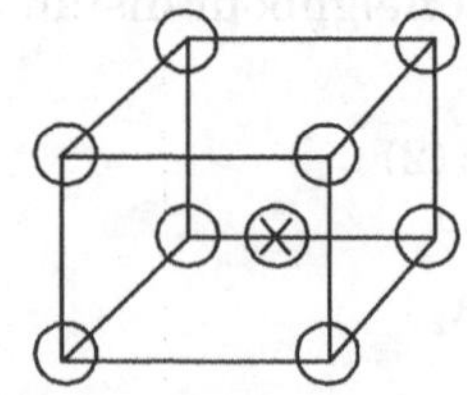

X → represent cubic void.

91. ccp (fcc) has maximum effective atoms (ions) packed = 4 $\left(8 \times \frac{1}{8} + 6 \times \frac{1}{2} = 4\right)$
(from corner) (from face centre)

But, in the formula itself (XY_3), the No. of Y^- ions = 3

So, $3Y^-$ ions are packed.

No. of Tetrahedral voids formed = 6

No. of Octahedral voids formed = 3

Now, X^{3+} ions (which is just one in numbers) occupies one octahedral void.

So, fraction of total void occupied $= \frac{1}{9}$

92. In fcc, $Z = 4 \left(\begin{array}{l} 8 \times \frac{1}{8} = 1 \text{ (from corners)} \\ 6 \times \frac{1}{2} = 3 \text{ (from face centre)} \end{array} \right)$

Total volume occupied $= 4 \times \frac{4}{3}\pi r^3 = \frac{16}{3}\pi r^3$

93. Let number of $Fe^{2+} = 100$

Let number of $O^{2-} = 100$

Now, 12% of 100 Fe^{2+} get replaced by Fe^{3+} i.e.

12 Fe^{2+} ions are replaced by Fe^{3+}.

Now, $3Fe^{2+}$ are replaced by Fe^{3+} = 2 (keeping charge balanced)

12 Fe^{2+} are replaced by Fe^{3+} = (keeping charge balanced) $\frac{2}{3} \times 12 = 8Fe^{3+}$

Hence, Fe^{2+} available now = 88 (100 – 12)

Number of Fe^{3+} available now = 8

Total Fe species = 96 (88 + 8)

$\therefore$ $Fe_{96}O_{100}$ or $Fe_{0.96}O_1$

94. For bcc,

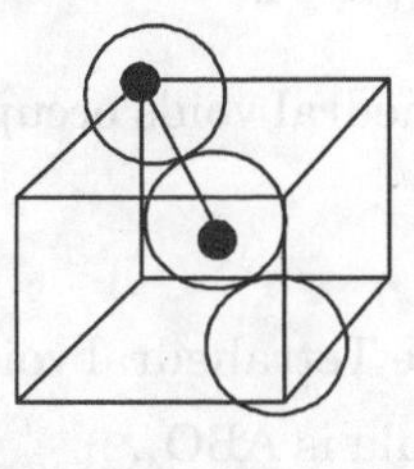

Nearest neighbour distance $= \frac{\sqrt{3}a}{2}$

Nearest neighbour distance given $= \sqrt{3}$ Å

$\therefore \frac{\sqrt{3}a}{2} = \sqrt{3}$ Å

$\boxed{a = 2Å}$

Apply, $\rho = \frac{Z \times M}{a^3 \times N_A} = \frac{2 \times 40 \times 10^{-3}}{(2 \times 10^{-10} m)^3} \times 6 \times 10^{23}$

$$\rho = \frac{2 \times 40 \times 10^{-3}}{8 \times 10^{-30} m^3 \times 6 \times 10^{23}} = \frac{10^{-2}}{6 \times 10^{-7}} kgm^{-3}$$

$= \frac{1}{6} \times 10^5$ kg m^{-3}

$= 0.166 \times 10^5 = 1.66 \times 10^4 = d \times 10^4$

$\boxed{\text{So, } d = 1.66}$

95. Let no. of metal ions in + 2 = y

Let no. of metal ions in + 3 = x – y

Total charge on metal ions in M_XO = + 2

$2y + 3(x - y) = +2$

$2y + 3x - 3y = +2$

$3x - y = 2$

$3x = 2 + y$

$\boxed{y = 3x - 2}$

No. of M^{2+} ions = 3x – 2

No. of M^{3+} ions = x – y

$= x - (3x - 2)$

$= x - 3x + 2 = 2 - 2x$

$$\text{Ratio} = \frac{\text{No. of } M^{3+} \text{ ions}}{\text{No. of } M^{2+} \text{ ions}} = \frac{2-2x}{3x-2} = \frac{2(1-x)}{3x-2}$$

96. Diamond has ZnS type structure.

'C' atoms at fcc locations & C atoms at alternate tetrahedral voids. So, total C atoms per unit cell = 8 (effective)

$$\rho = \frac{Z \times M}{a^3 \times N_A}$$

$$\rho_{initial} = \frac{8 \times 12}{a^3 \times N_A} \quad ...(1)$$

After atoms from body diagnol plane are removed

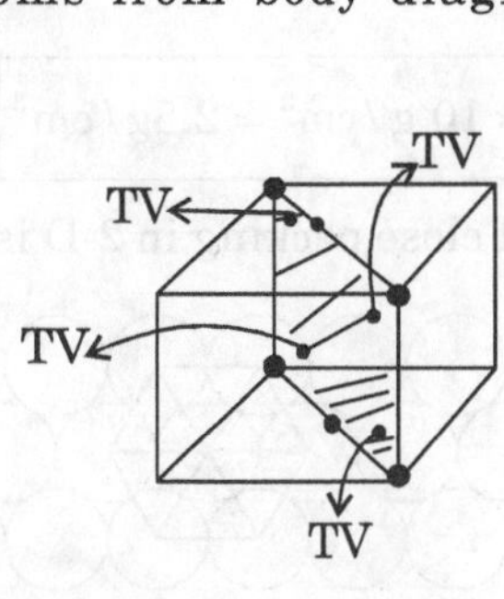

1. 4 corners are lost
2. 2 face centred atoms are lost.
3. 2 Tetrahedral voids are lost.

Now, effective No. of C atoms

$= 4 \times \frac{1}{8}$ (from corner) $+ 4 \times \frac{1}{2}$ (from face centre) + 2 (from tetrahedral voids)

So, No. of C atoms (effective)

$= \frac{1}{2} + 2 + 2 = \frac{9}{2}$ atoms

$$\rho_{final} = \frac{Z \times M}{a^3 \times N_A} = \frac{\frac{a}{2} \times M}{a^3 \times N_A} = \frac{4.5 \times 12}{a^3 \times N_A} \quad ...(2)$$

$$\% \text{ age redn.} = \frac{\frac{8 \times 12}{a^3 \times N_A} - \frac{4.5 \times 12}{a^3 \times N_A}}{\frac{8 \times 12}{a^3 \times N_A}} \times 100$$

$$= \frac{\frac{12}{a^3 \times N_A}(8 - 4.5)}{\frac{8 \times 12}{a^3 \times N_A}} \times 100$$

$$= \frac{3.5}{8} \times 100 = 43.75\%$$

97. No. of effective (atoms per unit cell = 8)

$$\rho(\text{density of unit cell}) = \frac{Z \times M}{a^3 \times N_A}$$

$$\rho = \frac{8 \times 12}{(0.4 \times 10^{-7}\text{cm})^3} \times \frac{1}{N_A}$$

$$\rho = \frac{96\text{g}}{(4 \times 10^{-8}\text{cm})^3 \times 6 \times 10^{23}}$$

$$\rho = \frac{96}{64 \times 10^{-24} \times 6 \times 10^{23}\text{cm}^3}\text{g}$$

$$\rho = \frac{96}{64 \times 6 \times 10^{-1}}\text{g/cm}^3$$

$$\boxed{\rho = \frac{6}{4 \times 6} \times 10\ \text{g/cm}^3 = 2.5\text{g/cm}^3}$$

98. Hexagonal close packing in 2-D is:

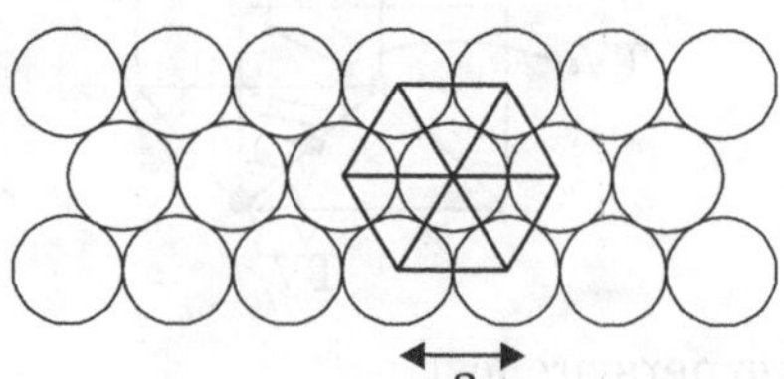

$$\text{Packing Fraction} = \frac{\text{Area of circles}}{\text{Total area}} = \frac{3 \times \pi r^2}{6 \times \frac{\sqrt{3}}{4}a^2}$$

(Total area involved is equivalent to the area of 6 equilateral triangles)

$$\text{P.F} = \frac{\pi r^2}{2 \times \frac{\sqrt{3}}{4}a^2} = \frac{\pi r^2}{\frac{\sqrt{3}(2r)^2}{2}} = \frac{\pi r^2}{\sqrt{3} \times 4r^2} \times 2$$

$$= \frac{\pi}{2\sqrt{3}} = 0.906$$

99. $\frac{\text{No. of } Fe^{3+}\text{ions}}{\text{No. of } Fe^{2+}\text{ion}} = \frac{15}{100}$ (given)

Along with 100 Fe^{2+}, 15 Fe^{3+} are also present.

Now, $2Fe^{3+}$ replace $Fe^{2+} = 3$

15 Fe^{3+} replace $Fe^{2+} = \frac{3}{2} \times 15 = 22.5$

So, total cationic sites = 100 + 22.5 = 122.5

Vacant voids = 22.5 – 15 = 7.5

Fraction of octahedral sites occupied by

$$\text{Vacancies} = \frac{7.5}{122.5} = 0.0612$$

100. O^{2-} ions are at → all corners $8 \times \frac{1}{8} = 1$; → all face centers $6 \times \frac{1}{2} = 3$

Total effective O^{2-} ions per unit cell = 4 → 8(T. Voids), 4(O. Voids)

25% octahedral voids means that 25% of 4 Octahedral voids are occupied.

So, 1 effective Octahedral voids is occupied $\left(\frac{25}{100} \times 4 = 1\right)$ by A.

No. of Tetrahedral voids occupied = 12.5% of 8

$$= \frac{12.5}{100} \times 8 = 1$$

So, 1 effective Tetrahedral void is occupied by B.

Hence, formula is ABO_4.

Now, O^{2-} at corner will have nearest neighbour as 'B' at (corner).

Tetrahedral void at a distance $\frac{\sqrt{3}a}{4}$ & next nearest neighbour as 'A' at $\frac{a}{2}$ distance in Octahedral void.

101. Ti^{4+} is placed in an octahedral void at the body centre. So, Co. No. = 6

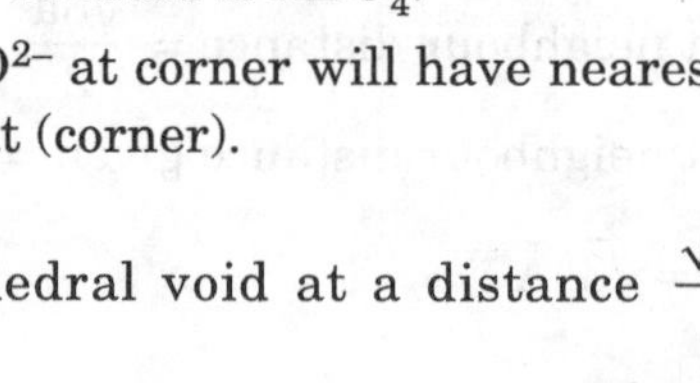

102. Nearest neighbour of S^{2-} are 4 Zn^{2+} ions at a distance = $\frac{\sqrt{3}a}{4}$.

Next nearest neighbour of S^{2-} are 12 S^{2-} at a distance = $\frac{a}{\sqrt{2}}$.

103.

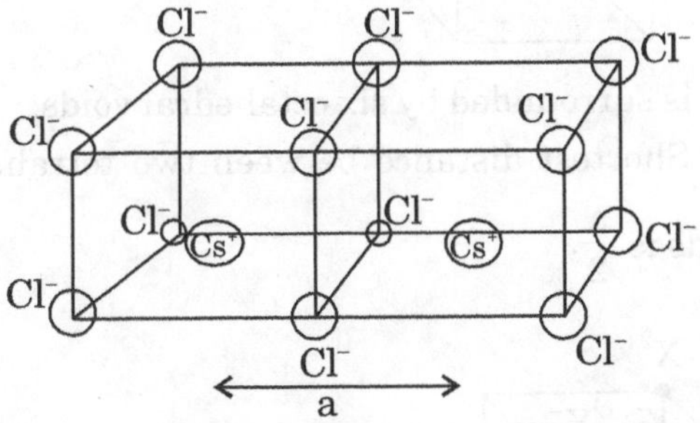

104.

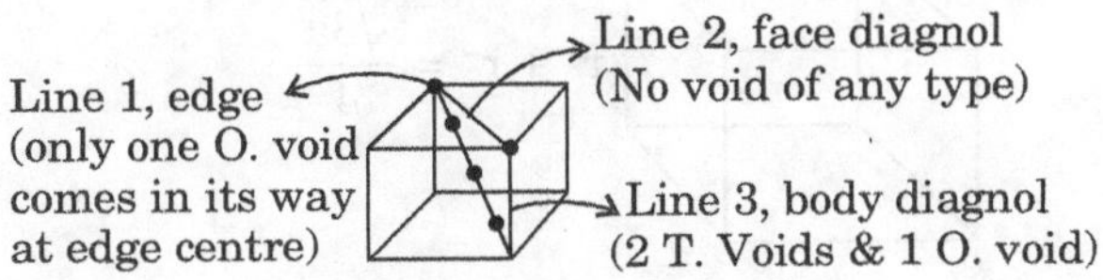

(fcc unit cell)

105. Apply, $\rho = \frac{Z \times M}{a^3 \times N_A}$

$$1g/cm^3 = \frac{Z \times 150g}{(10 \times 10^{-8} cm)^3} \times 6 \times 10^{23}$$

$$1 = \frac{Z \times 150}{10^{-21} \times 6 \times 10^{23}}$$

$$\frac{600}{150} = Z$$

$$\boxed{Z = 4}$$

Hence, it is fcc structure.

For fcc,

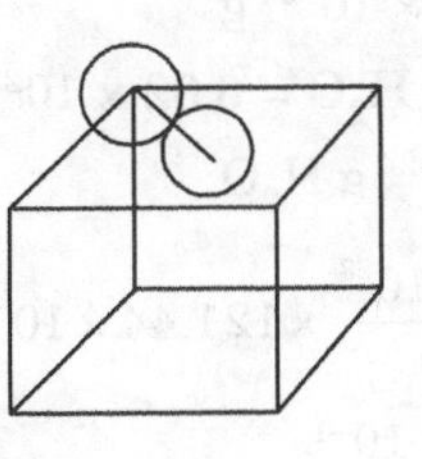

$$2r = \frac{\sqrt{2}a}{2}$$

$$r = \frac{\sqrt{2}a}{4} = \frac{\sqrt{2}}{4} \times 10 = 3.53 \text{ Å}$$

106. Structure of HCP unit cell is as follows:

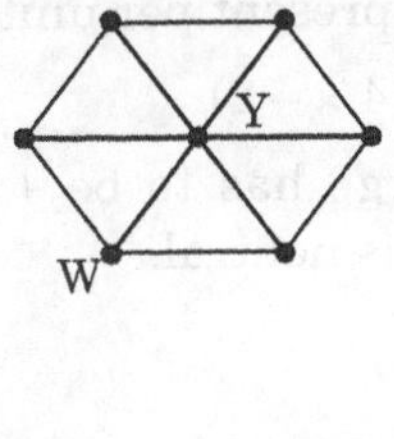

Contribution at corner in hcp = $\frac{1}{6}$

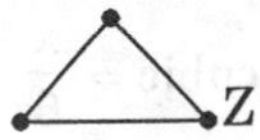

Effective No. of atoms at corners = $10 \times \frac{1}{6}$ ...(1)

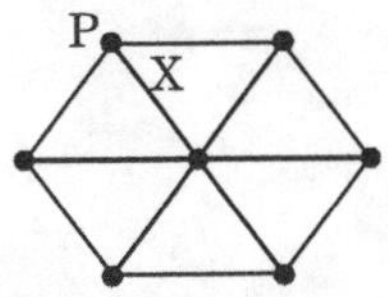

Effective No. of atoms of = 2 ...(2)

Total no. of effective atoms = $\frac{10}{6} + 2 = \frac{11}{3}$

107. The compound being formed has to be neutral.

Considering option (c),

Effective No. of Y^{2+} ions in hcp = 6

No. of octahedral voids = 6

Effective No. of X^+ ions in hcp = 6

(occupy all octahedral voids)

No. of tetrahedral voids = 2 × 6 = 12

Effective No. of Z^{3-} = 6

(occupy half of tetrahedral voids)

Total Cationic charge = + 12 (from 6 Y^{2+} ions) + 6 (from 6 X^+ ions) = + 18

Total Anionic charge = – 18 (from 6 Z^{3-} ions)

Hence, compound on the whole is neutral.

Considering Option (b)

Z^{3-} ions form ccp (i.e. effective no. of Z^{3-} = 4)

So, tetrahedral voids = 8

Y^{2+} ions occupy '4' tetrahedral voids.

Octahedral voids = 4

All are occupied by X^+ ions.

Hence, No. of X^+ ions = 4

No. of Y^{2+} ions = 4

No. of Z^{3-} ions = 4

Total cationic charge = + 4 (from four X^+ ions) + 8 (from four Y^{2+} ions) = + 12

Total anionic charge = – 12 (from four Z^{3-} ions)

Hence, compound is neutral.

108. Since the element is monoatomic, it must be existing in simple cubic arrangement where effective No. of atoms = 1.

Now, packing fraction in simple cubic = $\frac{\pi}{6}$.

(P. Fraction = Vol. occupied by atoms / Total vol. of cube)

$$P.F = \frac{1\times\frac{4}{3}\pi r^3}{a^3} = \frac{\frac{4}{3}\pi r^3}{(2r)^3}$$

(a = 2r for simple cubic)

$$P.F. = \frac{\pi}{6}$$

Now, $\frac{P.F}{\rho} = 0.1\ cm^3/gm$

$$\frac{P.F}{\rho} = \frac{\frac{\pi}{6}}{\frac{1\times M}{a^3\times N_A}} = 0.1\ cm^3\ gm^{-1}$$

$$\frac{\pi}{6}\times\frac{a^3\times N_A}{M} = 0.1\ cm^3\ gm^{-1} \quad ...(1)$$

Now, for simple cubic = a = 2 = 2 × 1 Å = 2Å

Putting the value of 'a' in equation (1)

$$\frac{\pi}{6}\times\frac{(2\times10^{-8}\,cm)^3\times6\times10^{23}}{M} = 0.1$$

$$\frac{\pi}{6}\times\frac{8\times10^{-24}\times6\times10^{23}}{0.1} = M$$

$$\boxed{8\pi = M}$$

109. Effective No. of atoms (Z) for 2D

$$hcp = 1+\frac{1}{3}\times6 = 3$$

Effective No. of atoms (Z) for 3D hcp

$= 12\times\frac{1}{6}$ (from corners)

+ 3 (from triangle inside hcp)

+ $2\times\frac{1}{2}$ (at face centre)

= 6

$$Ratio = \frac{3}{6} = \frac{1}{2}$$

110. In fluorite (CaF_2), cations occupy fcc locations where, as anions occupy all tetrahedral voids.

→ X^{2+} at corner is surrounded by 8 tetrahedral voids.

→ X^{2+} is at corner & face centre.

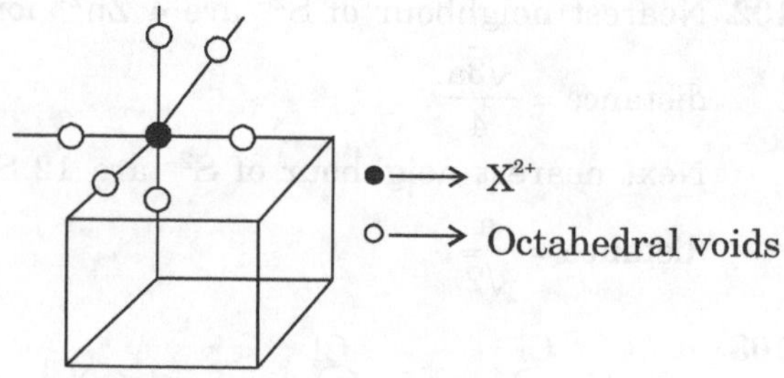

X^{2+} is surrounded by six octahedral voids.

→ Shortest distance between two tetrahedral voids is $\frac{a}{2}$.

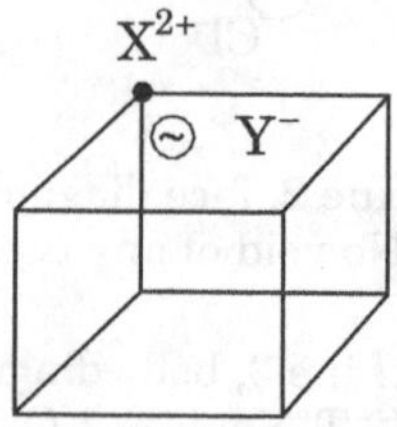

$$r^+ + r^- = \frac{\sqrt{3}a}{4}$$

So, statements a & d are WRONG.

111. Atoms A at corners → $8\times\frac{1}{8} = 1$

Atoms B at 5 face centres → $5\times\frac{1}{2} = \frac{5}{2}$

So, formula is $A_1\,B_{\frac{5}{2}} = A_2B_5$

112. Solutions not Given

113. From density,

1 cm^3 volume has weight of water = 0.92g

132 × 10^{-24} cm^3 has weight of water

= 0.92 × 132 × 10^{-24}g

= 121.44 × 10^{-24} g

Now, 18 gm H_2O = 6.02 × 10^{23} molecules of H_2O

121.44 × 10^{-24} g H_2O

$$= \frac{6.02\times10^{23}}{18}\times121.44\times10^{-24}$$

= 40.61 × 10^{-1}

= 4.061 ≈ 4 Ans.

114. O^{2-} ions located at → corners $\left(8\times\frac{1}{8}=1\right)$; → face centers $\left(6\times\frac{1}{2}=3\right)$

So, effective 4 O^{2-} ions are present per unit cell.

Total anionic charge = – 8 (4 × – 2)

Hence, total cationic charge has to be + 8 to ensure that the compound is neutral.

Na → at edge centres $\left(12 \times \frac{1}{4} = 3\right)$

Effective $Na^+ = 3$

Total charge carried by 3 Na^+ ions = + 3

Effective No. of W^{n+} ions = 1 (at body centre)

Charge on W = + 5

+ 5 (on W) + 3 (on $3Na^+$) = + 8

115. In ZnS, there are 4 effective Zn^{2+} and 4 effective S^{2-} ions.

$$\text{So, P.F.} = \frac{\left(\frac{4}{3}\pi r_+^3 + \frac{4}{3}\pi r_-^3\right)}{a^3} \times 4$$

$$\text{P.F.} = \frac{\frac{16}{3}\pi\left(r_+^3 + r_-^3\right)}{a^3}$$

Also, since the crystal is ideal, therefore anion-anion contact is maintained.

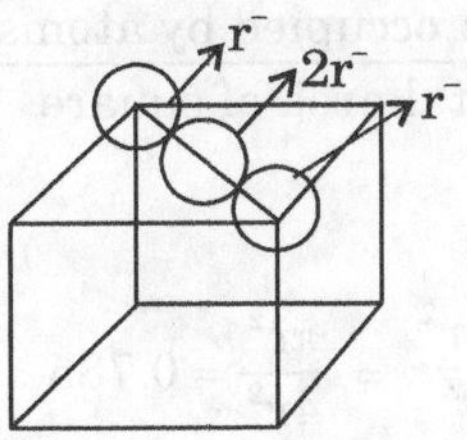

$$4r^- = \sqrt{2}a$$

$$\text{P.F.} = \frac{\frac{16}{3}\pi\left(r_+^3 + r_-^3\right)}{\left(\frac{4r_-}{\sqrt{2}}\right)^3}$$

$$= \frac{\pi}{3\sqrt{2}}\left(\left(\frac{r^+}{r^-}\right)^3 + 1\right)$$ (Limiting value for Tetrahedral void = $\frac{r^+}{r^-} = 0.225$)

$$= \frac{\pi}{3\sqrt{2}}((0.225)^3 + 1)$$

$$= 0.749$$

116. $\frac{r^+}{r^-} = \frac{90}{250} = 0.36$ which lies between 0.225 to 0.414.

So, it will slip easily in Tetrahedral void.

117.

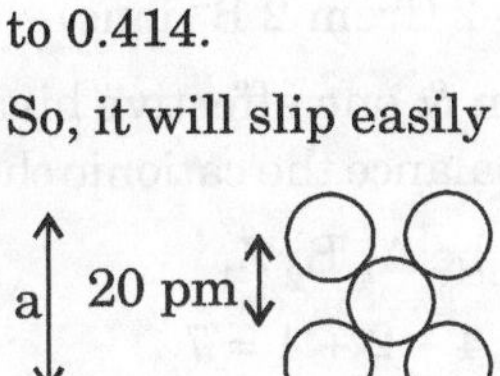

Now, 2r + 20 = a (from image) ...(1)

Also,

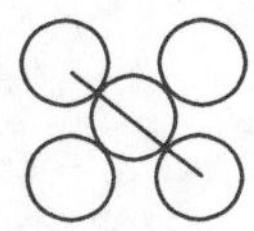

$4r = \sqrt{2}a$ (face diagonal)

$$r = \frac{\sqrt{2}a}{4}$$

Put value of 'r' in equation (1)

$$2 \times \frac{\sqrt{2}a}{4} + 20 = a$$

$$\frac{\sqrt{2}a}{2} + 20 = a$$

$$20 = a - \frac{a}{\sqrt{2}}$$

$$20 = a\left(1 - \frac{1}{\sqrt{2}}\right)$$

$$20 = a\left(1 - \frac{1}{1.414}\right)$$

a = 68.25 pm

118. 100 moles of NaCl are doped with $AlCl_3$

= 10^{-3} moles

1 mole of NaCl are doped with $AlCl_3$

$$= \frac{10^{-3}}{100} = 10^{-5} \text{ moles}$$

Concentration of cation vacancies is calculated per mole of NaCl.

10^{-5} moles of $AlCl_3 = 10^{-5} \times N_A$ molecules of $AlCl_3$

$= 10^{-5} \times N_A Al^{3+}$ ions

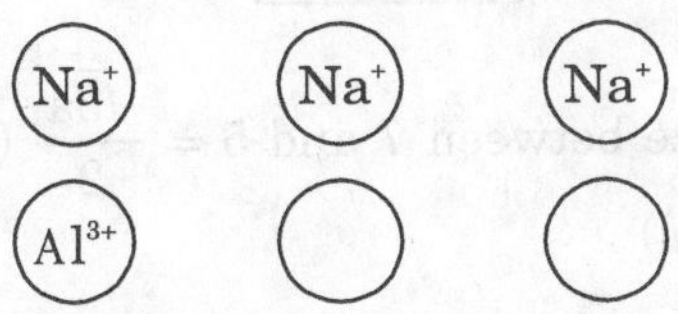

1 Al^{3+} creates cation vacancy = 2

$10^{-5} \times N_A$ Al^{3+} creates cation vacancy

$= 2 \times 10^{-5} \times N_A$

$= 2 \times 10^{-5} \times 6.02 \times 10^{23}$

$= 12.04 \times 10^{18}$

119.

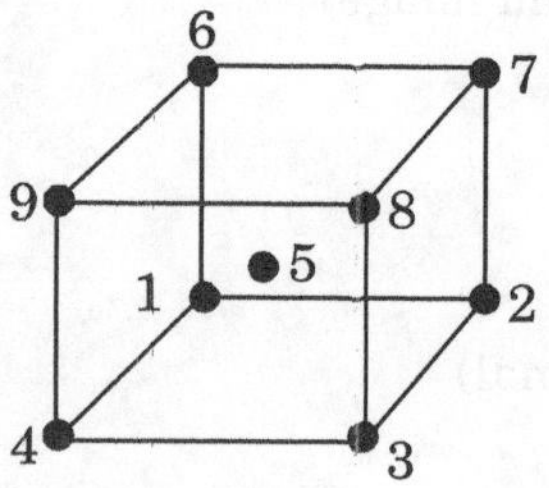

Wrt option a, atoms 6 and 7 are not in contact (in bcc)

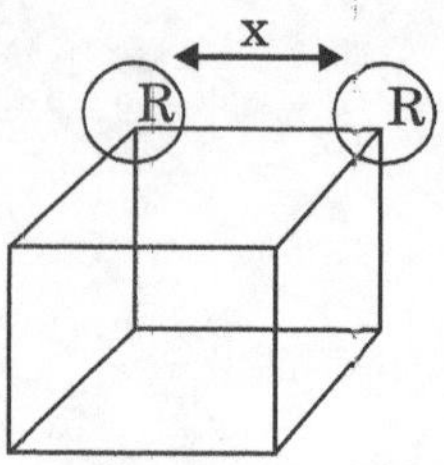

Here, $2R + x = a$

(bcc)

Wrt option b –

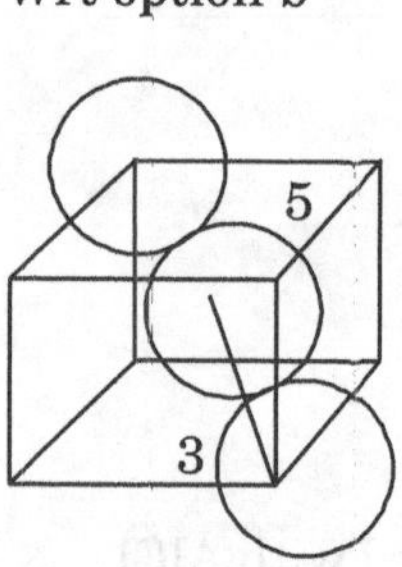

Distance between 5 and 3 = $\frac{\sqrt{3}a}{2} = 2R$

wrt option c,

Distance between 7 and 9 = $\sqrt{2}a$ (face diagonal)

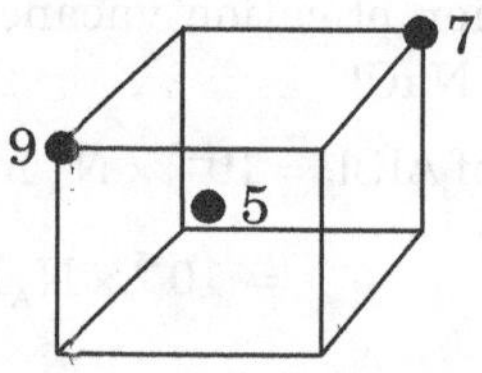

Distance between 7 and 5 = $\frac{\sqrt{3}a}{2}$ (half of body diagonal)

$$\text{Ratio} = \frac{\sqrt{2}a}{\frac{\sqrt{3}a}{2}} = \frac{\sqrt{2}a}{\sqrt{3}a} \times 2 = \frac{2\sqrt{2}}{\sqrt{3}} = \sqrt{\frac{8}{3}}$$

120. 5 mole% vacancies means that 1 mole of Na^+Cl^- when doped with $AlCl_3$ has 0.05 mole Cation Vacancies.

2 mole cation vacancies are created by Al^{3+} = 1 mole

0.05 mole cation vacancies are created by Al^{3+}

$= \frac{1}{2} \times 0.05$

$= 0.025$ mole

So, Al^{3+} present = 0.025 mole

1 mole Al^{3+} substitutes Na^+ = 3 mole

0.025 mole Al^{3+} substitutes $Na^+ = 3 \times 0.025$

$= 0.075$ mole Na^+

Moles of Na^+ present = 1 – 0.075 = 0.925

Moles of Al^{3+} present = 0.025

Mole of Cl^- present = 1

So, formula of the compound = $Na_{0.925}\,Al_{0.025}\,Cl_1$

121. Total atoms inside the square unit cell

$= \frac{1}{4} \times 4 + 1 = 2$

$$\text{P.F.} = \frac{\text{Area occupied by atoms}}{\text{Total area of square}} = \frac{1 \times \pi r^2}{a^2}$$

$a = 2r$

$$\text{P.F.} = \frac{1 \times \pi r^2}{(2r)^2} = \frac{\pi r^2}{4r^2} = 0.785$$

122.

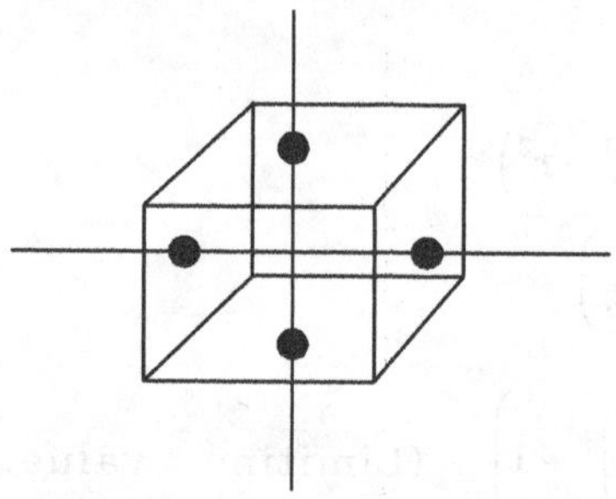

4 face centred S^{2-} ions are lost.

Effective S^{2-} ions lost = $\frac{1}{2} \times 4 = 2$

Effective A^+ = 4 (per unit cell)

Effective B^- ions = $8 \times \frac{1}{8} + 2 \times \frac{1}{2} = 2$ (corner + face centre)

Total cation charge = +4 (from 4 A^+ ions)

Total Anion charge = – 2 (from 2 B^- ions)

So, Z is a bivalent anion & one effective bivalent Z anions is required to balance the cationic charge.

Hence, formula should be $A_4\,B_2\,Z_1$

So, value of x + y + c = 4 + 2 + 1 = 7

124. 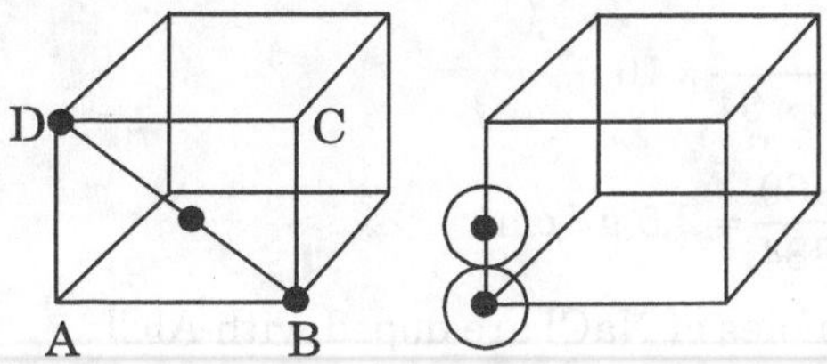

$$r^+ + r^- = \frac{a}{2}$$

No. of effective Na^+ ions = 4

No. of effective Cl^- ions $= 6 \times \frac{1}{8} + 5 \times \frac{1}{2}$

$$= \frac{3}{4} + \frac{5}{2} = \frac{3+10}{4} = \frac{13}{4}$$

$$\text{P.F.} = \frac{4 \times \frac{4}{3}\pi r_+^3 + \frac{13}{4} \times \frac{4}{3}\pi r_-^3}{a^3}$$

$$= \frac{4 \times \frac{4}{3}\pi r_+^3 + \frac{13}{4} \times \frac{4}{3}\pi r_-^3}{(2(r^+ + r^-))^3}$$

$$\text{P.F} = \frac{\frac{16}{3}\pi r_+^3 + \frac{13}{3}\pi r_-^3}{8(r^+ + r^-)^3}$$

125. $Fe_{0.93}\ O_{1.00}$

Let No. of Fe^{2+} = x

and No. of Fe^{3+} = 0.93–x

Total charge on Fe species = + 2

So, 2x + 3(0.93 – x) = + 2

2x + 2.79 – 3x = + 2

– x = – 0.79

$\boxed{x = 0.79}$

No. of Fe^{2+} ions = 0.79

No. of Fe^{3+} ions = 0.14

$$\boxed{\frac{\text{No. of } Fe^{3+}\text{ions}}{\text{No. of } Fe^{2+}\text{ions}} = \frac{0.14}{0.79} = 0.177}$$

Weight of Fe^{3+} = 0.14 × 56 = 7.84g

(where atomic weight of Fe = 56g)

126. $\frac{r^+}{r^-} = \frac{1.732}{1.414} - 1 = 0.225$

Which is exactly fitting in tetrahedral void.

Since, F^- ion occupies all tetrahedral voids, each Ca^{2+} will be surrounded by 8 F^- ions.

Also, since F^- exactly fits in the tetrahedral void, each Ca^{2+} will also touch 12 other Ca^{2+} ions.

127. Spinel is, a mineral, Mg Al_2 O_4 having general formula MM_2O_4, where divalent ions are occupied in tetrahedral void and trivalent ions in octahedral void and O^{2-} ions are arranged in fcc pattern.

Only $\frac{1}{8}$ th tetrahedral and $\frac{1}{2}$ of octahedral voids are occupied.

$$\frac{r_{Al3+}}{r_{O2-}} = 0.414, \quad \frac{r_{mg^{2+}}}{r_{O2-}} = 0.225$$

$$\text{P.F.} = \frac{\frac{4}{3}\pi\left(2 \times (r_{Al^{3+}})^3 + (r_{Mg^{2+}})^3 + (4r_{O^{2-}})^3\right)}{a^3}$$

Also, $4r_{O^{2-}} = \sqrt{2}a$

$\boxed{a = 2\sqrt{2}\ r_{O^{2-}}}$

$$\text{P.F.} = \frac{4}{3}\pi \frac{\left[2 \times (0.414\ r_{O^{2-}})^3 + (0.225\ r_{O^{2-}})^3 + (4r_{O^{2-}})^3\right]}{(2\sqrt{2}\ r_{O^{2-}})^3}$$

$$\therefore \text{P.F} = \frac{4}{3}\pi \frac{(2 \times (0.414)^3 + (0.225)^3 + 4)}{(2\sqrt{2})^3}$$

$\boxed{\text{P.F} = 0.768}$

128. 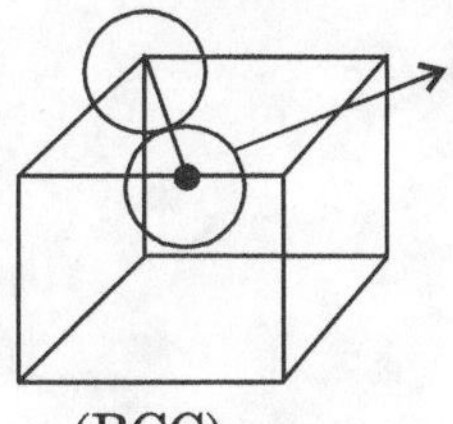

(BCC)

Nearest neighbour distance $= \frac{\sqrt{3}a}{2} = \frac{\sqrt{3}}{2} \times a = 433$

$$a = \frac{433 \times 2}{\sqrt{3}}$$

Next nearest neighbour distance = a

So, ans. $= \frac{433 \times 2}{\sqrt{3}} = 500\,\text{pm}$

129. $r = \frac{173.2}{2} = 86.6\,\text{pm}$

If it is ZnS type, both Zn^{2+} and S^{2-} ions are replaced by carbons. So, there are effective 8 C atoms per unit cell.

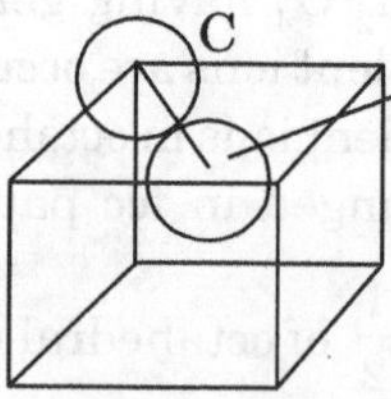

$$2r = \frac{\sqrt{3}a}{4}$$

$$\frac{8r}{\sqrt{3}} = a$$

$$\frac{8 \times 86.6}{\sqrt{3}} = a = 400 \text{ pm}$$

Now, apply

$$\rho = \frac{Z \times M}{a^3 \times N_A}$$

$$\rho = \frac{8 \times 12g}{(400 \times 10^{-10} cm)^3 \times 6 \times 10^{23}}$$

$$\rho = \frac{96g}{64 \times 10^{-24} \times 6 \times 10^{23}}$$

$$\rho = \frac{96}{6 \times 64} \times 10$$

$$\rho = \frac{960}{384} = 2.5 \text{ g / cm}^3$$

130. 100 moles of NaCl are doped with $AlCl_3$

$= 10^{-3}$ moles

1 moles of NaCl are doped with $AlCl_3 = 10^{-5}$ moles

(Concentration of cation vacanceis are calculated per mole)

1 mole Al^{3+} creates cation vacancies = 2 mole

10^{-5} mole Al^{3+} creates cation vacancies

$= 2 \times 10^{-5}$ mole

No. of cation vacancies

$= 2 \times 10^{-5} \times 6.02 \times 10^{23}$

$= 12.04 \times 10^{18}$

131.

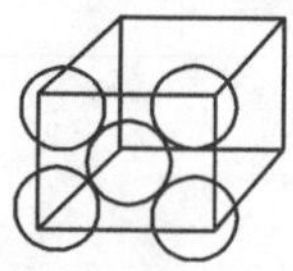

Face plane

■■

2

CHAPTER

Solutions

Concentration

1. The density (in g/ml) of a 3.6 M H_2SO_4 solution which is 29% by mass will be -

(*a*) 1.216 (*b*) 2.88

(*c*) 3.12 (*d*) 2.75

2. 5 molar, 1 L solution of an acid is divided in two equal volumes, then molarity of each half is -

(*a*) 1.25 M (*b*) 2.5 M

(*c*) 5 M (*d*) 7.5 M

3. 10 grams of a solute is dissolved in 'X' grams of a solvent to obtain a 10% (w/w) solution.Then, the value of 'X' is -

(*a*) 80 (*b*) 90

(*c*) 110 (*d*) 100

4. If an aqueous solution of urea is 6% (w/v), then the volume of solution containing 2 mole of urea is -

(*a*) 2 litre (*b*) 6 litre

(*c*) 4 litre (*d*) 1 litre

5. The amount of $CaCl_2$, which should be present in 50 ml of its solution to get a final concentration of 0.02 g/ml is -

(*a*) 1.5 g (*b*) 0.5 g

(*c*) 2.22 g (*d*) 1 g

6. What is molarity of K^+ in aqueous solution that contains 17.4 ppm of K_2SO_4? (M. Mass of K_2SO_4 is 174 g/mol)

(*a*) 2×10^{-4} m (*b*) 2×10^{-3} m

(*c*) 2×10^{-2} m (*d*) Unpredictable

7. A solution of $Al_2(SO_4)_3$ (1.25 gm/ml) is 34.2% (w/w). The molarity, normality & molality of the solution is, respectively -

(*a*) 1.25 M, 7.5 N, 1.519 molal

(*b*) 1.519 M, 75 N, 1.3 molal

(*c*) 7.5 M, 1.25 N, 1.5 molal

(*d*) None of these

8. The mole fraction of H_2O in 20% (w/w) aqueous solution of H_2O_2 is -

(*a*) $\frac{77}{68}$ (*b*) $\frac{68}{77}$

(*c*) $\frac{20}{80}$ (*d*) $\frac{80}{20}$

9. 171 g of cane sugar (mol. wt. = 342 g) are dissolved in 1000 g of water at 30°C. If the density of solution is 1.1 g/ml, then -

(*a*) molality > molarity

(*b*) molality = molarity

(*c*) molarity > molality

(*d*) None of these

10. A 'X' molal solution of a compound in benzene has mole fraction of solute equal to 0.2.

The value of 'X' is -

(*a*) 3·2

(*b*) 6·4

(*c*) 12·8

(*d*) 25·6

11. The molality of 1 litre solution of 93% H_2SO_4(w/v) is -

(given - the density of solution is 1.84 g/ml)

(*a*) 10.43 (*b*) 20.36

(*c*) 12.05 (*d*) 14.66

12. If 0·028 g of N_2 gas dissolves in 1 litre water at 'X' atm pressure of N_2 gas & the Henry's law Constant for the gas in water is 1×10^5 atm, then 'X' atm pressure of N_2 gas is equal to -

(*a*) 1·21 atm (*b*) 1·53 atm

(*c*) 1·80 atm (*d*) 2·13 atm

13. The quantity of CO_2 in 900 ml of soda water when packed under 1 atm CO_2 Pressure at 298 K is ($K_H = 2 \times 10^3$ atm) -

(*a*) 1·854 g (*b*) 1·102 g

(*c*) 2·335 g (*d*) 3·85 g

Ideal & Non-ideal Solutions

14. When acetone is added to chloroform, a hydrogen bond is formed between them. Then, solution shows, -

(*a*) Positive deviation from Raoult's law.

(*b*) Negative deviation from Raoult's law.

(*c*) No deviation from Raoult's law.

(d) Volume of solution is slightly increased.

15. Which of the following is WRONG for the solution of Chloroform & acetone?

(*a*) they form non - ideal solution

(*b*) entropy change on their mixing is positive.

(*c*) their solution appears to be cold on mixing.

(*d*) their mixing is an exothermic process.

16. Which of the following is a characteristic of water & ethanol mixture?

(*a*) $\Delta H_{sol} > 0$, $\Delta S_{sol.} = 0$

(*b*) $\Delta H_{sol} > 0$, $\Delta S_{sol.} > 0$

(*c*) $\Delta H_{sol.} < 0$, $\Delta V_{sol.} > 0$

(*d*) $\Delta H_{sol.} > 0$, $\Delta V_{sol.} < 0$

17. For an ideal binary solution with $P_A^0 > P_B^0$, which relation is correct?

(where X_A is mole fraction of A in liquid phase, X_B is mole fraction of B in liquid phase, Y_A is mole fraction of A in vapour phase & Y_B is the mole fraction of B in Vapour phase)

(*a*) $X_A = Y_A$ (*b*) $X_A > Y_A$

(*c*) $\frac{Y_A}{Y_B} > \frac{X_A}{X_B}$ (*d*) Both (a) & (b)

18. The solubility of N_2 in water at 300 K and 500 torr partial pressure is 0.01 gL^{-1}. The solubility in gL^{-1} at 750 torr partial pressure is

(*a*) 0.0075 (*b*) 0.005

(*c*) 0.02 (*d*) 0.015

19. Which of the following will form an ideal solution?

(*a*) $CHCl_3$ & acetone

(*b*) HNO_3 & water

(*c*) Benzene & Toluene

(*d*) None of these

20. Consider a binary mixture of volatile liquids. If at $X_A = 0{\cdot}4$, the vapour pressure of the solution is 580 torr then the mixture could be ($P_A^0 = 300$ torr, $P_B^0 = 800$ torr) :-

(*a*) Chloroform & acetone

(*b*) Chlorobenzene & Bromobenzene

(*c*) Benzene & toluene

(*d*) n-hexane & n-heptane

21. The total vapour presure of mixture of 1 mol of volatile component A ($P^0{}_A = 100$ mm Hg) & 3 mol of volatile component B ($P^0{}_B = 60$ mm Hg) is 75 mm. For such solution,

(*a*) there is +ve deviation from Raoult's law.

(*b*) V.P. is raised.

(*c*) B. pt. is lowered.

(*d*) All are correct.

22. The vapor pressure curves of the same solvent are shown. The curves do not intersect. The concentrations of solutions are in the order

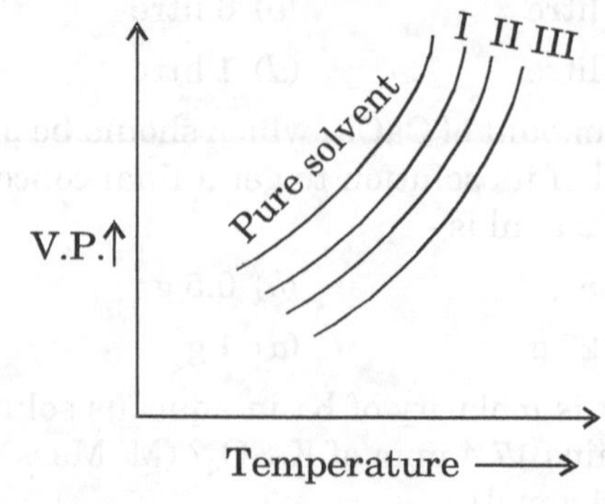

(*a*) III > II > I (*b*) I = II = III

(*c*) I > II > III (*d*) I > III > II

Colligative Properties

23. A mixture containing 0.25 mole fraction of component A having vapour pressure equal to 400 mmHg in pure state & component B having vapour pressure equal to 200 mmHg in pure state, the mole fraction of A in Vapour phase will be

(*a*) 0.4 (*b*) 0.6

(*c*) 0.75 (*d*) 0.25

24. A solution has a 1 : 4 mole ratio of pentane & hexane. The vapour pressure of pure pentane & pure hexane are 440 mm Hg & 120 mm Hg, respectively at 20°C. The mole fraction of pentane in the vapour phase will be

(*a*) 0.54 (*b*) 0.2

(*c*) 0.75 (*d*) 0.45

25. The vapour pressure of pure liquids A & B are 450 and 700 mm Hg respectively at 350 K. The composition of the liquid mixture if total vapour pressure is 600 mm Hg is

(Assuming ideal solution)

(*a*) $X_A = 0.4, X_B = 0.6$ (*b*) $X_A = 0.6, X_B = 0.4$

(*c*) $X_A = 0.3, X_B = 0.7$ (*d*) $X_A = 0.7, X_B = 0.3$

26. The vapour pressure of a solvent is decreased by 10 mm of Hg when a non-volatile solute was added to the solvent. The mole fraction of solute in the solution is 0.2. What would be the mole fraction of solvent if decrease in vapour pressure is 20 mm of Hg?

(*a*) 0.8 (*b*) 0.6

(*c*) 0.4 (*d*) 0.2

27. The lowering of vapour pressure due to a solute in 1 molal aqueous solution at 100°C is–

(*a*) 13.44 mm Hg (*b*) 14.12 mm Hg

(*c*) 31.2 mm Hg (*d*) 35.2 mm Hg

28. 3 gm urea is dissolved in 45 g of water. The relative lowering of vapour pressure is–

(*a*) 0.05 (*b*) 0.04

(*c*) 0.02 (*d*) 0.5

29. Two elements P & Q form compounds having molecular formula PQ_2 & PQ_4. When dissolved in 20 g of benzene (C_6H_6), 1g of PQ_2 lower freezing point by 2.3 K whereas 1g of PQ_4 lowers it by 1.3 K. Molal depression constant for benzene is 5.1 K kg/mol. Atomic masses of P & Q are, respectively.

(*a*) 56, 68 (*b*) 56, 56

(*c*) 25.5, 42.64 (*d*) 72, 68

30. Which of the following solutions will have the highest boiling point?

(*a*) 1% of glucose (w/w) in H_2O

(*b*) 1% of sucrose (w/w) in H_2O

(*c*) 1% NaCl (w/w) in H_2O

(*d*) 1% $CaCl_2$ (w/w) in H_2O

31. The osmotic pressure of 0.4% (w/v) urea solution is 1.66 atm & that of a solution of sugar of 3.42% (w/v) is 2.46 atm. When both the solutions are mixed in equal volume then the Osmotic pressure of the resultant solution will be -

(*a*) 1.64 atm (*b*) 2.46 atm

(*c*) 2.06 atm (*d*) 0.82 atm

32. At 300 K, the two solutions of glucose A & B with respective concentrations 0.01 M & 0.001 M are separated by semipermeable membrane. How much external pressure needs to be applied & on which solution so as to prevent osmosis?

(*a*) 0.2463 atm pressure is applied on solution B

(*b*) 0.2217 atm pressure is applied on solution A

(*c*) 0.0246 atm pressure is applied on solution B

(*d*) 0.0217 atm pressure is applied on solution A

33. Which of the following solutions will have the highest freezing point?

(assume molarity = molality)

(*a*) 0·10N $MgCl_2$

(*b*) 0·10N NaCl

(*c*) 0·10N Na_3PO_4

(*d*) All solutions have the same freezing point

34. By studying the elevation in boiling point of aqueous solution of glucose, the value of k_b for water is found to be 0.51 K Kg mol^{-1}. The value of k_b that can be expected from aqueous solution of $k_4[Fe(CN)_6]$ is -

(*a*) 0·51 (*b*) 2 × 0·51

(*c*) 3 × 0·51 (*d*) 5 × 0·51

35. The relative lowering in vapour pressure of an aqueous solution of NaCl is 0.167. The number of moles of NaCl present in 180g of water is -

(*a*) 1

(*b*) 2

(*c*) 3

(*d*) 4

36. Which of the following pairs of solutions at same temperature can be expected to be isotonic?

(a) 0.01 M KCl & 0·01M urea

(b) 0.01 M $MgCl_2$ & 0·01MkCl

(c) 0.1M $MgCl_2$ & 0.1M Na_2SO_4

(d) 0·1M $Ca(NO_3)_2$ & 0·5M acetic acid solution

37. 20 ml of $BaCl_2$ solution required 10 ml of 0·4M $AgNO_3$ solution for complete precipitation of AgCl. The Osmotic pressure of $BaCl_2$ solution assuming complete ionisation at 27°C will be-

(a) 7·38 atm (b) 4·5 atm

(c) 2·46 atm (d) None of these

38. The molecular weight of NaCl, determined by studying freezing point depression of its 0·5% aqueous solution is 30. The apparent degree of dissociation of NaCl is-

(a) 0·95 (b) 0·45

(c) 0·60 (d) 0·35

39. In a solution of A in B, 'A' tetramerises as $4A \rightarrow A_4$. If degree of association is 30%, the Van't Hoff Factor (i) is approximately.

(a) 0·775 (b) $\frac{1}{4}$

(c) 4 (d) None of these

40. Mixture of volatile components A & B has total vapour pressure (in torr)

$$P = 254 - 119X_A$$

where X_A is mole fraction of A in mixture. Assuming ideal solution, P_A^0 & P_B^0 are - (in torr)

(a) 254, 119 (b) 119, 254

(c) 135, 254 (d) 154, 119

41. The vapour pressure of the solution of two liquids A (P^o = 80 mmHg) & B (P^o = 120 mmHg) is found to be 100 mm when X_A = 0·4.

The result shows that -

(a) solution exhibits ideal behaviour.

(b) solution shows positive deviation.

(c) solution shows negative deviation.

(d) solution will show positive deviation for lower concentrations & negative deviation for higher concentrations.

42. Lowering in vapour pressure is highest for -

(a) 0·2 M Urea (b) 0·1 M glucose

(c) 0·1 M $MgSO_4$ (d) 0·1 M $BaCl_2$

43. The Van't Hoff factor for 0.1 M $Ba(NO_3)_2$ solution is 2.74. Then, the degree of dissociation is-

(a) 91.3% (b) 87%

(c) 100% (d) 74%

44. At 80°C, the vapour pressure of pure liquid 'A' is 520 mm Hg & that of pure liquid 'B' is 1000 mm Hg. If a mixture contains A & B & it boils at 80°C and 1 atm pressure, then the amount of 'A' in the mixture is-

(a) 50 mol percent (b) 70 mol percent

(c) 90 mol percent (d) 65 mol percent

45. The relative lowering of vapour pressure of an aqueous solution containing non-volatile solute is 0.0125. Calculate molality of the solution assuming solution to be very dilute.

(a) 0.70

(b) 0.55

(c) 0.45

(d) 0.0225

46. An aqueous solution of a compound AB freezes at −0.48°C. At this temperature, AB behaves as a non-electrolyte. The same solution boils at 100·26°C at a pressure of 1 atm. Also, for water, $\frac{k_f}{k_b} = 3 \cdot 7$. So, we can conclude that the compound AB, at the boiling point of solution-

(a) behaves as a non-electrolyte.

(b) ionises to the extent of 50%.

(c) behaves as a strong electrolyte.

(d) dimerises completely in the solution.

47. Match the K_b values for given solvents X, Y, and Z whose boiling points are 100, 27 and 253°C respectively. K_b values are randomly reported as 0.53, 0.98 and 0.68. The molecular weights of X, Y and Z are same. Assuming ΔS_V values for all the solvents are same. Then K_b for -

(1) X = 0.68, Y = 0.53; Z = 0.98

(2) X = 0.98, Y = 0.68; Z = 0.53

(3) X = 0.53, Y= 0.98; Z = 0.68

(4) None of these

48. 0.1M NaCl (aq.) & 0.2M $AgNO_3$ (aq.) solutions are mixed in 3 : 1 volume ratio. The freezing point of the resulting solution is -
(assume molarity = molality)

(*a*) 0.279 K (*b*) 272.8 K
(*c*) – 0.186°C (*d*) 271.3 K

49. The depression in freezing point of a 0.01 M solution of a solute in a particular solvent is 0.18. To this solution, an equal volume of 0.002 M solution of same solute in the same solvent is added. The depression in freezing point of the resultant solution is nearly- (assume M = m)

(*a*) 0.024 (*b*) 0.216
(*c*) 0.018 (*d*) 0.108

50. Vapour pressure of a highly dilute solution of a sparingly soluble salt AB is 20 mm of Hg at a temperature T, while pure water exerts a pressure of 20.005 mm Hg at the same temperature. The K_{sp} (solubility product constant) of AB at the same temperature is -

(*a*) 7.1×10^{-6} (*b*) 6.9×10^{-3}
(*c*) 2.4×10^{-10} (*d*) 4.9×10^{-5}

51. Equimolal solution of KCl & Compound 'X' in water shows depression in freezing point in the ratio 4 : 1. Assuming KCl to be completely ionized, Compound 'X' must-

(*a*) dissociate to the extent of 50%.
(*b*) dissociate to the extent of 75%
(*c*) dimerise to the extent of 50%
(*d*) trimerise to the extent of 75%

52. The osmotic pressure of a solution containing 0.02 moles of NaCl & 0.03 moles of glucose in 500 ml solution at 300 K is -

(*a*) 6.88 atm (*b*) 1.72 atm
(*c*) 3.44 atm (*d*) None of these

53. Which of the following relation is NOT correct for an aqueous dilute solution of K_3PO_4 if its degree of dissociation is α ?

(*a*) $\dfrac{\Delta P}{P^o}=\dfrac{\text{Molality}\times18\times(1+3\alpha)}{1000}$

(*b*) $\dfrac{\Delta P}{P^o}=\dfrac{\pi\text{ observed}\times18\times(1+3\alpha)}{RT\times1000}$

(*c*) $\dfrac{\Delta P}{P^o}=\dfrac{\Delta T_f(\text{observed})\times18}{K_f\times1000}$

(*d*) M.weight of K_3PO_4 = $\text{M.weight}_{\text{observed}}(1+3\alpha)$

54. The freezing point depression of a $0\cdot001$ molal solution of $Cr(NH_3)_4Br_3$ in water is $0\cdot0054$. If K_f for water is $1\cdot80$ K/molal, the correct formulation of the above complex molecule is -

(*a*) $[Cr(NH_3)_4Br_2]Br$ (*b*) $[Cr(NH_3)_4Br]Br_2$
(*c*) $[Cr(NH_3)_4]Br_3$ (*d*) $[Cr(NH_3)_3Br_3]$

55. Identify the correct statement(s).

(1) If HgI_2 is added to one mole of KI, the freezing point is raised.
(2) Depression in freezing point is a better colligative property than elevation in Boiling point to calculate molar masses of heavy solutes.
(3) At freezing point, the vapour pressure of liquid phase & solid phase becomes equal.
(4) Highly concentrated solution are ideal solutions.

(*a*) 1 & 2 only (*b*) 2, 3 & 4 only
(*c*) 1, 2 & 3 only (*d*) 3 only

56. The freezing point of an aqueous solution that contains 3% by mass urea, 7.45% by mass KCl and 9% by mass of glucose is
(given K_f of water = 1.86)

(*a*) 290 K (*b*) 285.5 K
(*b*) 266.073 K (*d*) 250 K

57. How many moles of sucrose should be dissolved in 500 gm of water so as to get a solution which has a difference of 104°C between boiling point & freezing point?

(*a*) 0.840 (*b*) 0.272
(*c*) 0.739 (*d*) 0.212

58. For the given electrolyte A_XB_Y, the degree of dissociation 'α' can be given as-

(*a*) $\alpha=\dfrac{i-1}{x+y-1}$ (*b*) $i=(1-\alpha)+x\alpha+y\alpha$

(*c*) $\alpha=\dfrac{1-i}{1-x-y}$ (*d*) All of these

59. The Osmotic pressure of a solution having $0\cdot1$M NaCl & $0\cdot2$M Na_2SO_4 & $0\cdot5$M HA (Weak acid having degree of dissociation 20% at 300 k) is-

(*a*) 3·486 atm (*b*) 7·241 atm
(*c*) 34·48 atm (*d*) 72·41 atm

60. CNS^- ions give red colour with Fe^{3+} ions in aqueous solution as-

$$Fe^{3+}(aq.) + 3CNS(aq.) \rightarrow Fe(CNS)_3(aq.)$$

If 0·1M KCNS solution is seperated from 0·1M $FeCl_3$ solution by means of a semi-permeable membrane, red colour will appear on-

(*a*) $FeCl_3$ solution side
(*b*) KCNS solution side
(*c*) Both sides simultaneously
(*d*) Neither side

61. The vapour pressure of two volatile liquid mixture is given by, $P_T = 5\cdot3 + 2X_B$ (in cm of Hg) where X_B is mole fraction of B in mixture. The ratio of mole fraction of A & B in vapour phase is-

(*a*) $\frac{73}{53}$ (*b*) $\frac{53}{73}$
(*c*) $\frac{73P_A^o}{53P_B^o}$ (*d*) $\frac{53X_A}{73X_B}$

62. Two 5 molal solutions are prepared by dissolving a non- electrolyte, non-volatile solute seperately in the solvents X & Y. The molecular weights of the solvents are M_x & M_y, respectively where $M_X = \frac{3}{4}M_Y$. The relative lowering of vapour pressure of the solution in X is 'M' times that of solution in Y. Given that the number of moles of solute is very small in comparison to that of solvent, the value of 'M' is-

(*a*) $\frac{3}{4}$ (*b*) $\frac{1}{2}$
(*c*) $\frac{1}{4}$ (*d*) $\frac{4}{3}$

63. An aqueous solution of a salt MX_2 at certain temperature has a Van't Hoff factor of 2. The degree of dissociation for this solution of the salt is -

(*a*) 0.50 (*b*) 0.33
(*c*) 0.67 (*d*) 0.80

64. The observed osmotic pressure for a 0.10 M solution of $Fe(NH_4)_2(SO_4)_2$ at 25°C is 10.8 atm. The expected & experimental (observed) values of Van't Hoff factor (i) will be respetively -

(*a*) 5 & 4.42 (*b*) 4 & 4
(*c*) 5 & 3.42 (*d*) 3 & 5.42

65. A molecule M associates in a given solvent according to the equation,

$$nM \rightleftharpoons (M)_n$$

For a certain concentration of M, the Van't Hoff factor was found to be 0.9 & the fraction of associated molecules was 0.2. Then, the values of n is -

(*a*) 3 (*b*) 5
(*c*) 2 (*d*) 4

66. A solution containing 0·85 g of $ZnCl_2$ in 125 gm of water freezes at –0·23°C. The apparent degree of dissociation of the salt is (K_f for H_2O = 1·86 k kg mol^{-1}, at. mass of Zn = 65·3 gm & Cl = 35·5 g)

(*a*) 1·36% (*b*) 73·9%
(*c*) 92% (*d*) 55%

67. Liquids A & B from an ideal solution. At 30°C, the total vapour pressure of a solution containing 1 mole of A & 2 mole of B is 250 mmHg. The total vapour pressure becomes 300 mmHg when 1 more mole of A is added to the first solution. The vapour pressure of pure A & pure B at the same temperature are-

(*a*) 150, 450 mmHg (*b*) 150 mmHg
(*c*) 450, 150 mmHg (*d*) 250, 300 mmHg

68. A non-volatile, non-electrolyte solute 'X' is dissolved in a suitable solvent & the osmotic pressure (π, in atm) of solutions of various concentrations 'C' in gm/ml is measured at 27°C. The slope of the plot π against 'C' is found to be 5×10^{-3}. Then the molecular weight of 'X' is

(*a*) $4{\cdot}9 \times 10^5$ (*b*) $4{\cdot}9 \times 10^3$
(*c*) $4{\cdot}9 \times 10^6$ (*d*) $4{\cdot}9 \times 10^4$

69. The empirical formula of a non-electrolyte is CH_2O. A solution containing 3g of this compound exerts the some osmotic pressure as that of 0·05 M glucose solution. Then, the molecular formula of compound is -

(*a*) CH_2O (*b*) $C_2H_4O_2$
(*c*) $C_3H_6O_3$ (*d*) $C_4H_8O_4$

70. If the amount of a non-electrolyte solute dissolved is doubled but that of solvent is quadrupled, the elevation in Boiling point will be -

(*a*) doubled (*b*) halved
(*c*) six times (*d*) unchanged

71. On dissolving 58·5 gm of NaCl in 9·9 moles of water, the vapour pressure of the solution is -

(Vapour pressure of pure H_2O is P^o)

(*a*) $0.83P^o$ (*b*) $0.45P^o$

(*c*) $1.2P^o$ (*d*) $0.90P^o$

72. Elevation in boiling point of 1 molar aqueous glucose solution (having density = 1·5 g/ml) is -

(*a*) K_b (*b*) $0·75\ K_b$

(*c*) $1·02\ K_b$ (*d*) $1·32\ k_b$

73. 60 g of urea is dissolved in 1100 g solution.

To keep $\Delta T_f / k_f$ as 1 mole/kg, water seperated in the form of ice is - (M. mass of urea = 60 g)

(*a*) 40 g (*b*) 60 g

(*c*) 100 g (*d*) 200 g

74. xg/L aqueous sucrose solution and yg/L aqueous NaCl solution are isotonic. Then x & Y, respectively can be

(a) 6.84, 0.585 (b) 3.42, 0.585

(c) 1.71, 0.18 (d) 1.71, 0.146

(*a*) both (a) & (d) (*b*) both (b) & (d)

(*c*) both (a) & (c) (*d*) (a), (b) & (c) only

75. Which one has the maximum freezing point?

(*a*) 6 g urea solution in 100 g H_2O

(*b*) 6 g acetic acid solution in 100 g H_2O

(*c*) 6 g NaCl solution in 100 g H_2O

(*d*) All have equal freezing point

76. Consider the following cases -

(I) 2M CH_3COOH solution in benzene at 27°C where there is a dimer formation to the extent of 100%.

(II) 0·5 M NaCl aqueous solution at 27°C (assuming 100% dissociation)

Which of the following statement (s) is/are true?

(*a*) both are isotonic

(*b*) I is hypertonic wrt II

(*c*) II is hypertonic wrt I

(*d*) I is hypertonic wrt II

77. A beaker containing 18 gram of glucose in 100 g water and another containing 18 g of urea in 100 g water are placed under a bell Jar & air is removed. After a course of time, when equilibrium reaches, how much water will be transferred from one beaker to the other?

(*a*) 12 g (*b*) 30 g

(*c*) 50 g (*d*) 26 g

78. A particular electrolyte M_XN_Y was dissolved in water. The degree of dissociation of salt in water was found to be 60%. Then, observed molar mass is given by the expression - (M = Normal molar mass of solute)

(*a*) $\dfrac{M}{0·6 + 0·4\,(x + y)}$

(*b*) M [0·6 + 0·4(x +y)]

(*c*) $\dfrac{M}{0·4 + 0·6\,(x + y)}$

(*d*) M [0·6 + 0·4(x – y)]

79. Certain mass say 'y' gm of urea is dissolved in 500 g of water and cooled upto – 0·5°C, whereby 128 g of ice separates out from the solution. If cryoscopic constant for water be 1.86 K kg mol^{-1}, the value of 'y' is -

(*a*) 12 g (*b*) 8 g

(*c*) 4 g (*d*) 6 g

80. 17·4% (w/v) solution of K_2SO_4 is isotonic with 5·85 % (w/v) solution of NaCl at 27°C. If NaCl is 100% ionised, what is the % age ionisation of K_2SO_4?

(atomic mass of K = 39, Na = 23)

(*a*) 40% (*b*) 50%

(*c*) 90% (*c*) 100%

81. Equal volume of 0·1 M urea & 0·1 M glucose is mixed. If the initial osmotic pressure of both was P atm, then the osmotic pressure of the mixture will be-

(*a*) less than P

(*b*) greater than P

(*c*) P

(*d*) 2 P

82. A solute 'X' trimerises to an extent of 20% and solute 'y' dimersises to an extent of 90%. Then, which of the following statement is/are true?

(assume solutions to be equi molal)

(*a*) Freezing point of X solution will be greater than freezing point of Y solution.

(*b*) Depression in freezing point of X is lower than in Y.

(*c*) Vapour pressure of X will be less than that of Y at same temperature.

(*d*) Osmotic pressure of X will be less than that of Y.

Brain Teasers

83. The vapour pressure of an aqueous solution is found to be 750 torr at certain temperature 'T'. If 'T' is the temperature at which pure water boils under atmospheric pressure & same solution shows elevation in Boiling point, $\Delta T_b = 1{\cdot}04\,K$, then the atmospheric pressure is -
($k_b = 0{\cdot}52$ K Kg mol^{-1})

(*a*) 777 torr (*b*) 325 torr
(*c*) 121 torr (*d*) None of these

84. When a solution containing non-volatile solute is diluted with water, its

(*a*) Osmotic pressure increases.
(*b*) Vapour pressure increases.
(*c*) freezing point increases.
(*d*) Both (b) & (c) are correct.

85. The freezing point order of the solution of different strength (by weight) of glucose is -

(*a*) 10% > 3% > 2% > 1%
(*b*) 1% > 2% > 3% > 10%
(*c*) 1% > 3% > 10% > 2%
(*d*) 10% > 1% > 3% > 2%

86. The boiling point of an aqueous solution of a non-volatile solute is 100·15°C. What is the freezing point of an aqueous solution obtained by diluting the above solution with an equal volume of water? The values of K_b & k_f for H_2O are 0·512°C molal^{-1} & 1·86°C molal^{-1},

(*a*) –0·544°C (*b*) –0·512°C
(*c*) –0·272°C (*d*) –1·86°C

87. Which of the following graphs is/are correct?

a. $T_b\uparrow$ (Boiling point of solution)

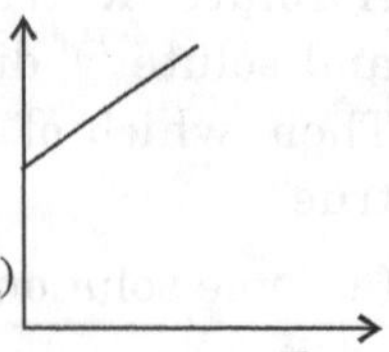

Molality of solution

b. V.P.↑

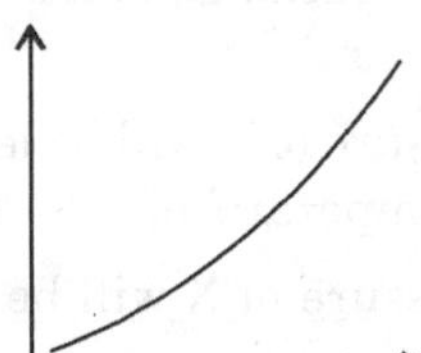

Temperature→

c. π ↑

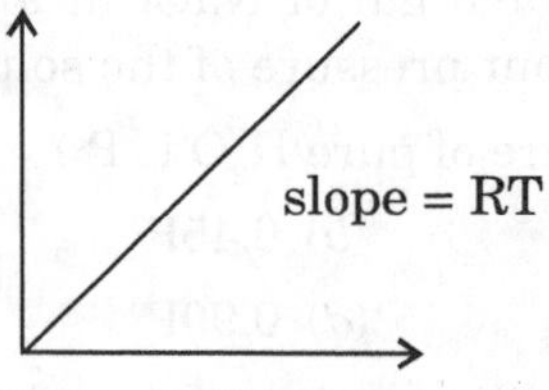

C →
(in g/ml)

d. V.P.↑

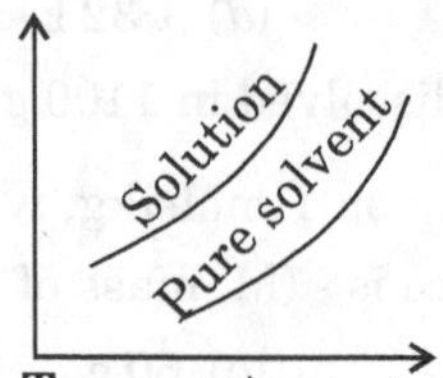

Temperature→

(*a*) a & b only (*b*) a, b & c only
(*c*) c & d only (*d*) b, c & d only

88. A quantity of 3·125 g of a mixture of KCl & NaCl dissolved in 1 kg of water produces a depression of 0·186°C in freezing point. The molar ratio of KCl to NaCl in the solution is (assuming complete dissociation of salts & $k_f = 1{\cdot}86$ k kg/mol) approx =

(*a*) 1 : 3 (*b*) 3 : 1
(*c*) 5 : 2 (*d*) 7 : 3

89. A cylinder fitted with a movable piston contains liquid water in equilibrium with water vapour at 25°C. Which of the following operation results in a decrease in equilibrium vapour pressure at 25°C?

(*a*) Removing small amount of vapour
(*b*) Removing small amount of liquid H_2O.
(*c*) Dissolving some salt in the water.
(*d*) All of these

90. A quantity of 10g of solute 'A' & 20 g of solute 'B' is dissolved in 500 ml water.

The solution is isotonic with the solution obtained by dissolving 6·67 g of 'A' & 30 g of 'B' in 500 ml water at the same temperature. The ratio of molar masses, $M_A : M_B$, is -

(*a*) 1 : 3
(*b*) 1 : 9
(*c*) 12 : 3
(*d*) 3 : 12

91. An aqueous solution of a non-volatile, nonelectrolyte solute (having molecular mass 150 g) boils at 373·26 k. The mass percentage of solute is (given kg of water = 0·52 k kg mol^{-1})

(*a*) 6·976% (*b*) 82%

(*c*) 82·5% (*d*) 80·175%

92. Equal masses of two aqueous solutions, one of 3·6 g glucose/100 g of water & other of 3·6 g urea/ 100 g of water are mixed. If the freezing point of resulting solution is –x°C, then the value of '10x' is -

(given k_f = 1·86 k kg mol^{-1})

(*a*) 7·44 (*b*) 744

3 74·4 (*d*) 0·744

93. Which of the following statement (s) is/are correct?

(*a*) At same temperature, the correct order of osmotic pressure for 0·5 M aqueous solution of each compound is $BaCl_2$ > NaCl > CH_3COOH > Sucrose.

(*b*) Benzene & Naphthalene form an ideal solution.

(*c*) Water will boil at 80°C at a pressure less than 1 atm.

(*d*) All are correct.

94. Which of the following binary mixtures will have same composition in liquid & vapour phase?

(1) Benzene - Toluene

(2) Water - nitric acid

(3) Water - ethanol

(4) n-hexane-n-heptane

(*a*) Both 1 & 4 (*b*) Both 1 & 3

(*c*) Both 2 & 3 (*d*) Both 3 & 4

95. 17.4% (w/v) solution of K_2SO_4 is isotonic with 5·85% (w/v) solution of NaCl at 27°C. If NaCl is 100% ionised, what is the percentage ionisation of K_2SO_4? (At. mass of K = 39, Na = 23)

(*a*) 40% (*b*) 50%

(*c*) 90% (*d*) 100%

96. A 20 ml sample of $CuSO_4$ solution was evaporated to dryness, leaving 0·967 g of residue. What was the molarity of the original solution?

(At. wt. of Cu = 63·5 g)

(*a*) 48·4 M (*b*) 0·303 M

(*c*) 0·75 M (*d*) None of these

97. Which represents incorrect difference?

I.

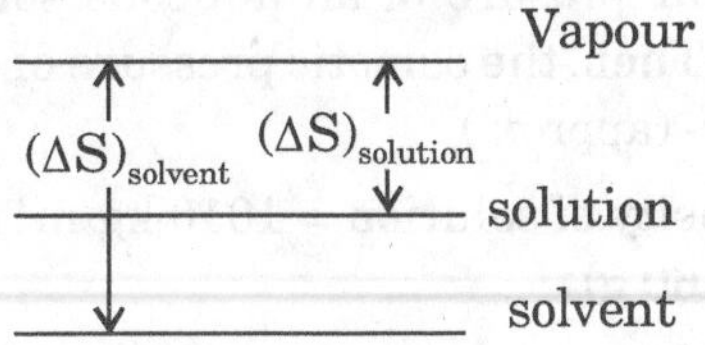

II.

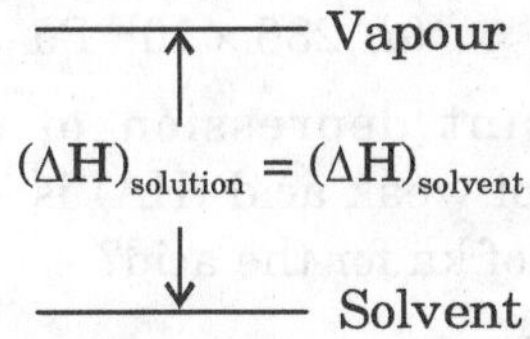

III.

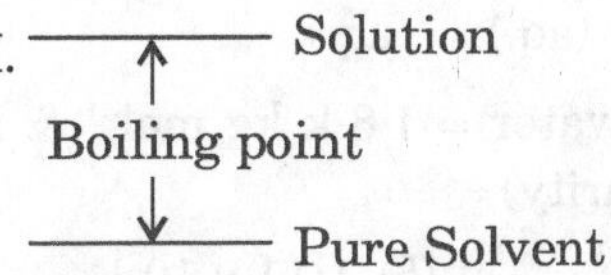

a) Only I b) Only II

c) All of these d) None of these

98. Which of the following statement (s) is/are correct for Van't Hoff factor (i) for a solution of weak electrolyte A_xB_y?

(*a*) $i = 1 - \alpha + X\alpha + Y\alpha$

(where α = degree of dissociation)

(*b*) i > 1 (at normal dilution)

(*c*) i increases more rapidly with dilution & attains a limiting value of (x + y) at infinite dilution.

(*d*) All are correct.

99. Which of the following aqueous solutions has greater osmotic pressure than 0·1M glucose aqueous solution?

(*a*) 0.1 M NaOH solution

(*b*) 23.3 g of $BaSO_4$ (mol. wt 233) added to 1 litre of water.

(*c*) 0.6 g urea in 100 ml solution

(*d*) Both (*a*) & (*b*)

100. When 400 g of a 20% (w/w) solution was cooled, 50 g of the solute got precipitated.

Then the percentage (by weight) of solute in the remaining solution is -

(*a*) 15%

(*b*) 7·5%

(*c*) 8·6%

(*d*) 11%

101. The vapour pressure of pure water at 293k is 2338 Pa & vapour presure of an aqueous solution is 2295·8 Pa. Then, the osmotic pressure of solution at 313 K is - (approx.)

(given, density of solution = 1010 kg/m³ & m·wt. of solute = 60 g)

(a) $2{\cdot}36 \times 10^6$ pa (b) 2360 Pa

(c) 236×10^8 Pa (d) 236×10^{10} Pa

102. The freezing point depression of a 0·1M aqueous solution of weak acid (HA) is –0·20°C. What is the value of ka for the acid?

$$\underset{(aq.)}{HA} \rightleftharpoons \underset{(aq.)}{H^+} + \underset{(aq.)}{A^-}$$

(Given : k_f for water = 1·8 k kg mol^{-1} & assume molality = molarity)

(a) $1{\cdot}35 \times 10^{-3}$ (b) $1{\cdot}11 \times 10^{-1}$

(c) $7{\cdot}6 \times 10^{-5}$ (d) $7{\cdot}45 \times 10^{-3}$

103. The solute 'A' is a ternary electrolyte & solute 'B' is a non-electrolyte. If 0·1 M solution of solute 'B' produces an Osmotic pressure of 2 P, then 0·05 M solution of A at same temperatue will produce an Osmotic pressure equal to -

(a) P (b) 1·5 P

(c) 2 P (d) 3 P

104. Select the correct statement (s).

(a) Lowering of vapour pressure of a solution is equal to the mole fraction of non - volatile solute present in it

(b) Vapour pressure of a liquid depends on the size of vessel.

(c) Addition of a non-volatile solute to water always lowers its vapour pressure.

(d) Molal depression constant is independent of the nature of solute as well as that of solvent.

105. Consider separate solutions of 0·5 M C_2H_5OH (aq.) 0·100 M $Mg_3(SO_4)_2$ (aq.), 0·250 M KBr (aq.) & 0·125 M Na_3PO_4 (aq.) at 25°C. Which statement is true about these solutions, assuming all salts to be strong electrolytes!

(a) 0·5 M C_2H_5OH (aq.) has the highest osmotic pressure.

(b) 0·1 M $Mg_3(PO_4)_2$ (aq.) has the highest osmotic pressure.

(c) 0·125 M $Na_3(PO_4)_2$ (aq.) has the highest osmotic pressure.

(d) All have same osmotic pressure.

106. In 100 g of Naphthalene, 2·423 g of sulphur was dissolved. Melting point of Naphthalene is 80·1°C. The latent heat of fusion of naphthalene is 35·7 Cal/g. Also, $\Delta T_f = 0{\cdot}661°C$. Then, molecular formula of sulphur is -

(a) S_2 (b) S_4

(c) S_6 (d) S_8

107. Identify the mismatch.

Column A		Column B
(a) Rast method	→	Camphor
(b) Antifreeze	→	Ethylene glycol
(c) 0·91% (w/v) NaCl	→	isotonic with blood
(d) C_2H_5OH & H_2O	→	maximum boiling azeotrope.

108. The Observed molecular mass of $AgNO_3$ is 92. Then the value of 1/i is -

(a) 0·48 (b) 0·54

(c) 1·85 (c) 0·85

109. The normal boiling point of water is 373 K. Vapour pressure of water at temperature T is 19 mm Hg. If the enthalpy of vaporisation is 40.67 kJ/ mol, then value of temperature T would be –

(a) 250 K (b) 291.1 K

(c) 302.27 K (d) 268.68 K

110. On addition of mercuric iodide to aqueous solution of potassium iodide, a compound 'X' is formed. Then vant Hoff factor for 'X' is – (assuming complete dissociation of X)

(a) 1 (b) 2

(c) 3 (d) 4

111. If M_C & M_0 are calculated molar mass of solute & observed molar mass of solute, respectively then these are related with α (degree of dissociation) as –

(a) $\alpha = \dfrac{M_C - M_O}{M_O(n-1)}$ (b) $\alpha = \dfrac{M_O - M_C}{M_C(n-1)}$

(c) $\alpha = \dfrac{M_C - M_O}{M_C(n-1)}$ (d) $\alpha = \dfrac{M_C - M_O}{M_C(1-n)}$

112. Select the correct statement (s).

(a) Value of i for an electrolyte is inversely related to the concentration of electrolyte.

(b) Value of i for NaCl at 0.001 molal concentration is greater than its value at 0.01 molal concentration.

(c) When NH_3 is added to $CuSO_4$, the value of vant Hoff factor i remains constant.

(d) All are correct.

113. Some substances can loose water of crystallization partially or completely on exposure to air. Such substances are called–

(a) Deliquescent substances

(b) Efflorescent substances

(c) Hygroscopic substances

(d) None of these

114. Two solutions of glucose have osmotic pressure 1.5 atm & 2.5 atm respectively. Now 1 litre of first solution is mixed with 2 liters of second solution, then the osmotic pressure of the resulting solution is –

(Assume temperature to be constant throughout)

(a) 1.62 atm (b) 6.12 atm

(c) 1.26 atm (d) 2.16 atm

115. pH of 0.1M BOH (a weak base) is found to be 12. The solution at temperature of T kelvin will display an osmotic pressure, equal to–

(a) 0.01 RT (b) 0.001 RT

(c) 0.11 RT (d) 0.1 RT

116. 17.4 % (w/v)K_2SO_4 (M.wt = 174 g / mol) solution at 27°C is isotonic to 4 % (w/v) NaOH solution at same temperature. If NaOH is 100 % ionised, what is the % age ionisation of K_2SO_4 in aqueous solution–

(a) 20 %

(b) 60 %

(c) 100 %

(d) 50 %

Answers

1. (a)	**2.** (c)	**3.** (b)	**4.** (a)	**5.** (d)	**6.** (a)	**7.** (a)	**8.** (b)	**9.** (a)	**10.** (a)
11. (a)	**12.** (c)	**13.** (b)	**14.** (b)	**15.** (c)	**16.** (b)	**17.** (c)	**18.** (d)	**19.** (c)	**20.** (a)
21. (d)	**22.** (a)	**23.** (a)	**24.** (d)	**25.** (a)	**26.** (b)	**27.** (a)	**28.** (c)	**29.** (c)	**30.** (c)
31. (c)	**32.** (b)	**33.** (c)	**34.** (a)	**35.** (a)	**36.** (c)	**37.** (a)	**38.** (a)	**39.** (a)	**40.** (c)
41. (c)	**42.** (d)	**43.** (b)	**44.** (a)	**45.** (a)	**46.** (c)	**47.** (a)	**48.** (b)	**49.** (d)	**50.** (d)
51. (d)	**52.** (c)	**53.** (b)	**54.** (b)	**55.** (c)	**56.** (b)	**57.** (a)	**58.** (d)	**59.** (c)	**60.** (d)
61. (d)	**62.** (a)	**63.** (a)	**64.** (a)	**65.** (c)	**66.** (b)	**67.** (c)	**68.** (c)	**69.** (b)	**70.** (b)
71. (a)	**72.** (b)	**73.** (a)	**74.** (a)	**75.** (a)	**76.** (a)	**77.** (c)	**78.** (c)	**79.** (d)	**80.** (b)
81. (c)	**82.** (c)	**83.** (a)	**84.** (d)	**85.** (b)	**86.** (c)	**87.** (b)	**88.** (a)	**89.** (c)	**90.** (a)
91. (a)	**92.** (a)	**93.** (d)	**94.** (c)	**95.** (b)	**96.** (b)	**97.** (d)	**98.** (d)	**99.** (a)	**100.** (c)
101. (a)	**102.** (a)	**103.** (d)	**104.** (c)	**105.** (d)	**106.** (d)	**107.** (d)	**108.** (b)	**109.** (b)	**110.** (c)
111. (a)	**112.** (d)	**113.** (b)	**114.** (d)	**115.** (c)	**116.** (d)				

Explanations

1. 3.6 M H_2SO_4 means that 3.6 moles of H_2SO_4 are present per litre of solution.

So, no. of moles of solute present

= 3.6 moles = 3.6 × 98 = 352.8 g

Volume of solution = 1 litre

29% by mass (w/w) H_2SO_4 solutions means that 29gm of H_2SO_4 is present in 100 gm of solution.

So, 29 gm H_2SO_4 is present in solution = 100 g

352.8 gm H_2SO_4 is present in solution

$$= \frac{100}{29} \times 352.8 = 1216.55 \text{ g}$$

So, weight of solution, when volume of solution is 1000 ml = 1216.55g

weight of solution, when volume of solution is

$$1\text{ml} = \frac{1216.55}{1000}\text{g}$$

$$= 1.216 \text{g/ml}$$

↓

density of solution.

2. 5 molar, 1 L solution of an acid means that 5 moles of solute are present per litre of solution.

When divided in two equal halves, each half will have volume = 0.5 L & will have 2.5 moles of acid in it.

$$\text{Now, } M = \frac{\text{Number of moles of Solute}}{\text{Volume of solution (in litres)}}$$

$$\boxed{M = \frac{2.5}{0.5} = 5M}$$

3. 10% (w/w) means that 10 g of solute is present in 100 g solution.

Which means that % age of solute in solution

= 10%

So, solvent present = 90 g

4. Urea solution is 6% (w/v) which means that 6 g of urea is present per 100 ml of a solution.

M . mass of urea = 60 g

$$\text{So, moles of urea present per 100 ml} = \frac{6}{60} = 0.1$$

0.1 moles of urea are present in solution with volume = 0.1 L (100 ml)

2 moles of urea are present in solution with

$$\text{volume} = \frac{0.1}{0.1} \times 2 = 2 \text{ L}$$

5. 1 ml solution has $CaCl_2$ = 0.02 g

50 ml solution should have $CaCl_2$ = 0.02 × 50 = 1 g

6. 17.4 ppm means that 17.4g of K_2SO_4 is present per 10^6 gm of solution.

weight of soln. = 10^6 gm

weight of K_2SO_4 = 17.4 g

weight of solvent (H_2O) = $10^6 - 17.4 \approx 10^6$ gm

Volume of solvent (H_2O) = 10^6 ml

$(\because \rho \text{ of } H_2O = 1\text{g/ml})$

Volume of solution ≃ 10^6 ml

(∵ amount of solute is very less in comparison to amount of solvent)

$$\text{Molarity of } K_2SO_4 = \frac{\text{Number of moles of solute}}{\text{Volume of solution (in litres)}}$$

$$M = \frac{\frac{17.4}{174}}{\frac{10^6}{1000}} = \frac{17.4}{174} \times \frac{1000}{10^6} = \underset{\text{Molarity of } K_2SO_4}{\underbrace{10^{-4} M}}$$

Now, $K_2SO_4 \rightarrow 2K^+ + SO_4^{2-}$

	K_2SO_4	$2K^+$	SO_4^{2-}
At t = 0	10^{-4}	0	0
At t = 0	0	2×10^{-4}	10^{-4}

$$\boxed{\therefore \text{ Molarity of } K^+ = 2 \times 10^{-4} M}$$

7. For $Al_2(SO_4)_3$: Molar mass

= 27 × 2 + 32 × 3 + 12 × 16

= 54 + 96 + 192 = 342 g

34.2% (w/w) means that 34.2 g of $Al_2(SO_4)_3$ is present in 100 gm of solution.

So, weight of solvent = 100 – 34.2 = 65.8 g.

$$\text{molality of solution} = \frac{\text{no. of moles of solute}}{\text{wt. of solvent (in kgs)}}$$

$$= \frac{\frac{34.2}{342}}{\frac{65.8}{1000}} = \frac{34.2}{342} \times \frac{1000}{65.8}$$

$$\boxed{m = 1.519 \text{ molal}}$$

For molarity of solution,

ρ of solution = 1.25 g/ml

weight of solutionvolume of solution.

$1.25\text{g} \rightarrow 1\text{ml}$

$$100\text{g} \rightarrow \frac{1}{1.25} \times 100 = 80\text{ml}$$

$$M = \frac{\text{Number of moles of solute}}{\text{Volume of solution (in litres)}}$$

$$M = \frac{\frac{34.2}{342}}{\frac{80}{1000}} = \frac{34.2}{342} \times \frac{1000}{80} \times 1 = 1.25M$$

For Normality: -

$$\boxed{N = M \times n\,\text{factor}}$$

For salts like $Al_2(SO_4)_3$, n factor = Total cationic charge or total anionic charge

$$Al_2(SO_4)_3 \rightarrow 2Al^{3+} + 3SO_4^{2-}$$

n factor = 6

N = M × n factor = 1.25 × 6 = 7.5 N

8. 20% (w/w) aq. H_2O_2 solution means that 20 g H_2O_2 is present in 100 gm of solution. So, amount of H_2O = 100 – 20 = 80 gm.

$$n_{H_2O_2} = \frac{20}{34}, \quad n_{H_2O} = \frac{80}{18}$$

$$x_{H_2O} = \frac{n_{H_2O}}{n_{H_2O} + n_{H_2O_2}} = \frac{\frac{80}{18}}{\frac{80}{18} + \frac{20}{34}}$$

$$\boxed{x_{H_2O} = \frac{68}{77}}$$

9. Given weight of cane sugar = 171 g

M. mass of cane sugar = 342 g

number of moles of cane sugar $\frac{171}{342} = 0.5$ moles

weight of solvent = 1000 g = 1 kg

So, number of moles of solute present per kg of solvent = 0.5

$$\boxed{\text{Hence, molality} = 0.5}$$

For molarity.

Also, ρ (density) of solution = 1.1 g/ml

Total weight of solution = 171 + 1000 = 1171 g

From density

1.1 g solution has volume = 1 ml

1171 g solution has volume $= \frac{1}{1.1} \times 1171\text{ml}$

= 1064.54 ml

$$M(\text{molarity}) = \frac{\text{Number of moles of solute}}{\text{Volume of solution}}$$

$$M = \frac{\frac{171}{342}}{\frac{1064.54}{1000}}$$

$$\boxed{M = \frac{171}{342} \times \frac{1000}{1064.54} = 0.469M}$$

∴ molality > molarity.

10. X_B (mole fraction of solute) = 0·2

$$X_B = \frac{2}{10} = \frac{n_B}{n_A + n_B}$$

It means for every total 10 moles in the solution, 2 moles are those of solute. So, 8 moles will be of solvent.

$$\text{So,} \quad \frac{\text{Number of moles of solute}}{\text{Number of moles of solvent}} = \frac{2}{8}\frac{1}{4}$$

Let number of moles of solute = x

Number of moles of solvent = 4x

$$\text{molality} = \frac{\text{Number of moles of solute}}{\text{Weight of solvent (in kgs)}}$$

$$M = \frac{x}{4x \times 78} \times 1000 = \frac{250}{78} = 3{\cdot}20$$

(where 78 is M. mass of C_6H_6)

11. 93% H_2SO_4 (w/v) means 93 gm of H_2SO_4 is present in 100 ml of solution.

100 ml solution has H_2SO_4 = 93 gm

1000 ml solution has $H_2SO_4 = \frac{93}{100} \times 1000 = 930\text{g}$

From $\rho = 1{\cdot}84\,\text{g/ml}$

1 ml of solution weighs = 1·84 g

1000 ml of solution weighs = 1·84 × 1000 = 1840g.

So, weight of 1 litre solution = 1840 g

weight of solute in 1 litre solution = 930 g

weight of solvent in 1 litre solution = 910 g

$$\text{Molality} = \frac{\text{Number of moles of solute}}{\text{Weight of solvent (in kgs)}}$$

$$M = \frac{\frac{930}{98}}{\frac{910}{1000}} = \frac{930}{98} \times \frac{100\cancel{0}}{91\cancel{0}}$$

$$M = \frac{93000}{98 \times 91} = 10 \cdot 43\,m$$

12. Apply, $P_{N_2} = K_H X_{N_2}$

$$x = 10^5 \times \frac{n_{N_2}}{n_{N_2} + n_{H_2O}} \quad (\rho \text{ of } H_2O = 1 \text{ g/ml})$$

Vol. of $H_2O \rightarrow$ WT. of H_2O

1 ml $\rightarrow$ 1g

1000 ml $\rightarrow$ 1000 g

$$x = 10^5 \times \frac{\frac{0{\cdot}028}{28}}{\frac{0{\cdot}028}{28} + \frac{1000}{18}} \quad 1000\,\text{ml} \rightarrow 1000\,\text{g}$$

$$x = \frac{0{\cdot}001}{0{\cdot}001 + 55{\cdot}5} \times 10^5$$

$$x = \frac{0{\cdot}001}{55{\cdot}5} \times 10^5$$

$$x = \frac{100}{55 \cdot 5} = 1 \cdot 80\,\text{atm}$$

13. Apply, Henry's law -

$$P_{CO_2} = K_H X_{CO_2}$$

Volume of K_H is high, So X_{CO2} in water is very very less. Hence, 900 ml soda water = 900 ml water.

$$P_{CO_2} = K_{H \times CO_2}$$

$$1\,\text{atm} = 2 \times 10^3\,\text{atm} \cdot \frac{n_{CO_2}}{n_{CO_2} + n_{H_2O}}$$

But $n_{CO_2} + n_{H_2O} = n_{H_2O}$ ($\because$ K_H is high)

$$1\,\text{atm} = 2 \times 10^3\,\text{atm} \cdot \frac{n_{CO_2}}{n_{H_2O}}$$

$$1\,\text{atm} = 2 \times 10^3\,\text{atm}. \frac{n_{CO_2}}{900/18}$$

$$\frac{1}{2 \times 10^3} = \frac{n_{CO_2}}{900} \times 18$$

$$\frac{50}{2 \times 10^3} = n_{CO_2}$$

$$\boxed{25 \times 10^{-3} = n_{CO_2}}$$

weight of CO_2 dissolved

$$= 25 \times 10^{-3} \times 44 = \frac{1100}{1000} = 1 \cdot 1\text{g}$$

15. Solution having chloroform & acetone shows negative deviation from Raoults' law. So, ΔH is –ve & energy is released. So, solution rather appears hot.

16. Water & ethanol mixture will show +ve deviation from Raoult's law. So, ΔH is +ve.

Also, $\Delta S_{sol.} = +ve$

If $\Delta S = -ve$

$$\Delta G = \Delta H - T\Delta S$$

$$= (+) - (+ \times -)$$

$$= (+) - (-)$$

$$= \Delta H + T\Delta S = +ve$$

Now, if ΔH is +ve & ΔS is -ve, ΔG will be +ve (T is temperature in Kelvin, always, +ve). So, process will not be possible. Hence, ΔS has to be +ve for solution.

17. $P_A = P_A^0 X_A$ (According to Raoult's law)

$P_A = P_{Total}\, Y_A$ (According to Dalton's law)

$$\therefore\ P_A^0 X_A = P_{Total} Y_A$$

$$P_A^0 = \frac{P_{Total}\, Y_A}{X_A} \quad (1)$$

Similarly,

$$P_B^0 = \frac{P_{Total}\, Y_B}{X_B} \quad (2)$$

Since, $P_A^0 > P_B^0$, therefore -

$$\frac{P_{Total}\, Y_A}{X_A} > \frac{P_{Total}\, Y_B}{X_B}$$

$$\therefore \frac{Y_A}{X_A} > \frac{Y_B}{X_B} \text{ or } \frac{Y_A}{Y_B} > \frac{X_A}{X_B}.$$

18. Apply Hensy's law

$$P\text{gas} = K_H X_{ges}$$

$$500 = k_H \cdot \frac{(n_{N_2})_I}{n_{N_2} + n_{H_2O}} \quad \text{...(1)}$$

$$750 = k_H \cdot \frac{(n_{N_2})_{II}}{n_{N_2} + n_{H_2O}} \quad \text{...(2)}$$

$$\frac{500}{750} = \frac{(n_{N_2})_I}{(n_{N_2})_{II}}$$

$$\frac{10}{15} = \frac{\frac{0.01}{M}}{\frac{n_{N_2}}{M}}$$

$$\frac{10}{15} = \frac{0.01}{n_{N_2}}$$

$$\boxed{\omega_{N_2} = \frac{15 \times 0.01}{10} = 0.015 \text{ g/L}}$$

20. $X_A = 0{\cdot}4$

$V{\cdot}P_{sol.} = 580$ torr

$P_S = P_A + P_B$

$$P_S = P_A^0X_A + P_B^0X_B$$
$$= 300 \times 0{\cdot}4 + 800 \times 0{\cdot}6$$
$$= 120 + 480 = 600 \text{ torr}$$

So, had the solution been ideal, the total V·P. Would have been 600 torr but actual V·P recorded is 580 torr, which is less than expected. Hence, the solution will show -ve deviation from Raoult's law. Hence Chloroform & acetone solution is answer.

21. Had solution been ideal -

$$P_{Total} = P_A + P_B$$
$$P_{Total} = P_A^0X_A + P_B^0X_B$$
$$P_{Total} = 100 \times \frac{1}{4} + 60 \times \frac{3}{4}$$
$$P_{Total} = 25 + 45 = 70 \text{ mm Hg}$$

OBSERVED $P_{TOTAL} = 75$ mmHg

Hence, solution shows positive deviation from Raoult's law.

22.

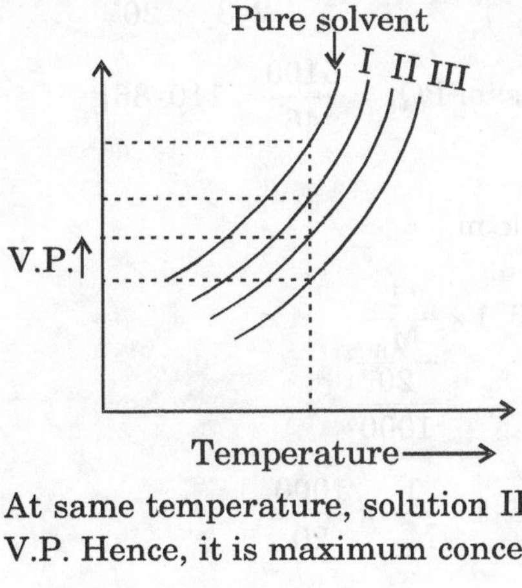

At same temperature, solution III has the least V.P. Hence, it is maximum concentrated.

23. $X_A = 0.25$

$P_A^0 = 400$ mm Hg

$X_B = 0.75$

$P_B^0 = 200$ mm Hg

Now, $P_A = P_{Total}\, Y_A$ (Dalton's law)

$$\frac{P_A}{P_{Total}} = Y_A$$

$$\frac{P_A^0X_A}{P_A + P_B} = Y_A \quad \text{(Raoult's law is used)}$$

$$\frac{P_A^0X_A}{P_A^0X_A + P_B^0X_B} = Y_A$$

$$\frac{400 \times 0.25}{40 \times 0.25 + 200 \times 0.75} = Y_A$$

$$\frac{100}{100 + 200 \times \frac{75}{100}} = Y_A$$

$$\frac{100}{100 + 150} = Y_A$$

$$\frac{100}{250} = Y_A$$

$$\boxed{Y_A = 0.4}$$

24. Let number of moles of pentane = x

So, number of moles of hexane = 4x

Let pentane be component 'A'.

$P_A = P_{total}\, Y_A$ (by Dalton's law)

$$\frac{P_A}{P_{Total}} = Y_A$$

$$\frac{P_A^0X_A}{P_A + P_B} = Y_A$$

$$\frac{P^0_{A\times A}}{P_A^0X_A + P_B^0X_B} = Y_A$$

$$\frac{400 \times \frac{x}{5x}}{400 \times \frac{x}{5x} + 120 \times \frac{4x}{5x}} = Y_A$$

$$\frac{80}{80 + 24 \times 4} = Y_A$$

$$\frac{80}{80 + 96} = Y_A$$

$$\frac{80}{176} = Y_A = 0.45$$

25. $P_A^0 = 450\,mm\,Hg$

$P_B^0 = 700\,mm\,Hg$

$P_{Total} = P_A + P_B$

$600 = P_A^0X_A + P_B^0X_B$

$600 = 450X_A + 700(1 - X_A)\ [\because X_A + X_B = 1]$

$600 = 450X_A + 700 - 700X_A$

$100 = 250X_A$

$\boxed{X_A = \frac{100}{250} = 0.4}$

$\boxed{X_B = 0.6}$

26. Apply, $\frac{P^0 - P_S}{P^0} = X_B \rightarrow$ mole fraction of solute

$P^0 - P_S = 10$

$\therefore\ \frac{10}{P^0} = 0.2$ (given $X_B = 0.2$)

$\boxed{P^0 = \frac{10}{0.2} = 50}$

Now, decrease in vapour pressure = 20 mm of Hg

$P^0 - P_S = 20$

$\frac{P^0 - P_S}{P^0} = X_B$

$\frac{20}{50} = X_B$ (mole fraction of solute)

$X_B = 0.4$

$\therefore\ X_A = 0.6$ Mole fraction of solvent

27. Apply, $\frac{P^\circ - P_S}{P^\circ} = X_B$

At 100°C (which is Boiling point of pure H_2O), the vapour pressure of pure H_2O = At mospheric pressure.

$\therefore\ P^\circ = 760$ mm Hg

Now, $\frac{P^\circ - P_S}{760} = X_B$ (mole fraction of solute)

(Molality of solution = 1)

$\therefore$ number of moles of solute = 1

wt. of solvent (in kgs) = 1 kg = 1000 g

So, $\frac{P^\circ - P_S}{760} = \frac{n_B}{n_A + n_B}$

$$\frac{P^\circ - P_S}{760} = \frac{1}{1 + \frac{1000}{8}}$$

$$\frac{P^\circ - P_S}{760} = \frac{1}{1 + 55.5}$$

$$\frac{P^\circ - P_S}{760} = \frac{1}{56.5}$$

$$P^\circ - P_S = \frac{760}{56.5} = 13.44 \text{ mm Hg}$$

28. Apply, $\frac{P^\circ - P_S}{P^\circ} = X_B$

i.e. relative lowering of vapour pressure = mole fraction of solute

$\therefore\ X_B = \frac{n_B}{n_A + n_B}$

Urea (NH_2CONH_2) has M.mass = 60 g

$$X_B = \frac{\frac{3}{60}}{\frac{3}{60} + \frac{45}{18}} = \frac{0.05}{0.05 + 2.5} = \frac{0.05}{2.55}$$

29. For PQ_2, $\Delta T_f = k_f m$

W_A (given weight of solvent) = 20 g

W_B (given weight of solute) = 1 g

Value of k_f (for benzene) = 5.1 k kg mol^{-1}

$\Delta T_f = 2.3k$

$$2\cdot3 = 5.1 \times \frac{\frac{1}{M_B}}{\frac{20}{1000}}$$

$$2\cdot3 = 5\cdot1 \times \frac{1}{M_B} \times \frac{1000}{20}$$

$$M_B(\text{molar mass of } PQ_2) = \frac{5\cdot1}{2\cdot3} \times \frac{1000}{20}$$

$$\text{Molar mass of } PQ_2 = \frac{5100}{46} = 110\cdot86\,g$$

For PQ_4,

$\Delta T_f = k_f m$

$$1\cdot3 = 5\cdot1 \times \frac{\frac{1}{M_B}}{\frac{20}{1000}}$$

$$1\cdot3 = 5\cdot1 \times \frac{1}{M_B} \times \frac{1000}{20}$$

$$M_B = \frac{5\cdot 1}{1\cdot 3} \times \frac{1000}{20}$$

$$M_B = \frac{51}{13} \times 50$$

$$(\text{Molar Mass of } PQ_4) = \frac{51 \times 50}{13} = 196.15\text{g}$$

$\therefore$ Molar mass of $PQ_2 = 110.86\text{g}$

Molar mass of PQ_4 = 196.15 g

Now, (for PQ_2)Atomic mass of P + 2 × Atomic mass of Q = 110.86 g (1)

(For PQ_4) Atomic mass of P + 4 × Atomic mass of Q = 196.15 g (2)

Subtracting both the equations, we get

– 2 × Atomic mass of Q = 110.86 – 196.15

– 2 × Atomic mass of Q = – 85.29 g

$$\boxed{\text{Atomic mass of } Q = \frac{85\cdot 29}{2} = 42.64\text{g}}$$

Putting this value in equation 1, Atomic mass of P = 25.5 g

30. For option 1 :

1% (w/w) glucose means -

1 gm of glucose is dissolved in 100 gm of solution.

$\therefore$ weight of solvent = 100 – 1 = 99gm

Apply $\Delta T_b = K_b\, m$

$$T_b^S - T_b^0 = k_b \times \frac{\frac{1}{180}}{\frac{99}{1000}}$$

(M. mass of glucose = 180g)

$$\boxed{T_b^S = k_b \times \frac{1}{180} \times \frac{1000}{99} + T_b^0} \quad (1)$$

For option 2 :

1% (w/w) sucrose in H_2O -

1 gm of sucrose is dissolved in 100 gm solution.

$\therefore$ weight of solvent = 100 – 1 = 99 gm

$$T_b^S - T_b^0 = k_b \times \frac{\frac{1}{342}}{\frac{99}{1000}} \text{ (M. mass of sucrose = 342)}$$

$$\boxed{T_b^S = k_b \times \frac{1}{342} \times \frac{1000}{99} + T_b^0} \quad (2)$$

For option 3 :

1% NaCl in H_2O

W_B (weight of solute) = 1 g

W_A (weight of solvent) = 99 g

Apply $\Delta T_b = i\, k_b m$

(i, Van't Hoff factor is applied because NaCl is an electrolyte)

$$T_b^S - T_b^0 = 2 \times k_b \times \frac{\frac{1}{58\cdot 5}}{\frac{99}{1000}}$$

$$T_b^S = 2 \times k_b \times \frac{1}{58\cdot 5} \times \frac{1000}{99} + T_b^0$$

$$\boxed{T_b^S = k_b \times \frac{1}{29\cdot 25} \times \frac{1000}{99} + T_b^0}$$

For option 4 :

1% $CaCl_2$ (w/w) in H_2O

1 gm of $CaCl_2$ is dissolved in 100 gm of solution

W_B = 1gm, W_A = 99 gm

For $CaCl_2$, i = 3 ($CaCl_2 \rightarrow Ca^{2+} + 2Cl^-$)

$\Delta T_b = ik_b m$

$$T_b^S - T_b^0 = 3 \times k_b \times \frac{\frac{1}{111}}{\frac{99}{1000}}$$

$$T_b^S - T_b^0 = k_b \times \frac{1}{111} \times \frac{1000}{99} \times 3$$

$$T_b^S = 3 \times k_b \times \frac{1}{111} \times \frac{1000}{99} \times T_b^0$$

$$\boxed{T_b^S = k_b \times \frac{1}{37} \times \frac{1000}{99} + T_b^0}$$

K_b and T_b^0 will be constant in all the four cases.

Considering all the four results, option 3 will have the highest boiling point.

31. When equal volumes of two solutions are mixed, then apply $\pi_3 = \frac{\pi_1 + \pi_2}{2}$

It can be derived as follows -

For 1st solution For 2nd solution

$$\pi_1 = \frac{n_1}{V} RT \quad (1) \qquad \pi_2 = \frac{n_2}{V} RT \quad (2)$$

After mixing, total no. of moles of solute = $n_1 + n_2$

After mixing, total volume of solution = 2 V

$$\pi_3 = \frac{n_1 + n_2}{2V} \times R \times T$$

$$\pi_3 \times 2V = (n_1 + n_2)RT$$

Put the values of n_1 & n_2 from equation 1 & 2

$$\pi_3 \times 2V = \left(\frac{\pi_1 V}{RT} + \frac{\pi_2 V}{RT}\right) \times RT$$

$$\pi_3 \times 2V = \pi_1 V + \pi_2 V$$

$$\pi_3 = \frac{\pi_1 V + \pi_2 V}{2V} = \frac{(\pi_1 + \pi_2)}{2V} V$$

$$\boxed{\pi_3 = \frac{\pi_1 + \pi_2}{2}}$$

Now, in this question also,

Urea solution = 0.4%(w/v)

(0.4 gm of urea in 100 ml solution)

sugar solution = 3.42% (w/v)

(3.42 gm of urea in 100 ml solution)

→ Equal volumes have been mixed

$$\therefore \text{ apply } \pi_3 = \frac{\pi_1 + \pi_2}{2} = \frac{1 \cdot 66 + 2 \cdot 46}{2} = 2 \cdot 06 \text{ atm}$$

32.

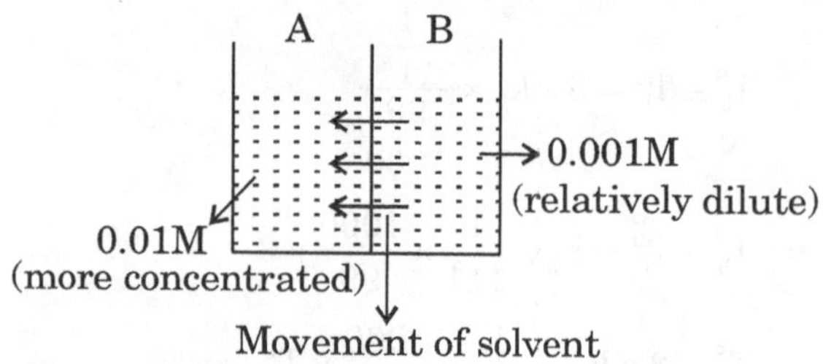

Now, to stop osmosis, Osmotic pressure has to be applied on solution A

$$\pi = (C_2 - C_1)RT$$

$$= (0 \cdot 01 - 0 \cdot 001) \times 0 \cdot 0821 \times 300$$

$$= 0 \cdot 009 \times 0 \cdot 0821 \times 300$$

$$\boxed{\pi = 0 \cdot 2217 \text{ atm}}$$

33. For $MgCl_2$, $MgCl_2 \rightarrow Mg^{2+} + 2Cl^-$

Total Cationic or anionic charge = 2

$\therefore$ n-factor = 2

N = M × n-factor

$$\boxed{\frac{0 \cdot 1}{2} = M}$$

i for $MgCl_2$ = 3 (assuming complete dissociation)

$$\Delta T_f = ik_f m$$

$$T_f^0 - T_f^S = 3 \times k_f \times \frac{0.1}{2}$$

$$\boxed{T_f^0 - \frac{3 \times k_f \times 0.1}{2} = T_f(s)} \quad (1)$$

For 2nd option

N = M × n factor

$0 \cdot 1 = M \times 1$ $\quad (NaCl \rightarrow Na^+ + Cl^-)$

$$\boxed{M = 0 \cdot 1}$$

i = 2

$$\Delta T_f = ik_f m$$

$$T_f^0 - T_f^S = 2 \times k_f \times 0 \cdot 1$$

$$\boxed{T_f^0 - 0 \cdot 2k_f = T_f^S} \quad (2)$$

For 3rd option

$$Na_3PO_4 \rightarrow 3Na^+ + PO_4^{3-}$$

N = M × n factor

$0 \cdot 1 = M \times 3$ (n-factor = 3 for Na_3PO_4)

$$\boxed{\frac{0 \cdot 1}{3} = M}$$

$$\Delta T_f = ik_f m \ (Na_3PO_4 \rightarrow 3Na^+ + PO_4^{3-})$$

$$T_f^0 - T_f^s = 4 \times k_f \times \frac{0 \cdot 1}{3}$$

$$\boxed{T_f^0 - \frac{0 \cdot 4}{3} k_f = T_{f(s)}} \quad (3)$$

Since solvent is same in all the three, T_f^0 & k_f are same. Comparing these 3 equations, Solution 3rd i.e. 0·1N Na_3PO_4 will have highest freezing point.

34. The value of kb depends on the nature of solvent only.

35. $$\frac{P^0 - P_S}{P^0} = \frac{in_B}{in_B + n_A}$$

$$0 \cdot 167 = \frac{2 \times n_B}{2 \times n_B + \frac{180}{18}} \quad (i = 2 \text{ for NaCl})$$

$$0 \cdot 167 = \frac{2n_B}{2n_B + 10}$$

$$0 \cdot 334 n_B + 1 \cdot 67 = 2n_B$$

$$1 \cdot 67 = 1 \cdot 67 n_B$$

$$\boxed{n_B = 1}$$

36. Isotonic solutions will have the same osmotic pressure.

In option 3,

$MgCl_2 \rightarrow Mg^{2+} + 2Cl^-$

$\boxed{i = 3}$

$\boxed{\pi = iCRT = 3 \times 0.1 \times R \times T = 0.3RT}$

$Na_2SO_4 \rightarrow 2Na^+ + SO_4^{2-}$

$\boxed{i = 3}$

$\boxed{\pi = iCRT = 3 \times 0.1 \times R \times T = 0.3RT}$

37. $BaCl_2 + 2AgNO_3 \rightarrow Ba(NO_3)_2 + 2AgCl$

20 ml, Conc = ? (for $BaCl_2$); 0.4 M, 10 ml (for $AgNO_3$)

$$\text{No. of moles of } AgNO_3 = \frac{0.4 \times 10}{1000} = 0.4 \times 10^{-2} = 0.004$$

No. of moles of $BaCl_2$ that would have reacted

$$\text{(from stoichiometry)} = 0.004 \times \frac{1}{2} = 0.002 \text{ moles}$$

So, moles of $BaCl_2$ = 0·002 moles

Volume = 20 ml

$$\text{Conc. of } BaCl_2 \text{ (M)} = \frac{0.002}{20} \times 1000 = 0.1M$$

$\pi = iCRT \quad (BaCl_2 \rightarrow Ba^{2+} + 2Cl^-)$

$i = 3$

$\pi = 3 \times 0.1 \times 0.0821 \times 300$

$\pi = 90 \times 0.0821 = 7.38 \text{atm}$

38. $$\text{Van't Hoff Factor}, i = \frac{\text{Normal molar mass of solute}}{\text{Abnormal molar mass of solute}}$$

$$\boxed{i = \frac{58.5}{30} = 1.95}$$

$$\alpha = \frac{i-1}{n-1} \qquad (NaCl \rightarrow Na^+ + Cl^-)$$

$$\alpha = \frac{1.95 - 1}{2-1} = 0.95$$

39. $nA \rightleftharpoons (A)_n$

For association, $i = 1 - \alpha + \frac{\alpha}{n}$

Here, $\alpha = 30\% = 0.3$

Now, $4A \rightleftharpoons (A)_4$

$$i = 1 - 0.3 + \frac{0.3}{4}$$

$i = 1 - 0·3 + 0·075 = 0·775$

40. Total vapour pressure of the solution is given by

$\boxed{P = 254 - 119X_A}$

To calculated P_A^0, $X_A = 1$

$\therefore \quad P = 254 - 119 \times 1 = 135$

$\boxed{P = P_A^0 = 135}$

To calculate $P_B^0, X_B = 1$

$X_A = 0$

$\boxed{P = P_B^0 = 254 - 119 \times 0 = 254}$

Also, alternative method

$P_T = P_A + P_B$

$P_T = P_A^0X_A + P_B^0X_B$

$P_T = P_A^0X_A + P_B^0(1 - X_A)$

$P_T = P_A^0X_A + P_B^0 - P_B^0X_A$

$P_T = P_B^0 + P_A^0X_A - P_B^0X_A$

$\boxed{P_T = P_B^0 + (P_A^0 - P_B^0)X_A}$

Now, relating this equation with equation of P_T given –

$\boxed{P = 254 - 119X_A}$

$\boxed{P_B^0 = 254}$

Also, $(P_A^0 - P_B^0)X_A = -119X_A$

$P_A^0 - P_B^0 = -119$

$P_A^0 - 254 = -119$

$\boxed{P_A^0 = +135}$

41. $P_{Total} = P_A + P_B$

$P_{Total} = P_A^0X_A + P_B^0X_B$

$P_{Total} = 80 \times 0.4 + 120 \times 0.6 \quad (X_A + X_B = 1)$

= 32 + 72

$\boxed{P_{Total} = 104}$

So, had it been an ideal solution, the vapour pressue of solution would have been 104 mm Hg but observed V.P. is less than expected i.e. 100 mm Hg. So, it's a case of negative deviation.

42. No. of solute particles will be maximum in 0·1 M $BaCl_2$ i.e. equal to 0·3. So, vapour pressure is maximum lowered.

$$BaCl_2 \rightarrow Ba^{2+} + 2Cl^-$$

0.1	0	0
0	0.1	0.2

$\Rightarrow 0·1 + 0·2 = 0·3$

43. $\alpha = \dfrac{i-1}{n-1}$

$(Ba(NO_3)_2 \rightarrow Ba^{2+} + 2NO_3^-)$

$$\alpha = \frac{2.74-1}{3-1} = \frac{1.74}{2} = 0.87 = 87\%$$

44. If a mixture boils at 80°C, it means its total V.P. at 80°C is equal to atmospheric P.

$$P_{Total} = P_A + P_B$$

$$760 = P_A^{\circ}X_A + P_B^{\circ}X_B$$

$$760 = 520X_A + 1000X_B$$

$$760 = 520X_A + 1000(1 - X_A)$$

$$760 = 520X_A + 1000 - 1000X_A$$

$$480X_A = 240$$

$$\boxed{X_A = \frac{240}{480} = 0.5}$$

i.e. 50 mol percent.

45. $\dfrac{P^{\circ} - Ps}{P^{\circ}} = X_B$

$$0.0125 = \frac{n_B}{n_A + n_B}$$

Since, solution is very dilute

$\therefore n_A + n_B \approx n_A$

$\therefore 0.0125 = \dfrac{n_B}{n_A}$ - (1)

Now, $m = \dfrac{n_B}{w_A(g)} \times 1000$ (n_B → number of moles of solute; $w_A(g)$ → weight of solvent)

$$\boxed{n_B = \frac{m \cdot w_A}{1000}}$$

Placing the value of n_B in equation (1)

$$0.0125 = \frac{\frac{M \cdot W_A}{1000}}{n_A}$$

$$0.0125 = \frac{\frac{M.W_A}{1000}}{\frac{W_A}{M_A}}$$

$$0.0125 = \frac{M \cdot W_A}{1000} \times \frac{M_A}{W_A}$$

Now, Solvent is water (aq.)

$\therefore M_A = 18g$

$$0.0125 = \frac{M \cdot W_A}{1000} \times \frac{18}{W_A}$$

$$\frac{0.0125 \times 1000}{18} = M$$

$$\boxed{0.70 \text{ molal}}$$

46. Apply, $\Delta T_f = K_f\, m$

$0.48 = K_f m$ (1)

Also, $\Delta T_b = iK_b \times m$

$0.26 = iK_b \times m$ (2)

Divide equation (1) by (2)

$$\frac{0.48}{0.26} = \frac{K_f \times m}{iK_b \times m}$$

$$\frac{48}{26} = \frac{3.7}{i} \qquad \left(\because \frac{K_f}{K_b} = 3.7\right)$$

$$i = \frac{3.7 \times 26}{48}$$

$$\boxed{i = 2}$$

Since, Van't Hoff factor is greater than 1. So, its a Case of dissociation & hence it acts as a strong electrolyte.

47. $K_b = \dfrac{M \times R \times (T_b^{o})^2}{\Delta H_{vap.} \times 1000}$

T_b^0 = Boiling point of pure solvent (in Kelvin)

Divide numerator & denominator by 'T_b^0'

$$K_b = \frac{M \times R \times T_b^{o}}{\frac{\Delta_V H}{T_b^{o}} \times 1000} = \frac{M \times R \times T_b^{o}}{\Delta S_{Vap.} \times 1000}$$

Now, $\Delta S_{Vap.}$ & Molar mass (M) of solvent is Constant.

So, $K_b \propto T_b^o$

Now, Boiling point is max. for z(253°C), So value of K_b for 'Z' is max. i.e. = 0.98

$K_b = 0.68$ for X

$K_b = 0.53$ for Y

48. $NaCl + AgNO_3 \rightarrow AgCl \downarrow + NaNO_3$

Let Vol. of $AgNO_3$ picked = 1 L

Molarity of $AgNO_3$ = 0.2 M

$\boxed{\text{So, moles of } AgNO_3 = 0.2}$

Now, Volume of NaCl = 3 L

Molarity of NaCl = 0.1 M

$\boxed{\text{So, moles of NaCl} = 0.3}$

Now, NaCl and $AgNO_3$ react in 1:1 mole ratio. So, 0.2 moles of $AgNO_3$ react with 0.2 moles of NaCl to form 0.2 moles of AgCl (which is precipitated and hence will not be considered as solute) and 0.2 moles of $NaNO_3$ (solute) Also, 0.1 mole of NaCl are left (solute).

$\Delta T_f = iK_f m$ for $NaNO_3$ for NaCl

$$\Delta T_f = 1.86 \times \frac{(2\times 0.2) + (2\times 0.1)}{4}$$

(Total volume of solution = 4 L)

$$T_f^o - T_f^s = 1.86 \times \frac{0.6}{4}$$

$$273 - T_f^s = 1.86 \times \frac{0.6}{4}$$

$$273 - T_f^s = 0.279$$

$$273 - 0.279 = T_f^s$$

$$\boxed{272.8\,K = T_f^s}$$

49. Apply, $\Delta T_f = K_f m$

$$0.18 = K_f \times 0.01$$

$$\frac{0.18}{0.01} = K_f$$

$$\boxed{18 = K_f}$$

After addition of solution,

Total no. of moles of solute = 0.002 + 0.01 = 0.012

Total volume of solution = 2 L

Apply, $\Delta T_f = K_f m$

$$\Delta T_f = 18 \times \frac{0.012}{2} \quad (K_f = 18 \quad \because \text{solvent is same})$$

$$\boxed{\Delta T_f = 0.108}$$

50. $P_S = 20$ mmHg

$P^o = 20.005$ mmHg

For highly dilute solutions,

$$\frac{P^o - P_s}{P^o} = \frac{in_B}{n_A}$$

$$\frac{20.005 - 20}{20.005} = \frac{in_B}{n_A} \qquad (1)$$

Now, $m = \frac{n_B}{w_A(g)} \times 1000$ (n_B → no. of moles of solvent; $w_A(g)$ → given weight of solvent)

Now, $n_B = \frac{m \cdot W_A}{1000}$

Putting the value of n_B in equation 1 -

$$\frac{0.005}{20{,}005} = i\frac{\frac{m\cdot W_A}{1000}}{\frac{W_A}{M_A}}$$

$$\frac{5}{20{,}005} = i\,m \cdot \frac{W_A}{1000} \times \frac{M_A}{W_A}$$

$$\frac{5}{20{,}005} = \frac{im}{1000} \times 18$$

(Molar mass of H_2O = 18 g)

$$\frac{5}{20{,}000} \times \frac{1000}{18} = m \times i$$

$$\frac{5000}{360090} = m \times i$$

Now for $AB \rightarrow A^+ + B^-$

i = 2

$$\frac{5000}{360090} = m \times 2$$

$$m = \frac{5000}{720180} = 0.00694$$

Since solution is highly dilute (aqueous),

∴ Molarity = molality

$$AB \rightleftharpoons A^+ + B^-$$

$K_{sp} = (A^+)'(B^-)' = (0.00694)(0.00694)$

$$\boxed{K_{sp} = 4.9 \times 10^{-5}}$$

51. For KCl,

$\Delta T_f = i K_f m$ (i = 2 for KCl)

$(\Delta T_f)_{KCl} = 2 \times K_f \times m$ (1)

For Compound X,

$\Delta T_f = i K_f m$

$(\Delta T_f)_X = i K_f \times m$ (2)

molalities of both the solutions are same -

Now, $\frac{(\Delta T_f)_{KCl}}{(\Delta T_f)_X} = \frac{4}{1}$ (given)

Divide equation (1) by (2)

$$\frac{(\Delta T_f)_{KCl}}{(\Delta T_f)_X} = \frac{2 \times K_f \times m}{i \times K_f \times m}$$

$$\frac{4}{1} = \frac{2}{i}$$

$$\boxed{i = \frac{2}{4} = \frac{1}{2} = 0.5}$$

Van't Hoff factor 'i' is less than 1, so its a case of association.

wrt option 4,

$3x \rightleftharpoons X_3$

Apply, $i = 1 - \alpha + \frac{\alpha}{n}$

$$i = 1 - 0.75 + \frac{0.75}{3}$$

$$i = 1 - 0.75 + 0.25$$

$$\boxed{i = 0.50}$$

52. $\pi = iCRT + CRT$
↓
for NaCl

$$\pi = 2 \times \frac{0.02}{0.5} \times R \times T + \frac{0.03}{0.5} \times R \times T$$

$$\pi = 0.0821 \times 300\left(\frac{0.04}{0.5} + \frac{0.03}{0.5}\right)$$

$$\pi = 0.0821 \times 300 \times \frac{0.07}{0.5}$$

$$\boxed{\pi = 3.44\,\text{atm}}$$

53. wrt option 1, apply

$$\frac{P^o - P_s}{P^o} = X_B$$

$$\frac{\Delta P}{p^o} = \frac{i n_B}{i n_B + n_A}$$

Since the solution is dilute aqueous,

$\frac{\Delta P}{p^o} = \frac{i n_B}{n_A}$ $(\because n_A > n_B)$ (1)

For K_3PO_4 $(K_3PO_4 \rightarrow 3K^+ + PO_4^{3-})$

Apply, $\alpha = \frac{i-1}{n-1}$

$$\alpha = \frac{i-1}{4-1}$$

$$\boxed{3\alpha + 1 = i}$$

Putting value of (i) in eqn. (1)

$\frac{\Delta P}{P^o} = (1+3\alpha)\frac{n_B}{n_A} \rightarrow$ weight of moles of solute (2)

$$m(\text{molality}) = \frac{n_B}{W_A(g)} \times 1000$$

Putting the value of n_B in eqn. (2) -

$$\frac{\Delta P}{P^o} = (1+3\alpha)\frac{\frac{m \cdot W_A}{1000}}{\frac{W_A}{M_A}}$$

$$\frac{\Delta P}{P^o} = (1+3\alpha) \cdot m \cdot \frac{W_A}{1000} \times \frac{M_A}{W_A}$$

Molar mass of solvent

$$\frac{\Delta P}{P^o} = (1+3\alpha)M \times \frac{18}{1000}$$

wrt 2nd option -

$\frac{\Delta P}{P^o} = \frac{i n_B}{n_A}$ (solution is dilute aqueous)

$\frac{\Delta P}{P^o} = (1+3\alpha) \cdot \frac{n_B}{n_A}$ (2)

$\pi = iCRT$

$\pi = \frac{i n_B}{V} \times R \times T$ (3)

Divide equation (2) by (3)

$$\frac{\Delta P}{P^o}\times\frac{1}{\pi}=\frac{(1+3\alpha)}{(1+3\alpha)}\times\frac{n_B}{n_A}\times\frac{V}{n_B}\times RT$$

$$\boxed{\frac{\Delta P}{P^o}\times\frac{1}{\pi}=\frac{V}{n_A\times RT}}$$

wrt 3rd option-

$$\frac{\Delta P}{P^o}=\frac{i n_B}{n_A} \quad (4)$$

$$\Delta T_f = i K_f m \quad (5)$$

Divide equation 4 to 5

$$\frac{\frac{\Delta P}{P^o}}{\frac{\Delta T_f}{1}}=\frac{\frac{i n_B}{n_A}}{i K_f m}$$

$$\frac{1}{\Delta T_f}\times\frac{\Delta P}{P^o}=i\cdot\frac{n_B}{n_A}\times\frac{1}{i K_f m}$$

$$\frac{\Delta P}{P^o}\times\frac{1}{\Delta T_f}=\frac{n_B}{n_A}\times\frac{1}{K_f}\times\frac{1}{\text{Molality}}$$

$$\frac{\Delta P}{P^o}\times\frac{1}{\Delta T_f}=\frac{n_B}{n_A}\times\frac{1}{K_f}\times\frac{1}{n_B}\times\frac{W_A}{1000}$$

$$\frac{\Delta P}{P^o}\times\frac{1}{\Delta T_f}=\frac{1}{W_A}\times\frac{18}{K_f}\times\frac{W_A}{1000}$$

$$\frac{\Delta P}{P^o}\times\frac{1}{\Delta T_f}=\frac{18}{K_f\times 1000}$$

$$\boxed{\frac{\Delta P}{P^o}\times\frac{18\times\Delta T_f}{K_f\times 1000}}$$

wrt option 4 :

$$i=\frac{\text{Normal M}\cdot\text{Mass of solute}}{\text{Observed Mass of solute}}$$

$$\boxed{(1+3\alpha)M\cdot w^t_{Obs.}=M\cdot wt_{normal}}$$

54. Apply,

$$\Delta T_f = i K_f m$$

$$0\cdot0054 = i\times 1.80\times 0.001$$

$$\frac{0\cdot0054}{0\cdot0018}=i$$

$$\boxed{i=3}$$

So, Complex is 2nd option i.e.

$$[Cr(NH_3)_4Br]Br_2 \to [Cr(NH_3)_4Br]^{2+} + 2Br^-$$

55. wrt statement 'a'

$$KI \to K^+ + I^-$$
(1 mole)

KI (1 mole), will furnish 2 moles of solute (i.e., one mole K^+ & one mole I^-)

After adding HgI_2^-

$$2KI + HgI_2 \to K_2[HgI_4]$$

Now, from stoichiometry -

2 moles of KI yield K_2 [HgI_4] = 1 mole

1 moles of KI yield K_2 [HgI_4] = $\frac{1}{2}$ mole

So, half mole of K_2 [HgI_4] is obtained.

It further dissociates as follows -

$$K_2[HgI_4] \to 2K^+ + (HgI_4)^{2-}$$

Now 1 mole K_2 [HgI_4], yield moles of ions = 3

$\frac{1}{2}$ mole K_2 [HgI_4], yield moles of ions = $3\times\frac{1}{2}=3/2$

So, finally, moles of solute get decreased from 2 to $3/2$, hence freezing point is raised.

wrt statement B,

K_f for a particular solvent is greater than K_b.

wrt statement C,

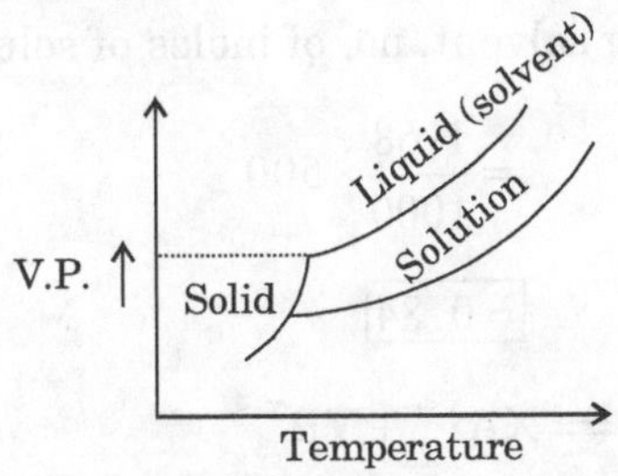

The V.P. of solid & liquid phases are same at freezing point.

wrt statement d, Highly 'dilute' solutions are ideal solutions.

56. Apply, $\Delta T_f = K_f m$

$$\Delta T_f = 1\cdot86\times\frac{\left(\frac{3}{60}+\frac{7\cdot45}{74\cdot5}\times2+\frac{9}{180}\right)}{\frac{80\cdot55}{1000}}$$

(Remember, only KCl is an electrolyte here. Also, weight of

solvent = 100 – 19·45 = 80·55g
↑
Total weight of solute

$$\Delta T_f = 1\cdot86 \times \frac{(0\cdot05+0\cdot2+0\cdot05)}{\frac{80\cdot55}{1000}}$$

$$\Delta T_f = 1\cdot86 \times \frac{0\cdot3}{80\cdot55} \times 1000$$

$273 - T_{f(s)} = 6\cdot927$

$273 - 6\cdot927 = T_{f(s)}$

$\boxed{266\cdot073\,k = T_{f(s)}}$

57. $\Delta T_f = k_f m$ (1)

$\Delta T_b = k_b m$ (2)

Perform 1 + 2 :-

$\Delta T_f + \Delta T_b = k_f m + k_b m$

$(T_f^o - T_f^s) + (T_b^s - T_b^o) = m(k_f + k_b)$

$273 - T_f^s + T_b^s - 373 = m(1.86 + 0.52)$ (1)

$\boxed{\text{Now, } T_b^s - T_f^s = 104}$

So, Placing the value in eqn. 1-

$273 + 104 - 373 = m \times 2.38$

$\frac{4}{2.38} = m$

1.68 = Molality of solution

So, in 1 kg solvent, no. of moles of solute = 1.68 in 500 g solvent, no. of moles of solute

$$= \frac{1\cdot68}{1000} \times 500$$

$\boxed{= 0\cdot84}$

58. $A_X B_Y \rightleftharpoons XA^{y+} + YB^{x-}$

At t = 0 1 0 0

At t = t $1-\alpha$ $X\alpha$ $Y\alpha$

$$i = \frac{\text{Observed no. of moles of solute}}{\text{Initial no. of moles of solute}}$$

$$\boxed{i = \frac{1-\alpha+x\alpha+y\alpha}{1}}$$

$i - 1 = x\alpha + y\alpha - \alpha$

$i - 1 = \alpha(x + y - 1)$

$$\boxed{\frac{i-1}{x+y-1} = \alpha}$$

Also, $\alpha = \frac{1-i}{1-x-y}$

59. Apply, $\pi = 2\times0\cdot1 + 3\times0\cdot2 + 1\cdot2\times0\cdot5RT$

[For 0.5 M HA, $HA \rightleftharpoons H^+ + A^-$]

$$\alpha = \frac{i=1}{n-1}$$

$$0\cdot2 = \frac{i-1}{2-1}$$

$\boxed{i = 1\cdot2}$

So, $\pi = (0\cdot2 + 0\cdot6 + 0\cdot6)0\cdot0821 \times 300$

$\pi = 1\cdot4 \times 0.0821 \times 300 = 34\cdot48\,\text{atm}$

60. Osmosis involves the movement of solvent only. Solute particles will not pass through the SPM. So, Fe^{3+} & CNS^- will never come in contact & hence, red color will not appear in ANY SIDE

61. $P_T = P_A + P_B$

$P_T = P_A^0 X_A + P_B^0 X_B$

$P_T = P_A^o(1 - X_B) + P_B^o X_B$

$P_T = P_A^o - P_A^o X_B + P_B^o X_B$

$\boxed{P_T = P_A^o + X_B\left(P_B^o - P_A^o\right)}$

Now, relating this equation with eqn. given i.e.

$\Rightarrow P_T = 5\cdot3 + 2X_B$

$\boxed{P_A^o = 5\cdot3}$ & $2X_B = X_B\left(P_B^o - P_A^o\right)$

i.e. $2X_B = XB\left(P_B^o - 5\cdot3\right)$

$2 = P_B^o - 5\cdot3$

$\boxed{7\cdot3 = P_B^o}$

So, $P_A^o = 5\cdot3$, $P_B^o = 7\cdot3$

$$Y_A = \frac{P_A^o X_A}{P_{Total}} = \frac{5\cdot3X_A}{P_{Total}} \quad (1)$$

$$Y_B = \frac{P_B^o X_B}{P_{Total}} = \frac{7\cdot3X_B}{P_{Total}} \quad (2)$$

$$\boxed{\frac{Y_A}{Y_B} = \frac{5\cdot3X_A}{P_{Total}} \times \frac{P_{Total}}{7\cdot3X_B} = \frac{5\cdot3X_A}{7\cdot3X_B}}$$

62. For solution in X-

$$\frac{P^o - P_s}{P_s} = \frac{n_B}{n_A} \quad (\because \text{ solution is highly dilute})$$

$$\left(\frac{n_B}{n_A}\right)_X = M\left(\frac{n_B}{n_A}\right)_Y$$

$$\frac{5}{W_X} \times M_X = M\left(\frac{5}{W_Y} \times M_Y\right)$$

Since given weight of solvents is

also same, $\boxed{w_x = w_y}$

$$M_X = M \cdot M_Y$$

$$\frac{M_x}{M_y} = M$$

$$\boxed{(\text{given})\frac{3}{4} = M}$$

63. $MX_2 \rightleftharpoons M^{2+} + 2X^-$

$$\alpha = \frac{i-1}{n-1}$$

$$\alpha = \frac{2-1}{3-1}$$

$$2\alpha = 1$$

$$\boxed{\alpha = ½ = 0.5}$$

64. $Fe(NH_4)_2(SO_4)_2 \rightarrow Fe^{2+} + 2NH_4^+ + 2SO_4^{2-}$

$\boxed{\text{Expected } i = 5}$

Apply,

$$\pi = iCRT$$

$$10.8 = i \times 0.1 \times 0.0821 \times 298$$

$$\boxed{i = 4.42}$$

↙

Observed

65. For association, apply -

$$i = 1 - \alpha + \frac{\alpha}{n}$$

$$\boxed{\alpha = 0 \cdot 2}$$

So, $0.9 = 1 - 0.2 + \dfrac{0.2}{n}$

$0.1 = \dfrac{0.2}{n}$ $\boxed{n = 2}$

66. $ZnCl_2 \rightleftharpoons Zn^{2+} + 2Cl^-$

Apply, $\Delta T_f = ik_fm$

$$0 - (-0{\cdot}23) = i \times 1{\cdot}86 \times m$$

$$0{\cdot}23 = i \times 1{\cdot}86 \times \frac{\frac{0{\cdot}85}{136{\cdot}3}}{\frac{125}{1000}}$$

$$0{\cdot}23 = i \times 1{\cdot}86 \times \frac{0{\cdot}85}{136{\cdot}3} \times \frac{1000}{125}$$

$$\frac{0{\cdot}23}{1{\cdot}86} \times \frac{136{\cdot}3 \times 125}{0{\cdot}85 \times 1000} = i$$

$$\boxed{i = 2{\cdot}47}$$

Apply, $\alpha = \dfrac{i-1}{n-1}$

$$\alpha = \frac{2{\cdot}478 - 1}{3-1}$$

$$\alpha = \frac{1{\cdot}478}{2} = 0{\cdot}739$$

$$\alpha = 73{\cdot}9\%$$

67. Apply Raoult's law

$$P_{Total} = P_A + P_B$$

$$250 = P_A^0 X_A + P_B^0 X_B$$

$$250 = P_A^0 \cdot \frac{1}{3} + P_B^0 \cdot \frac{2}{3} \quad (1)$$

After adding 1 mole of A -

$$P_{Total} = P_A + P_B$$

$$300 = P_A^0 \frac{2}{4} + P_B^0 \frac{2}{4} \quad (2)$$

From eqn. 1 -

$$750 = P_A^0 + 2P_B^0 \quad (4)$$

From eq. 2 -

$$600 = P_A^0 + P_B^0 \quad (5)$$

(Subtract 4 & 5) (–) (–) (–)

$$150 = P_B^0$$

Now, $P_A^0 + P_B^0 = 600$

$$P_A^0 + 150 = 600$$

$$\boxed{P_A^0 = 450}$$

68. Here, 'C' refers to concentration in g/ml. Then, Let C′ refer to concentration in mol/ltr.

$\therefore \quad \pi = C'RT$

$$\pi = \frac{n}{V}RT$$

$$\pi = \frac{W_B}{M_B} \times \frac{1000}{V_{(ml)}} \times R \times T$$

$$\pi = \frac{C}{M_B} \times 1000\,RT$$

$$\frac{\pi}{C} = \frac{1000\,RT}{M_B}$$

Slope of π v/s C $= \frac{\pi}{C} = \frac{1000\,RT}{M_B} = 5 \times 10^{-3}$ (given)

So, $\frac{1000\,RT}{M_B} = 5 \times 10^{-3}$

$$M_B = \frac{1000\,RT}{5 \times 10^{-3}} = \frac{1000 \times 0{\cdot}0821 \times 300}{5 \times 10^{-3}}$$

$$M_B = 60 \times 10^6 \times 0{\cdot}0821$$

$$\boxed{M_B = 4 \cdot 929 \times 10^6\ g}$$

69. Osmotic pressure (π) of 0·05 M glucose

$= 0{\cdot}05 \times R \times T$

$= 0{\cdot}05 \times RT$ (1)

$\therefore$ O·P· of this compound $= 0{\cdot}05 \times RT$

$C\,R\,T = 0{\cdot}05 \times RT$

$$\boxed{C = 0{\cdot}05}$$

$\therefore$ Concentration of unknown compound = 0·05 M

$$\text{Conc.(M)} = \frac{n}{V(L)}$$

$$0{\cdot}05 = \frac{\frac{3}{\text{Molar mass}}}{1_{(L)}}$$

Molar mass of solute $= \frac{3}{0{\cdot}05} = \frac{3}{5} \times 100 = 60\,g$

Empirical formula = CH_2O

Empirical formula mass = 30 g

Now, Empirical formula mass Xn = Mol. formula mass

$30 \times n = 60$

$n = 2$

$(E{\cdot}F{\cdot})_n = M{\cdot}F$

$(CH_2O)_2 = M.F$

$$\boxed{C_2H_4O_2 = \text{Molecular formula}}$$

70. On doubling the amount of solute, the no. of moles are doubled. Besides, the amount of solvent is quadrupled. So, molality of solution is halved. Hence, elevation in Boiling point is also halved.

71. Apply, $\frac{P^0 - P_s}{P^0} = \frac{in_B}{in_B + n_A}$

$$\frac{P^0 - P_s}{P^0} = \frac{2 \times 1}{2 \times 1 + 9{\cdot}9}$$

$$\frac{P^0}{P^0} - \frac{P_S}{P^0} = \frac{2}{11{\cdot}9}$$

$$1 - \frac{P_S}{P^0} = \frac{2}{11{\cdot}9}$$

$$0{\cdot}832 = \frac{P_S}{P^0}$$

$$\boxed{P_S = 0{\cdot}83P^0}$$

72. Molarity of glucose solution = 1 M which means that 1 mole of glucose is present in 1 litre of solution.

ρ (density of solution) = 1·5 g/ml

So, 1 ml of solution weights = 1·5 g

1000 ml of solution weights $= \frac{1{\cdot}5}{1} \times 1000 = 1500\,g$

Total weight of solution = 1500 g

weight of solute = 180 g (1 mole glucose)

weight of solvent = 1500 – 180 = 1320 g

So, molality of solution $= \frac{\text{Number of moles of solute}}{\text{weight of solvent [in kgs]}}$

$$\text{molality} = \frac{1}{1320} \times 1000 = 0{\cdot}757$$

$\therefore \Delta T_b = K_b m$

$\Delta T_b = k_b \times 0{\cdot}75$

$$\boxed{\Delta T_b = 0{\cdot}75K_b}$$

73. weight of solution = 1100 g

weight of solute (urea) = 60 g = 1 mole

$\therefore$ weight of solvent = 1100 – 60 = 1040 g

Now, $\Delta T_f = k_f m$

$$\frac{\Delta T_f}{k_f} = m$$

$$\boxed{\therefore m = 1\,\text{mole/kg}}$$

$\therefore$ amount of solvent in the solution

= 1 kg = 1000 g

So, amount of ice seperated = 1040 – 1000 = 40 g

74. Isotonic solutions have same osmotic pressures

$$\therefore \pi_{sucrose} = \pi_{NaCl}$$

$$(CRT)_{sucrose} = (iCRT)_{NaCl}$$

$$\left(\frac{n}{V_{(L)}}\right)_{sucrose} = 2\times\left(\frac{n}{V_{(L)}}\right)_{NaCl}$$

$$\frac{\omega_1}{342}\times\frac{1}{V_{(L)}} = 2\times\frac{\omega_2}{58.5}\times\frac{1}{V_{(L)}}$$

$$\frac{x}{342} = 2\times\frac{y}{58.5}$$

$$\frac{x}{y} = \frac{2\times 342}{58.5}$$

Then $\frac{x}{y}$ should have ratio equal to $\frac{684}{58.5}$

75. Wrt option 1,

No. of solute particles are less in 6g urea solution in 100g H_2O.

It is 1 molal urea solution & is a non-electrolyte.

Wrt option 2,

It is also 1 molal acetic acid solution & is a weak electrolyte. So, it will dissociate to some extent thereby increasing the number of solute particles.

Wrt option 3,

the molality of this solution is -

$$m = \frac{\frac{6}{58\cdot5}}{\frac{100}{1000}} = \frac{6}{58\cdot5}\times\frac{1000}{100} = \frac{60}{58\cdot5} = 1\cdot025 \text{ molal}$$

Also, the Van't Hoff factor for NaCl is 2. So, total particles of solute will be 2 × 1·025 = 2·050.

So, there will be max. depression in f·pt.

76. Osmotic pressure of CH_3COOH solution-

$$i = 1 - \alpha + \frac{\alpha}{n}$$

(for association)

$$i = 1 - 1 + \frac{1}{2}\left(\begin{matrix}\alpha = 100\% = 1\\ n = 2\end{matrix}\right)$$

$$\boxed{i = 1\cdot5 - 1 = 0\cdot5}$$

Apply, $\pi = iCRT$

$$\pi = 0\cdot5\times 2\times R\times T = 1\times R\times T$$

$$\boxed{\pi = RT}$$

For NaCl solution,

$\pi = iCRT$

$\pi = 2 \times 0.5\ RT$

$\pi = RT$

Both have same osmotic pressures, so both the solutions are isotonic.

77.

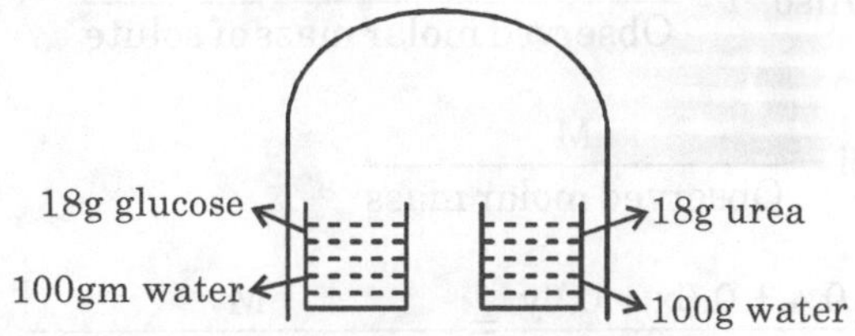

Conc. of glucose solution (molality)

$$= \frac{\frac{18}{180}}{\frac{100}{1000}} = \frac{18}{180}\times\frac{1000}{100} = 1\text{molal}$$

$$\text{Molality of urea solution} = \frac{\frac{18}{60}}{\frac{100}{1000}} = \frac{18}{60}\times\frac{1000}{100}$$

= 3 molal

So, urea solution is more concentrated.

Now, water will get transferred from glucose to urea solution until equilibrium is reached.

Let x gm water is transferred from glucose to urea solution & this will keep happening until conc. are equal.

$$\text{Now, } \frac{\frac{18}{180}}{\frac{100-x}{1000}} = \frac{\frac{18}{60}}{\frac{100+x}{1000}}$$

$$\frac{18}{180} \times \frac{1000}{100-x} = \frac{18}{60} \times \frac{2000}{100+x}$$

$$\frac{100}{100-x} = \frac{300}{100+x}$$

$$10000 + 100x = 30000 - 300x$$

$$400x = 20,000$$

$$x = \frac{20,000}{400}$$

78.

$$M_X N_Y \rightleftharpoons XM^{y+} + YN^{x-}$$

At, t = 0	1	0	0
At, t = t	$\frac{1-60}{100} \times 15$	0.6x	0.6y

$$i = \frac{\text{Observed no. of particles of solute}}{\text{Initial no. of particles of solute}}$$

$$i = \frac{0{\cdot}4 + 0{\cdot}6x + 0{\cdot}6y}{1}$$

$$\text{Also, } i = \frac{\text{Normal molar mass of solute}}{\text{Observed molar mass of solute}}$$

$$i = \frac{M}{\text{Observed molar mass}}$$

$$\frac{0.4 + 0.6x + 0.6y}{1} = \frac{M}{\text{Observed molar mass}}$$

$$\text{Observed molar mass} = \frac{M}{0{\cdot}4 + 0{\cdot}6(x+y)}$$

79. 128g of ice separated is not a part of solution because its freezing point did not get depressed. So, effective weight of solvent in the solution = 500 – 128 = 372 gm

Apply, $\Delta T_f = k_f\, m$

$$T_f^0 - T_f^{(s)} = 1{\cdot}86 \times \frac{\frac{y}{60}}{\frac{372}{1000}}$$

$$273 - T_{f(s)} = 1{\cdot}86 \times \frac{y}{60} \times \frac{1000}{372}$$

$$273 - 272{\cdot}5 = 1{\cdot}86 \times \frac{y}{60} \times \frac{1000}{372}$$

$$\frac{0{\cdot}5 \times 60 \times 372}{1{\cdot}86 \times 1000} = y$$

$$\boxed{y = 6 \text{ gm}}$$

80. Isotonic solutions have equal osmotic pressures.

$$\pi_{NaCl} = \pi_{K_2SO_4}$$

$$i_1 C_1 RT = i_2 C_2 RT$$

$$2 \times \frac{\frac{5{\cdot}85}{58{\cdot}5}}{\frac{100}{1000}} = i_2 \times \frac{\frac{17{\cdot}4}{174}}{\frac{100}{1000}}$$

$$2 \times \frac{5{\cdot}85}{58{\cdot}5} \times \frac{1000}{100} = i_2 \times \frac{17{\cdot}4}{174} \times \frac{1000}{100}$$

$$\boxed{2 = i_2}$$

Therefore, $\boxed{i_2 = 2}$

$$K_2SO_4 \rightarrow 2k^+ + SO_4^{2-}$$

$$\alpha = \frac{i-1}{n-1}$$

$$\alpha = \frac{2-1}{3-1} = \frac{1}{2}$$

$$\boxed{\alpha = 0{\cdot}5 = 50\%}$$

81.

For urea solution	For glucose solution
$\pi = CRT$	$\pi = CRT$
$P = 0{\cdot}1 \times R \times T$ -(1)	$P = 0{\cdot}1 \times R \times T$ -(2)

After mixing equal volumes -

Apply, $\pi = CRT$

Since equal volumes of 2 solutions are mixed,

$\therefore$ total no. of moles of solute = 0·2

Total volume = 2 L

$$\pi = \frac{n}{v} RT$$

$$\pi = \frac{0{\cdot}2}{2} \times R \times T = 0{\cdot}1RT$$

$$\boxed{\pi = 0{\cdot}1RT = P}$$

82. For association,

$$\boxed{i = 1 - \alpha + \frac{\alpha}{n}}$$

where α = degree of association.

For solute 'X'

apply, $i = 1 - \alpha + \frac{\alpha}{n}$

n = 3 (for trimerisation)

$\alpha = 20\% = 0{\cdot}2$

So, $i = 1 - 0{\cdot}2 + \frac{0{\cdot}2}{3}$

$i = 1 - 0{\cdot}2 + 0{\cdot}0666$

$\boxed{i = 0{\cdot}86}$

For solute 'Y'

apply, $i = 1 - \alpha + \frac{\alpha}{n}$

n = 2 (for dimerisation)

$\alpha = 90\% = 0{\cdot}9$

$i = 1 - 0{\cdot}9 + \frac{0{\cdot}9}{2}$

$i = 1 - 0{\cdot}9 + 0{\cdot}45$

$\boxed{i = 0{\cdot}55}$

For option 1 & 2.

For solution having solute 'X'

$\Delta T_f = ik_f m$

$T_f^0 - T_f^S = 0{\cdot}86 \times k_f \times m$ (1)

$\boxed{T_f^0 - 0{\cdot}86 k_f m = T_f^{(S)}}$ (2)

For solution having solute 'Y'

$\Delta T_f = ik_f M$

$T_f^0 - T_f^S = 0{\cdot}55 k_f M$ (3)

$\boxed{T_f^0 - 0{\cdot}55 k_f m = T_f^{(S)}}$ (4)

From 1 & 3

Solution having solute 'X' has greater depression in freezing point.

From 2 & 4

Solution having solute 'Y' has greater freezing point.

Wrt option 3,

Since Van't Hoff factor i is relatively greater for solute 'X', the no. of solute particles will be more & hence V.P. will be less.

83. $\Delta T_b = K_b.m$

$T_b^S - T_b^0 = K_b.m$

$1{\cdot}04 = 0{\cdot}52$ m

$\frac{1{\cdot}04}{0{\cdot}52} = m$

$\boxed{\text{molality} = 2\,\text{molal}}$

Apply,

$$\frac{P^0 - P_S}{P^0} = X_B$$

$$1 - \frac{P_S}{P^0} = X_B$$

$$1 - \frac{P_S}{P^0} = \frac{n_B}{n_A + n_B}$$

$$1 - \frac{750}{P^0} = \frac{2}{\frac{1000}{18} + 2}$$

(2 molal solution means that 2 moles of solute are dissolved per kg of solvent)

$$1 - \frac{750}{P^0} = \frac{2}{55{\cdot}5 + 2}$$

$$1 - \frac{750}{P^0} = \frac{2}{57{\cdot}5}$$

$$1 - 0{\cdot}0347 = \frac{750}{P^0}$$

$$0{\cdot}9653 = \frac{750}{P^0}$$

$$\boxed{P^0 = \frac{750}{0{\cdot}9653} = 777\,\text{torr}}$$

Now, since vapour pressure of pure H_2O is 777 torr at 'T' k & 'T' k is also the boiling point of water. Therefore,atmospheric P is equal to vapour pressure So, atmospheric pressure is also equal to 777 torr.

85. Greater the molality, greater is the freezing point depressed.

86. Apply, $\Delta T_b = k_b.m$

$T_b^S - T_b^0 = k_b.m$

$100{\cdot}15 - 100 = 0{\cdot}512$ m

$\frac{0{\cdot}15}{0{\cdot}512} = \text{molality}$

$\boxed{\text{molality} = 0{\cdot}293}$

$\boxed{m = 0{\cdot}293}$

Now, H_2O has $\rho = 1$g/ml. A 0·293 molal solution means 0·293 moles of solute are present per kg of solvent (water). Adding equal volume would mean adding equal weight of solvent.

So, now $m = {0.293}/{2}$.

$\Delta T_f = k_f m$

$T_f^0 - T_f^S = 1.86 \times \frac{0.293}{2}$

$T_f^0 - T_f^S = 0.272$

$\boxed{T_f^S = -0.272°C}$

87. Wrt graph a -

$\Delta T_b = k_b.m$

$T_b^S - T_b^0 = k_b.m$

$\boxed{T_b^S = k_b m + T_b^0}$

$y = mx + c$

Boiling point of solution is plotted on 'Y-axis' & molality of solution is plotted on 'X-axis'. Slope is +ve & equal to k_b. Intercept is equal to T_b^0.

wrt graph b

Graph is correct

Wrt graph c : Graph c is incorrect.

$\boxed{\text{slope} = \frac{1000\,RT}{M}}$

$\pi = C'RT$

$\pi = \frac{n}{V} RT$

$\pi = \frac{W}{M} \times \frac{1}{V} \times RT$

$\pi = \frac{W}{M} \times \frac{1}{V_{(ml)}} \times 1000\,RT$

$\pi = \frac{C}{M} \times 1000\,RT$

$\pi = \frac{1000\,RT}{M} \times C + O$

$\downarrow \qquad \downarrow \quad \downarrow$

$y = \qquad m \quad x + \quad c$

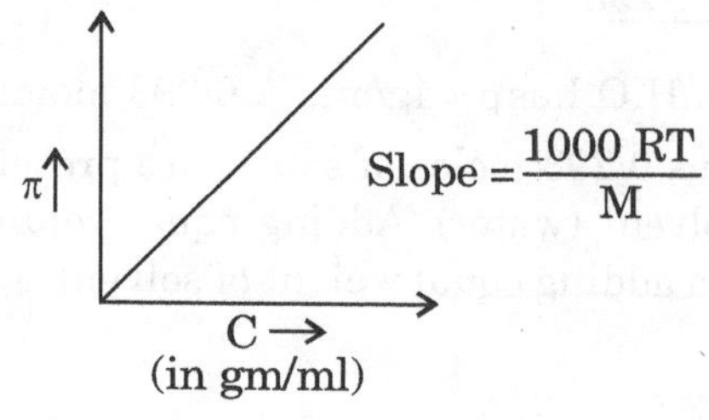

88. Apply $\Delta T_f = ik_f m$

$$0.186 = \frac{1.86 \times \left(2 \times \frac{x}{74.5} + 2 \times \frac{3.125 - x}{58.5}\right)}{1}$$

$$0.1 = \frac{2\left(\frac{x}{74.5} + \frac{3.125 - x}{58.5}\right)}{1}$$

$$\frac{0.1}{2} = \frac{x}{74.5} + \frac{3.125 - x}{58.5}$$

$0.05 = 0.0134x + 0.017(3.125 - x)$

$-0.0034 = -0.0036x$

$\boxed{x = 0.944}$

$\text{Moles of KCl} = \frac{0.944}{74.5}$

$\text{Moles of NaCl} = \frac{2.181}{58.5}$

$\boxed{\frac{n_{KCl}}{n_{NaCl}} = \frac{1}{3}}$

89. Addition of salt will decrease the vapour pressure because solute particles will increase.

90. Isotonic solutions have same osmotic pressure

$\pi_1 = \pi_2$

$C_1RT = C_2RT$

$C_1 = C_2$

$\frac{n_1}{V_1} = \frac{n_2}{V_2}$

$$\frac{\frac{10}{M_A} + \frac{20}{M_B}}{\frac{500}{1000}} = \frac{\frac{6.67}{M_A} + \frac{30}{M_B}}{\frac{500}{1000}}$$

$$\frac{10}{M_A} + \frac{20}{M_B} = \frac{6.67}{M_A} + \frac{30}{M_B}$$

$$\frac{10M_B + 20M_A}{M_A M_B} = \frac{6.67M_B + 30M_A}{M_A M_B}$$

$10\,M_B + 20\,M_A = 6.67\,M_B + 30\,M_A$

$3.33\,M_B = 10\,M_A$

$\frac{3.33}{10} = \frac{M_A}{M_B} = 0.33 = \frac{1}{3}$

91. Apply,

$$\Delta T_b = k_b m$$

$$T_b^S - T_b^0 = k_b \times m$$

$$373{\cdot}26 - 373 = 0{\cdot}52 \times m$$

$$\frac{0{\cdot}26}{0{\cdot}52} = m$$

$$\boxed{m = 0{\cdot}5}$$

Which means that 0·5 moles of solute are present per kg of solvent.

So, weight of solute = 0·5 × 150 = 75 g

weight of solvent = 1 kg = 1000 g

So, weight of solution = 75 + 1000 = 1075 g

weight percentage of solute

$$= \frac{75}{1075} \times 100 = 6{\cdot}976\%$$

92. $\Delta T_f = k_f m$

$$T_f^0 - T_f^s = k_f \times m$$

$$0 - (-x) = \frac{1{\cdot}86 \times \left(\frac{3{\cdot}6}{180} + \frac{3{\cdot}6}{60}\right)}{\frac{200}{1000}}$$

$$x = \frac{\frac{1.86 \times 3.6}{60}\left(\frac{1}{3} + \frac{1}{100}\right)}{\frac{200}{1000}}$$

$$x = \frac{1{\cdot}86 \times 3{\cdot}6}{60} \times \frac{4}{3} \times \frac{1000}{200}$$

$$x = \frac{1{\cdot}86 \times 3{\cdot}6}{9} = 0{\cdot}744$$

Volume of 10 x = 0·744 × 10 = 7·44

94. Azeotropes have same composition in liquid & vapour phase.

95. Isotonic solution have same osmotic pressure.

$$\pi_{K_2SO_4} = \pi_{NaCl}$$

$$i_1 c_1 RT = i_2 c_2 RT$$

$$i_1 c_1 = i_2 c_2$$

$$i_1 \times \frac{\frac{17{\cdot}4}{174}}{\frac{100}{1000}} = 2 \times \frac{\frac{5.85}{58.5}}{\frac{100}{1000}}$$

$$i_1 \times 0{\cdot}1 = 2 \times \frac{5{\cdot}85}{58{\cdot}5}$$

$$i_1 \times 0{\cdot}1 = 0{\cdot}2$$

$$\boxed{i_1 = 2}$$

$$K_2SO_4 \rightarrow 2k^+ + SO_4^{2-}$$

$$\alpha = \frac{i-1}{n-1} \text{ (for dissociation)}$$

$$\alpha = \frac{2-1}{3-1}$$

$$\boxed{\alpha = \frac{1}{2} = 0{\cdot}5 = 50\%}$$

96. $M = \frac{n}{V(L)}$

$$M = \frac{\frac{0{\cdot}967}{159{\cdot}5}}{\frac{20}{1000}} = \frac{0{\cdot}967}{159{\cdot}5} \times \frac{1000}{20} = 0{\cdot}303\,M$$

97. $A_X B_Y \rightleftharpoons XA^{y+} + y^{B^{x-}}$

At t = 0 1 0 0

At t = t $1-\alpha$ $X\alpha$ $y\alpha$

$$i = \frac{\text{Observed number of particles of solute}}{\text{Original number of particles of solute}}$$

$$i = \frac{1 - \alpha + x\alpha + y\alpha}{1}$$

99. O.P. of glucose solution = CRT = 0·1 RT

wrt option 1 -

$$\pi = icRT$$

$$\pi = 2 \times 0.1\,RT = 0.2\,RT$$

(NaOH is a strong base)

$$NaOH \rightarrow Na^+ + \overline{O}H$$

$$\boxed{i = 2}$$

wrt option 2, $BaSO_4$ in water will not from a solution because it is insoluble.

wrt option 3,

$$\pi = CRT = \frac{\frac{0{\cdot}6}{60}}{\frac{100}{1000}} \times RT$$

$$\boxed{\pi = \frac{0{\cdot}6}{60} \times \frac{1000}{100} \times RT = 0{\cdot}1\,RT}$$

So, answer is option 1.

100. 20% (w/w) means that 20 g of solute is present in 100 g of solution.

So,

weight of solutionweight of solute

100gm $\rightarrow$ 20gm

400gm $\rightarrow$ $\frac{20}{100} \times 400 = 80g$

Out of '80 g' solute, 50g solute got precipitated.

So, solute left = 30g

weight of solution, now = 400 – 50 = 350 g

So, percentage by weight of solute

$$= \frac{30}{350} \times 100 = 8.57\% = 8.6\%$$

101. Apply,

$$\frac{P^0 - P_s}{P^0} = X_B$$

$$\frac{2338 - 2295{\cdot}8}{2338} = X_B$$

$$\boxed{X_B = 0{\cdot}018}$$

$$X_B = 0{\cdot}018 = \frac{18}{1000}$$

which means out of every total 1000 moles (induding $\eta_{solute} + \eta_{solvent}$), 18 moles are of solute & 982 moles are of sovent.

$$\text{So, molality of solution} = \frac{\text{no. of moles of solute}}{\text{wt. of solvent (in kgs)}}$$

$$M = \frac{18}{982 \times 18/1000}$$

$$\boxed{M = \frac{18}{982 \times 18} \times 1000 = 1{\cdot}018}$$

Now, m = 1·018 which means that 1·018 moles of solute are present per kg of solvent.

So, wt. of solute = 1·018 × 60 = 61·099 g

wt. of solvent = 1000 g

Total wt. of solution = 61·099 + 1000

= 1061·099 g = 1·061 kg

Now, ρ of solution = 1010 kg/m³

weight of solutionVol. of solution

1010 kg $\rightarrow$ 1 m³

$$1{\cdot}061\,kg \rightarrow \frac{1}{1010} \times 1{\cdot}061 = 0{\cdot}00105\ M^3$$

Apply,

$$\pi = CRT$$

$$\pi = \frac{n}{V}RT$$

$$\pi = \frac{1{\cdot}018}{0{\cdot}00105} \times 8{\cdot}314 \times 293$$

$$\boxed{\pi = 2{\cdot}36 \times 10^6\ Pa}$$

102. Apply -

$$\Delta T_f = i k_f M$$

$$0 - (-0{\cdot}20) = i \times 1{\cdot}8 \times 0{\cdot}1$$

$$\frac{0{\cdot}20}{0{\cdot}18} = i$$

$$\boxed{i = 1{\cdot}11}$$

$$\text{For dissociation, } \alpha = \frac{i-1}{n-1}$$

$$\boxed{\alpha = \frac{1{\cdot}11 - 1}{2 - 1} = 0{\cdot}11}$$

$$\boxed{\alpha = 11\%}$$

Apply Ostwald's dilution law -

$$ka = \frac{c\alpha^2}{1-\alpha} = \frac{0{\cdot}1 \times (0{\cdot}11)^2}{1 - 0{\cdot}11}$$

$$Ka = \frac{0{\cdot}1 \times 0{\cdot}11 \times 0{\cdot}11}{0{\cdot}89}$$

$$\boxed{Ka = 0{\cdot}00135 = 1{\cdot}35 \times 10^{-3}}$$

103. For solute 'B'

Apply,

$$\pi = cRT$$

$$2P = 0{\cdot}1 \times R \times T \quad (1)$$

For Solute A.

$$\pi = icRT$$

$$\pi = 3 \times 0{\cdot}05 \times R \times T \quad (2)$$

(i = 3 for ternary electrolyte)

Divide equation 1 and 2

$$\frac{2P}{\pi} = \frac{0{\cdot}1RT}{0{\cdot}15RT}$$

$$\frac{2P}{\pi} = \frac{0{\cdot}1}{0{\cdot}15}$$

$$\frac{2P \times 0{\cdot}15}{0{\cdot}1} = \pi$$

$$\frac{P \times 15}{100 \times 1} \times 10 = \pi$$

$$\boxed{3P = \pi}$$

105. Apply, $\pi = icRT$

π (for C_2H_5OH solution) = 1 × 0·5 RT = 0·5 RT

π (for $Mg_3(PO_4)_2$ solution) = 5 × 0·1 RT = 0·5 RT

π (for KBr solution) = 2 × 0·25 RT = 0·5 RT

π (for Na_3PO_4) = 5 × 0·125 RT = 0·5 RT

So, all solutions have same osmotic pressure

106. $K_f = \dfrac{RT_f^{02}}{1000 L_f}$

$$\boxed{K_f = \frac{2 \times (353 \cdot 1)^2}{1000 \times 35 \cdot 7} = 6 \cdot 98}$$

$\Delta T_f = k_f \times m$

$$0 \cdot 661 = 6 \cdot 98 \times \frac{\frac{2 \cdot 423}{M_B}}{\frac{100}{1000}}$$

$$0 \cdot 661 = 6 \cdot 98 \times \frac{2 \cdot 423}{M_B} \times \frac{1000}{100}$$

$$M_B = \frac{6 \cdot 98 \times 2 \cdot 423 \times 10}{0 \cdot 661} = 256 \text{ g/mol}$$

$$\boxed{\text{Mol. formula of S} = \frac{256}{32} = 8}$$

So, correct formula is S_8.

108. $i = \dfrac{\text{Normal molar mass of solute}}{\text{Abnormal molar mass of solute}}$

$i = \dfrac{170}{92} = 1 \cdot 85$

(Normal molar mass of $AgNO_3$ = 108 + 14 + 48 = 170 g)

$\dfrac{1}{i} = \dfrac{1}{1 \cdot 85} = 0 \cdot 54$

109. The normal boiling point of water is 373K. At this temperature, the vapour pressure will equal atmospheric pressure.

Now, T_2 = 373 k

P_2 = 760 mm Hg

& T_1 = ?

P_1 = 19 mm Hg

Apply clausius clapeyron equation,

$$\log \frac{P_2}{P_1} = \frac{\Delta H_{Vap.}}{2.303 R} \frac{(T_2 - T_1)}{T_1 T_2}$$

$$\log \frac{760}{19} = \frac{40.67}{2.303 \times 8.314 \times 10^{-3}} \frac{(373 - T_1)}{373 \times T_1}$$

$$\log 40 = \frac{40.67 \times 1000}{2.303 \times 8.314} \frac{(373 - T_1)}{373 \times T_1}$$

$$1.6020 = \frac{40670}{2.303 \times 8.314} \frac{(373 - T_1)}{373 T_1}$$

$$\frac{1.6020 \times 2.303 \times 8.314}{10670} = \frac{(373 - T_1)}{373 T_1}$$

$$0.00075 = \frac{373 - T_1}{373 T_1}$$

$0.2813\, T_1 = 373 - T_1$

$1.2813\, T_1 = 373$

$$T_1 = \frac{373}{1.2813} = 291.1 K$$

110. $HgI_2 + 2KI \longrightarrow \underset{(X)}{K_2[HgI_4]}$

$K_2[HgI_4] \longrightarrow 2K^+ + HgI_4^{2-}$

For complete dissociation, i = n

$\boxed{\therefore i = 3}$

↓

Van't Hoff factor

111. For dissociation-

$$\alpha = \frac{i - 1}{n - 1} \quad ...(1)$$

$$\& \ i = \frac{M_c}{M_o}$$

put value of i in 1-

$$\alpha = \frac{\frac{M_c}{M_o} - 1}{n - 1}$$

$$\boxed{\alpha = \frac{M_c - M_o}{M_o(n - 1)}}$$

112. As dilution increases the number of ions value of Van't Hoff factor (i) is inversely related to Concentration of an electrolyte.

Value of i for NaCl, having 0.001 m Conc. = 1.98

Value of i for NaCl, having 0.01 m Conc. = 1.94

wrt option (c), assuming complete dissociation-

$$CuSO_4 \longrightarrow Cu^{2+} + SO_4^{2-}$$

$\boxed{i = 2}$

$$CuSO_4 + 4NH_3 \longrightarrow [Cu(NH_3)_4]SO_4$$

$$[Cu(NH_3)_4]SO_4 \longrightarrow [Cu(NH_3)_4]^{2+} + SO_4^{2-}$$

$\boxed{i = 2}$

114. Apply, $\pi_i = C_iRT$

$1.5 = C_1 RT$ ...(1)

Also, $\pi_2 = C_2 RT$

$2.5 = C_2 RT$ ...(2)

Divided by equation 1 to 2– $\frac{1.5}{2.5} = \frac{C_1}{C_2}$

$$\frac{15}{25} = \frac{C_1}{C_2}$$

$$\boxed{\frac{3}{5} = \frac{C_1}{C_2}}$$

Let initial Conc. = $3x = C_1$

New Conc. = $5x = C_2$

Now, $C_1 = 3xM$ & $C_2 = 5xM$

If 1 ltr of C_1 Solution is chosen, 3x moles of glucose will come as solute.

If 2 ltr of C_2 Solution is chosen, 10x moles of glucose will come as solute.

After mixing, total moles of glucose

= 10x + 3x = 13x

Total Volume of solution = 3L

π (osmotic p) = CRT $= \frac{13x}{3} \times RT$ ...(3)

Placing value of RT $= \frac{1.5}{C_1}$ from equation 1,

Also, $C_1 = 3x$

$$\therefore RT = \frac{1.5}{3x}$$

Putting value of RT in equation 3,

$$\pi = \frac{13x}{3} \times RT$$

$$= \frac{13x}{3} \times \frac{1.5}{3x} = \frac{13 \times 1.5}{3 \times 3}$$

$\boxed{\pi = 2.16 \text{ atm}}$

115. If = pH = 12

pOH = 2

Apply, pOH $= \frac{1}{2}(\text{pKb} - \log C)$

$2 \times 2 = \text{pKb}_b - \log 10^{-1}$

$4 = \text{pKb} + 1 \log 10$

$\boxed{3 = \text{pkb}}$

$kb = 10^{-3}$

Now, $\alpha = \sqrt{\frac{Kb}{C}}$

$$\alpha = \sqrt{\frac{10^{-3}}{10^{-1}}} = \sqrt{10^{-2}} = \sqrt{\frac{1}{100}} = \frac{1}{15} = 0.1$$

Apply (for dissociation)

$$\alpha = \frac{i-1}{n-1}$$

$$0.1 = \frac{i-1}{2-1} \quad (BOH \rightleftharpoons B^+ + \overline{O}H)$$

$0.1 = i - 1$

$\boxed{i = 1.1}$

Apply, $\pi = iCRT = 1.1 \times 0.1 \times RT$

$$= \frac{11}{100} \times RT = 0.11\ RT$$

116. Isotonic solution will have same osmotic pressure.

$$\pi_{K_2SO_4} = \pi_{NaOH}$$

$$i_1 \times \frac{n_1}{v_1} \times RT = i_2 \times \frac{n_2}{v_2} \times RT$$

$$i_1 \times \frac{\frac{17.4}{174}}{\frac{100}{1000}} = 2 \times \frac{\frac{4}{40}}{\frac{100}{1000}}$$

(For complete dissociation, i = n, ∴ i = 2 for NaOH)

$$i_1 \times \frac{17.4}{174} \times \frac{1000}{100} = 2 \times \frac{4}{40} \times \frac{1000}{100}$$

$$i_1 \times \frac{1}{10} = \frac{2}{10}$$

$\boxed{i_1 = 2}$

Now, $K_2SO_4 \longrightarrow 2K^+ + SO_4^{2-}$

$$\alpha = \frac{i-1}{n-1}$$

$$\alpha = \frac{2-1}{3-1} = \frac{1}{2} = 0.5 = 50\%$$

■■

3

CHAPTER

Electrochemistry

Electrochemistry (Faraday's Laws of Electrolysis)

1. Total charge required for the conversion of one mole Mn_3O_4 to MnO_4^{2-} in alkaline medium is
(a) 5F (b) 10 F
(c) 20 F (d) 15 F

2. 0.01 mole of electrons are passed through three cells connected in series, each containing aqueous solutions of KCl, $AgNO_3$ & H_2SO_4. The total volume of hydrogen evolved in the set–up at STP is
(a) 336 ml (b) 224 ml
(c) 33.67 ml (d) 22.4 ml

3. In the electrolysis of aq. solution of NaCl, 2.8 litres of chlorine gas at NTP, was liberated at anode. How much of hydrogen gas was liberated at cathode?
(a) 2.8 L (b) 5.6 L
(c) 11.2 L (d) 22.4 L

4. When 8040 coulombs of electricity is passed through a molten metal fluoride of the formula MF_2, 3.6 g of metal was deposited. Then the atomic weight of the metal is–
(a) 43.2 g (b) 67.6g
(c) 86.4 g (d) 55.4 g

5. A 250 ml sample of 0.2 M Cr^{3+} is electrolyzed with a current of 96.5 A. If the remaining (Cr^{3+}) is 0.1 M, then duration of the process is (assume no volume change)
(a) 25 seconds (b) 225 seconds
(c) 150 seconds (d) 75 seconds

6. Time required to coat a metal surface of 80 cm^2 with 5×10^{-3} cm thick layer of silver with the passage of 3 ampere current through a $AgNO_3$ solution is (ρ_{silver}(density of silver) = 1.05 g/cm^3)
(a) 115 seconds (b) 125 seconds
(c) 135 seconds (d) 145 seconds

7. When same quantity of electricity is passed for half an hour, the amount of copper & chromium deposited are respectively, 0.375 g & 0.30 g. The ratio of electrochemical equivalents of Cu & Cr is
(a) 0.8 (b) 1.25
(c) 2.5 (d) 1.62

8. The total volume of gases obtained at STP by electrolysis of aqueous sodium acetate, by passing 0.5A for 965 minutes is
(a) 10.7 litres (b) 20.8 litres
(c) 75.3 litres (d) 13.44 litres

9. The number of electrons passing per second through a cross section of aluminium wire carrying 10^{-5} A current per second is–
(a) 1.6×10^{-19} (b) 6.25×10^{-35}
(c) 6×10^{-16} (d) 6.25×10^{13}

10. Quantity of charge required to reduce 6.2 g of Nitrobenzene to Aniline is

(a) 29185 C (b) 57900 C

(c) 115800 C (d) 2895 C

11. In an experiment, 0.04F was passed through 400 ml of 1 M solution of NaCl. What would be the pH of the solution after electrolysis ? (Assume no change in volume)

(a) 8 (b) 10

(c) 13 (d) 6

12. One gram of metal M^{3+} was discharged by the passage of 18×10^{21} electrons. the atomic weight of metal is (approx.)

(a) 33.35 g (b) 133.4 g

(c) 66.7 g (d) 100 g

13. Electrolysis of aqueous solution of an electrolyte 'Y' using inert electrodes liberates H_2 at cathode and O_2 at anode. Then 'Y' is –

(1) $CuCl_2$ (2) KF

(3) NaOH (4) dil.HNO_3

(5) AgBr

(a) 2,3&4 (b) 1,2 & 3

(c) 1,2&4 (d) 1,3,4 &5

14. If cost of electricity for production of 'Y' litres of H_2 at NTP at cathode is rupees 'X' then the cost of production of 'Y' litres of O_2 at NTP at Anode will be Rs.

(a) 2X (b) 4X

(c) 16X (d) 32X

15. An electric current is passed through copper voltameter connected to a water voltameter. The cathode of copper voltameter weighed 0.03125 g more at the end of electrolysis, then the volume of oxygen evolved at STP is –

(a) 56 ml (b) 22.4 ml

(c) 5.6 ml (d) 11.2 ml

Electrolytic Conductance & Kohlrausch's Law

16. The molar conductivity of 0.025 mol L^{-1} methanoic acid is 46.1 S cm^2 mol^{-1}. Then its degree of dissociation is –

(Given $\lambda^{\infty}(H^+) = 349.6$ S cm^2 mol^{-1} and $\lambda^{\infty}(HCOO^-) = 54.6$ S cm^2 mol^{-1})

(a) 0.114 (b) 0.367

(c) 0.215 (d) 11.4

17. The specific conductance of a salt of 0.01 M concentration is 1.061×10^{-4} S cm^{-1}. Molar conductance of the same solution will be–

(a) $1.061 \times 10^{-4}\ \Omega^{-1}\ cm^2\ mol^{-1}$

(b) $1.061\ \Omega^{-1}\ cm^2\ mol^{-1}$

(c) $10.61\ \Omega^{-1}\ cm^2\ mol^{-1}$

(d) $106.1\ \Omega^{-1}\ cm^2\ mol^{-1}$

18. The equivalent conductance of a solution of weak monobasic acid having concentration $\frac{1}{32}$ M is 8 S cm^2 gm eq^{-1} & at infinite dilution, it is 400 S cm^2 gm eq^{-1}, the dissociation constant of the acid is–

(a) 1.25×10^{-4} (b) 1.25×10^{-5}

(c) 1.25×10^{-6} (d) 6.25×10^{-4}

19. The value of λ_m^{∞} of $Al_2(SO_4)_3$ is 858 S cm^2 mol^{-1} while λ_m^{∞} of SO_4^{2-} is 160 S cm^2 mol^{-1}. Then the equivalent conductance of Al^{3+} is–

(a) 63 S cm^2 gm eq^{-1} (b) 189 S cm^2 gm eq^{-1}

(c) 136 S cm^2 gm eq^{-1} (d) 378 S cm^2 gm eq^{-1}

20. The specific conductivity of a 0.5 M aq. solution of monobasic acid HA at 27°C is 0.006 S cm^{-1}. Its molar conductivity at infinite dilution is 200 S cm^2 mol^{-1}. The degree of dissociation of 0.5M HA (aq.) solution at 27°C is

(a) 1 (b) 0.06

(c) 0.2 (d) 0.6

21. The conductivity of 0.002 M CH_3COOH is 8×10^{-5} S cm^{-1}. If λ_m^{∞} of acetic acid is 392 S cm^2 mol^{-1}, then the pH of the solution is

(a) 3.69 (b) 4.30

(c) 2.69 (g) 2

22. If the conductance & specific conductance of a solution are equal, then cell constant of the cell is–

(a) 1 (b) 0.5

(c) 4 (d) 0

23. Molar conductance of a 0.5 M NH_4OH solution is 2.5×10^{-3} S m^2 mol^{-1}. Molar conductance of $Ba(OH)_2$, $BaCl_2$ & NH_4Cl at infinite dilutions are 525×10^{-4}, 280×10^{-4} & 130×10^{-4} S m^2 mol^{-1}, respectively. pH of the solution is

(a) 12.69 (b) 1.305

(c) 11.3010 (d) 2.695

24. In the plot of λ^c & $\sqrt{c}$, the slope is

(a) λ^∞ (b) –A

(c) $\frac{R}{2.303}$ (d) ∞

25. Equivalent conductance at infinite dilution of $BaCl_2$, H_2SO_4 & HCl aqueous solutions are x_1, x_2 & x_3 respectively. The equivalent conductance of $BaSO_4$ solution is

(a) $x_1 + x_2 - x_3$ (b) $x_1 - x_2 - x_3$

(c) $x_1 + x_2 - 2x_3$ (d) $x_1 - 2x_2 - x_3$

Electrochemical Series

26. The standard reduction potentials at 298 K for the following half cells are given–

$Fe^{3+}_{(aq.)} + e^- \rightleftharpoons Fe^{2+}_{(aq.)}; E° = 0.770V$

$2H^+ + 2e^- \rightleftharpoons H_{2(g)}$; E° = 0V

$Cr^{3+} + 3e^- \rightleftharpoons Cr_{(s)}$; E°= – 0.74V

$Zn^{2+}_{(aq)} + 2e^- \rightleftharpoons Zn_{(s)}; E° = -0.76V$

Which is the strongest reducing agent?

(a) $Zn_{(s)}$ (b) $Cr_{(s)}$

(c) $H_{2(g)}$ (d) $Fe^{2+}_{(aq)}$

27. Given,

$E°_{Cr^{3+}/Cr} = -0.74V$

$E°_{MnO_4^-/Mn^{2+}} = +1.51V$

$E°_{Cr_2O_7^{2-}/Cr^{3+}} = +1.33V$

$E°_{Cl/Cl^-} = 1.36V$

Based on the data given above strongest oxidising agent will be –

(a) Cl_2 (b) Cr^{3+}

(c) Mn^{2+} (d) MnO_4^-

28. The standard reduction potential values of three species A, B & C are 0.52, – 3.03V & – 1.18V respectively. The order of reducing power is –

(a) B > C > A (b) A > B > C

(c) C > A > B (d) B > A = C

29. A solution contains Fe^{2+}, Fe^{3+} & I^- ions. This solution was treated with iodine at 35°C. E°for Fe^{3+}/Fe^{2+} is + 0.77V & E° for I_2/I^- is 0.536V. The favorable redox reaction is–

(a) I^- will be oxidised to I_2

(b) I_2 will be reduced to I^-

(c) Fe^{2+} will get oxidised to Fe^{3+}

(d) There will be no redox reaction at all.

30. The standard reduction potentials for Zn^{2+}/Zn, Ni^{2+}/Ni & Fe^{2+}/Fe are – 0.76 V, –0.23V & – 0.44 V respectively. The reaction, $X + Y^{2+} \rightarrow X^{2+} + Y$ will be spontaneous when–

(a) X = Zn, Y = Ni (b) X = Ni, Y = Fe

(c) X = Ni, Y = Zn (d) X = Fe, Y = Zn

31. Standard reduction potentials of some half reactions are given below–

$F_{2(g)} + 2e^- \rightarrow 2F^-_{(aq.)}$; E° = +2.85V

$Cl_{2(g)} + 2e^- \rightarrow 2Cl^-_{(aq.)}$; E° = +1.36V

$Br_2 + 2e^- \rightarrow 2Br^-_{(aq.)}$; E° = +1.06V

$I_{2(s)} + 2e^- \rightarrow 2I^-_{(aq.)}$; E° = +0.53V

The strongest oxidising & reducing agents respectively are –

(a) Cl_2 & Br^- (b) Cl_2 & I_2

(c) F_2 & I^- (d) Br_2 & Cl^-

32. A button cell used in watches functions as follows–

$Zn_{(s)} + Ag_2O_{(s)} + H_2O_{(l)} \rightleftharpoons 2Ag(s) + Zn^{2+}_{(aq.)} + 2\overline{OH}_{(aq.)}$

The half cell potentials are –

$Zn^{2+}_{(aq.)} + 2e^- \rightarrow Zn_{(s)}$; E° = –0.76V

$Ag_2O_{(s)} + H_2O_{(l)} + 2e^- \rightarrow 2Ag_{(s)} + 2\overline{OH}_{(aq.)}$; E° = +0.34V

The cell potential is –

(a) 1.10 V (b) 0.42V

(c) 0.84 V (d) 1.34 V

33. E° for $F_2 + 2e^- \rightarrow 2F^-$ is 2.8 V, then E° for $\frac{1}{2}F_2 + e^- \rightarrow F^-$ is –

(a) 1.4 V (b) – 1.4

(c) 2.8 V (d) 5.6 V

34. Following are the values of some electrode potentials, which of these is most easily reduced?

(a) $Cu \rightarrow Cu^{2+} + 2e^-$; E° = – 0.345 V

(b) $Sn^{2+} + 2e^- \rightarrow Sn$; E° = +0.136V

(c) $Fe \rightarrow Fe^{2+} + 2e^-$; E° = + 0.440V

(d) $Zn \rightarrow Zn^{2+} + 2e^-$; E° = + 0.762 V

Which of the following metal ions is most easily reduced?

(a) Cu^{2+} (b) Sn^{2+}

(c) Fe^{2+} (d) Zn^{2+}

35. Given $E^\circ_{Cu^{2+}/Cu} = 0.337V$ & $E^\circ_{Sn^{2+}/Sn} = 0.136V$ then which of the following statement is correct

(a) Cu^{2+} ions can be reduced by $H_2(g)$.

(b) Cu can reduce Sn^{2+}

(c) Cu can be oxidised by H^+

(d) Sn^{2+} ions can be reduced by $H_2(g)$.

Nernst Equation

36. Which graph correctly corelates E_{cell} as function for the cell given below?

$Zn|Zn^{2+}_{(aq.)}||Cu^{2+}_{(aq.)}|Cu$;

$E^\circ_{Zn^{2+}/Zn} = -0.76V; E^\circ_{Cu^{2+}/Cu} = +0.34V$

Y–axis = E_{cell}

X–axis = log $(Zn^{2+})/(Cu^{2+})$

(a) 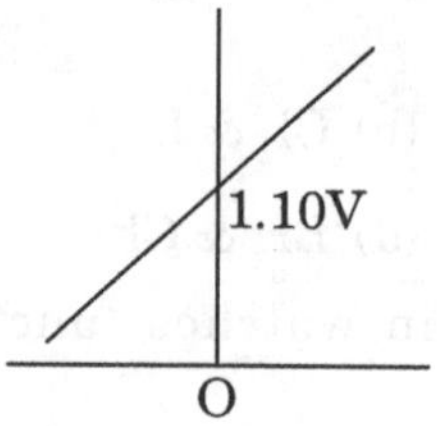

(b) 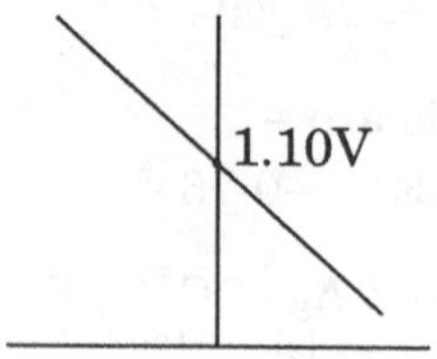

(c) 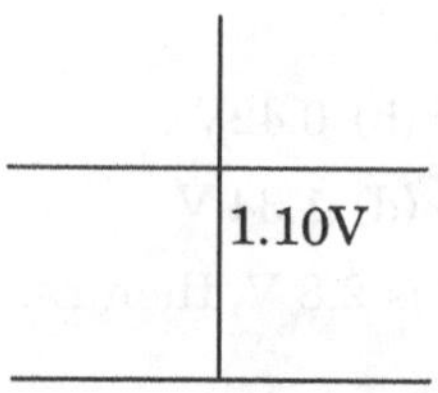

(d) None of these

37. The reduction potential of a hydrogen electrode containing a solution of pH = 4, is –

(a) 0.236 V (b) 4.059 V

(c) – 0.236 V (d) None of these

38. The emf of the following cell is –

$$Zn\,Zn^{2+}_{(1M)}\,||\,HCl_{(pH=2)}/H_{2(1atm)};Pt$$

Given $E^\circ_{Zn^{2+}/Zn} = -0.76V$

(a) 0.878V (b) 0.642V

(c) –0.878V (d) +0.701V

39. The value of E° at 25°C for the following reaction at the indicated concentrations is 1.50 V. Calculate ΔG° (in kJ) at 25°C– (approx)

$$Cr_{(s)} + 3Ag^+_{(aq,0.1m)} \rightarrow 3Ag_{(s)} + Cr^{3+}_{(aq.,0.1m)}$$

(a) –140.94 (b) –295

(c) –212 (d) –434

40. In the above question, the value of ΔG is–

(a) – 422.83 kJ (b) –494.77 kJ

(c) – 400 kJ (d) –512.87 kJ

41. The electrode potential of hydrogen electrode set up in 1M KCl & pH_2 = 1 atm, will be –

(a) –0.414 V (b) +0.414 V

(c) +0.236 V (d) None of these

42. Consider the following half reaction–

$$MnO_{2(s)} + 4H^+ + 2e^- \rightarrow Mn^{2+} + 2H_2O$$

If the pH of the solution is decreased by one unit then the reduction potential will change by–

(a) –0.118 V (b) +0.118 V

(c) 0.236 V (d) –0.236 V

43. The dissociation constant for $[Ag(NH_3)_2]^+$ into Ag^+ & NH_3 is 10^{-13} at 298 K. If $E^\circ_{Ag^+/Ag} = +0.8V$, then E° for the half cell $[Ag(NH_3)_2]^+ + e^- \rightarrow Ag + 2NH_3$ will be

(a) 0.33 V (b) –0.33 V

(c) –0.033 V (d) +0.033 V

44. The Gibbs energy for the decomposition of Al_2O_3 at 500°C is as follows–

$$\frac{2}{3}Al_2O_3 \rightarrow \frac{4}{3}Al + O_2; \Delta_rG = +965kJ.$$

The potential difference needed for electrolytic reduction of Al_2O_3 at 500°C is at least–

(a) 4.5 V (b) 3.0 V

(c) 2.5 V (d) 5.0 V

45. For the cell, $Tl/Tl^+_{(0.001M)}\,||\,Cu^{2+}_{(0.1M)}|Cu$, E_{cell} at 25°C is 0.83V. This can be increased–

(a) By increasing (Cu^{2+})

(b) By decreasing (Tl^+)

(c) By increasing (Tl^+)

(d) Both (a) & (b)

46. For the electrode Cu/Cu^{2+}, log (Cu^{2+}) (along X – axis) is plotted against E_{red} (along Y–axis). The plot obtained is shown in the fig. The electrode potential of the half cell Cu/Cu^{2+} (0.1 M) will be–

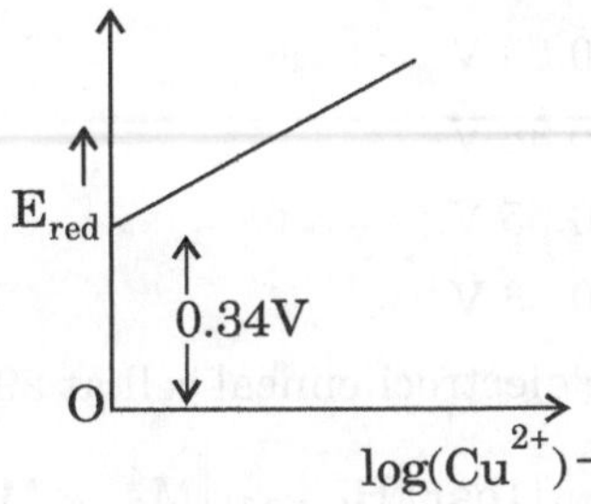

(a) $-0.34 + \frac{0.0591}{2}$ V (b) +0.34 V

(c) $0.34 + \frac{0.0591}{2}$ V (d) $-0.34 - \frac{0.0591}{2}$ V

47. How much will the reduction potential of a hydrogen electrode change when its solution initially at pH = O is neutralised to pH = 7?

(a) Increases by 0.059 V

(b) Decreases by 0.059 V

(c) Increases by 0.41 V

(d) Decreases by 0.41 V

48. Consider the following cell reaction –

$2Fe_{(s)} + O_{2(g)} + 4H^+_{(aq.)} \rightarrow 2Fe^{2+}_{(aq.)} + 2H_2O(l)$;

E° = 1.67 V

At $(Fe^{2+}) = 10^{-3}$M, $pO_2 = 0.1$ atm

& pH = 3, the cell potential at 25°C is–

(a) 1.47 V (b) 1.77 V

(c) 1.87 V (d) 1.57 V

49. The cell, $Zn\left|\underset{(1M)}{Zn^{2+}}\right|\left|\underset{(1M)}{Cu^{2+}}\right|Cu; [E_{cell} = 1.10V]$, was allowed to be completely discharged at 298 K. The relative concentration of Zn^{2+} to Cu^{2+}, $\frac{(Zn^{2+})}{(Cu^{2+})}$ is –

(a) 9.65×10^4 (b) anti log 24.08

(c) 37.3 (d) $10^{37.3}$

50. The equilibrium constant for the disproportionation reaction–

$2Cu^+_{(aq.)} \rightarrow Cu_{(s)} + Cu^{2+}_{(aq.)}$

at 25°C ($E^\circ_{Cu^+/Cu} = +0.52V$; $E^\circ_{Cu^{2+}/Cu^+} = 0.16$ V) is –

(a) 11.2×10^{-6} (b) 6×10^4

(c) 6×10^{12} (d) 1.2×10^6

Brain Teasers

51. Consider the following cell–

$Zn\left|\underset{(0.01M)}{Zn^{2+}}\right|\left|\underset{(1 Litre)}{HCl}\right|Pt; H_2(1\text{ atm})$

Minimum mass of NaOH required to be added in RHS to consume all the H^+ in the RHS of the above cell of Emf 0.701V at 25°C before its use, is

$\left(E^\circ_{Zn/Zn^{2+}} = +0.76V\right)$

(a) 0.0316 g (b) 0.001 g

(c) 0.4g (d) 1.264 g

52. $Zn\left|\underset{(aq.)}{ZnSO_4}\right|\left|\underset{(aq.)}{CuSO_4}\right|Cu$

For the above cell, when the concentration of Zn^{2+} is 10 times the concentration of Cu^{2+}, the expression for ΔG is ($E^\circ_{Cell = 1.1V}$)

(a) 2.303 RT + 1.1F (b) 2.303RT – 1.1 F

(c) 2.303 RT – 2.2 F (d) 2.2 F

53. The reduction potential of Cu^{2+} | Cu at pH = 10 is (ksp of $Cu(OH)_2 = 10^{-18}$ & $E^\circ_{Cu2+|Cu} = +0.34V$)

(a) 0.04 V (b) –0.04 V

(c) 0.31 V (d) – 0.31 V

54. Emf of cell, $Zn\left|\underset{(0.01M)}{Zn^{2+}}\right|\left|\underset{(0.001M)}{Fe^{2+}}\right|Fe$ at 298k is 0.2905 V. Then the magnitude of standard Gibb's energy for the cell reaction is

(a) 61.76 KJ (b) 56.9 KJ

(c) 70.45 KJ (d) 7.45 KJ

55. How long would a galvanic cell set up from a zinc bar weighing 32.65 g & 1 liter, 0.7 M $CuSO_4$ solution run, assuming that it delivers a steady current of one Ampere?

(At. wt. of Zn = 65.3, Cu = 63.5)

(a) 1.34 days (b) 2.35 days

(c) 0.9 day (d) 1.116 days

56. Consider the following reaction–

X→Y; $\Delta_r G^\circ = -193$ kJ/mol

All the energy released from the above reaction is used for oxidizing M^+ as $M^+ \rightarrow M^{3+} + 2e^-$, E° = – 0.25 volt

Under standard conditions, the no. of moles of M^+ oxidised when 1 mole of X is converted to Y is–

(a) 5 (b) 3

(c) 4 (d) 2

57. Two weak acid solutions HA_1 & HA_2 each with same concentration & having pKa values 3 & 5 respectively are placed in contact with hydrogen electrode (1atm at 25°C) & are interconnected through a salt bridge. The emf of the following cell

Pt, H_2(1 atm) | HA_2 | | HA_1 | H_2 (1atm); Pt

(a) 0.079V (b) 0.059V

(c) 0.118V (d) 0.029 V

58. The resistance of a 0.10 M weak acid HA in a Conductivity cell is 2×10^3 ohm. The cell constant of the cell is 0.78 cm^{-1} & λ_m^∞ of the acid is 390 S cm^2 mol^{-1}

Consider the following statements:–

(1) pH of the acid solution = 3

(2) pKa of the acid = 5

(3) degree of dissociation of the acid = 0.01 which of the statements given above are correct ?

(a) 1 & 2 only (b) 1 & 3 only

(c) 2 & 3 only (d) 1,2 & 3

59. The K_{sp} of $BaSO_4$ is 10^{-10}. If limiting ionic conductances of Ba^{2+} & SO_4^{2-} ions are 64 & 80 Ω^{-1} cm^2 mol^{-1}, then the value of specific conductance is–

(a) 144 × 10^{-8} Ω^{-1} cm^{-1} (b) 1.44×10^{-8} Ω^{-1} cm^{-1}

(c) 0.144 ×10^{-8} Ω^{-1} cm^{-1} (d) 14.4×10^{-8} Ω^{-1} cm^{-1}

60. The Electrochemical equivalent of a substance is 0.0006735. Its equivalent weight is–

(a) 65 (b) 26

(c) 25 (d) 21

61. Conductivity of a saturated solution of $AlCl_3$ type salt is 3.06 × 10^{-6} Ω^{-1} cm^{-1} while equivalent conductivity of the same salt is 1.02 Ω^{-1} cm^2 eq^{-1}. Then Ksp of this salt is–

(a) 2.7 × 10^{-11} (b) 0.27 × 10^{-11}

(c) 7.2×10^{-11} (d) None of these

62. Equal quantity of electricity is passed through three electrolytic cells containing aq. solutions of $FeSO_4$, $Fe_2(SO_4)_3$ & $Fe(NO_3)_3$. Then, Select the correct statement:

(a) Amount of Fe deposited in three cases is equal.

(b) Amount of Fe deposited in $Fe_2(SO_4)_3$ & $Fe(NO_3)_3$ is equal.

(c) Same gas is evolved in all at Anode.

(d) Both (b) & (c) are correct

63. By how much is the oxidising power of MnO_4^-/Mn^{2+} decreased if (H^+) is decreased from 1 M to 10^{-4}M at 25°C? Assume, (MnO_4^-) = (Mn^{2+}) = 1 M

(a) By 0.83 V

(b) By 0.38 V

(c) By 0.65 V

(d) By 0.56 V

64. For the electrochemical cell at 298k–

$$Pt_{(s)}\left|H_{2(g)}(1bar)\right|H^+_{(aq)1M}\left\|M^{4+}_{(aq.)},M^{2+}_{(aq.)}\right|Pt_{(s)}$$

$$E_{cell} = 0.092V \text{ When } \frac{M^{2+}_{(aq.)}}{M^{4+}_{(aq.)}} = 10^x$$

$$\text{Given} : E^\circ_{M^{4+}/M^{2+}} = 0.151V; \frac{2.303RT}{F} = 0.059$$

The value of x is –

(a) –2 (b) –1

(c) 1 (d) 2

65. The molar conductivity of a solution of a weak acid HA (0.01M) is 10 times smaller than the molar conductivity of a solution of a weak acid HB (0.10 M). If $\lambda^\infty_{m(A^-)} \approx \lambda^\infty_{m(B^-)}$, the difference in their pKa values ($pKa_{HA} - pKa_{HB}$) is (Consider α <<<1)

(a) 3 (b) – 4

(c) – 3 (d) 4

66. The standard reduction potential data at 25°C is given below –

E° (Fe^{3+}, Fe^{2+}) = + 0.77 V

E° (Fe^{2+}, Fe) = – 0.44 V

E° (Cu^{2+}, Cu) = + 0.34 V

E° (Cu^+, Cu) = + 0.52 V

E° (O_2+ 4 H^+ + 4e^-→2H_2O) = +1.23 V

E° (O_2+ 2H_2O+ 4e^-→4$\bar{O}H$) = +0.40 V

E° (Cr^{3+}, Cr) = – 0.74 V

E° (Cr^{2+}, Cr) = – 0.91 V

Match E°of the redox pair in list I with the values given in list II & select the correct answer using the code given below–

	List I		List II
P	E° (Fe^{3+}, Fe)	1.	0.18V
Q	E° ($4H_2O \rightleftharpoons 4H^+ + 4\bar{O}H$)	2.	–0.4V
R	E° (Cu^{2+}+Cu→ 2Cu^+)	3.	–0.036V
S	E°(Cr^{3+}, Cr^{3+})	4.	–0.83 V

Codes

	P	Q	R	S
(a)	4	1	2	3
(b)	2	3	4	1
(c)	1	2	3	4
(d)	3	4	1	2

67. The standard reduction potential for the reaction are given below : –

$$Ag^+ + e^- \rightarrow Ag; E^\circ_{RP} = +0.79V$$

$$[Ag(NH_3)_2]^+ + e^- \rightarrow Ag + 2NH_3; E^\circ_{RP} = +0.37V$$

What should be the k_f (formation constant) of $[Ag(NH_3)_2]^+$ ion ?

(a) 10^{-7} (b) 10^7

(c) 3×10^9 (d) 10^{-16}

68. A current of 4 A is passed for 8 hrs between the nickel electrodes in 0.5 L of 2 M solution of $Ni(NO_3)_2$. The molarity of Ni^{2+} at end of electrolysis is –

(a) 2M (b) 0.356 M

(c) 0.152 M (d) None of these

69. An Aq. solution containing 1 M each of $Cu(NO_3)_2$, $Mg(NO_3)_2$, $AgNO_3$, $Hg(NO_3)_2$ is being electrolysed using inert electrodes. The values of standard electrode potential are:

$Ag^+/Ag = +0.80$ V; $Hg^{2+}/Hg = 0.79$ V

$Cu^{2+}/Cu = +0.34$V; $Mg^{2+}/Mg = -2.37$ V

with increasing voltage the sequence of deposition of metals on the cathode is –

(a) Hg, Cu, Mg, Ag (b) Ag, Hg, Cu

(c) Ag, Hg, Cu, Mg, (d) None of these

70. A certain amount of charge is passed through acidulated water. A total of 504 ml of hydrogen & oxygen were collected at STP. Then the magnitude of charge passed is–

(a) 1600 C (b) 2895 C

(c) 3175 C (d) 3125 C

71. A current of 0.1 A was passed for 4 hrs through a solution of cupricyanide & 0.3745 g of copper was deposited on cathode. Calculate the current efficiency for copper deposition, (At. mass of Cu = 63.5 g)

(a) 79% (b) 39.5%

(c) 63.25% (d) 63.5 %

72. Which pair of electrolytes could not be distingui shed by the products of electrolysis using inert electrodes?

(a) 1 M KCl solution, 1 M KI solution

(b) 1 M KCl solution, 1 M NaCl solution

(c) 1 M $AgNO_3$ solution, 1 M $Cu(NO_3)_2$ solution

(d) 1 M $CuBr_2$ solution, 1 M $CuSO_4$ solution

73. The metal which cannot be obtained by electrolysis of an aqueous solution of its salt is

(a) Cr

(b) Ag

(c) Ca

(d) Cu

74. The electrode potentials for $Cu^{2+}_{(aq.)} + e^- \rightarrow Cu^+_{(aq.)}$ & $Cu^+_{(aq.)} + e^- \rightarrow Cu_{(s)}$ are +0.15V & + 0.50 V respectively. The value of $E^\circ Cu^{2+}/Cu$ is

(a) 0.150 V

(b) 0.5 V

(c) 0.325 V

(d) 0.650 V

75. Conductivity of all electrolytes decreases on dilution because–

(a) No. of ions per unit volume, increases

(b) No. of ions per unit volume, decreases

(c) No. of ions per unit volume remain same

(d) None of these

76. Select the correct statement

(a) Salt bridge helps to eliminate liquid Junction potential.

(b) Anode is –ve terminal in electrochemical cell.

(c) Anode is –ve terminal in electrolytic cell,

(d) Both (a) & (b) are correct.

77. Choose the INCORRECT statement.

(a) A dilute aq. solution of $CuSO_4$ will liberate O_2 at anode on electrolysis (using Pt electrodes)

(b) If Hg is used as cathode in the electrolysis of aq. NaCl soln. then Na^+ gets discharged at cathode in preference to H^+ ion.

(c) The products formed during the electrolysis of concentrated aq. NaCl include liberation of Cl_2 (at anode), H_2 (at cathode) & formation of NaOH in the electrolytic tank.

(d) None of these

78. Sodium– amalgam is prepared by the electrolysis of NaCl using Hg as cathode. How long should the current of 10 ampere be passed to produce 10% Na (by wt.) in Na–Hg on a cathode of 10 gm Hg ? (At. mass of Na = 23 gm)

(a) 7.77 min (b) 27 min
(c) 34 min (d) 16.25 min

79. $CuSO_4$ (aq.) solution undergoes electrolysis in the presence of copper electrodes, then–

(a) Cu^{2+} are reduced at cathode
(b) H^+ are reduced at cathode
(c) Cu gets oxidised at anode
(d) Both (a) & (c)

80. Choose the INCORRECT statement.

(a) Lead storage battery is an electrochemical cell but lacks a salt bridge.
(b) Molar conductivity increases on dilution.
(c) Potential of Hg cell remains almost constant because the overall cell reaction does not involve any ions
(d) None of these is INCORRECT.

81. What is true about $H_2 - O_2$ fuel cell?

(a) These are voltaic cells.
(b) This cell runs continuously as long as the reactants are fed.
(c) Efficiency (η) of fuel cell = $\dfrac{\Delta G}{\Delta H}$
(d) All are true

82. Electrolysis of an acetate solution produces ethane according to the reaction

$$2CH_3COO^{\ominus} \rightarrow C_2H_{6(g)} + 2CO_{2(g)} + 2e^-$$

What total volume of gases would be produced at 0°C & 1 atm, if a current of 0.5 A is passed through the solution for 482.5 min? Assume 80% current efficiency.

(a) 1.34 L (b) 2.68 L
(c) 4.03 L (d) 1.79 L

83. Resistance of 0.2 M solution of an electrolyte is 50 Ω. The specific conductance of the solution is 1.4 S m^{-1}. The resistance of 0.5 M solution of same electrolyte is 280 Ω. The molar conductivity of 0.5 M solution of electrolyte in S m^2 mol^{-1} is –

(a) 5×10^3 (b) 5×10^2
(c) 5×10^{-4} (d) 5×10^{-3}

84. A current of 3 A was passed for 1 hour through an electrolytic solution of $A_x B_y$ in water. If 2.977 gm of A (at. wt. = 106.4 g) is deposited at cathode & B is a monovalent ion, the formula of electrolyte is –

(a) AB_2 (b) AB
(c) AB_3 (d) AB_4

85. Electrode potential of an electrode–

$$\underset{(s)}{M} \rightarrow \underset{(2m)}{M^{n+}_{(aq.)}} + ne^-$$

is E_1. When the temperature is doubled & concentration of metal ion is made half, then the electrode potential becomes E_2. Select the correct relation.

(a) $E_2 > E_1$ (b) $E_1 > E_2$
(c) $E_1 = E_2$ (d) None of these

86. A lead storage battery has been used for one month i.e. 30 days at the rate of one hour per day by drawing a constant current of 2 amperes. moles of H_2SO_4 consumed are–

(a) 2.24 moles (b) 1.12 moles
(c) 3.36 moles (d) 4.48 moles

87. In a fuel cell, methanol is used as a fuel & oxygen gas is used as an oxidiser. The reaction is–

$$\underset{(l)}{CH_3OH} + \frac{3}{2}O_{2(g)} \rightarrow CO_{2(g)} + 2H_2O(l)$$

At 298 K, Standard Gibbs energy of formation for $CH_3OH_{(l)}$, $H_2O_{(l)}$ & $CO_{2(g)}$ are – 166.2, – 237.2 and – 394.4 kJ mol^{-1} respectively. If standard enthalpy of combustion of methanol is – 726 kJ mol^{-1}, the efficiency of the fuel cell is –

(a) 80%
(b) 87%
(c) 90%
(d) 97%

88. An oxide of a metal (At. wt. = 112) contains 12.5% Oxygen by weight and 0.965 ampere current was passed for a period of 1 minute through the molten liquid. The weight of metal deposited is –

(a) 0.0336 gm
(b) 0.0118 gm
(c) 0.0292 gm
(d) None of these

89. The dissociation constant of butanoic acid is 1.6×10^{-5} and the molar conductivity at infinite dilution is 380×10^{-4} Sm² mol⁻¹. Then, the conductivity of 0.01 M acid solution is –

(assume $\alpha <<<1$)

(a) 1.52×10^{-5} Sm⁻¹ (b) 1.52×10^{-2}Sm⁻¹

(c) 152×10^{-7} Sm⁻¹ (d) 15.2×10^{-6} Sm⁻¹

90. A galvanic cell is made up of S.H.E. and some other hydrogen electrode. The other hydrogen electrode should be dipped in which of the following solutions to get maximum value of emf ?

(a) 0.1 M HCl (b) 0.1 M CH_3 COOH

(c) 0.1 M H_2SO_4 (d) 0.1 M H_3 PO_4

91. When acidified zinc sulphate solution is elecrolysed between the zinc electrodes, it is zinc that is deposited at cathode because –

(a) Over voltage for H_2 evolution on zinc is quite large.

(2) Over voltage for Zn deposition on zinc is quite large

(3) Overvoltage for H_2 evolution on zinc is quite small

(4) Overvoltage has no role to play at all.

92. At 291k, saturated solution of $BaSO_4$ was found to have specific conductivity of $3.648 \times 10^{-6}\ \Omega^{-1}$ cm⁻¹, that of water used being $1.25 \times 10^{-6}\ \Omega^{-1}$ cm⁻¹. Ionic conductances of Ba^{2+} & SO_4^{2-} ions are 110 & 136.6 Ω^{-1} cm² mol⁻¹ respectively. Then, solubility of $BaSO_4$ is –

(At. mass of Ba = 137, S = 32, O = 16 gm)

(a) 22.66×10^{-3} g/L (b) 1.233×10^{-5} g/L

(c) 2.266×10^{-3} g/L (d) 12.33×10^{-5} g/L

93. The time required to liberate one gram equivalent of an element by passing one ampere current through its solution is

(a) 6.7 hrs (b) 13.4 hrs

(c) 19.9 hrs (d) 26.8 hrs

94. Select the correct statement (s).

(a) Leclanche cell & mercury cells are primary cells.

(b) H⁺ ion has a very high conductance due to Grotthuss conductance.

(c) Alkaline medium inhibits the rusting of iron as it consumes H⁺ ions which are other wise required for rusting.

(d) All are current

95. For the following cell with hydrogen electrodes at two different pressures, P_1 & P_2–

$$\underset{P_1}{Pt(H_2)}\Big|\underset{1M}{H^+_{(aq.)}}\Big|\underset{P_2}{Pt(H_2)}$$

Emf is given by –

(a) $\frac{RT}{F}\log_e\frac{P_1}{P_2}$

(b) $\frac{RT}{2F}\log_e\frac{P_1}{P_2}$

(c) $\frac{RT}{F}\log_e\frac{P_2}{P_1}$

(d) $\frac{RT}{2F}\log_e\frac{P_2}{P_1}$

96. An electrochemical cell can behave like an electrolytic cell when –

(a) $E_{cell} = 0$ (b) $E_{cell} > E_{ext}$

(c) $E_{ext} > E_{cell}$ (d) $E_{cell} = E_{ext}$

97. The standard free energies of formation (in kJ/mol) at 298 k are – 237.2, – 394.4 & –8.2 for H_2O (l), CO_2 (g) & pentane (g), respectively. The value of E°cell for pentane oxygen fuel cell is –

(a) 1.0968 V (b) 0.0968 V

(c) 1.968 V (d) 2.0968 V

98. K_a of weak acid in terms of λ_m^∞ & λ_m^c is given by expression–

(a) $K_a = \frac{C\Lambda_m^{c^2}}{\Lambda_m^\infty\left(\Lambda_m^\infty - \Lambda_m^c\right)}$

(b) $K_a = \frac{C\Lambda_m^{\infty^2}}{\Lambda_m^\infty\left(\Lambda_m^c - \Lambda_m^\infty\right)}$

(c) $K_a = \frac{C\Lambda_m^{\infty^2}}{\Lambda_m^c\left(\Lambda_m^c - \Lambda_m^\infty\right)}$

(d) None of these

99. When $CuCl_2$ solution was electrolysed using copper electrodes, the mass of cathode is increased by 3.18 gms. Then, at anode,–

(a) 0.1 mole of Cu dissolves as Cu^{2+}

(b) 0.05 mole of Cu dissolves as Cu^{2+}

(c) 0.22 litre of O_2 is liberated.

(d) None of these

100. Two amperes of current is passed for 16 min. & 5 seconds through 1000 ml of 2M aq. solution of $CuSO_4$ using Pt electrodes

Then,

(a) 0.635 gm of Cu is deposited at Cathode

(b) 1.2046×10^{22} electrons are passed from anode to cathode.

(c) The volume of O_2 gas liberated at anode is equal to O_2 liberated by the decomposition of 56 ml of 2 volume H_2O_2 solution at STP.

(d) All are correct

101. Which of the following methods are employed to prevent corrosion ?

(a) Galvanization

(b) Cathodic protection

(c) Using alkaline phosphates

(d) All of these

Answers

1. (b)	**2.** (b)	**3.** (a)	**4.** (c)	**5.** (d)	**6.** (b)	**7.** (b)	**8.** (d)	**9.** (d)	**10.** (a)
11. (c)	**12.** (d)	**13.** (a)	**14.** (a)	**15.** (c)	**16.** (a)	**17.** (c)	**18.** (b)	**19.** (a)	**20.** (b)
21. (a)	**22.** (a)	**23.** (a)	**24.** (b)	**25.** (a)	**26.** (a)	**27.** (d)	**28.** (a)	**29.** (a)	**30.** (a)
31. (c)	**32.** (a)	**33.** (c)	**34.** (a)	**35.** (a)	**36.** (b)	**37.** (c)	**38.** (b)	**39.** (d)	**40.** (a)
41. (a)	**42.** (b)	**43.** (d)	**44.** (c)	**45.** (d)	**46.** (a)	**47.** (d)	**48.** (d)	**49.** (d)	**50.** (d)
51. (c)	**52.** (c)	**53.** (a)	**54.** (a)	**55.** (d)	**56.** (c)	**57.** (b)	**58.** (d)	**59.** (a)	**60.** (a)
61. (a)	**62.** (d)	**63.** (b)	**64.** (d)	**65.** (a)	**66.** (d)	**67.** (b)	**68.** (a)	**69.** (b)	**70.** (b)
71. (a)	**72.** (b)	**73.** (c)	**74.** (c)	**75.** (b)	**76.** (d)	**77.** (d)	**78.** (a)	**79.** (d)	**80.** (d)
81. (d)	**82.** (c)	**83.** (c)	**84.** (d)	**85.** (a)	**86.** (a)	**87.** (d)	**88.** (a)	**89.** (b)	**90.** (b)
91. (a)	**92.** (c)	**93.** (d)	**94.** (d)	**95.** (b)	**96.** (c)	**97.** (a)	**98.** (a)	**99.** (b)	**100.** (d)
101. (d)									

Explanations

1. $16\bar{O}H + Mn_3O_4 \rightarrow 3MnO_4^{2-} + 10e^- + 8H_2O$

   It is evident from the equation that 10F charge is required for converting one mole Mn_3O_4 to MnO_4^{2-}

2. In aq. KCl, H^+ are reduced at cathode in preference to K^+.

   At Cathode $2H^+ + 2e^- \rightarrow H_2$

   2 mole of electrons evolve H_2 at STP = 22.4 L

   0.01 mole of electrons evolve H_2 at STP

   $$= \frac{22.4}{2} \times 0.01$$

   $$= 0.112 \text{ L}$$

   In aq. $AgNO_3$, Ag^+ are reduced at cathode in preference to H^+ (since E°_{RP} of $Ag^+ > E^\circ_{RP}$ of H^+), so no H_2 is evolved.

   In aq. H_2SO_4, H^+ are reduced at cathode, so H_2 is liberated at cathode.

   $2H^+ + 2e^- \rightarrow H_2 \uparrow$

   0.01 mole of electrons, will evolve H_2

   $$= 0.112 \text{ L (at STP)}$$

   Total volume of H_2 liberated

   $$= 0.112 + 0.112$$

   $$= 0.224 \text{ L}$$

   $$= 224 \text{ mL}$$

3. Amount of charge passed through anode & cathode will be same.

   At anode

   $2Cl^- \rightarrow Cl_2 + 2e^-$

   22.4L Chlorine is liberated by charge = 2 F

   2.8L Chlorine is liberated by charge

   $$= \frac{2}{22.4} \times 52.8F$$

   $$= 0.25F$$

   So, 0.25 F charge is passed through cathode also,

   At cathode

   $2H^+ + 2e^- \rightarrow H_2 \uparrow$

   2 F charge liberates H_2 = 22.4 L (at STP)

   0.25F charge liberates $H_2 = \frac{22.4}{2} \times 0.25 = 2.8L$

4. MF_2 dissociates as

   $MF_2 \rightarrow M^{2+} + 2F^-$

   At cathode

   $M^{2+} + 2e^- \rightarrow M$

   Apply, W = It

   It $w = \frac{Eq.wt}{F} It$ (IF = 96500C)

   $3.6 = \frac{Eq.wt}{96500} \times Q$ $(\because Q = It)$

   $96500 \times 3.6 = Eq.\ wt \times Q$

   $96500 \times 3.6 = Eq.\ wt \times 8040$

   $\boxed{\frac{96500 \times 3.6}{8040} = Eq.wt = 43.20}$

   Now, Eq. wt $= \frac{At.wt}{n\ factor}$

   n factor of M = 2 (from MF_2)

   $43.20 = \frac{At.wt}{2}$

   $43.20 \times 2 = At.wt$

   $\boxed{84.40g = At.wt}$

5. Conc. of Cr^{3+} solution = 0.2M

   Vol. = 250 ml = 0.25L

   Initial no. of moles of $Cr^{3+} = 0.2 \times 0.25 = 0.05$ (1)

   Now, conc. of Cr^{3+} = 0.1 M

   (After electrolysis)

   V = 0.25 L

   No. of moles of Cr^{3+} left in the solution

   $= 0.1 \times 0.25 = 0.025$ (2)

   So, no. of moles of Cr^{3+} deposited at cathode

   $= 0.05 - 0.025 = 0.025$

   At cathode

   $Cr^{3+} + 3e^- \rightarrow Cr$

   1 mole of Cr^{3+} get deposited by Q = 3 F

   0.025 mole of Cr^{3+} get deposited by Q

   $= 3 \times 0.025$

   $= 0.075\ F = 0.075 \times 96500\ C$

   $= 7237.5\ C$

   Now Q = It

   $7237.5 = 96.5 \times t$

   $\boxed{t = 75 \text{ seconds}}$

6. At cathode

$Ag^+ + e^- \rightarrow Ag$ (deposited at metal)

Volume of Ag to be deposited $= 80 \times 5 \times 10^{-3}$

$= 40 \times 10^{-2}$

$= 0.4\ cm^3$

From $\rho_{Ag} = 1.05\ g/cm^3$

$1\ cm^3$ Ag weighs = 1.05 g

$0.4\ cm^3$ Ag weighs $= 1.05 \times 0.4 = 0.42g$

Which means that 0.42 g of Ag needs to be deposited.

$Ag^+ + e^- \rightarrow Ag$

108 gm Ag deposited by Q = 1F

$$0.42\ gm = \frac{1}{108} \times 0.42 = 0.0038F$$

$= 0.0038 \times 96500\ C = 375.27C$

Now, apply Q = It

$375.27 = 3 \times t$

$$\frac{375.27}{3} = t$$

$\boxed{125 sec = t}$

7. 'Z' (Electrochemical equivalent) is defined as the weight of substance deposited when 1 ampere current is passed for a duration of 1 second i.e. when 1 C charge is passed.

Apply, w = zIt (for copper)

$0.375 = Z_{Cu} \times Q$ (1)

$0.30 = Z_{Cr} \times Q$ (2) (for chromium)

Divide eqn. (1) by (2) $\Rightarrow \frac{0.375}{0.30} = \frac{Z_{Cu}}{Z_{Cr}}$

$$\boxed{1.25 = \frac{Z_{Cu}}{Z_{Cr}}}$$

8. If electrolysis of aq. $CH_3COO^-Na^+$ is carried out,

$CH_3COO^-Na^+ \rightarrow CH_3COO^- + Na^+$

$H_2O \rightleftharpoons H^+ + \bar{O}H$

At Anode

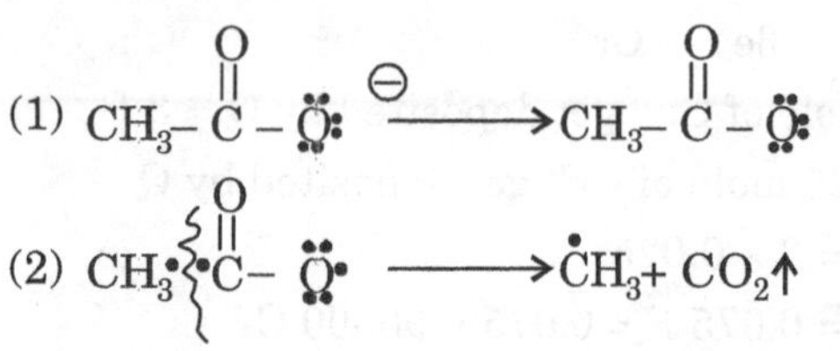

(3) $\dot{C}H_3 + \dot{C}H_3 \rightarrow C_2H_6$

So from 1,2 & 3

$$2CH_3-\overset{O}{\overset{||}{C}}-\ddot{O}^{\ominus} \longrightarrow C_2H_6 + CO_2\uparrow + 2e^- \quad ...(iv)$$

At cathode

$2H^+ + 2e^- \rightarrow H_2$ ...(5)

From equation (4) & (5)

2 F generates gaseous moles = 4 (2 mole CO_2, 1 mole C_2H_6, 1 Mole H_2)

2F generates gaseous volume = 4× 22.4 L

2 × 96500 C generates gaseous moles = 4 × 22.4 L

0.5 × 965 × 60C generates gaseous moles

$$= \frac{4 \times 22.4}{2 \times 96500} \times 0.5 \times 965 \times 60$$

9. Amount of charge passed, Q = It

$$Q = 10^{-5} \times 1sec = 10^{-5}C = \frac{10^{-5}}{96500}F$$

Now,

1F refers to e^- = 1 mole = N_A electroes

$$\frac{10^{-5}}{96500}F \quad " \quad " \quad " \quad = N_A \times \frac{10^{-5}}{96500}$$

$$= 6.02 \times 10^{23} \times \frac{10^{-5}}{96500} = 0.0062 \times 10^{16}$$

$$= \frac{62}{10,000} \times 10^{16} = 6.2 \times 10^{13}$$

10. $6H^+ + C_6H_5NO_2 + 6e^- \rightarrow C_6H_5NH_2 + 2H_2O$
(oxdn.state of N=+3) (oxdn.state of N=−3)

M. mass of $C_6H_5NO_2 = 12\times6+5+14+32$

= 77 + 46 = (Nitrobenzene) 123g

∴ Quantity of charge required to reduce 123 g $C_6H_5NO_2$ = 6 F

Quantity of charge required to reduce $C_6H_5NO_2$, 6.2g

$$= \frac{6}{123} \times 6.2 = 0.3024F$$

= 0.3024 × 96500 C

= 29185 C

11. At cathode

$$2H^+ + 2e^- \rightarrow H_2$$
$$2H_2O \rightarrow 2H^+ + 2\bar{O}H$$
$$\overline{2H_2O + 2e^- \rightarrow H_2 + 2\bar{O}H}$$

So 2 F charge deposits $\bar{O}H$ = 2 mols

0.04 F charge deposits $\bar{O}H = \frac{2}{2} \times 0.04$

= 0.04 mole

$$\text{Conc. of } (\bar{O}H) = \frac{0.04}{400} \times 1000$$

$(\bar{O}H) = 0.1M$

$pOH = -\log(\bar{O}H) = -\log(0.1)$

$pOH = -\log(10^{-1}) = -(-1)\log 10$

$\boxed{pOH = 1}$

$\boxed{pH = 14 - 1 = 13}$

12. $M^{3+} + 3e^- \rightarrow M$

18×10^{21} electrons deposit metal = 1 gm

6×10^{23} electrons deposit metal

$$= \frac{1}{18 \times 10^{21}} \times 6 \times 10^{23}\text{ gm}$$

(1 mole of electrons (1F charge) deposits wt. equal to equivalent wt. of a substance)

So, eqvt. wt. of metal $= \frac{6 \times 10^{23}}{18 \times 10^{21}} = \frac{100}{3}$ gm

Now, eqvt. wt. $= \frac{\text{At.wt.}}{\text{n factor}}$

$\frac{100}{3} = \frac{\text{At.wt}}{3}$ $(M^{3+}\text{has n factor} = 3)$

At. – wt. = 100 g

14. $2H^+ + 2e^- \rightarrow H_2$

22.4L H_2 is produced by charge = 2 F

YL H_2 is produced by charge $= \frac{2}{22.4} \times Y = \frac{Y}{11.2}F$

$\boxed{\text{So, cost of } \frac{Y}{11.2} \text{F charge} = \text{Rs.'X'}}$

Also, $4\bar{O}H \rightarrow 2H_2O + O_2 + 4e^-$

or $2\bar{O}H \rightarrow H_2O + \frac{1}{2}O_2 + 2e^-$

11.2 L O_2 is produced by Q = 2 F

Y L O_2 is produced by $= \frac{2}{11.2} \times YF = \boxed{\frac{Y}{5.6}F}$

Cost of $\frac{Y}{11.2}$ F charge = Rs X

Cost of $\frac{Y}{5.2}$F charge$= \frac{X}{\frac{Y}{11.2}} \times \frac{Y}{5.6}$

$$= \frac{X}{Y} \times 11.2 \times \frac{Y}{5.6} = \frac{11.2x}{5.6} = 2x$$

15. Amt. of copper deposited at cathode of copper voltameter = 0.03125 g

$Cu^{2+} + 2e^- \rightarrow Cu$

63.5 g Cu is deposited by Q = 2 F

0.03125 g Cu is deposited by Q

$$= \frac{2}{63.5} \times 0.03125$$

= 0.000984 F

= 0.000984 ×96500C

= 95C

Now, Vol. of O_2 liberated in water voltameter –

$4\bar{O}H \rightarrow 2H_2O + O_2 + 4e^-$

4 F evolves O_2 = 22400ml (at STP)

4 × 96500 C evolves O_2 = 22400 ml

95C evolves $O_2 = \frac{22400}{4 \times 96500} \times 95 = \frac{56 \times 95}{965}$ml

= 5.6 ml (approx)

16. Apply Kohlrausch's law–

$\lambda^\infty_{HCOOH} = \lambda^\infty H_{COO^-} + \lambda^\infty H^+ = 54.6 + 349.6$

$\boxed{\lambda^\infty_{m\,(HCOOH)} = 404.2 \text{ S cm}^2\text{mol}^{-1}}$

Then,

$$\alpha = \frac{\lambda^C_m}{\lambda^\infty_m} = \frac{46.1\text{S cm}^2\text{mol}^{-1}}{404.2\text{S cm}^2\text{mol}^{-1}} = 0.114$$

17. $K = 1.061 \times 10^{-4}$ s cm^{-1}

$\Lambda_m = K \times \boxed{V_{(ml)}} \longrightarrow$

It is the volume which contains 1 mole of an electrolyte.

C = 0.01 M

So, 0.01 moles are present in volume = 1 L

1 'moles are present in volume $= \frac{1}{0.01} = 100$L

= 100,000 ml

Now, $\Lambda_m = K \times V_{(ml)} = 1.061 \times 10^{-4} \times 10^5$

= 10.61 S cm^2 mol^{-1}

18. $\alpha = \frac{\Lambda^c}{\Lambda^\infty} = \frac{8}{400} = \frac{1}{50} = 0.02$

$$Ka = \frac{c\,\alpha^2}{1-\alpha} = \frac{\frac{1}{32} \times 0.02 \times 0.02}{1 - 0.02} = 1.25 \times 10^{-5}$$

19. Apply Kohlrausch's law–

$$\Lambda^\infty_m\ Al_2(SO_4)_3 = 2\lambda^\infty_{m\,(Al^{3+})} + 3\lambda^\infty_{m\,(SO_4^{2-})}$$

$$858 = 2 \times \lambda^\infty_{m\,(Al^{3+})} + 3 \times 160$$

$$858 = 2 \times \lambda^{\infty}_{m(Al^{3+})} + 480$$

$$378 = 2 \times \lambda^{\infty}_{m(Al^{3+})}$$

$$\frac{378}{2} = \lambda^{\infty}_{m(Al^{3+})}$$

$$189 = \lambda^{\infty}_{m(Al^{3+})}$$

$$\Lambda^{\infty}_{eq(Al^{3+})} = \frac{\Lambda^{\infty}_{m}}{\text{n-factor}} = \frac{189}{3} = 63.5\ cm^2 gm\ eq^{-1}$$

20. $K = 0.006\ S\ cm^{-1}$

$C = 0.5\ M$

$$\Lambda^{\infty}_{m} = 200\ S\ cm^2 mol^{-1}$$

$$\Lambda^{C}_{m} = \frac{K \times 1000}{M} = \frac{0.006 \times 1000}{0.5}$$

$$\alpha = \frac{\Lambda^{C}_{m}}{\Lambda^{\infty}_{m}} = \frac{\frac{0.006 \times 1000}{0.5}}{200} = \frac{6}{0.5} \times \frac{1}{200} = \frac{12}{200} = 0.06$$

21. $K = 8 \times 10^{-5}\ S\ cm^{-1}$

$C = 0.002\ m$

$$\Lambda^{C}_{m} = \frac{K \times 1000}{M} = \frac{8 \times 10^{-5} \times 1000}{0.002}$$

$$= \frac{8 \times 10^{-5} \times 10^{3} \times 10^{3}}{2}$$

$$\boxed{\Lambda^{C}_{m} = 40\ S cm^2\ mol^{-1}}$$

$$\alpha = \frac{\Lambda^{C}_{m}}{\Lambda^{\infty}_{m}} = \frac{40}{392} = 0.102$$

$$CH_3COOH_{(aq.)} \rightleftharpoons CH_3COO^-_{(aq.)} + H^+_{(aq.)}$$

C	0	0
$C - C\alpha$	$C\alpha$	$C\alpha$

$(H^+) = C\alpha = 0.002 \times 0.102$

$(H^+) = 0.000\ 20$

$$\left(H^+\right) = \frac{20}{100000} = 2 \times 10^{-4} M$$

$pH = -\log(H^+) = -\log(2 \times 10^{-4})$

$pH = -(\log 2 + \log 10^{-4})$

$pH = -(0.3010 - 4)$

$$\boxed{pH = 4 - 0.3010 = 3.69}$$

22. $R = \rho \frac{l}{a}$

$$\frac{1}{G} = \frac{1}{K}\frac{l}{a}$$

$$\boxed{K = G.\frac{l}{a}}$$

Now, K= G (given)

$$\boxed{\therefore \frac{l}{a} = 1}$$

23. $\Lambda^{\infty}_{m[Ba(OH)_2]} = 525 \times 10^{-4}$

$$\Lambda^{\infty}_{\frac{1}{2}Ba(OH)_2} = \frac{525 \times 10^{-4}}{2} \quad ...(1)$$

$$\Lambda^{\infty}_{\frac{1}{2}BaCl_2} = \frac{280 \times 10^{-4}}{2} \quad ...(2)$$

$$(1) - (2) \Rightarrow \frac{1}{2}\lambda^{\infty}_{m(Ba^{2+})} + \lambda^{\infty}_{m(\bar{O}H)} - \left(\frac{1}{2}\lambda^{\infty}_{m(Ba^{2+})} - \lambda^{\infty}_{m(Cl^-)}\right)$$

$$\Rightarrow \lambda^{\infty}_{m(\bar{O}H)} - \lambda^{\infty}_{m(Cl^-)} = \frac{525}{2} \times 10^{-4} - 140 \times 10^{-4} \quad ...(3)$$

$$\Lambda^{\infty}_{m}NH_4Cl = 130 \times 10^{-4} S\ m^2\ mol^{-1} \quad ...(4)$$

$$\lambda^{\infty}_{m\,NH_4^+} + \lambda^{\infty}_{m\,Cl^-} = 130 \times 10^{-4} \quad ...(5)$$

Add (3) + (5)

$$\lambda^{\infty}_{m(\bar{O}H)} - \lambda^{\infty}_{m(Cl^-)} + \lambda^{\infty}_{m(NH_4^+)} + \lambda^{\infty}_{m(Cl^-)} = \frac{525}{2} \times 10^{-4}$$

$$-140 \times 10^{-4} + 130 \times 10^{-4}$$

$$\Lambda^{\infty}_{m(NH_4OH)} = 10^{-4}\left(\frac{525}{2} - 140 + 130\right)$$

$$= 10^{-4}(262.5 - 140 + 130)$$

$$\boxed{\Lambda^{\infty}_{m(NH_4OH)} = 252.5 \times 10^{-4}\ S\ m^2 mol^{-1}}$$

$$\alpha = \frac{\Lambda^{C}_{m}}{\Lambda^{\infty}_{m}} = \frac{2.5 \times 10^{-3}}{252.5 \times 10^{-4}} = \frac{25}{252.5} = 0.099 \approx 0.1$$

$$NH_4 + \bar{O}H_{(aq.)} \rightleftharpoons NH^+_{4(aq.)} + \bar{O}H_{(aq.)}$$

C	0	0
$C - C\alpha$	$C\alpha$	$C\alpha$

$(\bar{O}H) = C\alpha = 0.5 \times 0.1 = 0.05\ M$

$pOH = -\log(\bar{O}H) = -\log(5 \times 10^{-2})$

$pOH = -(\log 5 + \log 10^{-2}) = -(0.6990 - 2)$

$pOH = 2 - 0.6990 = 1.301$

$pH = 14 - 1.301 = 12.69$

24. Debye Huckel Onsager's Eqn. is as follows–

$$\Lambda^C = \Lambda^\infty - A\sqrt{c}$$

$\downarrow$ y $\downarrow$ c $\downarrow$ mx

slope = –A

25. $\Lambda^\infty_{eq.(BaCl_2)} = \lambda^\infty_{eq.(Ba^{2+})} + \lambda^\infty_{eq.(Cl^-)}$ (1)

$\Lambda^\infty_{eq.(H_2SO_4)} = \lambda^\infty_{eq.(H^+)} + \lambda^\infty_{eq.(SO_4^{2-})}$ (2)

$\Lambda^\infty_{eq.(HCl)} = \lambda^\infty_{eq.(H^+)} + \lambda^\infty_{eq.(Cl^-)}$ (3)

Perform (1) + (2) – (3)

$$\lambda^\infty_{eq.(Ba^{2+})} + \lambda^\infty_{eq.(Cl^-)} + \lambda^\infty_{eq.(H^+)} + \lambda^\infty_{eq.(SO_4^{2-})} - \left(\lambda^\infty_{eq.(H^+)} + \lambda^\infty_{eq.(Cl^-)}\right)$$

$$= \Lambda^\infty_{eq.(BaSO_4)} = x_1 + x_2 - x_3$$

26. Strongest reducing agent will have the max. Oxidation potential.

'Zn' has max. O.P. i.e. + 0.76 V

27. Strongest Oxidising agent will have highest Redn. Potential i.e. 1.51 V.

28. Strongest reducing agent will have maximum Oxidation potential.

29. Reaction with + ve E_{cell} is spontaneous.

$2I^- \rightarrow I_2 + 2e^-; E^o_{Ox} = -0.536V$

Add $2Fe^{3+} + 2e^- \rightarrow 2Fe^{2+}; E^\circ_{red} = +0.770V$

$2I^- + 2Fe^{3+} \rightarrow 2Fe^{2+} + I_2; E^\circ_{cell} = +0.16V$

30. $Zn + Ni^{2+} \rightarrow Zn^{2+} + Ni$

$E^o_{cell} = E^o_{C(RP)} - E^o_{A(RP)} = -0.23 - (-0.76) =$

$-0.23 + 0.76 = 0.53V$

Here, $E^\circ_{cell} = \underset{\text{(which is +ve)}}{0.53V}$

32. $E_{cell} = E_{C(RP)} - E_{A(RP)} = 0.34 - (-0.76) = +1.10V$

33. E° is an intensive property.

35. H^+ has $E^\circ_{RP} = 0V$.

So, Cu^{2+} will get reduced because they have greater E°_{RP}

$Cu^{2+} + H_2 \rightarrow 2H^+ + Cu$

36. Anodic half reaction

$Zn \rightarrow Zn^{2+} + 2e^-$

Cathodic half reaction

$Cu^{2+} + 2e^- \rightarrow Cu$

Overall reaction $Zn + Cu^{2+} \rightarrow Zn^{2+} + Cu$

Apply NERNST equation

$$E_{cell} = E^\circ_{cell} - \frac{0.0591}{2} \log \frac{(Z_n^{2+})}{(Cu^{2+})}$$

- E_{cell} → y - axis
- E°_{cell} → C (intercept)
- $-\frac{0.0591}{2}$ → m (Slope)
- $\log \frac{(Z_n^{2+})}{(Cu^{2+})}$ → x - axis

$E^\circ_{cell} = E^\circ_{C(RP)} - E^\circ_{A(RP)} = +0.34 - (-0.76) = +1.10V$

Intercept = + 1.10 V slope = – ve

37. $2H^+ + 2e^- \rightarrow H_2$

$$E_{RP} = E^\circ_{RP} - \frac{0.0591}{2} \log \frac{(pH_2)}{(H^+)^2}$$

$$E_{RP} = 0 + \frac{0.0591}{2} \log \frac{(H^+)^2}{(pH_2)}$$

$$E_{RP} = \frac{0.0591}{2} \log \frac{(10^{-4})^2}{1}$$

$(H^+) = 10^{-4} M$

$\because pH = 4$ Given

$$E_{RP} = \frac{0.0591}{2} \log 10^{-8}$$

$$E_{RP} = \frac{0.0591}{2} \times (-8 \log 10)$$

$E_{RP} = -4 \times 0.0591$

$E_{RP} = -0.236 V$

38. $Zn \rightarrow \underset{1M}{Zn^{2+}} + 2e^-$

$2H^+ + 2e^- \rightarrow H_2$

$(10^{-2} M)$

$Zn + 2\underset{10^{-2}M}{H^+} \rightarrow \underset{(1M)}{Zn^{2+}} + H_2$

$E^\circ_{cell} = E^\circ_{C(RP)} - E^\circ_{A(RP)} = 0 - (-0.76) = +0.76V$

$$E_{cell} = E^{\circ}_{cell} - \frac{0.0591}{2}\log\frac{(Zn^{2+})(pH_2)^1}{(H^+)^2}$$

$$E_{cell} = 0.76 - \frac{0.0591}{2}\log\frac{(1)(1)}{(10^{-2})^2}$$

$$E_{cell} = 0.76 - \frac{0.0591}{2}\log\frac{1}{10^{-4}}$$

$$= 0.76 - \frac{0.0591}{2}\log 10^4$$

$$= 0.76 - \frac{0.0591}{2}\times 4\log 10$$

$$= 0.76 - 0.1182 = 0.6418 \approx 0.642\ V$$

39. $Cr \rightarrow Cr^{3+} + 3e^-$ (1)

$3Ag^+ + 3e^- \rightarrow 3Ag$ (2)

$Cr + 3Ag^+ \rightarrow Cr^{3+} + 3Ag$

Apply, $\Delta G^\circ = -nFE^\circ cell$

$\Delta G^\circ = -3\times 96500\times 1.50$

$= -96500\times 4.5$

$= -434250$ J

$= -434$ KJ

40. Apply

$\Delta G = \Delta G^\circ + RT\ln Qc$

$\Delta G = -nFE^\circ cell + RT\ln Qc$

$$\Delta G = -434 + 2.303RT\log\frac{(Cr^{3+})}{(Ag^+)^3}$$

$$\Delta G = -434 + 2.303\times\frac{8.314}{1000}\times 298\log\frac{(0.1)}{(0.1)^3}$$

$$\boxed{\Delta G = -422.83kJ}$$

41. $2H^+ + 2e^- \rightarrow H_2$

Apply NERNST eqn.

$$E = E^\circ - \frac{0.0591}{2}\log\frac{(pH_2)^1}{(H^+)^2}$$

$$E = 0 - \frac{0.0591}{2}\log\frac{1}{(H^+)^2}$$

(Since pH of KCl = 7, $\therefore$ $(H^+) = 10^{-7}$m)

$$E = -\frac{0.0591}{2}\log\frac{1}{(10^{-7})^2}$$

$$E = -\frac{0.0591}{2}\log 10^{14}$$

$$E = -\frac{0.0591}{2}\times 14\log 10$$

$$E = -\frac{0.0591}{2}\times 14$$

$$\boxed{E = -0.414V}$$

42. Apply, $E_{RP} = E^\circ_{RP} - \frac{0.0591}{2}\log\frac{(Mn^{2+})}{(H^+)^4}$

44. Apply, $\Delta G = -nFE_{cell}$

$1000\times 965 = -4\times 96500\times E_{cell}$

$$\frac{965000}{96500\times 4} = -E_{cell}$$

$$\boxed{E_{cell} = -2.5V}$$

46. $Cu^{2+} + 2e^- \rightarrow Cu$

$$E_{RP} = E^\circ_{RP} - \frac{0.0591}{2}\log\frac{1}{(Cu^{2+})}$$

$$E_{RP} = E^\circ_{RP} + \frac{0.0591}{2}\log(Cu^{2+})$$

↓ ↓ ↓

y – axis C mx – axis

Intercept = E°_{RP} = + 0.34 V

For Cu/Cu^{2+} (0.1 M)

$Cu \rightarrow Cu^{2+} + 2e^-$

$$E_{ox} = E^\circ_{ox} - \frac{0.0591}{2}\log(Cu^{2+})$$

$$E_{ox} = -0.34 - \frac{0.0591}{2}\log(10^{-1})$$

$$E_{ox} = -0.34 - \frac{0.0591}{2}\times(-1\log 10)$$

$$\boxed{E_{ox} = -0.34 + \frac{0.0591}{2}}$$

47. When pH = 0, (H^+) = 1M

$2H^+ + 2e^- \rightarrow H_2\uparrow$

$$E_{RP} = E^\circ_{RP} - \frac{0.0591}{2}\log\frac{(pH_2)^1}{(H^+)^2}$$

$$E_{RP} = 0 - \frac{0.0591}{2}\log\frac{1}{1}$$

$$\boxed{E_{RP} = 0V} \quad (1)$$

When pH = 7, $(H^+) = 10^{-7}$m

$$E_{RP} = E^\circ_{RP} - \frac{0.0591}{2}\log\frac{(pH_2)^1}{(H^+)^2}$$

$$E_{RP} = 0 - \frac{0.0591}{2}\log\frac{1}{(10^{-7})^2}$$

$$E_{RP} = -\frac{0.0591}{2}\log 10^{14}$$

$$E_{RP} = -\frac{0.0591}{2}\times 14$$

$$\boxed{E_{RP} = -0.4137V}$$

So reduction potential has decreased by 0.41 V.

48. $E = E^\circ - \frac{0.0591}{n}\log\frac{(Fe^{2+})^2}{(H^+)^4(pO_2)^1}$

$$2Fe \rightarrow 2Fe^{2+} + 4e^- \quad (1)$$

$$4H^+ + 4e^- + O_2 \rightarrow 2H_2O \quad (2)$$

$$\text{Add (1) \& (2)} \rightarrow 2Fe_{(s)} + O_{2(g)} + 4H^+_{(aq.)} \rightarrow 2Fe^{2+}_{aq.} + 2H_2O$$

$$E = 1.67 - \frac{0.0591}{4}\log\frac{(10^{-3})^2}{(10^{-3})^4(0.1)^1}$$

($\because H^+ = 10^{-3}M$)

$$E = 1.67 - \frac{0.0591}{4}\log\frac{10^{-6}}{10^{-12}\times 10^{-1}}$$

$$E = 1.67 - \frac{0.0591}{4}\log\frac{10^{-6}}{10^{-13}}$$

$$E = 1.67 - \frac{0.0591}{4}\times\log 10^7$$

$$E = 1.67 - \frac{0.0591}{4}\times 7\log 10$$

$$E = 1.67 - \frac{0.0591}{4}\times 7$$

$$E = 1.67 - 0.103$$

$$\boxed{E = 1.57V}$$

49.

$$Zn \rightarrow Zn^{2+} + 2e^-$$

$$Cu^{2+} + 2e^- \rightarrow Cu$$

$$Z_n + Cu^{2+} \rightarrow Zn^{2+} + Cu$$

Apply,

$$E_{cell} = E^\circ_{cell} - \frac{0.0591}{2}\log\frac{(Zn^{2+})}{(Cu^{2+})}$$

$$1.10 = E^\circ_{cell} - \frac{0.0591}{2}\log\frac{1}{1}$$

($\because \log 1 = 0$)

$$\boxed{1.10V = E^\circ_{cell}}$$

Onece it gets discharged, $E_{cell} = 0$

Apply,

$$E_{cell} = E^\circ_{cell} - \frac{0.0591}{2}\log\frac{(Zn^{2+})}{(Cu^{2+})}$$

$$0 = 1.10 - \frac{0.0591}{2}\log\frac{(Zn^{2+})}{(Cu^{2+})}$$

$$\frac{1.10\times 2}{0.0591} = \log\frac{(Zn^{2+})}{(Cu^{2+})}$$

$$37.3 = \log\frac{(Zn^{2+})}{(Cu^{2+})}$$

$$\boxed{\frac{(Zn^{2+})}{(Cu^{2+})} = 10^{37.3}}$$

50. $Cu^+ + e^- \rightarrow Cu \quad (1)$

$Cu^+ \rightarrow Cu^{2+} + e^- \quad (2)$

$$E_{cell} = E^\circ_{cell} - \frac{0.0591}{1}\log Q_c$$

At eqn. $Q_c = K_c$ & $E_{cell} = 0$

$$E^\circ_{cell} = \frac{0.0591}{1}\log K_c$$

$$E^\circ_{cell} = E^\circ_{\underset{(RP)}{C}} - E^\circ_{\underset{(RP)}{A}} = 0.52 - 0.16 = 0.36V$$

$\therefore 0.36 = 0.0591 \log Kc$

$$\log Kc = \frac{0.36}{0.0591} = 6.09$$

$$\boxed{K_c = 1.2\times 10^6}$$

51. $Zn \rightarrow \underset{(0.01m)}{Zn^{2+}} + 2e^- \Rightarrow$ Anodic Half reaction

$2H^+ + 2e^- \rightarrow H_{2(1atm)} \Rightarrow$ cathodic half reaction

$$Zn + 2H^+ \rightarrow \underset{(0.01m)}{Z^{2+}_n} + \underset{(1atm)}{H_2}$$

$$E_{cell} = E^\circ_{cell} - \frac{0.0591}{2}\log\frac{(Zn^{2+})(pH_2)}{(H^+)^2} \quad (1)$$

$$\boxed{E^\circ_{cell} = E^\circ_{\underset{(RP)}{c}} - E^\circ_{\underset{(RP)}{A}} = 0 - (-0.76) = +0.76V}$$

Place value of E°_{cell} in eqn. 1,

$$0.701 = 0.76 - \frac{0.0591}{2}\log\frac{(10^{-2})(1)}{(H^+)^2}$$

$$0.701 - 0.76 = -\frac{0.0591}{2}\log\frac{10^{-2}}{(H^+)^2}$$

$$-0.059 = -0.34 - \frac{0.0591}{2}\log\frac{10^{-2}}{(H^+)^2}$$

$$2 = \log\frac{10^{-2}}{(H^+)^2}$$

$2 = \log 10^{-2} - \log (H^+)^2$

$2 = -2 \log 10 - 2 \log (H^+)$

$4 = -2 \log (H^+)$

$-2 = \log (H^+)$

$$\boxed{(H^+) = 10^{-2}M}$$

To neutralise $(H^+) = 10^{-2}M$, $(\bar{O}H)$ reqd. $= 10^{-2}M$

So, moles of NaOH reqd. $= 10^{-2}$

$$1\text{mole} \xrightarrow{\text{weigh}} 40g$$

$$10^{-2}\text{mole} \xrightarrow{\text{weighs}} 40 \times 10^{-2} = \frac{40}{100} = 0.4g$$

52. $Zn \rightarrow Zn^{2+} + 2e^-$

$Cu^{2+} + 2e^- \rightarrow Cu$

$Zn + Cu^{2+} \rightarrow Zn^{2+} + Cu$

Apply,

$$E_{cell} = E^\circ_{cell} - \frac{2.303RT}{nF}\log\frac{(Zn^{2+})}{(Cu^{2+})}$$

$$E_{cell} = 1.1 - \frac{2.303RT}{2F}\log\frac{10(Cu^{2+})}{(Cu^{2+})}$$

$$\boxed{E_{cell} = 1.1 - \frac{2.303RT}{2F}}$$

Now, $\Delta G = -nF E_{cell}$

$$= -2 \times F\left(1.1 - \frac{2.303RT}{2F}\right)$$

$$= -2.2 F + 2.303 RT$$

53. $Cu^{2+} + 2e^- \rightarrow Cu$

$$E_{red} = E^\circ_{red} - \frac{0.0591}{2}\log\frac{1}{(Cu^{2+})} \qquad (1)$$

Also, $Ksp = (Cu^{2+})(\bar{O}H)^2$

$(pH = 10, pOH = 4, (\bar{O}H) = 10^{-4}M)$

$10^{-18} = (Cu^{2+})(10^{-4})^2$

$$\boxed{10^{-10}M = (Cu^{2+})}$$

Place the value in eqn. (1)

$$E_{red} = +0.34 - \frac{0.0591}{2}\log\frac{1}{10^{-10}}$$

$$E_{red} = +0.34 - \frac{0.0591}{2}\log 10^{10}$$

$$E_{red} = +0.34 - \frac{0.0591}{2} \times 10$$

$$\boxed{E_{red} = +0.04V}$$

54. $Zn \rightarrow Zn^{2+} + 2e^-$

$Fe^{2+} + 2e^- \rightarrow Fe$

$Zn + Fe^{2+} \rightarrow Zn^{2+} + Fe$

$E_{cell} = 0.2905$ V (given)

$$E_{cell} = E^\circ_{cell} - \frac{0.0591}{2}\log\frac{(Zn^{2+})}{(Fe^{2+})}$$

$$0.2905 = E^\circ_{cell} - \frac{0.0591}{2}\log\frac{10^{-2}}{10^{-3}}$$

$$0.2905 = E^\circ_{cell} - \frac{0.0591}{2}\log 10$$

$0.2905 = E^\circ_{cell} - 0.2955$

$$\boxed{E^\circ_{cell} = 0.32V}$$

Apply, $\Delta G^\circ = -nFE^\circ_{cell}$

$= -2 \times 96500 \times 0.32$

$= -96500 \times 0.64$

$= -61760J = -61.76$ kJ

55. $Zn + CuSO_4 \rightarrow ZnSO_4 + Cu$

No. of moles of zinc $= \frac{32.65}{65.3} = 0.5$moles

No. of moles of $CuSO_4 = 0.7 \times 1 = 0.7$ moles

$\therefore$ Zinc is the limiting reagent,

Cu deposited max. $= 0.545$ moles $= 0.5 \times 63.5$

$= 31.75$ g

Apply, w = Z It

$$31.75 = \frac{\text{Eq.wt.}}{96500} \times 1 \times t$$

$$31.75 \times 96500 = \frac{63.5}{2} \times 1 \times t$$

$$\frac{31.75 \times 96500 \times 2}{63.5} = t$$

t = 96500 sec = 1.116 days

56. $M^+ \rightarrow M^{3+} + 2e^-$

$E° = -0.25$ V

$\Delta G° = -2 \times F \times -0.25$

$= 0.5 \times 96500 = 48250$ J $= 48.25$ kJ

48.25 kJ oxidises moles of $M^+ = 1$

193 kJ oxidises moles of $M^+ = \frac{1}{48.25} \times 193 = 4$

57. $E°cell = 0$

Apply, $E_{cell} = 0 - \frac{0.059}{2} \log \frac{Ka_2}{Ka_1}$

58. Apply, $R = \rho \frac{l}{a}$

$$2 \times 10^3 = \frac{1}{K} \times \frac{l}{a}$$

$$2 \times 10^3 = \frac{1}{K} \times 0.78$$

$$K = \frac{0.78}{2000} \Omega^{-1} cm^{-1}$$

$$\Lambda_m^c = \frac{K \times 1000}{m}$$

$$= \frac{0.78}{2000} \times \frac{1000}{0.10} = \frac{78}{20}$$

$$= 3.9s\ cm^2 mol^{-1}$$

$$\boxed{\alpha = \frac{\Lambda_m^C}{\Lambda_m^\infty} = \frac{3.9}{390} = 0.01}$$

Also, $HA_{(aq.)} \rightleftharpoons H^+_{(aq.)} + A^-_{(aq.)}$

C	0	0
C–Cα	Cα	Cα

$(H^+) = C\alpha = 0.1 \times 0.01 = 10^{-3}$ M

$$\boxed{pH = -\log(H^+) = -\log(10^{-3}) = 3}$$

$Ka = C\alpha^2 = 0.1 \times (0.01)^2 = 10^{-1} \times 10^{-4} = 10^{-5}$

$pKa = -\log Ka = -\log 10^{-5} = -(-5) \log 10$

$$\boxed{pKa = 5}$$

59. $BaSO_4 \rightarrow Ba^{2+} + SO_4^{2-}$

S S

$$K_{sp} = (Ba^{2+})(SO_4^{2-})$$

$K_{sp} = S^2$

$10^{-10} = S^2$

$$\boxed{S = 10^{-5} mol/litre}$$

Apply,

$$\Lambda_m^\infty = \frac{K \times 1000}{Solubility}$$

$$144 = \frac{K \times 1000}{10^{-5}}$$

$$\boxed{144 \times 10^{-8} = K}$$

60. weight deposited by 1 C is electrochemical equivalent.
weight deposited by IF (96500 C) is called equivalent weight.
1C deposits weight = 0.0006735 g
96500 C deposits weight = 0.000 6735 × 96500
= 65 g

61. $K = 3.06 \times 10^{-6} \Omega^{-1} cm^{-1}$

$\Lambda_{eq.} = 1.02\ \Omega^{-1} cm^2 eq^{-1}$

Now,

$\Lambda_m = \Lambda_{eq.} \times$ n factor ($AB_3 \rightarrow A^{3+} + 3B^-$)

$\Lambda_m = 1.02 \times 3$ (n factor = 3)

$$\boxed{\Lambda_m = 3.06\ \Omega^{-1} cm^2 mol^{-1}}$$

$$\Lambda_m = \frac{K \times 1000}{Solubility}$$

$$3.06 = \frac{3.06 \times 10^{-6} \times 1000}{S}$$

$$\boxed{S = 10^{-3}}$$

$AB_3 \rightarrow A^{3+} + 3B^-$

S 3S

$K_{sp} = (A^{3+})(B^-)^3 = (S)(3S)^3 = 27S^4$

$= 27 \times (10^{-3})4 = 27 \times 10^{-12}$

63. $8H^+ + MnO_4^- + 5e^- \rightarrow Mn^{2+} + 4H_2O$

$$E_{RP} = E°_{RP} - \frac{0.0591}{5} \log \frac{(Mn^{2+})}{(MnO_4^-)(H^+)^8}$$

$$E_{RP} = E°_{RP} - \frac{0.0591}{5} \log \frac{(Mn^{2+})}{(MnO_4^-)} \left((H^+) = 1M\right)$$

$$E_{RP} = E°_{RP} - \frac{0.0591}{5} \log \frac{1}{1}$$

$$E_{RP} = E°_{RP} \quad (1)$$

$$E_{RP'} = E°_{RP} - \frac{0.0591}{5} \log \frac{1}{1 \times (10^{-4})^8}$$

$$E_{RP}' = E^\circ_{RP} - \frac{0.0591}{5}\log\frac{1}{10^{-32}}$$

$$E_{RP}' = E^\circ_{RP} - \frac{0.0591}{5}\log 10^{32}$$

$$E_{RP}' = E^\circ_{RP} - \frac{0.0591}{5}\times 32\log 10$$

$$E_{RP}' = E^\circ_{RP} - 0.378 \quad (2)$$

Comparing eqns. (1) & (2), the R.P. has decreased by 0.38V.

64. $H_2 \rightarrow 2H^+ + 2e^-$ (1)

$M^{4+} + 2e^- \rightarrow M^{2+}$ (2)

$M^{4+} + H_2 \rightarrow 2H^+ + M^{2+}$

$$E_{cell} = E^\circ_{cell} - \frac{2.303RT}{nF}\log\frac{(H^+)^2(M^{2+})}{(M^{4+})(pH_2)^1}$$

$$0.092 = 0.151 - \frac{2.303RT}{nF}\log\frac{1^2\times 10^x}{1}$$

$$0.092 = 0.151 - \frac{0.059}{n}\log 10^x$$

$$0.092 - 0.151 = -\frac{0.059}{2}\log 10^x$$

$$-0.059 = -\frac{0.059}{2}\log 10^x$$

$2 = \log 10^x$

$\boxed{x = 2}$

65. $\lambda^\infty_{A^-} \approx \lambda^\infty_{B^-}$

$\lambda^\infty_{H^+} + \lambda^\infty_{A^-} \approx \lambda^\infty_{H^+} + \lambda^\infty_{B^-}$

$\Rightarrow \lambda^\infty_{HA} \approx \lambda^\infty_{HB}$ (1)

Also, $\frac{\lambda^C_m}{\lambda^\infty_m} = \alpha$

So, $\lambda_m(HA) = \lambda^\infty_1\alpha_1$

$\lambda_m(HB) = \lambda^\infty_2\alpha_2$

Also, $\lambda_m(HB) = 10\lambda_m(HA)$

$\lambda^\infty_{m_2}\alpha_2 = 10\times\lambda^\infty_{m_1}\alpha_1$ (2)

$K_a = C\alpha^2 \ (\because \alpha <<< 1)$

$$\therefore \frac{Ka_{(HA)}}{Ka_{(HB)}} = \frac{0.01\times\alpha_1^2}{0.1\times\alpha_2^2} = \frac{0.01}{0.1}\times\left(\frac{\alpha_1}{\alpha_2}\right)^2$$

$$\frac{Ka_{(HA)}}{Ka_{(HB)}} = \frac{0.01}{0.1}\times\left(\frac{1}{10}\right)^2 = \frac{1}{1000}$$

$\Rightarrow \log[Ka_{(HA)} - Ka_{(HB)}] = -3$

$\log Ka_{HA} - \log Ka_{HB} = -3$

Multiply both sides with –ve

$-\log Ka_{(HA)} + \log Ka_{(HB)} = 3$

$\boxed{pKa_{(HA)} - pKa_{(HB)} = 3}$

66. For P

$Fe^{3+} + e^- \rightarrow Fe^{2+}$ (1)

$Fe^{2+} + 2e^- \rightarrow Fe$ (2)

Add $Fe^{3+} + 3e^- \rightarrow Fe$

Apply $\Delta_1\overset{\circ}{G} + \Delta_2\overset{\circ}{G} = \Delta\overset{\circ}{G}_3$

$-1\times F\times 0.77 + (-2\times F\times -0.44) = -3\times F\times E^\circ_{Fe^{3+}/Fe}$

$-1\times F\times 0.77 + 2\times F\times 0.44 = -3\times F\times E^\circ_{Fe^{3+}/Fe}$

$-0.77 + 0.88 = -3\times E^\circ_{Fe^{3+}/Fe}$

$-\frac{0.11}{3} = E^\circ_{Fe^{3+}/Fe}$

$\boxed{-0.036V = E^\circ_{Fe^{3+}/Fe}}$

For Q

Half reactions are–

$2H_2O \rightarrow O_2 + 4H^+ + 4e^-$; $E^\circ = -1.23V$

Add $4e^- + O_2 + 2H_2O \rightarrow \bar{O}H; E^\circ = +0.40V$

$4H_2O \rightarrow 4H^+ + 4\bar{O}H; E^\circ = ?$

For overall reaction

$E^\circ = -1.23 + 0.40$

$\boxed{E^\circ = -0.83V}$

For R

The half reactions & net reaction are as follows–

$Cu^{2+} + 2e^- \rightarrow Cu; E^\circ = +0.34V$

$2Cu \rightarrow 2Cu^+ + 2e^-; E^\circ = -0.52V$

$Cu^{2+} + Cu \rightarrow 2Cu^+; E^\circ = ?$

$\boxed{E^\circ = 0.34 - 0.52 = -0.18V}$

For S

The half reactions & net reaction are –

$Cr^{3+} + 3e^- \rightarrow Cr$

$Cr \rightarrow Cr^{2+} + 2e^-$

$Cr^{3+} + e^- \rightarrow Cr^{2+}$

For overall reaction,

$\Delta G_1^\circ + \Delta_2 G^\circ = \Delta_3 G^\circ$

$-3\times F\times -0.74 + (-2\times F\times 0.91) = -1\times F\times E^\circ_{Cr^{3+}/Cr^{2+}}$

$+2.22 - 1.82 = -E^\circ_{Cr^{3+}/Cr^{2+}}$

$0.40 = -E^\circ_{Cr^{3+}/Cr^{2+}}$

$\boxed{E^\circ = -0.4V}$

67. $Ag^+ + e^- \rightarrow Ag$; E° = + 0.79 V (1)

$[Ag(NH_3)_2]^+ + e^- \rightarrow Ag + 2NH_3$; E°= + 0.37 V (2)

Subtract (1) – (2)

$$Ag^+ - (Ag(NH_3)_2)^+ \rightarrow -2NH_3$$

$$Ag^+ + 2NH_3 \rightarrow (Ag(NH_3)_2)^+$$

$$\Delta G_1^\circ + \Delta G_2^\circ = \Delta G_3^\circ$$

$$-1\times F\times 0.79 - (-1\times F\times 0.37) = -1\times F\times E°$$

$$-0.79 + 0.37 = -E°$$

$$-0.42\ V = -E°$$

$$\boxed{E° = +0.42V}$$

Formation Constt is recorded at equation

$\therefore E_{cell} = 0$

$$E°_{cell} = \frac{0.06}{n}\log K_f$$

$$0.42 = \frac{0.06}{1}\log K_f$$

$$\frac{0.42}{0.06} = \log K_f$$

$\log K_f = 7$

$$\boxed{K_f = 10^7}$$

68. Since electrodes are of Ni (reactive electrode). Ni^{2+} which is reduced from solution is replenished by Ni electrode (anode). So, concentration remains the same.

69. H^+ will get reduced in preference to Mg^{2+}.

70. At cathode

$2H^+ + 2e^- \rightarrow H_2$ (1)

At anode

$$4\bar{O}H \rightarrow 2H_2O + O_2 + 4e^-$$

or

$$2\bar{O}H \rightarrow H_2O + \frac{1}{2}O_2 + 2e^- \quad (2)$$

Adding (1) & (2)

$$H_2O \rightarrow H_2 + \frac{1}{2}O_2$$

So, $\frac{3}{2}$ moles of gases (1 mole H_2 + $\frac{1}{2}$ mol O_2) are liberated by 2 F charge.

$\frac{3}{2}$ moles of gases are liberated by Q = 2 F

$\frac{3}{2}$ × 22.4 L (Volume) is liberated by Q = 2 F

$\frac{3}{2}$ × 22.400 ml (Volume) is liberated by Q = 2 F

504 ml (Volume) is liberated by Q

$$= \frac{2}{\frac{3}{2}\times 22400}\times 504$$

$$= \frac{2}{3\times 22400}\times 2\times 504$$

$$= \frac{4\times 504}{67200} = 0.03F$$

$= 0.03 \times 96500$ C = 2895 C

71. $Cu^{2+} + 2e^- \rightarrow Cu$

2F charge deposits copper = 63.5g

2 × 96500 C charge deposits copper = 63.5g

0.1 × 4 × 60 × 60 C charge deposits copper

$$= \frac{63.5}{2\times 96500}\times 0.4\times 60\times 60$$

$$= \frac{63.5\times 18\times 0.4}{965} = 0.473g$$

$$\%\ \text{current efficiency} = \frac{0.3745}{0.4737}\times 100\% = 79\%$$

72. KCl & NaCl solution will give same products at cathode & anode.

Solution of KCl will give H_2 at cathode & Cl_2 at anode.

Similarly, solution of NaCl will give H_2 at cathode & Cl_2 at anode.

73. H^+ will get reduced in preference to Ca^{2+}.

74. Add (1) & (2)

$$Cu^{2+} + e^- \longrightarrow Cu^+; E° = +0.15V \quad ...(1)$$

$$Cu^+ + e^- \longrightarrow Cu; E° = +0.50V \quad ...(2)$$

$$Cu^{2+} + 2e^- \longrightarrow Cu$$

Apply,

$$\Delta_1 G° + \Delta_2 G° + \Delta_3 G°$$

$$-1\times F\times 0.15 + (-1\times F\times 0.50) = -2\times F\times E°$$

$$-0.15 - 0.50 = -2E_o$$

$$\frac{-0.65}{-2} = E°$$

$$\boxed{E° = 0.325v}$$

78. $NaCl \xrightarrow{\text{electrolysis}} Na^+ + Cl^-$

At Cathode

$$Na^+ + e^- \longrightarrow Na$$

$$Na + Hg \longrightarrow Na(Hg)$$

$$Na^+ + e^- + Hg \longrightarrow Na(Hg)$$

Now, 90 gm Hg has 10 g Na on it.

Hg   Na

$90gm \longrightarrow 10gm$

$$10gm \longrightarrow \frac{10}{90} \times 10 = \frac{10}{9} gm\ Na$$

Apply, W = ZIt.

$$\frac{10}{9} = \frac{Eq.weight}{96500} \times 10 \times t$$

$$\frac{10}{9} = \frac{23}{96500} \times 10 \times t$$

$$\frac{10}{9} \times \frac{96500}{23 \times 10} = t = 7.77\,min.$$

82. 2F charge produces gaseous moles = 3

2 × 96500 C charge produces gaseous moles = 3

Charge passed through the solution (Q) =

It = 0.5 × 482.5 × 60 = 14,475 C

Current efficiency = 80%

Actual Q (charge) passed

$$= 14475 \times \frac{80}{100} = 11580\ C$$

Now, 2 × 96500 C produces gaseous moles = 3

11580 C produces gaseous moles

$$= \frac{3}{2 \times 96500} \times 11580$$

$$= \frac{3474}{19300} = 0.18$$

Vol. of gases produced = 0.18 × 22.4 = 4.032L

83. Resistance of 0.2M solution = 50Ω

$K = 1.4\ Sm^{-1}$

Apply, $R = \rho\frac{l}{a}$

$$R = \frac{1}{K}\frac{l}{a}$$

$$50\Omega = \frac{1}{1.4Sm^{-1}} \times \frac{l}{a}$$

$$50 \times 1.4m^{-1} = \frac{l}{a}$$

$$\boxed{70m^{-1} = \frac{l}{a}}$$

Now, cell constant $\left(\frac{l}{a}\right)$ will be a constant.

New Conc. of soln. = 0.5 M

Resistance = 280Ω

$$\frac{l}{a} = 70m^{-1}$$

Apply,

$$R = \rho\frac{l}{a}$$

$$R = \frac{1}{K}\frac{l}{a}$$

$$280\Omega = \frac{1}{K} \times 70m^{-1}$$

$$K = \frac{70m^{-1}}{280\Omega} = \frac{1}{4}\Omega^{-1}m^{-1} = 0.25\Omega^{-1}m^{-1}$$

$$\Lambda_m = K \times V_{(ml)} = 0.25\Omega^{-1}m^{-1}$$

[Vol. which contains 1 mole of electrolyte].

0.5 moles → 1 liter vol.

0.5 moles → 1000 cm^3

0.5 moles → $10^{-3}m^3$

$$1\ mole \rightarrow \frac{10^{-3}}{0.5}m^3 = 0.2 \times 10^{-2} = 2 \times 10^{-3}m^3$$

Now, $\Lambda_m = K \times V_{(ml)}$

$\Lambda_m = 0.25\ \Omega^{-1}m^{-1} \times 2 \times 10^{-3}m^3\ mol^{-1}$

$\Lambda_m = 0.50 \times 10^{-3}\ \Omega^{-1}m^2\ mol^{-1}$

$$\boxed{\Lambda_m = 5 \times 10^{-4}\Omega^{-1}m^2mol^{-1}}$$

84. Apply,

W = ZIt

$$2.977 = \frac{eq.wt.}{96500} \times 3 \times 1 \times 60 \times 60$$

$$\frac{2.977 \times 96500}{3 \times 60 \times 60} = \frac{At.wt.}{n\text{-factor}}$$

$$\frac{2.977 \times 96500}{3 \times 60 \times 60} = \frac{106.4}{n\text{-factor}}$$

$$n\text{-factor} = \frac{106.4 \times 3 \times 60 \times 60}{2.977 \times 96500}$$

n-factor = 4

4 ⤫ 1

A ⟵ ⟶ B

AB_4 → Formula

85. $M_{(s)} \rightarrow M^{n+}_{(aq.)} + ne^-$

$$E_1 = E° - \frac{2.303RT}{nF}\log(M^{n+})$$

$$E_1 = E° - \frac{2.303RT}{nF}\log 2$$

$$E_1 = E° - \frac{2.303RT}{nF} \times 0.3010$$

$$E_2 = E° - \frac{0.693RT}{nF} \quad (1)$$

Similarly,

$$E_2 = E^\circ - \frac{2.303RT}{nF \times 2}\log 1$$

$E_2 = E^\circ$ (2)

From (1) & (2)

$\boxed{E_2 > E_1}$

86. At anode

$$Pb \rightarrow Pb^{2+} + 2e^-$$
$$Pb^{2+} + SO_4^{2-} \rightarrow PbSO_4$$
$$\overline{Pb + SO_4^{2-} \rightarrow PbSO_4 + 2e^-}$$

At cathode

$$4H^+ + 2e^- + PbO_2 \rightarrow Pb^{2+} + 2H_2O$$
$$Pb^{2+} + SO_4^{2-} \rightarrow PbSO_4$$
$$\overline{4H^+ + 2e^- + PbO_2 + SO_4^{2-} \rightarrow PbSO_4 + 2H_2O}$$

Overall reaction –

$$Pb + SO_4^{2-} \rightarrow PbSO_4 + 2e^-$$
$$4H^+ + 2e^- + PbO_2 + SO_4^{2-} \rightarrow PbSO_4 + 2H_2O$$
$$\overline{Pb + 2SO_4^{2-} + 4H^+ + PbO_2 \rightarrow 2PbSO_4 + 2H_2O}$$

or

$Pb + 2H_2SO_4 + PbO_2 \rightarrow 2PbSO_4 + 2H_2O$

From eqns. it is evident that –

2 F charge consumes H_2SO_4 = 2 moles

2 × 96500 C charge consumes H_2SO_4 = 2 moles

3600 × 30 × 2C charge consumes H_2SO_4

$$= \frac{2}{2 \times 96500} \times 3600 \times 30 \times 2$$

= 2.24 moles

87. $\Delta_r G = [-394.4 + 2(-237.2)] - (-166.2)$

$\Delta_r G = -702.6$ kJ mol^{-1}

$$\text{Efficiency} = \frac{\Delta_r G}{\Delta H} = \frac{-702.6}{-726} \times 100 = 97\%$$

88. Let formula of metal oxide be M_2O_X.

At. wt. of metal = 112 gms

Now, weight percentage of oxygen = 12.5 %

$$\frac{16X}{224 + 15X} \times 100 = 12.5$$

1600 X = 12.5 (224 + 16 X)

1600 X = 12.5 × 224 + 16 × 12.5 X

1600 X = 2800 + 200 X

1400 X = 2800

$\boxed{X = 2}$

Apply, W = ZIt

$$W = \frac{\text{Eq.wt.}}{96500} \times 0.965 \times 1 \times 60 \times 60$$

$$W = \frac{\frac{112}{2}}{96500} \times 0.965 \times 3600$$

$$W = \frac{112}{2} \times \frac{1}{96500} \times 0.965 \times 60$$

$$W = 56 \times \frac{1}{96500} \times \frac{965}{1000} \times 60$$

$$W = \frac{56 \times 6}{10,000} = \frac{336}{10,000} = 0.0336\text{g}$$

89. $K_a = 1.6 \times 10^{-5}$

$K_a = C\alpha^2$ (from Ostwald's dilution law)

$1.6 \times 10^{-5} = 0.01 \times \alpha^2$

$1.6 \times 10^{-5} = 10^{-2} \times \alpha^2$

$1.6 \times 10^{-3} = \times\, \alpha^2$

$16 \times 10^{-4} = \alpha^2$

$\boxed{4 \times 10^{-2} = \alpha}$

$$\alpha = \frac{\Lambda_m^c}{\Lambda_m^\infty} = \frac{\Lambda_m^c}{380 \times 10^{-4}\,\text{Sm}^2\text{mol}^{-1}}$$

$$0.04 = \frac{\Lambda_m^c}{380 \times 10^{-4}}$$

$380 \times 10^{-4} \times 4 \times 10^{-2} = \Lambda_m^c$

$38 \times 4 \times 10^{-5} = \Lambda_m^c$

$\boxed{152 \times 10^{-5}\,\text{Sm}^2\text{mol}^{-1} = \Lambda_m}$

$\Lambda_m = K \times V_{(ml)}$

$152 \times 10^{-5} = K \times V_{(ml)}$ → Vol. which contains 1 mole of electrolyte

$152 \times 10^{-5} = K \times 10^5$ cm^3 mol^{-1}

152×10^{-5} Sm^2 mol^{-1} = K × $10^5 \times 10^{-6}$ m^3 mol^{-1}

152×10^{-5} Sm^2 mol^{-1} = K × 10^{-1} m^3 mol^{-1}

$\boxed{152 \times 10^{-4}\,\text{Sm}^{-1} = K}$

92. $K(BaSO_4) = K_{soln.} - K_{H_2O} = 10^{-6}(3.648 - 1.25)$
$= 2.398 \times 10^{-6}$

$$\text{Solubility} = \frac{K \times 1000}{\Lambda_m} = \frac{2.398 \times 10^{-6} \times 10^3}{(110 + 136.6)}\,\text{mol/ltr}$$

$$(\text{in gm/ltr}) = \frac{2.398 \times 10^{-3}}{246.6} \times 233 \text{ g/litre}$$

93. 1 gm eqvt. is deposited by 1 F (= 96500 C)

Q = It

96500 C = 1 × t

$$\boxed{t = 96500\,\text{sec}} = \frac{96500}{3600}\,\text{hrs} = 26.8\,\text{hrs}$$

95. It is electrode concentration cell.

At anode

$H_2 \rightarrow 2H^+ + 2e^-$

(P_1)

At cathode

$$\frac{2H^+ + 2e^- \rightarrow H_2(P_2)}{\underset{(P_1)}{H_2} \rightarrow \underset{(P_2)}{H_2}}$$

$E°_{cell} = 0$

$$E_{cell} = E°_{cell} - \frac{RT}{nF}\ln\frac{(P)}{(R)}$$

$$E_{cell} = -\frac{RT}{nF}\log_e\frac{P_2}{P_1}$$

n = 2 (electron change)

$$E_{cell} = -\frac{RT}{2F}\log_e\frac{P_2}{P_1}$$

$$\boxed{E_{cell} = \frac{RT}{2F}\log_e\frac{P_1}{P_2}}$$

97. Pentane oxygen fuel cell will involve the combustion of pentane.

$C_5H_{12} + 8O_2 \rightarrow 5CO_2 + 6H_2O$

$(16O + 32e^- \rightarrow 16O^{2-})$

n = 32

$\Delta_rG° = 5 \times (-394.5) + 6\,(-237.2) - (-8.2)$

$\Delta_rG° = -3387$ kJ/ mol

Now,

$\Delta G° = -n\,FE°_{cell}$

$-3387000 = -32 \times 96500 \times E°_{cell}$

$$\boxed{E°_{cell} = 1.0968V}$$

98. $K_a = \dfrac{C\alpha^2}{1-\alpha}$ (1)

$$\text{Now}, \alpha = \frac{\Lambda_m^c}{\Lambda_m^\infty}$$

Put the value of α in (1)–

$$K_a = \frac{C \times \left(\dfrac{\Lambda_m^c}{\Lambda_m^\infty}\right)^2}{1 - \dfrac{\Lambda_m^c}{\Lambda_m^\infty}} = \frac{C \times \dfrac{\Lambda_m^{c^2}}{\Lambda_m^{\infty^2}}}{\dfrac{\Lambda_m^\infty - \Lambda_m^c}{\Lambda_m^\infty}}$$

$$K_a = C \times \frac{\Lambda_m^{c^2}}{\Lambda_m^{\infty^2}} \times \frac{\Lambda_m^\infty}{\Lambda_m^\infty - \Lambda_m^c}$$

$$\boxed{K_a = C \times \frac{\Lambda_m^{c^2}}{\Lambda_m^\infty\left(\Lambda_m^\infty - \Lambda_m^c\right)}}$$

99. At cathode

$Cu^{2+} + 2e^- \rightarrow Cu$

63.5 g Cu is deposited by charge = 2 F

$$3.18 \text{ g Cu is deposited by charge} = \frac{2}{63.5} \times 3.18$$

$$= 0.1F$$

Same charge must have dissolved copper at anode.

$Cu \rightarrow Cu^{2+} + 2e-$

2 F dissolves copper = 1 mole

$$0.1 \text{ F dissolves copper } = \frac{1}{2} \times 0.1 = 0.05 \text{ moles}$$

4

CHAPTER

Chemical Kinetics

Rate, Rate Law, Rate Constant

1. A gaseous reaction is first order wrt A & B each. If the volume of the reaction vessel is reduced to one-fifth of the initial volume, the reaction rate becomes-

(a) 8 times (b) 5 times

(c) 0.2 times (d) 25 times

2. For the reaction, $H_2 + I_2 \longrightarrow 2HI$, the rate of disappearance of iodine is 10^{-6} mol litre^{-1} second^{-1}. what will be the rate of formation of HI?

(a) 10^{-6} (b) 2×10^{-6}

(c) $\frac{10^{-6}}{2}$ (d) 4×10^{-6}

3. The rate Constant is numerically the same for three reactions of first, second & third order respectively. Which one is true for rate of three reactions, if the concentration of reactants is same for all orders & is lesser than 1 M?

(a) $r_1 = r_2 = r_3$ (b) $r_1 > r_2 > r_3$

(c) $r_3 > r_2 > r_3$ (d) all of these

4. For a first order reaction, $A \rightarrow B$, the rate of reaction is 4×10^{-4} mol L^{-1} sec^{-1} when (A) = 2×10^{-2} mol litre^{-1}. What will be the value of rate constant, when (A) is increased to 4×10^{-2} mol litre^{-1}?

(a) 1×10^{-2} s^{-1} (b) 2×10^{-2} s^{-1}

(c) 4×10^{-2} s^{-1} (d) 4×10^{-4} s^{-1}

5. The reaction, $X \rightarrow Y$ follows third order kinetics. If the concentration of X is doubled, the rate of formation of Y will become-

(a) 2 times (b) 8 times

(c) 0.5 times (d) 0.125 times

6. The rate of disappearance of MnO_4^- in the following reaction is 4.56×10^{-3} Ms^{-1}. Then, rate of appearance of I_2 is-

$$2MnO_4^- + 10I^- + 6H^+ \longrightarrow 2Mn^{2+} + 5I_2 + 8H_2O$$

(a) 1.14×10^{-3} Ms^{-1}

(b) 5.7×10^{-3} Ms^{-1}

(c) 4.56×10^{-4} Ms^{-1}

(d) 1.14×10^{-2} Ms^{-1}

7. In a reaction, $3A + B \rightarrow A_3B$, the reactant A will disappear at-

(a) four times the rate at which B will disappear.

(b) the same rate at which B will disappear.

(c) thrice the rate at which B will disappear..

(d) one third the rate at which B will disappear.

8. Which of the following is INCORRECT about order of a reaction?

(a) It is Calculated experimentally.

(b) It is sum of powers of concentration terms in the rate law expression.

(c) The order of reaction cannot be fractional

(d) All of these are incorrect.

9. Given, rate of a reaction = $K (A)^0 (B)^1 (C)^2$. If the concentration of all the reactants is increased by 50% then the rate of reactant will be increased by-

(a) $\frac{3}{2}$ times (b) $\frac{9}{4}$ times

(c) $\frac{27}{8}$ times (d) $\frac{81}{16}$ times

10. For a reaction,

$$2NH_{3(g)} \longrightarrow N_{2(g)} + 3H_{2(g)}$$

it is given that, $\frac{-d}{dt}(NH_3) = K_1(NH_3)$,

$\frac{d}{dt}(N_2) = K_2(NH_3)$, $\frac{d}{dt}(H_2) = K_3(NH_3)$.

Then k_1, k_2 &k_3 can be related as-

(a) $k_1 = k_2 = k_3$ (b) $2k_1 = 3k_2 = 6k_3$

(c) $2k_1 = k_2 = 3k_3$ (d) $3k_1 = 6k_2 = 2k_3$

11. Consider the following reaction-

$2A + B \rightarrow C$

If initial rate of reaction is 0.3M/sec then on doubling the concentration of both A & B, rate becomes 2.4 M/sec. On doubling the concentration of A alone, rate becomes 0.6 M/sec, then

(a) order wrt A is 2

(b) order wrt B is 2

(c) overall order of reaction is 4

(d) order wrt B is 1.

12. Given, $\frac{d}{dt}(NH_3) = 34$ g/hr for the reaction

$N_2 + 3H_2 \rightleftharpoons 2NH_3$, then $\frac{-d}{dt}(H_2)$ in gm/hr is-

(a) 2 (b) 6

(c) 4 (d) 12

13. For given hypothetical reaction, $xA \rightarrow yB$ the rate expression is-

$\log\frac{(-d(A))}{dt} = \log\frac{d(B)}{dt} + 0.47$, then ratio of x : y is-

(a) 3 : 1 (b) 2 : 1

(c) 1 : 1 (d) 4 : 3

14. The experimental rate law for a reaction:-

$2A + B \rightarrow$ Product is Rate $\propto (A)(B)^{\frac{1}{2}}$. If the concentrations of both A & B are doubled, the rate increases by a factor of-

(a) $\sqrt{2}$ (b) 2

(c) $2\sqrt{2}$ (d) 4

15. For the reaction, $A + B \rightarrow$ Product, it is observed that

(1) On doubling the concentration of A only, the rate of reaction is also doubled.

(2) On doubling the initial concentration of both A & B, there is change by a factor of 8 in the rate of reaction.

Then, rate law expression is given by-

(a) rate = $K(A)(B)^2$ (b) rate = $k(A)^2(B)^2$

(c) rate = $K(A)(B)$ (d) rate = $K(A)^2(B)$

16. The rate law for a reaction between the substances A & B is given by-

$$\boxed{\text{Rate} = K(A)^n(B)^m}$$

On doubling the concentration of A & halving the concentration of B, the ratio of new rate to the earlier rate of reaction will be-

(a) m + n (b) n – m

(c) 2^{n-m} (d) $\frac{1}{2^{m+n}}$

17. Units of rate of reaction is-

(a) s^{-1} (b) $mol^{-1}\ L\ s^{-1}$

(c) mol ltr^{-1} sec^{-1} (d) Both a & b

Zero order & Ist order Questions

18. The time required for the completion of zero order reaction is-

(a) $\frac{(A)_o}{k}$ (b) $\frac{(A)_o}{2k}$

(c) $\frac{0.693}{k}$ (c) infinite

19. The ratio of $t_{7/8}$ & $t_{1/2}$ of a first order reaction, $2A \rightarrow B + C$ is-

(a) $\log\frac{2}{3}$ (b) 3

(c) $\frac{\log 7}{\log 2}$ (d) $\frac{\log 8}{\log 7}$

20. For a first order reaction, 3A → 2B, the concentration of A & B at the point of intersection is given in the figure-

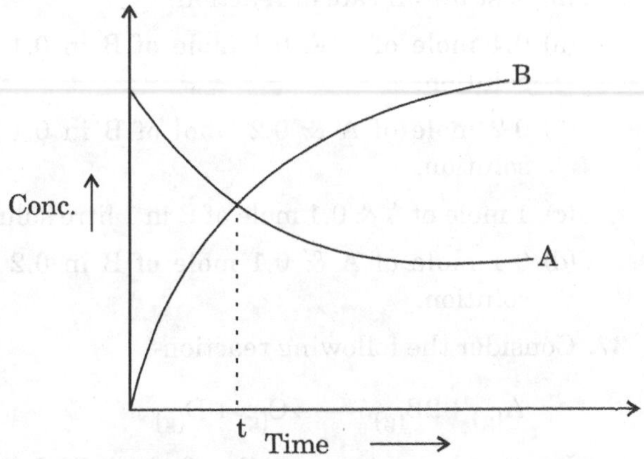

If A_o = 20 mol L^{-1} then Conc. of B at time t is equal to-

(a) 8 mol/L (b) 10 mol/L

(c) 4 mol/L (d) 13.3 mol/L

21. For the first order reaction-

$C_2H_4O_g \longrightarrow CH_{4(g)} + CO_{(g)}$

The initial pressure of $C_2H_4O(g)$ is 80 torr & total pressure at the end of 20 minutes is 120 torr. The time needed for 75% decomposition of C_2H_4O

(a) 20 minutes

(b) 40 minutes

(c) 80 minutes

(d) 120 minutes

22. The time taken for 99.9% of a first order reaction to complete is $7\frac{1}{2}$ hrs. The natural life time of this reaction is nearly-

(a) 45 minutes (b) 65 hours

(c) 1 hour 15 minutes (d) 1 hour 5 minutes

23. Concentration of Reactant in a I[st] order reaction is reduced to $\frac{1}{e^2}$ of initial concentration, after-

(a) 1 natural life time (b) 3 natural life times

(c) 2 natural life time (d) 4 natural life times

24. For the following first order reaction,

$SO_2Cl_2(g) \longrightarrow SO_2(g) + Cl_2(g)$, pressure was 0.8 atm after 100 seconds but one atm after a long time. Then the value of rate constant is-

(a) $\frac{0.009}{5}$ (c) $\frac{9}{5}$

(c) $\frac{0.09}{5}$ (d) none of these

25. 99% of a first order reaction was completed in 32 min. When will 99.9% of the reaction get completed?

(a) 50 min (b) 46 min

(c) 49 min (d) 48 min.

26. Two first order reactions have half lives in the ratio 3 :2. Calculate the ratio of time intervals $t_1 : t_2$. The time t_1 & t_2 are the time period for 25% & 75% completion for the first & second reaction, respectively-

(a) $\frac{3}{2} \times \frac{\log 1.33}{\log 4}$ (b) $\frac{3}{2} \times \frac{\log 2.8}{\log 3}$

(c) $\frac{2}{3} \times \frac{\log 1.33}{\log 4}$ (d) $\frac{2}{3} \times \frac{\log 5}{\log 3}$

27. For a reaction, mA → Product, rate equation can be written as, rate = $k[A]^m$. If the concentration is changed from 0.1 M to 0.15 M, then the rate becomes doubled, what will be the value of m?

(a) Zero (b) 1

(c) 1.7 (d) 2

28. For a first order reaction, A → 2B, the rate constant is 6.93×10^{-3} min^{-1} at 300 k. Percentage of A remaining at the end of 300 min. is-

(a) 75 (b) 50

(c) 25 (d) 12.5

29. Half life of a certain radioactive element is such that $\frac{7}{8}$ of a given quantity decays in 12 days. What fraction remains undecayed after 24 days?

(a) 0 (b) $\frac{1}{128}$

(c) $\frac{1}{64}$ (d) $\frac{1}{32}$

30. Rate constant of a reaction is 0.0693 min^{-1}. Starting with 10 mol L^{-1}, rate of reaction after 10 minutes will be-

(a) 0.0693 M min^{-1}

(b) 0.0693 × 5 M min^{-1}

(c) 0.0693 × 10 M min^{-1}

(d) None of these

31. Under the same reaction conditions, initial concentration of 1.386 mol dm^{-3} of a substance becomes half in 40 seconds & 20 seconds through first order & zero order respectively. Ratio $\left(\frac{k_1}{k_0}\right)$ of the rate constants for first order (k_1) & zero order (k_0) of the reactions is-

(a) 0.5 $mol^{-1}dm^3$ (b) 1 mol dm^{-3}

(c) 1.5 mol dm^{-3} (d) 2 $mol^{-1}dm^3$

32. The reaction, $x \rightarrow y$, follows first order kinetics. In 40 minutes, the concentration of x changes from 0.1 M to 0.025 M, then the rate of reaction when concentration of x is 0.01 M, is-

(a) 3.47×10^{-4} M/min (b) 62.3×10^{-11} M/min

(c) 34.7×10^{-7} M/min (d) 6.23×10^{-13} M/min

Determination of Orders of Reactions

33. The half life period for catalytic decomposition of XY_3 at 50 mm pressure is found to be 4 hrs & at 75 mm pressure is 2 hrs. Then, order of the reaction is-

(a) 3 (b) 1.7

(c) 2.7 (d) 1.5

34. For a reaction, $A \rightarrow nB$, at initial concentration of A = 3 mol/litre, rate is 6.4 mol L^{-1} sec^{-1}. When the concentration of A was 1.5 mol/litre, the rate is 1.6 mol L^{-1} sec^{-1}. The order of reaction wrt A is-

(a) 2.25 (b) 3

(c) 1.5 (d) 2

35. For n^{th} order reaction, $\frac{dx}{dt}$ = Rate = $k(A)^n$. Graph between log (rate) against log(A) is of the type

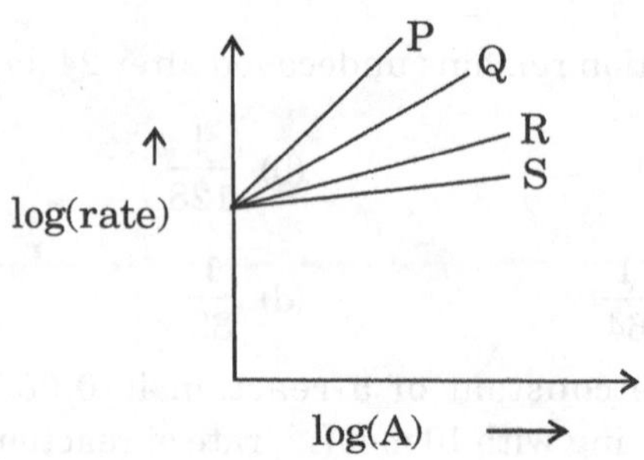

Axis P, Q, R, S are for the order

(a) 0 1 2 3

(b) 3 2 1 0

(c) 1 2 3 0

(d) 0 3 2 1

36. In a second order reaction, which is first order wrt each reactant A & B, which one of the following reaction mixtures will provide the highest initial rate of reaction?

(a) 0.1 mole of A & 0.1 mole of B in 0.1 litre solution.

(b) 0.2 mole of A & 0.2 mol of B in 0.1 litre solution.

(c) 1 mole of A & 0.1 mole of B in 1 litre solution.

(d) 0.1 mole of A & 0.1 mole of B in 0.2 litre solution.

37. Consider the following reaction-

$$A_{(g)} + 2B_{(g)} \longrightarrow C_{(g)} + D_{(g)}$$

It is an elementary reaction & the initial partial pressures of A & B are P_A = 0.60 & P_B = 0.80 atm. When P_C = 0.2 atm, the rate of reaction relative to initial rate is-

(a) $\frac{1}{48}$ (b) $\frac{1}{24}$

(c) $\frac{9}{16}$ (d) $\frac{1}{6}$

38. The following data pertains to a reaction between X & Y-

	[A] $(mol L^{-1})$	[B] $(mol L^{-1})$	Rate $(mol L^{-1} sec^{-1})$
I	1×10^{-2}	2×10^{-2}	2×10^{-4}
II	2×10^{-2}	2×10^{-2}	4×10^{-4}
III	2×10^{-2}	4×10^{-2}	8×10^{-4}

Which of the following inferences can be drawn from the above data?

(1) Rate constant of the reaction is 10^{-4}.

(2) Rate law of the reaction is k[A][B]

(3) Rate of reaction increases four times on doubling the concentration of both the reactants.

(a) 1, 2 & 3 (b) 1 & 2

(c) 2 & 3 (d) 3 only

39. The following data is for the reaction between A & B is first order wrt A & zero order wrt B

Experiment	(A) mol/L	(B) mol/L	rate
I	0.1	0.1	2×10^{-2}
II	Y	0.2	4×10^{-2}
III	0.4	0.4	Z

Then the values of y & z, respectively, are-

(a) 0.2, 0.4 (b) 0.2, 0.08

(c) 0.8, 0.2 (d) 0.4, 0.2

40. For the reaction, 2A + 3B → Products, A is in excess & on changing the concentration of B from 0.1 M to 0.4 M, rate gets doubled. So, rate law is-

(a) $\frac{dx}{dt} = k(A)^2(B)^3$ (b) $\frac{dx}{dt} = k(A)(B)$

(c) $\frac{dx}{dt} = k(A)^0(B)^2$ (d) $\frac{dx}{dt} = k(B)^{\frac{1}{2}}$

41. Consider the following data for the reaction given below-

A + B → Product

Expt.	$(A)_o$ (in mol/ltr)	$(B)_o$ (mol/ltr)	Rate $(R)_o$ $(mol\ ltr^{-1}\ sec^{-1})$
I	0.1	0.2	0.05
II	0.2	0.2	0.10
III	0.1	0.1	0.05

Then, the value of rate constant 'k' is

(a) 1.386 sec^{-1} (b) 13.86 sec^{-1}

(c) 26.72 sec^{-1} (d) None of these

42. The rate of a first order reaction is 0.04 mol ltr^{-1} sec^{-1} at 10 minutes & 0.03 mol $litre^{-1}$ sec^{-1} at 20 minutes after initiation. Then, $t_{1/2}$ of the reaction is-

(a) 2.406 min (b) 24.14 min

(c) 240.6 min (d) 0.204 min

Collision Theory & Arrhenius Equation

43. For a reaction occurring at 500 k, activation energy is found to be 1000 × $Jmol^{-1}$. The value of Boltzmann factor (b) is correctly represented as-

(a) $\log b = \frac{-2x}{2.303R}$ (b) $\log b = \frac{2000x}{2.303R}$

(c) $\log b = \frac{2x}{R}$ (d) $\log b = \frac{2x}{2.303R}$

44. According to Arrhenius equation, the graph of lnk v/s$\left(\frac{1}{T}\right)$ has slope equal to-

(a) $\frac{-E_a}{2.303R}$ (b) $\frac{-E_a}{R}$

(c) $\frac{E_a}{2.303R}$ (d) $\frac{+E_a}{R}$

45. Arrhenius equation is $K = Ae^{\frac{-E_a}{TR}}$. If activation energy is equal to RT, then-

(a) the rate of reaction does not depend on initial concentration.

(b) the rate constant becomes about 37% of the Arrhenius constant A.

(c) the rate constant becomes equal to 73% of the Arrhenius constant A.

(d) the rate of reaction becomes infinite.

46. A hydrogenation reaction is carried out at 500 k. If the same reaction is carried out in the presence of a catalyst at same rate, the temperature required is 400 k. If the catalyst lowers the activation energy by 20 KJ mol^{-1}, the activation energy of uncatalysed reaction at 500 k is-

(a) 40 KJ mol^{-1} (b) 60 KJ mol^{-1}

(c) 80 KJ mol^{-1} (d) 100 KJ mol^{-1}

47. Consider the following graphs-

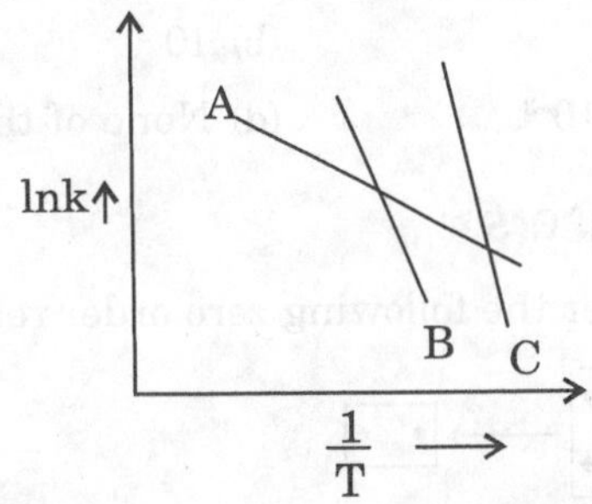

For the reactions A, B, C, the order of activation energy is-

(a) A > B > C (b) B > C > A

(c) C > B > A (d) A < B > C

48. The rate constant, the activation energy & the arrhenius parameter (A) of a chemical reaction at 25°C are 3 × 10^{-4} s^{-1}, 104.4KJ mol^{-1} & 6 × 10^{14} s^{-1} respectively. The value of rate constant where $E_a \to \infty$, is-

(a) Infinity (b) Zero

(c) 2 ×10^{18} s^{-1} (d) 6 ×10^{14} s^{-1}

49. The rate of a reaction doubles when its temperature changes from 300 k to 310 k. Activation energy of such reaction will be-

(a) 60.5 KJ mol^{-1}

(b) 53.6 KJ mol^{-1}

(c) 48.6 KJ mol^{-1}

(d) 58.5 KJ mol^{-1}

50. The rate constant of a first order reaction becomes six times when the temperature is raised from 350 k to 400 k. Then, the activation energy is-

(a) 4.17 KJ mol^{-1} (b) 41.7 KJ mol^{-1}

(c) 417 KJ mol^{-1} (d) 4170 KJ/mol

51. For a first order reaction, $R \rightarrow P$, the temperature (T) dependent rate constant (k) was found to follow the equation-

$$\log k = -2000\frac{1}{T} + 6$$

The pre-exponential factor A & activation energy (E_a), respectively are:-

(a) $10^6 S^{-1}$, 38.3 kJ mol^{-1} (b) $10^{-1} S^{-1}$, 16.6 kJ mol^{-1}

(c) $6 S^{-1}$, 16.6 kJ mol^{-1} (d) None of these

52. The activation energy for a reaction at temperature Tk was found to be 2.303 RTJmol^{-1}. The ratio of rate constant (k) to Arrhenius factor (A) is-

(a) 10^{-1} (b) 10^{-2}

(c) 2×10^{-3} (d) None of these.

Brain Teasers

53. Consider the following zero order reactions.

I. 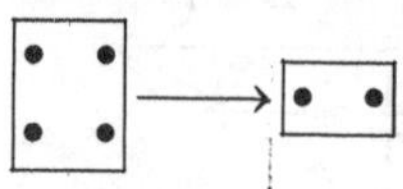

t = 0 t = 2 min

II. 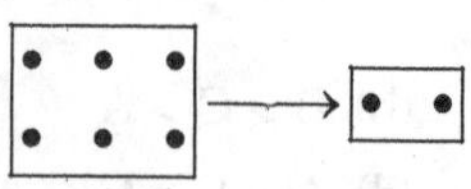

t = 0 t = x min

Then, the value of x is-

(a) 3 min

(b) 5 min

(c) 7 min

(d) None of these

54. Higher order reaction (>3) are rare due to-

(a) loss of active species on collision.

(b) low probability of simultaneous collision of all the reacting species.

(c) increase in entropy & activation energy as more molecules are involved.

(d) shifting of equilibrium towards reactants due to elastic collisions.

55. The rate constant of a first order reaction at 27°C is 10^{-3} min^{-1}. The temperature coefficient of this reaction is 2. what is the rate constant (in min^{-1}) at 17°C for this reaction?

(a) 10^{-3} (b) 5×10^{-4}

(c) 2×10^{-3} (d) 10^{-2}

56. A reaction, $2A + B \longrightarrow C + 2D$ is first order wrt A & second order wrt B. Initial concentration of A is 'x' while that of B is '2x'. The initial concentration of C & D is zero. If at t = 30 minutes, the concentration of C is $\frac{x}{4}$, the rate expression at t = 30 minutes is-

(a) Rate of reaction $= \frac{49x^3}{32} \times k$

(b) Rate of reaction $= \frac{7x^3}{32} \times k$

(c) Rate of reaction $= \frac{22x^3}{32} k$

(d) None of these

57. For the Non-equilibrium process, $A + B \rightarrow P$ the rate is I[st] order wrt A & 2nd order wrt B. If 1 mole each of A & B are introduced into a 1 L vessel & the initial rate was 1×10^{-2} mol L^{-1} sec^{-1}, rate, when half reactants have been turned into products, is-

(a) 1.25×10^{-3} mol L^{-1} sec^{-1}

(b) 1×10^{-2} mol L^{-1} sec^{-1}

(c) 2.50×10^{-3} mol L^{-1} sec^{-1}

(d) 2×10^{-2} mol L^{-1} sec^{-1}

58. An exothermic reaction, $A \rightarrow B$ has an activation energy of 17 kJ per mole of A. The heat of reaction is –40 kJ/mole. The E_a for the reverse reaction, $B \rightarrow A$ is-

(a) 75 kJ/mole (b) 57 kJ/mole

(c) 77 kJ/mole (d) 17 kJ/mole

59. Select the correct statement for zero order reaction.

(a) Quantity of product formed is directly proportional to time.

(b) Greater initial concentration of the reactant, greater is the half life period.

(c) If 50% reaction takes place in 100 minutes, 75% reaction will occur in 150 minutes.

(d) All are correct.

60. For $SO_2Cl_{2(g)} \longrightarrow SO_{2(g)} + Cl_{2(g)}$, pressures of SO_2Cl_2 at t = 0 & t = 20 minutes respectively are 700 mm & 350 mm of Hg. When $\log\left(\frac{P_o}{p}\right)$ is plotted against time (t), slope equal to- (assume Ist order kinetic)

(a) $1.505 \times 10^{-2}\ s^{-1}$

(b) $1.202 \times 10^{-3}\ min^{-1}$

(c) $1.505 \times 10^{-2}\ min^{-1}$

(d) $0.3465\ min^{-1}$

61. For the first order gaseous reaction-

$X_g \longrightarrow 2Y_{(g)} + Z_{(g)}$, the initial pressure, P_x = 90 mm Hg. The pressure after 10 minutes is 180 mm Hg. The rate constant of the reaction is-

(a) $2 \times 10^{-3}\ sec^{-1}$

(b) $2 \times 10^{3}\ sec^{-1}$

(c) $1.15 \times 10^{-3}\ sec^{-1}$

(d) $1.15 \times 10^{3}\ sec^{-1}$

62. For a parallel path reaction given below-

$$A \begin{cases} \xrightarrow{k_1} B \\ \xrightarrow{k_2} C \end{cases}$$

% age yield of B is given by

(a) $\frac{k_1}{k_2} \times 100$ (b) $\frac{k_2}{k_1} \times 100$

(c) $\frac{k_1}{k_1 + k_2} \times 100$ (d) $\frac{k_2}{k_1 + k_2} \times 100$

63. For a first order reaction

$$A \begin{cases} \xrightarrow{k_1} B \\ \xrightarrow{k_2} C \end{cases}$$

which of the following relation is INCORRECT?

(a) $k = k_1 + k_2$

(b) $\frac{1}{k} = \frac{1}{k_1} + \frac{1}{k_2}$

(c) $\frac{1}{t_{\frac{1}{2}}} = \frac{1}{\left(t_{\frac{1}{2}}\right)_1} + \frac{1}{\left(t_{\frac{1}{2}}\right)_2}$

(d) All of these are incorrect.

64. The rate of a reaction 'A', doubles on increasing the temperature from 300 to 310 k. By how much, the temperature of reaction 'B' Should be increased from 300k so that rate doubles if activation energy of reaction B is twice that of reaction A. (approx.)

(a) 10k (b) 5k

(c) 2.45 k (d) 19.67k

65. The % age increase in the rate constant of a reaction when its temperature is increased from 298k to 308k, is nearly (E_a = 12.68 kcal/mol)

(a) 63% (b) 50%

(c) 100% (d) 10%

66. For a first order reaction

$$F_{2(g)} \longrightarrow 2F_{(g)}$$

initially F_2 gas & Ne gas were taken at a pressure of 2000 mm Hg. After a long time, pressure is flask is 2400 mm Hg. If half life of decomposition of F_2 is 30 min. Then, the ratio of final pressure to initial pressure after 2 hrs is-

(a) 1.18 (b) 2

(c) 2.2 (d) None of these

67. If a first order reaction completes 'x%' in 20 minutes & 19% in 40 minutes, then the value of x is- (log 1.12 = 0.05) (approx)

(a) 11 (b) 40

(c) 20 (d) 30

68. The rate law equation for the reaction, $2A + B \rightarrow C$ is found to be, rate = $k(A)^1(B)^2$. The correct statement in relation to this reaction is that the-

(a) Unit of k must be sec^{-1}

(b) $t_{1/2}$ is a constant

(c) Rate of formation of C is twice the rate of disappearance of A.

(d) Value of k is independent of initial concentrations of A & B.

69. Value of $t_{1/2}$ for a first order reaction can change-

(a) By using catalyst

(b) By altering temperature

(c) By altering initial Concentration of reactant

(d) Both (a) & (b)

70. If E_a of a reaction is zero, then-

(a) increase in temperature will increase the rate constant.

(b) increase in temperature will decrease the rate constant.

(c) Temperature will have no effect on rate constant.

(d) None of these

71. The value of rate constant of a pseudo first order reaction-

(a) depends on the concentration of reactant present in small amount.

(b) depends on the concentration of reactants present in excess.

(c) is independent of Concentration of reactant

(d) depends only on temperature

72. If $E_f < E_b$, where E_f & E_b are the activation energies of forward & backward reactions respectively then the reaction-

(a) is endothermic

(b) is exothermic

(c) has $\Delta H = 0$

(d) Can be either exothermic or endothermic

73. For Arrhenius equation, $K = Ae^{\frac{-E_a}{RT}}$, match the following :

Quantity	Name
(a) K	(i) Arrhenius parameters
(b) A	(ii) Boltzmann's factor
(c) E_a	(iii) Frequency factor
(d) A & E_a collectively	(iv) Activation energy
(e) $e^{\frac{-E_a}{RT}}$	(v) Rate Constant

(a) a - iii, b - ii, c - v, d - i, e - iv

(b) a - v, b - ii, c - iv, d - i, e - iii

(c) a - v, b - iii, c - iv, d - i, e - ii

(d) a - iii, b - i, c - iv, d - ii, e - v

74. Identify the correct statement with respect to the collision theory.

(a) Every collision is an effective collision.

(b) Gas phase reactions are always of zero order.

(c) Collision of molecules is a pre - requisite for any reaction to occur.

(d) All are correct.

75. A drop of solution (volume 0.05 ml) contains 3×10^{-6} moles of H^+. If the rate constant of disappearance of H^+ is 10^7 mol ltr^{-1} sec^{-1}. How long would it take for H^+ in drop to disappear?

(a) 6×10^{-8} sec (b) 6×10^{-7} sec

(c) 6×10^{-9} sec (d) 6×10^{-10} sec

76. For a given reaction, energy of activation for forward reaction ($E_{a\ forward}$) is 80 kJ mol^{-1}, ΔH is –40 KJ mol^{-1} for the reaction. A catalyst lower $E_{a(forward)}$ to 20 KJ mol^{-1}. The ratio of Activation energy for reverse reaction before & after the addition of catalyst is-

(a) 1.0 (b) 0.5

(c) 1.2 (d) 2

77. Assuming gas phase decomposition of dimethyl ether follows I[st] order Kinetics.

$$\underset{(g)}{CH_3OCH_3} \longrightarrow \underset{(g)}{CH_4} + H_{2(g)} + CO_{(g)}$$

The reaction is carried out in a closed container with Constant volume at 500°C & has a half life of 14.5 minutes. Initially, only dimethyl ether is present at a pressure of 0.4 atm.

The total Pressure of the system after 12 mins is (given log 1.8 = 0.249)

(a) 0.74 atm (b) 2.56 atm

(c) 0.10 atm (d) 4.48 atm

78. For a given reaction of I[st] order, it takes 20 min. for concentration to drop from 1 mol/L to 0.6 mol/L. The time required for the concentration to drop from 0.6 mol L^{-1} to 0.36 mol L^{-1} is- (approx.)

(a) more than 40 min (b) less than 20 min

(c) equal to 20 min (d) infinity

79. If $\left(\frac{dx}{dt}\right) = k(H^+)^n$ & rate becomes 100 times when pH changes from 2 to 1. Hence, order is-

(a) 1 (b) 2

(c) 3 (d) 0

80. Consider the following reaction-

$${}^{M}_{Z}A_{(g)} \longrightarrow {}^{M-8}_{Z-4}B_{(g)} + \alpha - \text{particles}$$

(α – particles are helium nuclei, so will form the gas by trapping electrons)

The radioactive disintegration follows first order Kinetics. Starting with 1 mole of A in a 1 - litre closed flask at 27°C, total pressure set up after two half lives is approximately-

(a) 25 atm (b) 12 atm

(c) 61.5 atm (d) 40 atm

81. Consider the following reaction-

$Zn + 2H^+ \longrightarrow Zn^{2+} + H_2 \uparrow$

Half life period is independent of concentration of zinc at constant pH. For the constant concentration of Zn, rate becomes 100 times when pH is decreased from 3 to 2. Hence,

(a) $\frac{dx}{dt} = k(Zn)^\circ(H^+)^2$

(b) $\frac{dx}{dt} = k(Zn)(H^+)^2$

(c) rate is not affected if conc. of zinc is made four times & that of H^+ is halved.

(d) Both (b) & (c)

82. Select the correct statement (s).

(a) Order can be zero, negative or fractional but molecularity cannot be zero, negative or fractional.

(b) Order is determined for both, elementary and complex reactions but molecularity is determined for elementary reactions only.

(c) Order can change with conditions like change in pressure but molecularity does not change.

(d) All are correct

83. The chemical reaction, $2O_{3(g)} \longrightarrow 3O_{2(g)}$,

proceeds as follows-

$O_3 \rightleftharpoons O_2 + O\,(fast)$ ...(1)

$O + O_3 \longrightarrow 2O_2\,(slow)$ ...(2)

Correct Rate law expression is-

(a) $r = K(O_3)^2$

(b) $r = K(O_3)^2(O_2)^{-1}$

(c) $r = K(O_3)(O_2)^1$

(d) unpredictable

84. The rate constant of a reaction increases by 7% when its temperature is raised from 300 K to 310 K, while its equilibrium constant increases by 3%. Then the E_a for the forward & backwards reactions are, respectively- (log 1.07 = 0.0294) (log 1.03 = 0.0128)

(a) 5.23 KJ mol^{-1}, 2.95 KJ/mol

(b) 56.25 KJ mol^{-1}, 32.65 KJ/mol

(c) 32.65 KJ mol^{-1}, 56.25 KJ/mol

(d) 3.625 KJ mol^{-1}, 5.625 KJ/mol

85. Ethylene (C_2H_4) is produced as-

$C_4H_8 \longrightarrow 2C_2H_4$

Rate constant is $2.5 \times 10^{-5}\ sec^{-1}$. In what time will molar ratio of ethylene to cyclobutane attain the value of 1?

(a) 16213 sec (b) 20224 sec

(c) 4141 sec (d) 82 sec

86. For a hypothetical reaction, $R \longrightarrow P$, the E_a for forward & backward reactions are 15KJ mol^{-1} & 9 KJ mol^{-1}. Potential energy of R is 10 KJ mol^{-1}. Which of the following statement (s) is/are correct?

(a) The threshold energy for forward reaction is 25 KJ

(b) Potential Energy of P is 16 KJ

(c) $\Delta H_{reaction\,(forward)} = 6KJ$

(d) All are correct.

87. Consider the following reaction and its corresponding graph-

$R \longrightarrow P$

$\frac{dx}{dt} = K(R)^2$

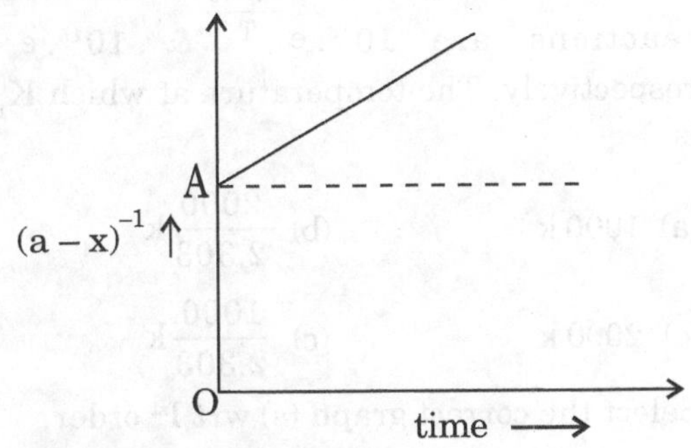

If $K = 10^{-2}\ L\ mol^{-1}\ min^{-1}$

OA = 0.10 L mol^{-1}

what is the rate of reaction at the start of reaction?

(a) 1 mol L^{-1} min^{-1} (b) 3 mol L^{-1} min^{-1}

(c) 1.75 mol L^{-1} min^{-1} (d) 3.75 mol L^{-1} min^{-1}

88. Find out the percentage of reactant molecules crossing over the activation energy barrier at 325 K, given that $\Delta H_{325\,K} = 0.12$ KCal and $E_{a(backward)} = +0.02$ kcal

(a) 80.65% (b) 67.67%

(c) 65.8% (d) 61.1%

89. Select the incorrect statement (s).

(a) For a Ist order reaction, the time required to reduce successively the concentration of reactant by a constant fraction is always same.

(b) As a Ist order reaction proceeds at constant. Temperature, the rate remains constant.

(c) Larger the values of ∊a, greater is the effect on the value of K for a given temperature change.

(d) Catalyst decreases E_a for both forward & backward reactions.

90. Which among the following represents correct expression for Ist order reaction?

(a) $(A)_o = (A)\,e^{-kt}$

(b) $(A) = (A)_o e^{-kt}$

(c) $kt = 2.303\log\frac{(A)_o}{(A)}$

(d) Both b & c

91. For two reactions having activation energies $E_{a_1} > E_{a_2}$, M_1 & M_2 are temperature coefficients respectively, then which is correct?

(a) $M_1 > M_2$ (b) $M_2 > M_1$

(c) $M_1 = M_2$ (d) None of these

92. The rate constants K_1 & K_2 for two different reactions are $10^{16}.e^{\frac{-2000}{T}}$ & $10^{15}.e^{\frac{-1000}{T}}$, respectively. The temperature at which $K_1 = K_2$ is-

(a) 1000 k (b) $\frac{2000}{2.303}$ k

(c) 2000 k (c) $\frac{1000}{2.303}$ k

93. Select the correct graph (s) wrt Ist order.

(a) Rate

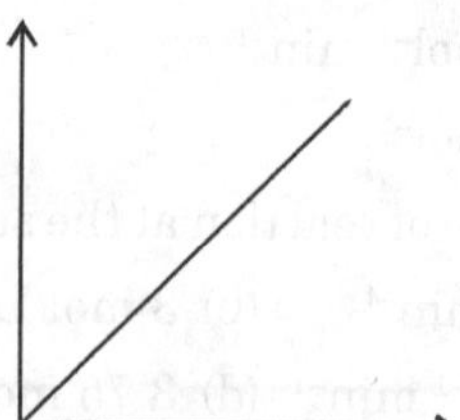

Conc. of Reactant. ⟶

(b) log(A)

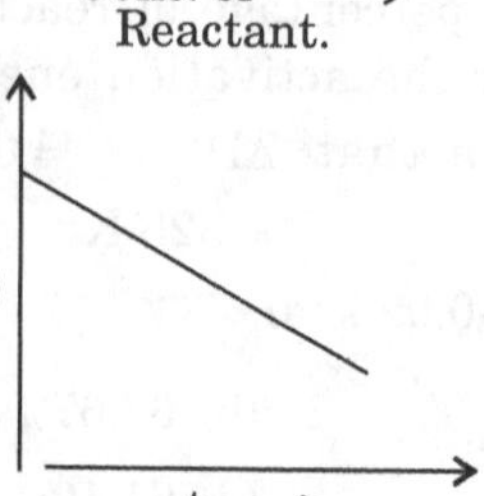

t ⟶

(A) = Conc. of reactant left

(c) $t_{1/2}$ ↑

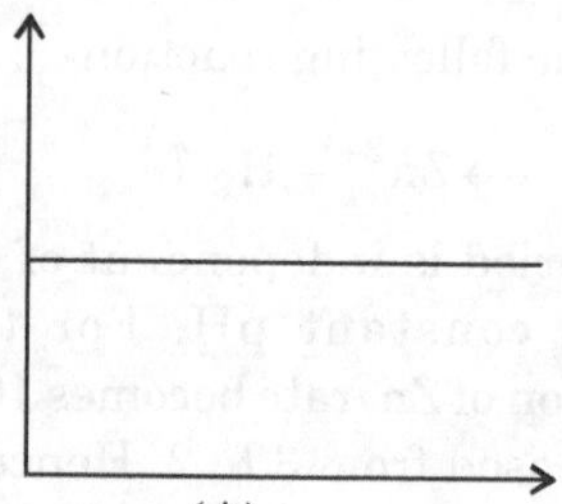

$(A)_o$ ⟶

$(A)_o$ = initial Conc. of Reactant

(d) All are correct

94. The temperature coefficient of a reaction is 2. The rate of this reaction, on raising the temperature by 15° shall increase approximately by-

(a) 3.2 times (b) 2.8 times

(c) 5.6 times (d) 4.2 times

95. For the first order reaction, concentration of reactant after two average lives is reduced to –

(a) $\frac{100}{e}\%$ (b) $\frac{10}{e}\%$

(c) $\frac{10}{e^2}\%$ (d) $\frac{100}{e^2}\%$

96. Graph between $\log t_{1/2}$ & $\log\frac{1}{(A)_0}$ for nth order reaction is as follows–

$\log t_{\frac{1}{2}}$ ↑

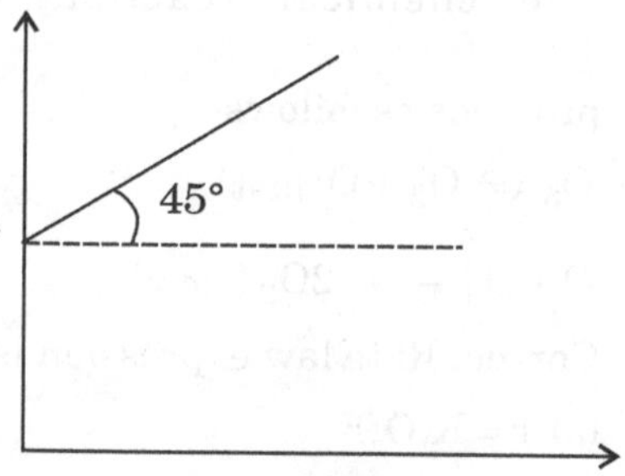

$\log\left(\frac{1}{A_0}\right)$ ⟶

Then, the value of n is –

(a) 2 (b) 1

(c) 0 (d) 0.5

97. Which of the following is/are correct regarding a catalyst ?

(a) A catalyst cannot initiate a reaction. It can only accelerate the rate of reaction.

(b) A catalyst does not alter ΔG of a reaction.

(c) A catalyst does not alter ΔH of a reaction

(d) All are correct.

98. The initial rates of a reaction :–
$3A + 2B + C \rightarrow$ Products, at different initial concentrations are given below –

Initial rate (Molar S^{-1})	$(A)_o$ (in M)	$(B)_o$ (in M)	$(C)_o$ (in M)
5×10^{-3}	0.010	0.005	0.010
5×10^{-3}	0.010	0.005	0.015
1×10^{-2}	0.010	0.010	0.010
1.25×10^{-3}	0.005	0.005	0.010

The correct rate law is –

(a) Rate of reaction = $k (A)^2 (B)^1 (C)^o$

(b) Rate of reaction = $k (A)^1 (B)^2 (C)^2$

(c) Rate of reaction = $k (A)^2 (B)^o (C)^1$

(d) Rate of reaction = $k (A)^1 (B)^1 (C)^1$

99. For the reaction $2A + B \rightarrow A_2B$, rate = $K(A)(B)^2$ with $K = 2 \times 10^{-6}$ mol^{-2} L^2 sec^{-1} & inital concentration of A is 0.1 mol L^{-1} & that of B is 0.2 mol L^{-1}. Then, the rate of reaction after (A) is reduced to 0.06 mol L^{-1}, is –

(a) 3.89×10^{-9} mol L^{-1} sec^{-1}

(b) 8×10^{-9} mol L^{-1} sec^{-1}

(c) 6.66×10^{-7} mol L^{-1} sec^{-1}

(d) 9×10^{-21} mol L^{-1} sec^{-1}

100. During decomposition of an activated complex –

(a) Energy is always released

(b) Energy is always absorbed

(c) Energy does not change

(d) Reactants may be formed

101. For an exothermic reaction occuring is two steps as follows, select the correct graph –

(1) $A + B \rightarrow X$ (slow)

(2) $X \rightarrow AB$ (fast)

(a)
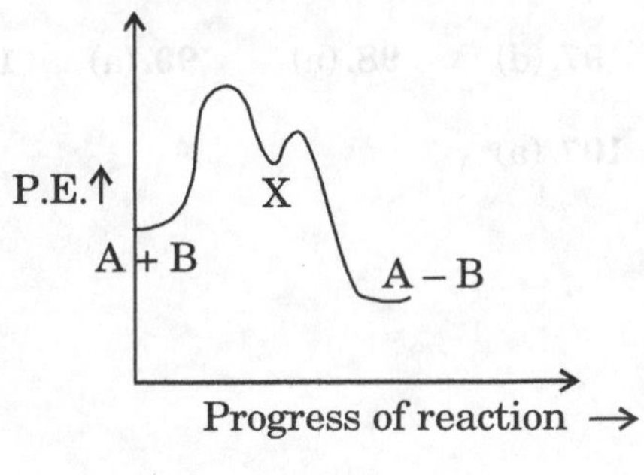

(b)
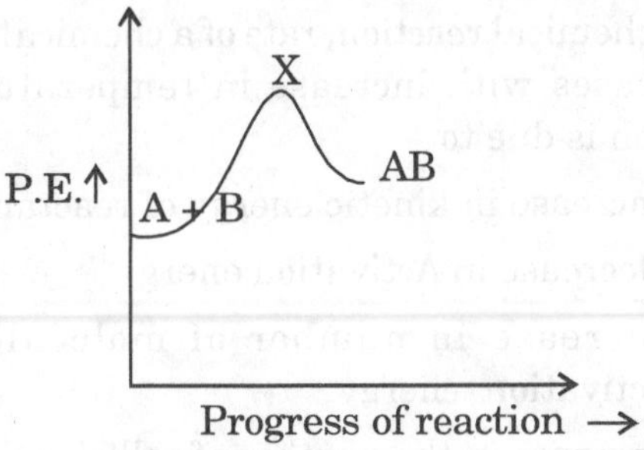

(c)
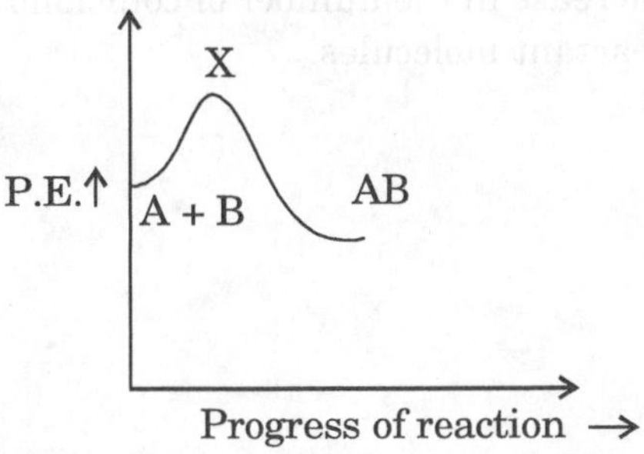

(d) None of these

102. For producing the effective collisions the colliding molecules must possess –

(a) Threshold energy & proper orientation

(b) Energy less then activation energy

(c) only proper orientation

(d) None of these

103. Arrhenius equation may be written as -

(a) $\frac{d}{dT} \ln k = \frac{Ea}{RT}$

(b) $\frac{d}{dT} \ln k = \frac{Ea}{RT^2}$

(c) $\frac{d}{dT} \ln k = \frac{-Ea}{RT^2}$

(d) None of these

104. Select the INCORRECT statement.

(a) Half life depends on the concentration of reactants for first order reaction.

(b) a fast reactant has a large value of rate constant.

(c) For first order reaction , the half life is independent of initial concentration of reactant.

(d) All are Incorrect.

105. Activation energy is dependent on–

(a) Pressure

(b) Concentration

(c) Nature of reactant

(d) all of these

106. In a chemical reaction, rate of a chemical reaction increases with increase in temperature. The reason is due to –

(a) Increase in kinetic energy of reactants.

(b) Decrease in Activation energy

(c) Increase in number of molecules with activation energy.

(d) Increase in the number of collisions between reactant molecules.

107. The rate of a reaction doubles when its temperature changes form 300 K to 310 K. Activation energy of such a reaction will be –

(a) 53.6 kJ mol^{-1}

(b) 48.6 kJ mol^{-1}

(c) 58.5 kJ mol^{-1}

(d) 60.5 kJ mol^{-1}

Answers

1. (d)	**2.** (b)	**3.** (b)	**4.** (d)	**5.** (b)	**6.** (d)	**7.** (c)	**8.** (c)	**9.** (c)	**10.** (d)
11. (b)	**12.** (b)	**13.** (a)	**14.** (c)	**15.** (a)	**16.** (c)	**17.** (c)	**18.** (a)	**19.** (b)	**20.** (a)
21. (b)	**22.** (d)	**23.** (c)	**24.** (d)	**25.** (d)	**26.** (a)	**27.** (c)	**28.** (d)	**29.** (c)	**30.** (b)
31. (a)	**32.** (a)	**33.** (c)	**34.** (d)	**35.** (b)	**36.** (b)	**37.** (d)	**38.** (c)	**39.** (b)	**40.** (d)
41. (a)	**42.** (b)	**43.** (a)	**44.** (d)	**45.** (b)	**46.** (d)	**47.** (c)	**48.** (b)	**49.** (b)	**50.** (b)
51. (a)	**52.** (a)	**53.** (d)	**54.** (b)	**55.** (b)	**56.** (a)	**57.** (a)	**58.** (b)	**59.** (d)	**60.** (c)
61. (c)	**62.** (c)	**63.** (b)	**64.** (b)	**65.** (c)	**66.** (a)	**67.** (a)	**68.** (d)	**69.** (d)	**70.** (c)
71. (b)	**72.** (b)	**73.** (c)	**74.** (c)	**75.** (c)	**76.** (d)	**77.** (a)	**78.** (c)	**79.** (b)	**80.** (c)
81. (d)	**82.** (d)	**83.** (b)	**84.** (a)	**85.** (a)	**86.** (d)	**87.** (a)	**88.** (a)	**89.** (b)	**90.** (d)
91. (a)	**92.** (d)	**93.** (d)	**94.** (b)	**95.** (d)	**96.** (a)	**97.** (d)	**98.** (a)	**99.** (a)	**100.** (a)
101. (a)	**102.** (a)	**103.** (b)	**104.** (a)	**105.** (c)	**106.** (c)	**107.** (a)			

Explanations

1. According to question, $r = k(A)^r(B)^r$ ...(1)

If 'v' is reduced to $\frac{1}{5}^{th}$, the concentration will become 5 times.

Now, $r' = k(5A)^r(5B)^r$ ...(2)

$$\frac{r}{r'} = \frac{k(A)^r(B)^r}{k(5A)^r(5B)^r}$$

$$\frac{r}{r'} = \frac{1}{25}$$

$$\boxed{25r = r'}$$

2. According to question,

$$\frac{-d(I_2)}{dt} = 10^{-6} \text{ mol litre}^{-1} \text{ second}^{-1}$$

$H_2 + I_2 \longrightarrow 2HI$ (given)

Rate of Reaction =

$$-\frac{d}{dt}(H_2) = \frac{-d}{dt}(I_2) = +\frac{1}{2}\frac{d}{dt}(HI)$$

$$10^{-6} = +\frac{1}{2}\frac{d}{dt}(HI)$$

$$\boxed{2 \times 10^{-6} = \frac{d}{dt}(HI)}$$

3. Rate of reaction$_1$ = $k(R)^1$ ...(1)

(for first order)

Rate of reaction$_2$ = $k(R)^2$ ...(2)

(for 2nd order)

Rate of reaction$_3$ = $k(R)^3$ ...(3)

(for 3rd order)

If Concentration of the Reactant is < 1 M, its cube will give the least value. So, rate will follow the order-

$r_1 > r_2 > r_3$

4. Value of rate constant 'k' does not depend on the concentration.

5. $x \rightarrow y$

Rate of reaction, $r = k(x)^3$

After concentration of x is doubled,

$r' = k(2x)^3$ ...(2)

$$\frac{r}{r'} = \frac{k(x)^3}{k(2x)^3}$$

$$\frac{r}{r'} = \frac{x^3}{8x^3}$$

$$\boxed{8r = r'}$$

So, rate of reaction becomes 8 times.

Also, rate of reaction $= \frac{-d(x)}{dt} = \frac{+d(y)}{dt}$

So, rate of formation of y = $\left(\frac{+dy}{dt}\right)$

= Rate of reaction

Since, rate of reaction has become 8 times, rate of formation of y also becomes 8 times.

6. According to the question,

Rate of Reaction $= -\frac{1}{2}\frac{d}{dt}(MnO_4^-) = +\frac{1}{5}\frac{d}{dt}(I_2)$

Now, rate of disappearance of

$$MnO_4^- = \frac{-d}{dt}(MnO_4^-) = 4.56 \times 10^{-3} Ms^{-1}$$

$$\text{So, } \frac{1}{2} \times 4.56 \times 10^{-3} = +\frac{1}{5}\frac{d}{dt}(I_2)$$

$$\frac{4.56 \times 5}{2} \times 10^{-3} = +\frac{d}{dt}(I_2)$$

$$\boxed{11.4 \times 10^{-3} = \frac{d}{dt}(I_2) \text{ or } 1.14 \times 10^{-2} Ms^{-1}}$$

7. $3A + B \longrightarrow A_3B$

$$\text{Rate of reaction} = \frac{-1}{3}\frac{d(A)}{dt} = \frac{-d(B)}{dt} = \frac{+d}{dt}(A_3B)$$

$$\text{So, } \frac{-d(A)}{dt} = 3 \times \frac{-d(B)}{dt}$$

It is evident that rate of disappearance of A is 3 times the rate of disappearance of B.

8. Order of a reaction can be fractional.

9. $r = k(A)^0(B)^1(C)^2$ ...(1)

$$r' = k\left(A + \frac{A}{2}\right)^0\left(B + \frac{B}{2}\right)^1\left(C + \frac{C}{2}\right)^2$$

$$r' = k\left(\frac{3A}{2}\right)^0\left(\frac{3B}{2}\right)^1\left(\frac{3C}{2}\right)^2 \quad ...(2)$$

$$\frac{r}{r'} = \frac{k(A)^0(B)^1(C)^2}{k\left(\frac{3A}{2}\right)^0\left(\frac{3B}{2}\right)^1\left(\frac{3C}{2}\right)^2}$$

$$\frac{r}{r'} = \frac{(B)^1(C)^2}{(3B)9C^2} \times 2 \times 4$$

$$\frac{r}{r'} = \frac{8}{27}$$

$$\boxed{r' = \frac{27}{8} r}$$

rate of reaction will be increased by $\frac{27}{8}$ times

10. Given,

$2NH_3 \rightleftharpoons N_2 + 3H_2$

Rate of reaction

$$= -\frac{1}{2}\frac{d}{dt}(NH_3) = +\frac{d}{dt}(N_2) = +\frac{1}{3}\frac{d}{dt}(H_2)$$

$$= \frac{k_1(NH_3)}{2} = k_2(NH_3) = \frac{1}{3} \times k_3(NH_3)$$

$$= \frac{1}{2}k_1 = k_2 = \frac{k_3}{3}$$

$= 3\,k_1 = 6\,k_2 = 2\,k_3$

11.

A	B	Rate of reaction
a	b	0.3
2a	2b	2.4
2a	b	0.6

Let rate law be

rate = $k(A)^x (B)^y$

$0.3 = k(a)^x (b)^y$ ...(1)

$2.4 = k(2a)^x (2b)^y$ ...(2)

$0.6 = k(2a)^x (b)^y$ ...(3)

Solving $\frac{1}{3} \Rightarrow \frac{1}{2} = \left(\frac{1}{2}\right)^x$

$\boxed{x = 1}$

Solving $\frac{2}{3} \Rightarrow 4 = (2)^y$

$\boxed{y = 2}$

Order wrt B is 2.

12. Consider the reaction,

$N_2 + 3H_2 \rightleftharpoons 2NH_3$

Rate of formation of

$NH_3 = \frac{d}{dt}(NH_3) = 34g/hr$

Now, $n = \frac{w}{M} = \frac{34}{17} = 2$ mole/hr

(no. of moles)

Rate of Reaction

$$= \frac{-d}{dt}(N_2) = \frac{-1}{3}\frac{d}{dt}(H_2) = \frac{+1}{2}\frac{d}{dt}(NH_3)$$

$$\boxed{+\frac{d}{dt}(NH_3) = 2\text{mol ltr}^{-1}\text{hr}^{-1}}$$

$$\frac{-d}{dt}(H_2) = \frac{3}{2} \times 2 = 3 \text{ mol ltr}^{-1}\text{ hr}^{-1}$$

For H_2–

1 mole weighs = 2 g

3 mole weighs = 3 × 2 = 6 g

So, $\frac{-d}{dt}(H_2) = 6\text{gm/hr}$

13. $xA \rightarrow yB$

Rate of reaction $= -\frac{1}{x}\frac{d(A)}{dt} = +\frac{1}{y}\frac{d(B)}{dt}$

$$\boxed{\frac{-d(A)}{dt} = \frac{+d(B)}{dt} \times \frac{x}{y}}$$

Take log on both sides-

$$\log\frac{-d(A)}{dt} = \log\left[+\frac{d(B)}{dt} \times \frac{x}{y}\right]$$

$$\log\frac{-d(A)}{dt} = \log\frac{d(B)}{dt} + \log\frac{x}{y} \quad ...(1)$$

Now, relating the equation given with equation '1', we get

$$\log\frac{x}{y} = 0.47$$

$\frac{x}{y} = 3$ ($\because$ log 3 = 0.47)

$\boxed{x : y = 3 : 1}$

14. Given

Rate of reaction $= k(A)(B)^{\frac{1}{2}}$ ...(1)

$r' = k(2A)(2B)^{\frac{1}{2}}$ ...(2)

$$\frac{r}{r'} = \frac{k(A)(B)^{\frac{1}{2}}}{k(2A)(2B)^{\frac{1}{2}}}$$

$$\frac{r}{r'} = \frac{1}{2} \times \left(\frac{1}{2}\right)^{\frac{1}{2}}$$

$$\frac{r}{r'} = \frac{1}{2\sqrt{2}}$$

$$\boxed{2\sqrt{2}\,r = r'}$$

15. Let rate law be-

rate = k(A)^m(B)^n ...(1)

2r = k(2A)^m (B)^n ...(2)

8r = k(2A)^m (2B)^n ...(3)

Solving 1, 2 & 3 we get-

$\boxed{m=1}$ $\boxed{n=2}$

$\boxed{\text{So, rate} = k(A)^1(B)^2}$

16. rate (r) = k(A)^n(B)^m ...(1)

$$r' = k(2A)^n \left(\frac{B}{2}\right)^m \quad ...(2)$$

$$\frac{r}{r'} = \left(\frac{1}{2}\right)^n (2)^m = 2^{m-n}$$

$$\boxed{\frac{r}{r'} = 2^{n-m}}$$

18. Integrated equation for zero order is as follows-

$kt = (A)_o - (A)$

Once reaction is completed, (A) = 0
↓
Concentration of reactant left

$\therefore\ kt = (A)_o$

$$\boxed{t = \frac{(A)_o}{k}}$$

19. $kt = 2.303 \log \frac{(A)_0}{(A)}$ — $(A)_0$ → initial concentration of the reactant; (A) → concentration of the reactant left after

$$kt_{\frac{7}{8}} = 2.303 \log \frac{(A)_0}{\frac{1}{8}(A)_0}$$

$$kt_{\frac{7}{8}} = 2.303 \ \log 8 \quad ...(1)$$

Also $kt_{\frac{1}{2}} = 0.693$ ...(2)

Divide 1 & 2-

$$\frac{t_{\frac{7}{8}}}{t_{\frac{1}{2}}} = \frac{2.303 \log 8}{0.693}$$

$$\frac{t_{\frac{7}{8}}}{t_{\frac{1}{2}}} = \frac{2.303 \log 8}{2.303 \times \log 2}$$

$$\frac{t_{\frac{7}{8}}}{t_{\frac{1}{2}}} = \frac{\log 8}{\log 2}$$

$$\frac{t_{\frac{7}{8}}}{t_{\frac{1}{2}}} = \frac{\log 2^3}{\log 2}$$

$$\frac{t_{\frac{7}{8}}}{t_{\frac{1}{2}}} = 3 \times \frac{\log 2}{\log 2}$$

$$\boxed{\frac{t_{\frac{7}{8}}}{t_{\frac{1}{2}}} = 3}$$

20.

	3A →	2B
At t = 0	20	0
At t = t	20 − x	$\frac{2}{3}$x

At time t, Concentration of A & B are equal

$$\therefore\ 20 - x = \frac{2}{3}x$$

$$20 = \frac{2}{3}x + x$$

$$20 = \frac{5x}{3}$$

$$\frac{60}{5} = x$$

$$\boxed{x = 12}$$

Concentration of B $= \frac{2}{3}x = \frac{2}{3} \times 12 = 8$ moles L^{-1}

21.

	$C_2H_4O_{(g)} \longrightarrow$	CH_4 (g)	+ $CO_{(g)}$
At t = 0	80	0	0
At t = 20 mins	80 − p	p	p

Now, $80 - p + p + p = 120$

$80 + p = 120$

$\boxed{p = 40}$

Since it is first order reaction and after 20 mins, half of the pressure of reactant is left.

So, $t_{\frac{1}{2}} = 20$ mins

$$t_{\frac{1}{2}} = \frac{0.693}{k}$$

$$20 = \frac{0.693}{k}$$

$$k = \frac{0.693}{20}$$

Apply, $kt = 2.303 \log\frac{(A)_o}{(A)}$

$$\frac{0.693}{20} \times t = 2.303 \log\frac{80}{\frac{25}{100} \times 80}$$

$$\frac{0.693}{20} \times t = 2.303 \log\frac{80}{20}$$

$$\frac{0.693}{20} \times t = 2.303 \log 4$$

$$\frac{2.303 \times 0.3010 \times t}{20} = 2.303 \times 2 \times 0.3010$$

$\boxed{t = 40 \text{ minutes}}$

22. Apply, $kt = 2.303 \log\frac{(A)_o}{(A)}$

$$k \times \frac{15}{2} = 2.303 \log\frac{(A)_o}{\frac{0.1(A)_o}{100}}$$

$$k \times \frac{15}{2} = 2.303 \log 1000$$

$$k \times \frac{15}{2} = 2.303 \log 10^3$$

$$k \times \frac{15}{2} = 2.303 \times 3 \log 10$$

$$\boxed{k = \frac{2.303 \times 3 \times 2}{15} = \frac{2.303 \times 2}{5}}$$

Av. life (natural life time) $= \frac{1}{k} = \frac{1}{2.303 \times \frac{2}{5}}$

Av. life $= \frac{5}{2.303 \times 2} = \frac{5}{4.606} = 1.085$ hrs

≈ 65 mins (1 hr 5 mins)

23. Apply, $(A) = (A)_o\, e^{-kt}$

Let time taken for Concentration of Reactant to get reduced to $\frac{1}{e^2}$ of initial Concentration = t & let 'n' natural life time in time t

$$1 \text{ natural life time} = \frac{1}{k}$$

$$n \text{ natural life time} = \frac{n}{k}$$

$$(A) = (A)_o\, e^{-kt}$$

$$\frac{1}{e^2} \times (A)_o = (A)_o\, e^{\frac{-k \times n}{k}}$$

$$\frac{1}{e^2} = e^{-n}$$

$$e^{-2} = e^{-n}$$

$\boxed{n = 2}$

24.

	$SO_2Cl_{2(g)} \longrightarrow$	$SO_{2(g)}$	$+ Cl_{2(g)}$
At = 0	P	0	0
At t = 100 sec	P – P′	P′	P′
After long time, t = ∞	0	P	P

At $t = \infty$

$2P = 1$ atm

$$\boxed{P = \frac{1}{2} = 0.5 \text{ atm}}$$

At t = 100 seconds

$P - P' + P' + P' = 0.8$

$P + P' = 0.8$

$0.5 + P' = 0.8$

$\boxed{P' = 0.3 \text{ atm}}$

For first 100 sec, apply first order integrated equation

$$kt = 2.303 \log\frac{P}{P - P'}$$

$$k \times 100 = 2.303 \log\frac{0.5}{0.5 - 0.3}$$

$$k \times 100 = 2.303 \log\frac{0.5}{0.2}$$

$$k = \frac{2.303}{100}\left(\log\frac{5}{2}\right)$$

$$k = \frac{2.303}{100}(\log 5 - \log 2)$$

$$k = \frac{2.303}{100}(0.6990 - 0.3010)$$

$$\boxed{k = 0.009\ s^{-1}}$$

25. Apply,

$$kt = 2.303 \log \frac{(A)_0}{(A)}$$

$$k \times t_{99\%} = 2.303 \log \frac{(A)_0}{\frac{1}{100}(A)_0}$$

$$k \times t_{99\%} = 2.303 \log \frac{(A)_0}{(A)_0} \times 100$$

$$k \times t_{99\%} = 2.303 = \log 10^2$$

$$k \times 32 = 2.303 \times 2 \log 10$$

$$k = \frac{2.303 \times 2}{32} = \frac{2.303}{16}$$

For 99.9% completion

$$k \times t_{99.9\%} = 2.303 \log \frac{(A)_0}{(A)}$$

$$k \times t_{99.9\%} = 2.303 \log \frac{(A)_0}{\frac{0.1}{100}(A)_0}$$

$$\frac{2.303}{16} \times t_{99.9\%} = 2.303 \log \frac{(A)_0}{0.1(A)_0} \times 100$$

$$\frac{2.303}{16} \times t_{99.9\%} = 2.303 \log 1000$$

$$\frac{2.303}{16} \times t_{99.9\%} = 2.303 \log 10^3$$

$$\frac{t_{99.9\%}}{16} = 3 \log 10$$

$$t_{99.9\%} = 3 \times 16 = 48 \text{ min.}$$

26. Reaction 1 $\left(t_{\frac{1}{2}}\right)_I = \frac{0.693}{k_1}$

Reaction 2 $\left(t_{\frac{1}{2}}\right)_{II} = \frac{0.693}{k_2}$

$$\frac{3}{2} = \frac{0.693}{k_1} \times \frac{k_2}{0.693}$$

$$\boxed{\frac{3}{2} = \frac{k_2}{k_1}}$$

I[st] reaction

25% completed

$$k\,t = 2.303 \log \frac{(A)_0}{(A)}$$

$$k_1 t_1 = 2.303 \log \frac{(A)_0}{\frac{75}{100}(A)_0}$$

$$k_1 t_1 = 2.303 \log \frac{100}{75}$$

$$k_1 t_1 = = 2.303 \log 1.33 \qquad ...(1)$$

IInd reaction

75% completed

$$k_2 t_2 = 2.303 \log \frac{(A)_0}{(A)}$$

$$k_2 t_2 = 2.303 \log \frac{(A)_0}{\frac{25}{100}(A)_0}$$

$$k_2 t_2 = 2.303 \log \frac{(A)_0}{25(A)_0} \times 100$$

$$k_2 t_2 = 2.303 \log 4 \qquad ...(2)$$

$$\frac{k_1 t_1}{k_2 t_2} = \frac{2.303}{2.303} \frac{\log 1.33}{\log 4}$$

$$\frac{2}{3} \times \frac{t_1}{t_2} = \frac{\log 1.33}{\log 4}$$

$$\boxed{\frac{t_1}{t_2} = \frac{3}{2} \times \frac{\log 1.33}{\log 4}}$$

27. According to question

$$r = k(0.1)^m \qquad ...(1)$$

$$2r = k(0.15)^m \qquad ...(2)$$

Divide both

$$\frac{1}{2} = \left(\frac{0.1}{0.15}\right)^m$$

Take log on both sides-

$$\log \frac{1}{2} = \log \left(\frac{10}{15}\right)^m$$

$$\log \frac{1}{2} = m \log \left(\frac{10}{15}\right)$$

$$\log \frac{1}{2} = m \log \frac{2}{3}$$

$$\log 1 - \log 2 = m(\log 2 - \log 3)$$

$$0 - 0.3010 = m(0.3010 - 0.4770)$$

$$\frac{-0.3010}{-0.176} = m$$

$$\boxed{1.7 = m}$$

28. $A \rightarrow 2B$

$k = 6.93 \times 10^{-3}\ min^{-1}$

$$t_{\frac{1}{2}} = \frac{0.693}{k} \text{ (for I}^{st}\text{ Order)}$$

$$t_{\frac{1}{2}} = \frac{0.693}{6.93 \times 10^{-3}}$$

$$t_{\frac{1}{2}} = \frac{0.693}{6.93} \times \frac{1000}{1000} \times 100 = 100 \text{ min}$$

$$\boxed{t_{\frac{1}{2}} = 100 \text{ min}}$$

$$\boxed{\text{No. of half lives after 300 min.} = 3}$$

Amount of reactant left, (A) after 3 half lives

$$= \frac{(A)_o}{2^3}$$

$$(A) = \frac{(A)_o}{8}$$

$$\therefore \frac{(A)}{(A)_o} = \frac{1}{3} = \text{fraction of reactant left}$$

$$\%\text{ age left undecayed} = \frac{1}{8} \times 100 = 12.5\%$$

29. Radioactivity follows first order kinetics.

Apply,

$$kt = 2.303 \log \frac{(A)_o}{(A)}$$

$$k \times 12 = 2.303 \log \frac{(A)_o}{\frac{1}{8}(A)_o}$$

$$k \times 12 = 2.303 \log \frac{(A)_o}{(A)_o} \times 8$$

$$k = \frac{2.303}{12} \times \log 2^3$$

$$k = \frac{2.303}{12} \times 3 \log 2 = \frac{2.303}{12} \times 3 \times 0.3010$$

$$k = \frac{0.693 \times 3}{12} = \frac{0.693}{4}$$

$$t_{\frac{1}{2}} = \frac{0.693}{k} = \frac{0.693}{\frac{0.693}{4}} = 4 \text{ days}$$

$$\boxed{t_{\frac{1}{2}} = 4 \text{ days}}$$

No. of half lives at end of 24 days = 6

Amount of reactant left, (A) after 6 half lives $= \frac{(A)_o}{2^6}$

$$(A) = \frac{(A)_o}{64}$$

$$\frac{(A)}{(A)_o} = \frac{1}{64} = \text{fraction left}$$

30. $k = 0.0693\ min^{-1}$

$$\boxed{t_{\frac{1}{2}} = \frac{0.693}{k} = \frac{0.693}{0.0693} = 10 \text{ mins}}$$

So, Concentration of reactant left after 10 mins

$$= \frac{10}{2} = 5 \text{ mol } L^{-1}$$

$R \rightarrow P$

Rate of Rxn. = $k\,[R]^1 = 0.0693 \times 5\ Mmin^{-1}$

31. $t_{\frac{1}{2}}$ for Ist order reaction = 40 seconds

$t_{\frac{1}{2}}$ for zero order reaction = 20 seconds

For Ist order,

$$t_{\frac{1}{2}} = \frac{0.693}{k_1}$$

$$40 = \frac{0.693}{k_1}$$

$$\boxed{k_1 = \frac{0.693}{40}} \quad ...(1)$$

For zero order,

$$t_{\frac{1}{2}} = \frac{(A)_o}{2k_o}$$

$$20 = \frac{1.386}{2k_o}$$

$$k_o = \frac{1.386}{40} \quad ...(2)$$

$$\frac{k_1}{k_o} = \frac{\frac{0.693}{40}}{\frac{1.386}{40}} = \frac{0.693}{40} \times \frac{40}{1.386} = \frac{0.693}{1.386} = 0.5$$

$mol^{-1}\ dm^3$

32. For 40 mins, $(A)_o = 0.1$ M

(A) = 0.025 M

$$\text{Apply, } kt = 2.303 \log \frac{(A)_o}{(A)}$$

$$k \times 40 = 2.303 \log \frac{0.1}{0.025}$$

$k \times 40 = 2 \times 303 \log 4$

$k \times 40 = 2.303 \log 2^2$

$k \times 40 = 2.303 \times 2 \log 2$

$$k = \frac{2.303 \times 2 \times 0.3010}{40}$$

$$\boxed{k = \frac{0.693}{20}}$$

Now, Rate of reaction = k[x]

$$= \frac{0.693}{20} \times 0.01 = 3.47 \times 10^{-4} \text{ m/min}$$

33. $t_{\frac{1}{2}} \propto \frac{1}{(A)_o^{n-1}}$ or $t_{\frac{1}{2}} \propto \frac{1}{(p_o)^{n-1}}$

where $(A)_o$ = initial Concentration of reactant

n = order of reaction

$$\left(t_{\frac{1}{2}}\right)_I (p_o)_I^{n-1} = \left(t_{\frac{1}{2}}\right)_{II} (p_o)_{II}^{n-1}$$

$4 \times (50)^{n-1} = 2 \times (75)^{n-1}$

$$\frac{4}{2} = \left(\frac{75}{50}\right)^{n-1}$$

$$2 = \left(\frac{17}{10}\right)^{n-1}$$

$$2 = \left(\frac{3}{2}\right)^{n-1}$$

$$\log 2 = \log\left(\frac{3}{2}\right)^{n-1}$$

$0.3010 = n - 1 (\log 3 - \log 2)$

$0.3010 = n - 1(0.4770 - 0.3010)$

$0.3010 = n - 1(0.1760)$

$$\frac{0.3010}{0.1760} = n - 1$$

$1.7 = n - 1$

$\boxed{n = 1.7 + 1 = 2.7}$

Order = 2.7

34. Rate of reaction = $k(A)^x$ (x = order of reaction)

$6.4 = k(3)^x$ ...(1)

$1.6 = k(1.5)^x$ ...(2)

$4 = (2)^x$

$\boxed{x = 2}$

35. Rate = $k(A)^n$

Take log on both sides-

log(rate) = log (k. $(A)^n$)

log(rate) = log k + log $(A)^n$

$$\boxed{\log(\text{rate}) = \log k + n \log(A)}$$

(log (rate) → y – axis; log k → c; n → m; log (A) → x – axis)

$\boxed{n = \text{order} = \text{slope}}$

So, greater the slope, higher is the order.

36. Rate of reaction = $k(A)^1 (B)^1$

For option (b), Rate of reaction

$$= k\left[\frac{0.2}{0.1}\right]\left[\frac{0.2}{0.1}\right]$$

= 4k

which is max.

37. $A + 2B \rightarrow C + D$

It is an elementary reaction. So, rate law is-

Rate of reaction = $k(A)^1 (B)^2$

Initial of reaction = $k[0.60]^1 [0.80]^2$ ...(1)

	A	+	2B	→	C	+ D
At t = 0	0.60		0.80		0	0
At t = t	0.60 – p		0.80 – 2p		P	P

$\boxed{P_C = P = 0.2}$

Now, $P_A = 0.60 - 0.2 = 0.40$ atm

$P_B = 0.80 - 2p = 0.80 - 2 \times 0.2$

$= 0.80 - 0.4 = 0.40$ atm

New rate of reaction = $k[A]^1 (B)^2$

New rate of reaction = $k(0.40)(0.40)^2$ ...(2)

$$\text{Ratio} = \frac{\text{New rate of reaction}}{\text{Initial rate of reaction}}$$

$$= \frac{k(0.4)(0.4)^2}{k(0.6)(0.8)^2}$$

$$= \frac{0.4 \times 0.16}{0.6 \times 0.64} = \frac{4}{6} \times \frac{1}{4} = \frac{1}{6}$$

38. Let Order wrt A = x

Order wrt B = y

From I

Rate = $k(A)^x (B)^y$

$2 \times 10^{-4} = k[1 \times 10^{-2}]^x [2 \times 10^{-2}]^y$ ...(1)

From II

$4 \times 10^{-4} = k[2 \times 10^{-2}]^x [2 \times 10^{-2}]^y$ ...(2)

Dividing (1) by (2)

$\frac{1}{2} = \left(\frac{1}{2}\right)^x$

$\boxed{\therefore x = 1}$

Similarly from II & III

$4 \times 10^{-4} = k[2 \times 10^{-2}]^x [2 \times 10^{-2}]^y$ ...(3)

$8 \times 10^{-4} = k[2 \times 10^{-2}]^x [4 \times 10^{-2}]^y$ ...(4)

$\frac{1}{2} = \left(\frac{1}{2}\right)^y$

$\boxed{y = 1}$

So, rate law is-

$\boxed{\text{Rate of reaction} = k[A]^1 [B]^1}$

From I

Rate $= k(A)'(B)'$

$2 \times 10^{-4} = k \times 2 \times 10^{-4}$

$\boxed{k = 1}$

So, statement (1) is wrong.

However, rate $= k(A)'(B)'$

On doubling the Conctant of both A & B, rate will become four times.

39. From (I) & II

Rate $= k[A]^1 [B]^0$

$2 \times 10^{-2} = k[0.1]^1 [0.1]^0$ ...(1)

$4 \times 10^{-2} = k[Y]^1 [0.2]^0$ ...(2)

Divide 1 & 2-

$\frac{1}{2} = \left(\frac{0.1}{Y}\right)$

$\boxed{Y = 0.2}$

From expt I, value of k can be calculated

$2 \times 10^{-2} = k[0.1]^1 [0.1]^0$

$2 \times 10^{-2} = k(10^{-1})$

$\boxed{k = 0.2}$

From expt. III

rate $= k(A)^1 (B)^0$

(z)

$z = 0.2(0.4)^1 (0.4)^0$

$\boxed{z = 0.08}$

40. Rate of reaction does not depend upon the concentration of reactant which is in excess. So, rate law is-

Rate of reaction $= k[B]^x$

(where x = order write B)

(r)rate $= k(0.1)^x$ ...(1)

$2r = k(0.4)^x$ ...(2)

Divide $\frac{1}{2}$

$\frac{r}{2r} = \left(\frac{1}{4}\right)^x$

$\frac{1}{2} = \left(\frac{1}{4}\right)^x$

$\frac{1}{2} = \left(\frac{1}{2}\right)^{2x}$

$2x = 1$

$\boxed{x = \frac{1}{2}}$

$\boxed{\text{So, rate} = \frac{dx}{dt} = k(B)^{\frac{1}{2}}}$

41. Let, Rate law be-

Rate of Reaction $= k[A]^x[B]^y$

From, I & II

$0.05 = k(0.1)^x(0.2)^y$ ...(1)

$0.10 = k(0.2)^x(0.2)^y$ ...(2)

Divide $\frac{1}{2}$

$\frac{1}{2} = \left(\frac{1}{2}\right)^x$

$\boxed{x = 1}$

Now, compare I & III

$0.05 = k[0.1]^1[0.2]^y$ ...(3)

$0.05 = k[0.1]^1[0.1]^y$ ...(4)

Divide these

$1 = (2)^y$

$(2)^0 = (2)^y$

$\boxed{y = 0}$

So, rate law is-

Rate of reaction $= k[A]^1[B]^0$

From any of the three data. 'k' can be calculated-from I

$0.05 = k[0.1]^1[0.2]^0$

$\frac{0.05}{0.1} = k$

$\boxed{0.5 = k}$

Now, $t_{\frac{1}{2}} = \frac{0.693}{k} = \frac{0.693}{0.5} = 1.386\,\text{sec}^{-1}$

42. $R \rightarrow P$

Rate of Reaction = $k[R]^1$

$0.04 = k[R]_1$ ...(1)

$0.03 = k[R]_2$ ...(2)

$$\frac{4}{3} = \frac{(R)_1}{(R)_2}$$

For those 10 minutes (between 10 minutes & 20 minutes, after initiation) I[st] order equation Can be applied,

$$kt = 2.303 \log\frac{(A)_o}{(A)}$$

$$k \times 10 = 2.303 \log\frac{4}{3}$$

$$k = \frac{2.303}{10}(\log 4 - \log s\ 3)$$

$$k = \frac{2.303}{10}(0.6020 - 0.4770)$$

$$\boxed{k = 0.0287}\ min^{-1}$$

$$t_{\frac{1}{2}} = \frac{0.693}{k} = \frac{0.693}{0.0287\ min^{-1}} = 24.14\ min$$

43. $E_a = 1000\,x\ J\ mol^{-1}$

$$b(\text{Boltzmann factor}) = e^{\frac{-E_a}{RT}}$$

$$b = e^{\frac{-1000x}{RT}}$$

Take ln on both sides

$$\ln b = \ln e^{\frac{-1000x}{RT}}$$

$$\ln b = \frac{-1000x}{RT}\ln e$$

(lne = 1)

$$\ln b = \frac{-1000x}{RT}$$

($\ln = 2.303 \log_{10}$)

$$2.303 \log_{10} b = \frac{-1000x}{RT}$$

$$\boxed{\log_{10} b = \frac{-1000x}{2.303RT}}$$

$$\log b = \frac{-1000x}{2.303R \times 500}$$

$$\boxed{\log b = \frac{-2x}{2.303R}}$$

44. $k = Ae^{\frac{-E_a}{RT}}$

$$\ln k = \ln\left[A.e^{\frac{-E_a}{RT}}\right]$$

$$\ln k = \ln A + \ln e^{\frac{-E_a}{RT}}$$

$$\ln k = \ln A - \frac{E_a}{RT}$$

$$\boxed{\ln K = \ln A - \frac{E_a}{R} \times \frac{1}{T}}$$

$\ln K \rightarrow y$, $\ln A \rightarrow c$, $\frac{E_a}{R} \times \frac{1}{T} \rightarrow mx$

$$\boxed{slope = \frac{-E_a}{R}}$$

45. $k = Ae^{\frac{-E_a}{RT}}$

$$\boxed{E_a = RT}$$

Now, $k = Ae^{\frac{-RT}{RT}}$

$$k = Ae^{-1}$$

$$\boxed{k = \frac{1}{e} \times A}$$

$$k = \frac{1}{2.713} \times A$$

$$\boxed{k = 0.37\ A}$$

$$\boxed{k = 37\%\ \text{of}\ A}$$

46. Without catalyst (at 500 k)

$$k = Ae^{\frac{-E_a}{RT}}$$

$$k = Ae^{\frac{-E_a}{R \times 500}}$$

$$k = Ae^{\frac{-E_a}{500R}} \quad ...(1)$$

At 400 k (with catalyst)

$$k = Ae^{\frac{-E_a}{RT}}$$

$$k = Ae^{\frac{-(E_a - 20)}{400\ R}} \quad ...(2)$$

Since rate is same (given), ∴ k is same

From (1) & (2)-

$$Ae^{\frac{-E_a}{500\,R}} = Ae^{\frac{20-E_a}{400R}}$$

$$e^{\frac{-E_a}{500\,R}} = e^{\frac{20-E_a}{400\,R}}$$

$$\frac{-E_a}{500\,R} = \frac{20-E_a}{400R}$$

$$-400\,E_a = 10{,}000 - 500\,E_a$$

$$100\,E_a = 10{,}000$$

$$\boxed{E_a = 100\text{ kJ}}$$

47. $\ln k = \ln A - \frac{E_a}{RT}$

$$\boxed{\ln K = \ln A - \frac{E_a}{R}\times\frac{1}{T}}$$

y c mx

$$\text{slope} = \frac{-E_a}{R}$$

Greater the slope, greater is the E_a.

48. Apply $k = Ae^{\frac{-E_a}{RT}}$

If $E_a \longrightarrow \infty, k = 0$

49. Rate constant. at 300 k = k

Rate constant. at 310 k = 2k

Apply, $\log\frac{k_2}{k_1} = \frac{E_a}{2.303\,R}\frac{(T_2 - T_1)}{T_1T_2}$

$$\log\frac{2k}{k} = \frac{E_a}{2.303\,R}\left(\frac{310-300}{310\times 300}\right)$$

$$\frac{\log 2\times 2.303R\times 310\times 300}{10} = E_a$$

$$\frac{0.3010\times 2.303\times 8.314\times 10^{-3}\times 310\times 300}{10} = E_a$$

$$\boxed{E_a = 53.3\text{kJ mol}^{-1}}$$

50. $k_2 = 6k_1$

Apply, $\log\frac{k_2}{k_1} = \frac{E_a}{2.303\,R}\frac{(T_2 - T_1)}{T_1T_2}$

$$\log\frac{6k_1}{k_1} = \frac{E_a}{2.303\times 8.314\times 10^{-3}}\left(\frac{400-350}{400\times 350}\right)$$

$$\boxed{E_a = 41.7\text{kJ mol}^{-1}}$$

51. $k = Ae^{\frac{-E_a}{RT}}$

$$\ln k = \ln A - \frac{E_a}{RT}$$

$$\boxed{\log_{10} k = \log_{10} A \frac{-E_a}{2.303\,RT}}$$

$$\boxed{\text{or } \log_{10} k = \frac{-E_a}{2.303\,RT} + \log_{10} A} \quad ...(1)$$

$$\text{Also, } \log k = \frac{-2000}{T} + 6 \quad ...(2)$$

Relating (1) & (2)-

$\log A = 6$

$$\boxed{A = 10^6\,s^{-1}}$$

$$\text{Also, } \frac{-E_a}{2.303RT} = \frac{-2000}{T}$$

$$E_a = 2000\times 2.303\times 8.314\times 10^{-3}$$

$$\boxed{E_a = 38.3\text{kJ mol}^{-1}}$$

52. $E_a = 2.303\text{ RT Jmol}^{-1}$

$$k = Ae^{\frac{-E_a}{RT}}$$

$$\frac{k}{A} = e^{\frac{-E_a}{RT}} = e^{\frac{-2.303RT}{RT}}$$

$$\frac{k}{A} = e^{-2.303}$$

$$\ln\frac{k}{A} = \ln e^{-2.303}$$

$$\ln\frac{k}{A} = -2.303\ln e$$

$$\ln\frac{k}{A} = -2.303$$

$$2.303\log_{10}\frac{k}{A} = -2.303$$

$$\log\frac{k}{A} = -1$$

$$\boxed{\frac{k}{A} = 10^{-1}}$$

$$\boxed{\frac{k}{A} = 0.1}$$

53. For I[st] set,

$kt = (A)_o - (A)$

$k \times 2 = 4 - 2$

$\boxed{k = 1}$

For IInd set,

$kt = (A)_o - (A)$

$1 \times x = 6 - 2$

$\boxed{x = 4}$

55. $\dfrac{k_2(\text{Rate constant at } 27°C)}{k_1(\text{Rate constant at } 17°C)} = 2$

$\dfrac{10^{-3}}{k_1} = 2$

$k_1 = \dfrac{1}{2} \times 10^{-3} = 0.5 \times 10^{-3} = 5 \times 10^{-4}$

56.

	2A +	B →	C +	2D
At t = 0	x	2x	0	0
Att = 30mins.	$\frac{x-x}{2}$	$\frac{2x-x}{4}$	$\frac{x}{4}$	$\frac{x}{2}$

At 30 mins, Rate of reaction = $k(A)(B)^2$

Rate of reaction $= k\left(\dfrac{x}{2}\right)\left(\dfrac{7x}{4}\right)^2$

Rate of reaction $= k\left(\dfrac{x}{2}\right)\left(\dfrac{49x^2}{16}\right)$

$\boxed{\text{Rate of reaction} = k\dfrac{49x^3}{32}}$

57.

	A	+ B	→ P
At t = 0	1	1	0
At t = t	1 – 0.5	1 – 0.5	0.5

Initial rate = 1×10^{-2} mol L^{-1} sec^{-1}

Rate = $k[A]^1 [B]^2$

$10^{-2} = k(1)(1)^2$

$\boxed{k = 10^{-2}}$

At time = t

Rate of reaction = $k[A][B]^2$

$= 10^{-2}(0.5)(0.5)^2$

$= 10^{-2} \times 0.5 \times 0.25$

$= 10^{-2} \times \dfrac{125}{1000}$

Rate of reaction = 125×10^{-5} or 1.25×10^{-3} mol L^{-1} sec^{-1}

58.

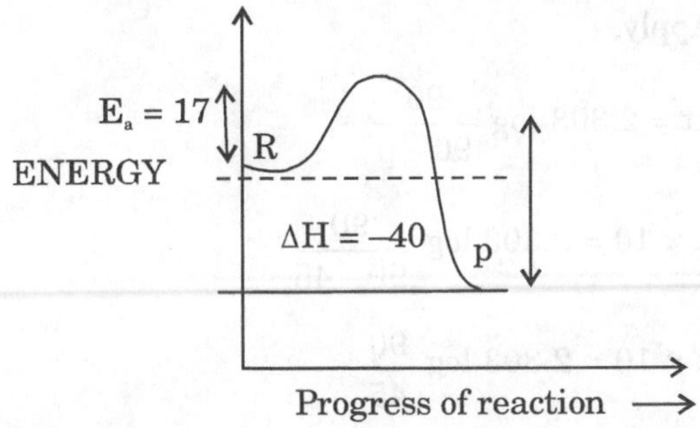

$\Delta H = E_{a_f} - E_{a_b}$

$-40 = 17 - E_b$

$-40 - 17 = -E_b$

$-57 = -E_b$

$\boxed{E_b = 57 kJ/mole}$

60. $SO_2Cl_{2(g)} \longrightarrow SO_{2(g)} + Cl_{2(g)}$

	SO_2Cl_2	SO_2	Cl_2
At t = 0	700	0	0
At t = 20 mins	700 – 350	350	350

$kt = 2.303 \log \dfrac{(p_o)}{(P)}$

$k \times 20 = 2.303 \log \dfrac{700}{350}$

$k = \dfrac{2.303}{20} \times 0.3010 = \dfrac{0.693}{20}$

Now, $kt = 2.303 \log \dfrac{(p_o)}{(p)}$

$\log \dfrac{p_o}{p} = \dfrac{kt}{2.303} + O$

↓

$y = mx + c$

$\text{slope} = \dfrac{k}{2.303} = \dfrac{\frac{0.693}{20}}{2.303} = \dfrac{0.693}{20} \times \dfrac{1}{2.303}$

$\text{slope} = \dfrac{2.303 \times 0.3010}{20 \times 2.303} = \dfrac{0.3010}{20} = 0.01505$

$= \dfrac{1505}{100000} = 1.505 \times 10^{-2} \text{ min}^{-1}$

61. $X_{(g)} \longrightarrow 2Y_{(g)} + Z_{(g)}$

	X	2Y	Z
At t = 0	90	0	0
At t = 10 mins	90 – p	2p	p

$90 - p + 2p + p = 180$

$90 + 2p = 180$

$2p = 90$

$\boxed{p = 45}$

Apply,

$$kt = 2.303 \log \frac{90}{90 - p}$$

$$k \times 10 = 2.303 \log \frac{90}{90 - 45}$$

$$k \times 10 = 2.303 \log \frac{90}{45}$$

$$k = \frac{0.693}{10} = 0.0693\,\text{min}^{-1}$$

$$k = \frac{0.693}{\text{min}} = \frac{0.0693}{60\,\text{sec}} = 0.001155\,\text{sec}^{-1}$$

$$\boxed{k = 1.15 \times 10^{-3}\,\text{sec}^{-1}}$$

64. $k_{300\,k} = k_1$

$k_{310\,k} = 2k_1$

$$\log \frac{k_2}{k_1} = \frac{E_a}{2.303R} \frac{(T_2 - T_1)}{T_1 T_2}$$

$$\log \frac{2k_1}{k_1} = \frac{E_a}{2.303R} \frac{(310 - 300)}{310 \times 300}$$

$$\frac{0.3010 \times 2.303 \times 8.314 \times 310 \times 300}{10} = E_a$$

53598 J/mole = E_a

or

53.59 kJ/mole = E_a

Now, $E_{a(B)} = 2E_{a(A)} = 2 \times 53.6 = 107.2$ kJ/mole

Apply, $\log \frac{k_2}{k_1} = \frac{E_a}{2.303R} \frac{(T_2 - T_1)}{T_1 T_2}$

$$\log \frac{2k_1}{k_1} = \frac{107.2}{2.303 \times 8.314 \times 10^{-3}} \frac{(T_2 - 300)}{T_2 \times 300}$$

$$\frac{0.3010 \times 2.303 \times 8.314 \times 10^{-3}}{107.2} = \frac{T_2 - 300}{300T_2}$$

$$0.0000537 = \frac{T_2 - 300}{300T_2}$$

$0.0161\, T_2 = T_2 - 300$

$300 = T_2 - 0.0161\, T_2$

$300 = 0.983\, T_2$

$$\boxed{T_2 = 305.18k}$$

$\Delta T = 305.18 - 300$

$$\boxed{\Delta T = 5.18k}$$

65. Apply,

$$\log \frac{k_2}{k_1} = \frac{E_a}{2.303R} \frac{(T_2 - T_1)}{T_1 T_2}$$

$$\log \frac{k_2}{k_1} = \frac{12.68}{2.303 \times 2 \times 10^{-3}} \frac{(308 - 298)}{308 \times 298}$$

$$\log \frac{k_2}{k_1} = \frac{12.68 \times 1000}{4.606} \frac{(10)}{308 \times 298}$$

$$\log \frac{k_2}{k_1} = \frac{12.68 \times 10{,}000}{4.606 \times 308 \times 298}$$

$$\log \frac{k_2}{k_1} = \frac{126800}{422757}$$

$$\log \frac{k_2}{k_1} = 0.3$$

$$\frac{k_2}{k_1} = 2$$

$$\boxed{k_2 = 2k_1}$$

$$\%\text{age increase} = \frac{k_2 - k_1}{k_1} \times 100 = \frac{2k_1 - k_1}{k_1} \times 100$$

$$= \frac{k_1}{k_1} \times 100 = 100\%$$

66. Let $p_{initial}$ of $F_2 = p$

$p_{Ne} = 2000 - p$

	$F_{2(g)} \longrightarrow$	$2F_{(g)}$
At t = 0	p	0
At t = 2 hrs	p – p′	2p′
After long time →	O	2 p

$2p + p_{Ne} = 2400$

$2p + 2000 - p = 2400$

$p + 2000 = 2400$

$$\boxed{p = 400\text{ mm Hg}}$$

Now, $t_{1/2} = 30$ min

$$t_{1/2} = \frac{0.693}{k}$$

$$k = \frac{0.693}{30} = 0.0231\,\text{min}^{-1}$$

For a period of 2 hrs, apply

$$kt = 2.303 \log \frac{P}{p - p'}$$

$$0.0231 \times 2 \times 60 = 2.303 \log \frac{P}{p - p'}$$

$$\log\frac{p}{p-p'} = 1.20$$

$$\frac{p}{p-p'} = 16$$

$$\frac{400}{400-p'} = 16$$

$400 = 6400 - 16p'$

$16p' = 6000$

$$\boxed{p' = \frac{6000}{16} = 375\text{mm Hg}}$$

Final p after 2 hrs $= P - p' + 2p' + P_{Ne}$

$= P + p' + (2000 - p)$

$= 400 + 375 + 2000 - 400$

$= 2375$ mm Hg

$$\text{Ratio} = \frac{p_{final}}{p_{initial}} = \frac{2375}{2000} = 1.18$$

67. Reaction is 19% completed in 40 minutes.

$$kt = 2.303\log\frac{(A)_o}{(A)}$$

$$k \times 40 = 2.303\log\frac{(A)_o}{\frac{81}{100}(A)_o}$$

$$k \times 40 = 2.303\log\frac{100}{81}$$

$$k = \frac{2.303}{40}(\log 100 - \log 81)$$

$\log 100 = \log 10^2 = 2\log 10 = 2$

$\log 81 = \log 3^4 = 4\log^3 = 4 \times 0.4770 = 1.90$

$$k = \frac{2.303}{40}(2 - 1.90)$$

$$k = \frac{2.303}{40} \times 0.1 = 0.00575$$

For 20 min

$$kt = 2.303\log\frac{(A)_o}{(A)}$$

$$0.00575 \times 20 = 2.303\log\frac{(A)_o}{(A)}$$

$$0.05 = \log\frac{(A)_o}{(A)}$$

$$\frac{(A)_o}{(A)} = 1.12$$

$$\frac{(A)}{(A)_o} = \frac{1}{1.12} = \frac{100}{112}$$

$$\text{fraction left } \frac{(A)}{(A)_o} = \frac{25}{28}$$

$$\text{fraction reacted} = 1 - \frac{25}{28} = \frac{3}{28}$$

$$\%\text{ age reacted} = \frac{3}{28} \times 100 \approx 10.7\%$$

69. $t_{\frac{1}{2}} = \frac{0.693}{k}$

'k' can change with temperature & catalyst (as catalyst alters E_a).

70. $k = Ae^{\frac{-E_a}{RT}}$

if $E_a = 0$

$\boxed{k = A}$

i.e. k is NOT dependent upon temperature

72.

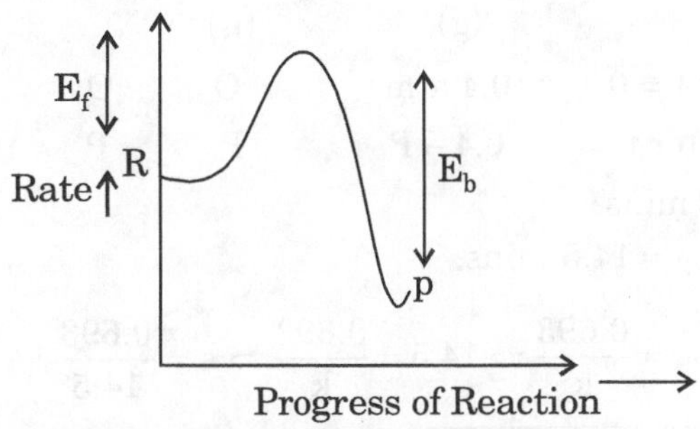

75. Units of k(mol ltr^{-1} sec^{-1}) convey that it is a zero order reaction.

∴ Apply

$kt = (A)_o - (A)$

$$10^7 \times t = \left(\frac{3 \times 10^{-6}}{0.05} \times 1000\right) - 0$$

$$t = \frac{3}{5} \times \frac{10^{-6} \times 10^3}{10^7} \times 100$$

$t = 0.6 \times 10^{-8}$

$t = 6 \times 10^{-9}$ sec

76.

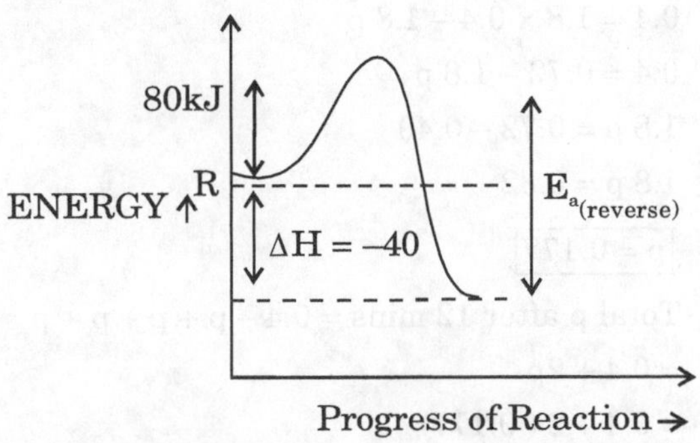

Before catalyst

E_a for reverse reaction $= 80 + 40 = 120$ kJ

After addition of catalyst

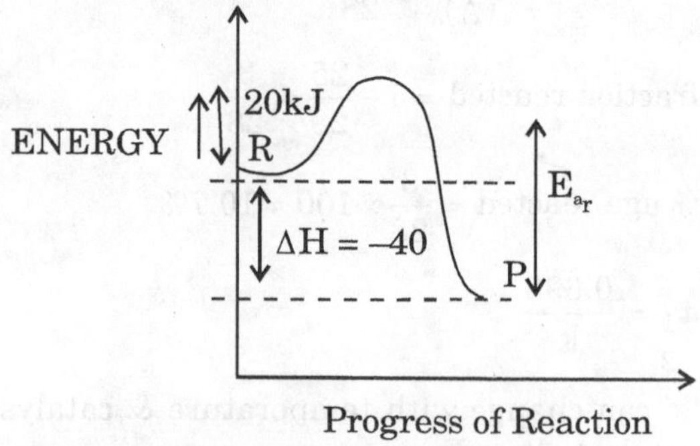

After catalyst E_a for reverse reaction

$= 20 + 40 = 60$ kJ

Ratio of $E_a = \frac{120}{60} = \frac{2}{1} = 2:1$

77. $CH_3OCH_3 \longrightarrow CH_4 + H_{2(g)} + CO_{(g)}$

(g) (g)

At t = 0	0.4 atm	O	O	O
After t = 12 mins	0.4 – P	P	P	P

$t_{1/2} = 14.5$ mins.

$t_{1/2} = \frac{0.693}{k} \Rightarrow 14.5 = \frac{0.693}{k} \Rightarrow k = \frac{0.693}{14.5}$

$\boxed{k = 0.0478 \text{ min}^{-1}}$

Apply, I[st] order equation for 12 mins-

$kt = 2.303 \log \frac{0.4}{0.4 - p}$

$0.0478 \times 12 = 2.303 \log \frac{0.4}{0.4 - p}$

$0.249 = \log \frac{0.4}{0.4 - p}$

$\frac{0.4}{0.4 - P} = 1.8$

$0.4 = 1.8 \times 0.4 - 1.8$ p

$0.4 = 0.72 - 1.8$ p

1.8 p $= 0.72 - 0.40$

1.8 p $= 0.32$

$\boxed{p = 0.177}$

Total p after 12 mins = 0.4 – p + p + p + p

= 0.4 + 2p

= 0.4 + 2 (0.177)

= 0.4 + 0.355 = 0.755 atm

78. Apply,

$kt = 2.303 \log \frac{(A)_o}{(A)}$

$k \times 20 = 2.303 \log \frac{1}{0.6}$

$k \times 20 = 2.303 \log \frac{5}{3}$

$k = \frac{2.303}{20}(\log 5 - \log 3)$

$k = \frac{2.303}{20}(0.6990 - 0.4770)$

$\boxed{k = \frac{2.303}{20} \times 0.222 = 0.025 \text{ min}^{-1}}$

Apply again,

$k = 0.025 \text{ min}^{-1}$

$kt = 2.303 \log \frac{(A)_o}{(A)}$

$0.025 \times t = 2.303 \log \frac{0.6}{0.36}$

$t = \frac{2.303}{0.025} \log \left(\frac{60}{36}\right)$

$t = \frac{2.303}{0.025} \log \frac{10}{6}$

$t = \frac{2.303}{0.025} (\log 10 - \log 6)$

$t = \frac{2.303}{0.025} (1 - 0.778)$

$\boxed{t = 20.45 \text{ min}}$

79. When pH = 2

$(H^+) = 10^{-2}$ M

rate, $r = k(10^{-2})^n$ ...(1)

When pH = 1

$r' = k(10^{-1})^n$ ($r' = 100$ r given)

$100 r = k(10^{-1})^n$ ...(2)

Divide equation (1) by (2)

$\frac{r}{100r} = \frac{10^{-2n}}{10^{-n}}$

$10^{-2} = 10^{-n}$

$\boxed{n = 2}$

80. $$^{M}_{Z}A_{(g)} \longrightarrow {}^{M-8}_{Z-4}B_{(g)} + 2\,{}^{4}_{2}He$$

At t = 0 1 0 0

After t = 2 half lives 1 – 0.75 0.75 1.5

Concentration of A left after 2 half lives = $\frac{(A)_0}{2^2} = \frac{1}{4} = 0.25$

Concentration of A reacted = 1 – 0.25 = 0.75

Total number of gaseous moles after two half lives = 1 – 0.75 + 0.75 + 1.5 = 2.5

Apply, PV = nRT

P × 1 = 2.5 × 0.0821 × 300

$\boxed{P = 61.575 \text{ atm}}$

81. Since $t_{1/2}$ is independent of Concentration of Zn (at constant. pH) so, it is first order wrt Concentration of Zn.

now, $r \propto (H^+)^n$

when pH = 3 $\longrightarrow (H^+) = 10^{-3}$ M

$r \propto (10^{-3})^n$ ...(1)

$100\,r \propto (10^{-2})^n$ ...(2)

$$\frac{r}{100\,r} = \left(\frac{10^{-3}}{10^{-2}}\right)^n$$

$$\frac{1}{100} = (10^{-1})^n$$

$10^{-2} = 10^{-n}$

$-n = -2$

$\boxed{n = 2}$

Rate of reaction $= \frac{dx}{dt} = k[Zn]^1[H^+]^2$

83. Slowest step is the rate determining step.

$\therefore$ rate = $k(O)'(O_3)'$ – (from slow step) ...(3)

Rate of reaction does not depend on the Concentration of intermediate.

$\therefore$ from equation (1) in question,

$$k_{eq.} = \frac{(O_2)'(O)'}{(O_3)'}$$

$$\frac{k_{eq.}(O_3)}{O_2} = (O)$$

Placing the concentration of O in equation(3)

$$\text{rate} = k\frac{k_{eq.}(O_3)}{O_2} \times (O_3)$$

$\boxed{\text{rate} = k'(O_3)^2(O_2)^{-1}}$

$\left(\boxed{k\,k_{eq.} = k_1}\right)$

84. k_{at} 300 k = k_1

k at 310 k $= k_1 + \frac{7}{100}k_1 = 1.07\,k_1$

Apply, Arrhenius equation

$$\log\frac{k_2}{k_1} = \frac{E_a}{2.303R}\frac{(T_2 - T_1)}{T_1 T_2}$$

$$\log\frac{1.07\,k_1}{k_1} = \frac{E_a}{2.303 \times 8.314 \times 10^{-3}}\left(\frac{310 - 300}{310 \times 300}\right)$$

$$\frac{0.0294 \times 2.303 \times 8.314 \times 10^{-3} \times 310 \times 300}{10} = E_a$$

$\boxed{E_a = 50.83 \text{ KJ/mol}}$

85. C_4H_8 (cyclobutane) → $2C_2H_4$ (ethylene)

At t = o a 0

at t = t a – x 2x

$\frac{a - x}{2x} = 1$ (given)

a – x = 2x

a = 3x

$x = \frac{a}{3}$

Rate constant unit indicate that it follows Ist order kinetics

$$kt = 2.303\log\frac{(A)_o}{(A)}$$

$$2.5 \times 10^{-5} \times t = 2.303\log\frac{a}{a - \frac{a}{3}}$$

$$2.5 \times 10^{-5} \times t = 2.303\log\frac{a}{\frac{2a}{3}}$$

$$2.5 \times 10^{-5} \times t = 2.303\log a \times \frac{3}{2a}$$

$$t = \frac{2.303}{2.5 \times 10^{-5}}(\log 3 - \log 2)$$

$$t = \frac{2.303 \times 0.1760}{2.5 \times 10^{-5}} = 16213.12 \text{sec}$$

Apply Van't Hoff Equation.

$$\log\frac{k_2}{k_1} = \frac{\Delta H}{2.303R}\frac{(T_2 - T_1)}{T_1 T_2}$$

$\boxed{k_1 \text{ Equilibrium Constant at } T_1}$

$$k_1 + \frac{3}{100}k_1 = \text{Equilibrium constant at } T_2$$

$\boxed{1.03k_1 = \text{Equilibrium constant at } T_2}$

$$\log\frac{1.03k_1}{k_1} = \frac{\Delta H}{2.303R}\left(\frac{310-300}{310\times300}\right)$$

$$\frac{10^{-3}\times0.0128\times2.303\times8.314\times310\times300}{10} = \Delta H$$

$\boxed{2.28 \text{ KJ/mol} = \Delta H}$

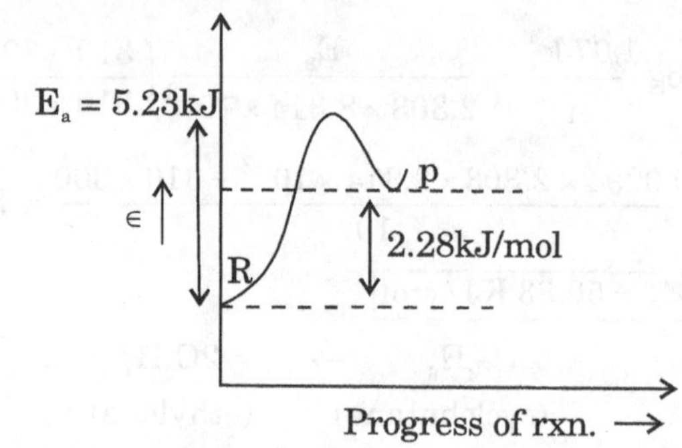

$$E_{a_f} - \Delta H = E_{a_b}$$

5.23 – 2.28 = 2.95 KJ/mol

86.

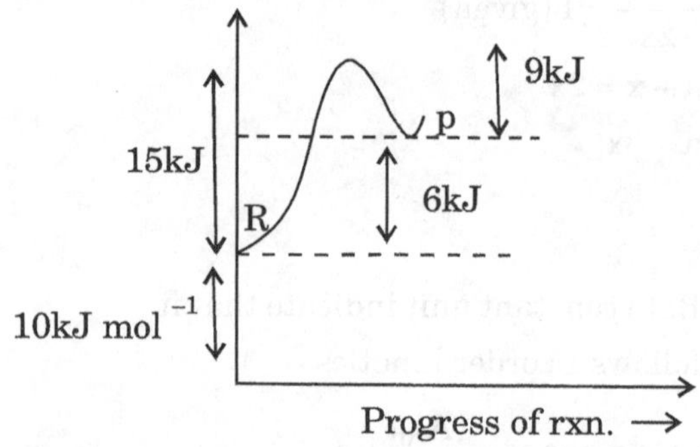

Threshold energy = 15 + 10 = 25 KJ mol^{-1}

87. Rate law suggests 2nd order reaction.

$$kt = \frac{1}{(A)} - \frac{1}{(A)_0}$$

$$kt = \frac{1}{(a-x)} - \frac{1}{a}$$

$$kt = (a-x)^{-1} - a^{-1}$$

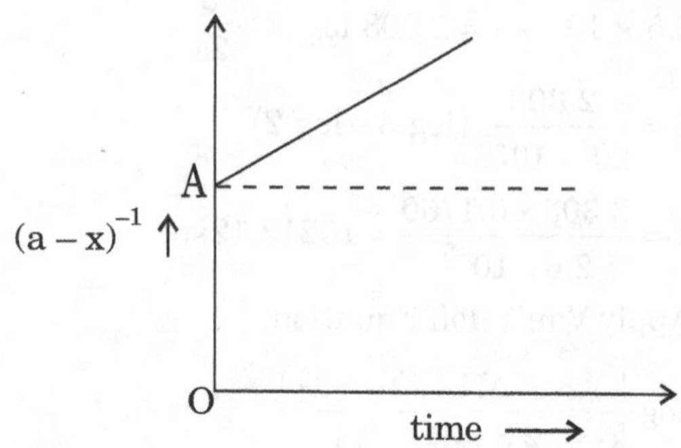

$$a^{-1} = 0.10$$

$$\frac{1}{a} = 0.10$$

$$\boxed{a = \frac{1}{0.1} = 10 \text{ mol L}^{-1}}$$

Rate of reaction = $k(R)^2 = 10^{-2}(10)^2$

$\boxed{\text{Rate of reaction} = 1 \text{ mol L}^{-1} \text{ min}^{-1}}$

88.

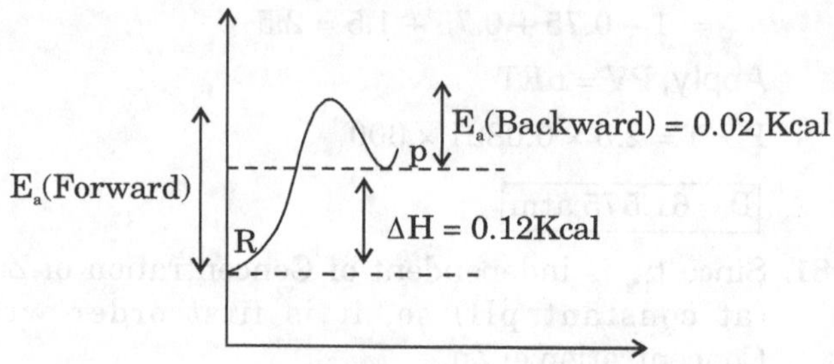

$E_{a(forward)}$ = 0.12 + 0.02 = 0.14 k cal

$E_{a(forward)}$ = 0.14 × 1000 cal = 140 cal

% age of reactant molecules crossing the energy

$$\text{barrier}(x) = e^{\frac{-E_a}{RT}} \times 100$$

$$x = e^{\frac{-140}{2\times325}} \times 100$$

$$x = e^{\frac{-140}{650}} \times 100$$

$$\ln x = \ln e^{\frac{-14}{65}} + \ln 100$$

$$\ln x = \frac{-14}{65} + 2.303\log_{10} 100$$

$$\ln x = \frac{-14}{65} + 2.303 \log 10^2$$

$$\ln x = \frac{-14}{65} + 2.303\times2$$

$$2.303 \log_{10} x = 4.391$$

$$\log x = 1.90$$

$\boxed{x = 80.65\%}$

91. Greater the E_a, greater is temperature coefficient.

92. $k_1 = k_2$

$$10^{16}.e^{\frac{-2000}{T}} = 10^{15}.e^{\frac{-1000}{T}}$$

$$10 = e^{\frac{1000}{T}}$$

$$\ln 10 = \ln e^{\frac{1000}{T}}$$

$$\ln 10 = \frac{1000}{T}$$

$$2.303 \log_{10} 10 = \frac{1000}{T}$$

$$\boxed{T = \frac{1000}{2.303} k}$$

94. Apply

$$\frac{k_2}{k_1} = \mu^{\frac{\Delta T}{10}}$$

where k_1 & k_2 are Rate constants.

μ is the temperature coefficient

$$\frac{k_2}{k_1} = 2^{\frac{15}{10}}$$

$$\frac{k_2}{k_1} = 2^{1.5}$$

$$\frac{k_2}{k_1} = 2^1 \times 2^{\frac{1}{2}}$$

$$\frac{k_2}{k_1} = 2 \times \sqrt{2} = 2 \times 1.4$$

$$\boxed{k_2 = 2.8k_1}$$

95. One average life $= \frac{1}{k}$

Two average lives $= \frac{2}{k}$

So, $t = \frac{2}{k}$

Apply, $(A) = (A)_o e^{-kt}$

$$(A) = (A)_o e^{-k \times \frac{2}{k}}$$

$$(A) = \frac{(A)_o}{e^2}$$

$$\%age = \frac{\frac{(A)_o}{e^2}}{(A)_o} \times 100 = \frac{(A)_o}{e^2} \times \frac{1}{(A)_o} \times 100 = \frac{100}{e^2}$$

96. $t_{\frac{1}{2}} \ \alpha \left(\frac{1}{A_o}\right)^{n-1}$

$$t_{\frac{1}{2}} = B\left(\frac{1}{A_o}\right)^{n-1} \quad \text{(where B is Constant)}$$

$$\log t_{\frac{1}{2}} = \log B + (n-1)\log\frac{1}{(A)_o}$$

slope = tan 45° = n – 1

1 = n – 1

$$\boxed{n = 2}$$

98. Let orders wrt A, B & C are x, y & z respectively.

Now,

$5 \times 10^{-3} = (0.010)^x (0.005)^y (0.010)^z$ ...(1)

$5 \times 10^{-3} = (0.010)^x (0.005)^y (0.015)^z$ ...(2)

$1 \times 10^{-2} = (0.010)^x (0.010)^y (0.010)^z$ ...(3)

$1.25 \times 10^{-3} = (0.005)^x (0.005)^y (0.010)^z$ ...(4)

Divide $\frac{1}{2}$ –

$$1 = \left(\frac{10}{15}\right)^z$$

$$1 = \left(\frac{2}{3}\right)^z$$

or

$$\left(\frac{2}{3}\right)^o = \left(\frac{2}{3}\right)^z$$

$$\boxed{\therefore z = 0}$$

Divide 3 to 2,

$$\frac{1 \times 10^{-2}}{5 \times 10^{-3}} = (2)^y \left(\frac{2}{3}\right)^z$$

Now, z = 0

So, $\frac{1 \times 10^{-2}}{5 \times 10^{-3}} = 2^y$

$2^1 = 2^y$

$$\boxed{y = 1}$$

Now, Divide $\frac{1}{4}$

$$\frac{5}{1.25} = 2^x$$

$4 = 2^x$

$2^2 = 2^x$

$$\boxed{x = 2}$$

So, Rate law is-

Rate of Reaction $= k(A)^2(B)^1(C)^0$

99.

	2A	+ B ⟶	A_2B
At t = 0	0.1	0.2	0
At t = t	0.1 – 0.04	0.2 – 0.02	0.02

Because (A) left = 0.06 M

∴ (A) reacted = 0.04 M

So, Conc. of A = 0.06 M

Conc. of B = 0.18 M

Rate of Reaction = k (A) $(B)^2$

$= 2 \times 10^{-6} (0.06)(0.18)^2$

$= 3.89 \times 10^{-9}$ mol L^{-1} sec^{-1}

100. Activated Complex is formed at threshold Energy level (i.e at max. energy)

When this decomposes, energy is released.

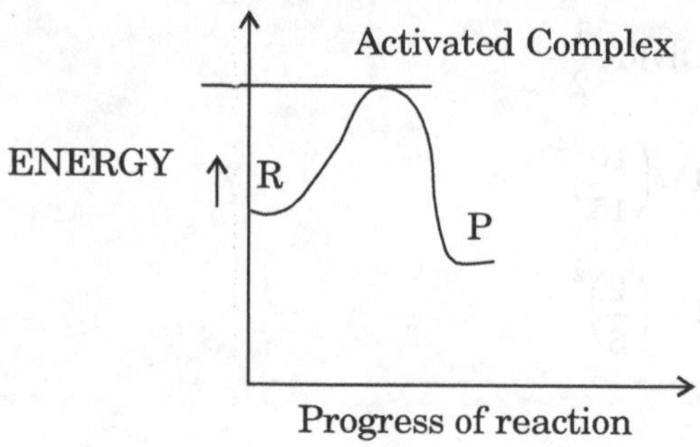

101.

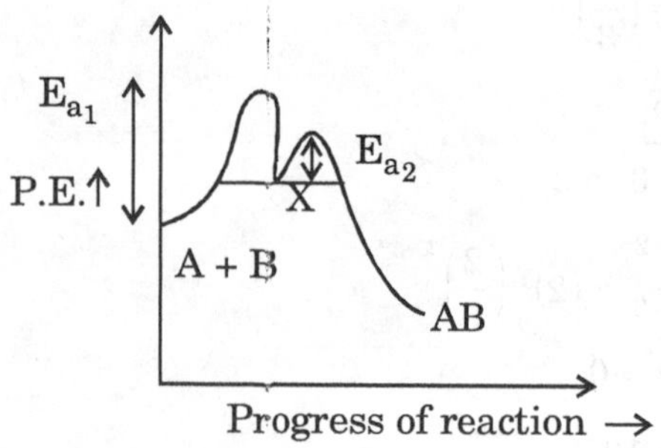

Clearly, $E_{a_1} > E_{a_2}$.

So, $A + B \xrightarrow{E_{a_1}} X(\text{slow})$

$X \xrightarrow{E_{a_2}} AB(\text{fast})$

103. $k = Ae^{\frac{-Ea}{RT}}$

$$\ln k = \ln A + \ln e^{\frac{-Ea}{RT}}$$

$$\ln k = \ln A + \left(\frac{-Ea}{RT}\right)\ln e$$

$$\ln k = \ln A - \frac{Ea}{RT} \quad (\because \ln e = 1)$$

Differentiating both sides-

$$\frac{d}{dT}\ln k = \frac{d}{dT}\ln A - \frac{d}{dT}\left(\frac{Ea}{RT}\right)$$

$$\frac{d}{dT}\ln k = O - \frac{Ea}{R}\frac{d}{dT}(T^{-1})$$

$$\frac{d}{dT}\ln k = -\frac{Ea}{R} \times -1(T^{-1-1})$$

$$\frac{d}{dT}\ln k = \frac{Ea}{R}T^{-2}$$

$$\boxed{\frac{d}{dT}\ln k = \frac{Ea}{RT^2}}$$

104. Reactants in gaseous phase will have lower activation energy in comparison to Reactants in solid phase.

107. Apply,

$$\log\frac{k_2}{k_1} = \frac{Ea}{2.303R}\left(\frac{T_2 - T_1}{T_1 T_2}\right)$$

$$\log\frac{2k_1}{k_1} = \frac{Ea}{2.303 \times 8.314 \times 10^{-3}}\left(\frac{310 - 300}{310 \times 300}\right)$$

$$\frac{0.3010 \times 2.303 \times 8.314 \times 10^{-3} \times 310 \times 300}{10} = Ea$$

$$\boxed{53.6 \text{ kJ mol}^{-1} = Ea}$$

5

CHAPTER

Surface Chemistry

1. Which of the following are characteristics of physisorption ?

A. Weak attractive interactions between adsorbent & adsorbate.

B. Monolayer formation of adsorbate on adsorbent.

C. It remains unaffected by change of temperature.

D. It decreases with increase of temperature.

(a) only A & B (b) only B & C

(c) only A & D (d) All of these

2. The correct order of adsorption of gases NH_3, HCl CO_2 & SO_2 on 1gm of charcoal is

(a) $SO_2 > NH_3 > HCl > CO_2$

(b) $SO_2 > HCl > NH_3 > CO_2$

(c) $NH_3 > HCl > CO_2 > SO_2$

(d) None of these

3. Consider the graph below between $\log \frac{x}{m}$ & log p which is straight line at an angle of 45° with an intercept equal to log 2.

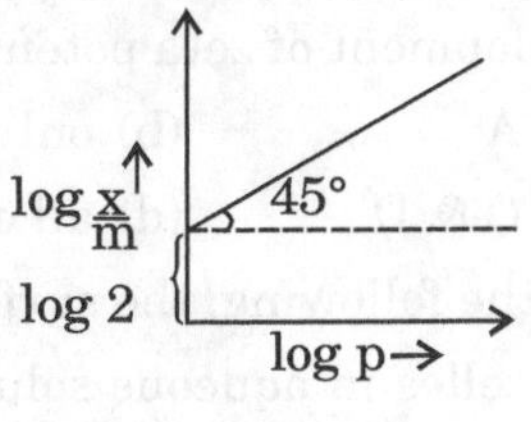

Then, the value of $\frac{x}{m}$ at a pressure of 2 atm is –

(a) 2 (b) 4

(c) 8 (d) 1

4. The incorrect relationship wrt adsorption process is –

(a) $\frac{x}{m} = f(P)$ at constant T

(b) $\frac{x}{m} = f(T)$ at constant P

(c) $P = f(T)$ at constant $(\frac{x}{m})$

(d) $\frac{x}{m} = P \times T$

5. In which of the following processes, both ΔH & ΔS are positive?

(a) Chemisorption of H_2 as H–atoms on the surface of glass.

(b) Adsorption of highly hydrated salts on the solid adsorbent.

(c) Adsorption of N_2 gas on charcoal

(d) Both (a) & (b)

6. Match the colloidal sols. in column – I with their characteristics in column – II

Column– I	**Column – II**
A. As_2S_3	P. Positively charged colloid.
B. Fe $(OH)_3$ sol	Q. negatively charged colloid
C. gold	R. can be formed by peptisation.
D. egg albumin	S. intrinsic colloid.

(a) A – Q, R; B – Q; C – P, D – S

(b) A – Q, R; B – P, R; C – Q; D – S

(c) A – P, R; B – Q,S; C – Q; D – R

(d) None of these

7. In which of the following pairs (both colloids), are an example of multi molecular colloids?

(a) Sulphur sol, gold sol

(b) Gold sol, soap

(c) Sulphur sol, nylon

(d) Nylon, soap

8. Match the entry in column – I with its corresponding entry in column – II.

Column – I	**Column – II**
A. Smoke	i) Aerosol of liquid
B. Milk	ii) Aerosol of solid
C. Cheese	iii) Emulsion
D. Fog	iv) Gel

	A	B	C	D
(a)	ii	i	iii	iv
(b)	iii	ii	iv	i
(c)	i	ii	iii	iv
(d)	ii	iii	iv	i

9. Which one of the following is/are correct?

(a) Movement of dispersion medium under the influence of electric field is termed as electro-osmosis

(b) Movement of colloidal particles under the influence of electric field is called electrodialysis

(c) As_2S_3 is a positively charged sol.

(d) Both (b) & (c) are correct.

10. Which of the following process will not coagulate a lyophobic colloid ?

(a) Persistent electrophoresis

(b) Persistent dialysis

(c) Addition of electrolyte

(d) Addition of lyophillic sol.

11. Lyophillic sols. are more stable than lyophobic sols. because in lyophillic sols.

(a) Colloidal particles have positive charge.

(b) Colloidal particles have negative charge.

(c) There is strong electrostatic repulsion between the dispersed phase & the dispersion medium

(d) Colloidal particles are solvated.

12. The correct order of coagulating power to cause the coagulation of ferric hydroxide sol is–

(a) $K_2CrO_4 > K_4[Fe(CN)_6] > KBr$

(b) $K_4(Fe(CN)_6) > K_2CrO_4 > KBr$

(c) $K_2CrO_4 > KBr > K_4[Fe(CN)_6]$

(d) none of these

13. Gold number is a measure of –

(a) Protective action performed by lyophillic colloid for lyophobic colloid.

(b) Protective action performed by lyophobic colloid for lyophilic colloid.

(c) Randomness of lyophilic colloid

(d) None of these

14. A freshly prepared $Fe(OH)_3$ precipitate is peptised by adding $FeCl_3$ solution. The charge on colloidal particles is due to preferential adsorption of

(a) Cl^- ions (b) Fe^{3+} ions

(d) $\bar{O}H$ ions (d) Both (a) & (c)

15. Colloidal particles carry charges. It can be shown by –

(a) Tyndall effect

(b) electrophoresis

(c) Brownian movement

(d) All of these

16. For A, B & C, the CMC values are 10^{-4} mol/ltr, 10^{-3} mol/ltr & 10^{-1} mol/ltr respectively. Micelles formation will be–

(a) fastest in A (b) fastest in B

(c) fastest in C (d) at same rate in A,B&C

17. Consider the following–

$$AgNO_3 + \underset{(excess)}{KI} \rightarrow \text{silver iodide sol.}$$

The correct statements wrt the above reaction are

A. fixed layer is formed by I^- ions.

B. the diffused layer is formed by K^+ ions.

C. the negative charge on the above colloid is due to preferential adsorption of I^- ions.

D. fixed & diffused layers lead to the development of zeta potential.

(a) only A (b) only B & C

(c) only C & D (d) all of these

18. Among the following, the surfactant that will form micelles in aqueous solution at the lowest molar concentration at ambient conditions is –

(a) $CH_3(CH_2)_{15}N^+(CH_3)_3Br^-$

(b) $CH_3(CH_2)_{11}OSO_3^-Na^+$

(c) $CH_3(CH_2)_6COO^-Na^+$

(d) $CH_3(CH_2)_{11}N^+(CH_3)_3Br^-$

19. In the experiment on electro–osmosis, in which of the following, the level of dispersion medium will fall on the cathode side

(a) Gold sol. (b) Starch sol.

(c) $Fe(OH)_3$ sol. (d) As_2S_3 sol.

20. When O_2 is adsorbed on a metallic surface, electron transfer occurs from metal to O_2. The true statement (s) regarding this adsorption is / are –

(a) Heat is released

(b) Occupancy of $\pi * 2p$ is increased

(c) Bond length of O_2 is increased

(d) All are true.

21. The Coagulation values in milli moles per liter of the electrolytes used for the coagulation of As_2S_3 are given below–

I. (NaCl) = 52, II. ($BaCl_2$) = 0.69,

III. ($MgSO_4$) = 0.22

The correct order of their coagulating power is –

(a) III > II > I (b) III > I > II

(c) I > II > III (d) II > I > III

22. The correct statement (s) pertaining to adsorption of a gas on solid surface is/are

(a) Adsorption is always exothermic

(b) Physisorption may transform into chemisorption at high temperature.

(c) Chemisorption is more exothermic than physisorption, however it is very slow due to greater activation energy.

(d) All are correct.

23. 3 gm of activated charcoal was added to 50 ml of acetic acid solution (0.06 N) in a flask, After an hour, it was filtered & the strength of the filterate was found to be 0.042 N. The amount of acetic acid adsorbed per gm of charcoal is – (assume same volume)

(a) 42 mg (b) 54 mg

(c) 18 mg (d) 36 mg

24. The dispersed phase in colloidal Iron (III) hydroxide & colloidal gold is positively & negatively charged, respectively. Which of the following statements is not correct?

(a) Magnesium chloride solution coagulates the gold sol. more readily than iron (III) hydroxide.

(b) Sodium sulphate solution causes coagulation in both sols.

(c) Mixing the sols. has no effect.

(d) Coagulation in both sols. can be brought about by electrophoresis

25. Gold No.'s of protective colloids A, B, C & D are 0.50, 0.01, 0.10 & 0.005 respectively. The correct order of their protective powers is –

(a) D > B > C > A (b) A > B > C > D

(c) B > D > C > A (d) C > B > A > D

26. Which of the following is INCORRECT ?

(a) Colloidal solution of graphite in H_2O : Aquadag

(b) Colloidal solution of graphite in Oil : Oildag

(c) Colloidal solution of gold : Purple of cassius

(d) None of these

27. Identify the mismatch.

(a) Milk → Emulsion

(b) Cheese → Gel

(c) Muddy water → sol

(d) Hair cream → sol

28. Bredig's arc method is employed for obtaining colloidal solutions of metals like –

(a) Gold (b) Silver

(c) Platinum (d) All of these

29. The stability of colloidal solutions is mainly due to –

(a) Presence of similar charges on colloidal particles.

(b) Brownian motion

(c) Solvation of colloidal particles

(d) All of these

30. Select the correct application.

(a) Colloidal antimony is used to cure Kala azar.

(b) Milk of magnesia is used for stomach disorders.

(c) Argyrol is used as eye lotion.

(d) Colloidal gold is used to treat Arsenic poisoning

31. Select the correct statement (s)

(a) If $FeCl_3$ is added to excess of hot water, a +vely charged sol. of hydrated ferric oxide is formed due to adsorption of Fe^{3+} ions.

(b) When $FeCl_3$ is added to NaOH, a negatively charged sol. is obtained with adsorption of $\bar{O}H$ ions

(c) Metal hydroxide sols like $Al(OH)_3$, $Cr(OH)_3$ are + vely charged.

(d) All are correct.

32. Which of the following is NOT a lyophobic colloid?
(a) Starch sol
(b) Gold sol
(d) As_2S_3 sol
(d) $Fe(OH)_3$ sol

33. Which one of the following does not involve coagulation?
(a) Peptization
(b) Formation of delta
(c) Treatment of drinking water by potash alum
(d) Clotting of blood by $FeCl_3$.

34. Which of the following kinds of catalysis can be explained by the adsorption theory ?
(a) Heterogenous catalysis
(b) Homogenous catalysis
(c) Acid base catalysis
(d) Enzyme catalysis

35. Match the entry in Column –I with its corresponding entry in Column – II.

Column - I	Column - II
(i) Occlusion	A. Adsorption of gas on metal surface.
(ii) Coagulation	B. Conversion of precipitate to colloid.
(iii) Gelatin	C. Lyophillic colloid
(iv) Peptisation	D. Conversion of latex of rubber

(a) (i) – A, (ii) – D, (iii) – C, (iv) – B
(b) (i) – B, (ii) – D, (iii) – A, (iv) – C
(c) (i) – B, (ii) – A, (iii) – C, (iv) – D
(d) none of these

36. The function of ice in Bredig's arc method is to–
(a) Increase the vapour pressure
(b) Increases the temperature of apparatus
(c) Fetch water
(d) Condense the metal vapours.

37. The substances, which at low concentrations behave as strong electrolytes but at higher concentrations exhibit colloidal behavior are –
(a) Associated colloids
(b) Multi molecular colloids
(c) Macro molecular colloids
(d) All of these

38. Cottrell precipitator (Smoke Precipitator) works on the principle of –
(a) absorption
(b) centrifugation
(c) neutralization of charges on colloids
(d) addition of electrolytes

39. To coagulate 100 ml of a colloid, 1 litre of 0.03 N $MgCl_2$ is required. Then flocculation value of $MgCl_2$ is –
(a) 150 (b) 300
(c) 100 (d) 600

40. A colloidal sol of a substance 'X' is a reversible sol & is highly stable towards coagulation by addition of electrolyte. 'X' may be colloidal sol of –
(a) Metal (b) Metal sulphide
(c) Gum (d) Sulphur

41. On addition of 1 ml solution of 10% NaCl to 10 ml gold sol in the presence of 0.5 gm of starch, the coagulation is Just prevented. The gold number of starch is-
(a) 50 (b) 500
(c) 0.5 (d) 250

42. The ability of an ion to bring about coagulation of a given colloid depends upon-
(a) its size
(b) magnitude of its charge only
(c) sign of its charge
(d) both magnitude & sign of its charge.

43. On addition of a catalyst to a reversible reaction,
(a) value of equilibrium constant is increased.
(b) value of equilibrium constant is decreased.
(c) equilibrium concentrations are changed.
(d) equilibrium concentrations remain the same.

44. Under the influence of an electric field, the particles in a sol migrate towards cathode. The coagulation of the same sol is studied using NaCl, Na_2SO_4 and Na_3PO_4 solutions of same molarity. Coagulation value will be maximum for-
(a) NaCl (b) Na_2SO_4
(c) Na_3PO_4 (d) Same for all

45. Which of the following colloids act as an emulsifier for ice cream?
(a) Starch (b) Cellulose
(c) Casein (d) Gelatin

46. Which of the following is based upon Tyndall effect?

A. Tail of comet B. Delta formation

C. Blue colour of sky D. Coagulation

(a) both A & B (b) both A & C

(c) both B & C (d) both C & D

47. 500 ml of 0.3 M $AgNO_3$ is added to 600 ml of 0.5 MKI solution. The species which will move towards cathode & anode, respectively are-

(a) $\frac{AgI}{I^-}$ & NO_3^- (b) $\frac{AgI}{I}$ & K^+

(c) K^+ & $\frac{AgI}{I^-}$ (d) $\frac{AgI}{K^+}$ & I^-

48. Gold number of gum arabic is 0.15. The amount of gum arabic required to protect 100 ml of red gold sol from coagulation by 10 ml of 10% NaCl solution is-

(a) 0.15 millimoles (b) 0.15 mg

(d) 15 mg (d) None of these

49. Which of the following graphs is/are correct?

(a)

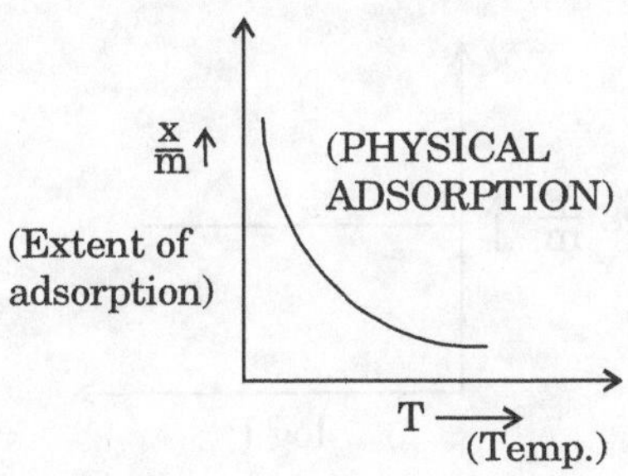

(b)

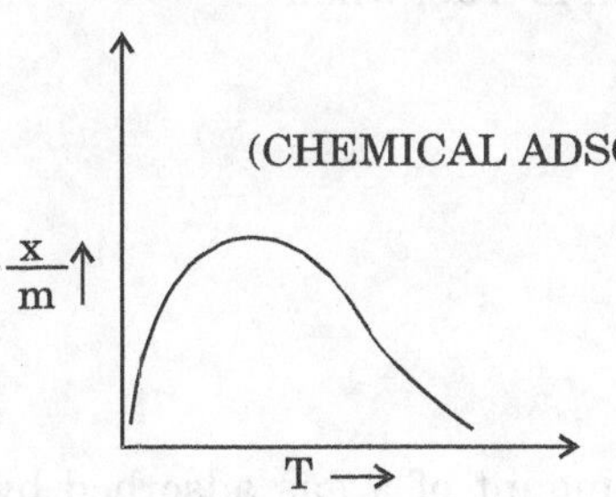

(c)

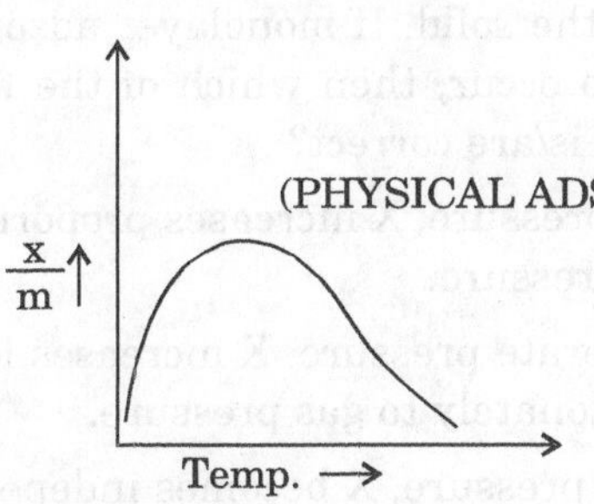

(d) Both (a) & (b) are correct.

50. Which one of the following is a man made macromolecule?

(a) Starch (b) Cellulose

(c) Protein (d) Nylon

51. Which of the following will show Tyndall effect?

(a) Aq. solution of soap below CMC value.

(b) Aq. solution of soap above critical micellisation concentration.

(c) Aq. solution of NaCl

(d) Aq. solution of sugar

52. Which of the following Curves is in accordance with Freundlich adsorption isotherm?

(a)

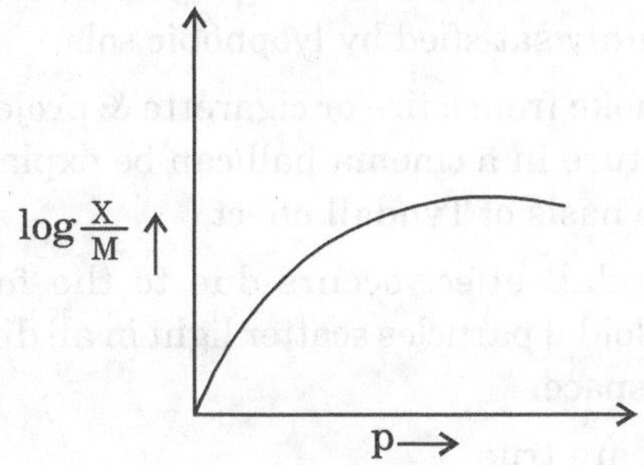

(b)

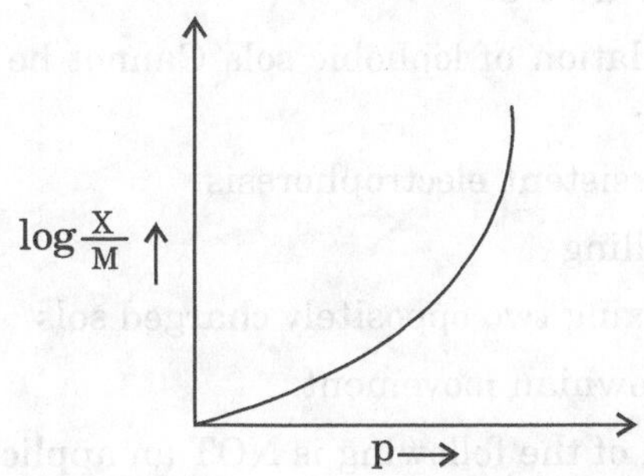

(c)

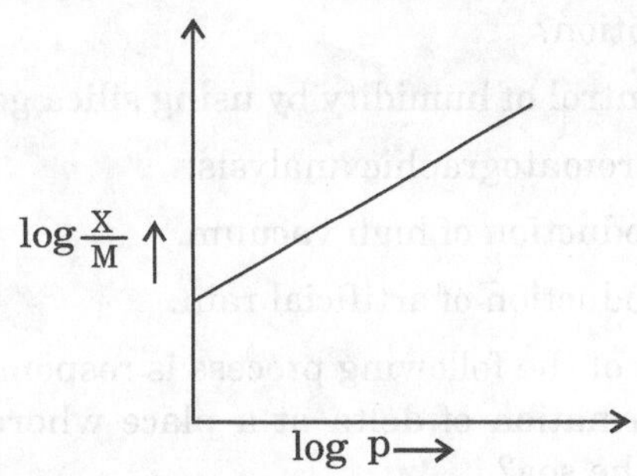

(c) None of these

53. Select the true statement (s).

(a) The temperature above which micelle formation occurs is called Kraft temperature.

(b) Lyophilic colloids (Reversible Colloids) cannot be coagulated easily

(c) Lyophobic sol can be protected by lyophilic sol from coagulation.

(d) All are correct.

54. Variation of adsorption with pressure at different constant temperatures is shown-

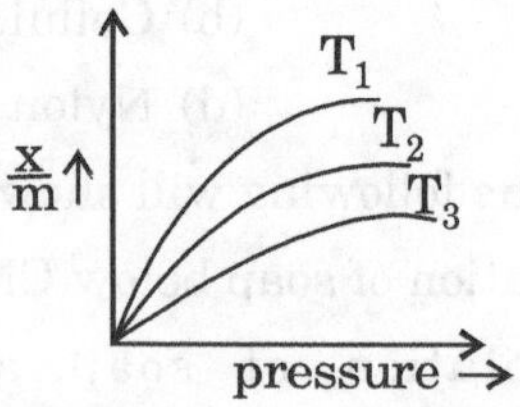

T_1, T_2 & T_3 respectively can be-

(a) 195K, 224K, 273K (b) 224K, 195K, 273K

(c) 225K, 223K, 373K (d) 225K, 161K, 273K

55. What is true about Tyndall effect?

(a) Conditions for showing Tyndall effect are mainly satisfied by lyophobic sols.

(b) Smoke from a fire or cigarette & projection of picture in a cinema hall can be explained on the basis of Tyndall effect

(c) Tyndall effect occurs due to the fact that colloidal particles scatter light in all directions in space.

(d) All are true

56. Coagulation of lophobic sols Cannot be carried out by-

(a) Persistent electrophoresis

(b) Boiling

(c) Mixing two oppositely charged sols

(d) Brownian movement

57. Which of the following is NOT an application of adsorption?

(a) Control of humidity by using silica gels.

(b) Chromatographic analysis.

(c) Production of high vacuum.

(d) Production of artificial rain.

58. Which of the following process is responsible for the formation of delta at a place where rivers meet the sea?

(a) Emulsification (b) Colloid formation

(c) Coagulation (d) Peptisation

59. Select the incorrect statement.

(a) A liquid dispersed in a solid is called gel.

(b) A liquid dispersed in a liquid is called emulsion.

(c) Collodion refers to colloidal sol of cellulose nitrate in a mixture of ethyl alcohol & ether.

(d) None of these

60. In Freundlich adsorption isotherm, the value of $\frac{1}{n}$ is-

(a) between 0 & 1 in all cases.

(b) between 2 & 4 in all cases.

(c) 1 in case of physical adsorption.

(d) Both (b) & (c)

61. Which of the following factors affect adsorption of gases by solids?

(a) Surface area of the adsorbent

(b) Nature of gas being adsorbed

(c) Temperature & Pressure

(d) All of these

62. Bredig's arc method involves-

(a) Dispersion of metal

(b) Condensation of metal

(c) Dispersion as well as condensation

(d) None of these

63. Consider the following graph between log $\frac{x}{m}$ & log P.

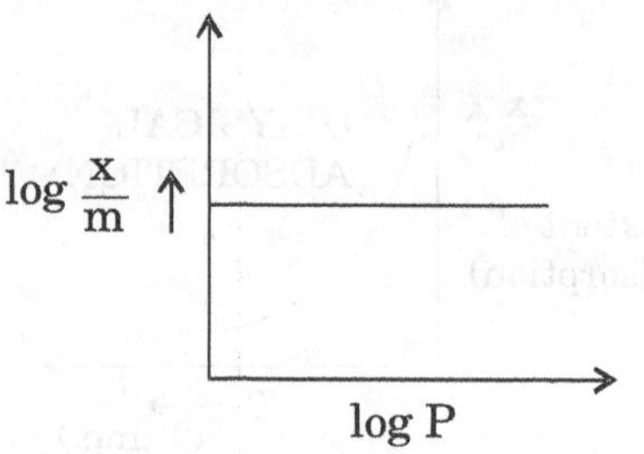

Above graph is true, when-

(a) P = 0

(b) P = 1

(c) $\frac{1}{n} = 1$

(d) $\frac{1}{n} = 0$

64. 'X' is the amount of a gas adsorbed by a fixed amount of the solid. If monolayer adsorption is supposed to occur, then which of the following statements is/are correct?

(a) At low pressure, X increases proportionately to gas pressure.

(b) At moderate pressure, X increases less than proportionately to gas pressure.

(c) At high pressure, X becomes independent of gas pressure.

(d) All are correct.

65. The number of moles of lead nitrate needed to coagulate 2 moles of colloidal AgI is/are-

(a) 2 (b) 1

(c) $\frac{1}{2}$ (d) $\frac{2}{3}$

66. 1 mole of (AgI) Ag^+ sol. is exactly coagulated by-

(a) 1 mole of KI (b) 500 ml of 1 M K_2SO_4

(c) Both (a) & (b) (d) 2 moles of KI

67. SnO_2 is shaken with a small amount of NaOH solution to form a colloidal sol of sodium stannate. The sol thus obtained can be coagulated most easily by-

(a) Na_3PO_4 (b) $AlCl_3$

(c) $K_4[Fe(CN)_6]$ (d) HCl

68. The dispersed phase, dispersion medium & the nature of colloidal solution of 'gold sol' respectively are-

(a) Solid, solid, lyophobic

(b) liquid, liquid, lyophobic

(c) solid, liquid, lyophobic

(d) solid, solid, lyophillic

69. Gels, on standing, exude small amount of liquid. This phenomenon is called-

(a) Efflorescence (b) Syneresis

(c) Thixotropy (d) Adsorption

70. The potential difference between the fixed charged layer & the diffused layer having opposite charge, is called-

(a) Zeta potential

(b) Colloidal potential

(c) Electrokinetic potential

(d) Both (a) & (c)

71. In both, dialysis and osmosis, which particles do not pass through a semipermeable membrane-

(a) water (b) colloids

(c) small molecules (d) All of these

72. Gas masks containing activated charcoal removes poisonous gases from atmosphere & it acts on the principle of-

(a) adsorption

(b) absorption

(c) occlusion

(d) None of these

73. In homogenous catalysis, the catalyst & the reactant are in the same-

(a) Energy (b) System

(c) Physical state (d) None of these

74. Water, carrying impurities is purified by addition of potash alum. Al^{3+} of the potash alum causes-

(a) Peptisation of –vely charged turbidity.

(b) Coagulation of –vely charged turbidity.

(c) Peptisation of +vely charged turbidity

(d) Coagulation of +vely charged turbidity

75. 3.6 gm of oxygen is adsorbed on 1.2 g of metal powder, what volume of oxygen is adsorbed per gram of adsorbent at STP is-

(a) 2.1 L (b) 6.7 L

(c) 5.4 L (d) 9.2 L

76. A detergent having molecular formula $C_{12}H_{25}SO_4^-Na^+$ forms a solution and becomes a colloidal sol at a concentration of 10^{-3} M. On an average, 10^{13} colloidal particles are present in 1 mm^3. The average number of ions present in one colloidal particle (micelle) is-

(a) 50 (b) 60

(c) 40 (d) 30

77. Protective action is performed by 'A' colloids for 'B' colloids. So, A & B are, respectively

(a) lyophillic and lyophillic

(b) lyophillic and lyophobic

(c) lyophobic and lyophillic

(d) lyophobic and lyophobic

78. Match the entry in column-I with its corresponding entry in column-II.

Column-I	Column – II
i. ZSM – 5	x. Test of charge on colloidal particle.
ii. Gas mask	y. Freundlich adsorption isotherm
iii. Electrophoresis	z. Methanol to gasoline
iv. $\frac{x}{m} = Kp^{\frac{1}{n}}$	t. Activated charcoal

	(i)	(ii)	(iii)	(iv)
(a)	t	z	x	y
(b)	x	t	y	z
(c)	z	t	x	y
(d)	y	z	x	t

79. Match the following

	Column-I	Column-II
A.	Physical adsorption	1) $\frac{x}{m} = Kp^{\frac{1}{n}}$
B.	Chemisorption	2) Bulk phenomenon
C.	Freundlich adsorption isotherm	3) Multilayered
D.	Absorption	4) Unilayered

	A	B	C	D
(a)	1	2	3	4
(b)	3	4	1	2
(c)	2	3	1	4
(d)	3	4	2	1

80. A substance which forms micelles in the solution, contains-

(a) carboxylic group

(b) alkyl groups

(c) water insoluble long hydrocarbon group & water soluble polar group

(d) water soluble hydrocarbon group & water insoluble polar group.

81. On adding $AgNO_3$ solution into KI solution, a negatively charged colloidal sol is obtained when they are mixed as follows-

(a) 100 ml of 0.1M $AgNO_3$ + 100 ml of 0.1 M KI

(b) 100 ml of 0.1M $AgNO_3$ + 100 ml of 0.2 M KI

(c) 100 ml of 0.2M $AgNO_3$ + 100 ml of 0.1 M KI

(d) None of these

82. Chemisorption initially increases with increasing temperature. It is attributed to the reason that chemisorption involves-

(a) low value of ΔH

(b) +ve value of enthalpy change

(c) low activation energy

(d) high activation energy

83. In an experiment, addition of 4ml of 0.005 M $BaCl_2$ to 16 ml of As_2S_3 sol. just causes coagulation in 2 hrs. The effective ion & its coagulating value is-

(a) Ba^{2+}, 1.25

(b) Cl^-, 2.25

(c) Cl^-, 1.75

(d) Ba^{2+}, 2

84. Which of the following reactions will result in the formation of gold sol?

(a) $AuCl_3 + SnCl_2 \longrightarrow$

(b) $AuCl_3 + HCHO + H_2O \longrightarrow$

(c) $AuCl_3 + NH_2NH_2 \longrightarrow$

(d) All of these

85. Which of the following is an associated colloid?

(a) Rubber (b) Nylon

(c) Gold sol (d) Soap sol

86. Select the Macromolecular colloid.

(a) starch

(b) gold sol

(c) sulphur sol

(d) both (b) and (c)

87. Select the incorrect match

(a) Solid (D.P.) & Gas (D. M.) $\rightarrow$ Aerosol

(b) Solid(D.P.) & solid (D.M.) $\rightarrow$ Solid sol

(c) Liquid (D.P.) & solid (D.M.) $\rightarrow$ Gel

(d) None of these

88. Which of the following statement is/are correct?

(a) lyophillic sols are reversible in nature.

(b) lyophillic sols are usually formed by organic substances like starch & proteins.

(c) lyophobic sols are usually formed by inorganic materials like metals, their sulphides

(d) All are correct.

89. Tyndall effect-

(1) refers to scattering of light by colloidal particles

(2) helps to confirm the heterogeneous nature of colloidal solutions.

(3) is observed when there is large difference in the refractive indices of dispersed phase

(4) is observed when diameter of dispersed particles is not much smaller as compared to wavelength of light used.

(a) only 1, 2 & 3 are correct

(b) only 2 & 3 are correct

(c) only 3 & 4 are correct

(d) All are correct.

90. What happens when a lyophilic sol is added to a lyophobic sol?

(a) Lyopohilic sol is protected

(b) Lyophobic sol is protected

(c) Film of lyophilic sol is formed over lyophobic sol.

(d) Both (b) & (c)

91. Which of the following will precipitate the negatively charged emulsions?

(a) urea (b) glucose

(c) KCl (d) All of these

92. A solid adsorbent can be activated by-

(a) making the surface of adsorbent rough

(b) crushing the adsorbent into small pieces

(c) removing the gases already adsorbed

(d) All of these acts.

93. Which of the following forms an intrinsic colloid?

(a) sulphur (b) As_2S_3

(c) $Fe(OH)_3$ (d) None of these

94. Under the influence of an electric field, the particles in a sol migrate towards cathode. The coagulation of the same sol is studied using NaCl, Na_2SO_4 & Na_3PO_4 solutions. Their coagulating values will be in the order:-

(a) $NaCl > Na_2SO_4 > Na_3PO_4$

(b) $Na_2SO_4 > Na_3PO_4 > NaCl$

(c) $Na_3PO_4 > Na_2SO_4 > NaCl$

(d) None of these

95. Which of the following is/are Heterogenous?

(a) True solutions (b) Colloidal solutions

(c) suspension (d) Both (b) & (c)

96. What is true about chemisorption?

(a) It is always reversible.

(b) It forms multimolecular layer.

(c) It does not require any activation energy.

(d) It is specific in nature.

97. The colour of colloidal particles depend upon-

(a) wavelength of scattered light

(b) size & shape of colloidal particles

(c) The manner in which observer receives the light

(d) All of these

98. Bredig's arc method is employed for preparation of colloidal sol of-

(a) Sodium (b) Silver

(c) Gold (d) All of these

99. Gold number refers to-

(a) amount of gold in lyophillic colloid.

(b) volume of gold

(c) weight of lyophillic colloid in kgs.

(d) weight of lyophillic colloid in milli grams.

100. Flocculation value of a coagulating electrolyte is expressed in-

(a) millimoles L^{-1} (b) mol L^{-1}

(c) mg K^{-1} (d) microgram L^{-1}

101. Emulsifier, in milk is-

(a) Fat

(b) Lactic acid

(d) Salicylic acid

(d) Casein

102. For the coagulation of particular colloidal solution, the order of coagulation power of some electrolytes is in the order of $Na_3PO_4 > BaSO_4 > AlCl_3$. Then, in electrophoresis, the dispersed phase particles migrate towards:-

(a) anode

(b) remains stationary at place

(c) migrate randomly

(d) Cathode

103. Which among the following is an incorrect statement?

(1) Milk is oil in liquid type of emulsion.

(2) Gold sol is solid in liquid type of colloid.

(3) Process of converting fresh precipitate into colloid is called peptisation.

(4) Chemical adsorption is multilayered

Brain Teasers

104. The solution of rubber is an example of

(a) Liquid aerosol

(b) Multimolecular colloid

(c) Associated colloid

(d) Macromolecular colloid

Answers

1. (c)	**2.** (a)	**3.** (b)	**4.** (d)	**5.** (d)	**6.** (b)	**7.** (a)	**8.** (d)	**9.** (a)	**10.** (d)
11. (d)	**12.** (b)	**13.** (a)	**14.** (b)	**15.** (b)	**16.** (a)	**17.** (d)	**18.** (a)	**19.** (c)	**20.** (d)
21. (a)	**22.** (d)	**23.** (c)	**24.** (c)	**25.** (a)	**26.** (d)	**27.** (d)	**28.** (d)	**29.** (d)	**30.** (d)
31. (d)	**32.** (a)	**33.** (a)	**34.** (a)	**35.** (a)	**36.** (d)	**37.** (a)	**38.** (c)	**39.** (a)	**40.** (b)
41. (b)	**42.** (d)	**43.** (d)	**44.** (a)	**45.** (d)	**46.** (b)	**47.** (c)	**48.** (a)	**49.** (d)	**50.** (d)
51. (b)	**52.** (c)	**53.** (d)	**54.** (a)	**55.** (d)	**56.** (d)	**57.** (d)	**58.** (c)	**59.** (d)	**60.** (a)
61. (d)	**62.** (c)	**63.** (d)	**64.** (d)	**65.** (b)	**66.** (c)	**67.** (b)	**68.** (c)	**69.** (b)	**70.** (d)
71. (b)	**72.** (a)	**73.** (c)	**74.** (b)	**75.** (a)	**76.** (b)	**77.** (b)	**78.** (c)	**79.** (b)	**80.** (c)
81. (b)	**82.** (d)	**83.** (a)	**84.** (d)	**85.** (d)	**86.** (a)	**87.** (d)	**88.** (d)	**89.** (d)	**90.** (d)
91. (c)	**92.** (d)	**93.** (d)	**94.** (a)	**95.** (d)	**96.** (d)	**97.** (d)	**98.** (a)	**99.** (d)	**100.** (a)
101. (d)	**102.** (d)	**103.** (d)	**104.** (d)						

Explanations

2. Greater the attractive forces, greater is T_c & greater is extent of adsorption.

5. Wrt freundlich's adsorption isotherm,

$$\frac{x}{m} = K P^{\frac{1}{n}}$$

$$\log \frac{x}{m} = \log K + \log P^{\frac{1}{n}}$$

$$\log \frac{x}{m} = \log K + \frac{1}{n} \log P$$

$$\downarrow \qquad \qquad \downarrow$$

$$y = c + m x$$

So, $\log K = \log 2$

$\boxed{K = 2}$

$$\text{Slope} = \frac{1}{n} = \tan 45°$$

$\boxed{n = 1}$

Apply,

$$\frac{x}{m} = KP^{\frac{1}{n}}$$

$$\frac{x}{m} = 2 \times 2^{\frac{1}{1}} = 4$$

12. $Fe(OH)_3$ is a +vely charged colloid. According to HARDY SCHULZE Rule, greater the valence (charge) on ion, greater is its coagulating power. $[Fe(CN)_6]^{4-}$ will have max. coagulating power, followed by CrO_4^{2-} & then Br^-.

16. CMC value is the concentration above which micelle formation occurs.

17. $AgNO_3 + \underset{(excess)}{KI} \longrightarrow AgI\downarrow + KNO_3$

$$\begin{array}{l|l} Ag\,I & I^- \quad K^+ \\ Ag\,I & I^- \quad K^+ \rightarrow \text{diffused layer} \\ Ag\,I & I^- \quad K^+ \end{array}$$

$\downarrow$

fixed layer

18. Greater the hydrophobic part, lesser is the solubility in water & greater is the tendency to form micelles.

19. $Fe(OH)_3$ sol is a +vely charged sol & the dispersion medium will be –vely charged & hence move towards anode (which is +ve). So, dispersion medium will fall on cathode side.

21. Coagulation values & coagulating power are inversely related.

23. Milli eqvt. of acetic acid initially = $0.06 \times 50 = 3$

Milli eqvt. left = $0.042 \times 50 = 2.1$

Milli eqvt. of acetic acid adsorbed = $3 - 2.1 = 0.9$
weight of acetic acid adsorbed = $0.9 \times 60 = 54$ mg

Acetic acid adsorbed on 3g charcoal = 54

Acetic acid adsorbed on 1g charcoal = $\frac{54}{3} = 18\text{mg}$

25. Gold No.'s & protective power are inversely related.

27. Hair Cream is an emulsion.

30. Colloidal gold is used for inter-muscular injections.

31. Wrt option (a) & (b)-

$Fe_2O_3.\ xH_2O/Fe^{3+}$

+vely charged

$Fe_2O_3 . \times H_2O / \overline{O}H$

–vely charged

39. For $MgCl_2$, n factor = 2

N = M × n factor

$0.03 = M \times 2$

$\boxed{M = 0.015\,M}$

Volume of $MgCl_2$ chosen = 1 ltr

So, no. of moles of $MgCl_2$ = 0.015

Millimoles of $MgCl_2 = 0.015 \times 1000 = 15$ milli moles

To coagulate 100 ml colloid, milli moles of $MgCl_2$ req. = 15

To Coagulate 1000 ml colloid, milli moles of $MgCl_2$

req. $= \frac{15}{100} \times 1000 = 150$

40. lyophilic sols are reversible.

41. Gold no. refers to wt. of lyophillic colloid (Starch) in milligrams.

∴ Weight of starch = $0.5 \times 1000 = 500$ mg

44. Since the sol particles migrate towards cathode, sol particles must be +vely charged & to coagulate it, Cl^- (from NaCl), SO_4^{2-} (from Na_2SO_4) & PO_4^{3-} (from Na_3PO_4), will participate.

Now, Coagulating power follows the order-

$PO_4^{3-} > SO_4^{2-} > Cl^-$

∴ Coagulating value follows the order-

$Cl^- > SO_4^{2-} > PO_4^{3-}$

47. No. of moles of $AgNO_3 = 0.3 \times \frac{500}{1000} = 0.15$

No. of moles of KI $= 0.5 \times \frac{600}{1000} = 0.3$

So, KI is in excess

$$\underset{}{AgNO_3} + \underset{(\text{excess})}{KI} \longrightarrow AgI \downarrow + KNO_3$$

AgI will preferentially adsorb common ions i.e. I^- ions from medium.

∴ AgI/I (–vely Charged colloid) ↓ Migrate towards anode & K^+ ↓ Migrate towards cathode

48. According to definition,

The amount required for 10 ml of gold sol = 0.15 mg

∴ the amount required for 100 ml of gold sol

$= \frac{0.15}{10} \times 100 = 1.5$ mg

49. Physical adsorption decreases with increase in temperature.

Chemical adsorption first increases, reaches maximum & then decreases, with increase in temperature.

52. According to freundlich's adsorption isotherm-

$$\frac{x}{m} = K P^{\frac{1}{n}}$$

$$\log \frac{x}{m} = \log K + \log P^{\frac{1}{n}}$$

$$\boxed{\log \frac{x}{m} = \log K + \frac{1}{n} \log P}$$ FIG

$$y = c + m\,x$$

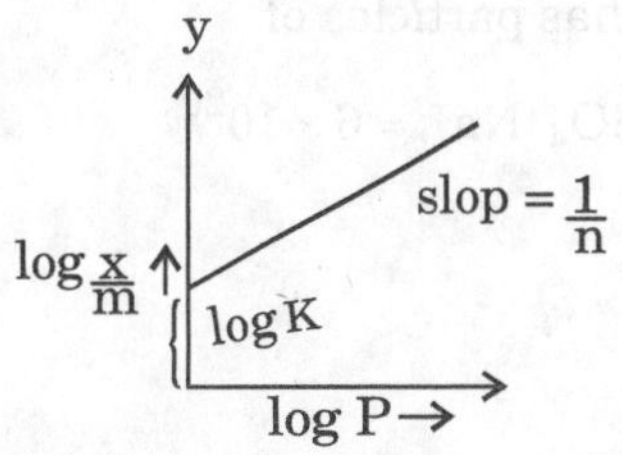

54. extent of adsorption will be max. at low temperature.

63. Apply, $\log \frac{x}{m} = \log K + \frac{1}{n} \log P$

Slope of graph $= \frac{1}{n} = 0$

64. Follow Freundlich's adsorption isotherm.

65. $Pb(NO_3)_2 + 2AgI \longrightarrow 2AgNO_3 + PbI_2$

From equation, it is evident that 1 mole of $Pb(NO_3)_2$ is needed to coagulate 2 moles of AgI.

66. $(AgI)\,Ag^+$ is a +vely charged colloid.

1 mole of KI will furnish 1 mole of I^- which will coagulate the sol.

Also, 500 ml of 1 M K_2SO_4 means 0.5 moles of K_2SO_4 which will in turn furnish 0.5 moles of SO_4^{2-} reqd. to coagulate 1 mole of $(AgI)\,Ag^+$.

$$(AgI)Ag^+ + KI \longrightarrow AgI\downarrow + AgI\downarrow + K^+$$

$$2(AgI)Ag^+ + K_2SO_4 \longrightarrow AgI + Ag_2SO_4$$

67. $SnO_2 + 2NaOH \longrightarrow Na_2SnO_3 + H_2O$

$$SnO_2 + SnO_3{}^{2-} \longrightarrow \underset{\text{negatively charged colloid}}{\underbrace{(SnO_2)\,SnO_3^{2-}}}$$

Now, in order to coagulate a negatively charged colloid, cation with max. +ve charge is required according to HARDY SCHULZE Rule.

So, among the given options, Al^{3+} will coagulate it most easily.

75. 1.2 gm adsorbent, absorbs O_2 = 3.6 gm

1 gm adsorbent, absorbs $O_2 = \frac{3.6}{1.2} = 3g$

Now, 32 gm O_2 at STP = 22.4 L

3gm O_2 at STP $= \frac{22.4}{32} \times 3 = 2.1$ L

76. No. of particles of

$C_{12}H_{25}SO_4^-\,Na^+ = 10^{-3} \times 6 \times 10^{23} = 6 \times 10^{20}$.

So, 1 ltr has particles of

$C_{12}H_{25}SO_4^-\,Na^+ = 6 \times 10^{20}$ or

1000 ml has particles of

$C_{12}H_{25}SO_4^-\,Na^+ = 6 \times 10^{20}$

1000×10^3 mm³ has particles of

$C_{12}H_{25}SO_4^-\,Na^+ = \frac{6 \times 10^{20}}{1000 \times 10^3}$

1 mm³ has particles of

$C_{12}H_{25}SO_4^-\,Na^+ = 6 \times 10^{14}$

No. of colloidal particles per mm³ = 10^{13}.

So, number of ions per colloidal particle

$= \frac{6 \times 10^{14}}{10^{13}} = 60$

83. Millimoles of $BaCl_2$ added = 0.005 × 4 = 0.02

16 ml of As_2S_3 is coagulated by $BaCl_2$ = 0.02 milli moles

1000 ml of As_2S_3 is coagulated by $BaCl_2$

$= \frac{0.02}{16} \times 1000 = 1.25$

As_2S_3 is a –vely charged colloid, so cation is required to coagulate it.

84. $2AuCl_3 + 3SnCl_2 \longrightarrow 2Au + 3SnCl_4$

$2AuCl_3 + 3HCHO + 3H_2O \longrightarrow 2Au + 3HCOOH + 6HCl$

$4AuCl_3 + 3NH_2NH_2 \longrightarrow 4Au + 3N_2 + 12HCl$

94. If colloidal particles migrate towards cathode, they will themselves be +vely charged.

To coagulate, +vely charged particles, anion is required.

Coagulating power:-

$PO_4^{3-} > SO_4^{2-} > Cl^-$

Coagulating value

$Cl^- > SO_4^{2-} > PO_4^{3-}$

102. If coagulating power is in order, $PO_4^{3-} > SO_4^{2-} > Cl^-$, then it must be a positively charged colloid i.e. the dispersed phase particles must be carrying +ve charge, so will migrate towards cathode.

103. Chemical adsorption is monolayered

6

CHAPTER

General Principles and Process of Isolation of Elements

Extraction of Metals Ores, Concentration of Ores

1. Which of the following minerals contains Titanium?

(a) Cassiterite (b) Rutile

(c) Haematite (d) Spodumene

2. Cinnabar is generally concentrated by

(a) froth floatation (b) roasting

(c) gravity separation (d) reduction by carbon

3. Aluminium is present in bauxite as well as beryl, but generally it is extracted from bauxite and not from beryl because

(a) bauxite is an ore where as beryl is a mineral

(b) beryl is an ore where as bauxite is a mineral

(c) it can be extracted profitably from bauxite and not from beryl

(d) both (a) & (c)

4. Leaching of silver is carried out by heating it with a dilute solution of

(a) NaCN (b) HCI

(c) NaOH (d) NaCN in presence of O_2

5. Which of the following salts is least likely to be found in minerals?

(a) Chloride (b) Sulphate

(c) Sulphide (d) Nitrate

6. Which of the following ores is best concentrated by froth floatation method ?

(a) Magnetite (b) Cassiterite

(c) Cinnabar (d) Malachite

7. Metal which can be extracted from dolomite, magnesite and carnallite is

(a) Na (b) K

(c) Mg (d) Ca

8. Which of the following substances consists of only one element?

(a) Chalk (b) Quartz

(c) Graphite (d) Tin stone

9. Which of the following is an example of halide ore?

(a) Fluorspar (b) Sylvine

(c) Carnallite (d) All of these

10. Iron is mainly extracted from

(a) haematite (b) siderite

(c) pyrites (d) malachite

11. An example of an oxide ore is

(a) copper glance (b) malachite

(c) cuprite (d) feldspar

12. Which of the following represents the formula of the ore cryolite?

(a) $Na_2Al_2O_3$ (b) Na_3AlF_6

(c) CaF_2 (d) $KAlSi_3O_8$

13. Sulphide ores are generally concentrated by
(a) froth floatation process
(b) magnetic separation
(c) gravity separation
(d) leaching

14. Which of the following ores can be concentrated by magnetic separation?
(a) Galena (b) Cinnabar
(c) Haematite (d) Cuprite

15. Mac Arthur forest cyanide process is used in the extraction of
A. gold
B. silver
C. platinum
(a) both A & C (b) A only
(c) both B & C (d) both A & B

16. Which of the following method is used to concentrate Cassiterite ore?
(a) Leaching
(b) Electromagnetic separation
(c) Froth Floatation
(d) Smelting

17. Froth floatation process used for the concentration of ores is a practical application of
(a) coagulation (b) liquation
(c) absorption (d) adsorption

18. Wolframite and tin stone can be seperated by
(a) magnetic separation
(b) froth floatation
(c) leaching method
(d) gravity separation

19. Froth-floatation method is successful in separating impurities from ores because
(a) pure ore is lighter than water
(b) pure ore is insoluble in pine oil, fatty acid etc.
(c) impurities are soluble in water containing additives like pine oil, fatty acid etc.
(d) pure ore is not as easily wetted by water as by pine oil, fatty acid etc

20. The ore zinc blende is concentrated by
(a) froth floatation
(b) magnetic separation
(c) chemical separation
(d) hydraulic washing

21. The method of concentrating the ore which makes use of the difference in density between ore and impurities is called
A. Liquifaction B. Hydraulic washing
C. Levigation
(a) both A & C (b) A only
(c) both A & B (d) both B & C

22. A high melting compound, which is mixed with the ore for removal of acidic impurities, is
(a) SiO_2 (b) CaO
(c) HgO (d) $Na_2B_4O_7$

23. The extraction of which of the following metals involves complex formation?
A. Au B. Cu
C. Ag
(a) both B & C (b) A only
(c) both A & B (d) both A & C

24. In metallurgy, benefaction process involves the removal of
(a) slag (b) flux
(c) gangue (d) ore

25. Metallurgy of which of the following ores generally involves roasting as one of the step?
(a) Sulphide ores (b) Carbonate ores
(c) Oxide ores (d) Silicate ores

26. Heating of copper pyrites in oxygen for oxidation of sulphur is called
(a) roasting (b) calcination
(c) smelting (d) slagging

27. The function of calcination in metallurgical operations is
A. to remove moisture
B. to decompose carbonate
C. to remove volatile impurities of S, As, P
(a) A, B & C (b) both B & C
(c) both A & B (d) both A & C

Reduction, Ellingham Diagram

28. The element which is most difficult to be extracted from its oxide using Coke as a reducing agent is
(a) Ag (b) Mg
(c) Hg (d) Si

Directions (Q. 29-31) : Ellingham diagram.

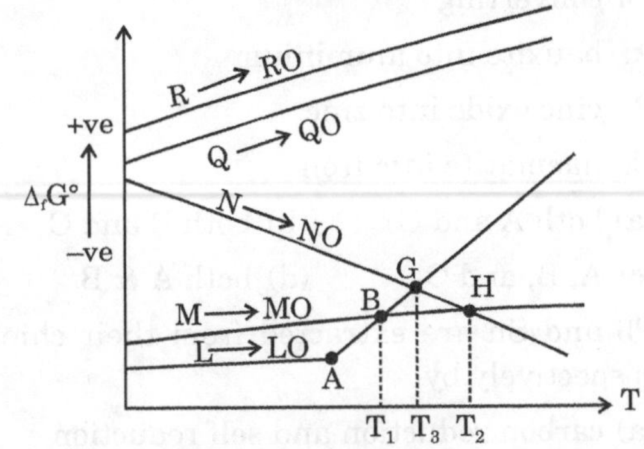

29. Which of the following can act as strongest reducing agent below T_3K?

(a) L (b) M
(c) Q (d) R

30. What is not true above T_3 K?

(a) LO can be reduced with N
(b) MO can not be reduced with Q
(c) MO can be reduced with L
(d) QO can be reduced with M

31. Which of the following oxides may decompose easily on heating?

(a) NO (b) LO
(c) RO (d) MO

32. The basic flux among the following is

(a) silica (b) borax
(c) magnesite (d) galena

33. The main purpose of smelting of an ore is

(a) oxidation of metal
(b) reduction of metal oxide
(c) removal of volatile impurities
(d) to obtain metal in the molten form

34. The reaction which represents the process of smelting is

(a) $CaCO_3 \rightarrow CaO + CO_2$
(b) $2PbS + 3O_2 \rightarrow 2PbO + 2SO_2$
(c) $Fe_2O_3 + 3C \rightarrow 2Fe + 3CO$
(d) $Al_2O_3.2H_2O \rightarrow Al_2O_3 + 2H_2O$

35. The main purpose of adding flux to an ore in the blast furnace is to convert

(a) infusible impurities to fusible material
(b) soluble impurities to insoluble impurities
(c) fusible impurities to infusible impurities
(c) mineral into silicate

36.

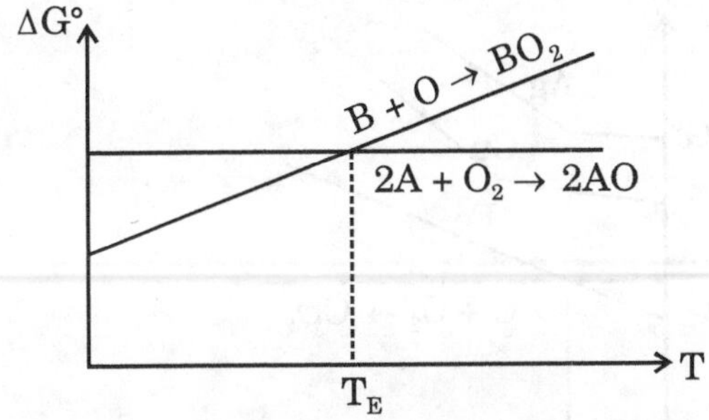

In the ellingham diagram for the solid metals A and B and gaseous oxides BO_2 and AO

A. at $T < T_E$, BO_2 is more stable than AO
B. at $T > T_E$, AO is more stable than BO_2
C. at $T = T_E, \Delta G°_{reduction}$ is equal to zero
D. ΔS is zero for oxidation of A

(a) both A and C (b) both B and D
(c) A, B, and C (d) all are correct

37. A metal which can not be obtained directly by auto reduction of its sulphide ore is

(a) Cu (b) Pb
(c) Hg (d) Zn

38. The highest temperature zone in blast furnace is

(a) reduction zone (b) heat absorption zone
(c) fusion zone (d) combustion zone

39. Which of the following metals is extracted using electrometallurgical process?

(a) Fe (b) Pb
(c) Na (d) Ag

40. The substance used in the thermite process of reducing metal ores is

(a) aluminium (b) hydrogen
(c) tungsten (d) carbon

41. The most suitable method for the extraction of sodium is electrolysis of its molten salt like NaCl. This is because

A. Na is highly electropositive
B. Na is a strong reducing agent
C. Electrolysis of aq.NaCl liberates H_2(g) at cathode

(a) both A and C
(b) both B and C
(c) A, B, and C
(d) both A & B

42. 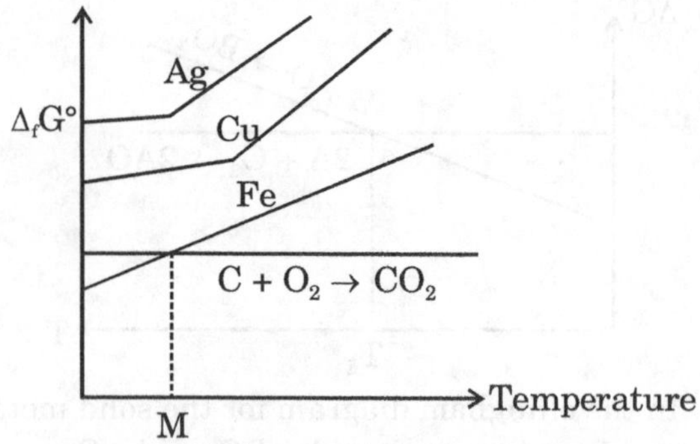

Consider the diagram and choose the INCORRECT statement

(a) Above point M, Ag can reduce oxide of Fe

(b) Fe and C do not show any phase transition

(c) At high temperature, C is the best reducing agent for oxides of Ag, Cu, Fe

(d) Below point M, Cu can reduce oxide of Ag

43. Which of the following statements is not correct about Ellingham diagram?

(a) $\Delta_fG°$ increases with an increase in temperature

(b) It consists of plots of $\Delta_fG°$ versus temperature for formation of oxides

(c) Most of Ellingham curves show positive slope

(d) It expresses the kinetics of the reduction processes

44. Metal that cannot be extracted by carbon reduction process is

(a) Fe (b) Al

(c) Cu (d) Zn

45. $\Delta G°$ vs T plot in the Ellingham diagram slopes downward for the reaction

(a) $Mg + \frac{1}{2}O_2 \rightarrow MgO$

(b) $2Ag + \frac{1}{2}O_2 \rightarrow Ag_2O$

(c) $2C + O_2 \rightarrow 2CO$

(d) $CO + \frac{1}{2}O_2 \rightarrow CO_2$

46. The group of oxides, that cannot be reduced by carbon to give the respective metals, is

(a) Cu_2O, K_2O

(b) Fe_2O_3, ZnO

(c) CaO, K_2O

(d) PbO, Fe_3O_4

47. Pyrometallurgical process of extraction is suitable for converting

A. bauxite into aluminium

B. zinc oxide into zinc

C. haematite into iron

(a) both A and C (b) both B and C

(c) A, B, and C (d) both A & B

48. Pb and Sn are extracted from their chief ores respectively by

(a) carbon reduction and self reduction

(b) self reduction and carbon reduction

(c) electrolysis and self reduction

(d) self reduction and electrolysis

49. After partial roasting, the sulphide of copper is reduced by

(a) reduction by carbon

(b) electrolysis

(c) self-reduction

(d) cyanide process

Methods of Refining and Extraction of Elements

50. One of the following metals forms a volatile compound and the advantage of this property is taken for its purification. This metal can be

A. Titanium

B. Nickel

C. Cobalt

(a) both A and C (b) both A and B

(c) A, B, and C (d) both B & C

51. Which of the following oxides is not removed by reduction in reduction zone of blast furnance during extraction of iron from haematite?

(a) SiO_2 (b) CaO

(c) MnO_2 (d) P_4O_{10}

52. In the extraction of copper from copper pyrites, the molten matte contains

(a) Fe only (b) Cu_2S only

(c) Cu_2S and FeS (d) CuS and Fe_2S_2

53. Which of the following process(es)is not used for purification of Bauxite ore?

(a) Halls process (b) Serpeck's process

(c) Baeyer's process (d) Mond's process

54. During the extraction of iron from haemetite in the blast furnace, the calcium ion ends in the form of

(a) slag (b) gangue
(c) calcium metal (d) CaO

55. The method of zone refining of metals is based on the principle of

(a) greater mobility of pure metal than that of the impurity
(b) higher melting point of the impurity than that of the pure metal
(c) greater noble character of the solid metal than that of the impurity
(d) greater solubility of the impurity in the molten state than in the solid

56. Which of the following processes is not involved in smelting of iron in the blast furnace?

(a) Oxidation (b) Reduction
(c) Decomposition (d) Sublimation

57. The main constituent of slag, obtained during the extraction of copper from copper pyrites, is

(a) $CaSiO_3$ (b) $FeSiO_3$
(c) $CuSiO_3$ (d) SiO_2

58. Which of the following reactions is involved in the final step for the extraction of copper from copper pyrite in Bessemer converter?

(a) $4Cu_2O + FeS \rightarrow 8Cu + FeSO_4$
(b) $Cu_2S + 2Cu_2O \rightarrow 6Cu + SO_2$
(c) $2Cu_2O + FeS \rightarrow 4Cu + Fe + SO_2$
(d) $Cu_2O + 2FeO \rightarrow 2Cu + 2Fe + O_2$

59. In blast furnace, iron oxide can be reduced by

A. Coke above 1073 K B. CO above 1073 K
C. CO below 1073 K

(a) both A and C (b) both A and C
(c) A, B, and C (d) both B and C

60. In alumino-thermite process, aluminium is used as

(a) oxidising agent (b) flux
(c) reducing agent (d) slag

61. Aluminium is prepared in large quantities by

(a) heating cryolite in a limited quantity of air
(b) reduction of alumina with coke
(c) reduction of alumina with sodium
(d) electrolysis of alumina dissolved in cryolite

62. Copper metal is refined by

(a) liquation (b) hydrogen reduction
(c) electrolysis (d) distillation

63. To obtain tungsten from tungsten oxide (WO_3) the method used is

(a) alumino-thermite process
(b) electrolytic reduction
(c) carbon reduction
(d) reduction with hydrogen

64. Gold is extracted by hydrometallurgical process based on its property

(a) of being electro positive
(b) of being less reactive
(c) to form complexes which are water soluble
(d) to form salts which are water soluble

65. Copper metal, from low grade copper ores, can be extracted using

(a) electrometallurgy (b) smelting
(c) pyrometallurgy (d) hydrometallurgy

66. For obtaining highly pure Silicon which is used as a semiconductor material, the method used is

(a) Mond's process
(b) Van Arkel process
(c) Hall's process
(d) Zone refining

Brain Teasers

67. MgO is used as a refractory material in furnaces because

(a) it possesses great structural strength
(b) it can withstand high temperature
(c) it gives oxygen on heating
(d) it is not affected by acids

68. A metal exists as high grade sulphide ore. Which of the following is the correct sequence of steps involved in the preparation of metal from its ore?

(a) froth floatation → roasting → auto reduction → electrolytic refining
(b) leaching → calcination → smelting → liquation
(c) froth floatation → roasting → calcination → electrolytic refining
(d) gravity separation → roasting → reduction with H_2 → poling

69. In a lime kiln, to get higher yield of CO_2, the measure that can be taken is

(a) removal of CaO

(b) addition of more $CaCO_3$

(c) increase of temperature

(c) increase of pressure

70. In the Froth Floatation process, zinc sulphide and lead sulphide can be separated by

(i) using collectors

(ii) adjusting the proportion of oil to water

(iii) using depressant

(iv) using froth stabilisers

(a) both (ii) & (iv) (b) both (i) & (ii)

(c) both (i) & (iv) (d) both (ii) and (iii)

71. Identify the mismatch

(a) Bauxite : aluminium

(b) Magnetite : Iron

(c) Sylvine : NaCl

(d) Fluorspar : CaF_2

72. Match the entries in column-I with their corresponding entries in column-II

Column-I	Column-II
i. Malachite	a. Carbonates
ii. Calamine	b. Oxides
iii. Zincite	c. Sulphides
iv. Sphalerite	d. Both iron &copper
v. Copper pyrites	

(a) i-a, d ; ii-c ; iii-b ; iv-c ; v-c

(b) i-a ; ii-a ; iii-b ; iv-c ; v-c, d

(c) i-b ; ii-a ; iii-b, d ; iv-c ; v-d

(d) i-c ; ii-c, d ; iii-b ; iv-c ; v-a

73. Which are correct statements about the role of substances added in the froth floation process?

(i) Collectors enhance the non-wett ability of the mineral particles

(ii) Collectors enhance the wettability of gangue particles

(iii) By using depressants in the process two sulphide ores can be separated

(iv) Froth stabilisers decrease wettability of gangue

(a) both (ii) & (iv) (b) both (i) & (ii)

(c) both (i) & (iv) (d) both (i) and (iii)

74. Identify the incorrect statement

(a) Cinnabar mainly contains mercuric chloride

(b) Gold is found in native State

(c) Silver glance mainly contains silver sulphide

(d) Copper pyrites is $CuFeS_2$

75. Which of the following ores is a double salt?

A. Dolomite B. Borax

C. Malachite D. Magnesite

E. Carnalite

(a) A, C and E (b) B, C and D

(c) both A and E (d) Both B and D

76. Identify the incorrect statements

A. Aluminium can reduce MgO above 1623K

B. ZnO can be reduced with CO at a high temperature

C. Carbon is used to reduce even the stable oxides like Al_2O_3 and MgO at a high temperature when it gets converted to CO

D. Mg is mostly used to reduce Al_2O_3 below 1623 K

(a) only B (b) B and C

(c) A and D (d) A, B, C and D

77. 'A' is carefully chosen to combine with 'B' present in tho ore to produce easily fusible 'C' to carry away the Impurities. A, B and C respectively are

(a) slag, gangue, flux (b) flux, gangue, slag

(c) gangue, flux, slag (d) slag,

78.

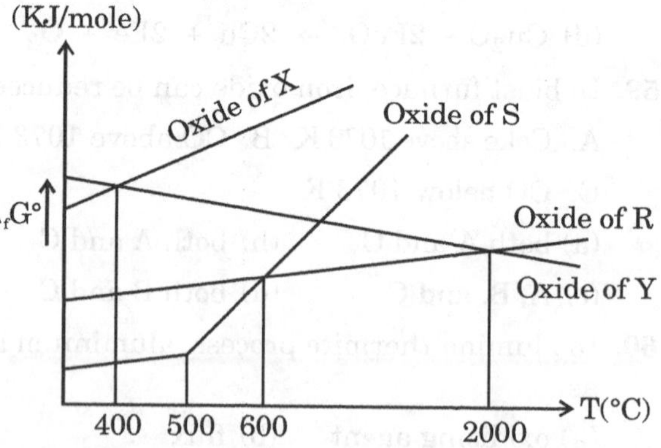

In the above Ellingham diagram

(a) oxide of X can be reduced at any temperature by Y

(b) below 600°C, R can reduce S from its oxide

(c) S can reduce all oxides below 500°C

(d) X can reduce oxides of Y above 600°C

79. Free energy of formation $\Delta_f \overset{\circ}{G}$ of MgO(s) and CO(g) at 1273 K and 2273 K are given below

(i) $\Delta \overset{\circ}{G}_f$[MgO(s)] = –941 kJ/mol at 1273 K

(ii) $\Delta \overset{\circ}{G}_f$[MgO(s)] = –341 kJ / mol at 2273 K

(iii) $\Delta \overset{\circ}{G}_f$CO(g) = –439 kJ / mol at 1273 K

(iv) $\Delta \overset{\circ}{G}_f$CO(g) = –628 kJ / mol at 2273 K

The temperature at which carbon can be used as reducing agent for MgO(s) is

(a) 2273 K (b) 1273 K
(c) < 2273 K (d) data insufficient

80. Why lime stone is added in the extraction of lead from galena?

A. It removes the impurity of silica as fusible slag

B. It converts lead silicate to lead

C. It removes the impurity of iron oxides as fusible slag

(a) only A (b) both A and B
(c) both B and C (d) both A and C

81. If $\Delta_f G°$ is plotted against T, then it is a straight line

A. passing through origin with slope -R In K

B. with intercept ΔH and slope –ΔS

C. with intercept ΔH and slope ΔS

D. passing through orgin with slope -2.303 R log K

(a) only A (b) only B
(c) both C and D (d) A, B and D

82. $CuFeS_2 + O_2 \rightarrow (A) + (B) + SO_2$

$(B) + O_2 \rightarrow (C) + SO_2$

$(C) + SiO_2 \rightarrow (D)$

In the above reactions occurring during extraction of Cu from copper pyrites, which of the following is INCORRECT?

(a) A : Cu_2S (b) B : FeS
(c) C : Fe_2O_3 (d) D : $FeSiO_3$

83. Match the items of Column I with the items of Column II and assign the correct

a. Coloured bands	p. Zone refining
b. Impure metal to volatile complex	q. Fractional distillation
c. Purification of Ge & Si	r. Mond Process
d. Purification of mercury	s. Chromatography
	t. Liquation

(a) a-r, b-s, c-t, d-q (b) a-s, b-r, c-p, d-q
(c) a-p, b-q, c-t, d-r (d) a-q, b-s, c-t, d-r

84. A metal ore is a magnetic oxide ore. The metal obtained by its metallurgical process contains impurities that are lesser fusible than the metal itself. Which of the following processes might not have been employed in its extraction?

(a) Magnetic separation
(b) Liquation
(c) Calcination
(d) Auto reduction

85. Choose the incorrect combination

(a) flux used in extraction of iron : SiO_2
(b) hydrometallurgy :leaching by bacteria
(c) anode mud during electrolytic refining of Cu : Contains Au, Ag etc.
(d) zone refining : Si, Ge

86. Choose the set of correct statements among the following

A. Ellingham diagram is plot $\Delta_f G°$ per mole of oxide formed versus temperature

B. The line C → CO slopes downwards and so C is used as reducing agent for all the metal oxides

C. Slag is easily fusible material which melts at temperature of furnace, soluble in the molten metal

D. Hydrometallurgy involves precipitation of Cu^2 ions from solution in presence of scrap Fe

E. Liquation is used when melting point of metal is lower than impurities

(a) A, B and E (b) D and E
(c) C, D and E (d) A, D and E

87. Match the items of column-1 with the items of column-ll.

Column-1	Column-ll
a. Blisterred Cu	p. Aluminium
b. Blast furnace	q. $2Cu_2O + Cu_2S \rightarrow 6Cu + SO_2$
c. Reverberatory furnance	r. Iron
d. Hall-Heroult process	s. $FeO + SiO_2 \rightarrow FeSiO_3$
	t. $2Cu_2S + 3O_2 \rightarrow 2Cu_2O + 2SO_2$

(a) a-r, b-s, c-t, d-q (b) a-q, b-t, c-s, d-r
(c) a-p, b-q, c-t, d-r (d) a-q, b-r, c-s, d-p

Answers

1. (b) 2. (a) 3. (d) 4. (d) 5. (d) 6. (c) 7. (c) 8. (c) 9. (d) 10. (a)
11. (c) 12. (b) 13. (a) 14. (c) 15. (d) 16. (b) 17. (d) 18. (a) 19. (d) 20. (a)
21. (d) 22. (b) 23. (d) 24. (c) 25. (a) 26. (a) 27. (a) 28. (b) 29. (a) 30. (c)
31. (c) 32. (c) 33. (b) 34. (c) 35. (a) 36. (c) 37. (d) 38. (d) 39. (c) 40. (a)
41. (c) 42. (a) 43. (d) 44. (b) 45. (c) 46. (c) 47. (b) 48. (b) 49. (c) 50. (b)
51. (b) 52. (c) 53. (d) 54. (a) 55. (d) 56. (d) 57. (b) 58. (b) 59. (a) 60. (c)
61. (d) 62. (c) 63. (d) 64. (c) 65. (d) 66. (d) 67. (b) 68. (a) 69. (c) 70. (d)
71. (c) 72. (b) 73. (d) 74. (a) 75. (c) 76. (b) 77. (b) 78. (c) 79. (a) 80. (b)
81. (d) 82. (c) 83. (b) 84. (d) 85. (a) 86. (b) 87. (d)

Explanations

1. Rutile has the formula TiO_2.

2. Cinnabar has formula, HgS and since its a sulphide ore, it is concentrated by froth floatation process.

7. Carnallite has formula, KCl. $MgCl_2$. $6H_2O$ magnesite is $MgCO_3$ and dolomite is $MgCO_3$ $CaCO_3$.

So, Mg can be extracted from all the three

8. Graphite has carbon only.

9. Fluorspar is CaF_2, sylvine is KCl & carnallite has composition KCl. $MgCl_2$. $6H_2O$. so all of these contain halide.

11. Copper glance is a sulphide ore (Cu_2S). Malachite has formula $CuCO_3.Cu(OH)_2$.

Cuprite is Cu_2O & feldspar has the formula $KAl\,Si_3O_8$.

14. Haematite (Fe_2O_3) is on ore of iron.

So, it can be extracted by magnetic seperation.

15. Mac–Arthur forest cyanide process is used for the extraction of silver & gold.

Both silver and gold particles dissolve in dilute solution of NaCN in presence of oxygen of air forming complex cyanides.

$$4\,Ag + 8\,NaCN + 2H_2O + O_2 \rightarrow 4Na\,[Ag\,(CN)_2] + 4NaOH$$

$$4\,Au + 8\,NaCN + 2H_2O + O_2 \rightarrow 4Na\,[Au\,(CN)_2] + 4NaOH$$

Ag or Au is recovered from the solution by the addition of electropositive metal like zinc.

$$2Na\,[Ag(CN)_2] + Zn \rightarrow Na_2\,[Zn(CN)_4] + 2Ag\downarrow$$

$$2Na\,[Au(CN)_2] + Zn \rightarrow Na_2\,[Zn(CN)_4] + 2Au\downarrow$$

18. Wolframite is an ore of iron i.e. $FeWO_4$, a magnetic are & is separated from non–magnetic ore, cassiterite (SnO_2) by electromagnetic seperation.

36. More $\Delta G°$ is – ve, more is the stability of oxide.

37. Zinc is a relatively reactive metal, not directly obtained by auto reduction of sulphide ore.

46. Oxides of reactive metals cannot be reduced by Carbon.

50. Nickel is obtained by mond's process.

MOND'S PROCESS

$$\text{Impure Ni} + CO \xrightarrow{60-80°C} Ni(CO)_4 \xrightarrow{180°C} Ni + 4CO$$

(CO is recycled from the last step back to the first.)

Pure Titanium is obtained by VANARKEL PROCESS.

$$\text{Impure metal} + I_2 \rightarrow \underset{\text{vapours}}{\text{Metal iodide}} \xrightarrow[\text{Tungsten filament}]{\text{heating}} \text{Pure metal} + I_2$$

(I_2 is recycled back to the first step.)

$$\text{Impure } Ti(s) + 2I_{2(g)} \xrightarrow{523K} TiI_4(g)$$

$$TiI_{4(g)} \xrightarrow{1700k} Ti + 2I_2(g)$$

VAN ARKEL method is quite expensive & Ti, Zr, Hf, Si are refined by this method.

7

CHAPTER

p-Block Elements

Group-15

1. Which of the following statements is /are true about nitrogen molecule?

(a) N_2 is inert at room temperature.

(b) CO, $\overline{C}N$ & $N\overset{+}{O}$ are isoelectronic with N_2.

(c) CO, $\overline{C}N$ & $N\overset{+}{O}$ have partly polar bonds whereas it is not the case in N_2.

(d) All are correct.

2. Select the incorrect statement(s) about phosphorous & its allotropes.

1. Phosphorous exists as a solid at room temperature.
2. White phosphorous shows the phenomenon of Chemiluminescence
3. White phosphorous is highly reactive & it is therefore stored under water.
4. White phosphorous is thermodynamically, the most stable allotrope of phosphorous

(a) Only 1 is correct

(b) Only 2, 3 & 4 are correct

(c) Only 1, 2 & 3 are correct

(d) All statements are correct

3. SbF_3 & BiF_3 exist as

(a) Covalent solids (b) Covalent liquids

(c) Ionic solids (d) None of these

4. Nitrogen can exist as N_2 molecule because –

(a) It can form strong 2pπ – 2pπ multiple bonds

(b) It can form strong 3pπ – 3pπ multiple bonds

(c) Of its lower ionization energy

(d) None of these

5. Which of the following statement is correct?

(a) Oxides of nitrogen as N_2O_3 & N_2O_5 are monomeric because nitrogen can form multiple bonds.

(b) N & P are non–metals whereas Bi is a true metal.

(c) Ammonia is a colourless gas & is quite poisonous

(d) All are correct

6. Which of the following ammonium salts upon heating will liberate ammonia?

(a) $NH_4^+Cl^- \xrightarrow{\Delta}$

(b) $(NH_4)_2SO_4 \xrightarrow{\Delta}$

(c) $NH_4^+NO_3^- \xrightarrow{\Delta}$

(d) Both (a) & (b)

7. Select 'WRONG' statement about Phosphine.

(a) It can be formed when Ca_3P_2 is hydrolysed

(b) It is extremely toxic gas

(c) Unlike NH_3 it is not very soluble in water

(d) None of these

8. Which one of the following is an INCORRECT reaction?

(a) $PCl_3 + 3H_2O \rightarrow H_3PO_3 + 3HCl$

(b) $NH_3 + HCl \rightarrow NH_4Cl$

(c) $PCl_5 + 4H_2O \rightarrow H_3PO_4 + 5HCl$

(d) $NF_3 + 3\,H_2O \rightarrow HNO_3 + 3\,HF$

9. Among the following the least basic nitrogen trihalide is

(a) NF_3 (b) NCl_3

(d) NBr_3 (d) NI_3

10. Among the following, ease of hydrolysis is maximum for

(a) $AsCl_3$ (b) $SbCl_3$

(c) PF_3 (d) NF_3

11. Very pure N_2 can be prepared by heating

(a) $NH_4\,NO_3$ (b) $(NH_4)_2\,Cr_2\,O_7$

(c) $Ba\,(N_3)_2$ (d) Both (a) & (b)

12. Which one of the following does not exist?

(a) NI_3 (b) NCl_3

(c) $SbCl_3$ (d) NCl_5

13. Phosphonium iodide on reaction with KOH forms

(a) PH_3 (b) NH_3

(c) P_4O_6 (d) P_4O_{10}

14. HNO_3 when reacts with P_4O_{10}, it gives

(a) NO_2 (b) N_2O_3

(c) N_2O_4 (d) N_2O_5

15. Which statement is WRONG about N_2O_5?

(a) It is anhydride of HNO_3

(b) In solid state, it exists as $NO_2^+NO_3^-$

(c) It can be prepared by heating HNO_3 over $P_4\,O_{10}$

(d) None of these

16. Which one of the following is called phosphinic acid?

(a) H_3PO_3 (b) H_3PO_2

(c) H_3PO_4 (d) $H_4P_2O_7$

17. Which one of the following is not an acidic salt?

(a) NaH_2PO_3 (b) NaH_2PO_2

(c) $Na_3HP_2O_6$ (d) Na_2HPO_4

18. In which of the following reactions, oxidation state of nitrogen in the reactant & the product is same?

(a) Reaction of Ca_3N_2 with HCl

(b) Heating $NH_4^+NO_3^-$

(c) Heating $NH_4^+NO_2^-$

(d) Heating $(NH_4)_2Cr_2O_7$

19. Which of the following statements are true about the allotropes of phosphorous ?

(a) White phosphorous is reactive because of angle strain.

(b) White phosphorous shows phosphorescence

(c) Red phosphorous has a polymeric structure.

(d) Phossy Jaw is caused by red phosphorous.

(a) a, b & c only (b) a, b & d only

(c) both b & c only (d) All are correct.

20. Concentrated nitric acid, upon long standing turns yellow brown due to the formation of

(a) NO_2 (b) N_2O

(c) NO (d) None of these

21. Consider the following reaction

$CaCN_2 + H_2O \rightarrow$ Solid + gas

The same gas can also be produced by which of the following reaction–

(a) $NH_4^+NO_2^- \xrightarrow{\Delta}$

(b) $NH_4^+NO_3^- \xrightarrow{\Delta}$

(c) $(NH_4)_2\,Cr_2O_7 \xrightarrow{\Delta}$

(d) $(NH_4)_2\,SO_4 \xrightarrow{\Delta}$

22. Which of the following oxides of 'N' is /are neutral?

(a) N_2O (b) NO

(c) N_2O_5 (d) Both (a) & (b)

23. Select the correct statement about NH_3

(a) It is obtained by the reaction of $(NH_4)_2\,SO_4$ with NaOH.

(b) With Nessler's reagent (alkaline K_2HgI_4), it forms a reddish brown precipitate of colouration due to formation of iodide of millions base

(c) $\ddot{N}H_3$ can act as a ligand.

(d) All are correct

24. An orange solid A on heating gives a colourless gas B. Gas B in dry condition is passed over heated Ca to give a solid C. The solid C futher reacts with water to produce a gas D which forms a blue colored compound on reaction with $CuSO_4$. Then A, B, C, D & E respectively are

(a) $(NH_4)_2Cr_2O_7$, N_2, $Ca_3\,N_2$, NH_3, $[Cu\,(NH_3)_4]\,SO_4$

(b) $NH_4^+NO_3^-$, N_2O, $Ca_3\,N_2$, N_2, NH_3

(c) $NH_4^+Cl^-$, N_2, $Ca_3\,N_2$, NH_3, N_2O_5

(d) $NH_4\,NO_2$, N_2O, Ca_3N_2, NH_3, $CuSO_4$

25. The high reactivity of white phosphorous is due to –
(a) Tetrahedrally arranged P_4 units
(b) bond angle of 60° increases strain factor
(c) weak vander waals forces of attraction
(d) both (b) & (c)

Group-16

26. Which of the following statements are correct about group 16 elements?
1. Tendency to form pπ – pπ bonds decreases down the group.
2. They can form both dioxides & trioxides.
3. SO_3 can exist as monomers as well as trimer.

(a) both (1) & (2)
(b) both (2) & (3)
(c) both (1) & (3)
(d) all statements are correct.

27. SF_6 exists but OF_6 does not because-
(a) the difference in electronegativity is less between O & F.
(b) sulphur has a larger ionisation energy than oxygen.
(c) sulphur has more electron gain enthalpy than oxygen.
(d) sulphur can expand its covalency & octet.

28. The gas which can be absorbed by alkaline pyrogallol solution is-
(a) O_3 (b) O_2
(c) SO_2 (d) N_2O

29. Boiling point of H_2Te is more than that of H_2S because of-
(a) weaker H-bonding in H_2Te
(b) lower electronegativity of Te than S.
(c) strong Van der Waals interaction in H_2Te.
(d) more metallic character of Te than S.

30. Which of the following statements is INCORRECT about ozone?
(a) O_3 is used as a germicide for purification of air.
(b) In O_3, O-O bond length is identical with that of molecular oxygen.
(c) O_3 molecule is angular in shape
(d) It is a bleaching agent & causes permanent bleaching.

31. In the reaction, 2 Hg + O_3 → A + B, A & B respectively are-
(a) O_2 & Hg_2O (b) O_2 & Hg
(c) O_2 & HgO (d) O_2 & Hg_2O_2

32. The yellow colored crystalline substance gave a colourless gas 'X' on reaction with fluorine. X is thermally stable & has octahedral geometry. X can be-
(a) SF_6 (b) SF_4
(c) S_2F_2 (d) S_2F_6

33. Which of the following reactions do not result in the formation of SO_4^{2-} ion?
(a) $SO_2 + MnO_4^- \xrightarrow{H^+}$
(b) $SO_2 + Cr_2O_7^{2-} \xrightarrow{H^+}$
(c) $SO_2 + Fe^{3+} \xrightarrow{H^+}$
(d) $SO_2 + Ba(OH)_2 \longrightarrow$

34. Which of the following reactions is NOT involved in CONTACT process?
(a) $S + O_2 \longrightarrow SO_2$
(b) $2SO_2 + O_2 \xrightarrow{V_2O_5} 2SO_3$
(c) $SO_3 + H_2O \longrightarrow H_2SO_4$
(d) $H_2S_2O_7 + H_2O \longrightarrow 2H_2SO_4$

35. An element 'X' burns in air to form corresponding dioxide 'A'. When solution of 'A' is treated with gaseous hydride 'B' of X, yellow solution of X is obtained. A & B are respectively-
(a) H_2S & SO_2 (b) SO_3 & SO_2
(c) SO_2 & H_2S (d) CO_2 & CH_4

36. Sulphuric acid cannot act as–
(a) dehydrating agent
(b) pickling agent
(c) reducing agent
(d) moderate oxidising agent

37. Sulphuric acid cannot act as a dehydrating agent for-
(a) $H_2C_2O_4$
(b) HCOOH
(c) $C_{12}H_{22}O_{11}$
(d) NH_3

38. A certain compound on burning gave three oxides. The first turned lime water milky, the second turned cobalt chloride paper pink & the third formed an aqueous solution of pH nearly equal to three. The elements present in the compound are-

(a) C, H, Na (b) C, S, O

(c) C, H, S (d) C, H, O

39. Which of the following reactions is incorrect?

(a) $2KClO_{3(s)} \xrightarrow[420K]{MnO_2} 2KCl_{(s)} + 3O_{2(g)}$

(b) $2Na_2O_{2(s)} + 2H_2O_{(l)} \longrightarrow \underset{(aq.)}{4NaOH} + O_{2(g)}$

(c) $Ag_2O_{(s)} \xrightarrow{\Delta} 2Ag_{(s)} + \frac{1}{2}O_2(g)$

(d) $2KNO_{3(s)} \xrightarrow{\Delta} 2KO_{2(s)} + 2NO_2(g)$

40. Correct order of dissociation constants (K_a) of following hydrides in aqueous solution at 298 k is-

(a) $H_2O > H_2S > H_2Se > H_2Te$

(b) $H_2Te > H_2Se > H_2S > H_2O$

(c) $H_2Te > H_2O > H_2Se > H_2S$

(d) $H_2O > H_2Te > H_2Se > H_2S$

41. Select the incorrect statement about group 16 elements.

(a) sulphur has a greater tendency to catenate than oxygen.

(b) OF_2 is called fluoride of oxygen & not oxide of fluorine.

(c) monohalides of sulphur are dimeric.

(d) sulphur is sp^2 hybridised in H_2SO_4.

42. Consider the following reaction-

$O_3 + H_2O_2 \rightarrow$

In the above reaction-

(a) O_3 acts as an oxidising agent.

(b) H_2O_2 acts as a reducing agent.

(c) H_2O_2 acts as an oxidising agent.

(d) Both (a) & (b) are correct.

43. Which of the following is/are correct tests for ozone?

(a) O_3 converts moist I_2 to HIO_2.

(b) A filter paper soaked in a alcoholic benzidine

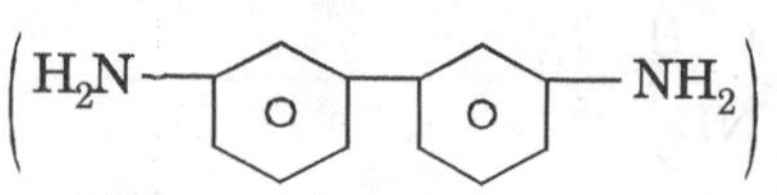

becomes brown when in contact with O_3.

(c) Pure Hg (a mobile liquid) when brought in contact with O_3, starts sticking to glass surface forming a type of tail due to dissolution of Hg_2O in Hg.

(d) Both (b) & (c)

44. Select the correct statement about oxides.

(a) Cl_2O_7 & Mn_2O_7 are acidic oxides.

(b) Cr_2O_3 & PbO are amphoteric oxide.

(c) Pb_3O_4, Fe_3O_4 & Mn_3O_4 are mixed oxides.

(d) All are correct

45. Which one of the following chalcogens is strongly radioactive?

(a) O (b) S

(c) Te (d) Po

46. Select correct statement about O_3?

(a) It is the triatomic allotrope of oxygen.

(b) It is unstable & decomposes to O_2.

(c) O_3 is angular with bond angle equal to 117° (approx) & both the O - O bond lengths are equal.

(d) All statements are correct.

47. Which of the following Oxo acids have sulphur linkage with lowest & highest oxidation state of sulphur?

(a) Pyrosulphurous acid

(b) Thiosulphuric acid

(c) Dithionous acid

(d) Marshall's acid

48. Which of the following statement is correct about sodium thiosulphate ?

(a) It can be prepared by boiling sulphur in sodium sulphite.

(b) It can be used as an antichlor.

(c) It gets oxidised by $KMnO_4$.

(d) All are correct.

Group-17

49. Concentrated H_2SO_4 cannot be used to prepare HBr from NaBr, because it

(a) reduces HBr

(b) oxidises HBr

(c) disproportionates HBr

(d) reacts slowly with NaBr

50. Which one of the following is NOT a pseudohalide?

(a) $CNO^{\ominus}$ (b) $OCN^{\ominus}$

(c) N_3^- (d) $RCOO^{\ominus}$

51. Select the incorrect order against the property mentioned.

(a) $Cl_2 > Br_2 > F_2 > I_2$: Bond dissociation Enthalpy

(b) $Cl > F > Br > I$: Electron affinity

(c) $F_2 > Cl_2 > Br_2 > I_2$: Overall reactivity of halogens

(d) None of these

52. Which one of the following cannot undergo disproportionation reaction?

(a) F_2 (b) Cl_2

(c) Br_2 (d) I_2.

53. Which of the following is NON-SPONTANEOUS?

(a) $F_2 + H_2O \longrightarrow HF + O_2$

(b) $Cl_2 + H_2O \longrightarrow HCl + HOCl$

(c) $Br_2 + H_2O \longrightarrow HBr + HOBr$

(d) $I_2 + H_2O \longrightarrow HI + HOI$

54. Which one of the following statement is correct?

(a) Cl_2 gas can be prepared by the reaction of NaCl & Conc H_2SO_4.

(b) ClO_2 does not dimerise but Cl_2O_4 exists.

(c) Bond angle in Cl_2O is greater than 109°28′.

(d) With excess NH_3, chlorine gives N_2 & NH_4Cl.

55. A gas X is passed through water to form a saturated solution. The aqueous solution, on treatment with $AgNO_3$ gives a white precipitate. The saturated aqueous solution also dissolve magnesium ribbon with the evolution of colorless gas y, 'x & 'y' are, respectively-

(a) CO_2, Cl_2 (b) Cl_2, CO_2

(c) Cl_2, H_2 (d) H_2, Cl_2

56. When Cl_2 reacts with hot concentrated KOH solution, it gives a compound of type MXO_3. Hybridisation, number of lone pairs & geometry of central atom 'X' is-

(a) Sp^3d, one lone pair & Triagonal bipyramidal.

(b) Sp^3, one lone pair tetrahedral.

(c) Sp^3d^2, two lone pair & octahedral.

(d) Sp^3, two lone pair & tetrahedral.

57. Which one of the following is the strongest acid?

(a) $HClO_4$ (b) $HClO_3$

(c) $HClO_2$ (d) HClO

58. A greenish yellow gas reacts with an alkali metal hydroxide to form a halate which can be used in fireworks & safety matches. The gas & the halate are-

(a) Br_2, $KBrO_3$ (b) Cl_2, $KClO_3$

(c) I_2, $NaIO_3$ (d) I_2, KIO_3

59. The halogen which reacts vigorously with water to give a mixture of O_2 & O_3 is-

(a) F_2 (b) Cl_2

(c) Br_2 (d) I_2

60. When I^- is oxidised by MnO_4^- in an alkaline medium, I^- converts into-

(a) IO_3^- (b) I_2

(c) IO^- (d) IO_4^-

61. Upon ionisation of matter $(ICl_3)_2$, a cation (x) & an anion (y) are formed. The hybridisation of central atom in x & y, are respectively-

(a) Sp^3d^2 & sp^3 (b) Sp^3d & sp^3

(c) Sp^3 & sp^3d^2 (d) Sp^3 & sp^3d

62. Select the correct option.

(a) ClO_2 is the mixed anhydride of $HClO_2$ & $HClO_3$.

(b) ClO_3 is the mixed anhydride of $HClO_3$ & $HClO_4$.

(c) Halogens form anions readily.

(d) All are correct.

63. In the preparation of HBr or HI, NaX (X = Br, I) is treated with H_3PO_4 & not with concentrated H_2SO_4 since-

(a) H_2SO_4 makes the reaction reversible.

(b) H_2SO_4 oxidises HX to X_2 (Br_2, I_2)

(c) Na_2SO_4 is water soluble & Na_3PO_4 is water insoluble.

(d) All of these

64. Which of the following is/are correct?

(a) $MnO_2 + 4HCl \longrightarrow MnCl_2 + Cl_2 + 2H_2O$

(b) $KMnO_4 + 16HCl \longrightarrow 2KCl + 2MnCl_2 + 8H_2O + Cl_2$

(c) $4HCl + O_2 \xrightarrow[723k]{CuCl_2} 2H_2O + Cl_2$ (Deacon's process)

(d) All are correct

65. In which of the following interhalogen compounds, chlorine has a positive oxidation state?

(a) ICl (b) ICl_3
(c) ClF (d) Both (a) & (b)

66. The hybrid state of Iodine in I_2Cl_6 is-

(a) Sp (b) Sp^2
(c) Sp^3 (d) Sp^3d^2

67. Which of the following polyhalides does not exist?

(a) ICl_2^- (b) I_3^-
(c) F_3^- (d) ICl_4^-

68. In which of the following reaction Cl_2/H_2O is acting as an Oxidising agent?

(a) $Na_2SO_3 + Cl_2 + H_2O \longrightarrow Na_2SO_4 + 2HCl$

(b) $SO_2 + Cl_2 + 2H_2O \longrightarrow H_2SO_4 + 2HCl$

(c) $I_2 + 6H_2O + 5Cl_2 \longrightarrow 2HIO_3 + 10HCl$

(d) All are these

69. Which one of the following reaction is incorrect wrt preparation of HI?

(a) $H_3PO_4 + NaI \longrightarrow HI + NaH_2PO_4$

(b) $H_2SO_4 + NaI \longrightarrow HI + NaHSO_4$

(c) $2P + 3I_2 \longrightarrow 2PI_3 \xrightarrow{+6H_2O} 6HI + 2H_3PO_3$

(d) All of these are incorrect

70. $\bar{C}N$ is a pseudohalide. It resembles Cl^-, Br^- & I^- in which of the following respects:-

(a) It forms an acid like H CN.

(b) It can be oxidised to form a molecule $(CN)_2$ (cyanogen)

(c) It forms insoluble salts with Ag^+, Pb^{2+} & Hg^{2+}.

(d) In all the above respects.

Group-18

71. Which is the most abundant group 18 element in air?

(a) Xe (b) He
(c) Kr (d) Ar

72. In the clathrates of xenon with water, the nature of bonding between xenon & water molecule is:-

(a) dipole-induced dipole interaction

(b) hydrogen bonding

(c) covalent bonding

(d) coordinate bonding

73. The correct products x & y, in the following reactions, are respectively

(a) $CsF + XeF_6 \longrightarrow x$

(b) $PF_5 + XeF_2 \longrightarrow y$

(a) $Cs^+(XeF_7)^-$, $(XeF_5)^+(PF_6)^-$

(b) $(CsF_2)^-(XeF_5)^+$, $(XeF_3)^+(PF_4)^-$

(c) $Cs^-(XeF_7)^+$, $(XeF_6)F^-$

(d) None of these

74. Select the correct statement (s).

(a) The structure of XeF_6 is a distorted octahedron.

(b) XeO_3, in alkaline solution (above pH = 10.5), forms the Xenate ion $(H\,XeO_4)^-$.

(c) XeO_3 is an explosive white hygroscoic solid.

(d) All are correct.

75. Which of the following do not form clathrate compounds?

(a) He (b) Ne
(c) Kr (d) Both (a) & (b)

76. Which of the following is NOT obtained by the direct reaction of constituent elements?

(a) XeF_2 (b) XeO_3
(c) XeF_4 (d) XeF_6

77. He gas is used as a diluent for oxygen in modern diving apparatus because of its-

(a) light weight

(b) Non inflammable nature

(c) inertness for blood

(d) very low solubility in blood.

78. Which of the following does not exist?

(a) XeO_2F_2 (b) XeF_6
(c) $XeCl_3$ (d) XeF_2

79. Which one of the following is least adsorbed on charcoal?

(a) He (b) Ne
(c) Ar (d) Kr

80. In the reaction given below, O_2F_2 acts as-

$XeF_4 + O_2F_2 \longrightarrow$

(a) an oxidising agent

(b) a reducing agent

(c) both oxidising & reducing agent

(d) None of these

81. Select the correct statement (s).

1. XeO_6^{4-} (Perxenate ion) is a powerful oxidising agent.
2. XeF_2 undergoes hydrolysis to form Xe, HF & O_2.
3. XeF_4 reacts violently with water and undergoes disproportionation to form Xe & O_3.
4. XeF_6 undergoes complete hydrolysis to form XeO_3 & HF.
5. Hybridisation of Xe in XeF_2 is Sp^3.

(a) only 1, 2 & 3 are correct
(b) only 4, 5 are correct
(c) only 1, 2, 3, & 4 are correct
(d) All are correct.

82. Select the incorrect order-
(a) Rn > Xe > Kr > Ar > Ne > He (Boiling point)
(b) Rn > Xe > Kr > Ar > Ne > He (Ease of liquefaction)
(c) Rn > Xe > Kr > Ar > Ne > He (solubility)
(d) None of these is incorrect.

83. Which of the following aerogen is least polarisable?
(a) He (b) Ar
(c) Ne (d) Xe

84. Which one of the following is isostructural with NH_3?
(a) XeO_3 (b) XeF_2
(c) $XeOF_4$ (d) XeO_2F_2

85. In which one of the following options, the 2nd compound has more numbers of pπ-dπ bonds than the first one?
(a) XeO_2F_2, $XeOF_4$ (b) XeO_2F_4, XeO_4
(c) XeO_3F_2, XeO_2F_2 (d) XeO_4, XeO_2F_2

Brain Teasers

86. Select the correct order of acidic strength.
(a) $N_2O_5 > P_4O_{10} > As_4O_{10} > Sb_4O_{10}$
(b) $As_4O_{10} > P_4O_{10} > N_2O_5 > Sb_4O_{10}$
(c) $P_4O_{10} > N_2O_5 > As_4O_{10} > Sb_4O_{10}$
(d) $Sb_4O_{10} > As_4O_{10} > P_4O_{10} > N_2O_5$

87. Which of the following reaction is referred to as VOLCANO EXPERIMENT?
(a) $N_2 + O_2 \rightleftharpoons 2NO$
(b) $(NH_4)_2Cr_2O_7 \xrightarrow{\Delta} N_2 + Cr_2O_3 + 4H_2O$
(c) $NaN_3 \xrightarrow{\Delta} Na + N_2$
(d) None of these

88. The component of aqua regia which can dissolve noble metals is-
(a) Nitrosyl chloride (b) nascent chlorine
(c) H_2O (d) All of these

89. Thermodynamically the most stable form of phosphorous is-
(a) White phosphorous
(b) Yellow phosphorous
(c) Red phosphorous
(d) Black phosphorous

90. Important components in holme's signal are-
(a) $Al_4C_3 + CaC_2$ (b) $CaC_2 + Ca_3P_2$
(c) $Ca_3P_2 + Al_4C_3$ (d) $Al_4C_3 + Be_2C$

91. A translucent white waxy solid (A) on heating in an inert atmosphere is converted into its allotropic form (B). Allotrope (A) on reaction with dilute aq. KOH liberates a highly poisonous gas (C) having rotten fish like smell. With excess of Chlorine, (C) forms (D) which hydrolyses to compound (E). Then, (A), (B), (C), (D) & E are, respectively-
(a) Red P, white P, PH_3, PCl_3, H_3PO_4
(b) White P, red P, PH_3, PCl_5, H_3PO_4
(c) Red P, white P, PH_3, PCl_5, H_3PO_3
(d) Monoclinic S, rhombic S, SO_2, SO_2Cl_2, H_2SO_3

92. The most stable form of sulphur is-
(a) Rhombic-sulphur
(b) Octahedral sulphur
(c) Monoclinic or prismatic sulphur
(d) Both (a) & (b)

93. Select the correct statement about SO_2.
(a) It is an acidic oxide.
(b) It turns lime water milky.
(c) A solution of SO_2 in water when treated with H_2S, turns yellow.
(d) All are correct.

94. The state of hybridisation in the anionic part of solid Cl_2O_6 is-
(a) Sp^3d^2 (b) Sp^3
(c) Sp^3d (d) Sp^2

95. In which of the following reactions is $PbSO_4$ formed?
(a) $PbO_2 + SO_2$
(b) $PbS + O_3$
(c) $PbS + H_2O_2$
(d) All of the above

96. N_2 is passed through CaC_2 (heated). Then, which of the following statement is correct for the product formed?

(1) Hybridisation of C is sp.

(2) Urea is an intermediate formed during hydrolysis of the above product.

(3) Anion present in the product is not a pseudo halide ion.

(4) Hydrolysis of the product gives rise to NH_3 gas.

(a) Only 1 & 2 are correct

(b) Only 3 & 4 are correct

(c) Only 1, 2 & 4 are correct.

(d) All are correct.

97. Copper metal on treatment with dilute HNO_3 produces a gas 'A'. 'A' when passed through acidic solution of stannous chloride, a nitrogen containing compound 'B' is obtained. 'B' on reaction with HNO_2 produces a gas C. Then, A, B & C, respectively are-

(a) NO, NH_2OH, N_2O (b) NO_2, N_2O, NH_2OH

(c) NO, NH_3, NO_2 (d) NO, NO_2, NH_3

98. Match the products in the following reactions-

List-I	List-II
1. $PCl_5 + H_2O \longrightarrow$ (ltd.)	(a) $N_3P_3Cl_6 + 12HCl$
2. $PCl_5 + H_2O \longrightarrow$ (excess)	(b) $(PCl_4)^+(AlCl_4)^-$
3. $PCl_5 + AlCl_3 \longrightarrow$	(c) $H_3PO_4 + HCl$
4. $PCl_5 + NH_4Cl \longrightarrow$	(d) $POCl_3 + HCl$

(a) 1-d, 2-c, 3-b, 4-a (b) 1-c, 2-d, 3-a, 4-b

(c) 1-d, 2-a, 3-b, 4-d (d) 1-c, 2-a, 3-d, 4-b

99. Select the incorrect statement.

(a) Solid N_2O_5 is ionic & exists as $(NO_2)^+(NO_3)^-$.

(b) Correct order of acidic strength of oxoacids follows the order, $H_3PO_2 > H_3PO_3 > H_3PO_4$.

(c) Contrary to electronegativity, PF_3 acts as a strong donor due to pπ-dπ back bonding from F → P.

(d) None of these

100. The maximum covalency of N is-

(a) 5 (b) 4

(c) 6 (d) 3

101. Which of the following are amphoteric oxides?

(a) Al_2O_3

(b) ZnO

(c) BeO

(d) All of these are amphoteric oxides.

102. Which of the following orders of given properties is incorrect?

(a) $PF_3 > PCl_3$ (Basic character)

(b) $(CH_3)_3N > (SiH_3)_3N$ (Basic character)

(c) $CHCl_3 > CHF_3$ (Acidic Character)

(d) $SiH_3–OH > CH_3 – OH$ (Acidic character)

Answers

1. (d)	2. (c)	3. (c)	4. (a)	5. (d)	6. (d)	7. (d)	8. (d)	9. (a)	10. (a)
11. (c)	12. (d)	13. (a)	14. (d)	15. (d)	16. (b)	17. (b)	18. (*)	19. (b)	20. (a)
21. (d)	22. (d)	23. (d)	24. (a)	25. (b)	26. (d)	27. (d)	28. (b)	29. (c)	30. (b)
31. (a)	32. (a)	33. (d)	34. (c)	35. (c)	36. (c)	37. (d)	38. (c)	39. (d)	40. (b)
41. (d)	42. (d)	43. (d)	44. (d)	45. (d)	46. (d)	47. (b)	48. (d)	49. (b)	50. (b)
51. (d)	52. (a)	53. (d)	54. (b)	55. (c)	56. (b)	57. (a)	58. (b)	59. (a)	60. (a)
61. (*)	62. (d)	63. (b)	64. (d)	65. (c)	66. (d)	67. (c)	68. (d)	69. (b)	70. (d)
71. (d)	72. (a)	73. (a)	74. (d)	75. (d)	76. (b)	77. (d)	78. (c)	79. (a)	80. (a)
81. (c)	82. (d)	83. (a)	84. (a)	85. (b)	86. (a)	87. (b)	88. (b)	89. (d)	90. (b)
91. (b)	92. (d)	93. (d)	94. (b)	95. (d)	96. (c)	97. (a)	98. (a)	99. (d)	100. (b)
101. (d)	102. (d)								

Explanations

1. N_2 molecules contains a triple bond with a short bond length of 1.09A, so, this bond is stable & N_2 is inert.

2. Thermodynamically, the most stable of allotrope of phosphorous is black phosphorous.

4. $N \equiv N$ Two π bonds are formed by $2p\pi - 2p\pi$ overlap (which is a better over lap in comparison to 3p – 3p overlap)

6. If anion of ammonium salt is not oxidizing as Cl^- or SO_4^{2-} then upon heating, ammonia is evolved.

So, $NH_4^+Cl^- \xrightarrow{\Delta} NH_3 + HCl$

$$(NH_4)_2SO_4 \xrightarrow{\Delta} 2NH_3 + H_2SO_4$$

If anion is oxidising as NO_3^-, N_2O results

$$\overset{-3}{N}H_4\overset{+5}{N}O_3 \rightarrow \overset{+1}{N_2}O + 2H_2O$$

7. $Ca_3P_2 + 6H_2O \rightarrow 2PH_3 + 3Ca(OH)_2$

wrt (c) option,

NH_3 can form H–bonds with H_2O but PH_3 can't.

8. NF_3 cannot undergo hydrolysis as both N & F lacks vacant d–orbitals. So H_2O can't attack NF_3

9.

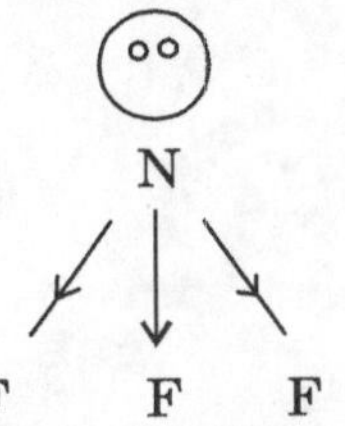

In NF_3, the three fluorine atoms decrease the electron charge density on nitrogen thereby making it least basic.

10. Out of given options, NF_3 cannot be hydrolysed because both N & F lack vacant orbitals. In PF_3, there is $2p\pi - 3p\pi$ back bonding thereby making P – F bond stronger & making its hydrolysis difficult.

Out of $AsCl_3$ & $SbCl_3$, $AsCl_3$ is most easily hydrolysed because as has greater effective nuclear charge thereby inviting water to attack.

11. $Ba(N_3)_2 \xrightarrow{\Delta} Ba + N_2 \uparrow$

Barium azide

12. 'N' cannot show covalency of five i.e., 'N' cannot afford to form five covalent bonds because it lacks vacant d – orbitals.

13. $PH_4^+I^- + KOH \rightarrow PH_3 + H_2O + KI$

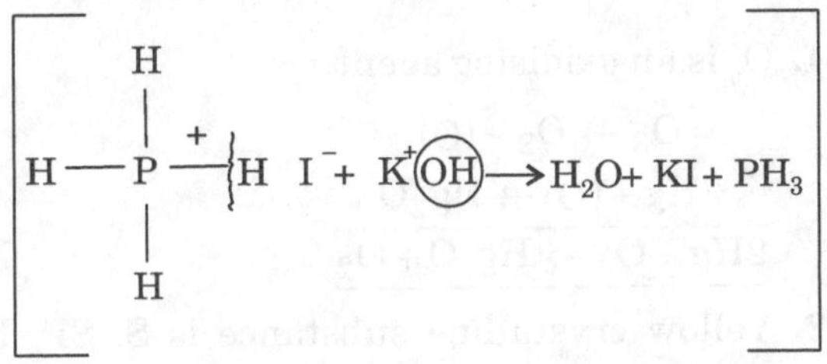

14. P_4O_{10} acts as a dehydrating agent & results in the formation of N_2O_5

$$HNO_3 \xrightarrow{-H_2O} N_2O_5$$

HNO_3

16. H_3PO_2 (hypo phosphorous acid) is also called phosphinic acid

17. $Na^+\bar{O}H + \underset{\text{(monobasic acid)}}{H_3PO_2} \rightarrow \underset{\text{(Salt lacks acidic H)}}{NaH_2PO_2} + H_2O$

18. $\underset{\text{N is in -3 oxidation, state}}{Ca_3N_2} + 6HCl \rightarrow 3CaCl_2 + \underset{\text{N is in -3 oxidation, state}}{2NH_3}$

21. $CaCN_2 + 3H_2O \rightarrow \underset{\text{(Solid)}}{CaCO_3} + \underset{\text{(gas)}}{2NH_3}$

$$(NH_4)_2SO_4 \xrightarrow{\Delta} 2NH_3 + H_2SO_4$$

22. N_2O_5 is an acidic oxide. It is anhydride of HNO_3.

23. Ammonium salts on reaction with base yield NH_3

Wrt option 1,

$(NH_4)_2SO_4 + 2NaOH \rightarrow Na_2SO_4 + 2H_2O + 2NH_3$

Both options (b) & (c) are also correct

24. $(NH_4)_2Cr_2O_7 \xrightarrow{\Delta} N_2 + Cr_2O_3 + 4H_2O$

orange solid (A)   (B) Color less gas

$\underset{}{Ca} + \underset{(B)}{N_2} \rightarrow \underset{(C)}{Ca_3N_2}$

$Ca_3N_2 + H_2O \rightarrow Ca(OH)_2 + \underset{(D)}{NH_3}$

$\underset{\text{(aq.)}}{CuSO_4} + \underset{\text{(aq.) (D)}}{NH_3} \rightarrow \underset{\text{(Blue colored)}}{[Cu(NH_3)_4]SO_4\text{(aq.)}}$

26.

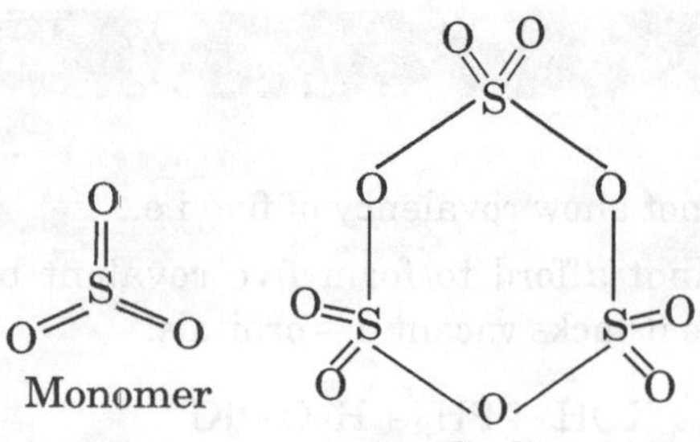

Monomer Cyclic trimen of SO_3

31. O_3 is an oxidising agent.

$$O_3 \rightarrow O_2 + (O)$$
$$2Hg + (O) \rightarrow Hg_2O$$
$$\overline{2Hg + O_3 \rightarrow Hg_2O + O_2}$$

32. Yellow crystalline substance is S. SF_6 has an octahedral geometry.

33. $SO_2 + Ba(OH)_2 \longrightarrow BaSO_3 + H_2O$

(Barium sulphite)

34. H_2O is not directly added to SO_3 because H_2SO_4 obtained from this reaction is in vapour state & further requires condensation.

35. $S + O_2 \longrightarrow SO_2$

$SO_2 + 2H_2S \longrightarrow 3S + 2H_2O$

(moist) (yellow)

37. H_2SO_4 cannot be used as dehydrating agent for NH_3 as acid-base reaction will occur resulting in salt (ammonium sulphate) formation.

38. CO_2 turns lime water milky.

H_2O turns cobalt chloride paper pink.

Oxide of sulphur will form an aqueous solution of pH nearly equal to three (since it forms acidic oxides)

39. $KNO_3 \xrightarrow{\Delta} KNO_2 + \frac{1}{2}O_2 \uparrow$

(strong heating)

40. H_2Te is max. acidic among all hydrides & hence has a greater ka.

42. $2H^+ + 2e^- + O_3 \longrightarrow O_2 + H_2O$

$$H_2O_2 \longrightarrow O_2 + 2H^+ + 2e^-$$
$$\overline{O_3 + H_2O_2 \longrightarrow 2O_2 + H_2O}$$

(O. Agent) (R. Agent)

It is also supported by the fact that standard reduction potential of Ozone is higher (+ 2.07v) than standard reduction potential of H_2O_2 (+ 1.77 v) So, O_3 is a stronger oxidising agent than H_2O_2.

44. Acidic oxides react with water to produces acids.

$Cl_2O_7 + H_2O \longrightarrow 2HClO_4$

$Mn_2O_7 + H_2O \longrightarrow 2HMnO_4$

Cr_2O_3 & PbO, both are amphoteric oxides.

$PbO + 2H_2SO_4 \longrightarrow PbSO_4H_2O$

$PbO + 2NaOH \longrightarrow Na_2PbO_2 + H_2O$

$PbO + H_2SO4 \longrightarrow PbSO_4 + H_2O$

$Cr_2O_3 + 2NaOH \longrightarrow Na_2CrO_4 + H_2O$

$Cr_2O_3 + 3H_2SO_4 \longrightarrow Cr_2(SO_4)_3 + 3H_2O$

Pb_3O_4 (2 $PbO.PbO_2$), Fe_3O_4 ($FeO.Fe_2O_3$) & Mn_3O_4 (2 $MnO.MnO_2$) are mixed oxides.

47. Pyrosulphurous acid

($H_2S_2O_5$)

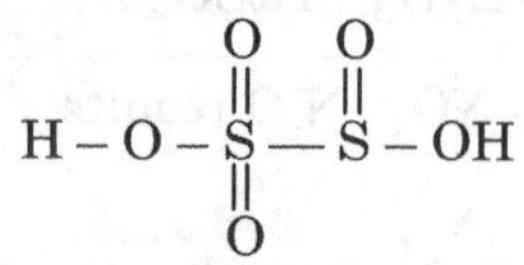

S(+ V), S(+ III)

Thiosulphuric acid

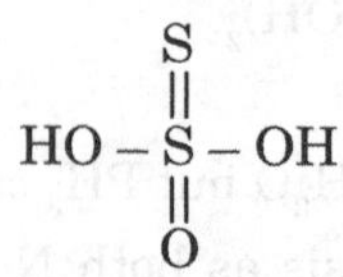

S(+ VI), S(– II)

Dithionous acid

$H_2S_2O_4$

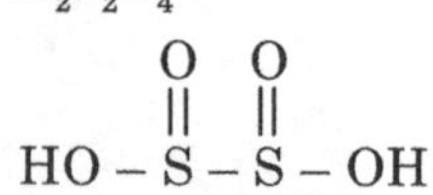

S(+ III)

Marshall's acid

$H_2S_2O_8$

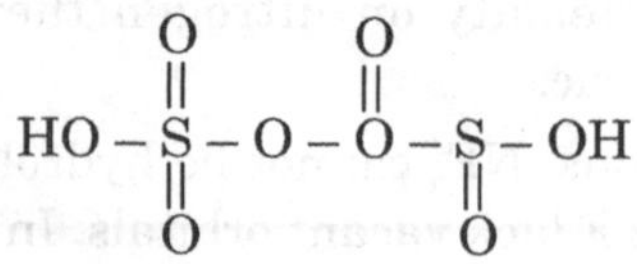

S(+ VI)

48. wrt option (a),

$Na_2SO_3 + S \xrightarrow[\text{in absence of air}]{\text{boiled}} Na_2S_2O_3$

wrt option b, sodium thiosulphate removes chlorine from surface of fibres while dyeing according to following reaction-

$Na_2SO_3 + 4Cl_2 + 5H_2O \longrightarrow 2NaHSO_4 + 8HCl$

So, it is antichlor.

wrt option c,

$2KMnO_4 + Na_2S_2O_3 \longrightarrow K_2SO_4 + Na_2SO_2 + Mn_2O_3$

49. Conc. H_2SO_4 will oxidise HBr to Br_2.

50. All pseudohalide ions have 'N' as one of the element.

52. Fluorine cannot exhibit +ve oxidation state.

53. The reaction of I_2 with water is Nonspontaneous. In fact, I^- can be oxidised by oxygen in acidic medium.

$$4I^- + 4H^+ + O_2 \longrightarrow \underset{(s)}{2I_2} + \underset{(l)}{2H_2O}$$

56. $\underset{(hot)}{KOH} + Cl_2 \longrightarrow KCl + KClO_3 + H_2O$

$KClO_3$ will exist as

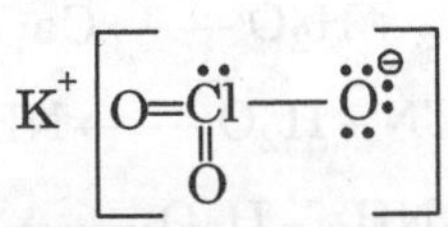

So, Cl has one lone pair, its hybridisation is sp^3 & geometry is tetrahedral.

57. $HClO_4$ is the strongest acid among the given option because its Conjugate base i.e. ClO_4^- is maximum stabilised by resonance.

58. The halate used in fireworks & safety matches is $KClO_3$ & the greenish yellow gas is chlorine.

$3Cl_2 + 6KOH \longrightarrow KClO_3 + 5KCl + 3H_2O$

59. $2F_2 + 2H_2O \xrightarrow{dark} 4HF + O_2$

$F_2 + 3H_2O \longrightarrow 6HF + O_3$

61. $2ICl_3 \rightleftharpoons \underset{sp^3}{ICl_2^+} + \underset{sp^3d^2}{ICl_4^-}$

65. 'F' is more electro –ve then Cl, so 'F' has –ve oxidation state while chlorine has a positive oxidation state.

66.

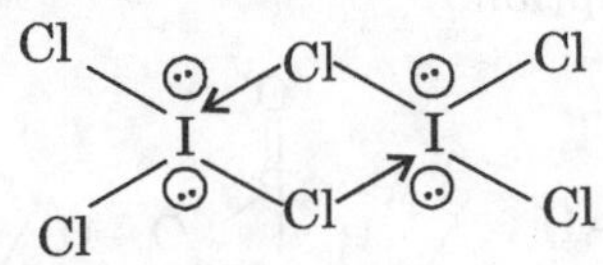

67. F_3^- does not exist because 'F' cannot expand its octet.

69. Concentration H_2SO_4 is an oxidising agent & will oxidise HI to I_2.

73. With metallic fluorides like CsF, XeF_6 acts as a F^- ion acceptor.

with nonmetallic fluorides like PF_5, Xefluorides act as F^- ion donors.

74. wrt option b,

$$XeO_3 + NaOH \longrightarrow \underset{\text{Sodium Xenate}}{Na^+[HXeO_4]^-}$$

75. Smaller noble gases He & Ne do not form clathrate compounds because the gas atoms are small enough to escape from cavities.

80.

$$\underset{+4}{XeF_4} + \underset{+1}{O_2F_2} \longrightarrow \underset{+6}{XeF_6} + \underset{0}{O_2}$$

(Oxidising agent)

81. Hybridisation of Xe in XeF_2 is sp^3d.

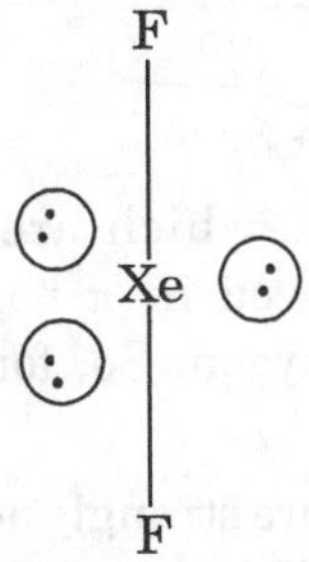

83. He is smallest in size among all aerogens & is hence, least polarisable.

84.

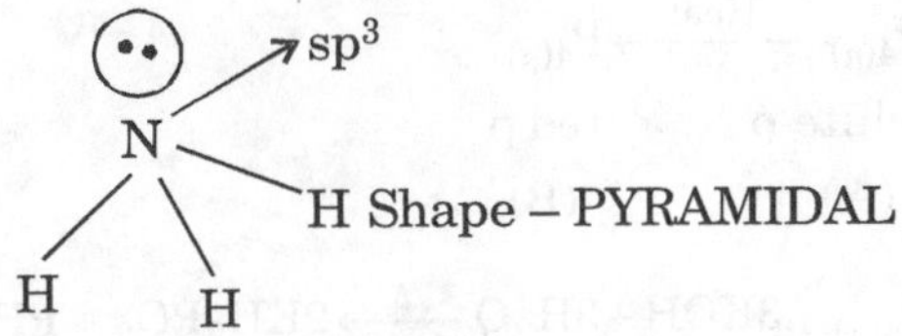

Shape – PYRAMIDAL

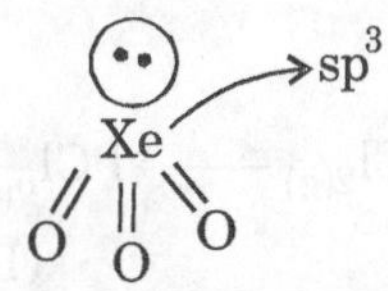

Shape – PYRAMIDAL

85. wrt b option

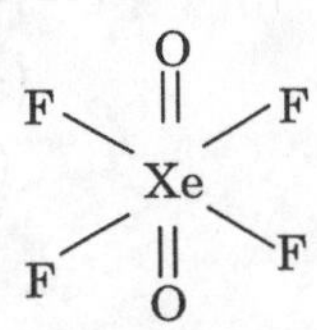

Xe (54):- (Kr)4 d^{10} $5s^2$ $5p^6$ (4 Ground state)

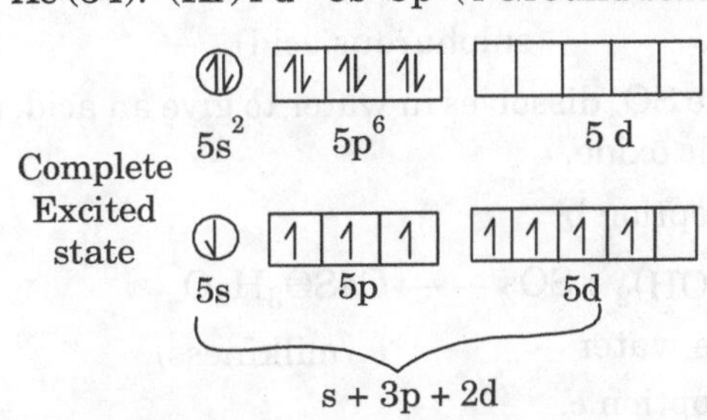

Hybridisation of Xe is sp^3d^2. So, two d-orbitals remain unhybridised & will be involved in π bonding 'O' has p-orbitals for π bond formation- So, 2 pπ–dπ bonds are here.

For XeO_4

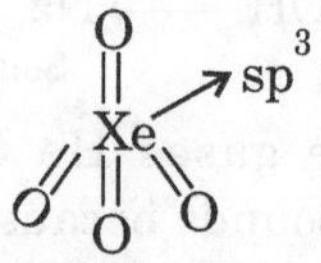

Xe (54):– (Kr)$4d^{10}5s^2 5p^6$ (G.S.)

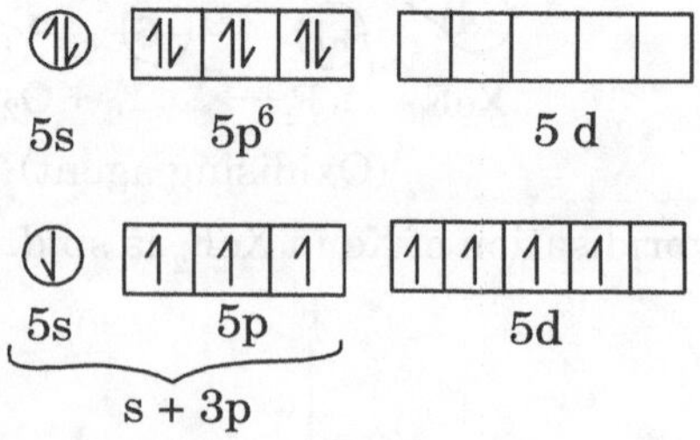

Four d-orbitals which are left unhybridised with get involved in π bond formation with p-orbitals of oxygen. So, four $p\pi$–$d\pi$ bonds are there in XeO_4.

86. All pentoxides are strongly acidic in nature & the strength of acidic character decreases down the group.

91. (a) $P_{4(s)} \xrightarrow{\text{Heat}} P_{4(s)}$
white p (A) red p (B)

(b) $P_{4(s)} + 3KOH + 3H_2O \xrightarrow{\Delta} 2KH_2PO_2 + PH_{3_g}$
white P (C)

(c) $PH_{3(g)} + 4Cl_{2(g)} \longrightarrow PCl_{5(s)} + 3HCl_{(g)}$
(C) (D)

(d) $PCl_5 + 4H_2O_{(l)} \longrightarrow H_3PO_4 + SHCl_{(aq)}$
(D) (aq) (E)

93. wrt option a,

$SO_2 + H_2O \longrightarrow H_2SO_3$
(sulphurous acid)

Since SO_2 dissolves in water to give an acid, it an acidic oxide.

wrt option b,

$Ca(OH)_2 + SO_2 \longrightarrow CaSO_3H_2O$
lime water (milkiness)

wrt option c,

$SO_2 + 2H_2S \longrightarrow 3S + 2H_2O$
(moist)

94. Cl_2O_6 in solid exists as $(ClO_2)^+(ClO_4)^-$.
In ClO_4^-. Cl is sp^3 hybridised.

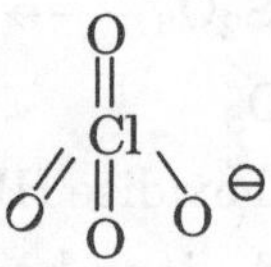

96. $CaC_2 + N_2 \xrightarrow[1378\,k]{1273-} \underbrace{CaCN_2 + C(\text{graphite})}_{\text{NITROLIM}}$

wrt statement; hybridisation of C in CN_2^{2-} (cyanamide ion) its sp.

$$:\overset{\ominus}{\ddot{N}} = C = \ddot{N}:^{\ominus}$$

Hydrolysis of $CaCN_2$

$$CaCN_2 + H_2O \longrightarrow CaO + H_2NCN$$
$$H_2NCN + H_2O \longrightarrow NH_2CONH_2$$
$$NH_2CONH_2 + H_2O \longrightarrow 2NH_3 + CO_2$$
$$CaO + CO_2 \longrightarrow CaCO_3$$
$$\overline{CaCN_2 + 3H_2O \longrightarrow CaCO_3 + 2NH_3}$$

97. $3Cu + 8HNO_3 \longrightarrow 3Cu(NO_3)_2 + 4H_2O + 2NO$
(A)

$3SnCl_2 + 6HCl + 2NO \longrightarrow 3SnCl_4 + 2NH_2OH$
(A) (B)

$NH_2OH + HNO_2 \longrightarrow N_2O + 2H_2O$
(C)

98. $PCl_5 + H_2O \longrightarrow POCl_3 + 2HCl$
$PCl_5 + 4H_2O \longrightarrow H_3PO_4 + 5HCl$
$PCl_5 + AlCl_3 \longrightarrow (PCl_4)^+(AlCl_4)^-$
$3PCl_3 + 3NH_4Cl \longrightarrow N_3P_3Cl_6 + 12HCl$

99. wrt b option,

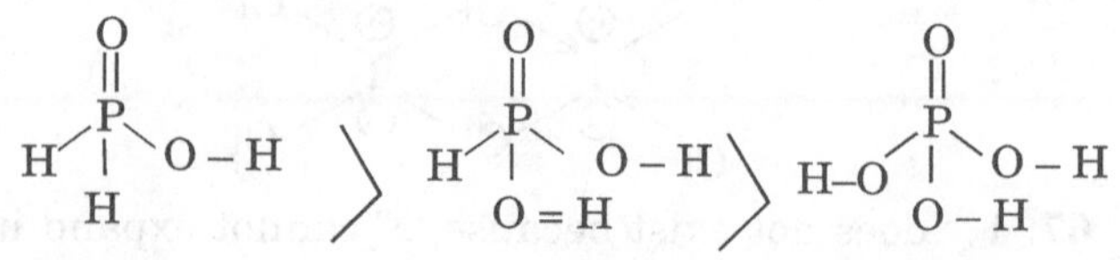

H_3PO_2 H_3PO_3 H_3PO_4

The inductive effect of the single oxygen atom acts on the single –O–H in H_3PO_2 but it is distributed over two & three O–H bonds in H_3PO_3 & H_3PO_4, respectively.

100. The maximum covalency of N is 4 (Max three pure covalent bonds & one dative bond can be formed by N)

102. wrt option (a),

$PCl_3 > PF_3$ (basic character)

Because –I exerted by F is greater than that of chlorine & it will decrease electron density on phosphorous making it less basic.

wrt option (b),

In $(SiH_3)_3N$, there is $p\pi - d\pi$ back bonding due to which lone pair on 'N' gets delocalised making it less basic.

wrt option (c),

Conjugate base of $CHCl_3$ i.e. $\ddot{C}Cl_3^{\ominus}$, is stabilised by d-orbital resonance. So, $CHCl_3$ is more acidic than CHF_3.

wrt option (d),

Conjugate base of $SiH_3 - OH$ is stabilised by $p\pi - d\pi$ bonding. So, it is more acidic than CH_3OH.

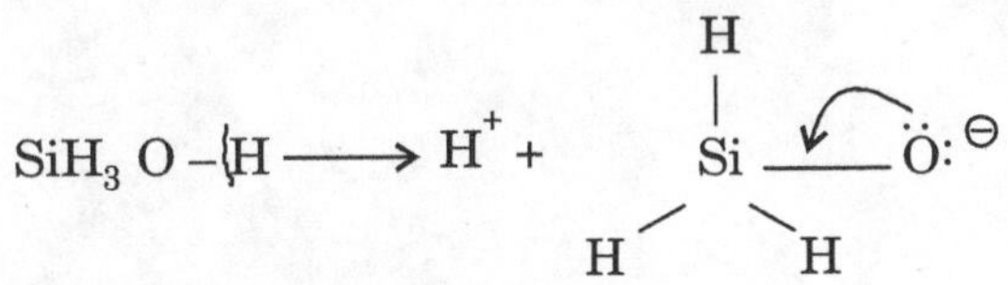

Alkyl & Aryl halides

(Aryl halides)

8

CHAPTER

d- and f-Block Elements

1. Which of the following is/are NOT Transition elements?

(a) Zn (b) Cd

(c) Hg (d) All of these

2. Which of the following transition metal does not show variable oxidation state ?

(a) Fe (b) Ti

(c) Sc (d) All of these

3. Select the correct statement (s) about d-block elements.

(a) Atomic radii decreases irregularly with increases in atomic number in a series.

(b) Towards the middle of 3d series the nuclear charge factor and the screening effect by addition of d-electrons almost neutralise each other.

(c) In case of Cr, Mo & W, there are six unpaired electrons involved in metallic bonding.

(d) All are correct.

4. Select the WRONG statement.

(a) Mn in the first transition series & Tc in the 2nd series shows exceptionally low melting points.

(b) In Zn, Cd & Hg the number of unpaired electrons are zero & so they exhibit weakest metallic bonding.

(c) d-block elements, in general, show higher melting points in comparison to s-block elements.

(d) None of these is INCORRECT.

5. Transition metals-

(a) exhibit only diamagnetism.

(b) show inert pair effect.

(c) do not form alloys

(d) show variable oxidation states

6. Which of the following statement is/are incorrect regarding Cr & S,

(a) Both SO_3 &CrO_3 are acidic oxides.

(b) Both can form $X_2O_7^{2-}$ type of compounds

(c) Structure of CrO_3 & SO_3 is different.

(d) All of these are incorrect.

7. E° values for Cr^{3+}/Cr^{2+} & Mn^{3+}/Mn^{2+} are −0.41V & +1.51V, respectively Considering these, select the correct option from the following statement.

(a) Cr^{2+} acts as a reducing agent & Mn^{2+} acts as an oxidising agent in their aqueous solutions

(b) $Cr^{2+}_{(aq.)}$ is more stable than $Cr^{3+}_{(aq.)}$

(c) $Mn^{3+}{}_{(aq.)}$ is more stable than $Mn^{2+}{}_{(aq.)}$

(d) None of these

8. Which one of the following characteristics of the transition metals is associated with their catalytic activity?

(a) Colour of hydrated ions

(b) Variable oxidation states

(c) High enthalpy of atomisation

(d) Paramagnetic behaviour.

9. Which of the following alloys 'do not' contain silver ?

(a) Coinage alloy

(b) Silver solder

(c) Silver Copper alloy

(d) German silver

10. Which of the following statement is/are correct?

(a) $K_2[NiCl_4]$ exists but K_2 $[PtCl_4]$ does not.

(b) $K_2[PtCl_6]$ exists but $K_2[NiCl_6]$ does not.

(c) Both $K_2[PtCl_4]$ & $K_2[NiCl_6]$ are highly stable.

(d) Both (a) & (b) are correct

11. Which of the following does not belong to 3d series of transition elements?

(a) Ti (b) Fe

(c) Pd (d) V

12. The stability of particular oxidation state of a metal in aqueous solution is determined by-

(a) enthalpy of sublimation of the metal

(b) ionisation energy

(c) enthalpy of hydration of the metal ions

(d) All of these

13. Match the properties given in Column I with the transition elements given in Column II.

Column I (Property)	**Column II** (Transition element)
(A) Highest oxidation state	(p) Cr
(B) Highest density	(q) Os
(C) Element with maximum unpaired electrons.	(r) Tc
(D) Radioactive transition element.	(s) Ru

(a) A-q, s; B-q; C-p; D-r

(b) A-q, r; B-s; C-p; D-r

(c) A-p, q; B-p; C-r; D-s

(d) None of these

14. A transition element M forms the oxides MO, M_2O_3, MO_3 & M_2O_7 then which of the following statement about these oxides is true?

(a) MO is most acidic

(b) M_2O_3 is most likely to be a strong oxidising agent

(c) MO_3 is most acidic

(d) M_2O_7 can not act as a reducing agent.

15. Which of following is wrong?

(a) Cr > Fe > Mn (order of M.pt)

(b) IE_3 of Mn > IE_3 of Fe

(c) Cu > Ni > Zn (order of IE_2)

(d) None of these is wrong

16. Metal-Metal bonding is more frequent in 4d or 5d series than in 3d series. This is due to-

(a) their greater enthalpies of atomisation.

(b) their ability to involve both ns & (n – 1)d electrons in bond formation.

(c) Comparable sizes of 4d & 5d series elements.

(d) All the these.

17. Value of $E^{\circ}_{Zn^{2+}/Zn}$ is more negative than expected because-

(a) of very high enthalpy of atomisation of Zn.

(b) of stability of Zn^{2+} due to d^{10} configuration.

(c) of very low ionisation energy of Zn^{2+}.

(d) Both (a) & (c)

18. Select the correct statement (s).

(a) Chromate, in acidic medium tends to get converted into dichromate whereas in basic medium dichromate tends to get converted into chromate.

(b) CrO_3 give H_2CrO_4 & $H_2Cr_2O_7$ on reacting with water.

(c) All 3d elements form oxides with formula MO, except Sc.

(d) All are correct.

19. What is true about chromyl chloride test?

(a) It indicates the presence of chloride radical.

(b) Chloride of Ag, Hg, Pb do not give the test.

(c) Red colored vapours of CrO_2Cl_2 are evolved.

(d) All statement are correct.

20. Which of the following forms stable +4 oxidation state?

(a) La(Z = 57) (b) Eu(Z = 63)

(c) Ce (Z = 58) (c) Gd (Z = 64)

21. A metal M on heating in nitrogen gas gives Y. Y on treatment with H_2O gives a colorless gas which when passed through $CuSO_4$ solution gives a blue colour . Y is-

(a) NH_3 (b) $Mg(NO_3)$

(c) Mg_3N_2 (d) MgO

22. Which statement is INCORRECT ? (Z of Ce = 58, Lu = 71, La = 57, Yb = 70)

(a) Color of Yb^{3+} ion is pink.

(b) La^{3+} is diamagnetic

(c) Ce^{4+} has f^0 configuration.

(d) Lu^{3+} has f^{14} configuration

23. When a small amount of $KMnO_4$ is added to concentrated H_2SO_4, a green oily compound is obtained, which is highly explosive in nature. The compound may be-

(a) $MnSO_4$ (b) Mn_2O_7

(c) MnO_2 (d) Mn_2O_3

24. When a chromite Ore (A) is fused with Na_2CO_3 in free excess air & the product is dissolved in H_2O, a yellow solution of compound (B) is obtained. After treatment of this yellow solution with H_2SO_4, compound (C) can be crystallised from the solution. When compound (C) is treated with KCl, orange crystals of compound (D) crystallise out. Then, D is-

(a) $FeCr_2O_4$ (b) Na_2CrO_4

(c) $Na_2Cr_2O_7$ (d) $K_2Cr_2O_7$

25. Identify 'B' in the following reaction-

$$KMnO_4 \xrightarrow{\Delta} K_2MnO_4 + B + O_2$$

'B' is insoluble in water & is obtained as a black residue.

(a) Mn_2O_7 (b) MnO_4^-

(c) MnO_2 (d) Mn_2O_3

26. Select the correct statement (s).

(a) CuI_2 is not KNOWN.

(b) It is difficult to separate Zr & Hf.

(c) Copper Cannot liberate H_2 from acids.

(d) All are correct.

27. Four successive members of first row transition elements are listed below with atomic numbers. Which one of them is expected to have the highest $E^\circ_{M^{3+}/M^{2+}}$ value?

(a) Co(Z = 27) (b) Cr(Z = 24)

(c) Mn(Z = 25) (d) Fe (Z = 26)

28. In context with transition elements, which of following statements is INCORRECT?

(a) In the highest oxidation states, the transition metals show basic character & form cationic complexes.

(b) Once the d^5 configuration is exceeded, the tendency to involve all the 3d electrons in bonding decreases.

(c) Oxidation state of Ni in $Ni(CO)_4$ is zero.

(d) Both (b) & (c) are incorrect.

29. Among the oxides, Mn_2O_7 (I), V_2O_3 (II), V_2O_5 (III), CrO (IV) & Cr_2O_3 (V), the basic oxides are-

(a) I & II (b) II & III

(c) III & IV (d) II & IV

30. The electronic configuration of Eu(Z = 63); Gd(Z = 64) & Tb(Z = 65) are,

(a) $(Xe)4f^65d^16s^2$, $(Xe)4f^75d^16s^2$ & $(Xe)4f^85d^16s^2$

(b) $(Xe)4f^76s^2$, $(Xe)4f^75d^16s^2$ & $(Xe)4f^96s^2$

(c) $(Xe)4f^76s^2$, $(Xe)4f^86s^2$ & $(Xe)4f^85d^16s^2$

(d) None of these

31. Which of the following is NOT an actinoid?

(a) Curium (Z = 96)

(b) Californium (Z = 98)

(c) Uranium (Z = 92)

(d) Terbium (Z = 65)

32. $KMnO_4$ can be prepared from K_2MnO_4 as per the reaction:-

$$3\,MnO_4^{2-} + 2\,H_2O \rightleftharpoons 2\,MnO_4^- + MnO_2 + 4\bar{O}H$$

The reaction can go to completion by removing $\bar{O}H$ ions by adding-

(a) HCl

(b) KOH

(c) CO_2

(d) SO_2

33. Which one of the following does not correctly represent the correct order of the property indicated against it?

(a) Ti < V < Cr < Mn ; increasing melting point

(b) Ti < V < Mn < Cr ; increasing 2nd ionisation enthalpy

(c) Ti < V < Cr < Mn ; increasing number of oxidation states.

(d) $Ti^{3+} < V^{3+} < Cr^{3+} < Mn^{3+}$; increasing magnetic moment

34. The bonds present in the structure of dichromate ion are-

(a) 4 equivalent Cr – O bonds only.

(b) 6 equivalent Cr – O bonds & one O – O bond.

(c) 6 equivalent Cr – O bonds & one Cr – Cr bond.

(d) 6 equivalent Cr – O bonds & one Cr – O – Cr bond.

35. Select the correct statement (s).

(a) $K_2Cr_2O_7$ is preferred over $Na_2Cr_2O_7$ as primary standard in volumetric estimation because $Na_2Cr_2O_7$ is hygroscopic in nature but $K_2Cr_2O_7$ is not.

(b) $FeCr_2O_4$ is used as a starting material for preparation of $K_2Cr_2O_7$.

(c) $K_2Cr_2O_7$ is a good reducing agent

(d) Both (a) & (b) are correct.

36. Amount of oxalic acid present in a solution can be determined by its titration with $KMnO_4$ solution in the presence of H_2SO_4. The titration gives unsatisfactory result when carried out the presence of HCl because HCl-

(a) reduces MnO_4^- to Mn^{2+}.

(b) oxidises oxalic acid to CO_2 & H_2O.

(c) gets oxidised by oxalic acid to chlorine.

(d) furnishes H^+ ions in addition to those from oxalic acid.

37. $KMnO_4$ acts as an oxidising agent in alkaline medium. When alkaline $KMnO_4$ is treated with KI, iodide is oxidised to-

(a) I_2

(b) IO^-

(c) IO_3^-

(d) IO_4^-

38. Which of the following compound does not exist?

(a) CoF_2

(b) Mn_2O_7

(c) MnO_3F

(d) MnF_7

39. Which of the statement (s) given below wrt Lanthanoids & actinides is/are WRONG?

(a) Actinides can show higher oxidation states (till + 7 also) in comparison to Lanthanoids.

(b) Actinides have a great tendency to form oxo-ions & complexes in comparison to lanthanoids.

(c) Actinides are radioactive whereas lanthanoids, except promethium are NON-Radioactive.

(d) None of these is WRONG.

40. The stability of $Cu^{2+}_{(aq.)}$ rather than Cu^+ (aq.) is due to-

(a) Much more negative $\Delta H_{hyd.}$ of $Cu^{2+}_{(aq.)}$ than Cu^+ (aq.)

(b) Much more positive $\Delta H_{hyd.}$ of $Cu^{2+}_{(aq.)}$ than $Cu^{2+}_{(aq.)}$

(c) Zero $\Delta H_{hyd.}$ of $Cu^{2+}_{(aq.)}$

(d) None of these.

41. When H_2O_2 is added to an acidified solution of a dichromate, then which statement (s) is/are correct?

(a) deep blue-violet colored peroxo compound, $CrO(O_2)_2$ or CrO_5 is formed.

(b) This peroxo compound form adduct with pyridine.

(c) The adduct formed has an approximately pentagonal pyramidal structure.

(d) All are correct.

42. What is true regarding Cr_2O_3?

(a) It is a green solid.

(b) It is prepared by heating $(NH_4)_2Cr_2O_7$, also called volcano experiment.

(c) It is used as a pigment

(d) All are true.

43. Which of the following is NOT a consequence of the lanthanoid contraction?

(a) 5d elements have higher IE_1 than 3d or 4d elements.

(b) Zr & Hf have comparable sizes.

(c) High density of 6th period elements.

(d) All of these

44. Trends in ionisation along the 3d series is irregular. A sudden dip is seen in the ionisation energy of Ni, (IE_1) because-

(a) there is great increase in coulombic exchange energy.

(b) there is great decrease in coulombic exchange energy.

(c) greater lattice energy is involved.

(d) exchange energy has nothing to do with it.

45. The ability of oxygen to stabilise high oxidation states exceeds that of fluorine because-

(a) O is more electro negative than F.

(b) F can form multiple bonds but O cannot.

(c) O can form multiple bonds but F cannot.

(d) Both (a) & (b) are correct reasons.

46. Copper, Tin & Zinc are the components of which of the following alloys?

(a) Gun metal (b) monel metal

(c) Invar (d) Stainless steel.

47. Which of the following is false?

(a) $TiCl_4$ is a colorless compound because Ti^{4+} ion has no unpaired electron.

(b) The colour of transition metal ion in a complex can arise due to d - d transition.

(c) Colour of certain oxy salts of transition metals is due to change transfer.

(d) $K_2Cr_2O_7$ is colored due to d - d transition.

48. Identify the incorrect statement.

(a) Scandium (III) is more stable than Sc (II) or Sc (I)

(b) Cr (VI) in the form of dichromate in acidic medium is a strong oxidising agent

(c) In gp. 6, Mo (VI) is more stable than Cr (VI).

(d) Cr (I) is the most stable oxidation state of chromium as it has half filled subshell.

49. Which of the following has oxygen in –1 oxidation state?

(a) $Cr_2O_7^{2-}$ (b) CrO_4^{2-}

(c) MnO_4^{2-} (d) CrO_5

50. Acidified $K_2Cr_2O_7$ solution turns green when Na_2SO_3 is added to it. This is due to the formation of-

(a) $CrSO_4$ (d) $Cr_2(SO_4)_3$

(c) CrO_4^{-2} (d) $Cr_2(SO_3)_3$

51. Select the correct statement.

(a) $La(OH)_3$ is less basic than $Lu(OH)_3$.

(b) Lanthanum is actually a d-block element.

(c) Atomic radii of Zr &Hf are same because they belong to same period.

(d) All are correct.

52. $KMnO_4$ is fused with hot KOH, then the product formed is-

(a) black MnO_2

(b) brown Mn_2O_3

(c) green K_2MnO_4

(d) purple $KMnO_4$

53. A violet compound of manganese (A) decomposes on heating to liberate oxygen & compound (B) and (C) of manganese are formed. Compound (C) reacts with KOH in presence of kNO_3 to give compound (B). On heating (C) with Conc. H_2SO_4 & NaCl, chlorine gas is liberated & a compound (D) of manganese along with other products is formed. The A, B, C & D, respectively, are -

(a) $KMnO_4$, K_2MnO_4, MnO_2, $MnCl_2$

(b) $KMnO_4$, K_2MnO_4, $MnCl_2$, MnO_2

(c) K_2MnO_4, $KMnO_4$, $MnCl_2$, MnO_2

(d) K_2MnO_4, $KMnO_4$, Mn_2O_7, MnO_2

54. VO_2^+, CrO_4^{2-} & MnO_4^- are pale yellow, strong yellow & intense purple respectively in aqueous solution. Then, the darkening of colour is due to-

(a) ligand to metal charge transfer

(b) d-d transition

(c) half filled d-subshells

(d) increasing number of unpaired electrons.

55. Which of the following increasing order of oxidising power is correct for the following species?

VO_2^+ , MnO_4^-, $Cr_2O_7^{2-}$

(a) $MnO_4^- > Cr_2O_7^{2-} > VO_2^+$

(b) $Cr_2O_7^{2-} > MnO_4^- > VO_2^+$

(c) $MnO_4^- > VO_2^+ > Cr_2O_7^{2-}$

(d) $VO_2^+ > MNO_4^- > Cr_2O_7^{2-}$

56. $KMnO_4$ acts as an oxidant in neutral, alkaline as well as acidic media. The final products obtained from it in three conditions are respectively-

(a) MnO_2, MnO_2^+, Mn^{3+} (b) MnO_2, MnO_2 & Mn^{2+}

(c) MnO, MO_2^+ & Mn^{3+} (d) MnO_4^{2-}, Mn^{3+} & Mn^{2+}

57. Which of the following can exist?

(a) CoF_3 (b) $CoCl_3$

(c) $CoBr_3$ (d) CoI_3

58. Select the WRONG statement about K_2MnO_4.

(a) It is tetrahedral, paramagnetic & a green colored compound.

(b) In it, $2p\pi$-$3p\pi$ bonding is present

(c) In acidic medium, it disproportionates into $KMnO_4$ & MnO_2.

(d) It is prepared by reacting pyrolusite with KOH & air.

59. In which of the following oxoions, all the M-O bond lengths are not identical?

(a) CrO_4^{2-} (b) MnO_4^-

(c) MnO_4^{2-} (d) $Cr_2O_7^{2-}$

60. Which of the following cannot be oxidised by acidified $KMnO_4$?

(a) $C_2O_4^{2-}$

(b) NO_2^-

(c) S^{2-}

(d) All of these can be oxidised

61. Lanthanides & Actinoids resemble each other in-

(a) Electronic configuration

(b) Common oxidation state

(c) Ionisation energy

(d) Formation of a complex.

62. Which of the following characteristics of lanthanides is correct?

(a) Reducing property of lanthanides decreases from La to Lu.

(b) Complex forming ability of Lanthanides increases from La to Lu.

(c) Lanthanides form stable compounds in +3 oxidation state.

(d) All the correct.

63. The oxidation potential of the transition elements are lower than oxidation potential of s-block elements because-

(a) the hydration energy of transition metal cations are high.

(b) The I.E. of transition elements are higher than that of corresponding s-block elements.

(c) I.E. of transition elements are lower than that of corresponding s-block elements.

(d) The M.pt. of s-block elements are low.

64. Select the correct statement.

(a) Vanadium exhibits its highest oxidation state in VF_5.

(b) Other halides of vanadium undergo hydrolysis to give oxohalides of formula VOX_3.

(c) Hg_2Cl_2 is known as calomel & $HgCl_2$ is called corrosive sublimate.

(d) All are correct.

65. The compound that gets oxidised even on exposure to atmosphere is-

(a) $Cr_2(SO_4)_3$ (b) $NiSO_4$

(c) $KMnO_4$ (d) $FeSO_4$

66. When CO_2 is passed into aqueous-

(a) Na_2CrO_4 solution, its yellow colour changes to orange.

(b) K_2MnO_4 solution, it disproportionates to $KMnO_4$ & MnO_2.

(c) $KMnO_4$ solution, its pink colour changes to green.

(d) Both (a) & (b)

67. One of the products formed due to reaction between $KMnO_4$ & HCl is-

(a) red liquid, CrO_2Cl_2

(b) Black powder, MnO_2

(c) greenish yellow gas, Cl_2

(d) colourless liquid, $HClO_4$

68. In which of the following oxoanions, the oxidation state of central atom is not same as that of its group number in the periodic table?

(a) MnO_4^- (b) $Cr_2O_7^{2-}$

(c) VO_4^{3-} (d) FeO_4^{2-}

69. Conversion of K_2MnO_4 into $KMnO_4$, can be brought about by-

(a) O_3 (b) Cl_2

(d) CO_2 (d) All of these

70. In the reaction given below, peroxodisulphate ions act as-

$2Mn^{2+} + S_2O_8^{2-} + 8H_2O \longrightarrow 2MnO_4^- + 10SO_4^{2-} + 16H^+$

(a) oxidising agent (b) reducing agent

(c) reductant (d) None of these

71. The equivalent weight of $KMnO_4$, when it is acting as an oxidising agent in acidic medium, is -

(M. mass of $KMnO_4$ = 158.5g)

(a) 158 (b) 31.6

(c) 52.16 (d) 79

72. If n_1 moles of alkaline $KMnO_4$ are required to Oxidise 1 mole of KI & n_2 moles of acidified $KMnO_4$ are required to oxidise 1 mole of KI, then the ratio of n_1 to n_2 is :-

(a) 1 : 1 (b) 1 : 10

(c) 2 : 5 (d) 10 : 1

73. A red solid is insoluble in water. However, it becomes soluble if some KI is added to water Heating the red solid in a test tube results in liberation of some violet coloured fumes & droplets of a metal appear on the cooler parts of the test tube, Then, the red solid is-

(a) HgI_2 (b) HgO

(c) Pb_3O_4 (d) $(NH_4)_2Cr_2O_7$

74. The maximum oxidation state shown by V(Z = 23), Cr(Z = 24), Co(Z = 27) & Sc(Z = 21) are respectively

(a) +5, +6, +3, +3 (b) +3, +4, +5, +2

(c) +5, +3, +2, +1 (d) +4 in each case.

75. The yellow colour solution of Na_2CrO_4 changes to orange red on passing CO_2 gas due to formation of-

(a) $Na_2Cr_2O_7$ (b) CrO_3

(c) CrO_5 (d) Na_3CrO_8.

76. Which of the following oxide (s) of transition metals is/are amphoteric in nature?

(a) Cr_2O_3 (b) V_2O_5

(c) ZnO (d) All of these

77. The dip in the boiling point of manganese in 3d series is due to-

(a) large size of atom

(b) less electronegativity of Mn

(c) less delocalisation of valence electrons owing to extra stability of half filled configuration

(d) All of these

78. Which of the following is/are mixed oxides?

(a) Pb_3O_4 (b) Fe_3O_4

(c) Mn_3O_4 (d) All of these

79. Ammoniacal Cu_2Cl_2 absorbs-

(a) CO_2 (b) CO

(c) Both CO & CO_2 (d) CCl_4

80. Which of the following can undergo disproportionation?

(a) Zn^{2+}

(b) Mn^{2+}

(c) Cu^+

(d) All of these

Brain Teasers

81. The lanthanoid contraction is responsible for the fact that –

(a) Zr & Y have about same radius

(b) Zr & Nb have similar oxidation states.

(c) Zr & Hf have about the same radius

(d) Zr & Zn have same oxidation state.

Answers

1. (d)	2. (c)	3. (d)	4. (d)	5. (d)	6. (c)	7. (a)	8. (b)	9. (d)	10. (d)
11. (c)	12. (d)	13. (a)	14. (d)	15. (d)	16. (a)	17. (b)	18. (d)	19. (d)	20. (c)
21. (c)	22. (a)	23. (b)	24. (d)	25. (c)	26. (d)	27. (a)	28. (a)	29. (d)	30. (b)
31. (d)	32. (c)	33. (a)	34. (d)	35. (d)	36. (a)	37. (c)	38. (d)	39. (d)	40. (a)
41. (d)	42. (d)	43. (c)	44. (a)	45. (c)	46. (a)	47. (d)	48. (d)	49. (d)	50. (b)
51. (b)	52. (c)	53. (a)	54. (a)	55. (a)	56. (b)	57. (a)	58. (b)	59. (d)	60. (d)
61. (b)	62. (d)	63. (b)	64. (d)	65. (d)	66. (d)	67. (c)	68. (d)	69. (d)	70. (a)
71. (b)	72. (d)	73. (a)	74. (a)	75. (a)	76. (d)	77. (c)	78. (d)	79. (b)	80. (c)
81. (c)									

Explanations

1. Transition elements are those which have incompletely filled (n – 1)d orbitals in its ground state or in any one of its oxidation state.

$Zn(30):(Ar)4s^2 3d^{10}$	$Cd(48):4d^{10}\,5s^2$
$Zn^{2+}:(Ar)\,3d^{10}$	$Cd^{2+}:4d^{10}$

Hg (80) : $5d^{10}\,6s^2$, Hg^{2+} : $5d^{10}$.

2. Sc show only +3 oxidation state.

5. d-block elements can show variable oxidation states because of small energy difference in (n – 1)d & ns orbitals, so both the orbitals can be used for bond formation.

7. Configuration of Cr^{2+} changes from d^4 to d^3 on losing an electron which gives it a half filled t_{2g} level.

To change from Mn^{3+} to Mn^{2+} results in d^5 configuration.

8. Reaction $2I^- + S_2O_8^{2-} \longrightarrow I_2SO_4^{2-}$

Mechanism: -

(1) $2Fe^{3+} + 2I^- \longrightarrow 2Fe^{2+} + I_2$

(2) $2Fe^{2+} + S_2O_8^{2-} \longrightarrow 2Fe^{3+} + 2SO_4^{2-}$

Here, Fe^{3+} is acting as a catalyst.

9. German silver has Cu, Zn & Ni

10. Sum of IE_1, & IE_2 for Ni is 2.49×10^3 kJ/mol while for Pt is 2.66×10^3 kJ/Mol.

$\therefore$ Ni in +2 is more stable than Pt^{2+}.

Also, sum of IE_1, IE_2, IE_3 & IE_4 is 11.29×10^3 KJ/mol for Ni where as it is 9.36×10^3 KJ/mol. for Pt

So, Pt^{4+} is more stable than Ni^{4+}.

13. RuO_4 & OsO_4 have respective metals in +8 oxidation states.

18. wrt option a,

$$\underset{\text{(Chromate ion)}}{CrO_4^{2-}} \underset{^-OH}{\overset{H^+}{\rightleftharpoons}} \underset{\text{(dichromate ion)}}{Cr_2O_7^{2-}}$$

19. $K_2Cr_2O_7 + 4NaCl + 6H_2SO_4 \longrightarrow 2KHSO_4 + 4NaHSO_4 + 2\,CrO_2Cl_2 + 3H_2O$

20. Formation of Ce^{4+} is favored by its noble gas configuration.

21. $\underset{M}{3Mg} + N_2 \longrightarrow \underset{Y}{Mg_3\,N_2}$

$\underset{Y}{Mg_3N_2} + 6H_2O \longrightarrow 3Mg(OH)_2 + \underset{\text{Colorless}}{2NH_3\uparrow}$

$CuSO_4 + 4NH_3 \longrightarrow \underset{\text{Blue complex}}{(Cu(NH_3)_4)SO_4}$

22. Yb^{3+} is a colorless ion.

23. $KMnO_4 + H_2SO_4 \longrightarrow KHSO_4 + Mn_2O_7 + H_2O$
Cold conc.

24. $\underset{(A)}{4FeCr_2O_4} + 8Na_2CO_3 + 7O_2$

$$\longrightarrow \underset{(B)}{8Na_2CrO_4} + 2Fe_2O_3 + 8CO_2\uparrow$$

$$2Na_2CrO_4 + H_2SO_4 \longrightarrow \underset{(C)}{Na_2Cr_2O_7} + Na_2SO_4 + H_2O$$

$$\underset{(C)}{Na_2Cr_2O_7} + 2KCl \longrightarrow \underset{(D)}{K_2Cr_2O_7} + 2NaCl$$

26. wrt option a–

CuI_2 is not known because Cu^{2+} oxidises I^- to iodine.

wrt option b–

Zr & Hf have nearly same sizes & hence are difficult to separate.

wrt option c–

$Cu + 2HCl \longrightarrow CuCl_2 + H_2\uparrow$

It is because $E^\circ_{Cu^{2+}/Cu} = +0.34V$ whereas

$$E^\circ_{H^+/H_2} = 0.V$$

27. Based upon their electrode potentials.

28. In highest oxidation states, acidic character is shown & not basic.

31. Terbium is a lanthanoid

32. $\overline{O}H$ will react with CO_2 to form CO_3^{2-} ions

33. wrt option 1, order is incorrect as Cr will have maximum melting point.

34.

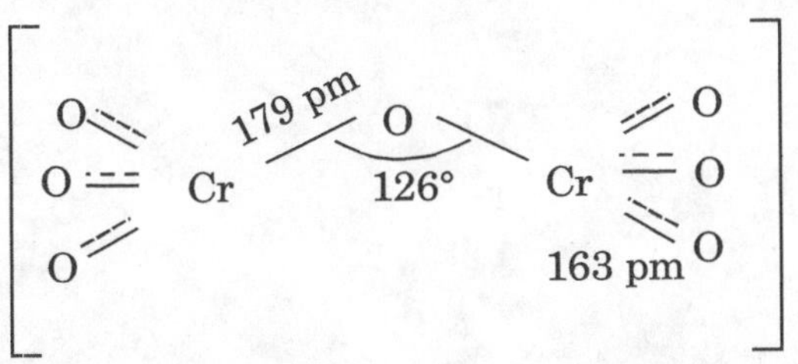

36. When acidified with H_2SO_4, $KMnO_4$ oxidises oxalic acid to CO_2 but when acidified with HCl, $KMnO_4$ will oxidise oxalic acid to CO_2 & also Cl^- to Cl_2.

38. Highest Mn fluoride known is MnF_4.

39. Greater range of oxidation states is possible for actinides because there is not much difference in energies of 5f, 6d & 7s. Also, 5f orbitals are not as buried as 4f orbitals & hence 5f electrons can participate in bonding also. Removal of electrons is possible from all the three i.e. 5f, 6d & 7s.

41. $Cr_2O_7^{2-} + 2H^+ + 4H_2O_2 \longrightarrow 2CrO(O_2)_2 + 5H_2O$

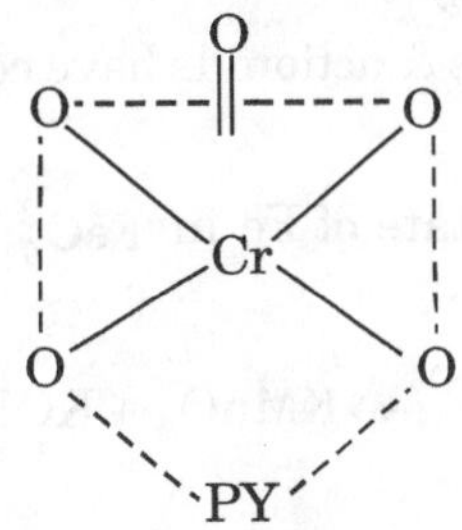

42. $(NH_4)_2Cr_2O_7 \xrightarrow{\Delta} \underset{(Green)}{Cr_2O_3} + N_2 + 4H_2O$

44. Ni has configuration (Ar) $3d^8 4s^2$ where exchange energy is 13E & in Ni^+, configuration is (Ar) $3d^8 4s^1$ which after reorganisation becomes (Ar) $3d^9$ & exchange energy becomes 16E. This sudden increase in exchange energy lowers its I.E.

47. d-d transition is not possible $K_2Cr_2O_7$ because Cr is in +6 oxidation state & lacks d-electrons.

49. CrO_5

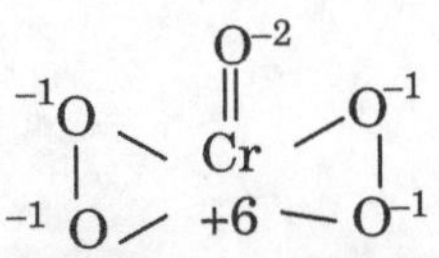

52. $4KMnO_4 + 4KOH \longrightarrow 4K_2MnO_4 + O_2 + 2H_2O$

53. $\underset{(A)}{2KMnO_4} \xrightarrow{\Delta} \underset{(B)}{K_2MnO_4} + \underset{(C)}{MnO_2 + O_2}$

$2MnO_2 + 4KOH + O_2 \longrightarrow 2K_2MnO_4 + 2H_2O$

$MnO_2 + 4NaCl + 4H_2SO_4 \longrightarrow MnCl_2 + 2NaHSO_4 + 2H_2O + Cl_2$.

55. It is because of increasing stability of the lower species to which they are reduced. MnO_4^- will be reduced to Mn^{2+} which has stable half filed configuration.

Also, $Cr_2O_7^{2-}$ is reduced to Cr^{3+} which has half filed t_{2g} level.

VO_2^+ is reduced to V^{3+} which has configuration (Ar) $3d^2$.

stability follows order : - $Mn^{2+} > Cr^{3+} > V^{3+}$.

Oxidising power follow order : -

$MnO_4^- > Cr_2O_7^{2-} > VO_2^+$

56. $MnO_4^- + 2H_2O + 3e^- \rightarrow MnO_2 + 4\overline{O}H$(neutral)

$MnO_4^- + 2H_2O + 3e^- \rightarrow MnO_2 + 4\overline{O}H$(dil. alkaline)

$MnO_4^- + 8H^+ + 5e^- \rightarrow Mn^{2+} + 4H_2O$(acidic)

57. In CoF_3, Co is in +3 oxidation state & F^- Can stabilise its +3 oxidation state by means of high lattice energy.

61. Lanthanoids & actionids have common oxidation state of +3.

68. Oxidation state of Fe in FeO_4^{2-} is 6 whereas it gp. No in 8.

69. $K_2MnO_4 \xrightarrow{O_3} KMnO_4 + KOH + O_2$

$\xrightarrow{Cl_2} KMnO_4 + KCl$

$\xrightarrow{CO_2} KMnO_4 + K_2CO_3 + MnO_2$

71. Eq. wt. $= \dfrac{\text{M.wt}}{\text{n factor}}$

$8H^+ + MnO_4^- + 5e^- \longrightarrow Mn^{2+} + 4H_2O$

Eq.wt $= \dfrac{158.5}{5} = 31.6$

72. In alkaline medium,

$3H_2O + 6MnO_4^- + 3I^- \rightarrow 6MnO_2 + 3IO_3^- + 6\overline{O}H$

3 moles of KI are oxidised by $KMnO_4$ = 6 moles

1 mole of KI are oxidised by $KMnO_4 = \dfrac{6}{3} = 2$

$\therefore\ n_1 = 2$

In acidic medium

$8H^+ + MnO_4^- + 5I^- \longrightarrow Mn^{2+} + 5I_2 + 4H_2O$

5 moles of KI are oxidised by $KMnO_4$ = 1 moles

1 mole of KI are oxidised by $KMnO_4$

$= \dfrac{1}{5}$ moles = 0.2 moles

$\therefore\ n_2 = 0.2$

Now, $\dfrac{n_1}{n_2} = \dfrac{2}{0.2}$

$\dfrac{2 \times 10}{0.2} = 10 : 1$

78. 2PbO.PbO_2, FeO. Fe_2O_3; 2MnO. MnO_2.

80. $2Cu^{2+} + 4I^- \longrightarrow Cu_2I_2 + I_2$

9

CHAPTER

Co-ordination Compounds

Basic Terms and Nomenclature

1. Which of the following cannot act as a ligand ?

(a) PH_3 (b) Cl^-

(c) O_2^- (d) $\overset{+}{N}H_4$

2. Which of the following ligands will not form a metal nitrogen bond when bonded with a metal atom ?

(a) EDTA

(b) ethane-1, 2-diamine

(c) glycinato

(d) acetylacetonato

3. Match the entry in column-I with its corrresponding entry in column-II.

Column-I	Column-II
A. $[Pt(NH_3)_2Cl(NO_2)]$	(i) diammine chloridonitrito-N platinum (II)
B. $[Co(NH_3)_5(CO_3)]Cl$	(ii) Pentaammine carbonato cobalt (III) chloride
C. $K_2[Zn(OH)_4]$	(iii) Potassium tetrahydroxo zincate (II)
D. $K_3[Cr(C_2O_4)_3]$	(iv) Potassium trioxalato chromate (III)

(a) A - iv, B - iii, C - i, D - ii

(b) A - ii, B - iii, C - i, D - iv

(c) A - iv, B - i, C - ii, D - iii

(d) A - i, B - ii, C - iii, D - iv

4. The correct IUPAC name of the following complex is :

$$[PtCl_2(NH_3)_4]\ [PtCl_4]$$

(a) tetra amminedichlorido platinum (IV) tetrachlorido platinate (II)

(b) tetra amminedichlorido platinum (II) tetrachlorido platinate (IV)

(c) tetra ammine dichlorido platinum (III) tetrachlorido platinate (III)

(d) Both (b) & (c)

5. Which one of the following is a bidentate ligand?

(a) 2, 2-dipyridyl (b) dmg

(c) Oxalate (d) All of these

6. The correct IUPAC name of the following compound is :

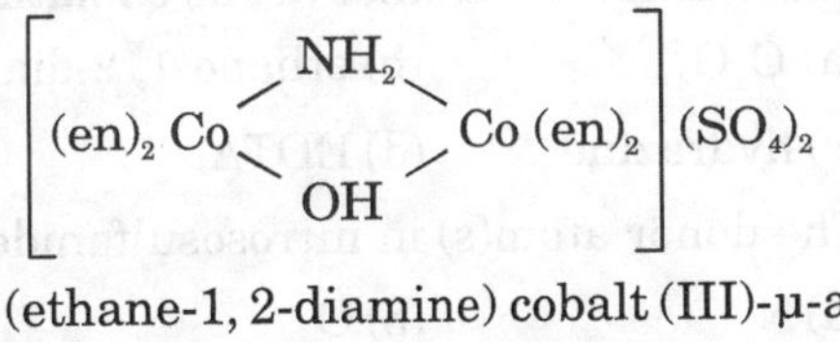

(a) bis (ethane-1, 2-diamine) cobalt (III)-μ-amido-μ- hydroxobis (ethane-1, 2-diamine) cobalt (III) sulphate.

(b) bis (ethane-1, 2-diamine) cobalt (III)-μ-hydroxo-μ-imidobis (ethane-1, 2-diamine) cobalt (III) sulphate.

(c) bis (ethane-1, 2-diamine)-μ-imido-μ-hydroxo bis(ethane-1, 2-diamine) dicobalt (III) sulphate.

(d) None of these

7. Which one of the following is a bidentate & an ambidentate ligand?

(a) $\bar{O}CN$ (b) $\bar{S}CN$

(c) NOS^- (d) $C_2S_2O_2^{2-}$

8. Which of the following statement is/are correct wrt complexes given below ?

Complex I : $[Co(NH_3)_4 CO_3]Br$

Complex II : $[Co(NH_3)_5 CO_3]Br$

1. The oxidation state of cobalt in both the complexes is +3.
2. The co-ordination number of Co in both the complexes is six.
3. Carbonate acts as a bidentate ligand in both the complexes.
4. Ammonia is a neutral ligand in both the complexes.

(a) Only 1 & 2 are correct

(b) Only 2 & 3 are correct

(c) 1, 2 & 4 only are correct

(d) Only 3 is correct

9. The correct IUPAC name of the following compound is :

$$[Cr(H_2O)_4 Cl_2]Cl \cdot 2H_2O$$

(a) tetra aquadichlorido chromium (III) chloride-2-water

(b) tetra aquadichlorido chromium (III) chloride dihydrate.

(c) Dichlorido tetraqua chromium (III) chloride dihydrate.

(d) Both (a) & (b)

10. A ligand that can form a ring structure with central atom is called a chelating ligand. Which of the following cannot act as chelating ligand.

(a) $C_2O_4^{2-}$ (b) ethane-1, 2-diamine

(c) hydrazine (d) EDTA

11. The donor atom(s) in nitrososulfanide is/are :

(a) N (b) O

(c) S (d) All of these

12. Which of the following cannot act as ambidentate ligand?

(a) thiosulphate ion

(b) selenocyanide ion

(c) thiocyanate ion

(d) None of these

13. Which of the following can act as pie acceptor ligand(s)?

(1) CO (2) $\bar{C}N$

(3) $\overset{+}{N}O$ (4) PPh_3

(5) C_2H_4

(a) Only 1, 2 & 3 (b) Only 1, 2 & 4

(c) Only 2, 3 & 5 (d) All of these

14. Which of the following will give test of Fe^{2+} in aqueous solution ?

(a) $(NH_4)_2 SO_4 \cdot FeSO_4 \cdot 24H_2O$

(b) $(NH_4)_2 SO_4 \cdot Fe_2(SO_4)_3 \cdot 24H_2O$

(c) $K_4[Fe(CN)_6]$

(d) $K_3[Fe(CN)_6]$

15. The correct formula of the complex named tris (ethane-1, 2-diamine) cobalt (III) sulphate is :

(a) $[Co(en)_3]SO_4$ (b) $[Co(en)_2]SO_4$

(c) $[Co(en)_3]_2 SO_4$ (d) $[Co(en)_3]_2 (SO_4)_3$

16. The number of bridging ligands and the number of bromine atoms per molecule in the compound, pentaammine chromium (III)-μ-hydroxo pentaammine chromium (III) bromide respectively are :

(a) 1, 5

(b) 2, 6

(c) 1, 4

(d) 1, 3

17. The correct IUPAC name for

$[(CO)_3 Fe(CO)_3 Fe(CO)_3]$ is :

(a) tri-μ-hexacarbonyl iron (II)

(b) tri-μ-carbonyl-bis tricarbonyl iron (o)

(c) tri-μ-nanocarbonyl iron (III)

(d) hexa-μ-tricarbonyl ferrate (o)

18. The correct formula for tetraamminedichlorido cobalt (III) hexa cyanochromate (III) is :

(a) $[Co(NH_3)_4 Cl_2][Cr(CN)_5]$

(b) $[Co(NH_3)_4 Cl_2]_3 [Cr(CN)_6]$

(c) $[Cr(NH_3)_4 Cl_2][Co(CN)_6]$

(d) $[Cr(NH_3)_2 Cl_2 (CN)_2][Co(NH_3)_2 (CN)_4]$

19. Select the ligand(s) with INCORRECT IUPAC Name(s).

Ligand	IUPAC
(a) $\leftarrow \bar{N}O_2$ (N donor)	Nitro
(b) $\leftarrow \overset{\ominus}{O}NO$ (O donor)	Nitrito
(c) $\leftarrow \overset{\ominus}{N}CS$ (N donor)	isothiocyanato

(d) None of these are incorrect.

20. Select the complex where name of metal has suffix '–ate'?

(a) $[Co(NH_3)_6]Cl_3$ (b) $[Ni(CO)_4]$

(c) $Li[AlH_4]$ (d) All of these

Isomerism

21. The total number of possible isomers for the complex $[Co(en)_2Cl_2]Cl$ is/are :

(a) 1 (b) 2
(c) 3 (d) 4

22. $[Co(NH_3)_5NO_3]SO_4$ & $[Co(NH_3)_5SO_4]NO_3$ exhibit :

(a) co-ordination isomerism
(b) linkage isomerism
(c) ionisation isomerism
(d) optical isomerism

23. Match the complex in list-I with the type of isomerism in list-II.

List-I	List-II
A. $[Pt(NH_3)_2Cl_2]$	(i) Optical
B. cis$[Co(en)_2Cl_2]$	(ii) Ionisation
C. trans $[Co(en)_2(NO_2)Cl]SCN$	(iii) co-ordination
D. $[Co(NH_3)_6][Cr(CN)_6]$	(iv) Geometrical

(a) A - ii, B - iv, C - iii, D - i
(b) A - iii, B - iv, C - ii, D - i
(c) A - iv, B - i, C - ii, D - iii
(d) A - ii, B - i, C - iii, D - iv

24. For the complex $[Co(H_2O)_2(NH_3)_2Cl_2]^+$, the total number of stereoisomers is/are :

(a) 5 (b) 4
(c) 7 (d) 6

25. Which of the following isomerism(s) is/are exhibited by the compound shown below ?

$$[Co(SCN)_2(NH_3)_4]Cl$$

(a) Geometrical isomerism
(b) Ionisation isomerism
(c) Linkage isomerism
(d) All of these

26. Which of the following complex ion has geometrical isomers?

(a) $[Ni(NH_3)_5Br]^+$

(b) $[Co(NH_3)_2(en)_2]^{3+}$

(c) $[Cr(NH_3)_4 en]^{3+}$

(d) $[Co(en)_3]^{3+}$

27. The number of geometric isomers that can exist for sq. planar $[Pt(Cl)(Py)(NH_3)(NH_2OH)]^+$ is :

(Py = Pyridine)

(a) 2 (b) 3
(c) 4 (d) 6

28. The ionization isomers of $[Cr(H_2O)_4Cl(NO_2)]Cl$ is :

(a) $[Cr(H_2O)_4(O_2N)]Cl_2$

(b) $[Cr(H_2O)_4Cl_2]NO_2$

(c) $[Cr(H_2O)_4Cl(ONO)]Cl$

(d) $[Cr(H_2O)_4Cl_2(NO_2)]\cdot H_2O$

29. Which of the following complexes has same number of stereoisomeric structures in both tetrahedral & sq. planar forms?

(a) $[M(gly)_2]$

(b) $[MI_3]^-$

(c) [MABCD]

(d) $[M(NH_3)_4]$

Where A, B, C & D are monodentate ligands.

30. Select the correct statement(s) among the following :

(a) $\left[Fe(H_2O)_5(NH_3)\right]CO_3$ cannot show ionisation isomerism.

(b) $[MA_3B_3]$ cannot show optical isomerism. (where A & B are monodentate ligands)

(c) $\left[Co(en)_2(NO_2)Cl\right]SCN$ has 5 sturctural & 3 stereoisomers.

(d) All are correct.

31. The type of isomerism observed in $\left[Pt(NH_3)_2 Cl_2\right]$, is also observed in :

(a) $\left[Co(en)_3\right]^{3+}$ (b) $\left[PtCl_3(ONO)\right]^{2-}$

(c) $\left[PtCl_2Br_2\right]^{2-}$ (d) All of these

32. The pair(s) of co-ordination complexes/ions which can show the same kind of isomerism is/are :

(a) $\left[Cr(NH_3)_5 Cl\right]Cl_2$ & $\left[Cr(NH_3)_4 Cl_2\right]Cl$

(b) $\left[Co(NH_3)_4 Cl_2\right]^+$ & $\left[Pt(NH_3)(H_2O)Cl\right]^+$

(c) $\left[Pt(NH_3)_3(NO_3)\right]Cl$ & $\left[Pt(NH_3)_3 Cl\right]Br$

(d) Both (b) & (c)

33. Which of the following complexes have 4 isomers ?

(a) $\left[Pt(NH_3)_2 Cl_2\right]$ (b) $\left[Ni(CO)_4\right]$

(c) $\left[CO(en)_3\right]Cl_3$ (d) $\left[Co(en)_2 Cl_2\right]Br$

34. The complex $\left[ZnCl_2(NH_3)_2\right]$ will exhibit :

(a) Linkage isomerism

(b) Geometrical isomerism

(c) Optical isomerism

(d) No isomerism

35. Match the entry in column-I with corresponding correct choice in column-II.

Column-I (co-ordination complex)	Column-II (Isomerism)
(i) $\left[Co(NH_3)_5 NO_2\right]Cl_2$	1. Linkage
(ii) $\left[Co(NH_3)_5 Br\right]SO_4$	2. Geometrical
(iii) $\left[Co(en)_2 Cl_2\right]Cl$	3. Ionisation
(iv) $\left[Pt(gly)_2\right]$	4. Optical

(a) i - 1; ii - 3; iii - 2; iv - 4

(b) i - 1, 2; ii - 3; iii - 3, 4; iv - 2, 4

(c) i - 1, 3; ii - 3; iii - 2, 4; iv - 2

(d) i - 3; ii - 1; iii - 3, 4; iv - 1, 2

36. The type of isomerism(s) shown by $\left[Cr(NH_3)_2(OH)_2 Cl_2\right]^{-1}$ is/are :

(a) Hydrate (b) Geometrical

(c) Optical (d) Both (b) & (c)

37. The term facial & meridional is associated with which of the following complexes.

(a) $[MA_3 B_3]$ (b) $[M(AB)_3]$

(c) [M AB CD] (d) Both (a) & (b)

Where A, B, C & D are monodentate ligands & AB is unsymmetrical bidentate ligand.

38. Which of the following shows optical isomerism but no geometrical isomerism?

(a) $\left[Co(OX)_3\right]^{3-}$ (b) $\left[Co(NH_3)_4 Cl_2\right]^+$

(c) $\left[Co(en)_2 Cl_2\right]^+$ (d) $\left[Co(NH_3)_2 Cl_2(en)\right]^+$

39. The total number of possible stereoisomers for MABCDEF is/are :

(a) 15 (b) 12

(c) 30 (d) 35

40. The possible number of isomers for $\left[Co(NH_3)_6\right]\left[Cr(NO_2)_6\right]$ is/are :

(a) 3 (b) 4

(c) 5 (d) 6

41. How many optical isomers are possible for the complex $\left[Ni(H_2O)(Cl)(NH_3)(NH_2OH)\right]NO_2$ with magnetic moment 2.82 B.M. ?

(a) 2 (b) 5

(c) 0 (d) 3

42. Consider the following arrangments of the octahedral complex ion $\left[Co(NH_3)_4 Cl_2\right]^+$

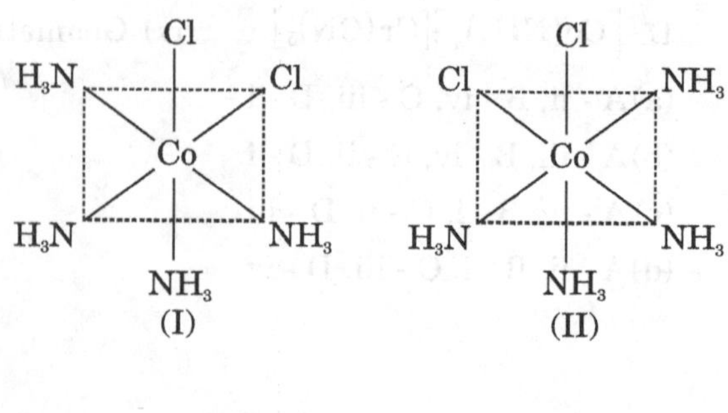

(I) (II)

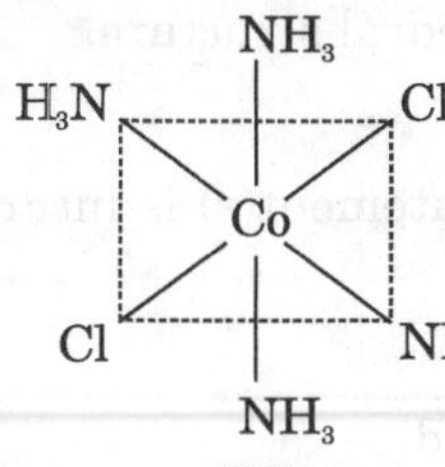

(III)

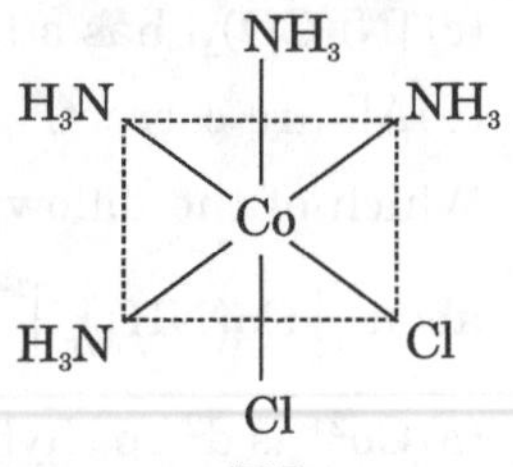

(IV)

Which of the following statements is/are incorrect?

(a) II & III are *cis* & *trans* isomers respectively.

(b) III & IV are *trans* & *cis* isomers respectively.

(c) II & IV are identical

(d) I & II are enantiomers

43. A complex has 2 optical isomers. Their correct structures are :

(a) 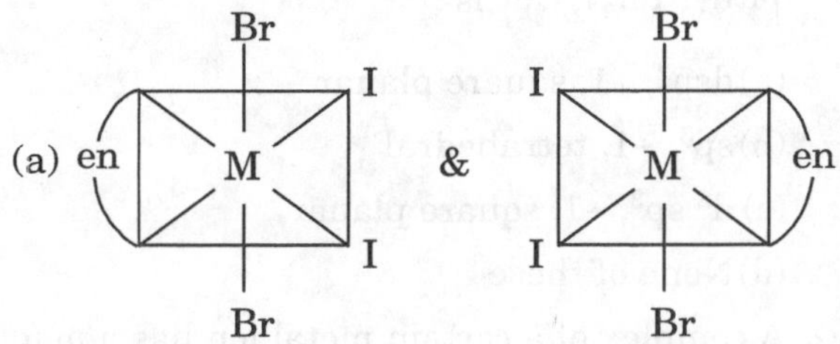

(b) 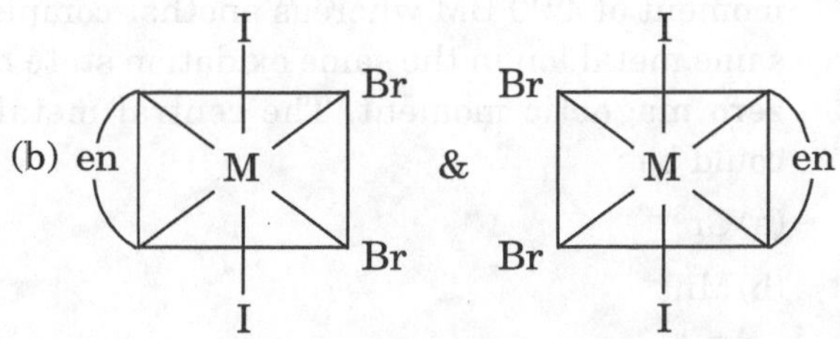

(c) 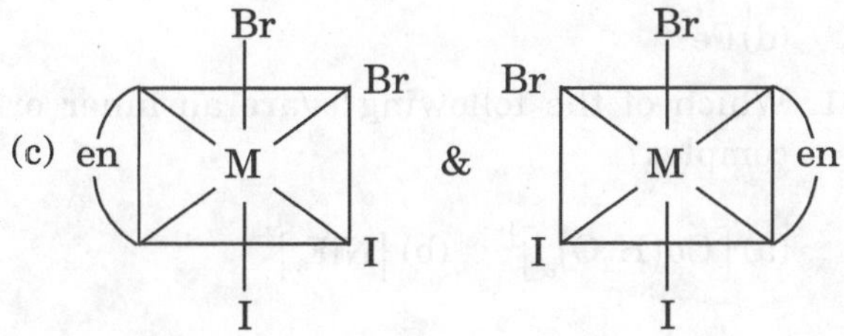

(d) All of these

44. Consider the following reaction :

$$[M(gly)(en)]^{+} \xrightarrow[-en]{+gly^{-}} [M(gly)_2]^{0}$$

If reactant has no stereoisomer but product exists in two stereoisomeric forms, then hybridisation of metal M, in product, is

(a) sp^3

(b) dsp^2

(c) either dsp^2 or sp^3

(d) either d^2sp^3 or sp^3d^2

45. In which of the following pairs, both the complexes show optical isomerism?

(a) cis – $[Cr(C_2O_4)_2Cl_2]^{3-}$; cis – $[Co(NH_3)_4Cl_2]$

(b) $[Co(en)_3]Cl_3$, cis – $[Co(en)_2Cl_2]Cl$

(c) $[PtCl(dien)]Cl$, $[NiCl_2Br_2]^{2-}$

(d) $[Co(NH_3)_3(NO_3)_3]$, cis – $[Pt(en)_2Cl_2]$

46. The number of geometrical isomers for octahedral $[Co(NH_3)_2Cl_4]^-$ and $[AuCl_2Br_2]^-$, $[Pt(en)Cl_2]$ (both square planar) are respectively,

(a) 2, 2, 2 (b) 2, 2, no isomerism

(c) 3, 2, 2 (d) 2, 3, no isomerism

47. Which of the following will not show geometrical isomerism?

(a) $[Cr(NH_3)_4Cl_2]Cl$

(b) $[Co(en)_2Cl_2]Cl$

(c) $[Ni(NH_3)_2Cl_2]$

(d) $[Pt(NH_3)_2Cl_2]$

Valence Bond Theory (VBT)

48. Octahedral complex of Ni(II) must be

(a) inner orbital

(b) outer orbital

(c) either (a) or (b) depending upon the ligand strength

(d) None of these

49. Which one of the following has square planar structure :

(a) $[NiCl_4]^{2-}$

(b) $[Zn(NH_3)_4]^{2+}$

(c) $[Ni(CN)_4]^{2-}$

(d) Both (a) & (b)

50. The total number of unpaired electron(s) in $[Mn(CN)_6]^{3-}$ is/are (according to VBT)

(a) 1

(b) 2

(c) 3

(d) zero

51. Which one of the following statement is/are correct about $[Ni(NH_3)_6]^{2+}$?

(a) It is a diamagnetic complex.

(b) Ni is in +2 oxidation state.

(c) Hybridised state of Ni^{2+} is $sp^3 d^2$ & it is paramagnetic.

(d) both (b) & (c) are correct.

52. Which of the following is/are outer orbital complex(es)?

(a) $[Co(C_2O_4)_3]^{3-}$ (b) $[V(H_2O)_6]^{3+}$

(c) $[Cr(NH_3)_6]^{3+}$ (d) None of these

53. Ni^{2+} in alkaline medium is treated with 'A' to give a complex 'B' which gives rosy red precipitate. Then the INCORRECT statement about A and B is :

(a) A is a bidentate ligand

(b) Co-ordination number of Ni in 'B' is 6

(c) B is square planar in shape

(d) B is diamagnetic.

54. Which of the following have square planar structure?

(a) $[PdCl_4]^{2-}$

(b) $[PtCl_4]^{2-}$

(c) $[Ni(CN)_4]^{2-}$

(d) All of these are square planar

55. In which of the following, atleast 5 atoms including the metal itself, are linear?

(a) $[Ag(NH_3)_2]^+$ (b) $[Ag(CN)_2]^-$

(c) $[Ni(CO)_4]$ (d) $[Ni(H_2O)_4]^{2+}$

56. Amongst the following ions, which one has the highest paramagnetism?

(a) $[Cr(H_2O)_6]^{3+}$ (b) $[Fe(H_2O)_6]^{2+}$

(c) $[Zn(H_2O)_6]^{2+}$ (d) $[Cu(H_2O)_6]^{2+}$

57. Select the correct statement(s).

(a) In d^3 type configuration, no pairing occurs whether the ligand is strong or weak.

(b) In d^4 type configuration, only one pairing occurs if the ligand is strong.

(c) $[Ni(CO)_4]$ has a tetrahedral structure.

(d) All are correct.

58. Which of the following statement(s) is incorrect about $[Co(NH_3)_6]^{2+}$?

(a) Co^{2+} is $d^2 sp^3$ hybridised.

(b) Complex is paramagnetic corresponding to one unpaired electron.

(c) It involves promotion of an electron from 3d to 5s or 4d, which becomes loosely bonded & hence it is easily oxidised to $[Co(NH_3)_6]^{3+}$.

(d) None of these are incorrect.

59. The hybridisation, oxidation number of central metal ion & shape of wilkinsons catalyst $[Rh(PPh_3)_3 Cl]$ is :

(a) dsp^2, +1, square planar

(b) sp^3, +1, tetrahedral

(c) $d^2 sp^3$, +1, square planar

(d) None of these

60. A complex of a certain metal ion has a magnetic moment of 4.90 BM whereas another complex of same metal ion in the same oxidation state has a zero magnetic moment. The central metal ion could be :

(a) Cr^{3+}

(b) Mn^{2+}

(c) Fe^{3+}

(d) Fe^{2+}

61. Which of the following is/are an inner orbital complex?

(a) $[Co(H_2O)_6]^{3+}$ (b) $[NiF_6]^{2-}$

(c) $[Ni(NH_3)_6]^{2+}$ (d) Both (a) & (b)

62. Which of the following statement(s) is/are correct wrt Tetrahedral complexes?

(a) Tetrahedral geometry is favoured by metal ion with noble gas configuration (eg. Be^{2+}), pseudonoble gas configuration (eg Zn^{2+}) with large ligands like Cl^-, Br^-, I^- etc.

(b) Tetrahedral complexes do not show geometrical isomerism.

(c) Complexes with tetrahderal geometry have metal ions with co-ordination No. = 4.

(d) All are correct.

63. Consider the following statements :

(1) Square planar complexes are less favored sterically than tetrahedral complexes & are prohibitively crowded by large ligands.

(2) Square planar complexes are commonly formed by d^8 species such as Ni^{2+}, Pd^{2+}, Pt^{2+} & Au^{3+}.

(3) The requirement for the stability of square planar complexes is the presence of nonbulky, strong field ligands which can act as π acceptor also. These conditions are relaxed for heavy metal ion like Pt, Pd etc.

(4) $[PtCl_4]^{2-}$ is a tetrahedral complex.

INCORRECT statement(s) amongst the above statements is/are :

(a) 1, 2 & 3 only (b) 4 only

(c) 2, 3 & 4 only (d) All of these

64. Identify the mismatch

Complex ions	**Hybridisation**
(a) $[Ti(H_2O)_6]^{2+}, [CrF_6]^{3-}$	$\rightarrow d^2sp^3$
(b) $[Co(H_2O)_6]^{3+}, [CoF_6]^{3-}$	$\rightarrow sp^3d^2$
(c) $[NiCl_4]^{2-}, [Zn(NH_3)_4]^{2+}$	$\rightarrow sp^3$

(d) None of these

65. Select the correct statement about sodium nitroprusside, $Na_2[Fe(CN)_5NO]$.

(1) Here Fe has oxidation state +2.

(2) $\overset{+}{N}O$ present here is a strong field ligand.

(3) It is an inner orbital complex.

(4) It is an outer orbital complex.

Correct statement(s) is/are :

(a) 1 only (b) 2, & 3 only

(c) 1, 2 & 3 only (d) All are correct.

66. Select the correct statement(s) about brown ring complex formed during the detection of NO_3^- ion.

(1) Brown ring complex has the formula $[Fe(H_2O)_5NO]SO_4$.

(2) The colour is due to charge transfer.

(3) This complex formally contains Fe(+1) & $\overset{+}{N}O$ since Fe^{2+} gains one electron from NO, which then changes to $\overset{+}{N}O$.

(4) Its magnetic moment is 3.87 B.M. confirming the presence of 3 unpaired electrons.

(5) Hybridisation of Fe in this complex is sp^3d^2.

(a) Only 1 & 2 are correct

(b) Only 2, 3 & 4 are correct

(c) Only 4 & 5 are correct

(d) All are correct.

67. Which of the following pairs contain only tetrahedral complexes?

(a) $[ZnCl_4]^{2-}$ & $[MnCl_4]^{2-}$

(b) $[Zn(NH_3)_4]^{2+}$ & $[Cu(NH_3)_4]^{2+}$

(c) $[MnCl_4]^{2-}$ & $[Ni(CN)_4]^{2-}$

(d) $[ZnCl_4]^{2-}$ & $[Ni(CN)_4]^{2-}$

CFT

68. What is the correct configuration for a metal ion with d^7 for octahedral complex in the presence of strong field ligands?

(a) $t_{2g}^6\ eg^1$ (b) $t_{2g}^5\ eg^2$

(c) $t_{2g}^3\ eg^4$ (d) $t_{2g}^4\ eg^3$

69. Which one of the following in correct ?

(a) $[Co(NH_3)_6]^{2+}$ is readily oxidised to $[Co(NH_3)_6]^{3+}$

(b) $\Delta_t = \frac{4}{9}\Delta_0$

(c) $d_{x^2-y^2}$ & d_{z^2} suffer greater repulsions than other three orbitals in octahedral geometry.

(d) All are correct.

70. Tetrahedral complexes are less stable than octahedral or square planar complexes because in tetrahedral complexes.

(a) the crystal field splitting is smaller, so the lower set of energy levels is stabilised less than in other geometries.

(b) The lower energy set of levels is only doubly degenerate i.e., lesser no. of electrons are placed in lower energy level.

(c) 6 monodentate ligands approach the metal ion.

(d) Both (a) & (b) are correct.

71. Crystal field splitting in tetrahedral complexes is less than in octahedral complexes because.
(a) In tetrahedral complexes there are four monodentate ligands instead of six as in case of octahedral complexes.
(b) In tetrahedral complexes there are six monodentate ligands instead of four as in case of octahedral complexes.
(c) Direction of orbitals does not coincide with the direction of ligands in tetrahedral field.
(d) Both (a) & (c)

72. Which of the following are correct statements about crystal field splitting ?
(a) Ligands carrying greater charge density cause greater splitting.
(b) Among uncharged ligands the ones which are less basic cause greater splitting.
(c) C donors are weak field ligands.
(d) Both (a) & (c) are correct.

73. Crystal field splitting is maximum in :
(a) $[Co(NH_3)_6]^{3+}$
(b) $[Rh(NH_3)_6]^{3+}$
(c) $[Ir(NH_3)_6]^{3+}$
(d) All show equal splitting

74. Spin only magnetic moment for an octahedral complex having CFSE = $-0.6\ \Delta_0$ and sorrounded by weak field ligands can be :
(a) 4.9 B.M. (b) 1.73 B.M.
(c) 3.7 B.M. (d) Both (a) & (b)

75. CFSE for high spin d^4 octahedral complex is :
(a) $-1.8\ \Delta_0$ (b) $-1.6\ \Delta_0 + P$
(c) $-1.2\ \Delta_0$ (d) $-0.6\ \Delta_0$

76. CFSE for octahedral complexes is zero in :
(a) d^8 configuration
(b) d^{10} configuration
(c) high spin d^5 configuration
(d) Both (b) & (c)

77. According to CFT, wave number obtained is 20,300 cm^{-1} for $t_{2g} \rightarrow$ eg. The CFSE (in kJ/mol) for the complex $[Ti(H_2O)_6]^{3+}$ is :
(a) –242 kJ/mol (b) –96.8 kJ/mol
(c) –194 kJ/mol (d) –109 kJ/mol

EAN & Werner's Theory (Effective Atomic Number)

78. In which of the following molecules/ions the effective atomic no. of metal is 36?
(a) $[Cr(CO)_6]$ (b) $[Fe(CN)_6]^{3-}$
(c) $[Co(CN)_6]^{4-}$ (d) $[Ni(NH_3)_6]^{2+}$

79. Consider the following complexes :
(1) K_2PtCl_6 (2) $PtCl_4 \cdot 2NH_3$
(3) $PtCl_4 \cdot 3NH_3$ (4) $PtCl_4 \cdot 5NH_3$
Their respectively electrical conductance in aqueous solution are :
(a) 256, 0, 97, 404 (b) 404, 0, 97, 256
(c) 256, 97, 0, 404 (d) 404, 97, 256, 0

80. EAN for 'Fe' in the complex $[Fe(CO)_2(NO)_2]$ is
(a) 35 (b) 36
(c) 33 (d) 31

81. Which one of the following do not have EAN equal to 36?
(a) $[V(CO)_6]^-$
(b) $[Fe(\pi-C_5H_5)_2]$
(c) $[Fe(CO)_5]$
(d) $[Ti(\sigma-C_5H_5)_2(\pi-C_5H_5)_2]$

82. $CoCl_3.3NH_3$ does not form any precipitate with excess $AgNO_3$ solution, whereas 1 mole of $CoCl_3.5NH_3$ gives two moles of AgCl with excess $AgNO_3$. The van't Hoff factor for both the compounds (assuming 100% ionisation) respectively, are :
(a) 0 & 2 (b) 0 & 3
(c) 1 & 3 (d) 1 & 2

83. The ratio of primary valency & secondary valency of the metal ion is the co-ordination compound, $K_2[Ni(CN)_4]$ is :
(a) 1 : 2
(b) 1 : 3
(c) 2 : 1
(d) 3 : 1

84. A solution containing 0.319 gm of complex $CrCl_3.6H_2O$ was passed through a cation exchanger & the solution given out was neutralised by 28.5 ml of 0.125 M NaOH. The correct formula of the complex will be :

(molecular wt. of complex = 266.5)

(a) $[CrCl(H_2O)_5]Cl_2 \cdot H_2O$

(b) $[Cr(H_2O)_6]Cl_3$

(c) $[CrCl_2(H_2O)_4]Cl \cdot 2H_2O$

(d) All are correct

85. EAN Rule is strictly followed by :

(a) Cyano complexes

(b) Fluoro complexes

(c) Carbonyl complexes

(d) All of these

86. X, Y, Z are three complexes of chromium (III) with the empirical formula $CrCl_3H_{12}O_6$. All the three complexes have water or chloride ion as ligands. Complex (A) does not react with conc. H_2SO_4 whereas complexes (B) and (C) lost 6.75% & 13.5% of their original weight, respectively on treatment with conc. H_2SO_4. Correct formulae of A, B, & C respectively are :

(a) $[Cr(H_2O)_6]Cl_3$, $[Cr(H_2O)_5Cl]Cl_2 \cdot H_2O$, $[Cr(H_2O)_4Cl_2]Cl.2H_2O$

(b) $[Cr(H_2O)_5Cl]Cl_2 \cdot H_2O$, $[Cr(H_2O)_6]Cl_3$, $[Cr(H_2O)_4Cl_2]Cl \cdot 2H_2O$

(c) $[Cr(H_2O)_5Cl] \cdot H_2O$, $[Cr(H_2O)_6]Cl_3$, $[Cr(H_2O)_4Cl_2]Cl \cdot 2H_2O$

(d) None of these

87. The number of precipitable halide ions in the complex chloropentaamminecobalt (III) chloride is :

(a) 2

(b) 3

(c) 4

(d) 1

Metal Carbonyls and Organometallic Compounds

88. Which one of the following is a π-acceptor ligand?

(1) CO (2) $\bar{C}N$

(3) $\overset{+}{N}O$ (4) PF_3

(5) C_2H_4

(a) Only 1, 2 & 3 (b) Only 2, 3 & 5

(c) Only 3 & 4 (d) All of these

89. The hapticity of the following ligand before & after the removal of 'marked' Hydrogen ion (H^-) is :

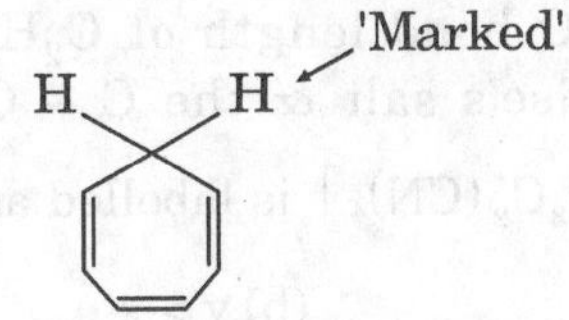

(a) 6, 7 (b) 7, 6

(c) 5, 4 (d) 4, 5

90. Which of the following is a σ-bonded organometallic compound?

(a) Zeise's salt

(b) Ferrocene

(c) bis (benzene) chromium/dibenzene chromium

(d) Grignards' reagent

91. Keeping 18-electron rule in mind, which of the following statement is/are correct for the complex given below?

$$[W(CO)_2(C_5H_5)_2]$$

(a) Both C_5H_5 ligands are pentahapto

(b) Both C_5H_5 ligands are trihapto

(c) One of the C_5H_5 ligands is pentahapto whereas other is trihapto.

(d) None of these

92. Which of the following statement is/are correct about zeises salt ?

(1) It's formula is $K[PtCl_3(\eta^2 - C_2H_4)]$

(2) Here, C – C axis is perpendicular to the platinum ligand plane.

(3) C_2H_4 here acts as a π-acceptor ligand.

(4) Relative to free ethylene the C – C bond is lengthened slightly.

(5) The bond between the ethylene molecule & the metal ion may be considered as a sigma dative bond.

(a) Only 1 is correct

(b) Only 2 & 3 are correct

(c) 1, 2, & 4 only are correct

(d) All statements are correct.

93. Which of the following statement is WRONG about $Mn_2(CO)_{10}$?

(a) It is made up of two square pyramidal $Mn(CO)_5$ units joined by a Mn – Mn bond.

(b) EAN of Mn in $Mn_2(CO)_{10}$ is 36.

(c) Oxidation state of Mn in $[Mn_2(CO)_{10}]$ is zero.

(d) None of the these is INCORRECT

94. If C – C bond length of C_2H_4 is labelled as x in zeise's salt & the C – C of $C_2(CN)_4$ in $K[PtCl_3C_2(CN)_4]$ is labelled as y, then :

(a) x > y (b) y > x

(c) x = y (d) None of these

95. Select the INCORRECT statement about ferrocene ?

(1) Its correct formula is $[Fe(\eta^5 - C_5H_5)_2]$

(2) Oxidation state of Fe in ferrocene is +2.

(3) EAN of metal ion in ferrocene is 36.

(4) All the five C atoms in cyclopentadienyl ring are equidistant from Fe.

(5) All the C – C bond lengths are equal in ferrocene.

(6) Ferrocene undergoes friedal crafts acylation.

(a) Only 1, 2 & 3 are correct

(b) Only 2, 3 & 4 are correct

(c) Only 6 is correct

(d) All statments are correct

96. Select the correct order of M – C bond order in the following species :

(1) $[Ni(CO)_4]$ (2) $[Co(CO)_4]^-$

(3) $[Fe(CO)_4]^{2-}$

(a) 3 > 2 > 1 (b) 3 = 2 = 1

(c) 2 > 1 > 3 (d) 1 > 2 > 3

97. Jahn Teller distortion is not observed in high spin octahedral complexes of :

(a) d^9 configuration

(b) d^7 configuration

(c) d^8 configuration

(d) d^4 configuration

98. Which one of the following ligand substitution reaction can occur ?

(a) Cis $-[CoCl_2(en)_2] \xrightarrow{en}$

(b) trans $-[CoCl_2(en)_2] \xrightarrow{en}$

(c) trans $-[Pt(NH_3)_2Cl] \xrightarrow{H_2C_2O_4}$

(d) Both (b) & (c)

99. Correct statement(s) about metal carbonyls is/are:

(a) They involve synergic bonding.

(b) $V(CO)_6$ will behave as oxidising agent.

(c) σ bond is formed by donation of lone pair of electrons of C into vacant d-orbitals of metal whereas π bond results by donation of electrons from filled d-orbitals of metal into vacant antibonding π* orbital of CO.

(d) All are correct.

100. WRONG statement amongst the folloiwng is :

(a) $[Co(NH_3)_6][Cr(NO_2)_6]$ can be distinguished from $[Cr(NH_3)_6][Co(NO_2)_6]$ by electrolysis of their aqueous solution.

(b) $[Cr(NH_3)_6][Cr(NO_2)_6]$ can be distinguished from $[Cr(NH_3)_4(NO_2)_2][Cr(NH_3)_2(NO_2)_4]$ by conductivity measurements.

(c) PPh_3 is a strong field ligand.

(d) None of these

Brain Teasers

101. The octahedral complex of a metal ion M^{3+} with four monodentate ligands L_1, L_2, L_3 & L_4 absorb wavelength in the region of red, green, yellow & blue respectively. The correct order of ligand strength of four ligands is :

(a) $L_1 > L_4 > L_2 > L_3$ (b) $L_3 > L_4 > L_2 > L_1$

(c) $L_1 > L_2 > L_3 > L_4$ (d) $L_4 > L_2 > L_3 > L_1$

102. Select the correct statement(s).

(a) In $K_4[Fe(CN)_6]$, the ligand has satisfied only the 2° valency (secondary valency)

(b) In $K_3[Fe(CN)_6]$, the ligand has satisfied both 1° & 2° valencies of metal ion in complex.

(c) In $[Cu(NH_3)_4]SO_4$, the ligand has satisfied only the 2° valency of copper ion.

(d) Both (b) & (c) are correct.

103. Which of the following is/are correct order of stability ?

(a) $\left[Fe(C_2O_4)_3\right]^{3-} > \left[Fe(H_2O)_5\right]^{3+}$

(b) $[Fe(edta)]^- > [Fe(en)_3]^{3+}$

(c) $\left[Fe(CN)_6\right]^{3-} > [Fe(CN)_6]^{4-}$

(d) All orders of stability are correct.

104. Consider the following reaction

$$[Ma_3b_2c]^{n+} \xrightarrow{-b/+d} [Ma_3bcd]^{n+}$$

(a, b, c are monodentate ligands)

Then, which of the following statement is/are correct.

(a) The number of pairs of enantiomers is increased by one.

(b) The number of geometrical isomers in the final product are four.

(c) The number of geometrical isomers in the final product are six.

(d) Both (a) & (b) are correct.

105. Consider the following reactions :

(1) $K_2[PtCl_4] + 2K\ gly \rightarrow X + 4KCl$

(2) $\left[Pt(NH_3)_4\right](NO_3)_2 + 2K\ gly \rightarrow Y + 2KNO_3$

Where K gly is potassium glycinate.

'X' is soluble is polar solvent while 'Y' is soluble in non-polar solvent. Then,

(a) X is cis $\left[Pt(gly)_2\right]$, Y is cis $\left[Pt(gly)_2\right]$

(b) X is cis $\left[Pt(gly)_2\right]$, Y is trans $\left[Pt(gly)_2\right]$

(c) X is trans $\left[Pt(gly)_2\right]$, Y is trans $\left[Pt(gly)_2\right]$

(d) X is trans $\left[Pt(gly)_2\right]$, Y is cis $\left[Pt(gly)_2\right]$

106. A metal complex having composition $Cr(NH_3)_4IBr_2$ was isolated in two forms X & Y. Also,

(1) X reacts with $AgNO_3$ to give pale yellow ppt. which is partially soluble in NH_4OH.

(2) Y reacts with $AgNO_3$ to give yellow ppt which is insoluble in NH_4OH.

Then, correct statement is/are

(a) Cis form of X is optically inactive whereas cis form of Y is optically active.

(b) Cis form of X & trans form of Y are optically active.

(c) Cis form of X & trans form of Y are optically inactive.

(d) None of these is/are correct.

107. Consider the following reactions :

(1) $\left[M(H_2O)_4\right]^{2+} + 4CH_3NH_2 \underset{}{\overset{k_1}{\rightleftharpoons}} A; \Delta_1 \overset{o}{G}$

(2) $\left[M(H_2O)_4\right] + 2en \underset{}{\overset{k_2}{\rightleftharpoons}} B; \Delta_2 \overset{o}{G}$

where en is $\begin{array}{l} CH_2-NH_2 \\ | \\ CH_2-NH_2 \end{array}$

wrt the above reactions, the correct statement(s) is/are :

(1) $\Delta_2 \overset{o}{G}$ is more negative then $\Delta_1 \overset{o}{G}$

(2) Complex A is optically inactive

(3) entropy change is higher for reaction of formation of complex B.

(4) formation constant k_2 is greater than formation constant k_1.

(a) 1, 3, & 4 but not 2

(b) 1 & 2 but not 3 & 4

(c) 1, 2, 3 & 4 are true

(d) 3 & 4 but not 1 & 2

108. Maximum number of atoms which are in the same plane in $[Ni(CO)_4]$ are :

(a) 3 (b) 2

(c) 4 (d) 5

109. The ratio of complexed silver to uncomplexed silver in 0.1 M NH_3 solution is :

(stability constant for $[Ag(NH_3)_2]^+ = 1.7 \times 10^7$)

(a) 1.7×10^6 (b) 1.7×10^5

(c) 0.59×10^5 (d) 0.59×10^{-9}

110. The correct statement on the isomerism associated with the following complex ions,

A. $\left[Ni(H_2O)_5NH_3\right]^{2+}$

B. $\left[Ni(H_2O)_4(NH_3)_2\right]^{2+}$ &

C. $\left[Ni(H_2O)_3(NH_3)_3\right]^{2+}$ is:

(a) A & B show only geometrical isomerism

(b) A & B show only geometrical & optical isomerism

(c) B & C show only geometrical & Optical isomerism

(d) B & C show only geometrical isomerism

111. Select the correct statement(s).

(a) $Cs_2[CuCl_4]$ is tetrahedral but $(NH_4)_2[CuCl_4]$ is square planar.

(b) Acetylacetone complexes in general are more stable then ethylene diamine complexes.

(c) All the complexes of Pt(+II) & Au(+III) with strong field as well as with weak field ligands are square planar.

(d) All are correct.

112. Which of the following statements is true for the complex $[Ni(PPh_3)_2Br_2]$?

(a) Hybridisation is same as in $[Ni(CN)_4]^{2-}$

(b) Hybridisation is same as in $[Ni(CO)_4]$

(c) Hybridisation is same as in $[NiCl_4]^{2-}$

(d) Both (b) & (c)

113. An octahedral complex of Co^{3+} is diamagnetic. The hybridisation involved in the formation of complex is :

(a) sp^3d^2 (b) dsp^2
(c) d^2sp^3 (d) sp^3d

114. An octahedral complex with molecular composition $M.5NH_3.ClSO_4$ has two isomers, A & B. The solution of A gives a white precipitate with $AgNO_3$ solution & solution of B gives white precipitate with $BaCl_2$ solution. The type of isomerism exhibited by the complex is :

(a) Linkage isomerism

(b) Ionisation isomerism

(c) Coordinate isomerism

(d) geometrical isomerism

115. Which of the following statement(s) is/are correct?

(a) cis – $[Pt(NH_3)_2Cl_2]$ will have some dipole moment.

(b) cis – $[Pt(NH_3)_2Cl_2]$ will show optical isomerism

(c) cis – $[CrCl_2(C_2O_4)_2]$ is a chiral molecule

(d) Both (a) & (c) are correct.

116. Consider the following statements :

(1) Zn(+2) has zero CFSE for octahedral geometry.

(2) All tetrahedral complexes are mainly high spin & low spin are rarely observed.

(3) In the reaction, $[CoCl_2(NH_3)_4]^+ + Cl^- \rightarrow [CoCl_3(NH_3)_3]^+ + NH_3$, if the reactant is in cis form, then two isomers of the product are obtained.

(4) $[Ni(PF_3)_4]$ is a diamagnetic, tetrahedral complex

(5) $[Sc(H_2O)_6]^{3+}$ & $[Ti(H_2O)_6]^{3+}$, both are colourless

(a) Only 4 & 5 are correct

(b) Only 1, 2 & 3 are correct

(c) Only 2 is correct

(d) Only 1, 2, 3 & 4 are correct

117. The octahedral complex $[Rh(en)_2(NO_2)SCN]^+$ can exist in 'X' total no. of isomeric forms including stereoisomers. Hence, 'X' is :

(a) 6 (b) 8
(c) 10 (d) 12

118. Which of the following is inner orbital & high spin complex ?

(a) $[Cr(NH_3)_6]^{3+}$ (b) $(V(H_2O)_6)^{3+}$
(c) $[Co(H_2O)_6]^{3+}$ (d) All of these

119. Which of the following complex has minimum magnitude of Δ_o?

(a) $[Cr(CN)_6]^{3-}$ (b) $[Co(NH_3)_6]^{3+}$
(c) $[CrCl_6]^{3-}$ (d) $[Cr(H_2O)_6]^{3+}$

120. A chelating ligand has 2 or more than two donor atoms to bind to a single metal ion-which of the following is NOT a chelating ligand?

(a) Thiosulphato

(b) Oxalato

(c) Ethane –1,2–diamine

(d) Glylcinato

121. Which of the following metal carbonyl is paramagnetic?

(a) $[Ni(CO)_4]$ (b) $[Fe(CO)_5]$
(c) $[V(CO)_6]$ (d) $[Cr(CO)_6]$

122. Which of the following will have more than two stereoisomeric forms ?

(1) $[CrCl_3(NH_3)_3]$ (2) $[Cr(en)_3]^{3+}$
(3) $[CoCl_2(en)_2]^+$ (4) $[CoBrCl(ox)_2]^{3-}$

(a) 1 & 3 (b) 1 & 2
(c) 3 & 4 (d) All of these

123. Calculate EAN of Ag in $[Ag(CN)_2]^-$

(a) 50 (b) 92
(c) 66 (d) 34

Answers

1. (d)	**2.** (d)	**3.** (d)	**4.** (a)	**5.** (d)	**6.** (a)	**7.** (d)	**8.** (c)	**9.** (d)	**10.** (c)
11. (d)	**12.** (d)	**13.** (d)	**14.** (a)	**15.** (d)	**16.** (a)	**17.** (b)	**18.** (b)	**19.** (d)	**20.** (c)
21. (c)	**22.** (c)	**23.** (c)	**24.** (d)	**25.** (d)	**26.** (b)	**27.** (b)	**28.** (b)	**29.** (a)	**30.** (d)
31. (c)	**32.** (d)	**33.** (d)	**34.** (d)	**35.** (c)	**36.** (d)	**37.** (d)	**38.** (a)	**39.** (c)	**40.** (d)
41. (a)	**42.** (d)	**43.** (c)	**44.** (c)	**45.** (b)	**46.** (b)	**47.** (c)	**48.** (b)	**49.** (c)	**50.** (b)
51. (d)	**52.** (d)	**53.** (b)	**54.** (d)	**55.** (b)	**56.** (b)	**57.** (d)	**58.** (d)	**59.** (a)	**60.** (d)
61. (d)	**62.** (d)	**63.** (b)	**64.** (d)	**65.** (c)	**66.** (d)	**67.** (a)	**68.** (a)	**69.** (d)	**70.** (d)
71. (d)	**72.** (a)	**73.** (c)	**74.** (d)	**75.** (d)	**76.** (d)	**77.** (b)	**78.** (a)	**79.** (a)	**80.** (b)
81. (d)	**82.** (c)	**83.** (a)	**84.** (b)	**85.** (c)	**86.** (a)	**87.** (a)	**88.** (d)	**89.** (a)	**90.** (d)
91. (c)	**92.** (d)	**93.** (d)	**94.** (b)	**95.** (d)	**96.** (a)	**97.** (c)	**98.** (a)	**99.** (d)	**100.** (d)
101. (d)	**102.** (d)	**103.** (d)	**104.** (d)	**105.** (b)	**106.** (c)	**107.** (c)	**108.** (d)	**109.** (b)	**110.** (d)
111. (d)	**112.** (d)	**113.** (c)	**114.** (b)	**115.** (d)	**116.** (d)	**117.** (d)	**118.** (d)	**119.** (c)	**120.** (a)
121. (c)	**122.** (c)	**123.** (a)							

Explanations

1. $NH_3 + H^+ \rightarrow \overset{+}{N}H_4$

In ammonium ion (i.e. $\overset{+}{N}H_4$) N atom lacks a lone pair & hence cannot act as ligand (e^- donor)

2.

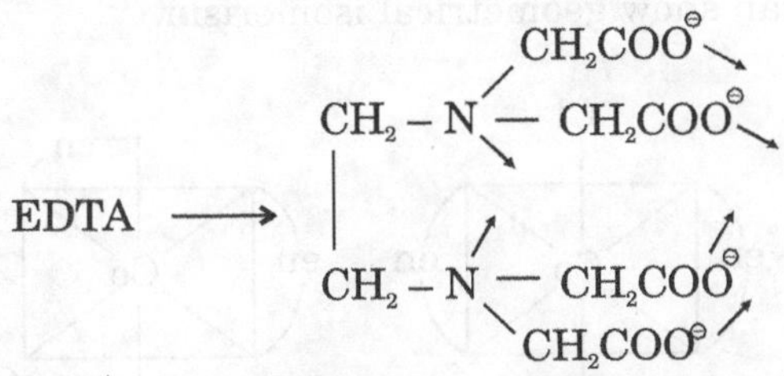

EDTA donates from 4 'O' atoms & 2 'N' atom. Hence, metal nitrogen bond can be formed.

•

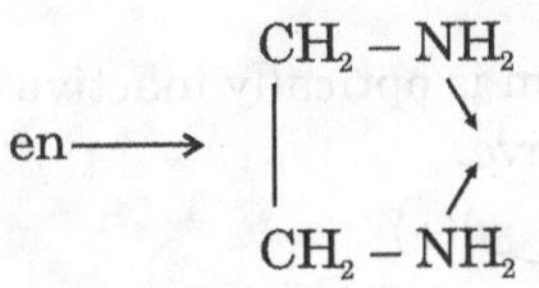

(ethane-1, 2-diamine)

It is also a N donor, so a metal nitrogen bond is formed

• glycinate has the formula →

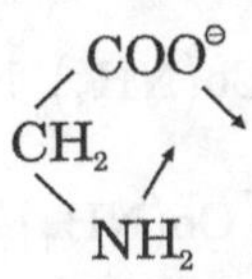

It has one 'O' atom & one 'N' atom as donor. So, a metal-N bond can be formed here as well.

• Acetylacetonato has the following formula :

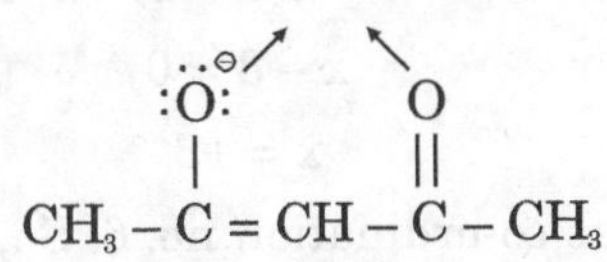

It is 'O' donor, so metal–N bond can't be formed.

5. (1)

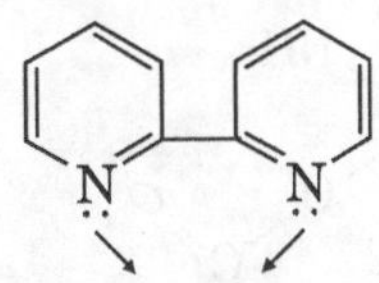

2, 2-Dipyridyl (Bidentate ligand)

(2) dmg

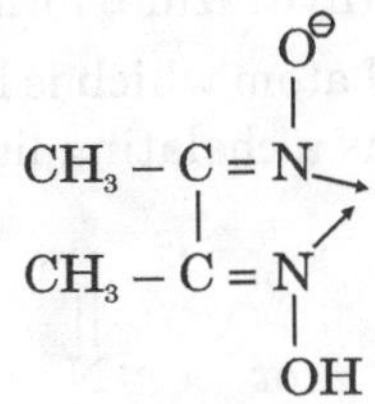

(3) Oxalate

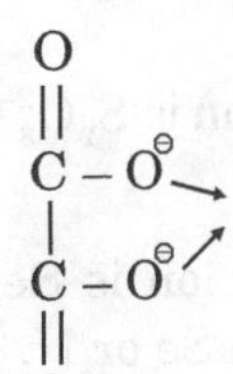

7. Option (d) is dithioxalate

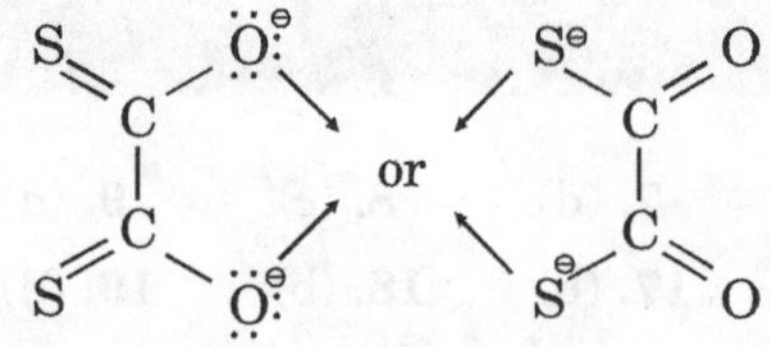

8. Complex I is $[Co(NH_3)_4CO_3]Br$.

Here, Co is in +3 oxidation state.

$$x + 4 \times 0 + (-2) + (-1) = 0$$
$$x + 0 - 2 - 1 = 0$$
$$x - 3 = 0$$
$$\boxed{x = +3}$$

Co^{3+} shows Co.No. 6. So, here CO_3^{2-} acts as a bidentate ligand.

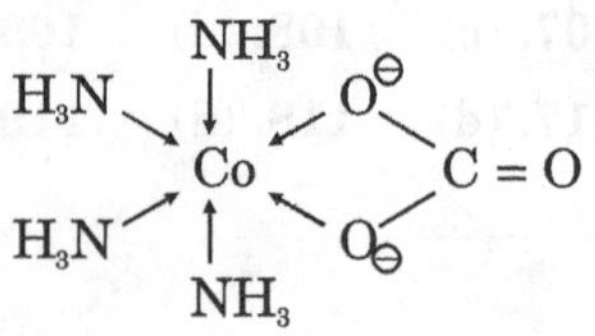

In Complex - II

$$[Co(NH_3)_5CO_3]Br$$

Co has +3 oxidation state

$$x + 5 \times 0 + (-2) + (-1) = 0$$
$$x - 3 = 0$$
$$x = +3$$

Co^{3+} has co-ordination no. 6. So, here CO_3^{2-} acts as a monodentate ligand.

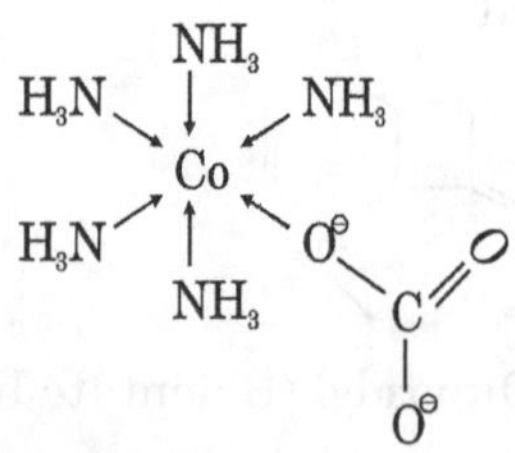

10. $\dot{N}H_2 - \dot{N}H_2$ (hydrazine) forms a 3 membered ring with central atom which is highly strained. So, it cannot act as a chelating ligand.

11.

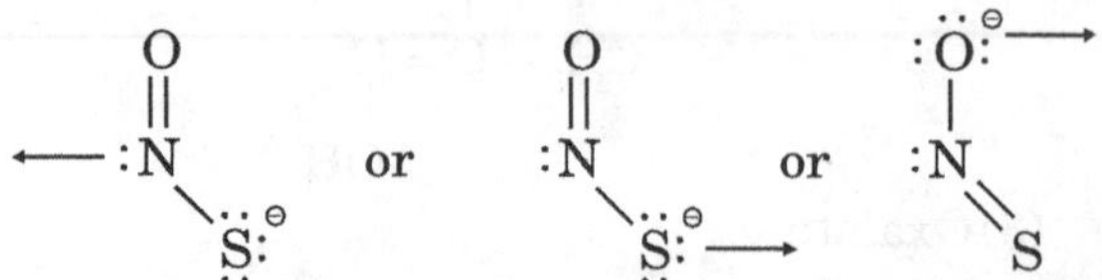

12. Thiosulphate ion is $S_2O_3^{2-}$ where donor atom could be S or O.

Selenocyanide ion is $SeCN^-$ where donor atom could either be Se or N.

Thiocyanate ion is SCN^- where donor atom could be S or N.

14. Option (a) has Fe^{2+} in $FeSO_4$.

Also, option (c) has Fe^{2+} but they are in co-ordination sphere & can't be isolated.

15. In option (d)

$$[Co(en)_3]_2(SO_4)_3$$

Let oxidation state of Co = x

$$2x + 6 \times 0 + (-6) = 0$$
$$2x - 6 = 0$$
$$2x = +6$$
$$\boxed{x = +3}$$

16. $[(H_3N)_5Cr-OH-Cr(NH_3)_5]Br_5$

17.

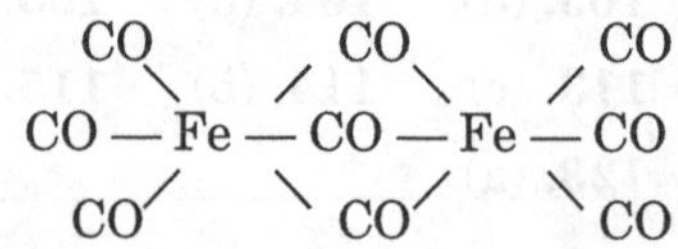

20. Correct IUPAC Name

(1) $[Co(NH_3)_6]Cl_3 \rightarrow$ Hexaammine cobalt (III) Chloride

(2) $[Ni(CO)_4] \rightarrow$ Tetracarbonyl Nickel (o)

(3) $Li(AlH_4) \rightarrow$ Lithium tetrahydrido aluminate (III)

21. It can show geometrical isomerism.

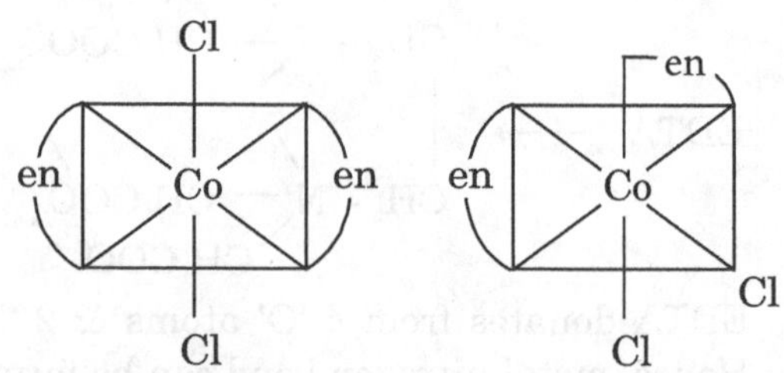

Trans form cis form

Also, trans form is optically inactive whereas cis is optically active.

So, cis form → d(+), l(–)

22. They exhibit ionisation isomerism as they furnish different ions.

$$[Co(NH_3)_5NO_3]SO_4 \rightarrow [Co(NH_3)_5NO_3]^{2+} + SO_4^{2-}$$

$$[Co(NH_3)_5SO_4]NO_3 \rightarrow [Co(NH_3)_5SO_4]^{+} + NO_3^{-}$$

23. For a, $\left(Pt(NH_3)_2Cl_2\right)$ is a square planar complex which can exhibit geometrical isomerism.

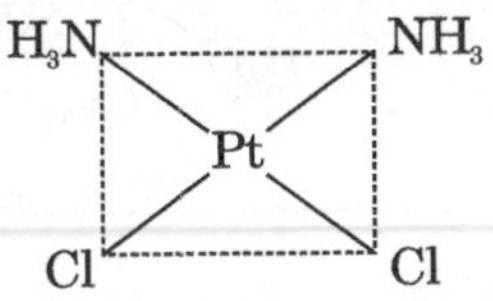
Cis

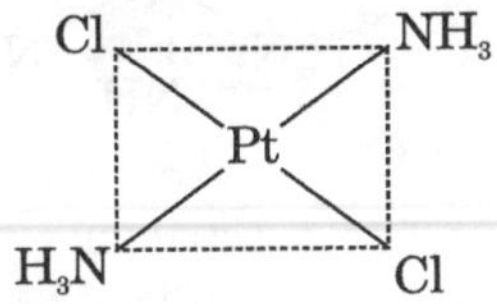
Trans

For option (b) i.e., cis$\left[Co(en)_2Cl_2\right]$, it can show optical isomerism as it lacks plane of symmetry.

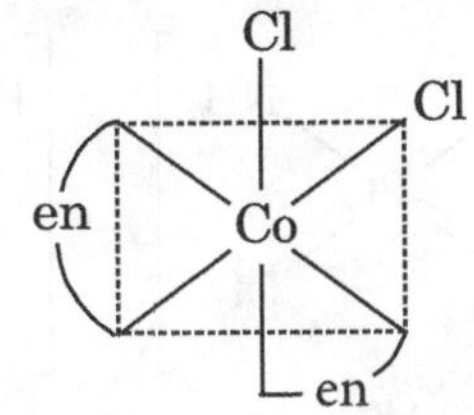

For option (c) i.e., trans $\left[Co(en)_2(NO_2)Cl\right]SCN$, it can show ionisation isomerism because Cl^- can act as counter ion & $\overline{S}CN$ as ligand.

For option (d), i.e., $\left[Co(NH_3)_6\right]^{3+}\left[Cr(CN)_6\right]^{3-}$, both cationic and anionic parts are complexes & hence can show co-ordination isomerism (by exchange of ligands).

24.

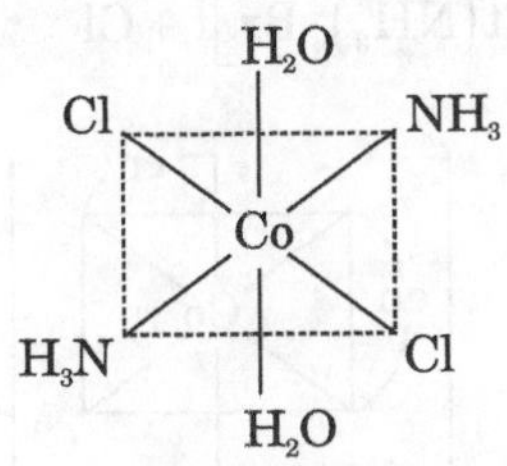
(I)
(All Trans)

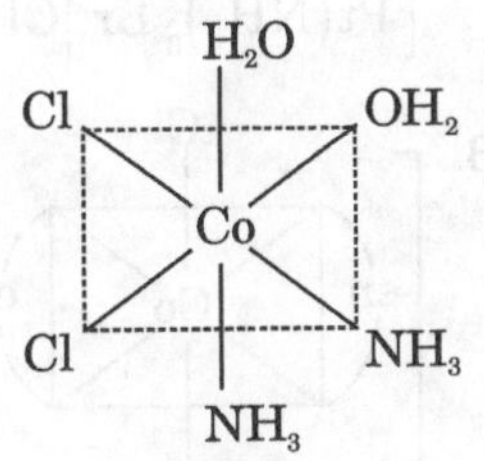
(II)
(All Cis)

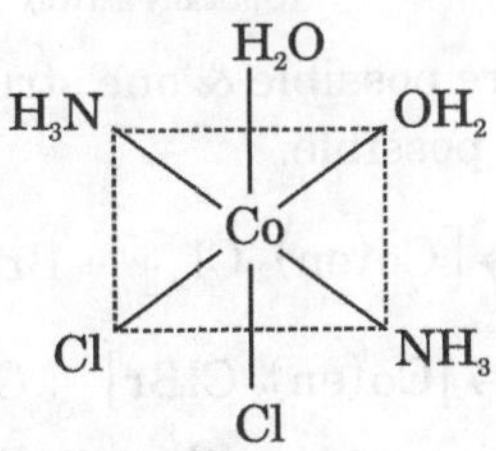
(III)

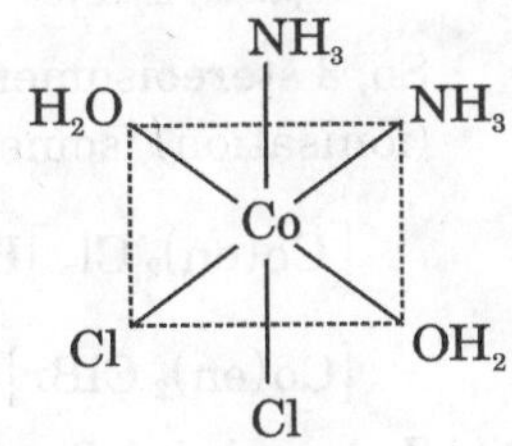
(IV)

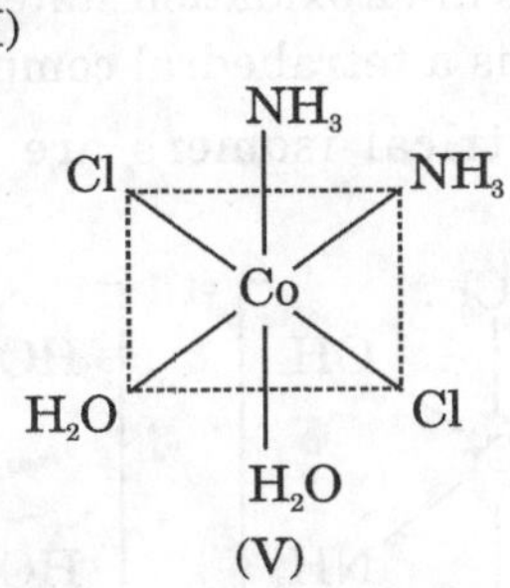
(V)

Among all these, molecule II (with all gps in cis) is optically active. So, total stereoisomers = 6.

25.

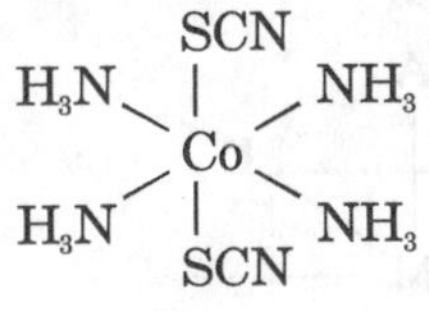
Trans

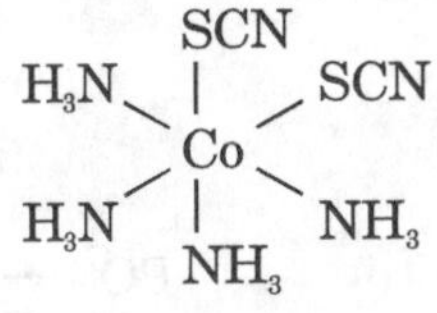
Cis

Also, it can show ionisation isomerism.

(a) $\left[Co(SCN)_2(NH_3)_4\right]Cl \rightarrow$

$$\left[Co(SCN)_2(NH_3)_4\right]^+ + Cl^-$$

(b) $\left[Co(SCN)Cl(NH_3)_4\right]SCN \rightarrow$

$$\left[Co(SCN)Cl(NH_3)_4\right]^+ + \overline{S}CN$$

Linkage isomerism can also be shown by the compound because $\overline{S}CN$ is an ambidentate ligand i.e., it can act as 'S donor' as well as 'N donor'.

26.

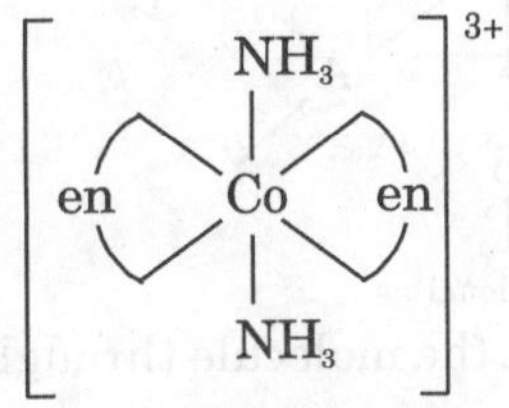
Trans

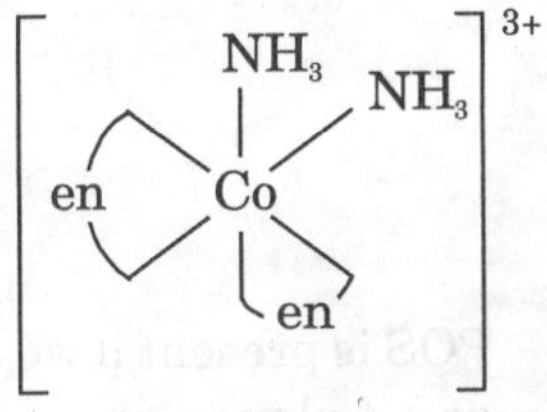
cis

27. It is [MABCD] type :

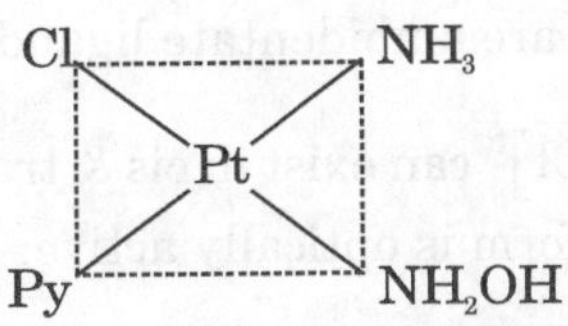
(I)

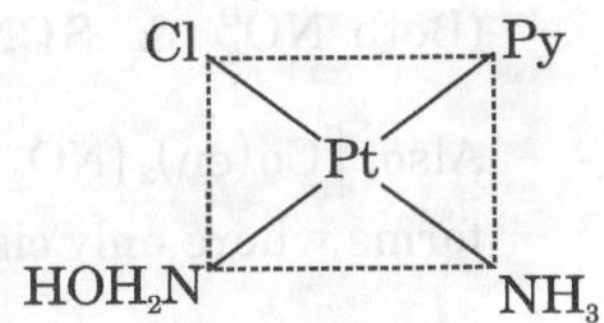
(II)

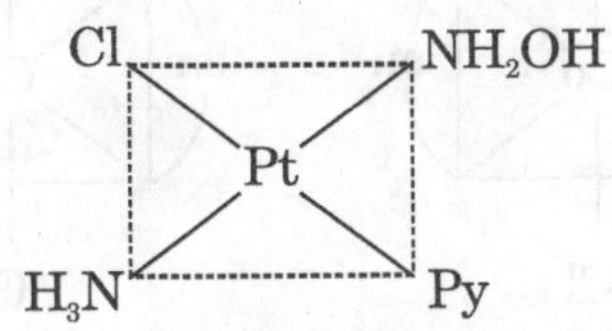
(III)

2 cis & 1 trans isomers are possible.

28. Ionisation isomers furnish different ions.

30. wrt option (a) i.e., $\left[Fe(H_2O)_5(NH_3)\right]CO_3$, ionisation isomerism is NOT possible ∵ none of the ligands are charged & hence cannot act as counter ion.

w.r.t. option (b), $[MA_3B_3]$ exist in 2 geometrical isomeric forms (Facial & Meridional) but NONE of them will show optical activity due to presence of plane of symmetry.

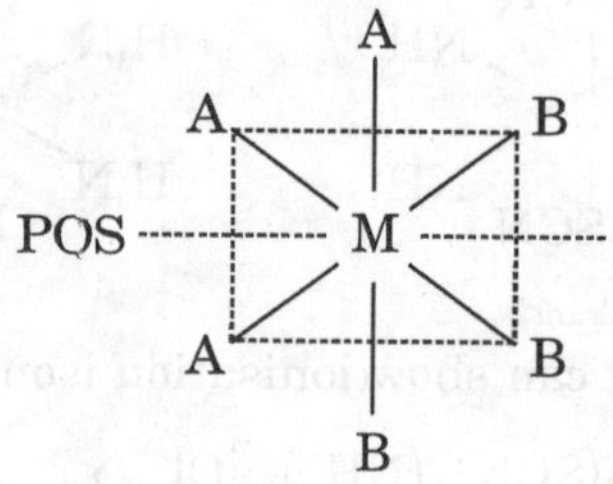

Facial

(POS is present along the plane going through A, which is placed perpendicular, to the horizontal plane, M & B, placed below the plane).

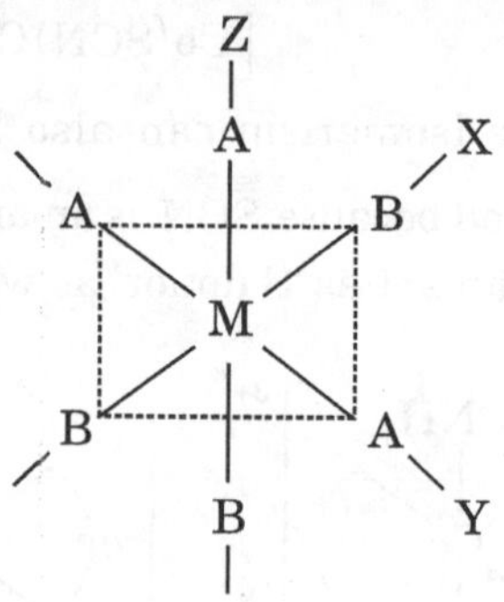

Meridional

POS is present if we cut the molecule through YZ or XZ plane.

w.r.t. option (c), it has 3 ionisation & 2 linkage isomers (structural isomers, 3 + 2 = 5).

(Both $NO_2^{\ominus}$ & $\overset{\ominus}{S}CN$ are ambidentate ligands)

Also, $[Co(en)_2(NO_2)Cl]^+$ can exist in cis & trans forms where only cis form is optically active.

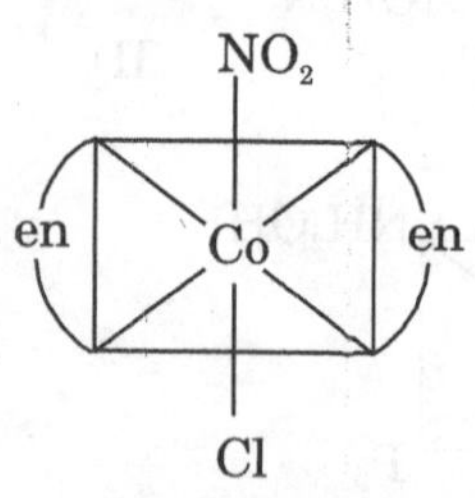

Trans (has POS)
(Optically inactive)

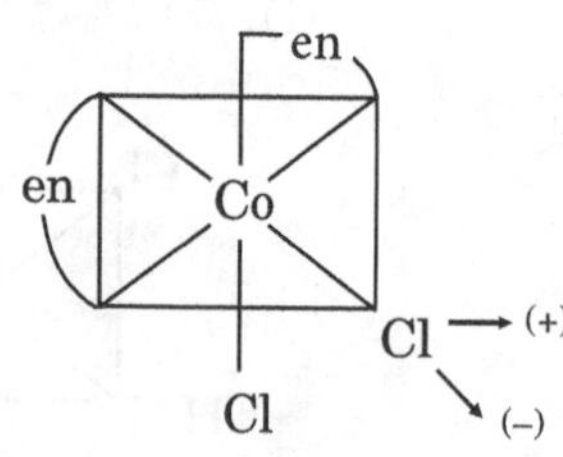

cis
(Optically active)

31. $[Pt(NH_3)_2Cl_2]$ is square planar & exhibits geometrical isomerism. It is also shown by $[PtCl_2Br_2]^{2-}$.

32. wrt option (b), both the complexes will show geometrical isomerism.

$[Co(NH_3)_4Cl_2]^+$ is an octahedral complex which can shown geometrical isomerism.

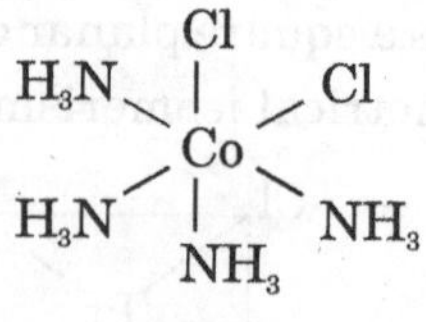

Cis
(wrt Cl)

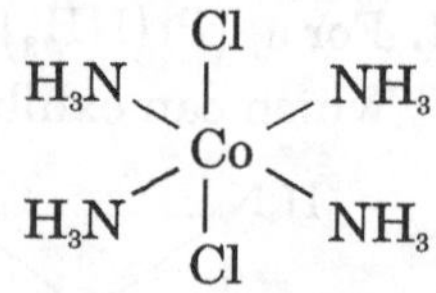

Trans

$[Pt(NH_3)_2(H_2O)Cl]^+$

(Pt^{2+} with co-ordination No. 4 forms sq. planar complexes).

So,

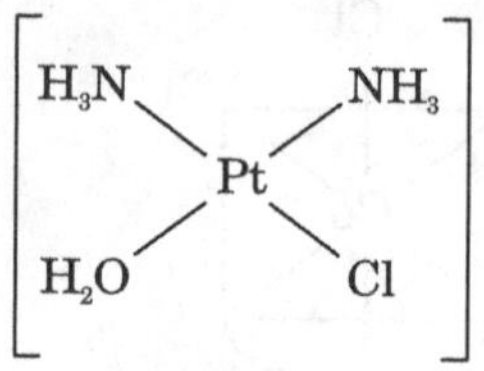

Cis

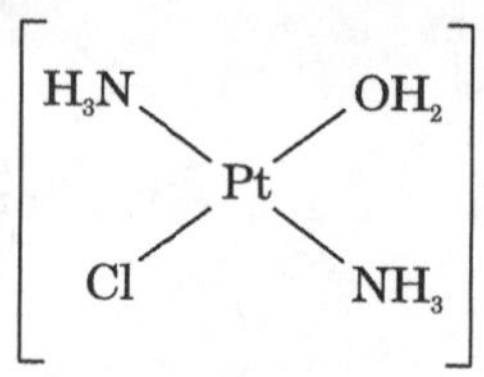

Trans

- wrt option (c) both the complexes can show ionisation isomerism.

(I) $[Pt(NH_3)_3NO_3]Cl \rightarrow [Pt(NH_3)_3NO_3]^+ + Cl^-$

(II) $[Pt(NH_3)_3Cl]NO_3 \rightarrow [Pt(NH_3)_3Cl]^+ + NO_3^-$

Also, $[Pt(NH_3)_3Cl]Br \rightarrow [Pt(NH_3)_3Cl]^+ + Br^-$

$[Pt(NH_3)_3Br]Cl \rightarrow [Pt(NH_3)_3Br]^+ + Cl^-$

33.

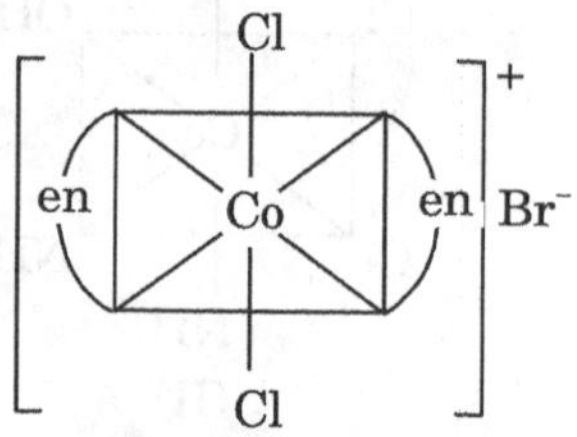

Trans
(Optically inactive)

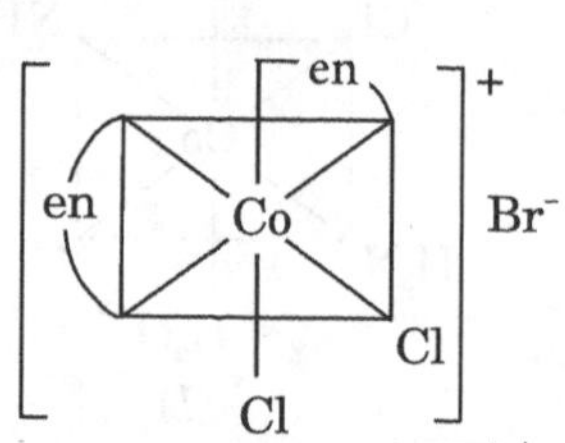

cis
(Optically active)

So, 3 stereoisomers are possible & one structural (ionisation) isomer is possible.

$[Co(en)_2Cl_2]Br \rightarrow [Co(en)_2Cl_2]^+ + Br^-$

$[Co(en)_2ClBr]Cl \rightarrow [Co(en)_2ClBr]^+ + Cl^-$

34. Zn here is in +2 oxidation state with co-ordination No. 4. It is a tetrahedral complex.

36. 5 geometrical isomers are possible for this complex.

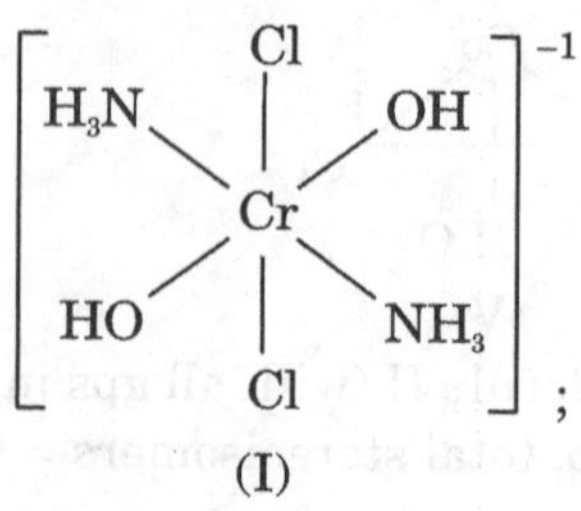

(I)

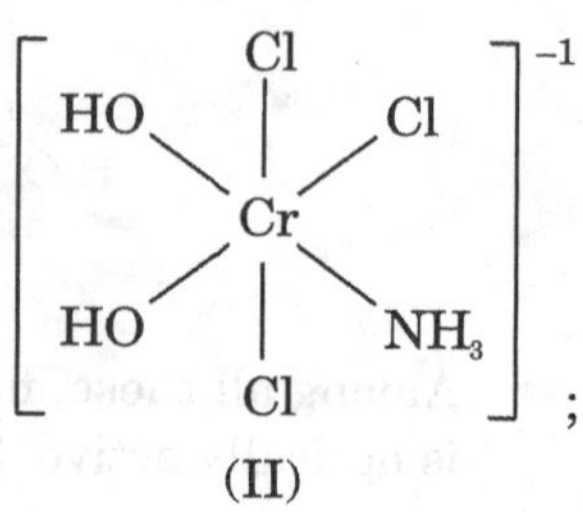

(II)

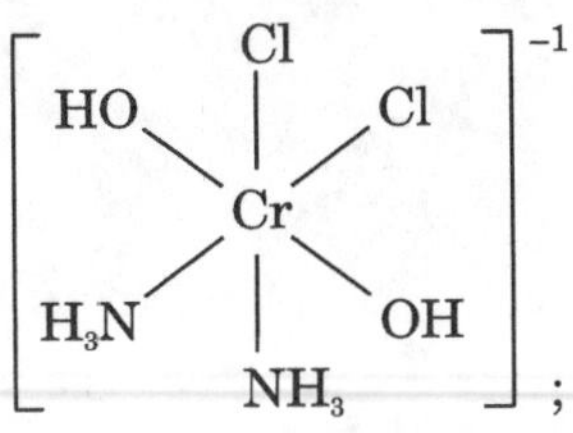

(III)

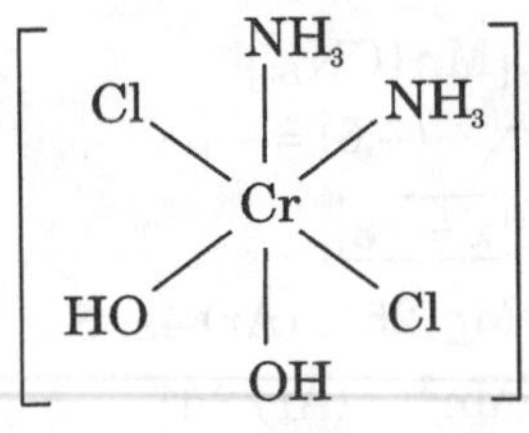

(IV)

&

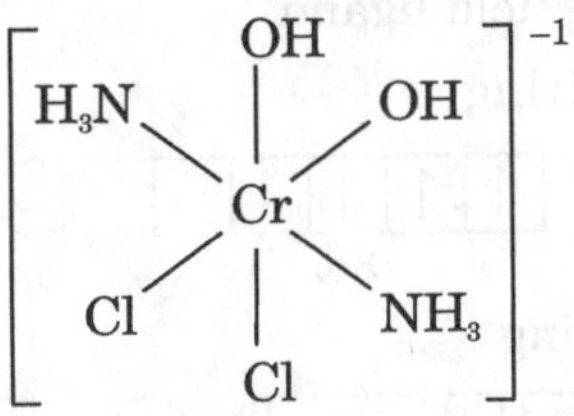

(V)

Out of these 5, only isomer numbered II, is optically active.

37. wrt option a :

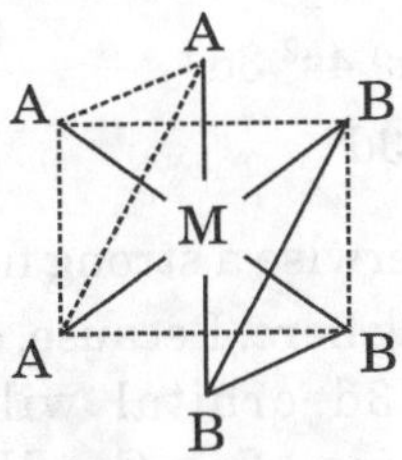

On joining same ligands, face of an octahedron is formed. So, it is facial.

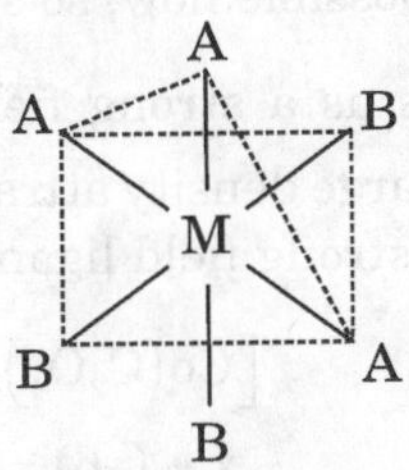

On joining same ligands, the plane passes through the molecule in-between, it is meridional.

wrt option (b), $[M(AB)_3] \approx [M(gly)_3]$

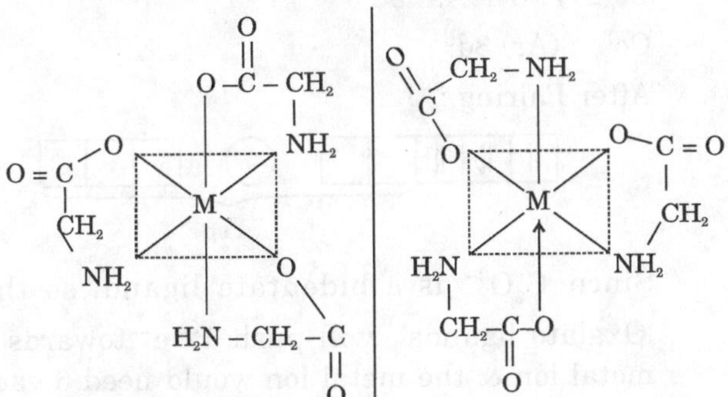

Meridional Facial

[On connecting 'N' atoms of the ligand, glycinato, face of an octahedron is formed].

39. 15 enantiomer pairs & 15 geometrical isomer is are possible.

40. (1) $[Co(NH_3)_6]^{3+}[Cr(NO_2)_6]^{3-}$

(2) $[Co(NH_3)_5(NO_2)]^{2+}[Cr(NO_2)_5(NH_3)]^{2-}$

(3) $[Co(NH_3)_4(NO_2)_2]^{+1}[Cr(NO_2)_4(NH_3)_2]^{-1}$

(4) $[Co(NH_3)_3(NO_2)_3]^{0}[Cr(NO_2)_3(NH_3)_3]^{0}$

(5) $[Co(NH_3)_2(NO_2)_4]^{-1}[Cr(NO_2)_2(NH_3)_4]^{+1}$

(6) $[Co(NH_3)(NO_2)_5]^{-2}[Cr(NO_2)(NH_3)_5]^{+2}$

(7) $[Co(NO_2)_6]^{3-}[Cr(NH_3)_6]^{3+}$

The molecules numbered '4' cannot exist because there is neither cation nor anion to bind the two complexes.

41. $[Ni(H_2O)(Cl)(NH_3)(NH_2OH)]NO_2$

$$x + 0 + (-1) + 0 + 0 + (-1) = 0$$

$$\boxed{x = +2}$$

Ni (28) : (Ar) $4s^2\ 3d^8$

Ni^{2+} : (Ar) $3d^8$

Magnetic moment (2.82 B.M.) Suggests that Ni^{2+} has 2 unpaired e^- i.e., pairing did not occur. Here Ni^{2+} has Co. No. 4 & hence will have sp^3 hybridisation. So, it [MABCD] type complex is (tetrahedral) which is optically active & hence can exist as 2 optical isomers (d & l).

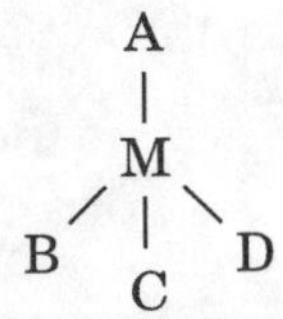

42. I & II cannot are not enantiomers ($\because$ they possess plane of symmetry), so they are not optically active.

Rather, they (I & II) are identical because all angles are same (equal).

$\angle Cl - Co - Cl = 90°$ (in both I & II)

$\angle Cl - Co - NH_3 = 90°$ (in both I & II)

$\angle NH_3 - Co - NH_3 = 90°$ (in both I & II)

43. POS is absent in (c) option.

44. In $[M(gly)_2]$, if M^{2+} is sp^3 hybridised, the complex will exist in 2 stereoisomeric forms (dextro & laevo) i.e., it will be optically active.

In $[M(gly)_2]$; if dsp^2 hybridisation is there, even then it will exist in two stereoisomeric forms i.e., cis & trans.

45. In option (b), both the complexes are optically active.

46. $[Co(NH_3)_2Cl_4]^-$ has 2 geometrical isomers (cis & trans)

In $[AuCl_2Br_2^-]^-$, cis & trans forms are possible.

No isomerism is possible in $[Pt(en)Cl_2]$.

47. Option (c) i.e., $[Ni(NH_3)_2Cl_2]$ has a tetrahedral geometry. So, it will not show geometrical isomerism.

48. Electronic configuration can be given as :

Ni(28) : (Ar) $4s^2\ 3d^8$

Ni^{2+} : (Ar) $3d^8$

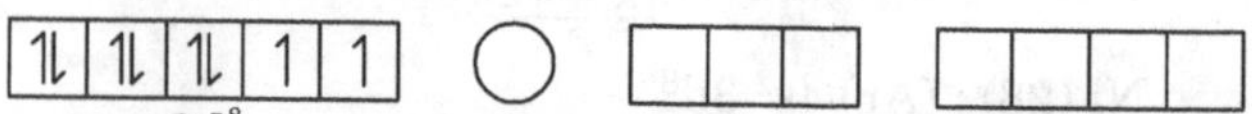

$3d^8$ 4s 4p 4d

Octahedral complex has M in sp^3d^2/d^2sp^3 hybridisation. As is evident from d^8 configuration, even after pairing, two 3d orbitals will not still be available to give $d^2\ sp^3$ hybridisation. Hence, $sp^3\ d^2$ hybridisation is only possible.

49. wrt option (c), $\bar{C}N$ is a strong field & Ni is in +2 oxidation state.

$[Ni(CN)_4]^{2-}$

$x + (-4) = -2$

$x - 4 = -2$

$\boxed{x = +2}$

Ni(28) : (Ar) $4s^2\ 3d^8$

Ni^{2+} : (Ar) $3d^8$

^-CN will force pairing of electrons.

Before pairing :

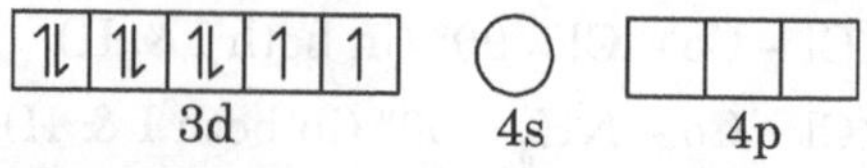

3d 4s 4p

After pairing :

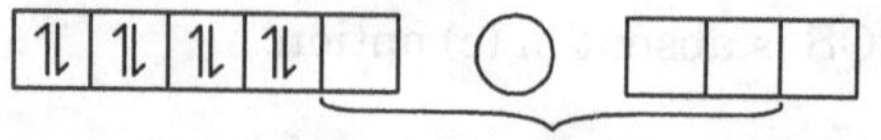

dsp^2 (diamagnetic)

50. $[Mn(CN)_6]^{3-}$

$x + (-6) = -3$

$\boxed{x = +3}$

Mn(25) : (Ar) $4s^2\ 3d^5$

Mn^{3+} : (Ar) $3d^4$

Co-ordination number of manganese is 6 and ^-CN is a strong field ligand.

Before pairing :

$Mn^{3+} \rightarrow$ 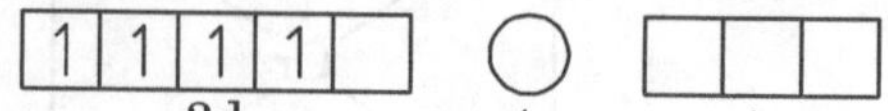

3d 4s 4p

After pairing :

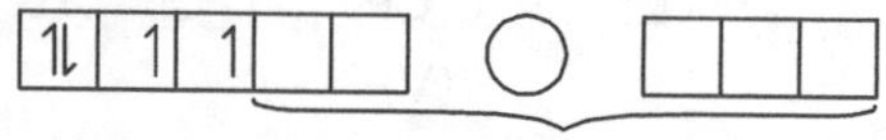

d^2sp^3

'NOT' All the electrons get paired up.

51. In $[Ni(NH_3)_6]^{2+}$, Ni is in +2 oxidation state.

Ni(28) : (Ar) $4s^2\ 3d^8$

Ni^{2+} : (Ar) $3d^8$

$\ddot{N}H_3$ is otherwise a strong field ligand but cannot force pairing here. Because, even if pairing occurs, only one 3d orbital will be available for hybridisation. For Co. No. 6, hybridisation required. is either $d^2\ sp^3$ or $sp^3\ d^2$. However, $d^2\ sp^3$ is not possible now, so $sp^3\ d^2$ should occur.

52. $C_2O_4^{2-}$ acts as a strong field ligand with Co^{3+}. Greater charge density attracts oxalato & it turns into SFL. (strong field ligand)

$[Co(C_2O_4)_3]^{3-}$

$x + (-6) = -3$

$x - 6 = -3$

$\boxed{x = +3}$

Co(27) : (Ar) $4s^2\ 3d^7$

Co^{3+} : (Ar) $3d^6$

After Pairing :

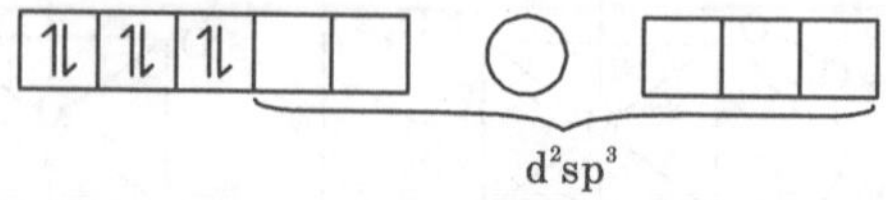

d^2sp^3

Since $C_2O_4^{2-}$ is a bidentate ligand, so three 'Oxalato ligands' will push 12 e^- towards the metal ion & the metal ion would need 6 vacant orbitals to accomodate those electrons. Hence, hybridisation achieved is $d^2\ sp^3$.

'b' option is $[V(H_2O)_6]^{3+}$

It is an octahedral complex with co-ordination No. 6 & V in +3 oxidation state. Hybridisation will be either $d^2 sp^3$ or $sp^3 d^2$.

V(23) : (Ar) $4s^2 3d^3$

V^{3+} : (Ar) $3d^2$

No pairing occurs because H_2O is a weak field ligand :

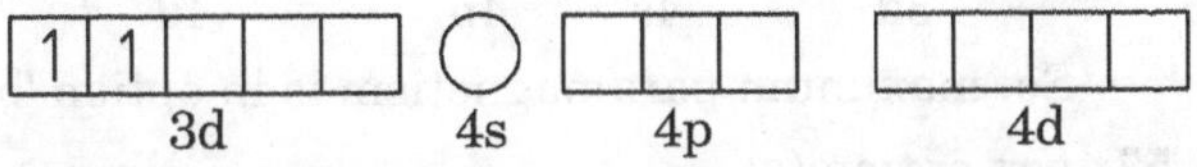

3d or 4d orbitals could be utilised for hybridisation. Six vacant orbitals are required because $6H_2O$ molecules will force 12 e^- towards metal ion. Hybridisation could be $sp^3 d^2$ or $d^2 sp^3$. But the preferred hybridisation will be $d^2 sp^3$ i.e., 3d orbitals will preferably participate in hybridisation. It is because :

1. 4d orbitals are extended more in space than 3d orbitals. So, $sp^3 d^2$ hybridised orbitals will cause the bond length to increase the between the metal & the ligand. So, bond length in outer orbital octahedral complexes is comparatively longer & so, they are less stable.
2. Also, the order of energies of various orbitals is 4d > 5s > 4p > 3d > 4s. Energy gap between 4s & 4d is large. So, it is tougher to hybridise 4s & 4d. In comparision, it is preferable to hybridise 3d & 4s.

So, in $\left[V(H_2O)_6\right]^{3+}$, the hybridisation is $d^2 sp^3$.

Also, wrt 'c' option i.e., $\left[Cr(NH_3)_6\right]^{3+}$

Cr is in +3 oxidation state & the complex is octahedral.

Cr(24) : (Ar) $4s^1 3d^5$

Cr^{3+} : (Ar) $3d^3$

'No pairing of electrons is required here because $d^2 sp^3$ hybridisation can be achieved other wise also.'

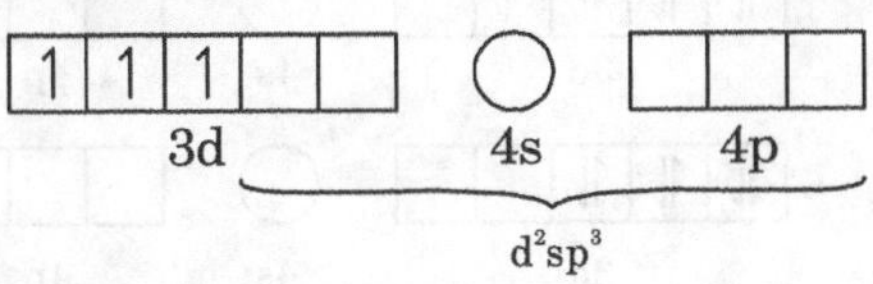

Number of unpaired e^- = 3

Now, since hybridisation in all the three complexes is $d^2 sp^3$, all are INNER ORBITAL COMPLEXES.

53. $Ni^{2+} + dmg + NH_4OH \rightarrow Ni(dmg)_2$

Now, in $\left[Ni(dmg)_2\right]$ Ni is in +2 oxidation state

$$x + (-2) = 0$$

$$\boxed{x = +2}$$

Ni (28) : (Ar) $4s^2 3d^8$

Ni^{2+} : (Ar) $3d^8$

'dmg' is a nitrogen donor & hence a strong field ligand. It will force pairing of electrons. Co-ordination number of Ni^{2+} here is 4 ∵ dmg is a bidentate ligand.

Before pairing :

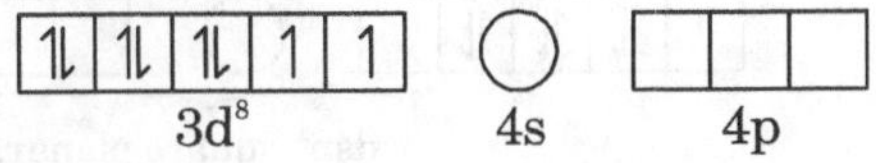

After pairing :

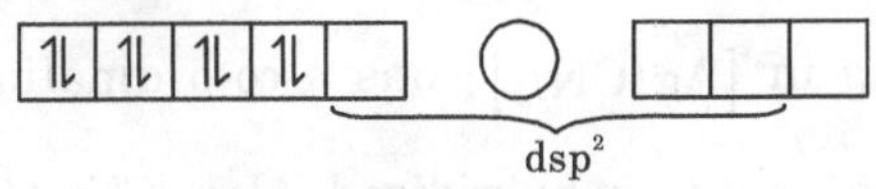

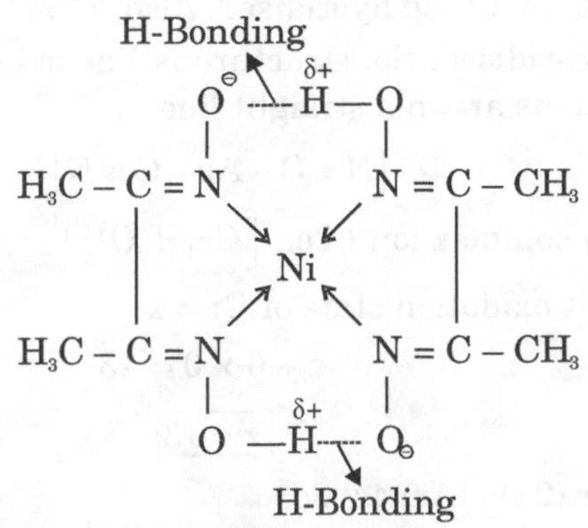

B is (dimethyl glyoximato) nickel (II) or

B is (2, 3 – butanedionedioximato) nickel (II).

54. wrt $\left[PdCl_4\right]^{2-}$

$$x + (-4) = -2$$

$$x - 4 = -2$$

$$\boxed{x = +2}$$

Pd^{2+} : [Kr] $4d^8$ 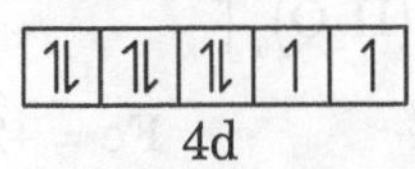

'4d & 5d' orbitals are bigger in size & extend farther into space causing greater interactions with the ligands creating more repulsions & hence pairing of electrons results (as is caused by strong field ligand).

After pairing :

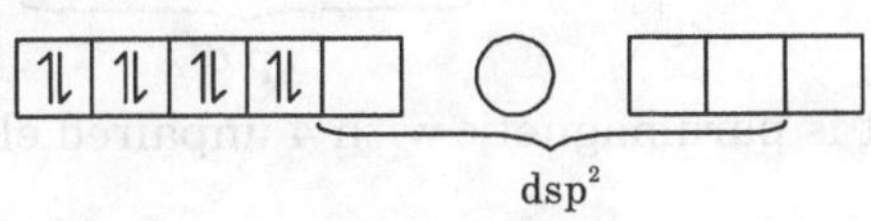

square planar, diamagnetic.

SAME CONCEPT stands valid for $\left[PtCl_4\right]^{2-}$.

Pt^{2+} : [Xe] $4f^{14} 5d^8$

After pairing in 5d :

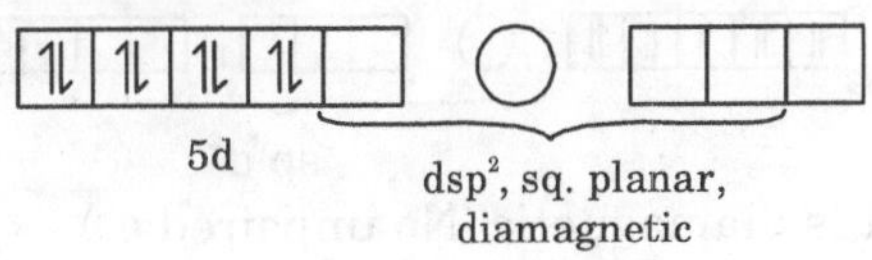

wrt $[Ni(CN)_4]^{2-}$

Here, Ni is in +2 oxidation state.

Ni (28) : (Ar) $4s^2\ 3d^8$

Ni^{2+} : (Ar) $3d^8$

$\bar{C}N$ is a strong field ligand resulting in pairing.

After pairing :

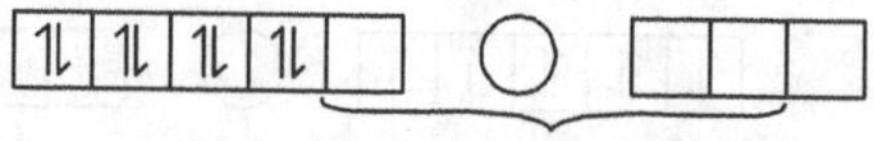

dsp^2, square planar, diamagnetic

55. Ag in $[Ag(CN)_2]^-$ has a co-ordination No. 2 & hence it is sp hybridised. Also, 'C' in '$\bar{C} \equiv N$' is sp hybridised. So, structure is linear i.e., all the 5 atoms are in a straight line.

$$[N \equiv C - Ag - C \equiv N]^-$$

56. In complex ion I i.e., $[Cr(H_2O)_6]^{3+}$

Let oxidation state of Cr = x

$$x + 6 \times 0 = +3$$

$$\boxed{x = +3}$$

Cr (24) : (Ar) $4s^1\ 3d^5$

Cr^{3+} : (Ar) $3d^3$

'No pairing occurs'

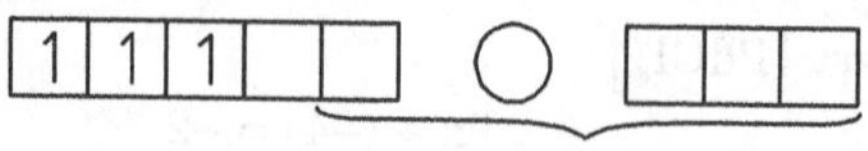

d^2sp^3

It is paramagnetic having 3 unpaired electrons.

(2) In $[Fe(H_2O)_6]^{2+}$

Fe = +2

Fe (26) : (Ar) $4s^2\ 3d^6$

Fe^{2+} : (Ar) $3d^6$

H_2O is a weak field ligand. No pairing occurs

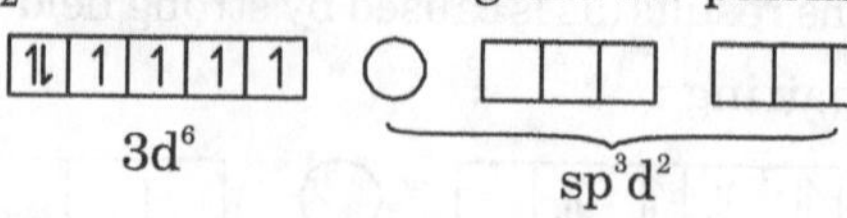

sp^3d^2

It is paramagnetic with 4 unpaired electrons.

(3) $[Zn(H_2O)_6]^{2+}$

Zn is in +2 oxidation state.

Zn (30) : (Ar) $4s^2\ 3d^{12}$

Zn^{2+} : (Ar) $3d^{10}$

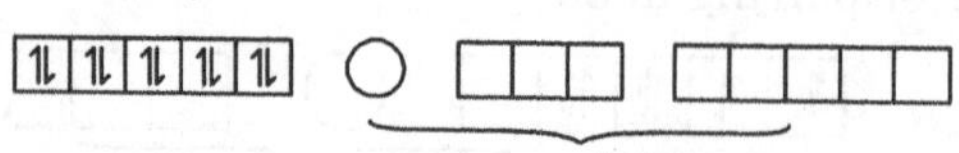

sp^3d^2

It is diamagnetic (No unpaired e^-)

(4) $[Cu(H_2O)_6]^{2+}$

Cu = + 2

Cu (29) : (Ar) $4s^1\ 3d^{10}$

Cu^{2+} : (Ar) $3d^9$

It has one unpaired e^-.

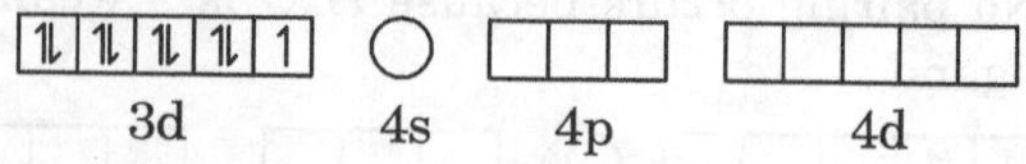

So, maximum paramagnetism is in option 'b'.

57. wrt option (c),

$[Ni(CO)_4]$

Oxidation state of Ni = 0

Ni (28) : (Ar) $4s^2\ 3d^8$

CO is a strong field ligand which will force pairing.

Now, (Ar) $4s^2\ 3d^8$

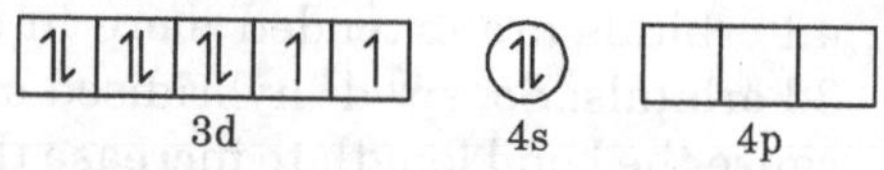

Energy difference between 3d & 4s is less, so electron pair from 4s enters 3d causing sp3 hybridisation.

After pairing :

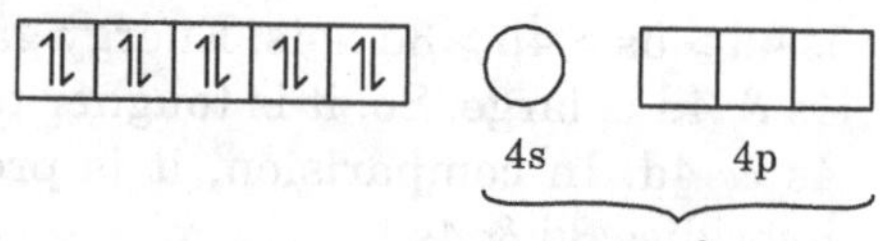

sp^3

58. $[Co(NH_3)_6]^{2+}$

Oxidation state of Co = +2

Co (27) : (Ar) $4s^2\ 3d^7$

Co^{2+} : (Ar) $3d^7$

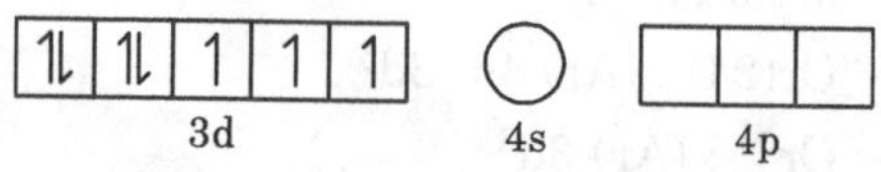

NH_3 is a strong field ligand, forces pairing.

After pairing :

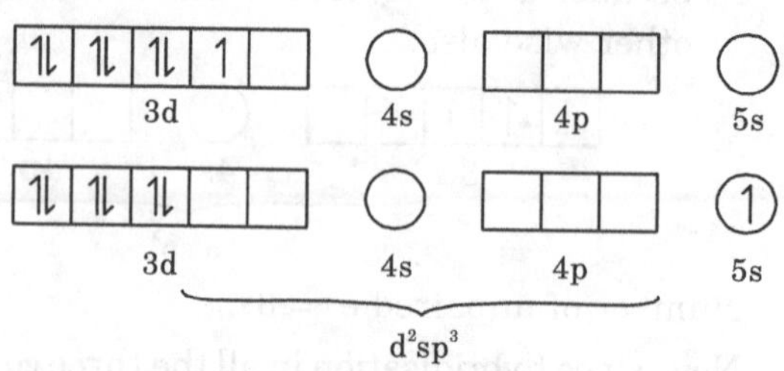

d^2sp^3

59. PPh_3 is a neutral ligand.

$$[Rh(PPh_3)_3Cl]$$

$$x + 3 \times 0 + (-1) = 0$$

$$x - 1 = 0$$

$$\boxed{x = +1}$$

Rh (45) : (Kr) $4d^8\ 5s^1$

Rh^+ : (Kr) $4d^8$

Before pairing :

4d: [⥮ | ⥮ | ⥮ | 1 | 1]   5s: ( )   5p: [| |]

PPh_3 is a strong field ligand which forces pairing of electrons.

After pairing :

[⥮ | ⥮ | ⥮ | ⥮ |]   ( )   [| |] — dsp²

Its a square planar complex.

60. $\mu = \sqrt{n(n+2)}$ B.M.

$4.90 = \sqrt{n(n+2)}$

No. of unpaired electrons. $\boxed{n = 4}$

Fe (26) : (Ar) $4s^2\ 3d^6$

Fe^{2+} : (Ar) $3d^6$

[⥮ | 1 | 1 | 1 | 1]

$\boxed{n = 4}$

If all e^- get paired up :

[⥮ | ⥮ | ⥮ | |]

$\boxed{n = 0}$

61. H_2O acts as a strong field ligand with Co^{3+} & forces pairing of electrons.

Co (27) : (Ar) $4s^2\ 3d^7$

Co^{3+} : (Ar) $3d^6$

Before pairing :

[⥮ | 1 | 1 | 1 | 1]

After pairing :

[⥮ | ⥮ | ⥮ | |]   ( )   [| |]

d^2sp^3, Diamagnetic

- For $[NiF_6]^{2-}$

  F^- acts as SFL with Ni^{4+}.

Due to greater charge density on Ni^{4+}, F^- comes very close & causes greater splitting.

Ni (28) : (Ar) $4s^2\ 3d^8$

Ni^{4+} : (Ar) $3d^6$

Before pairing :

3d: [⥮ | 1 | 1 | 1 | 1]   4s: ( )   4p: [| |]

After pairing :

[⥮ | ⥮ | ⥮ | |]   ( )   [| |]

d^2sp^3, Diamagnetic

For $[Ni(NH_3)_6]^{2+}$, Ni is in +2 oxidation state here.

Ni (28) : (Ar) $4s^2\ 3d^8$

Ni^{2+} : (Ar) $3d^8$

NH_3 is undoubtedly a SFL but will NOT force pairing here because even after pairing, only a single 3d orbital will be vacant & $d^2\ sp^3$ hybridisation will still NOT be achieved. So, NO PAIRING OF electrons occurs here.

3d: [⥮ | ⥮ | ⥮ | 1 | 1]   4s: ( )   4p: [| |]   4d: [| |]

sp^3d^2

PARAMAGNETIC COMPLEX.

63. $(PtCl_4)^{2-}$ is a square planar complex.

65. $Na_2[Fe(CN)_5NO]$

$+2 + x + (-5) + 1 = 0$

$x - 3 + 1 = 0$

$x - 2 = 0$

$\boxed{x = +2}$

Fe (26) : (Ar) $4s^2\ 3d^6$

Fe^{2+} : (Ar) $3d^6$

Since all ligands are strong field, pairing will occur.

After pairing :

3d: [⥮ | ⥮ | ⥮ | |]   4s: ( )   4p: [| |]

d^2sp^3, DIAMAGNETIC

67. $[ZnCl_4]^{2-}$

Let oxidation State of Zn = x

$x + (-4) = -2$

$x - 4 = -2$

$\boxed{x = -2 + 4 = +2}$

Zn (30) : (Ar) $4s^2\ 3d^{10}$

Zn^{2+} : (Ar) $3d^{10}$

[⥮ | ⥮ | ⥮ | ⥮ | ⥮]   ( )   [| |]

sp^3

For $[MnCl_4]^{2-}$

Let oxidation state of Mn = x

$$x + (-4) = -2$$

$$x - 4 = -2$$

$$\boxed{x = +2}$$

Mn (25) : (Ar) $4s^2\ 3d^5$

Mn^{2+} : (Ar) $3d^5$

Cl^- is a weak field ligand

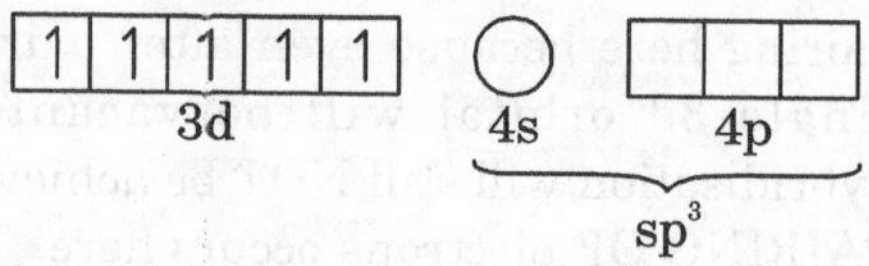

68. Splitting is large in case of strong field ligands ($\Delta_0 > P$).

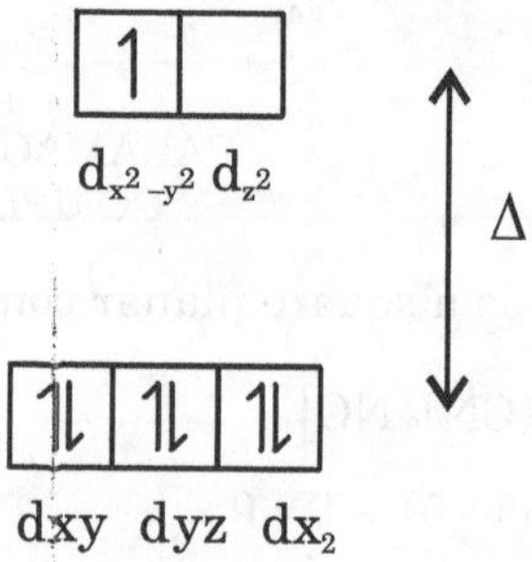

Δ_0 is large.

69. $[Co(NH_3)_6]^{2+}$ is readily oxidised to $[Co(NH_3)_6]^{3+}$ due to higher –ve value of CFSE (Crystal field stabilisation energy).

$[Co(NH_3)_6]^{2+}$

Co is in +2 oxidation state.

Co (27) : (Ar) $4s^2\ 3d^7$

Co^{2+} : (Ar) $3d^7$

with SFL(NH_3), configuration is $t_{2g}^6\ eg^1$

CFSE = $(-0.4x + 0.6y)\ \Delta_0$

where x = No. of e^- in t_{2g}

y = No. of e^- in eg

CFSE = $(-0.4 \times 6 + 0.6 \times 1)\Delta_0$

CFSE = $(-2.4 + 0.6)\Delta_0 = -1.8\ \Delta_0$

For $[Co(NH_3)_6]^{3+}$

Co^{3+} : (Ar) $3d^6$

with NH_3(SFL), configuration is $t_{2g}^6\ eg^0$

CFSE = $(-0.4x + 0.6\ y)\Delta_0$

$= (-0.4 \times 6 + 0.6 \times 0)\ \Delta_0$

$= -2.4\ \Delta_0$

72. Ligands carrying greater charge density cause greater splitting. Eg. F^- causes greater splitting than Cl^-.

Among uncharged ligands, the ones which are more basic cause greater splitting. Eg. NH_3 causes more splitting than H_2O.
(donors are strong field ligands.)

73. Order of splitting for metal ions follows the order

$$\underset{(Ir)}{5d} > \underset{(Rh)}{4d} > \underset{(Co)}{3d}$$

74. CFSE = $-0.6\ \Delta_0$

Can be achieved in two configurations namely :

$t_{2g}^3\ eg^1$

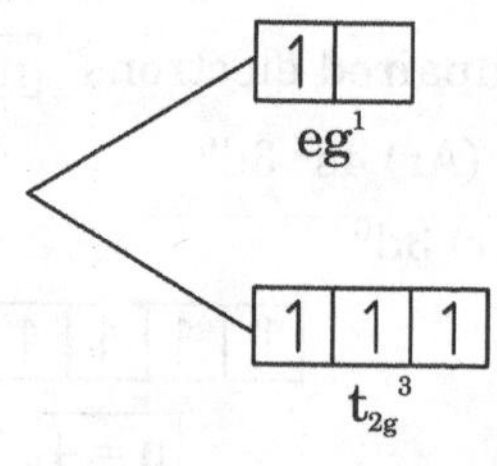

CFSE = $(-0.4 \times + 0.6\ y)\ \Delta_0$

$= (-0.4 \times 3 + 0.6 \times 1)\ \Delta_0$

$= -0.6\ \Delta_0$

No. of unpaired e^- = 4

$\mu = \sqrt{n(n+2)}$

$= \sqrt{4(4+2)} = \sqrt{24}$ B.M.

= 4.9 B.M.

Another possible configuration is $t_{2g}^6\ eg^3$.

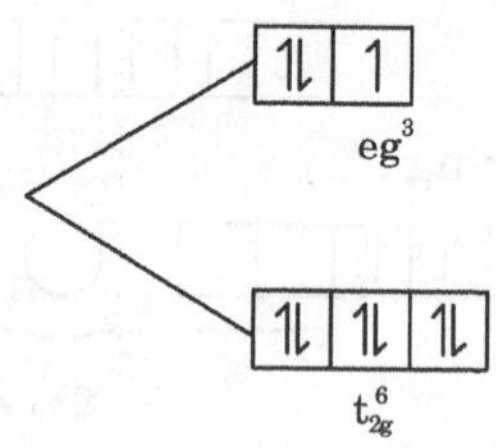

CFSE = $(-0.4 \times +0.6\ y)\Delta_0$

$= (-0.4 \times 6 + 0.6 + 3)\Delta_0$

$= (-2.4 + 1.8)\Delta_0$

$= -0.6\ \Delta_0$

No. of unpaired e^- = 1

$\mu = \sqrt{n(n+2)}$

$= \sqrt{1(1+2)}$

$= \sqrt{3} = 1.73$ B.M.

75. CFSE = $(-0.4 \times +0.6\ y)\ \Delta_0$

For high spin d^4, configuration is

$t_{2g}{}^3\ eg^1$.

x = 3 (No. of e^- in t_{2g})

y = 1 (No. of e^- in eg)

CFSE = $(-0.4 \times 3 + 0.6 \times 1)\Delta_0$

$= (-1.2 + 0.6)\Delta_0 = -0.6\Delta_0$

76. For d^{10} configuration , arrangement is $t_{2g}{}^6\ eg^4$.

CFSE = $(-0.4x + 0.6y)\ \Delta_0$

$= (-0.4 \times 6 + 0.6 \times 4)\ \Delta_0$

$= (-2.4 + 2.4)\ \ \Delta_0 = 0$

For high spin d^5, arrangement is $t_{2g}{}^3\ eg^2$.

CFSE = $(-0.4 \times +0.6y)\ \Delta_0$

$= (-0.4 \times 3 + 0.6 \times 2)\ \Delta_0$

$= 0$

77. In $[Ti(H_2O)_6]^{3+}$, Ti is in +3 oxidation state.

Ti (22) : (Ar) $4s^2\ 3d^2$

Ti^{3+} : (Ar) $3d^1$

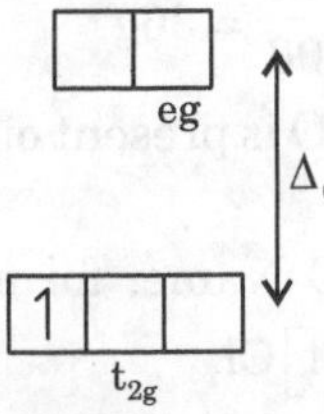

CFSE = $(-0.4x + 0.6y)\Delta_0$

$= (-0.4 \times 1 + 0.6 \times 0)\Delta_0$

CFSE = $-0.4\ \Delta_0$ ... (i)

$\bar{\nu} = 20{,}300\ cm^{-1} = \frac{1}{\lambda}$

When this single e^- will transit from t_{2g} to eg & then return, photon released will have energy = Δ_0.

So, $\Delta_0 = E = \frac{hc}{\lambda} = hc \times 20{,}300\ cm^{-1}$

$\Delta_0 = hc \times 20{,}300 \times 10^2\ m^{-1}$

$\Delta_0 = 6.626 \times 10^{-34}\ Js \times 3 \times 10^8\ ms^{-1} \times 20{,}300 \times 100\ m^{-1}$

$\Delta_0 = 6.626 \times 3 \times 20{,}300 \times 10^{-34} \times 10^8 \times 100$ J

$\Delta_0 = 6.626 \times 3 \times 20{,}300 \times 10^{-24}$ J

$$\boxed{\Delta_0 = 403523.4 \times 10^{-24}\ J}$$

Placing the value of Δ_0 in eqn 1

CFSE = $-0.4\Delta_0$

CFSE = $-0.4 \times 403523.4 \times 10^{-24}$ J

But answer is demanded in kJ/mol,

$\therefore$ CFSE = $-0.4 \times 403523.4 \times 10^{-24} \times 10^{-3} \times 6 \times 10^{23}$ kJ/mole

CFSE = $-0.4 \times 403523.4 \times 6 \times 10^{-27} \times 10^{23}$ kJ/mole

$= -2.4 \times 403523.4 \times 10^{-4}$ kJ/mole

$= -968456 \times 10^{-4}$ kJ/mole

$= -96.8$ kJ/mole

78. $[Cr(CO)_6]$

EAN = At. No. – oxidation state + 2 × Coordination No.

EAN = 24 – 0 + 2 × 6

= 24 + 12 = 36

79. Pt everywhere is in +4 oxidation state. It shows coordination number 6 when is +4.

(1) $K_2[PtCl_6] \xrightleftharpoons{aq.} 2K^+_{(aq)} + [PtCl_6]^{2-}_{(aq.)}$

(2) $[Pt(NH_3)_2\ Cl_4] \xrightleftharpoons{aq.} [Pt(NH_3)_2\ Cl_4]_{(aq.)}$

(3) $[Pt(NH_3)_3\ Cl_3]Cl \xrightleftharpoons{aq.} [Pt(NH_3)_3\ Cl_3]^+_{(aq.)} + Cl^-_{(aq.)}$

(4) $[Pt(NH_3)_5\ Cl]Cl_3 \xrightleftharpoons{aq.} [Pt(NH_3)_5\ Cl]^{3+}_{(aq.)} + 3Cl^-_{(aq.)}$

80. For complex, $[Fe(CO)_2\ (NO)_2]$

NO is a 3 e^- donor.

EAN = At. No. – oxidation state + 2x coordination No.

= 26 – 0 + 4 + 6

$\boxed{EAN = 36}$

81. For $[V(CO)_6]^-$

EAN = 23 – (–1) + 2 × 6

= 23 + 1 + 12

= 36

For $[Fe(\pi - C_5H_5)_2]$

C_5H_5 is cyclopentadienyl ion.

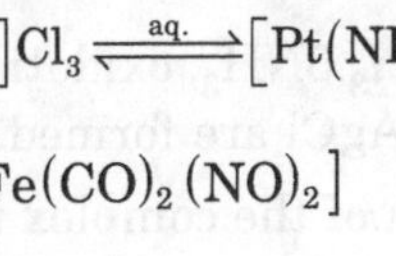

x + (–2) = 0

Oxidation state of Fe is +2

Cyclopentadienyl anion is aromatic and $6\pi\ e^-$ donor here.

So, EAN = 26 – 2 + 2 × 6

= 26 – 2 + 12 = 36

For $[Fe(CO)_5]$

EAN = 26 – 0 + 5 × 2 = 36

For $\left[Ti(\sigma-C_5H_5)_2(\pi-C_5H_5)_2\right]$

$x + (-2) + (-2) = 0$

$\boxed{x = +4}$

Oxidation state of Ti = +4

Here, two cyclopentadienyl rings act as $2e^-$ donor each (which show σ donation) & the rest two rings act as $6e^-$ donor (which show π donation)

EAN = 22 – 4 + 2 × 2 + 6 × 2

= 22 – 4 + 4 + 12

= 34

82. In $CoCl_3.3NH_3$, oxidation state of Co = +3

Co^{3+} shows coordination – No. = 6

So, complex is $[CoCl_3(NH_3)_3]$ and since there is no 'Cl' outside the co-ordination sphere, no ppt. of AgCl is formed.

Also in $CoCl_3.5NH_3$, oxidation state of Co = + 3 & 2 moles of AgCl are formed.

So, formula of the complex is

$[Co(NH_3)_5Cl]Cl_2$.

Now, the two complexes have been identified.

(1) $[CoCl_3(NH_3)_3] \rightarrow$ non-ionisable complex van't Hoff factor (i) = 1

(2) $[Co(NH_3)_5Cl]Cl_2 \rightarrow [Co(NH_3)_5Cl]^{2+} + 2Cl^-$

$\boxed{i = 3}$

83. 1° valency is oxidation No. & 2° valency is Coordination-No.

So, in $K_2[Ni(CN)_4]$

1° valency/oxidation state of Ni = +2

2° valency/Co-ordination No. = 4

Ratio = 1 : 2

84. $nCl^- + nH^+ \rightarrow nHCl$

1 mole of complex will form n moles of HCl which will further require n moles of NaOH.

$$\text{moles of complex} = \frac{0.319}{266.5} = 0.0012$$

$$\text{moles of NaOH used} = \frac{28.5 \times 0.125}{1000} = 0.0036$$

Now, moles of NaOH = moles of HCl

So, 0.0012 moles of complex = 0.0036 moles of HCl

1 mole of complex = 3 moles of HCl

So, n = 3

86. 'A' has to be $[Cr(H_2O)_6]Cl_3$ because it is not reacting with conc. H_2SO_4. Had there been some H_2O molecules outside the co-ordination sphere, it would have got dehydrated with conc. H_2SO_4.

For complex B on reacting with conc. H_2SO_4, if it is losing 6.75% of its mass, it means that percentage of H_2O (by mass) = 6.75%.

Molar mass of complex = 266.5

6.75% of 266.5 = weight of H_2O

$$\frac{6.75}{100} \times 266.5 = 18g(\text{weight of } H_2O)$$

It means one mole H_2O is outside the coordination sphere in complex B.

Similarly, for C

$$266.5 \times \frac{13.5}{100} = 36g$$

So, 2 mole H_2O is present outside the co-ordination sphere.

87. From IUPAC Name, formula of the complex is $[Co(NH_3)_5Cl]Cl_2$

So, precipitable halide ions = 2

89. 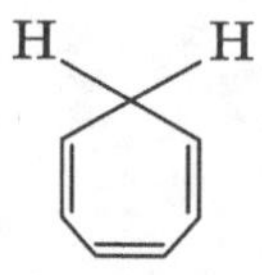

6π electrons will resonate & move between 6C's. so, hapticity of this organic ligand is 6.

Once H^- is removed,

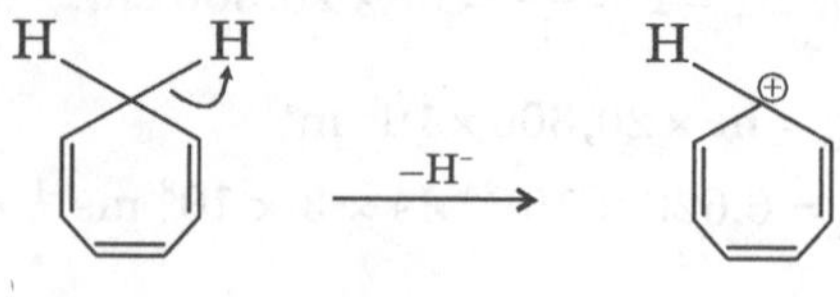

Now, in 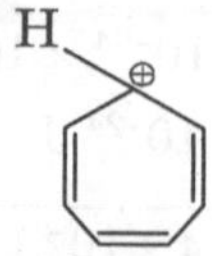 the six πe's can now move between 7 C's, so its hapticity is 7.

90. Compounds having M–C bond are called organometallic compounds.

In R-MgX (Grignard's reagent), there is a bond between C & Mg.

91. 'W' here has oxidation state of +2. It is because

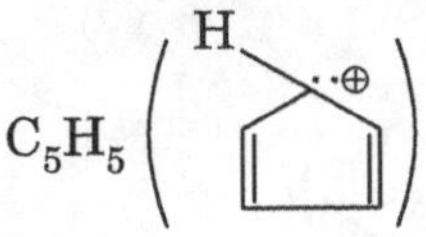 carries a uninegative charge.

W has configuration :

[Xe] $4f^{14}\ 5d^4\ 6s^2$

W^{2+} : (Xe) $4f^{14}\ 5d^4$

It has 4 valence e^-.

So, 4 + 6 (from pentahapto) + 4(from trihapto) + 2 × 2 = 18 (from CO.)

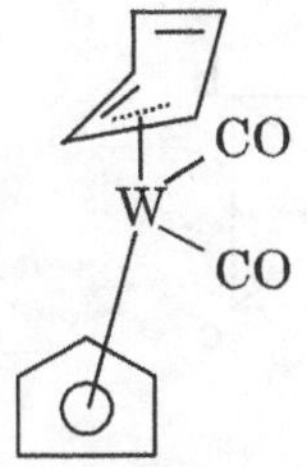

93. 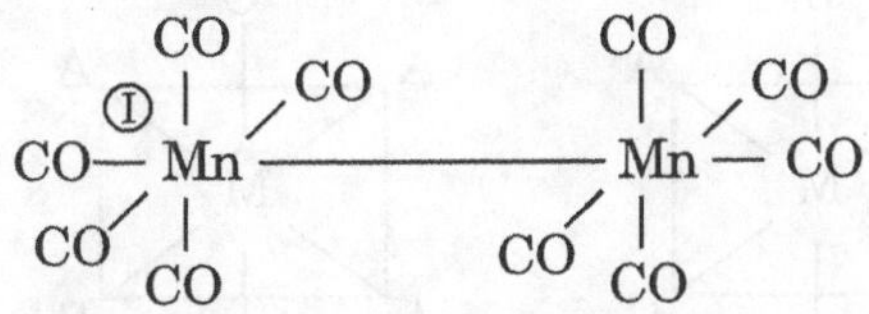

wrt Mn labelled I, 5 CO donate $2e^-$ each & Mn shares 1 e^- of the adjacent placed Mn.

So, total e^- wrt Mn labelled I = 25 + 10 + 1 = 36

94. 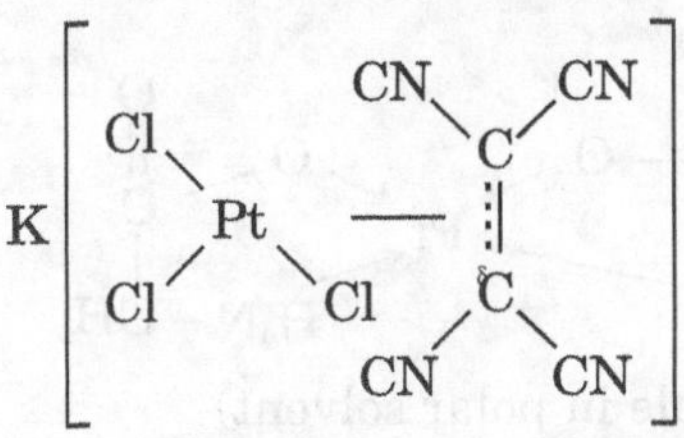

$\bar{C}N$ will exert - I effect creating partial +ve charge on C atom. So, C will accept more electrons from metal cation. So, C – C bond length increases.

95. C_5H_5 in ferrocene is 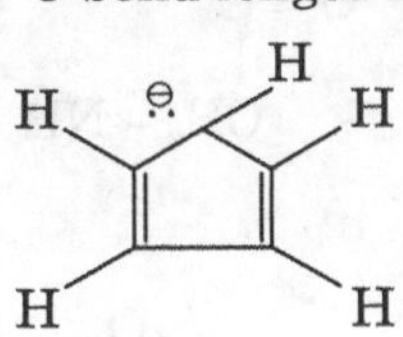

$\left[Fe(\eta^5 - C_5H_5)_2\right]$ x + (–2) = 0

x = + 2

Each cyclopentadienyl anion is a 6π e^- donor.

EAN = 26 – 2 + 2 × 6 = 36

Also, $(\eta^5 - C_5H_5)_2Fe + CH_3COCl \rightarrow$

$(\eta^5 - C_5H_4COCH_3)(\eta^5 - C_5H_5)Fe + HCl$

96. Higher the –ve charge density on central metal ion, higher will be the extent of back donation from metal to ligand (CO) & therefore metal-carbon bond order will increase.

97. for d^9 configuration, t_{2g} is symmetrically filled but eg is unsymmetrically filled. So, $d_{x^2-y^2}$ & d_{z^2} will suffer unequal repulsions leading to distortion

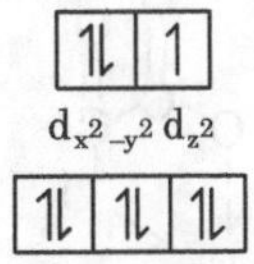

for d^7 configuration, t_{2g} level is unsymmetrically filled, So some distortion in octahedral geometry will surely occur.

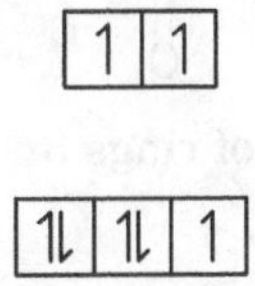

For d^8 configuration, t_{2g} & eg both are symmetrically filled

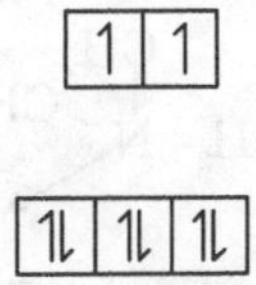

99. EAN of V in $[V(CO)_6]$ is 35. So, it intends to get reduced to reach 36 and hence acts like a good oxidising agent.

$$\boxed{EAN = 23 - 0 + 12 = 35}$$

100. $\left[Co(NH_3)_6\right]^{3+}\left[Cr(NO_2)_6\right]^{3-}$ can be distinguished from $\left[Cr(NH_3)_6\right]^{3+}\left[Co(NO_2)_6\right]^{3-}$ by electrolysis.

In one case cobalt (III) complex will go towards –ve' electrode. In other case, chromium (III) complex will go towards –ve electrode

For option b,

$\left[Cr(NH_3)_6\right]^{3+}\left[Co(NO_2)_6\right]^{3-}$ is carrying +3, –3 charge & $\left[Cr(NH_3)_4(NO_2)_2\right]^{+}\left[Cr(NH_3)_2(NO_2)_4\right]^{-}$ is carrying (+1, –1) charge. So, they can be distinguished by conductivity measurements. Also, PPh_3 is a phosphorous donor & a strong field ligand.

101. Photon of red λ will have min. energy. It means the extent of splitting is least with L_1. Hence, L_1 is the weakest ligand.

Photon of blue λ has max. energy. So, more energy might have been required to excite electron. So, splitting should have been more. Hence, L_4 is the strongest ligand of all.

102. Solutions not Given

103. In option (a), both $C_2O_4^{2-}$ & H_2O are 'O' donors. There is a difference in Δ_0 but not much because they belong to same class of ligands i.e., 'O' donors. So, chelation plays a major role in determining the stabilities of complexes.

For option (a) :

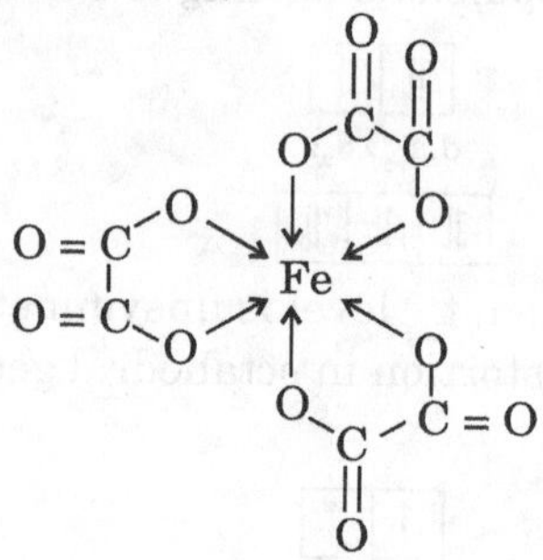

No. of rings 3

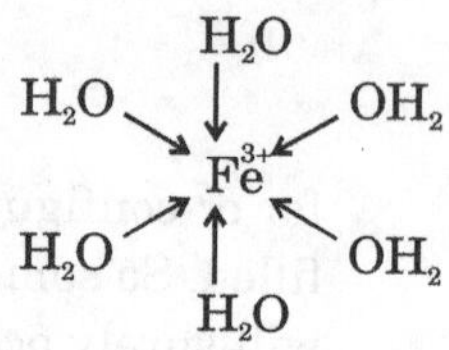

No Chelation

For option (b),

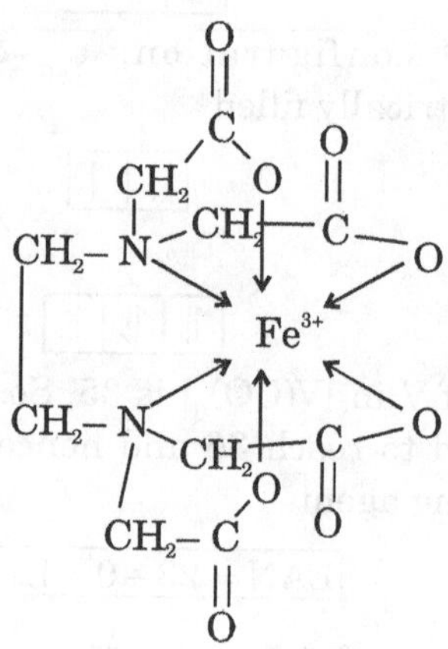

No. of rings = 5

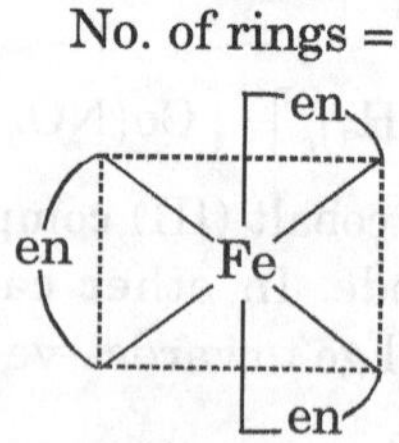

No. of rings = 3

For option (c), the ligands are same

But in $[Fe(CN)_6]^{3-}$, Fe is in +3 oxidation state, (which is higher), so Δ_0 is more.

104. In $[Ma_3b_2c]^{n+}$

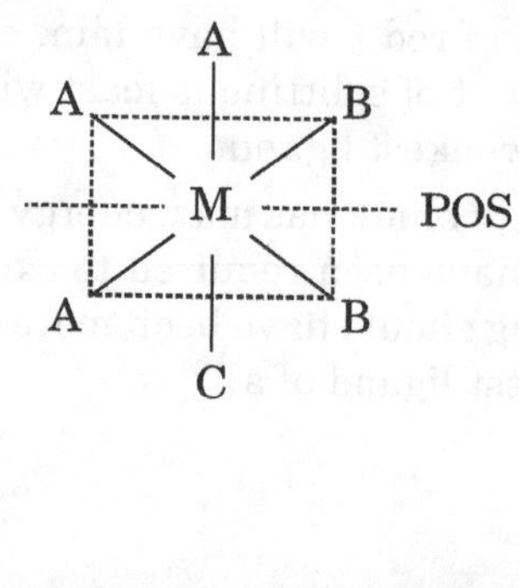

Optically inactive (No optical isomer)

$[Ma_3bcd]^{n+}$

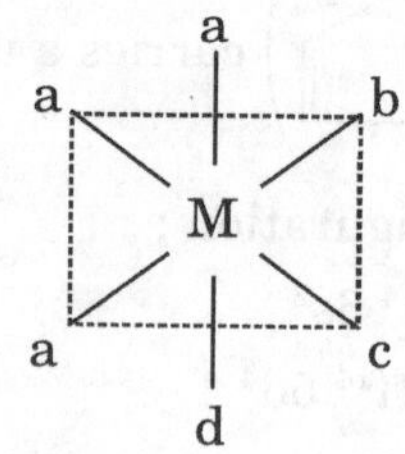

No. of enantiomeric pair = 1

Geometrical isomers in Ma_3bcd

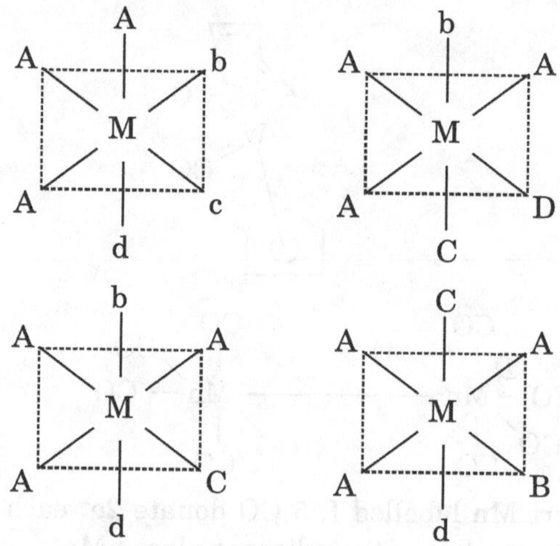

105. X is cis $[Pt(gly)_2]$

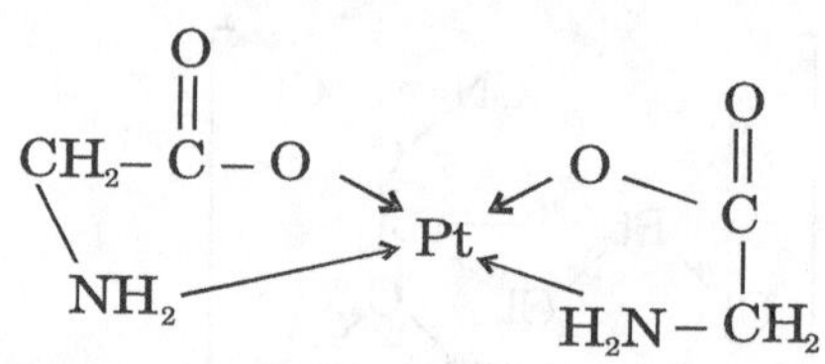

Polar (So, soluble in polar solvent)

Y is trans $[Pt(gly)_2]$

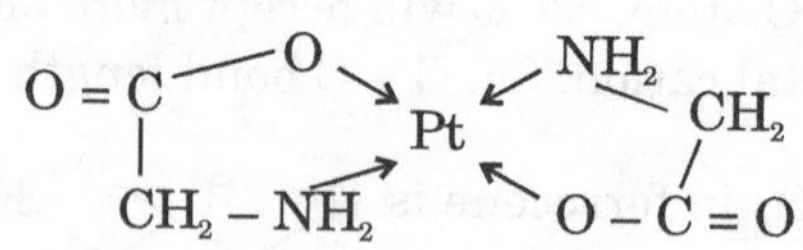

Trans

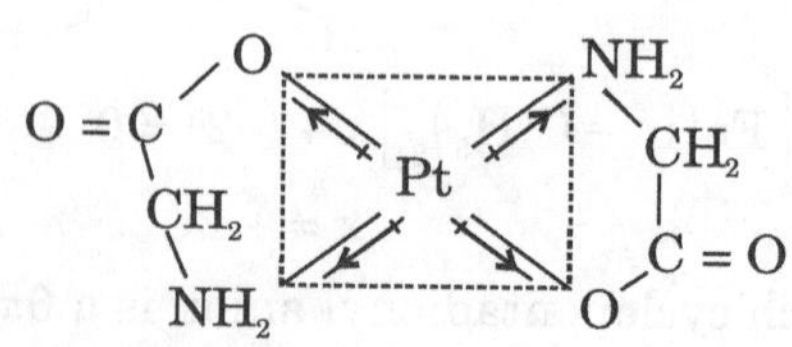

Non-polar trans form

(Soluble in non-polar solvent)

106. AgBr has pale yellow ppt. So, complex 'X' will be

$$\underset{'X'}{\left[Cr(NH_3)_4\, I\, Br\right]Br} + AgNO_3 \rightarrow \left[Cr(NH_3)_4\, IBr\right]NO_3 + \underset{\text{(Pale yellow)}}{AgBr}$$

AgI gives yellow ppt. So, complex 'Y' will be :

$$\underset{'Y'}{\left[Cr(NH_3)_4\, Br_2\right]I} + AgNO_3 \rightarrow \left[Cr(NH_3)_4\, Br_2\right]NO_3 + \underset{\text{(yellow ppt)}}{AgI}$$

X is $\left[Cr(NH_3)_4\, I\, Br\right]Br$ & Y is $\left[Cr(NH_3)_4 Br_2\right]I$

wrt option (a)

cis form of X :

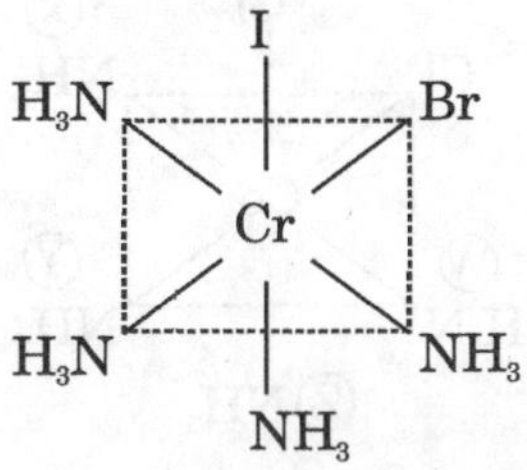

(has POS, optically inactive)

Cis form of Y :

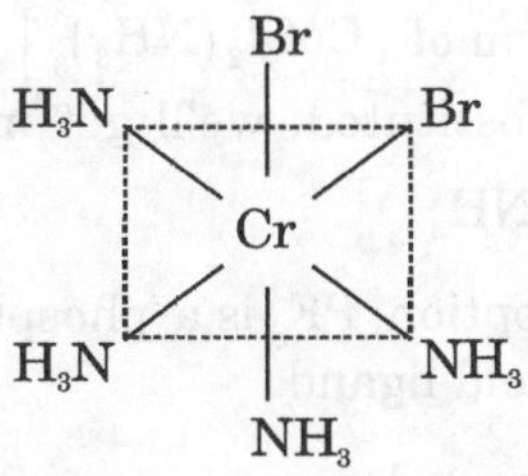

(has POS, optically inactive)

wrt option (b) :

cis form of X – trans form of Y –

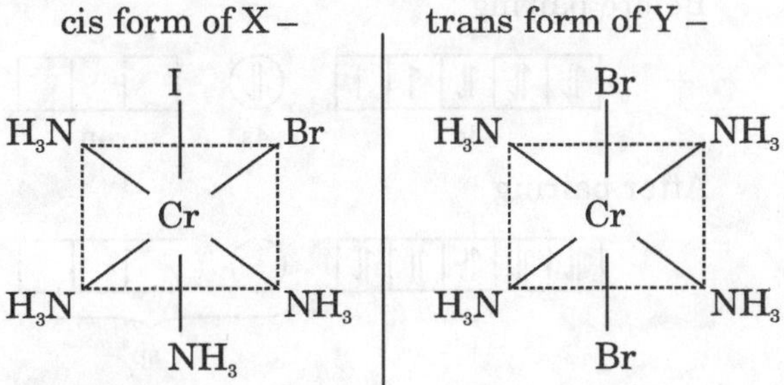

Optically inactive Optically inactive

wrt option (c) :

Both are optically inactive.

107. Consider reaction;

$$\left[M(H_2O)_4\right]^{2+} + 4CH_3NH_2 \rightleftharpoons \left[M(CH_3NH_2)_4\right]^{2+} + 4H_2O$$

Here, entropy charge is negligible because total number of moles of reactant are equal to those of product (5 moles of reactant & 5 moles of products).

Consider reaction 2,

$$\left[M(H_2O)_4\right]^{2+} + 2en \rightleftharpoons \left[M(en)_2\right]^{2+} + 4H_2O$$

Entropy change is +ve here (from 3 moles of reactants to 5 moles of product).

$\Delta_2 \overset{o}{G}$ is more –ve.

Also, $\left[M(en)_2\right]^{2+}$ is more stable than $\left[M(NH_2CH_3)_4\right]^{2+}$ due to chelation in the former complex.

108. $[Ni(CO)_4]$ is tetrahedral atoms 'ticked' are in same plane.

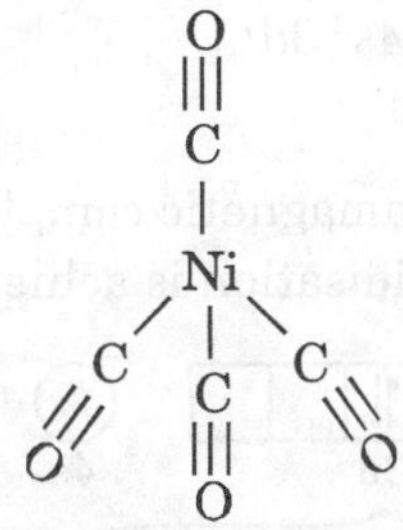

109. $Ag^+ + 2NH_3 \rightleftharpoons \left[Ag(NH_3)_2\right]^+$

$$K = \frac{\left[Ag(NH_3)_2\right]^+}{(Ag^+)(NH_3)^2}$$

$$1.7 \times 10^7 = \frac{\left[Ag(NH_3)_2\right]^+}{(Ag^+)(0.1)^2}$$

$$1.7 \times 10^7 \times 10^{-2} = \frac{\left[Ag(NH_3)_2\right]^+}{(Ag^+)}$$

$$\boxed{1.7 \times 10^5 = \frac{\left[Ag(NH_3)_2\right]^+}{(Ag^+)}}$$

110. B & C show only geometrical isomerism

(B) is $\left[Ni(H_2O)_4(NH_3)_2\right]^{2+}$

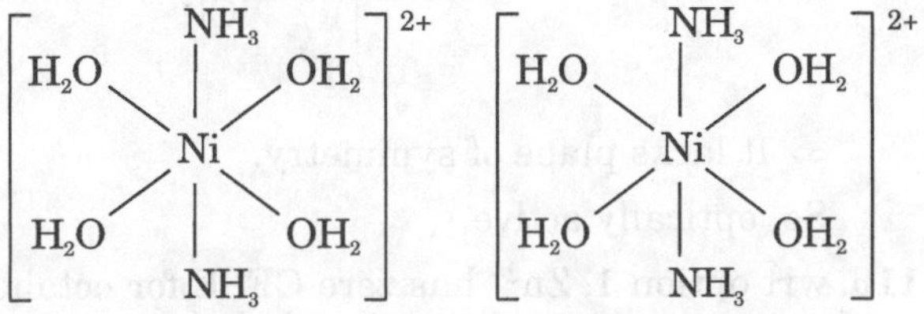

Trans Cis

111. wrt b option, acetylacetone complexes of the metal ions contain a six membered conjugate chelate ring & the resonance in its chelate ion is an additional factor contributing to its stability.

wrt c option :

The value of Δ_0 is larger for 2nd & 3rd row transition elements. The larger value of Δ_0 energetically favours the pairing of electrons resulting in square planar geometry.

112. In $[Ni(PPh_3)_2 Br_2]$, Ni is in +2 oxidation state.

With all four strong field ligands, geometry is square planar but here geometry is tetrahedral.

Similar geometry is in option (b) & (c).

113. Co (27) : (Ar) $4s^2\ 3d^7$

Co^{3+} : (Ar) $3d^6$

since, its a diamagnetic complex, pairing occurs & $d^2\ sp^3$ hybridisation is achieved.

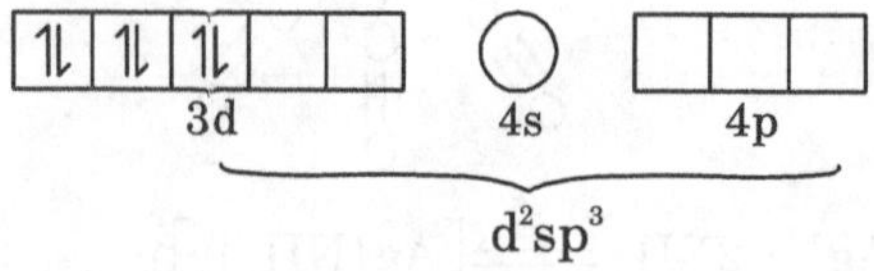

114. The two possible isomers for the given octahedral complex are

$$[M(NH_3)_5 SO_4]Cl \ \& \ [M(NH_3)_5 Cl]SO_4$$

115.

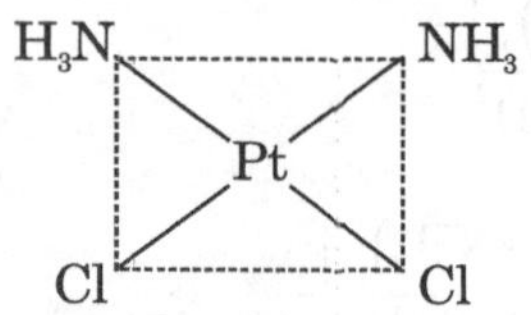

Cis
(will have some dipole moment)

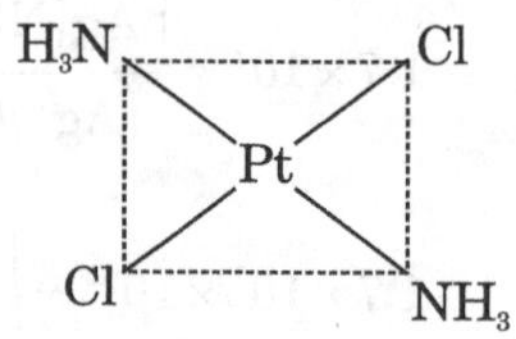

Trans
(has $\mu = 0$)

Also, wrt option c

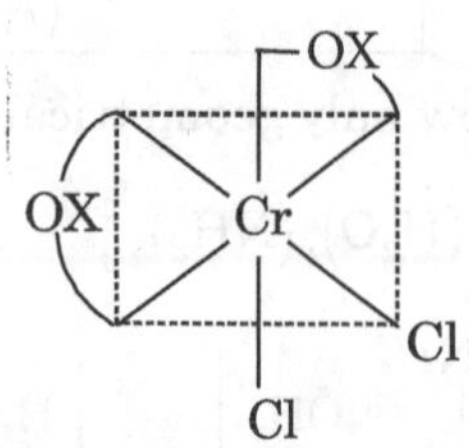

$\Rightarrow$ It lacks plane of symmetry.

So, optically active.

116. wrt option 1, Zn^{2+} has zero CFSE for octahedral geometry.

Zn^{2+} : (Ar) $3d^{10}$

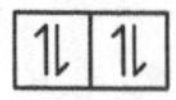

CFSE = $(-0.4x + 0.6\ y)\ \Delta_0$

$= (-0.4 \times 6 + 0.6 \times 4)\ \Delta_0$

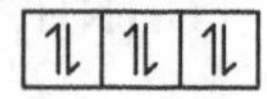

$= (-2.4 + 2.4)\ \Delta_0 = 0$

wrt 2nd option :

Δ_t is always much smaller even with strong field ligands & it is never energetically favorable to pair up the electrons.

For 3rd option :

$$[CoCl_2(NH_3)_4]^+ + Cl^- \rightarrow [CoCl_3(NH_3)_3] + NH_3$$

Reactant

If reactant is in cis form

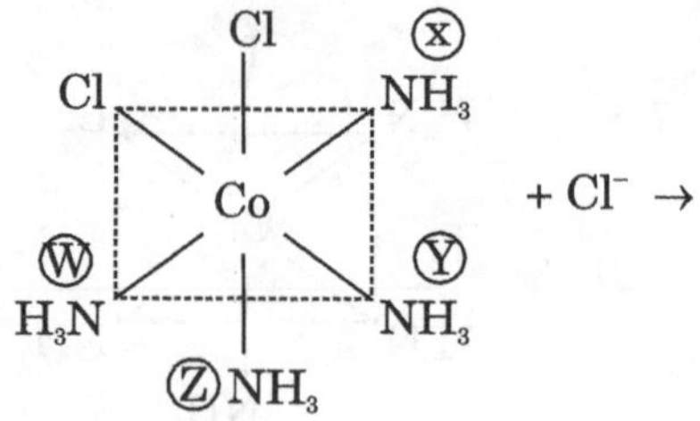

(cis wrt Cl)

Here, if 'NH_3' labelled 'W' is substituted, we'll get facial form of $[CoCl_3(NH_3)_3]$ & if 'NH_3' labelled 'Y' is substituted, we'll get meridional form of $[CoCl_3(NH_3)_3]$.

wrt 4th option, PF_3 is a 'phosphorous donor', so a strong field ligand.

In $[Ni(PF_3)_4]$, oxidation state of Ni = 0

Ni (28) : (Ar) $4s^2\ 3d^8$

Before pairing :

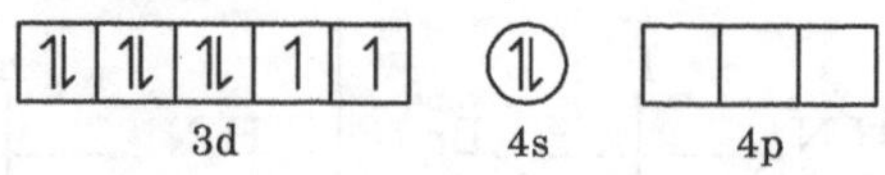

After pairing :

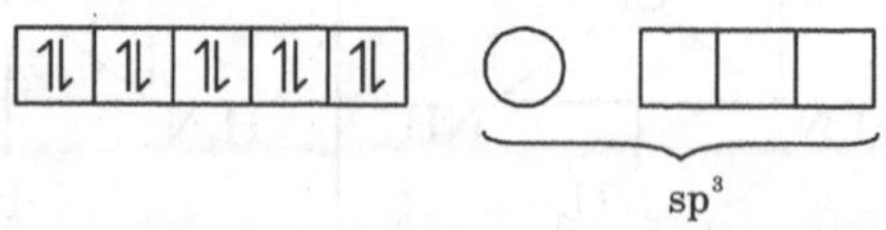

An e^- pair shifts from 4s to 3d resulting in diamagnetic, tetrahedral complex.

wrt 5th option :

$[Sc(H_2O)_6]^{3+}$ is colorless because Sc^{3+} lacks d-electrons $[Sc^{3+} : (Ar)]$ & hence d-d transition is NOT POSSIBLE.

117. It shows linkage, geometrical & Optical isomerism

(a) 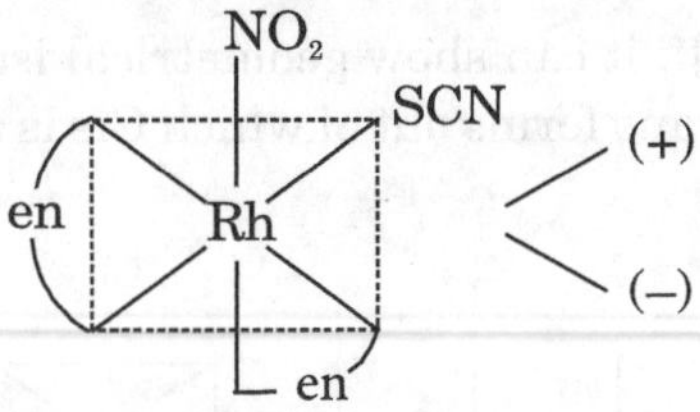

(It can show optical also)

(b) 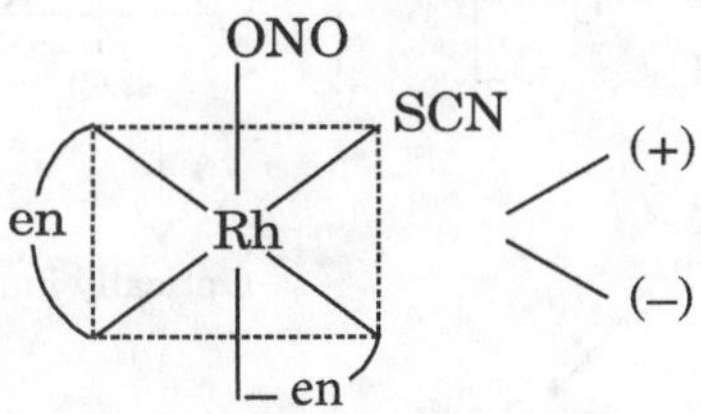

(It can show optical isomerism)

(c) 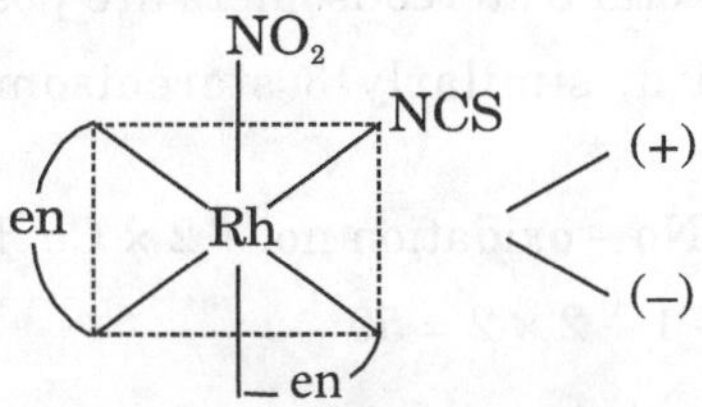

(Can show optical isomerism)

(d) 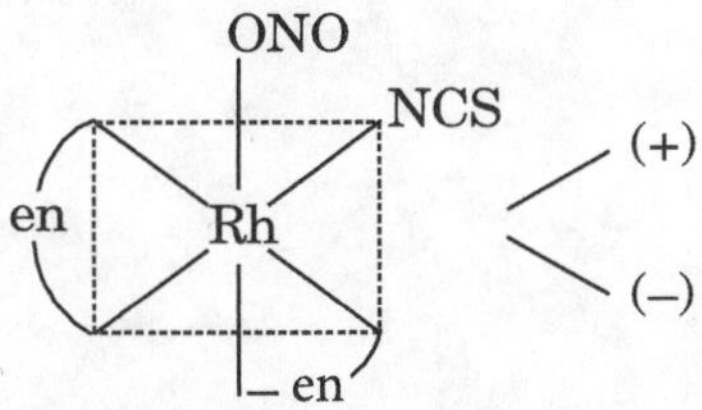

(Can show optical isomerism)

(e) 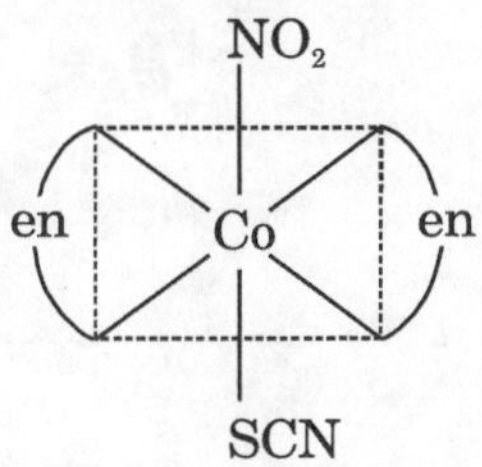

(No optical)

(f) 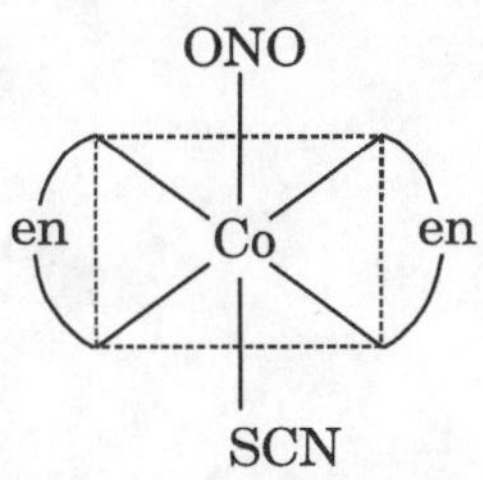

(No optical)

(g) 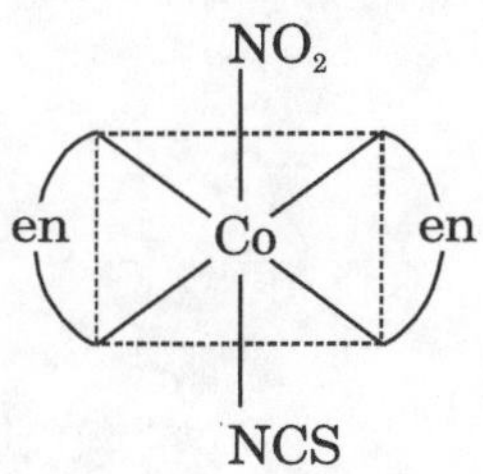

(No optical)

(h) 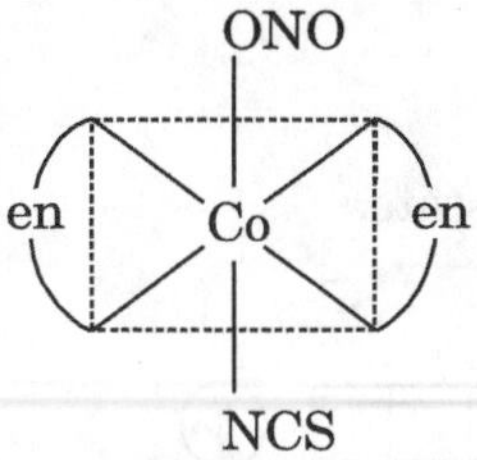

(No optical)

Total no. of isomers = 2 + 2 + 2 + 2 + 1 + 1 + 1 + 1

= 12

118. For $[Cr(NH_3)_6]^{3+}$

oxidation state of Cr = +3

Cr (24): (Ar) $4s^1$ $3d^5$

Cr^{3+}: – (Ar) $3d^3$

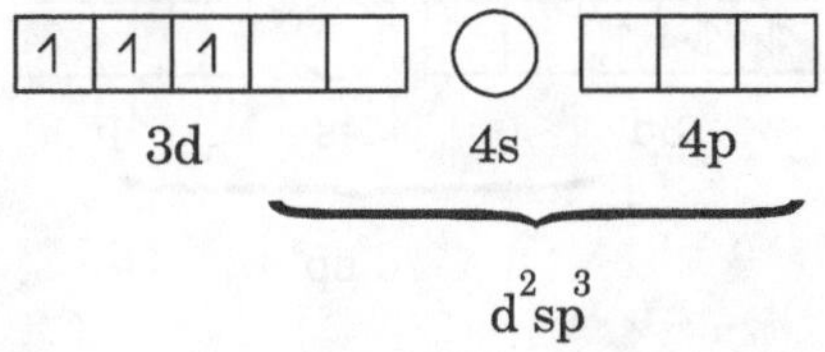

it is inner orbital & high spin complex

For $[V(H_2O)_6]^{3+}$

V = +3

V(23): (Ar) $4s^2$ $3d^3$

V^{3+}:- (Ar) $3d^2$

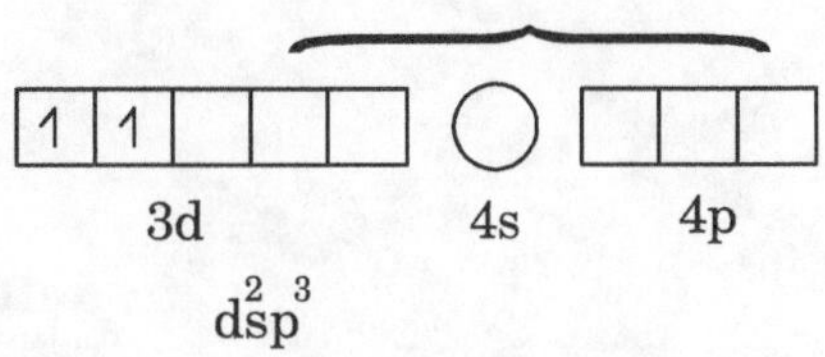

(inner orbital & high spin complex)

For $[Cr(H_2O)_6]^{3+}$

Cr = +3

Cr(24) : (Ar)$4s^1$ $3d^5$

Cr^{3+}:- (Ar)$3d^3$

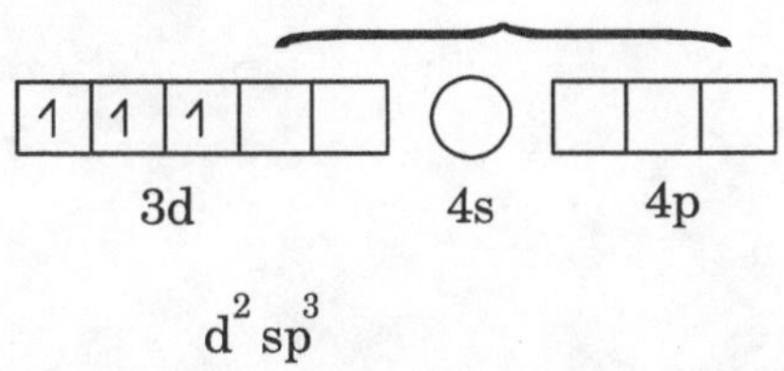

119. Geometry & oxidation state of metal ion is same everywhere (+3). Cl^- ion is the weakest ligand among these, So, Δ_o will be min,

120. $\overline{S}CN$ is not a chelating ligand.

121. wrt option (c),

$[V(CO)_6]$

V is in '0' oxidation state.

V(23): (Ar) $4s^2\ 3d^3$

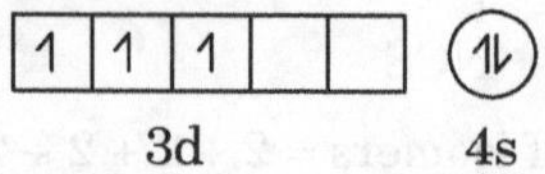

Since CO is a strong field ligand & energy difference between 3d & 4s is less, electron pair will shift from 4s to 3d to perform or aid in Back bonding.

After pairing

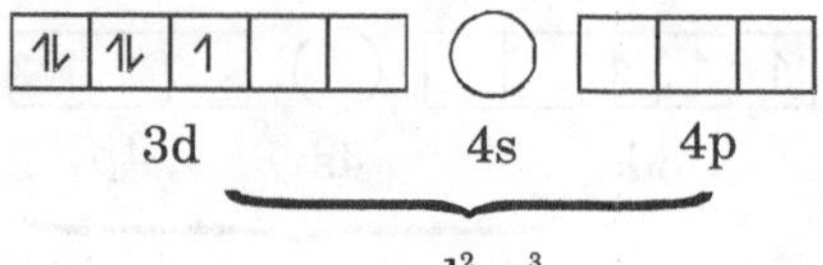

122. wrt option (c),

$[CoCl_2(en)_2]^+$, it can show geometrical isomerism i.e. Cis & trans forms out of which Cis is optically active.

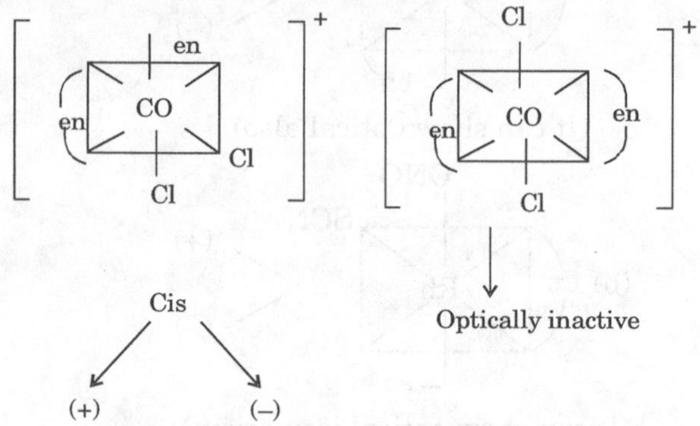

Therefore, total 3 stereo isomers are possible.

wrt option d, similarly 3 stereoisomers are possible.

123. EAN = At. No – oxidation no. + 2 × Co. No.

$= 47 - 1 + 2 \times 2 = 50$

CHAPTER 10

Haloalkanes and Haloarenes

Nucleophilicity and Basicity

1. Identify incorrect order against the property mentioned

(a) $CH_3COO^{\ominus} < \overset{\ominus}{O}H$ (nucleophilicity)

(b) $\overset{\ominus}{N}H_2 > \bar{O}H$ (basicity)

(c) $(CH_3)_2CHO^{\ominus} < (CH_3)_3CO^{\ominus}$ (basicity)

(d) $\overset{\ominus}{S}H > \bar{O}H$ (basicity)

2. Which one of the following is least basic?

(a) F^- (b) Br^-

(c) $\overset{\ominus}{N}H_2$ (d) $\overset{\ominus}{C}H_3$

3. Arange the following in decreasing order of their nucleophilicity in polar protic solvent

(1) $CH_3CH_2O^{\ominus}$ (2) $CH_3CH_2S^{\ominus}$

(3) $CH_3-\overset{O}{\overset{||}{C}}-O^{\ominus}$

(a) 2 > 1 > 3

(b) 3 > 1 >2

(b) 1 > 2 > 3

(d) 3 = 1 > 2

4. Which one of the following is the best leaving group?

(a) $CF_3SO_3^{\ominus}$ (b) $C_6H_5O^{\ominus}$

(c) $C_6H_5SO_3^{\ominus}$ (d) $CH_3COO^{\ominus}$

5. Select the INCORRECT STATEMENT?

(a) Among halide ions, F^- is the strongest nucleophile in aprotic solvent.

(b) Among halide ions, I^- is the strongest nucleophile in polar protic solvent.

(c) Fluoride ion is a stronger base than iodide ion.

(d) NH_3 is a stronger nucleophile than hydrazine (NH_2NH_2)

6. Select the correct decreasing order of nucleophilicity

(a) $\overset{\ominus}{O}H > C_6H_5O^{\ominus} > C_2H_5O^{\ominus} > CH_3COO^{\ominus} > H_2O$

(b) $C_2H_5O^{\ominus} > \overset{\ominus}{O}H > C_6H_5O^{\ominus} > CH_3COO^{\ominus} > H_2O$

(c) $C_6H_5O^{\ominus} > \overset{\ominus}{O}H > C_2H_5O^{\ominus} > H_2O > CH_3COO^{\ominus}$

(d) None of these

7. Which one of the following is the 'BEST LEAVING GROUP?'

(a) N_2 (b) $CF_3-SO_3^{\ominus}$

(c) $F_9C_4-\overset{O}{\underset{O}{\overset{||}{\underset{||}{S}}}}-O^{\ominus}$ (d) $\overset{\ominus}{O}H$

8. Select the 'CORRECT OPTION' against the property, mentioned.

(a) $(CH_3)_3CO^{\ominus} > CH_3CH_2O^{\ominus}$ (Basicity)

(b) $CH_3CH_2O^{\ominus} > (CH_3)_3CO^{\ominus}$ (Nucleophilicity)

(c) $RCOO^{\ominus} > RSO_3^{\ominus}$ (Nucleophilicity)

(d) All are correct

9. 'How many' of the following are strong nucleophiles in polar protic solvent?

$\overset{\ominus}{S}H, I^-, \bar{C}N, \bar{O}H, CH_3OH$

(a) 4 (b) 3

(c) 5 (d) 1

10. Which of the following represents the correct order of leavability of halide ions).

(a) $F^- > Cl^- > Br^- > I^-$

(b) $Br^- > I^- > F^- > Cl^-$

(c) $I^- > Br^- > Cl^- > F^-$

(d) None of these

11. Arrange the following nucleophiles in the decreasing order of nucleophillicity? (in water)

(a) $\overset{\ominus}{C}H_3 > \overset{\ominus}{N}H_2 > \overset{\ominus}{O}H > F^-$

(b) $\overset{\ominus}{N}H_2 > \overset{\ominus}{O}H > F^- > \bar{C}H_3$

(c) $F^- > \overset{\ominus}{C}H_3 > \overset{\ominus}{N}H_2 > \bar{O}H$

(d) None of these

12. The correct leaving group ability order is

(a) $\bar{O}H > H_2O$

(b) $\bar{O}H > \overset{\ominus}{S}H$

(c) $CH_3-\overset{O}{\overset{||}{C}}-O^\ominus > CH_3CH_2O^\ominus$

(d) $Cl^- > I^-$

13. The correct decreasing order of relative nucleophilicity of the following nucleophiles (in protic solvent) is

(a) $\overset{\ominus}{S}H > \bar{O}H > H_2O > AcO^\ominus > PhO^\ominus$

(b) $\overset{\ominus}{S}H > \overset{\ominus}{O}H > PhO^\ominus > AcO^\ominus > H_2O$

(c) $\overset{\ominus}{S}H > PhO^\ominus > \overset{\ominus}{O}H > H_2O > AcO^\ominus$

(d) None of these

14. The correct order of nucleophilicity is/are

(a) $CH_3S^\ominus > CH_3SH$

(b) $CH_3-CH_2-O^\ominus > (CH_3)_3CO^\ominus$

(c) $(CH_3CH_2)_3P > (CH_3CH_2)N$

(d) None are correct

15. The correct order/orders of leaving ability is/are

(a) 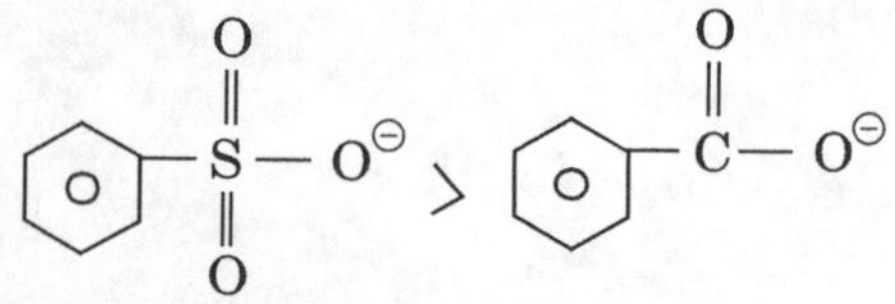

(b) $F_3CSO_3^\ominus > CCl_3SO_3^\ominus$

(c) $\overset{\ominus}{O}H > \overset{\ominus}{N}H_2$

(d) All are correct.

Methods of Preparation of Alkyl Halides

16. Propan-1-ol can be converted into n-propyl chloride by reacting it with-

(a) PCl_5 (b) $COCl_2$

(c) HCl (d) Both (a) & (b)

17. Following compounds are prepared by using suitable reagents. Identify the mismatch.

	Reagents	Compounds (Products)
(a)	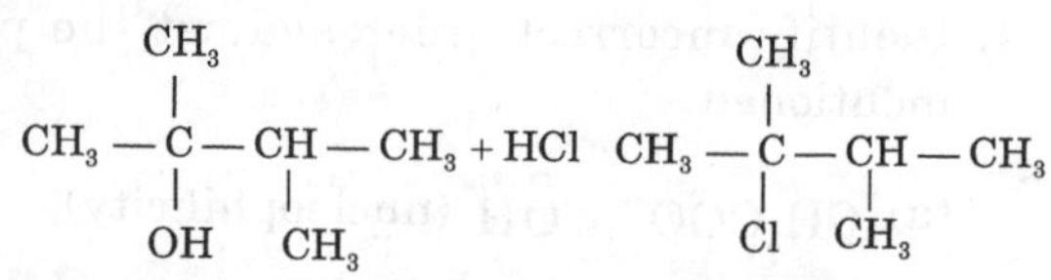	
(b)	$3CH_3CH_2OH + PBr_3$	$3CH_3CH_2Br$
(c)	$CH_3CH_2\ Cl + AgF$	CH_3CH_2F
(d)	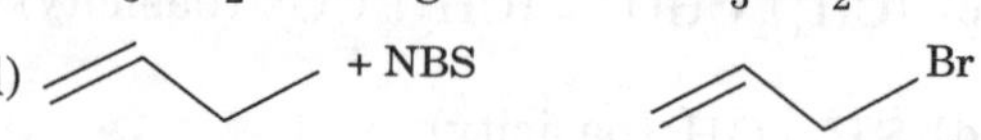	

18. The total number of optically active isomers obtained on monohalogenation of the following compound is

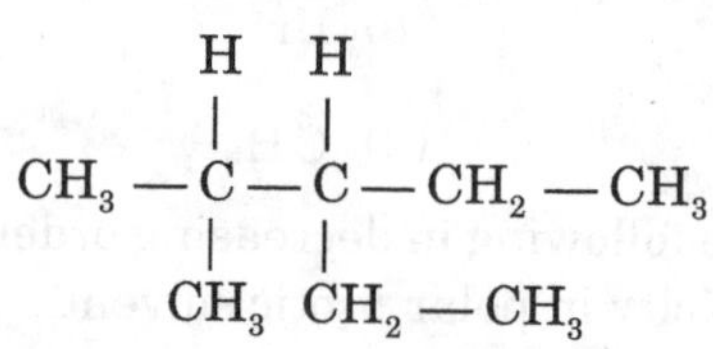

(a) 2 (b) 4

(c) 8 (d) 10

19. An alcohol gives turbidity with lucas reagent only on heating. The alcohol is

(a) 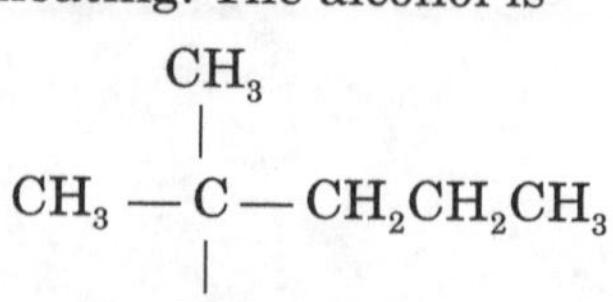

(b) 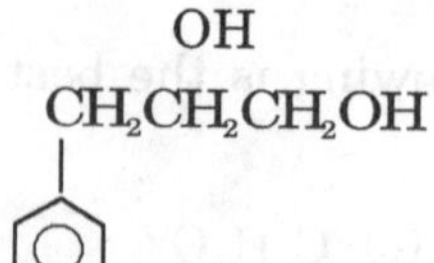

(c) 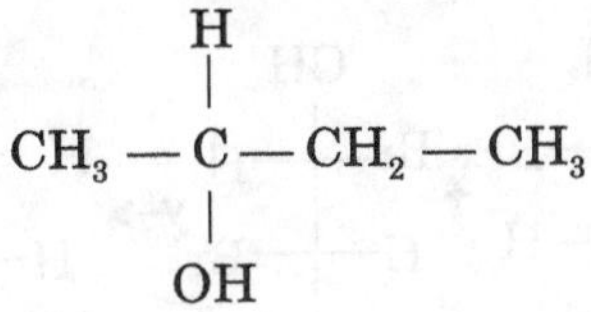

(d) Both (a) & (c)

20. Which of the following compounds can undergo bromination 'in dark' as well as 'in light'?

(a) $CH_3—CH_2—CH_3$ (b) CH_4

(c) $CH_2 = CH_2$ (d) $CH_3—CH=CH_2$

21. What is the major product 'X' in the following reaction).

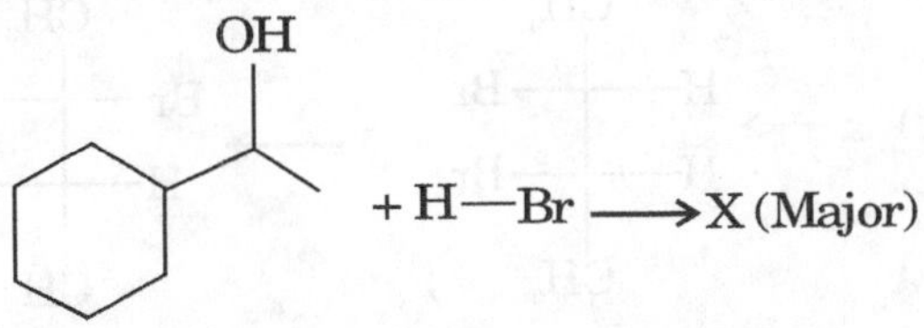

(a) 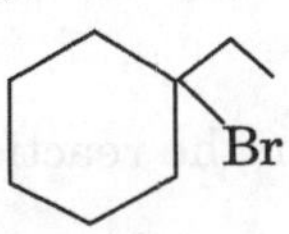 (b) 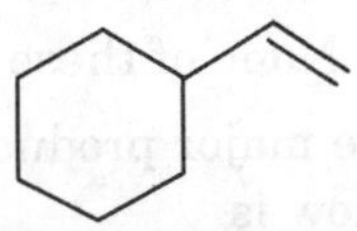

(c) 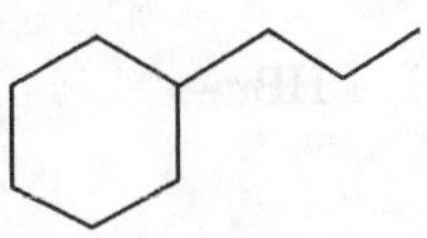 (d) Both (b) & (c)

22.

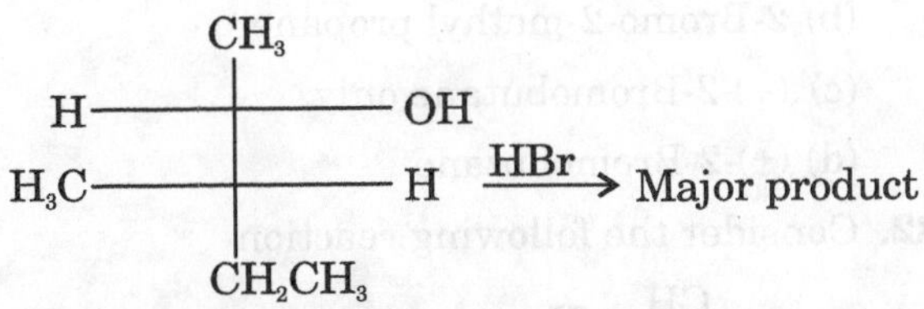

Which of the following structures represent the correct major product?

(a) 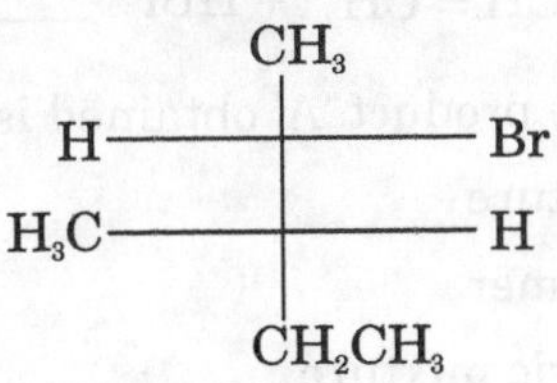

(b) 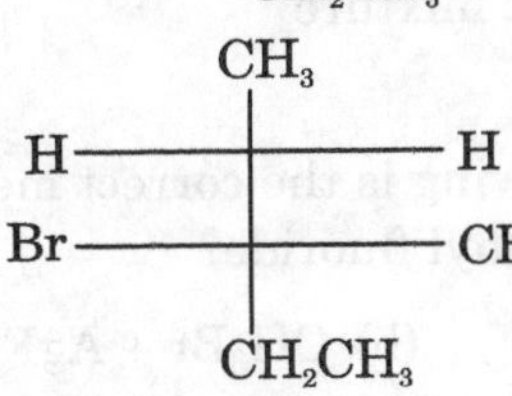

(c) 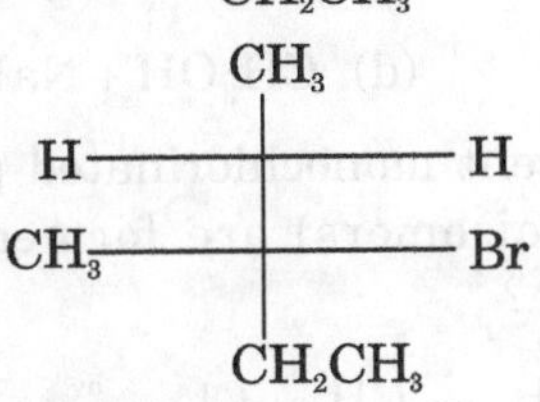

(d) Both (b) & (c)

23. $CH_3—CH_2—CH_2—CH_2—OH \xrightarrow[H_2SO_4]{NaBr,} x.$

Identify 'x' and the mechanism of reaction-

(a) $CH_3—CH_2-CH_2-CH_2—Br$, & S_N1

(b) $CH_3—CH_2-CH_2-CH_2Br$ & S_N2

(c) 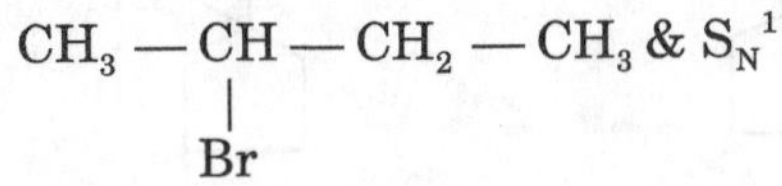

(d) 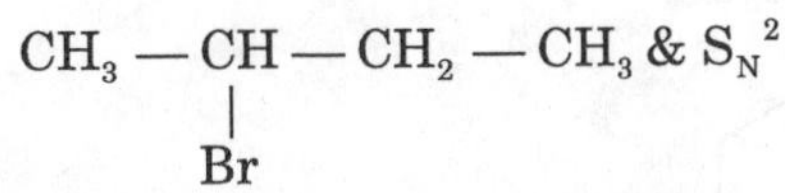

24.

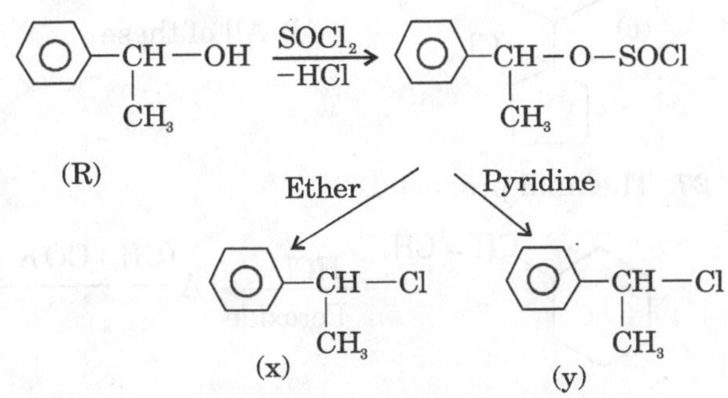

Which configuration will be adopted by x & y respectively?

(a) R, R

(b) R, S

(c) S, R

(d) R, Z

25. Anti - Markovnikov's addition of HBr is followed in which of the following alkenes?

(a) 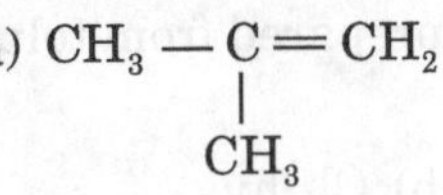

(b) $CH_2 = CH—CF_3$

(c) $CH_2 = CH—\overset{\oplus}{N}(CH_3)_3$

(d) both b & c

26.

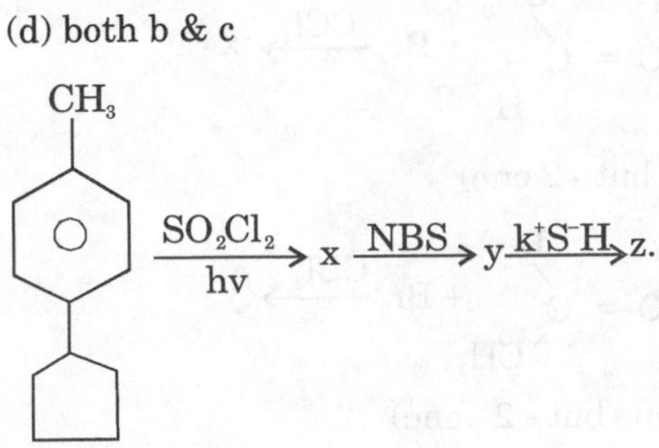

The final product 'z' is

(a) 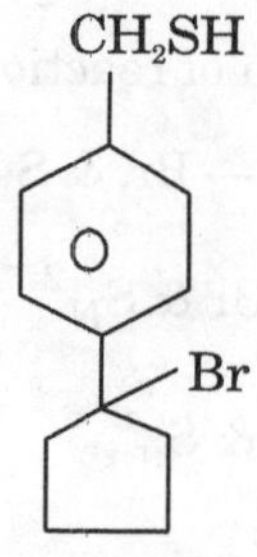

(b) 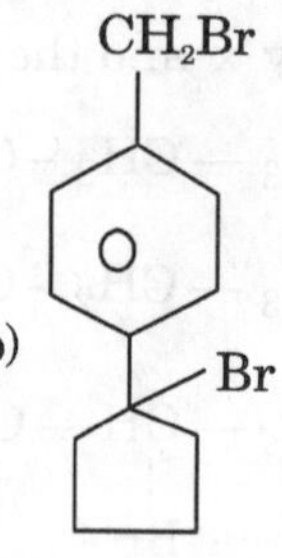

(c) 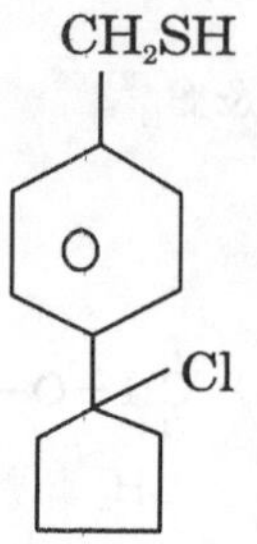

(d) All of these

27. The final product 'B' is -

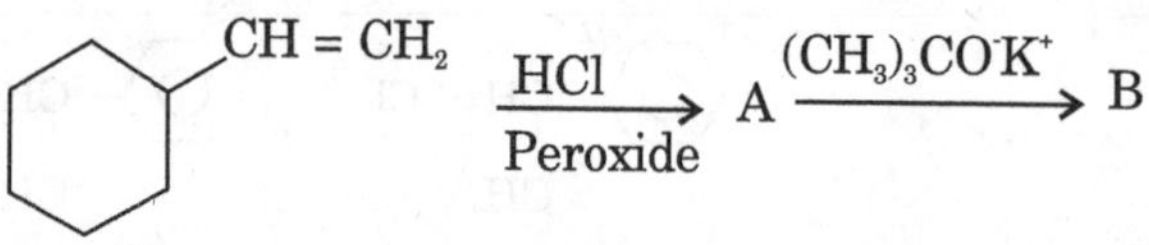

(a) 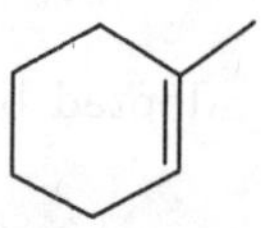

(b) 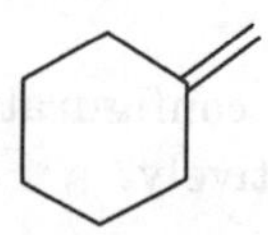

(c) 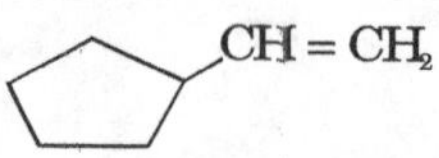

(d) 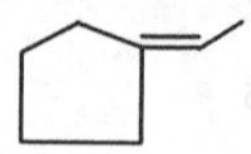

28. The compound which can decolourise Br_2/H_2O solution is/are -

(a) $CH_3—CH_2—CH_3$ (b) C_6H_6

(c) $CH_3—CH=CH_2$ (d) Both (a) & (b)

29. Benzyl chloride can be prepared from toluene by chlorination with

(a) SO_2Cl_2 (b) Cl_2/hv

(c) $SOCl_2$ (d) Both (a) & (b)

30. Consider the following reactions

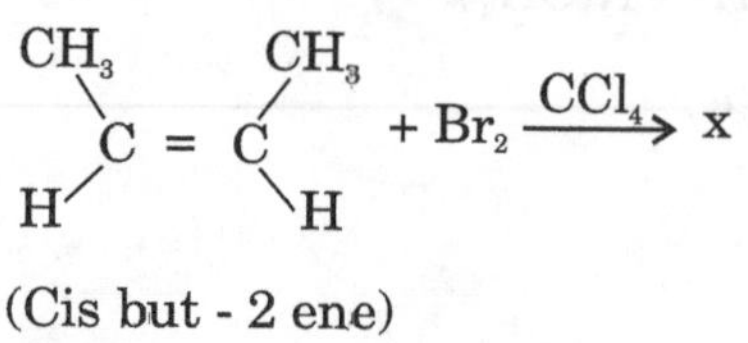

(Cis but - 2 ene)

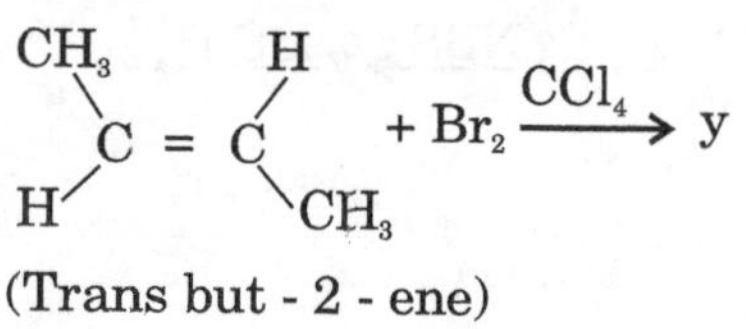

(Trans but - 2 - ene)

x & y in the above reaction are

(a) 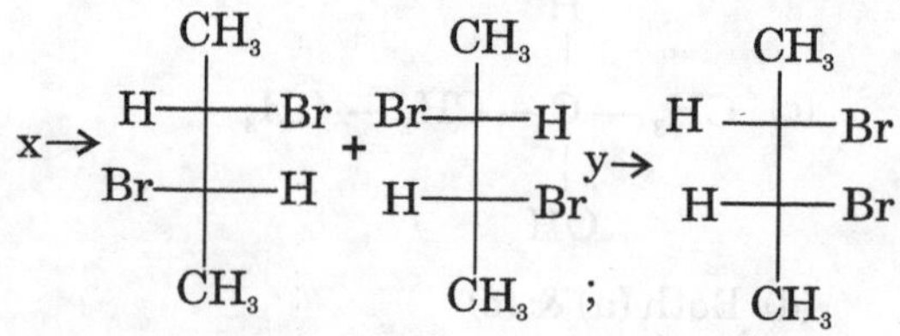

(b) 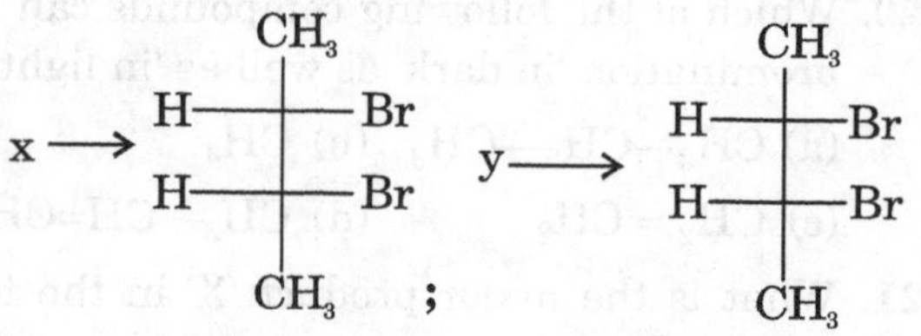

(c) 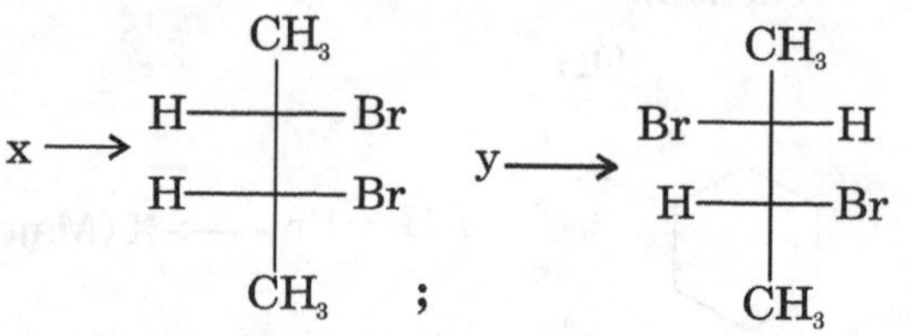

(d) None of these

31. The major product formed in the reaction given below is

$CH_3—CH_2—CH=CH_2 + HBr \rightarrow$

(a) 1-Bromobutane

(b) 2-Bromo-2-methyl propane

(c) (+)-2-Bromobutane only

(d) (±)-2-Bromobutane

32. Consider the following reaction-

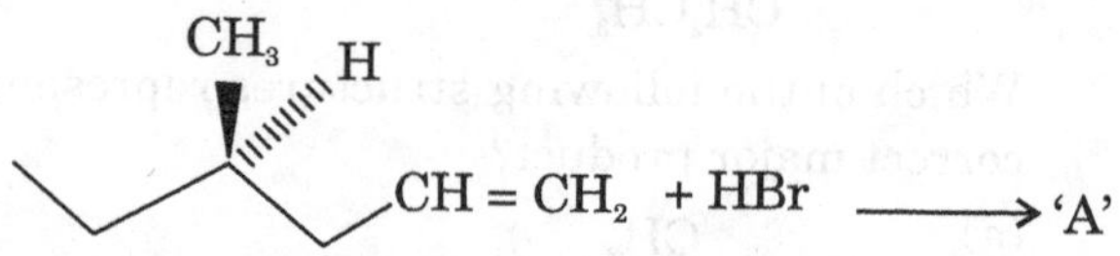

The final (major) product 'A' obtained is

(a) Racemic mixture

(b) Pure enantiomer

(c) Diastereomeric mixture

(d) None of these

33. Which of the following is the correct method for preparation of methyl fluoride?

(a) $CH_4 + HF \rightarrow$ (b) $CH_3Br + AgF$

(c) $CH_4 + F_2 \rightarrow$ (d) $CH_3OH + NaF \rightarrow$

34. How many different monochlorinated products (including stereoisomers) are formed in the following reaction?

$CH_3—CH_2—CH_2—CH_3 + Cl_2 \xrightarrow{hv}$

(a) 2 (b) 3

(c) 4 (d) 1

35. The % age yield of 2-chlorobutane in the following reaction is

$CH_3-CH_2-CH_2-CH_3 + Cl_2 \xrightarrow{hv}$

(a) 23% (b) 75.83%

(c) 92% (d) 71.69%

36. Which of the following is correct about FINKELSTEIN'S REACTION?

$CH_3-CH_2-Br + NaI \xrightarrow{Acetone} CH_3-CH_2I + NaBr$

(a) It is also called halide exchange method.

(b) It occurs via SN2 mechanism.

(c) NaCl or NaBr being less soluble than NaI in acetone gets deposited during course of reaction & hence according to Le-chatelier's principle, the equilibrium shifts forward.

(d) All are correct

37. Which of the following statement is/are true about the reaction below?

$CH_3CH_2COOAg + Br_2 \xrightarrow{CCl_4} CH_3-CH_2-Br + CO_2 + AgBr$

(1) It is called Borodine Hunsdiecker's reaction.

(2) The reaction follows free radical mechanism.

(3) The yield of alkyl halide follows the order :

Primary halide > 2° halide > 3° halide

(4) Acyl hypobromite is formed during the reaction.

(a) Only option 1 is correct.

(b) Only options 1, 2 & 3 are correct but 4 is wrong.

(c) Only option 4 is correct.

(d) All options are correct.

38. Iodination of alkanes is generally carried out in the presence of-

(a) Conc. HNO_3 (b) HIO_3

(c) HgO (d) All of these

39. Direct fluorination of hydrocarbons with pure F_2 gas occurs explosively because-

(a) of low bond dissociation energy of F_2 molecule

(b) of high bond dissociation energy of F_2 molecule

(c) of strongly exothermic nature of one of the termination steps ($R° + F° \rightarrow RF$)

(d) Both (a) & (c) are correct

40. Consider the following reaction-

$CH_3CH_2OH + KI + H_3PO_4 \xrightarrow{\Delta} CH_3-CH_2-I + KH_2PO_4 + H_2O$

Rather than using H_3PO_4 if we use H_2SO_4, then

(a) yield of the product is enhanced

(b) H_2SO_4 accelerates the rate of reaction to give alkyl iodide in maximum amount.

(c) H_2SO_4 is an oxidising agent & oxidises HI to HIO_3.

(d) H_2SO_4 is an oxidising agent & oxidises HI to I_2 & thus prevents the reaction between an alcohol & HI to form alkyl iodide.

41. 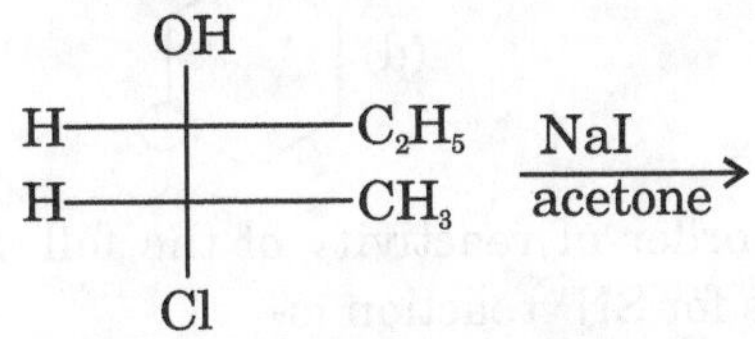

In the above reaction, the product is-

(1) 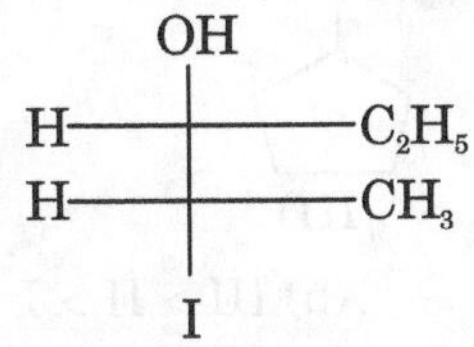

(2) 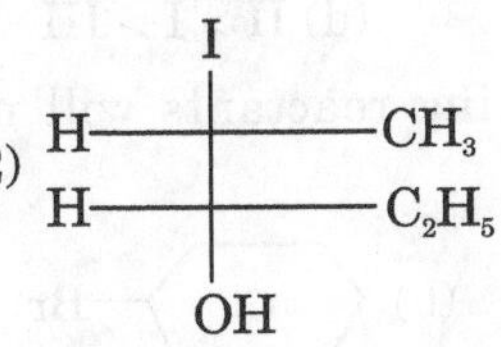

(3) 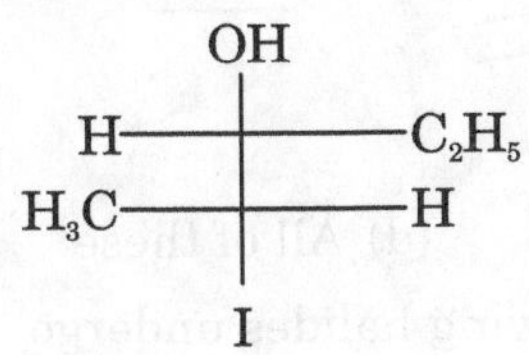

(4) 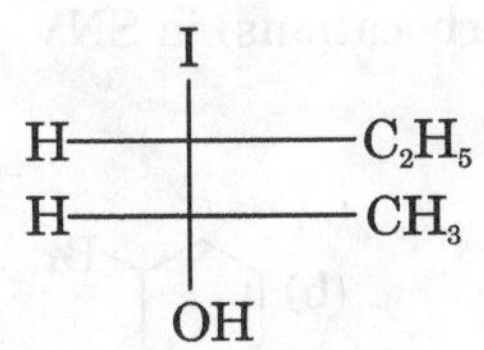

SN¹ & SN²

42. What is not true for SN² reactions?

(1) It is concerted mechanism.

(2) Rate of reaction increases as the concentration of nucleophile increases.

(3) Its rate is independent of concentration of R—X.

(4) In SN² reaction, the hybrid state of C (bearing the leaving group) changes from sp^3 to sp^2 & then returns back to sp^3 in the product.

43. Which one of the following compounds will be most reactive for SN^1 reaction?

(a) 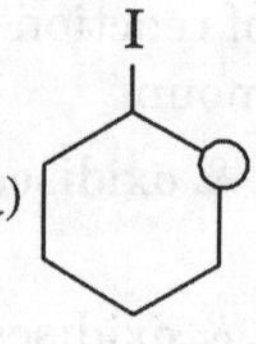 (b) 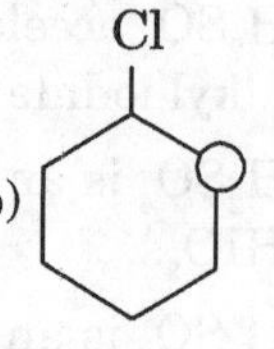

(c) 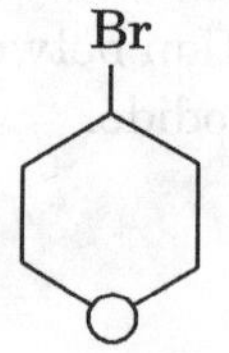 (d) 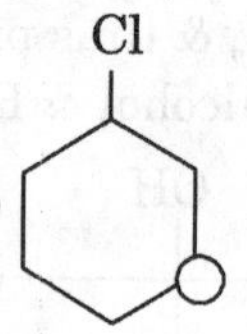

44. The correct order of reactivity of the following alkyl halides for SN^1 reaction is-

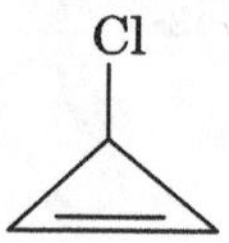
(I)

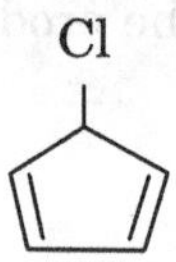
(II)

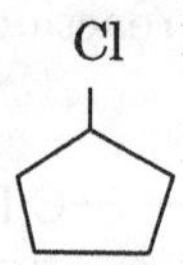
(III)

(a) I > II > III (b) III > II > I

(c) I > III > II (d) II > I > III

45. Which of the following reactants will neither favour SN^1 nor SN^2?

(a) 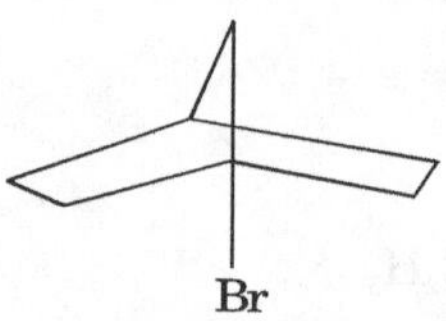 (b) 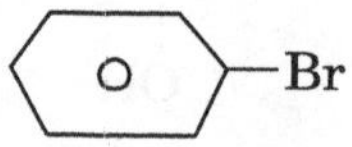

(c) $CH_2 = CH—Br$ (d) All of these

46. Which of the following halides undergo rearrangment (in carbocations) in SN^1 reaction?

(a) $CH_3—C(CH_3)_2—CH_2Br$ (b) 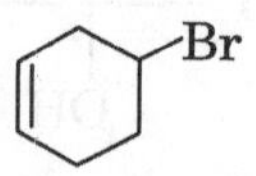

(c) 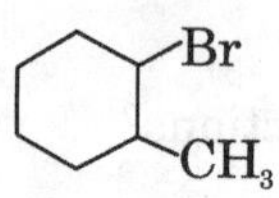 (d) All of these

47. 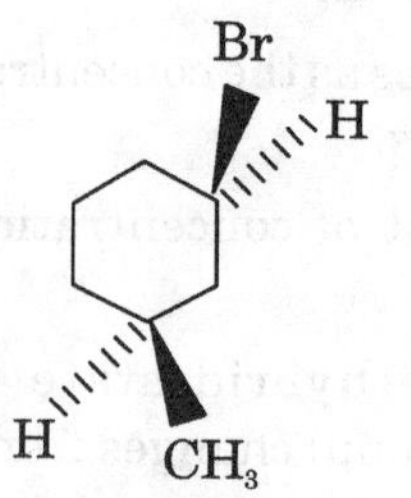 + KOH (aq) $\xrightarrow{SN^2}$ A

(1R, 3S) Cis 1-Bromo-3-Methyl Cyclohexane

The product 'A' formed in the above reaction is-

(a) (1S, 3S) - Trans -3- methyl cyclohexanol

(b) (1R, 3R) - Trans -3- methyl cyclohexanol

(c) (1S, 3R) - Cis -3- methyl cyclohexanol

(d) None of these

48. Identify the mismatch

(a) $CH_3Br + \bar{O}H \rightarrow CH_3OH + Br^-; SN^2$

(b) $(CH_3)_2CHBr + H_2O \rightarrow (CH_3)_2CHOH + HBr; SN^1$

(c) $(CH_3)_2CHBr + \bar{O}H \rightarrow (CH_3)OH + Br^-, SN^2$

(d) $(CH_3)_3CBr + \bar{O}H \rightarrow (CH_3)_3COH + Br^-; SN^2$

49. The correct order of reactivity of different bromide via SN^2 mechanism is-

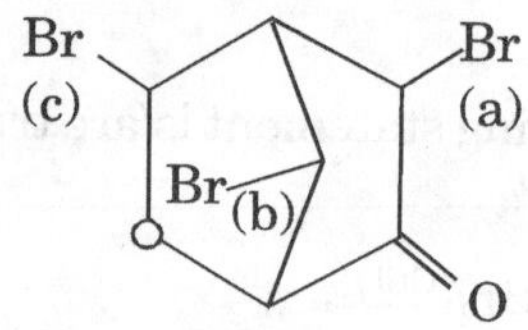

(a) a>b>c (b) b>a>c

(c) c>b>a (d) a>c>b

50. Which one of the halide is most reactive for SN^2 reaction?

(a) $CH_2 = CH - CH_2 - Cl$

(b) $C_6H_5 - CH_2 - Cl$

(c) $CH_3 - C(=O) - CH_2Cl$

(d) $CH_3 - O - CH_2Cl$

51. Which of the following molecules is maximum reactive towards S_N'?

(a) $CH_3 - C(CH_3)_2 - Cl$

(b) $CH_3 - C(=O) - CH_2 - Cl$

(c) $CH_3 - O - CH_2 - Br$

(d) $CH_3 - C(CH_3)_2 - Br$

52. 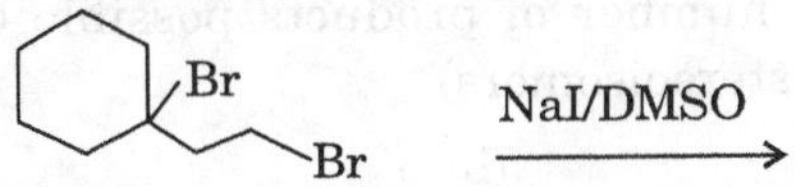

(a) 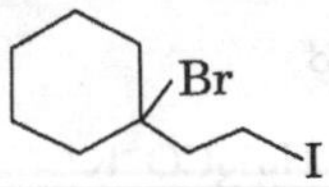 (b) 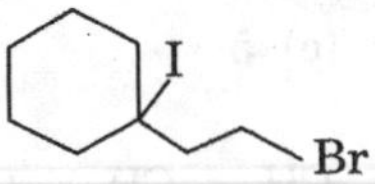

(c) 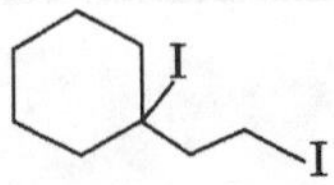 (d) None of these

53. Select the INCORRECT

(a) 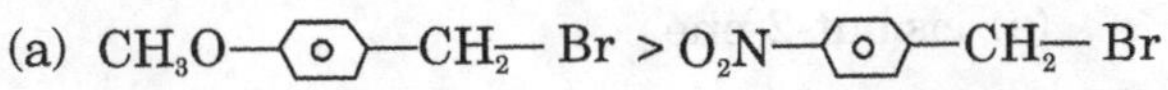
(reactivity towards SN[1])

(b) 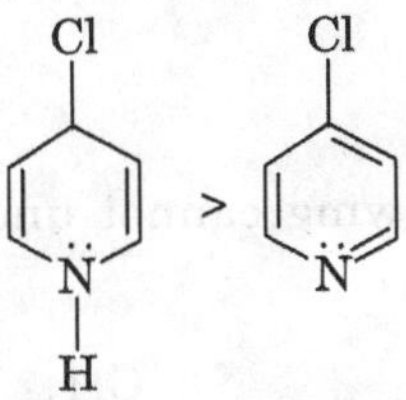 (reactivity towards SN[1])

(c) 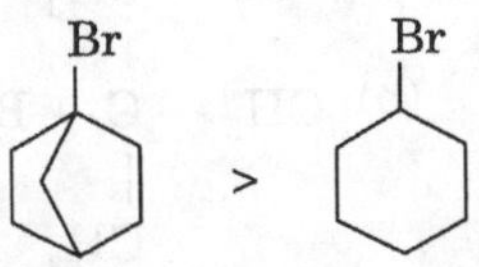 (reactivity towards SN[1])

(d) $CH_2 = CH—CH_2—Cl > CH_2 = CH—Cl$
(Reactivity towards SN[2])

54. In which of the following reactions will racenisation occur?

(a) 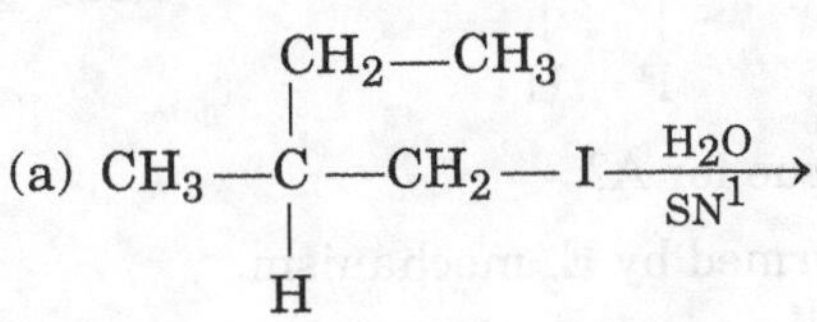

(b) 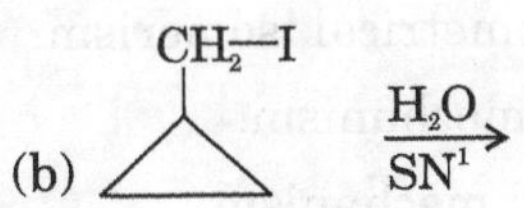

(c) 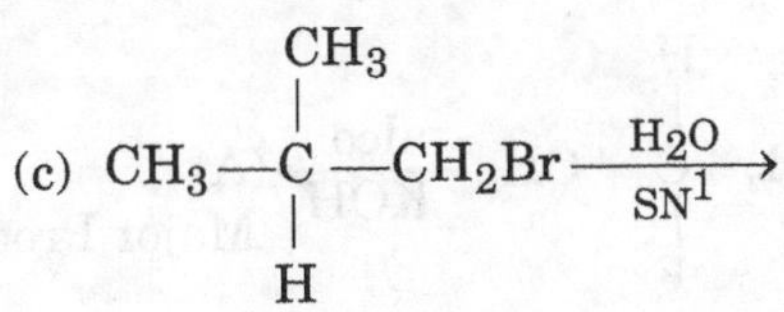

(d) 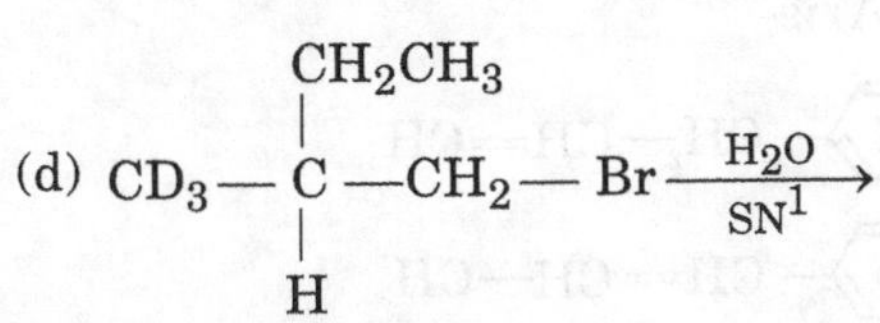

55. Which of the following statement is NOT CORRECT for S_N1?

(a) It generally involves partial racemisation.

(b) It is favoured by polar protic solvents.

(c) Carbocation is the reaction intermediate.

(d) None of the above

56. Select the correct match:

Column A (Substrate)	Column B (Mechanism followed)
(1) Benzyl & allyl Chloride	(a) Only SN[1]
(2) $R—\overset{O}{\overset{\|\|}{C}}—CH_2Cl$	(b) Only SN[2]
(3) $CH_3—O—CH_2Cl$	(c) Both SN[1] & SN[2]
(4) 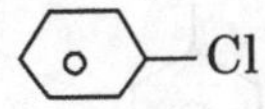	(d) Neither SN[1] nor SN[2]

(a) 1-c; 2-b; 3-c; 4-d (b) 1-d; 2-a; 3-c; 4-b

(c) 1-c; 2-c, 3-d, 4-a (d) 1-d, 2-b, 3-b, 4-a

57. 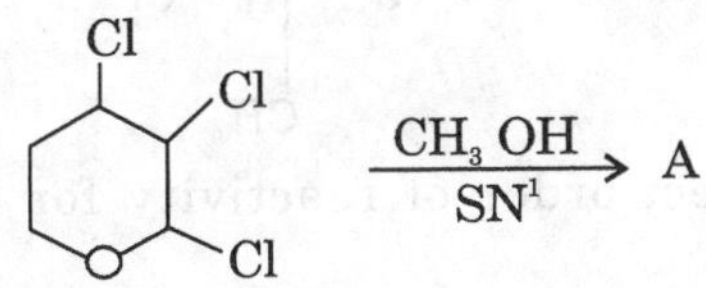

The major product 'A' in the above reaction is-

(a) 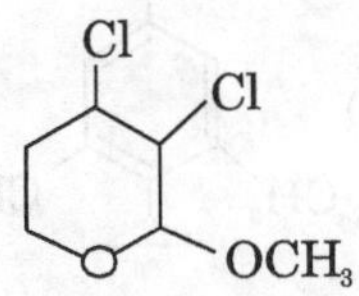 (b) 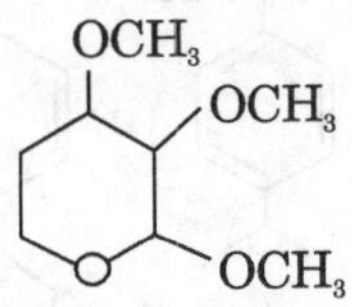

(c) 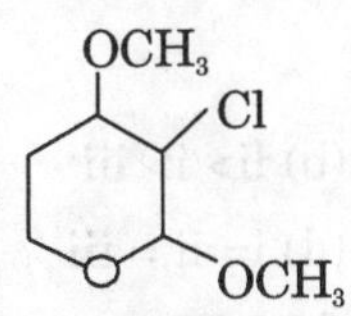 (d) None of these

58. Consider the following reaction-

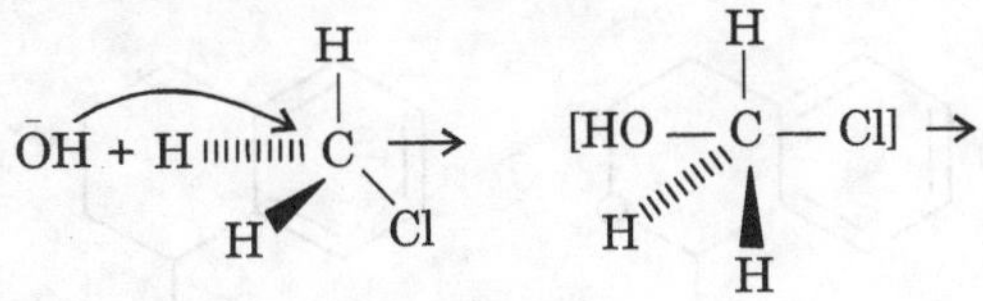

(A) (B)

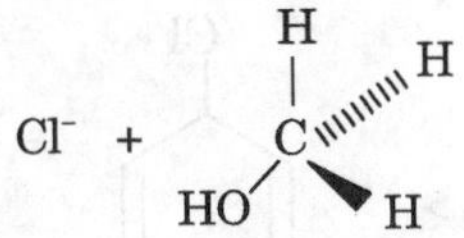

(C)

which of the following statement is correct?

(a) In the Transition state labelled 'B', the attacking Nucleophile, Carbon atom bearing the leaving group & the leaving group are collinear.

(b) The hybrid state of Carbon in 'A' is sp^3, in 'B' is sp^2.

(c) The reaction is favored by polar aprotic solvents.

(d) All are correct.

59. Under identified conditions, SN^1 in which of the following will lead to maximum racemisation?

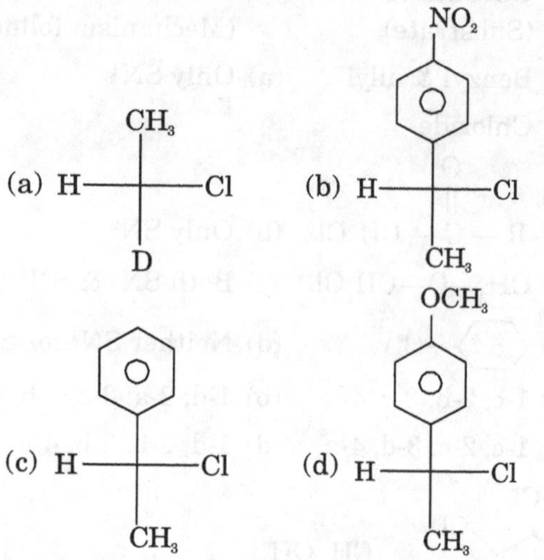

60. Identify correct order of reactivity for SN^1 reaction-

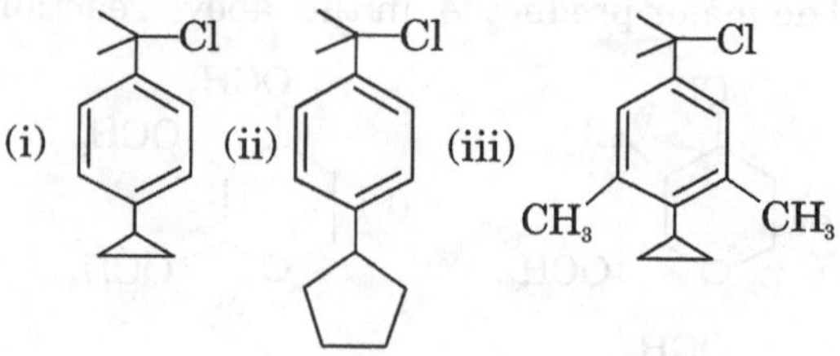

(a) i> iii> ii (b) ii> i> iii

(c) i> ii> iii (d) i= ii = iii

61. Select the INCORRECT ORDER towards SN^1 Reactivity-

(a) 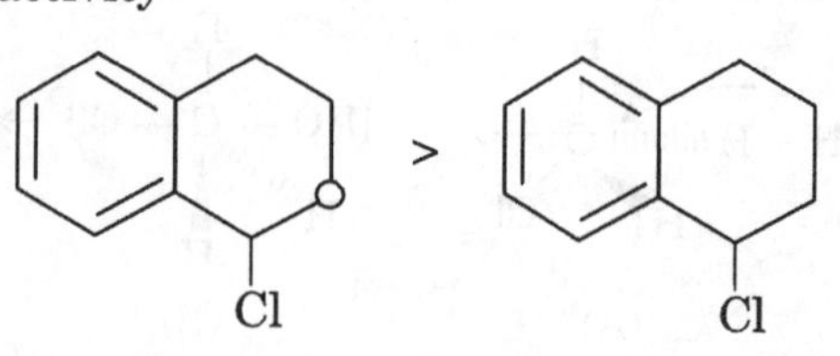

(b) 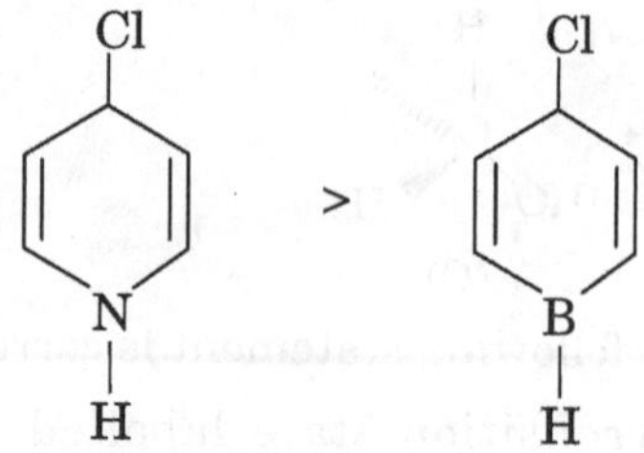

(c) 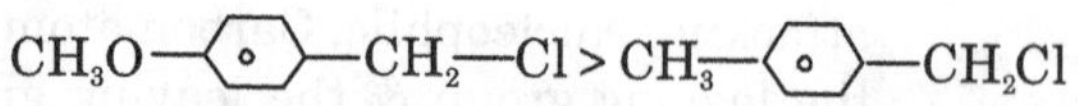

(d) None of these is incorrect

62. $CH_3-CH_2-C(CH_3)(Cl)-CH_2-CH_2-CH_3 \xrightarrow[KOH]{alc.}$ 'A'

(E_2 elimination)

Find total number of products possible (A) - (including stereoisomers)

(a) 4 (b) 6

(c) 5 (d) 3

63. $CH_3-CH_2-CH(Cl)-CH_3 \xrightarrow{(CH_3)_3CO^-K^+}$ A(major)

What is A?

(a) cis but-2-ene

(b) Trans But-2-ene

(c) But-1-ene

(d) Butane

64. Which one of the following cannot undergo E_2 elimination reaction?

(a) CH_3-CH_2-Br (b) $CH_3-C(CH_3)_2-Br$

(c) $(CH_3)_3CCH_2Br$ (d) CH_3-CH_2-Cl

65. $CH_3-CH_2-C(H)(F)-C(H)(H)-H \xrightarrow{RO^\ominus}$ A (major) + B (minor)

What is true for A?

(a) It is formed by E_2 mechanism.

(b) It can't exhibit geometrical isomerism.

(c) It is formed by E_1 mechanism.

(d) It is formed by SN^1 mechanism.

66. 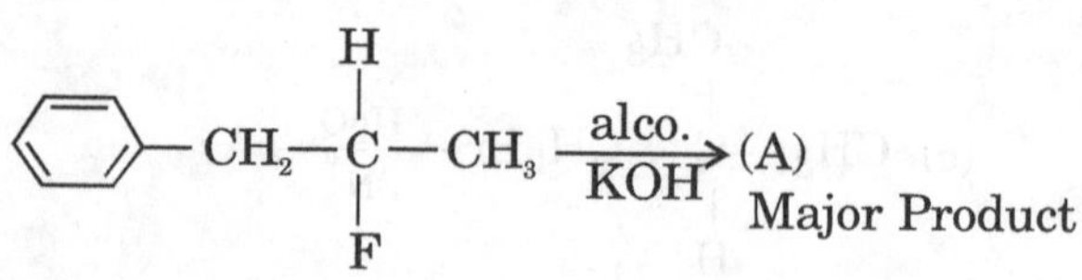

Then, (A) is-

(a) 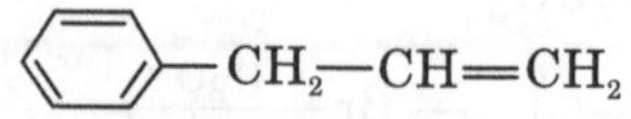

(b) 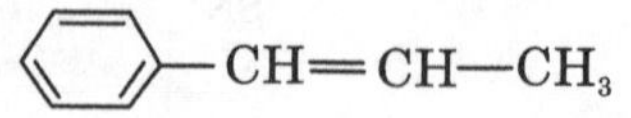

(c) 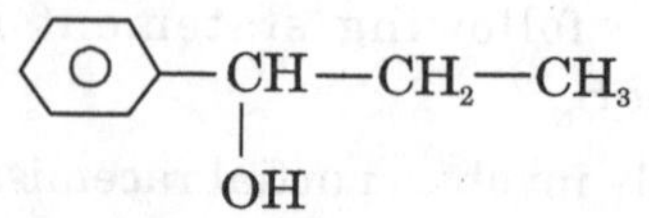

(d) 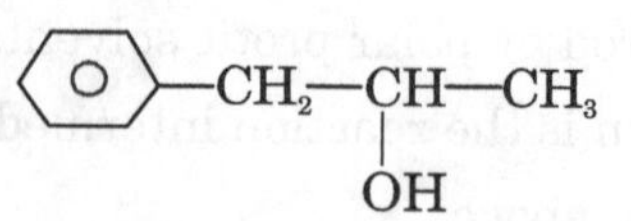

67. Select the correct order of reactivity.

(a) 3° halide > 2° halide > 1° halide (reactivity to wards E_1 reaction)

(b) 3° halide > 2° halide > 1° halide (reactivity to wards E_2 reaction)

(c) 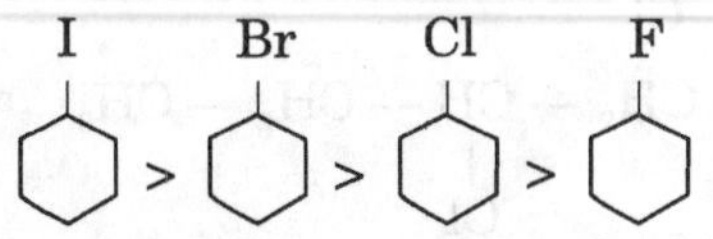 (reactivity towards E_2)

(d) All orders are correct.

68. The major products 'x' in the following reaction is-

$$CH_3-\overset{\displaystyle CH_3}{\underset{\displaystyle CH_3}{\overset{|}{\underset{|}{C}}}}-CH_2-Br\xrightarrow{E_1}'x'$$

(a) $CH_3-\overset{\displaystyle CH_3}{\overset{|}{C}}=CH-CH_3$

(b) $CH_3-\overset{\displaystyle CH_3}{\underset{\displaystyle CH_3}{\overset{|}{\underset{|}{C}}}}=CH_2$

(c) 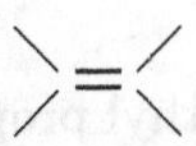

(d) Both (b) & (c)

69. The correct order of reactivity of following molecules towards E_2 reaction is-

(1) 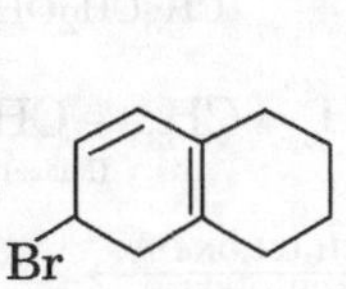 (2) 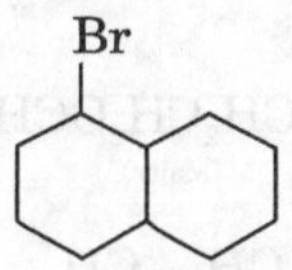 (3) 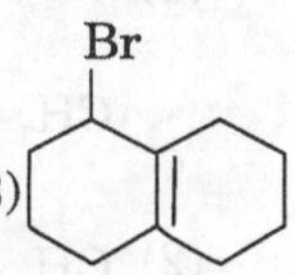

(a) 1 > 3 > 2 (b) 1 > 2 > 3

(c) 3 > 2 > 1 (d) None of these

70. Identify the correct reactivity order towards E_2 with alc. KOH.

(1) 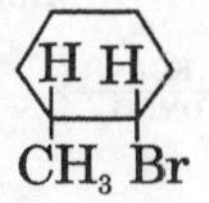 (2) 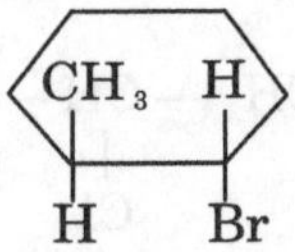

(3) 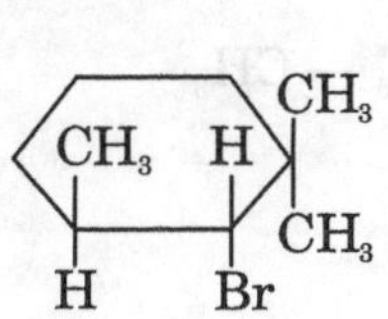

(a) 1 > 2 > 3 (b) 2 > 1 > 3

(c) 3 > 1 > 2 (d) 3 = 1 > 2

71. Which of the following order is/are Correct for the rate of E_2 reaction with alc. KOH?

(a) 2-Bromo-1-phenylbutane > 3-Bromo-1-phenylbutane

(b) 3-Bromocyclohexene > Bromocyclohexene

(c) 3-Bromo-2-methyl pentane > 2 Bromo – 4 – methylpentane

(d) All are correct

72. Select the correct reaction(s)-

(1) $CH_3-CH_2-\underset{\displaystyle F}{\underset{|}{CH}}-CH_3+CH_3O^{\ominus}$

$\rightarrow \underset{(Major)}{CH_3-CH_2-CH=CH_2}$

$+\underset{(Minor)}{CH_3-CH=CH-CH_3}$

(2) $CH_3-\overset{\displaystyle CH_3}{\underset{\displaystyle Br}{\overset{|}{\underset{|}{C}}}}-CH_2-CH_3+CH_3-\overset{\displaystyle CH_3}{\underset{\displaystyle CH_3}{\overset{|}{\underset{|}{C}}}}-O^{\ominus}$ (Bulky base)

$\rightarrow CH_2=\underset{\displaystyle CH_3}{\underset{|}{C}}-CH_2-CH_3$ (Major)

$+CH_3-\underset{(Minor)}{CH}=CH-CH_3$

(3) $CH_3-\overset{\displaystyle CH_3}{\underset{\displaystyle CH_3}{\overset{|}{\underset{|}{C}}}}-CH_2-\overset{\displaystyle CH_3}{\underset{\displaystyle Br}{\overset{|}{\underset{|}{C}}}}-CH_3+C_2H_5O^{\ominus}$

$\rightarrow CH_3-\overset{\displaystyle CH_3}{\underset{\displaystyle CH_3}{\overset{|}{\underset{|}{C}}}}-CH=\underset{\displaystyle Br}{\underset{|}{C}}-CH_3$ (Minor)

$+CH_3-\overset{\displaystyle CH_3}{\underset{\displaystyle CH_3}{\overset{|}{\underset{|}{C}}}}-CH_2-\underset{\displaystyle CH_3}{\underset{|}{C}}=CH_2$ (Major)

(4)

$$CH_2=CH-CH_2-\underset{\displaystyle Br}{\underset{|}{CH}}-\overset{\displaystyle CH_3}{\overset{|}{CH}}-CH_3+CH_3O^{\ominus}$$

$$\rightarrow \underset{(Major)}{CH_2=CH-CH=CH-\overset{\displaystyle CH_3}{\overset{|}{\underset{\displaystyle CH_3}{\underset{|}{CH}}}}}$$

$$+\underset{(Minor)}{CH_2=CH-CH_2-CH=\overset{\displaystyle CH_3}{\overset{|}{\underset{\displaystyle CH_3}{\underset{|}{C}}}}}$$

(a) Only 1 is correct

(b) Only 2 & 3 is correct

(c) Only 2, 3, 4 are correct

(d) All are correct

73. Which one is more easily dehydrohalogenated?

(a) 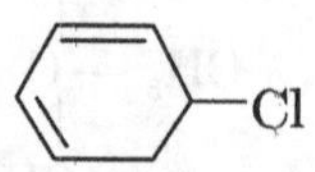 (b) 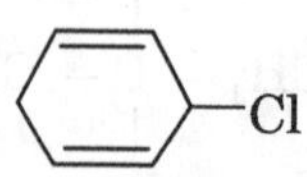

(c) 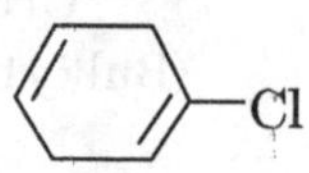 (d) All with same ease

74. Match the following-

Column I

(a) $CH_3-CHBr-CD_3$ on treatment with alc. KOH gives $CH_2=CH-CD_3$ as major product.

(b) $Ph-CHBr-CH_3$ reacts faster than Ph-$CHBr$-CD_3

(c) $Ph-CH_2-CH_2Br$ on $CH_3OD/CH_3O^{\ominus}$ gives treatment with $Ph-CD=CH_2$ as major product.

(d) $Ph-CH_2-CH_2Br$ & $PhCD_2CH_2Br$ react with same rate.

Column II

(P) E_1 reaction

(Q) E_2 reaction

(R) E_1 cb reaction

(S) First order reaction.

(a) A-Q; B-Q; C-R, S; D-P,S

(b) B-P; A-S; C-Q; D-Q

(c) A-Q; B-Q; C-P, R; D-S

(d) None of these

75. Which of the following will give only one alkene on dehydrohalogenation? (including all isomers)

(a) $CH_3-\underset{\displaystyle Cl}{\underset{|}{CH}}-CH_2-CH_2-CH_3$

(b) $CH_3-CH_2-\underset{\displaystyle Cl}{\underset{|}{CH}}-CH_2-CH_3$

(c) $CH_3-CH_2-CH_2-Cl$

(d) Both (a) & (b)

76. Rank the following molecules in decreasing order of reactivity towards E_2 reaction.

(1) 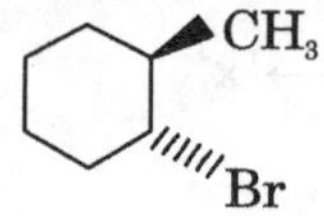 (2) 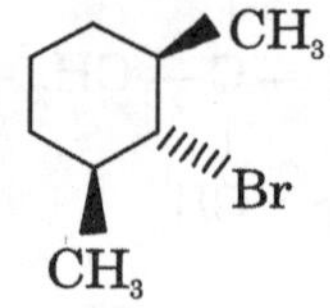

(3) 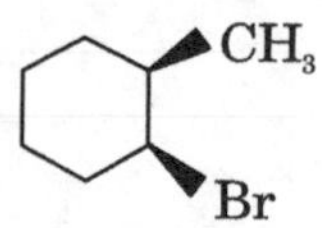

(a) 3 > 1 > 2 (b) 2 >1 > 3

(c) 1 > 2 > 3 (d) 2 > 3 > 1

Elimination V/s Substitution

77. Reaction of t-butyl bromide with Sodium methoxide produces-

(1) Isobutane (2) 2-Methyl propene

(3) t-butyl ethyl ether (4) None of these

78. Select the correct reaction (s)-

(1) $CH_3-CH_2-CH_2-Br \xrightarrow[CH_3CH_2OH,\,55°C]{CH_3CH_2ONa}$

$\underset{(Major)}{CH_3-CH_2CH_2OCH_2CH_3} + \underset{(Minor)}{CH_3-CH=CH_2}$

(2) $CH_3-\underset{\displaystyle Br}{\underset{|}{CH}}-CH_3 \xrightarrow[CH_3CH_2OH,\,55°C]{CH_3CH_2ONa}$

$\underset{(Major)}{CH_3-CH=CH_3} + \underset{(Minor)}{CH_3-\underset{\displaystyle OCH_2CH_3}{\underset{|}{CH}}-CH_3}$

(3) $CH_3-\underset{\displaystyle Cl}{\underset{|}{CH}}-(CH_2)_6CH_3 \xrightarrow[DMSO]{KCN}$

$\underset{(Major)}{CH_3-\underset{\displaystyle CN}{\underset{|}{CH}}-(CH_2)_6-CH_3}$

(4) All are correct

79. Identify the major product of the following reaction

$$CH_3-\underset{H}{\overset{CH_3}{C}}-\underset{H}{\overset{Cl}{C}}-CH_3 \xrightarrow{H_2O}$$

(a) $CH_3-\underset{H}{\overset{CH_3}{C}}-\underset{OH}{CH}-CH_3$

(b) $CH_3-\underset{CH_3}{\overset{H}{C}}-CH_2-CH_2-OH$

(c) $CH_3-\underset{OH}{\overset{CH_3}{C}}-CH_2CH_3$

(d) None of these

80. Which of the following would give a higher substitution/elimination ratio, when reacted with isopropyl bromide in ethanol?

(a) $CH_3S^{\ominus}$ (b) $CH_3O^{\ominus}$

(c) $(CH_3)_3CO^{\ominus}$ (d) $(CH_3)_3CS^{\ominus}$

81. The total number of SN^1 & E_1, products including geometrical isomers in the following reaction are

$$C_6H_5-\underset{H}{\overset{CH_3}{C}}-\underset{Br}{\overset{H}{C}}-CH_3 \xrightarrow{CH_3\ddot{O}H}$$

(a) 6 (b) 8

(c) 10 (d) 12

82. Which of the following reactions represent the major product?

(a) $CH_3-CH_2-\underset{F}{\overset{CH_3}{C}}-CH_2-CH_3 \xrightarrow[DMSO]{CH_3CH_2O^-Na^+} CH_3-CH_2-\overset{CH_2}{\overset{\|}{C}}-CH_2-CH_3$

(b) $CH_3-\underset{CH_3}{\overset{H}{C}}-\underset{H}{\overset{CH_3}{C}}-\underset{Br}{CH}-CH_3 \xrightarrow[DMF]{CH_3CH_2O^{\ominus}} CH_3-\underset{CH_3}{\overset{H}{C}}-\overset{CH_3}{C}=\overset{CH_3}{C}-H$

(c) $H_3C-\underset{CH_3}{\overset{H}{C}}-\underset{Br}{\overset{CH_3}{C}}-\underset{H}{\overset{CH_3}{C}}-CH_3 \xrightarrow[DMSO]{CH_3-\underset{CH_3}{\overset{CH_3}{C}}-O^{\ominus}} CH_3-\underset{CH_3}{\overset{H}{C}}-\overset{CH_2}{\overset{\|}{C}}-\underset{CH_3}{\overset{H}{C}}-CH_3$

(d) All of these

83. Select the incorrect reaction

(a) $CH_3-\underset{H}{\overset{CH_3}{C}}-CH_2Br \xrightarrow{CH_3CH_2\ddot{O}H} CH_3-\underset{:\ddot{O}CH_2CH_3}{\overset{CH_3}{C}}-CH_3$ (Major product)

(b) $CH_3-\underset{Cl}{\overset{CH_3}{C}}-CH_2-CH_3 + NaOH \xrightarrow[\Delta]{H_2O}$

$CH_3-\overset{CH_3}{C}=CH-CH_3$

(Major Product)

(c) $CH_3-CH_2-CH_2-Br + (C_2H_5)_3N \rightarrow$

$CH_3-CH_2-\underset{CH_2CH_3}{\overset{CH_2CH_3}{N^+}}-CH_2CH_2CH_3\ Br^-$

(Major Product)

(d) None of these is incorrect.

Aryl Halides

84. Benzochloride on reacting with Fe, Br_2 (1 equivalent) mainly gives-

(a) 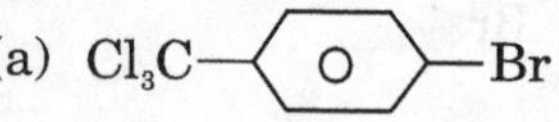

(b) 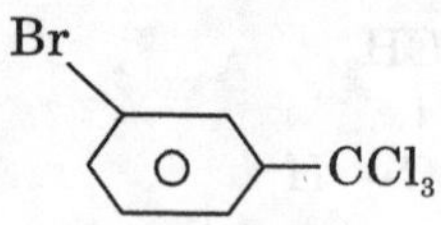

(c) 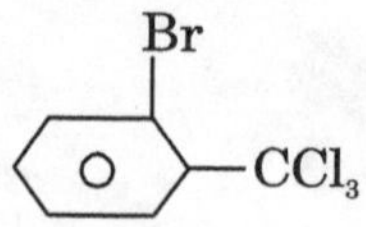

(d) Both (a) & (b)

85. 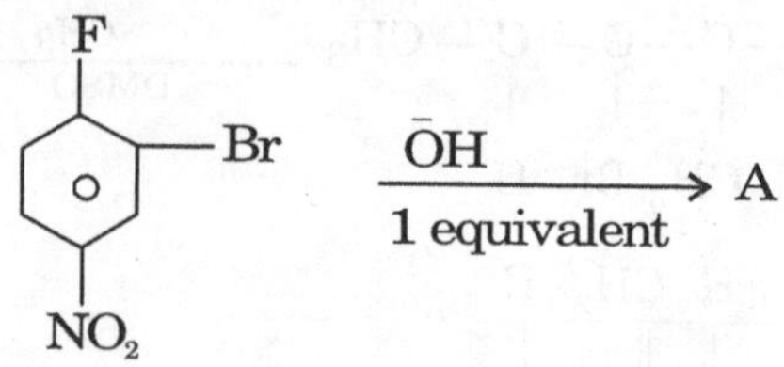

The Product 'A' is-

(a) 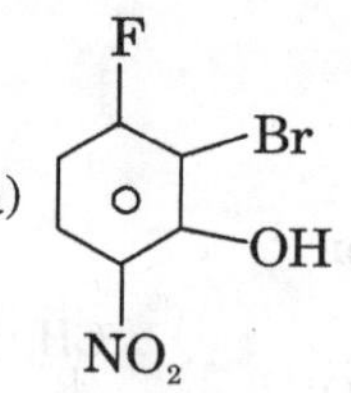

(b) 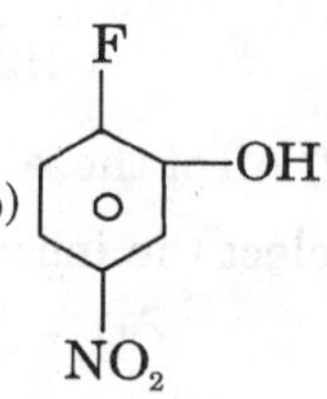

(c) 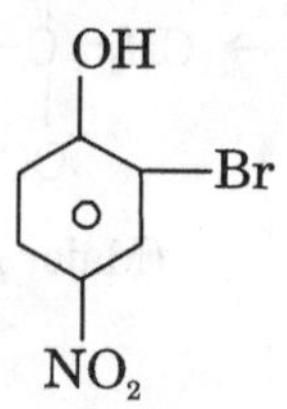

(d) 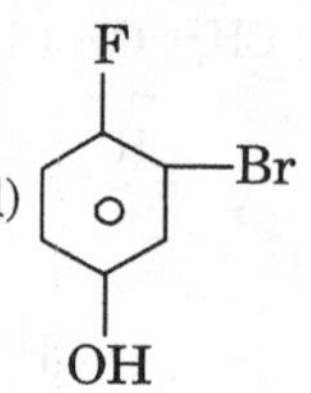

86. Consider the following reactions-

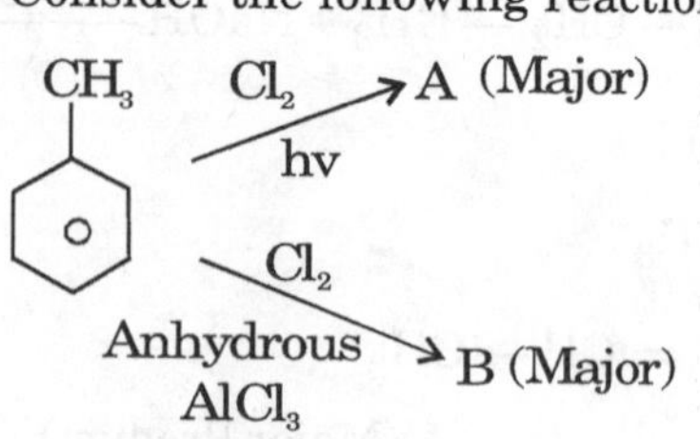

A & B, respectively are-

(a) 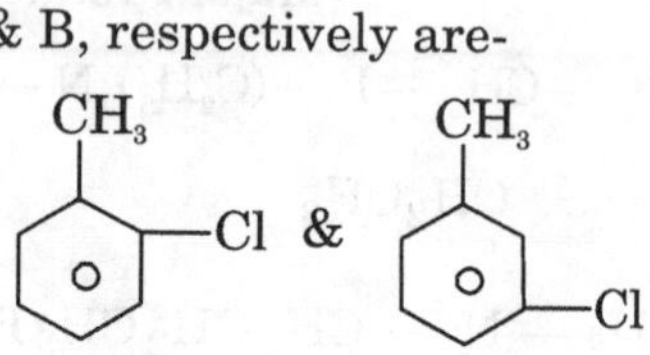

(b) 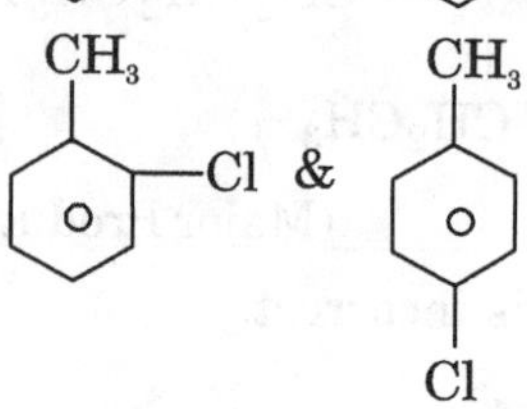

(c) 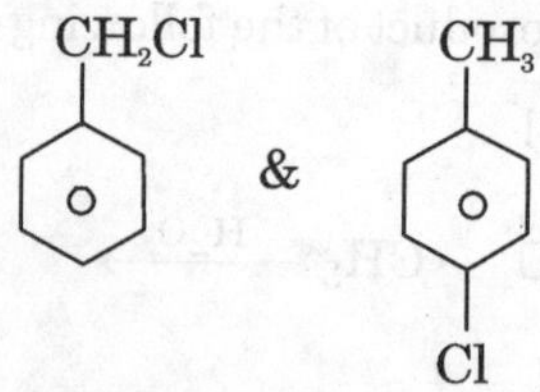

(d) 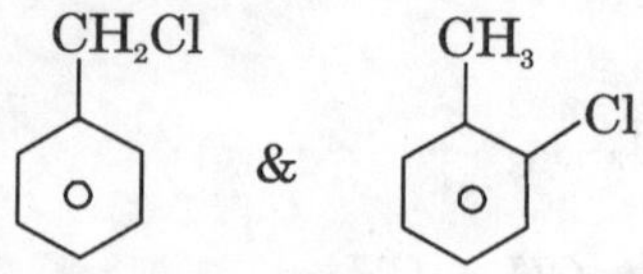

87. Which of the following will give Aryl SN[2] reaction?

(a) 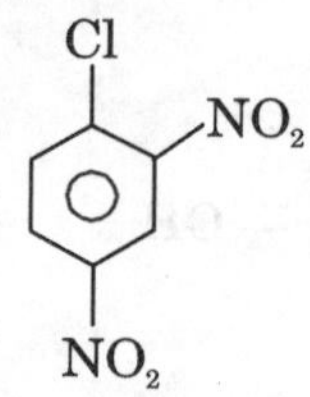

(b) 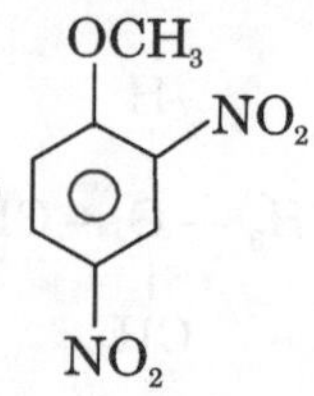

(c) 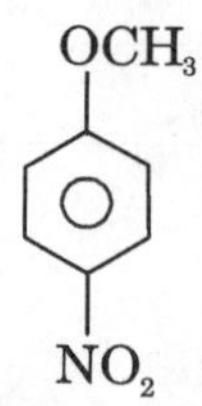

(d) All of above

88. Which of the following substrate fail to undergo elimination addition (benzyne) mechanism?

(a) 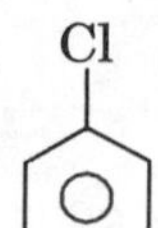

(b) 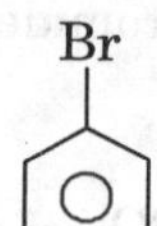

(c) 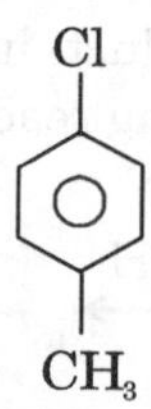

(d) 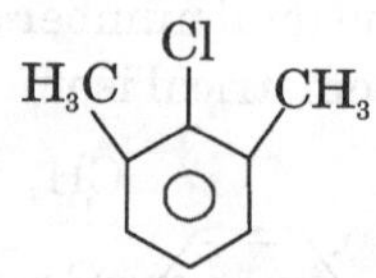

89. The major product 'X' in the following reaction is-

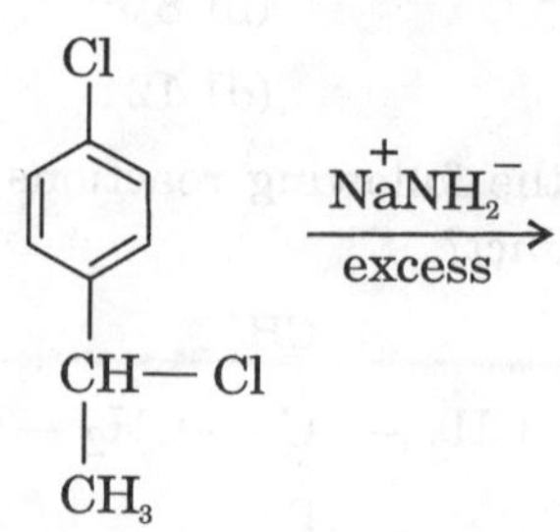

(a) 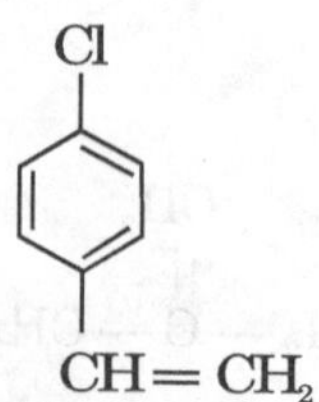

(b) 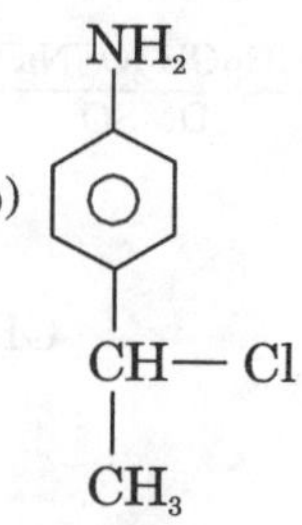

(c) 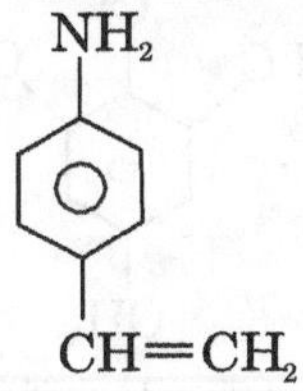

(d) Both a & b.

90. Which one of the following is least reactive for aryl SN^2 (addition - elimination)?

(a) 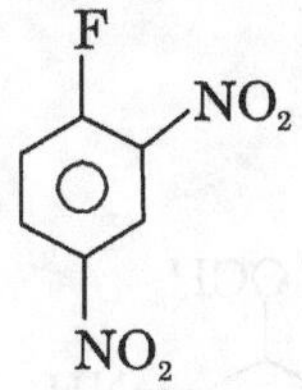

(b) 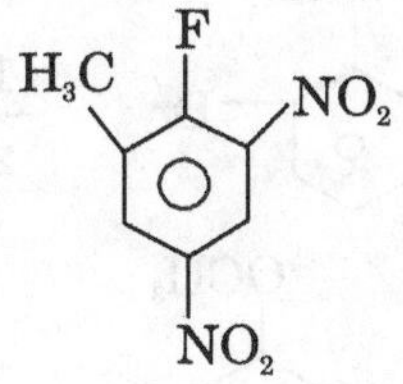

(c) 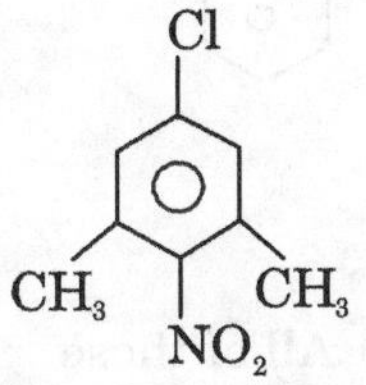

(d) 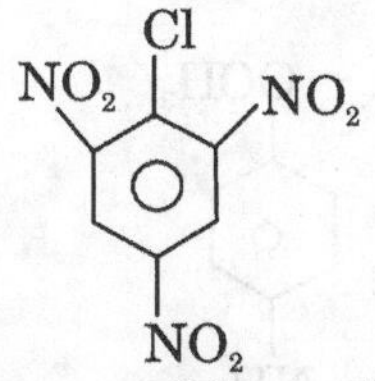

91. Which of the following are possible products of the reaction given below?

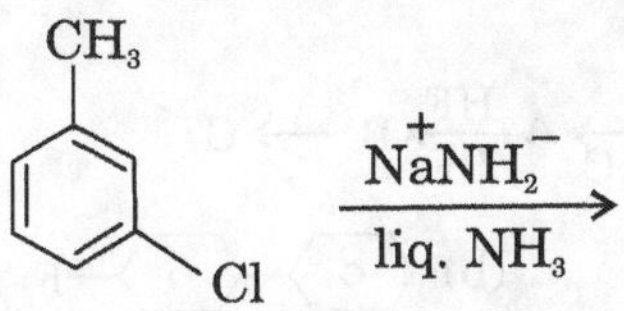

(a) 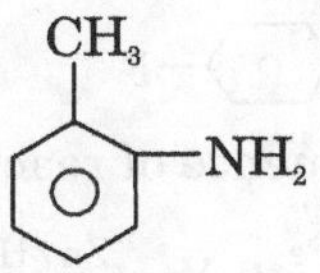

(b) 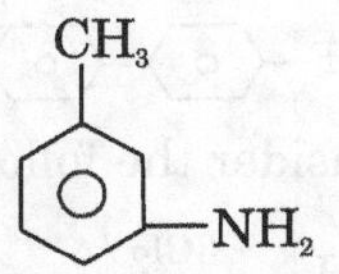

(c) 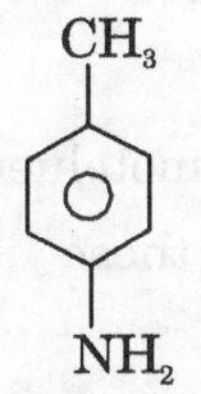

(d) All of these

92. Which of the following is most stable?

(a) 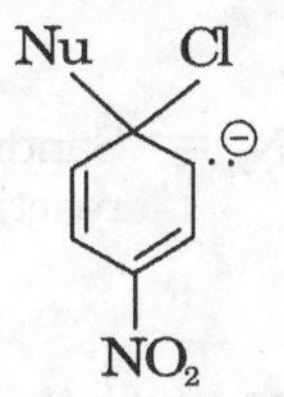

(b) 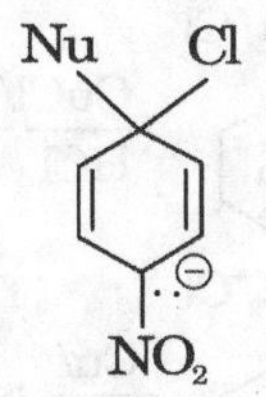

(c) 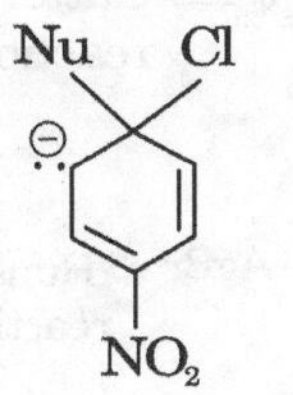

(d) 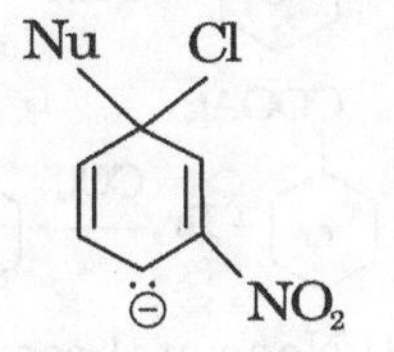

93. Consider the reaction-

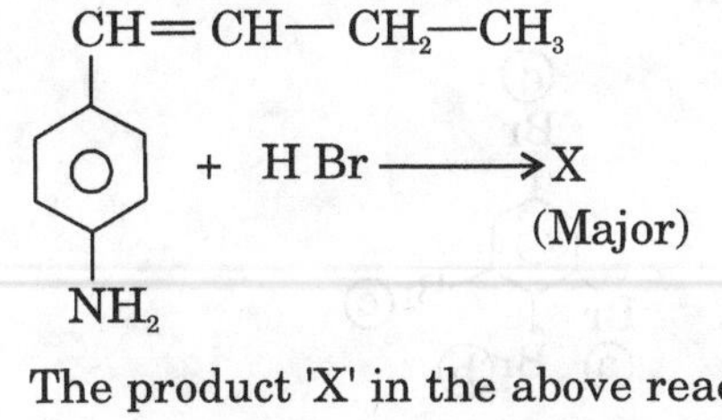

The product 'X' in the above reaction is -

(a) 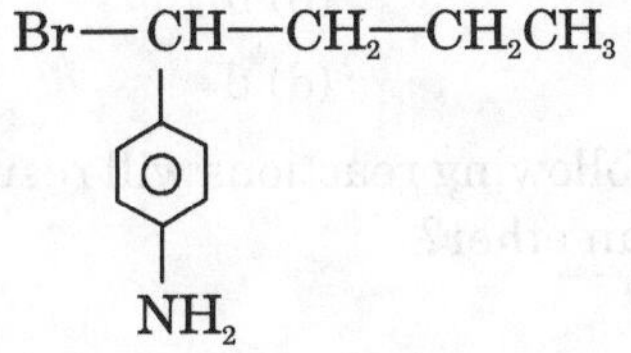

(b) 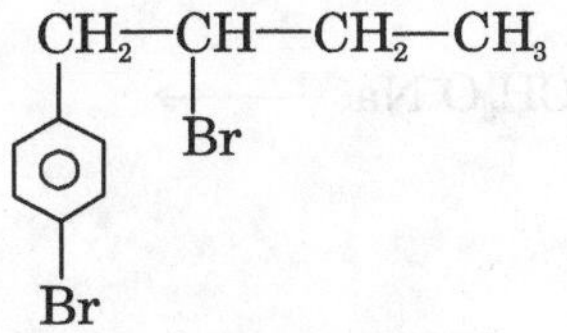

(c) 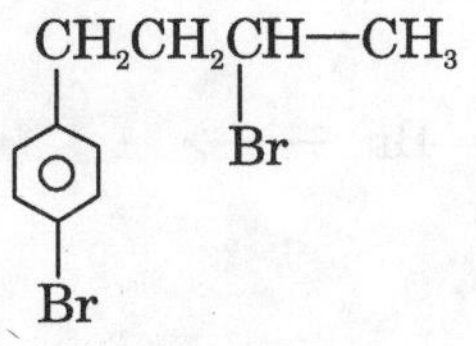

(d) 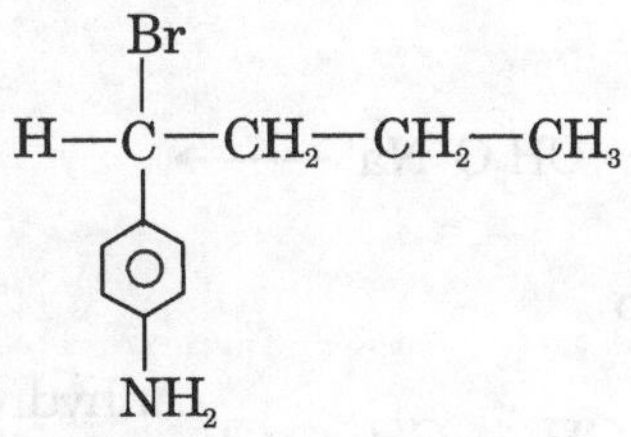

94. 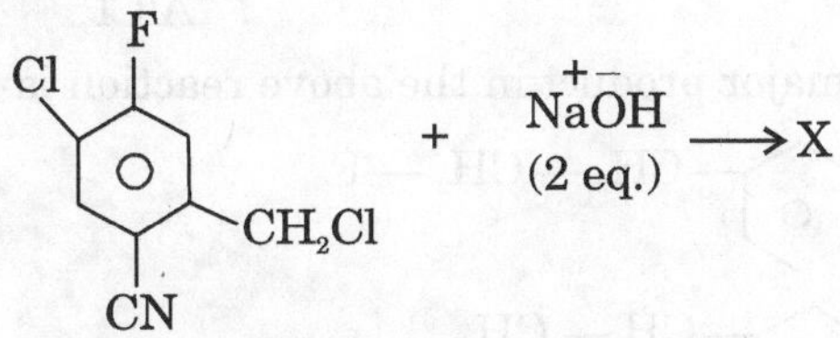

The major product 'X' in the above reaction is-

(a) 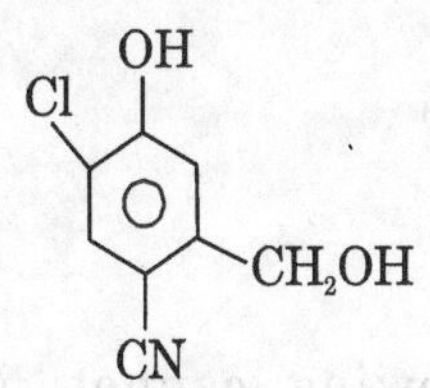

(b) 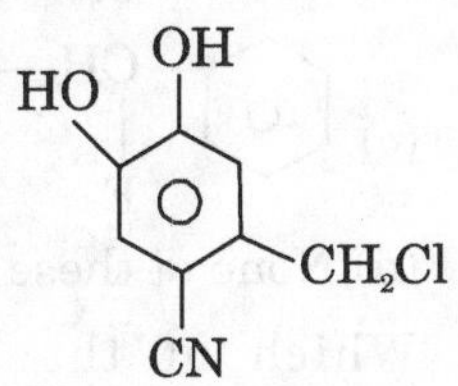

(c) 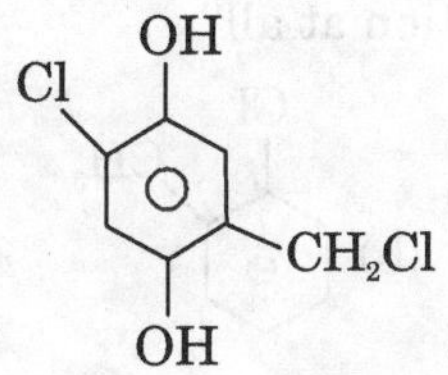

(d) None of these

95. Which halogen is substituted first in addition-elimination?

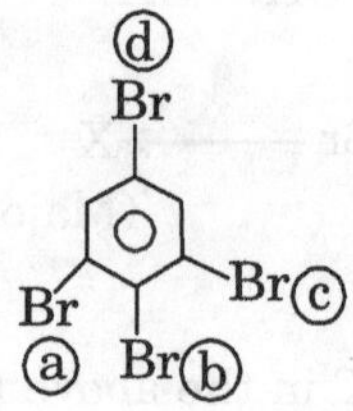

(a) a (b) b
(c) c (d) d

96. Which of the following reactions will result in the formation of an ether?

(a) 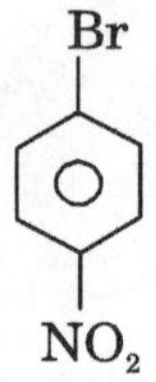 + $CH_3O^-Na^+ \longrightarrow$

(b) 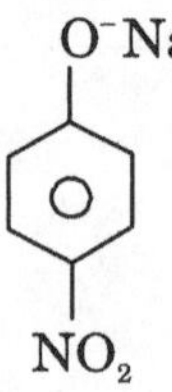 + CH_3—Br $\longrightarrow$

(c) 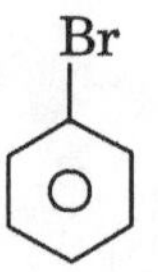 + $CH_3O^-Na^+ \longrightarrow$

(d) Both a & b

97. 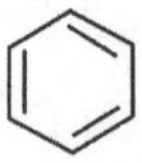 + F—CH_2—CH_2—Cl $\xrightarrow[AlCl_3]{\text{Anhydrous}}$

The major product in the above reaction is-

(a) 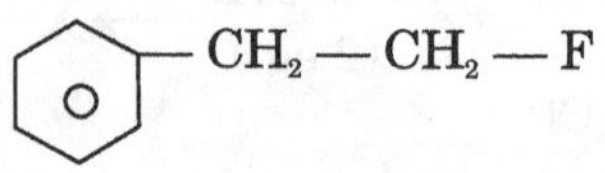

(b) 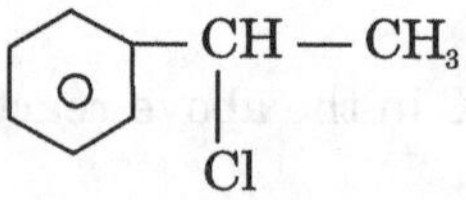

(c) 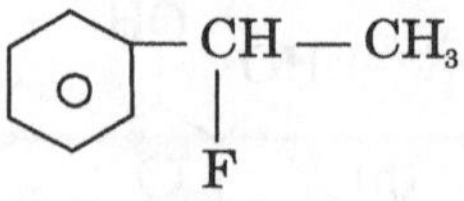

(d) None of these

98. Which of the following cannot undergo nucleophilic substitution at all?

(a) 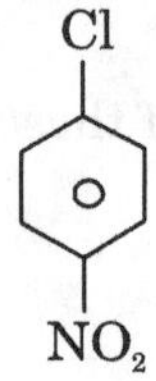 (b) 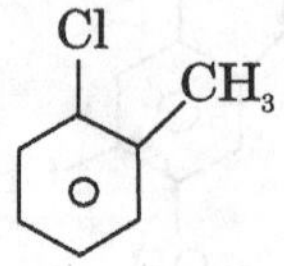

(c) 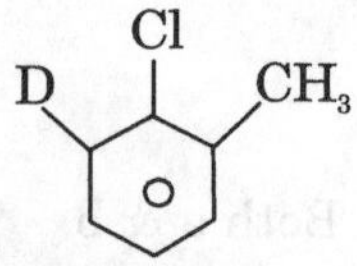 (d) 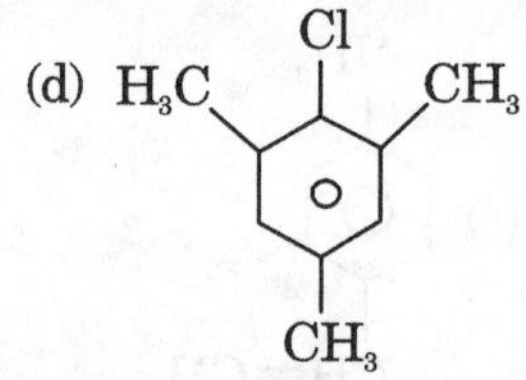

99. Identify the major product in the following reaction-

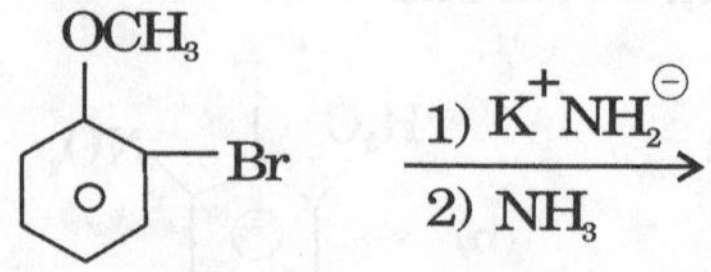

(a) 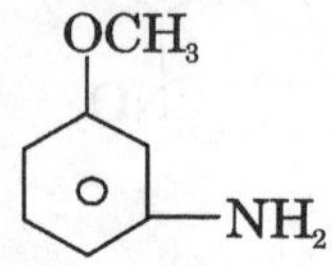 (b) 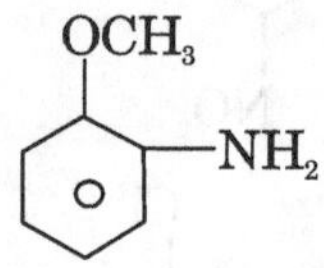

(c) 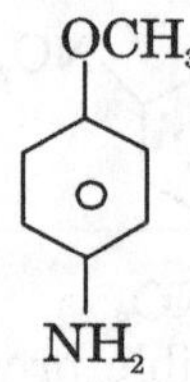 (d) All of these

100. Identify the correct product 'C' in the following reaction-

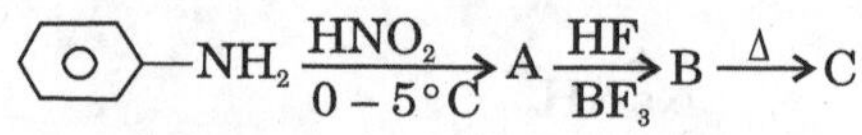

(a) 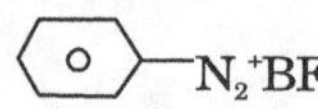 (b) 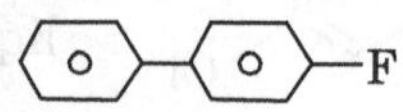

(c) 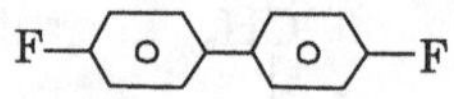 (d) 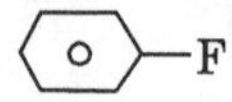

101. Consider the following sequence of reactions-

$C_7H_8 \xrightarrow{3Cl_2/\Delta} X \xrightarrow{Br_2/Fe} Y \xrightarrow{Zn/HCl} Z$

The compound Z is-

(a) m-Bromotoluene (b) o-Bromotoluene
(c) p-Bromotoluene (d) All of these

102. Identify the mismatch.

Reaction	Name
(a) 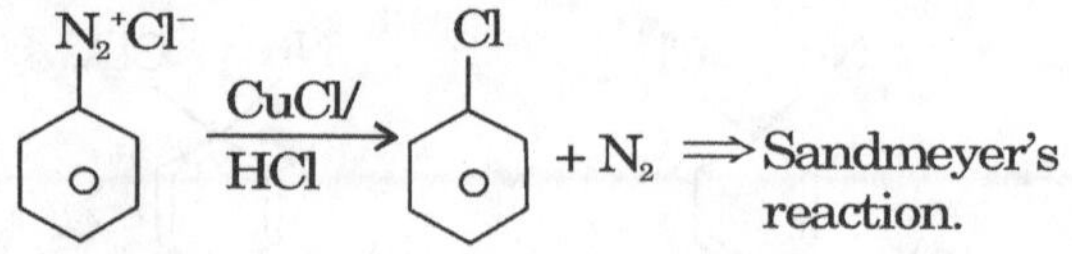	⇒ Sandmeyer's reaction.
(b) 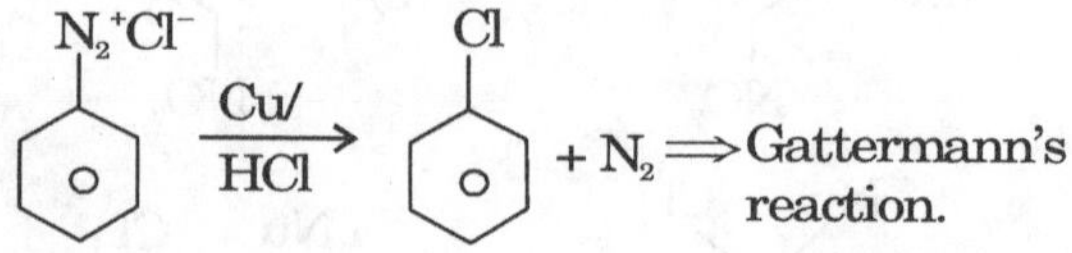	⇒ Gattermann's reaction.
(c) 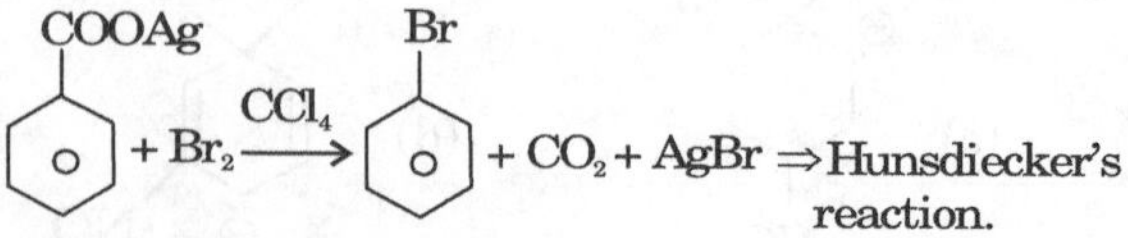	⇒ Hunsdiecker's reaction.

(d) None of these

103. 1-chloro-4-methyl benzene will undergo-
(a) electrophilic addition & nucleophilic addition
(b) electrophilic addition & nucleophilic substitution.
(c) electrophilic aromatic substitution & aromatic nucleophilic substitution
(d) Both a & b

104. The hybridisation of triple bonded 'C' in benzyne is

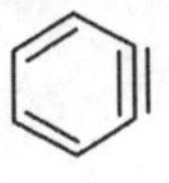

(a) sp (b) sp^2
(c) sp^3 (d) sp^3d

Brain Teasers

105. Select the correct order of leavability
(a) $R-\overset{\oplus}{N_2} > R-OSO_2C_4F_9 > R-OSO_2CF_3 > R-OTS > R-I > R-Br > R-\overset{\oplus}{OH_2}$
(b) $R-\overset{\oplus}{OH_2} > R-I > R-Br > R-OSO_2CF_3 > R-OTS > R-\overset{\oplus}{N_2}$
(c) $R-\overset{\oplus}{N_2} > R-I > R-Br > R-OSO_2CF_3 > R-\overset{\oplus}{OH_2} > R-O-SO_2C_4F_9$
(d) None of these

106. Select the correct order of reactivity towards SN^2
(a) 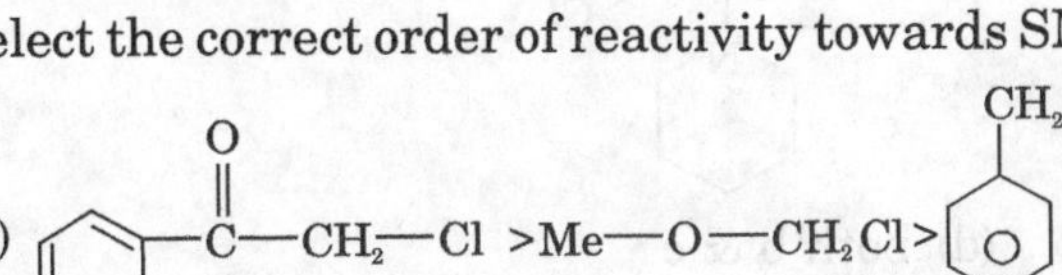
(b) 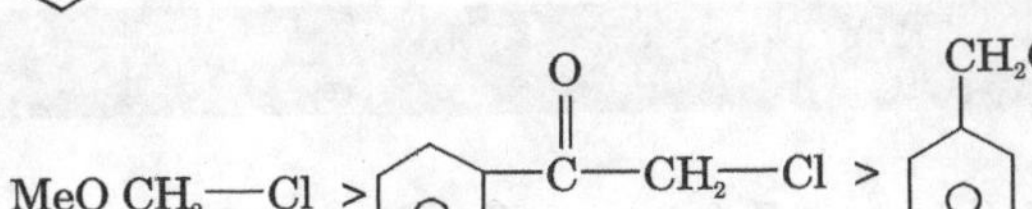
(c) 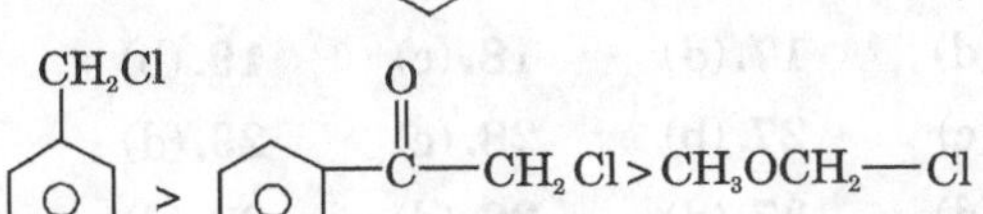
(d) 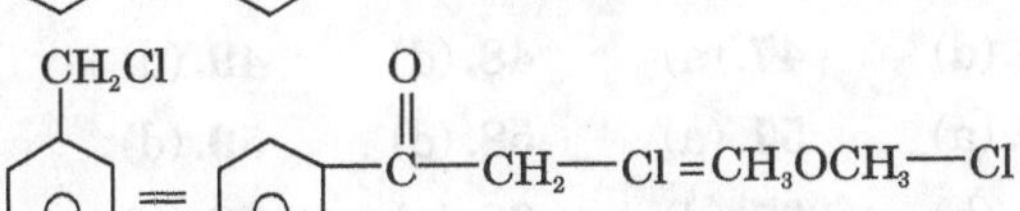

107. Following two reactions are given. Select the correct mechanisms for these reactions, respectively.

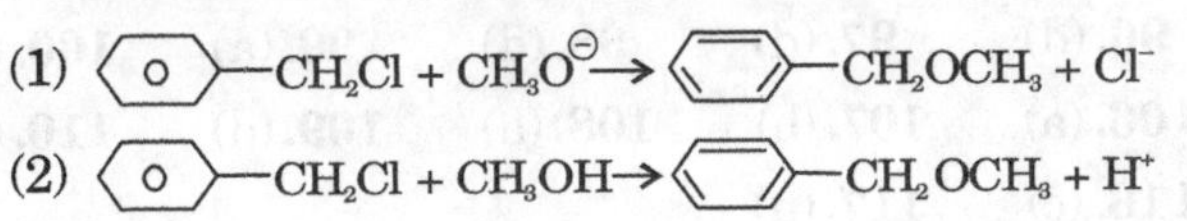

(a) SN^2, SN^2 (b) SN^2, SN^1
(c) SN^1, SN^1 (d) SN^2, E_1

108. Give the decreasing order of reactivity of alkyl halides towards SN^2-
(1) $(CH_3)_3CCH_2Br$ (2) $BrCH_2CH{=}CH_2$
(3) $ClCH_2CH_2CH_3$ (4) $BrCH_2CH_2CH_3$
(a) 2 > 4 > 3 > 1 (b) 4 > 2 > 3 > 1
(b) 1 > 2 > 3 > 4 (d) 4 > 3 > 2 > 1

109. Benzyl chloride can be prepared from toluene by chlorination with
(a) Cl_2/hv (b) SO_2Cl_2/peroxide
(c) $SOCl_2$ (d) Both a & b

110. Select the correct order of nucleophilicity
(a) 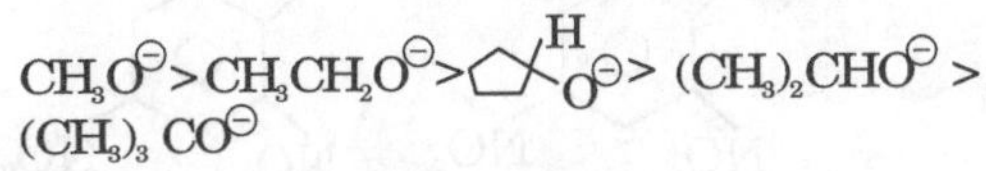
(b) 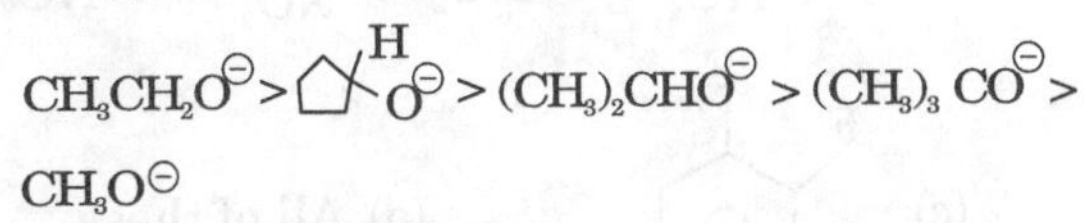
(c) 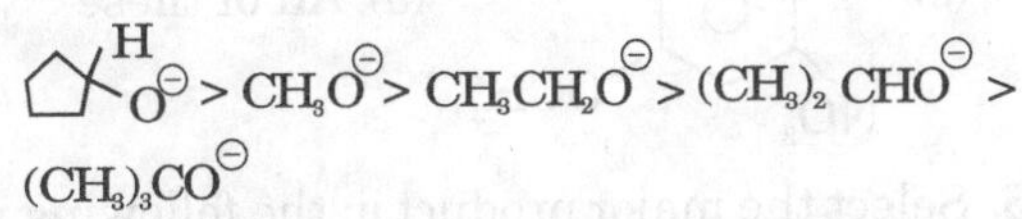
(d) None of these

111. The correct order of reactivity of various alkyl halides in the formation of grignards reagents is
(a) R—I > R—Br > R—Cl
(b) R—Cl > R—Br > R—I
(c) R—I > R—Cl > R—Br
(d) R—Br > R—I > R—Cl

112. Which one of the following is a β-elimination reaction?
(a) $CH_3-\underset{\displaystyle Cl}{\underset{|}{CH}}-CH_2-CH_3 \xrightarrow[\text{KOH}]{\text{alc.}}$
(b) $CH_3-\underset{\displaystyle OH}{\underset{|}{CH}}-CH_2-CH_3 \xrightarrow[H_3PO_4]{\text{Conc.}}$
(c) $CH_3-\underset{\displaystyle Cl}{\underset{|}{CH}}-\overset{\displaystyle Cl}{\overset{|}{CH}}-CH_3 \xrightarrow[\Delta]{Zn}$
(d) All of these

113. The correct reactivity order of following molecules towards E_2 is

(1) 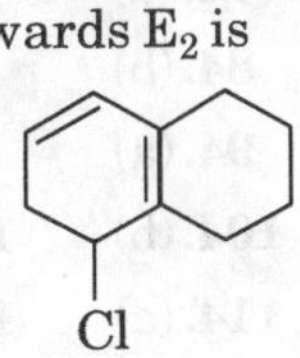 (2) 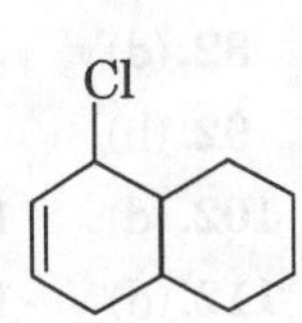

(3) 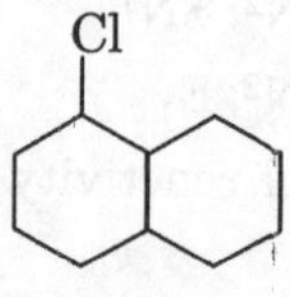

(a) 1 > 2 > 3 (b) 3 > 2 > 1

(c) 2 > 1 > 3 (d) 2 = 1 = 3

114. Select the major product in the following reaction

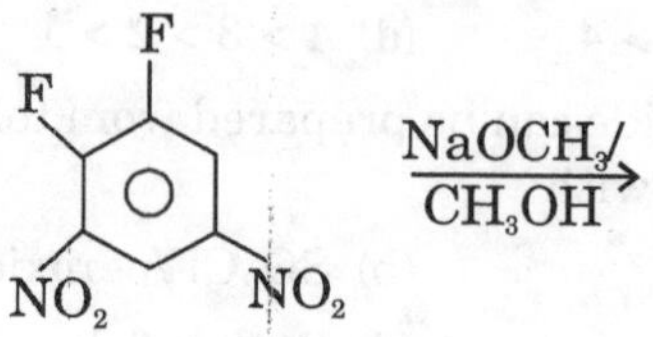

(a) 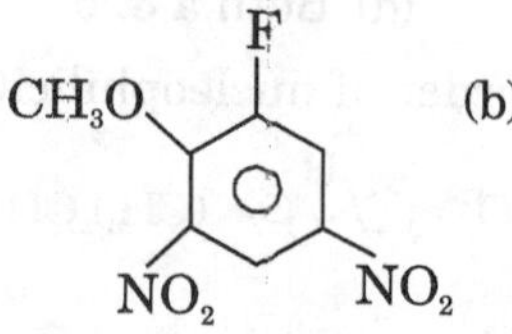 (b) 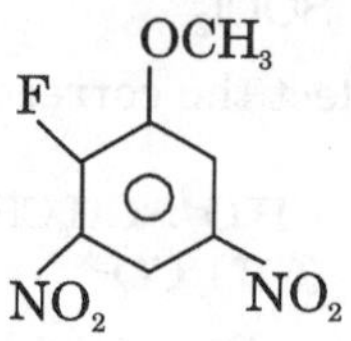

(c) 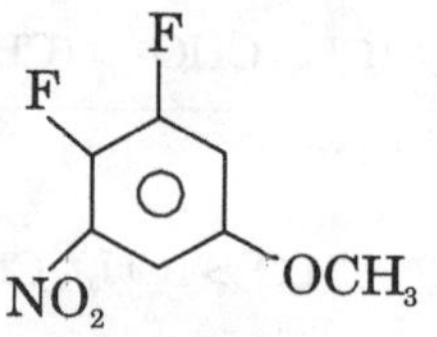 (d) All of these

115. Select the major product in the following reaction

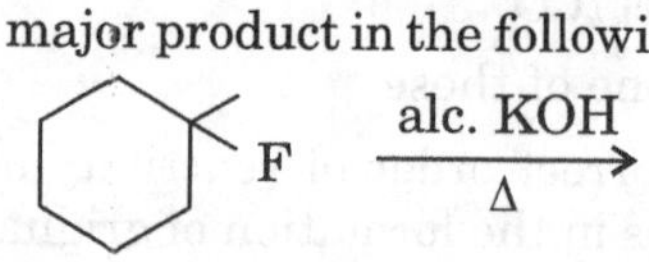

(a) 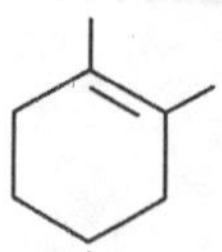 (b) 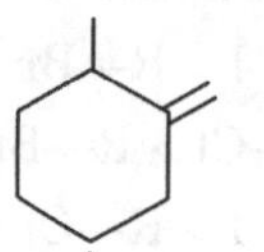

(c) 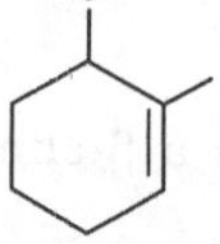 (d) 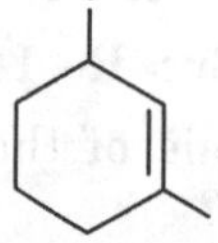

116. Which of the following is maximum reactive towards $S_N{}^1$ reaction ?

(a) 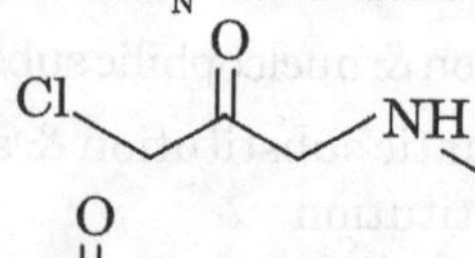

(b) 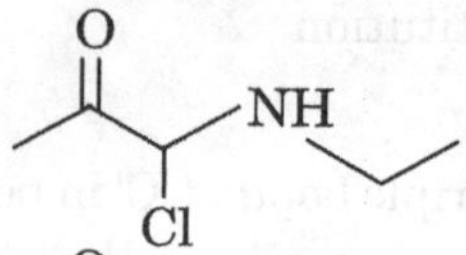

(c) 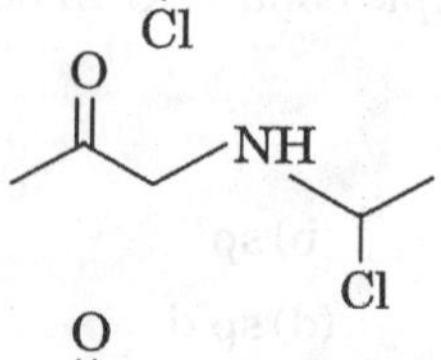

(d) 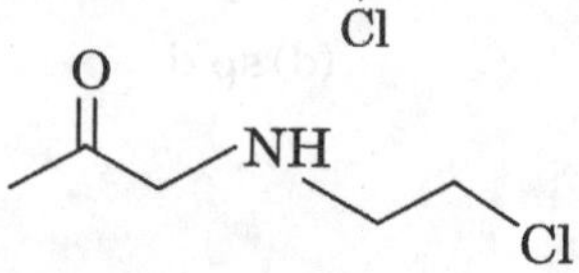

117. The major product of the following reaction will be

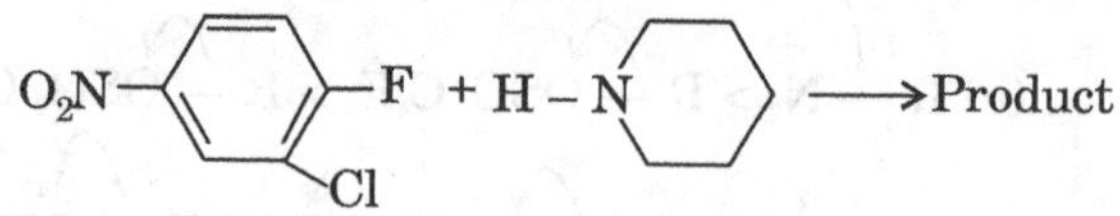

(a) 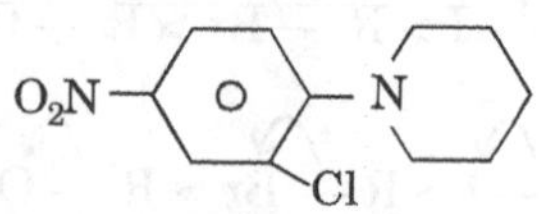

(b) 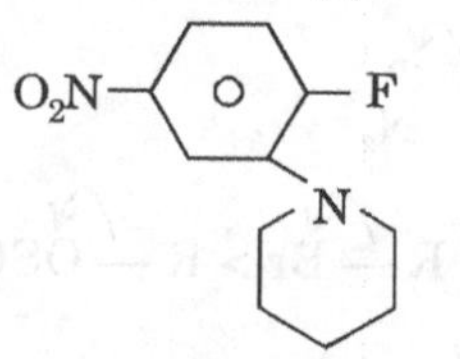

(c) 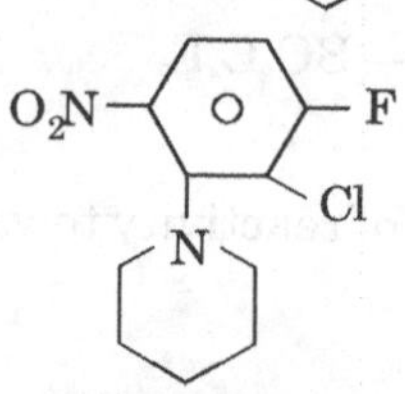

(d) both b & c

Answers

1. (d)	**2.** (b)	**3.** (a)	**4.** (a)	**5.** (d)	**6.** (b)	**7.** (a)	**8.** (d)	**9.** (a)	**10.** (c)
11. (a)	**12.** (c)	**13.** (b)	**14.** (d)	**15.** (d)	**16.** (d)	**17.** (d)	**18.** (c)	**19.** (b)	**20.** (d)
21. (a)	**22.** (d)	**23.** (b)	**24.** (b)	**25.** (d)	**26.** (c)	**27.** (b)	**28.** (c)	**29.** (d)	**30.** (a)
31. (d)	**32.** (c)	**33.** (b)	**34.** (b)	**35.** (d)	**36.** (d)	**37.** (d)	**38.** (d)	**39.** (d)	**40.** (d)
41. (c)	**42.** (c)	**43.** (a)	**44.** (c)	**45.** (d)	**46.** (d)	**47.** (a)	**48.** (d)	**49.** (d)	**50.** (c)
51. (c)	**52.** (a)	**53.** (c)	**54.** (d)	**55.** (d)	**56.** (a)	**57.** (a)	**58.** (d)	**59.** (d)	**60.** (a)
61. (d)	**62.** (c)	**63.** (c)	**64.** (c)	**65.** (b)	**66.** (b)	**67.** (d)	**68.** (a)	**69.** (a)	**70.** (a)
71. (d)	**72.** (d)	**73.** (a)	**74.** (a)	**75.** (c)	**76.** (a)	**77.** (b)	**78.** (d)	**79.** (c)	**80.** (a)
81. (a)	**82.** (d)	**83.** (d)	**84.** (b)	**85.** (c)	**86.** (c)	**87.** (d)	**88.** (d)	**89.** (c)	**90.** (c)
91. (d)	**92.** (b)	**93.** (d)	**94.** (a)	**95.** (b)	**96.** (d)	**97.** (d)	**98.** (d)	**99.** (a)	**100.** (d)
101. (a)	**102.** (d)	**103.** (c)	**104.** (b)	**105.** (a)	**106.** (a)	**107.** (b)	**108.** (a)	**109.** (d)	**110.** (a)
111. (a)	**112.** (d)	**113.** (a)	**114.** (a)	**115.** (b)	**116.** (c)	**117.** (a)			

Explanations

1. Nucleophilicity is kinetically controlled whereas basicity is thermodynamic property

   (a) In $CH_3COO^{\ominus}$, the –ve charge on 'O' is delocalised due to resonance. So, charge density on each 'O' is relatively decreased & hence it turns to be a weaker nucleophide than $\overset{\ominus}{O}H$.

   (b) H_2O is a stronger acid than NH_3. So, its conjugate base i.e. $\bar{O}H$ will be a weaker base.

   (c) Out of isopropyl alcohol

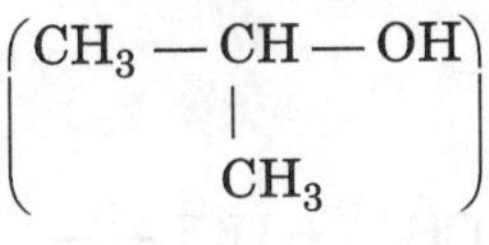

& ter-butyl alcohol

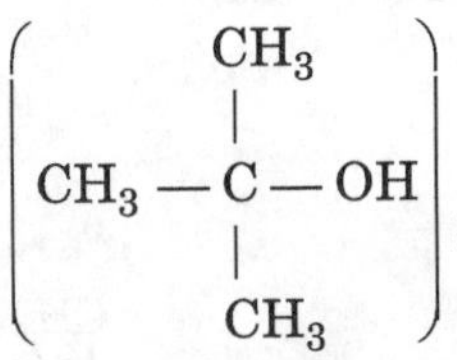

;

   ter-butyl alcohol is a weaker acid (because of greater +I effect). Hence, its conjugate base i.e. $(CH_3)_3O^{\ominus}$, will be a stronger base.

   (d) Out of H_2S & H_2O, H_2S is more acidic & hence its conjugate base i.e. $\overset{\ominus}{S}H$ will be a weaker base rather, $\bar{O}H$ should be more basic than $\bar{S}H$. So, option (d) is incorrect.

2. Acidic strength of their conjugate acids, follows the order

   H—Br > H—F > NH_3 > CH_4

   ∴ Br^- is least basic.

3. In polar protic solvent,

$$\text{Nucleophilicity} \propto \frac{1}{\text{Electronegativity}}$$

   Since 'S' is less electro –ve than 'O', so $CH_3CH_2S^{\ominus}$ is more nucleophilic.

   Among 1 & 3, (3) i.e. $CH_3COO^{\ominus}$ is resonance stabilised. So, it is relatively weaker nucleophilic

4. Among these ions, $CF_3—\overset{O}{\overset{\|}{\underset{\underset{O}{\|}}{S}}}—O^{\ominus}$ (Triflate ion) is the weakest base & weak bases are excellent leaving groups.

5. For option (a) & (b):

   In polar protic solvent

   Order of nucleophilicity: -

   $I^- > Br^- > Cl^- > F^-$

   (it is because F^- gets H-bonded with proton of protic solvent & –ve charge density on fluoride ion is lowered, turning it into a weaker nucleophile)

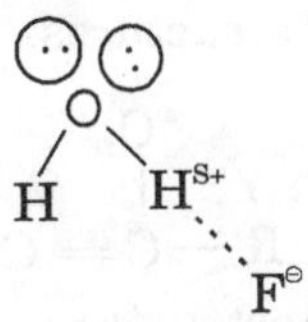

   In aprotic solvent

   Order of nucleophilicity → $F^- > Cl^- > Br^- > I^-$

   For (c) option :

   H – I > H – F (acidic strength)

   So, F^- is a stronger base than I^-.

   For Option (d):

   If an atom containing one or more unshared pairs is adjacent to the attacking atom on the nucleophile, the nucleophilicity is enhanced.

   Eg:- $HO_2^{\ominus}(H—\ddot{O}—\ddot{O}^{\ominus}:)$, $\ddot{N}H_2—\ddot{N}H_2$.

   It is referred to as alpha effect (α-effect)

6. For a given atom type or within a period of the periodic table, nucleophilicity parallels basicity.

7. N_2, being maximum stable is an excellent leaving group.

   N ≡ N → Triple Covalent bond makes it highly stable & hence, an excellent leaving group.

8. For option (1),

   Tertiary butoxide is a stronger base than ethoxide ion. It is because ter-butyl alcohol is a weaker acid than ethanol.

   Acidic strength

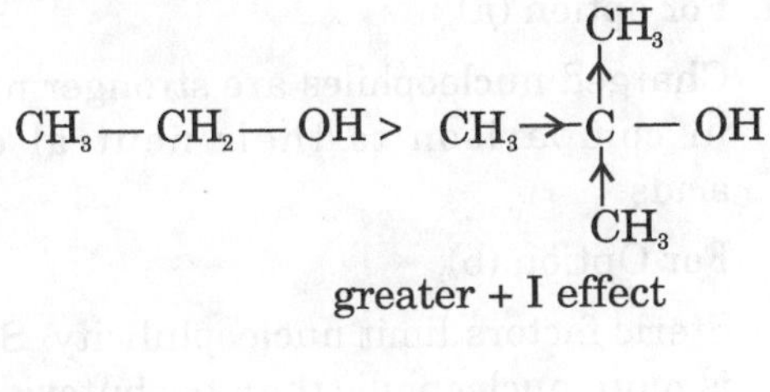

   greater + I effect

For option (b)

Steric factors limit nucleophilicity. So, ter-butoxide is a weaker nucleophile than ethoxide.

For option (c)

$RSO_3^{\ominus}$ is more resonance stabilised than $RCOO^{\ominus}$.

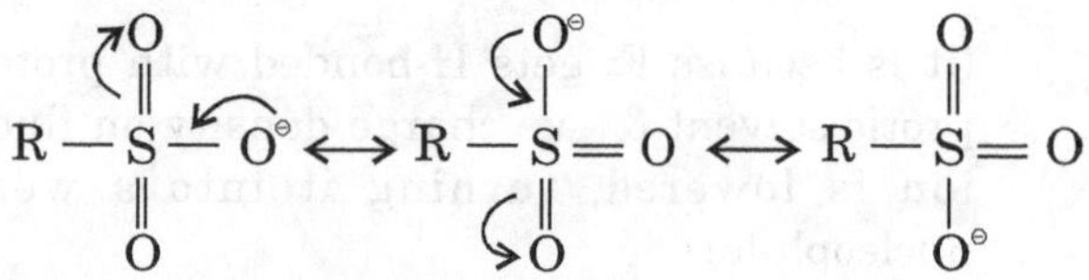

Three equally contributing structures.

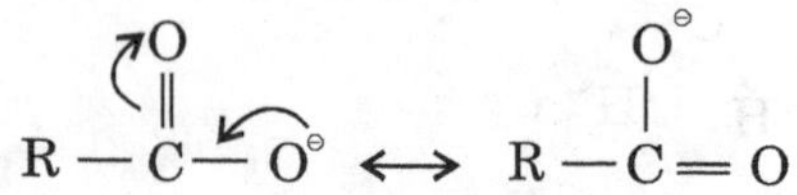

→ Two equally contributing structures.

9. All except CH_3OH are strong Nucleophiles.

10. Halogen acids follow the given order for acidic strength

H—I > H—Br > H—Cl > H—F

So, basic strength would follow the order.

$F^- > Cl^- > Br^- > I^-$ (Basic strength)

(weak acids have strong conjugate bases)

→ Order of leaving ability

$I^- > Br^- > Cl^- > F^-$

(weak bases are good leaving groups)

11. If active atoms of nucleophiles fall in a period then nucleophilicity decreases form left to right.

$$\text{Nucleophilicity} \propto \frac{1}{\text{Electro negativity}}.$$

12. Weaker bases are better leaving groups.

13. Among, $\overset{\ominus}{S}H$ & $\bar{O}H$, $\bar{S}H$ is more nucleophillic (since 'S' is less electro –ve than 'O'). $PhO^{\ominus}$ & $AcO^{\ominus}$, both are stabilised by resonance but $AcO^{\ominus}(CH_3COO^-)$ is stabilised more. Hence its less nucleophilic. H_2O comes last as it is a neutral molecule.

14. For option (a),

Charged nucleophiles are stronger nucleophiles in comparison to their neutral congugate acids.

For Option (b),

Steric factors limit nucleophilicity. So, ethoxide is more nucleophilic than ter-butoxide.

For Option (c),

A lone pair each, rests on P & N. But P has a bigger size & hence the e^- cloud is easily polarizable.

16. $CH_3—CH_2—OH + HCl \xrightarrow{?}$

1° alcohols need the presence of lewis acid like anhyd. $ZnCl_2$ to accompalish this reaction. Primary alcohols do not react appreciably at room temperature with Lucas reagent i.e. anhyd. $ZnCl_2/HCl$.

17. 3° alcohols can react with HCl even in the absence of lewis acid like anhyd. $ZnCl_2$.

Option (a)

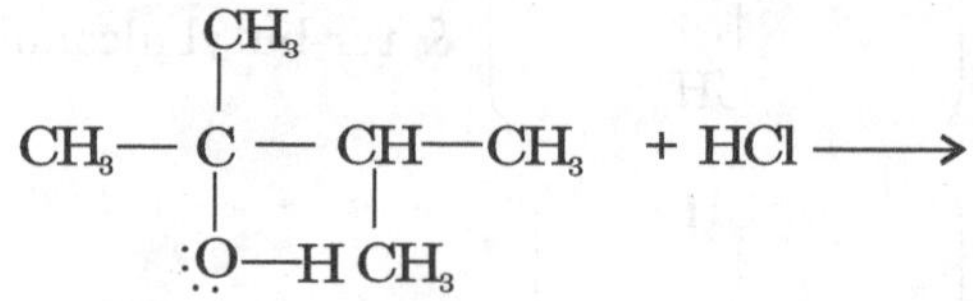

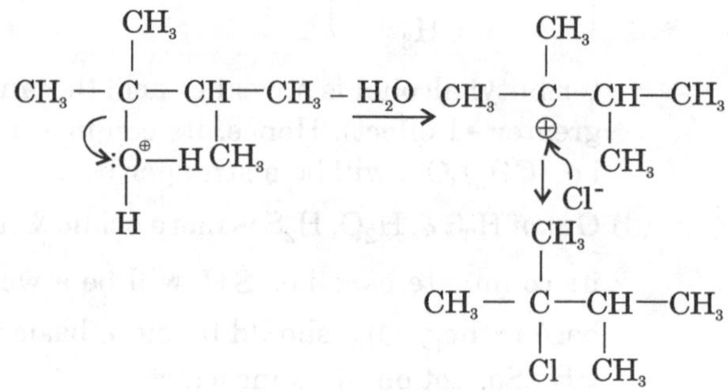

For Option (b).

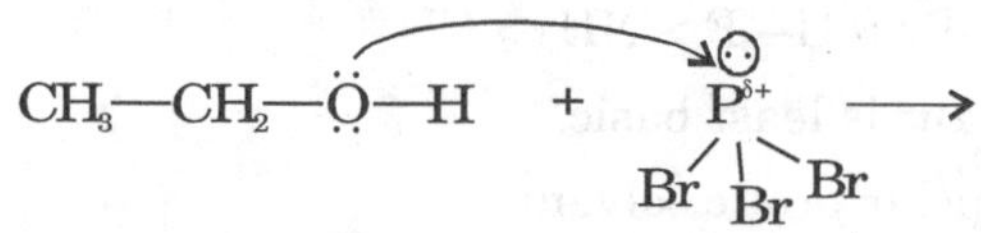

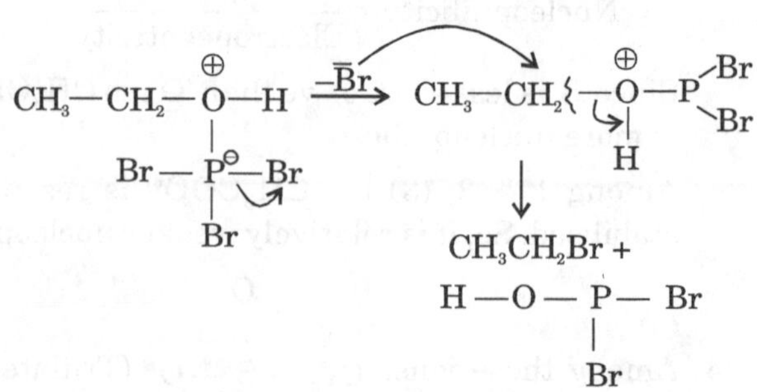

Similarly, again CH_3CH_2OH attacks vacant orbital of 'P' in $HOPBr_2$ twice to yield H_3PO_3.

For option (c)

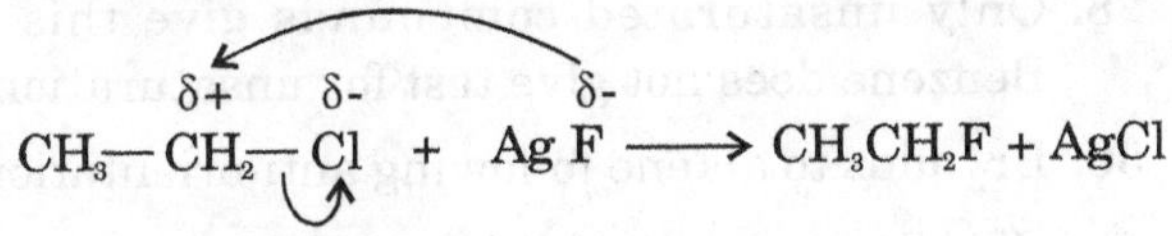

'Swarts reaction'.

For option (d).

$$CH_2=CH-CH_2-CH_3 \xrightarrow{NBS} CH_2=CH-\underset{\displaystyle Br}{\underset{|}{CH}}-CH_3$$

(Free radical halogenation at allylic C)

18.

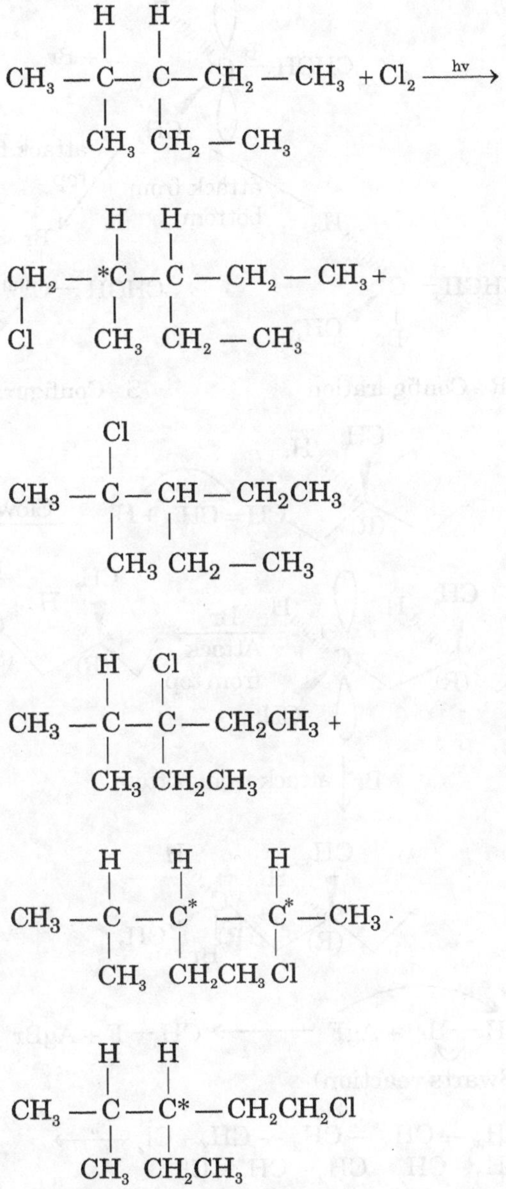

19. 1° alcohols require heating to react with Lucas reagent.

20.

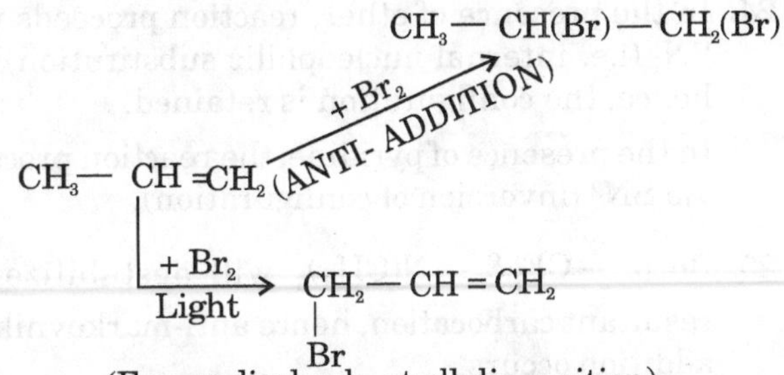

(Free radical sub. at allylic position).

21.

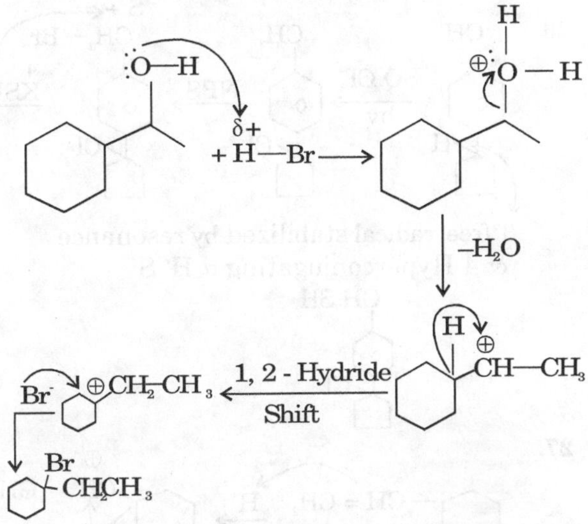

22.

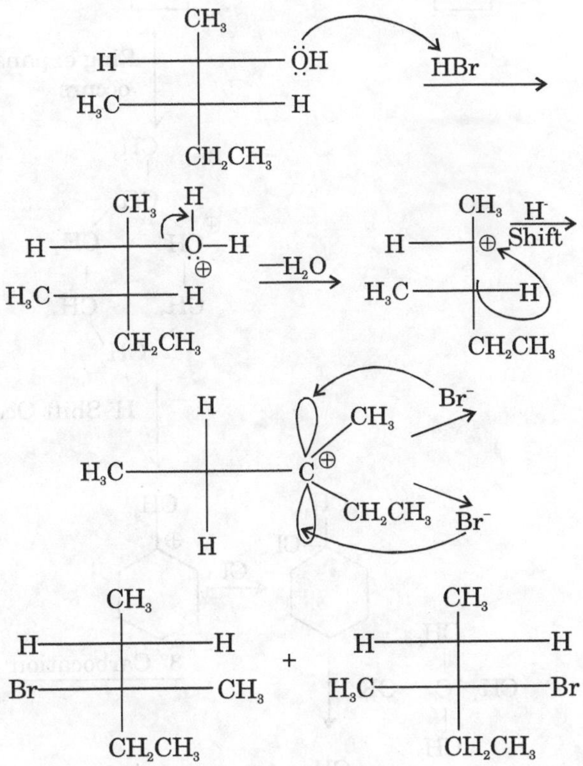

23. $NaBr + H_2SO_4 \rightarrow HBr + Na_2SO_4$

HBr is generated in situ which then attack at butanol via S_N^2.

24. In the presence of ether, reaction proceeds with SN_i (i.e. internal nucleophilic substitution) and hence, the configuration is retained.

In the presence of pyridine, the reaction proceeds via SN^2 (inversion of configuration).

25. Both $-CF_3$ & $-\overset{\oplus}{N}(CH_3)_3$ will destabilize the resultant carbocation, hence anti-markovnikov's addition occurs.

26.

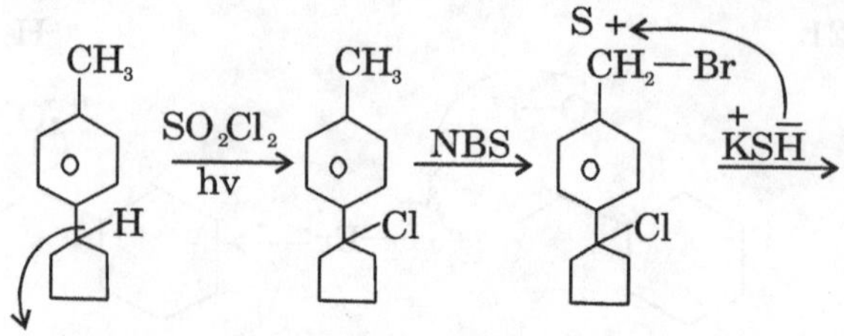

3°free radical stabilized by resonance & 4 Hyperconjugating α H′ S

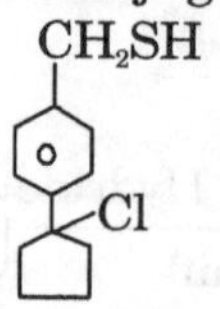

27.

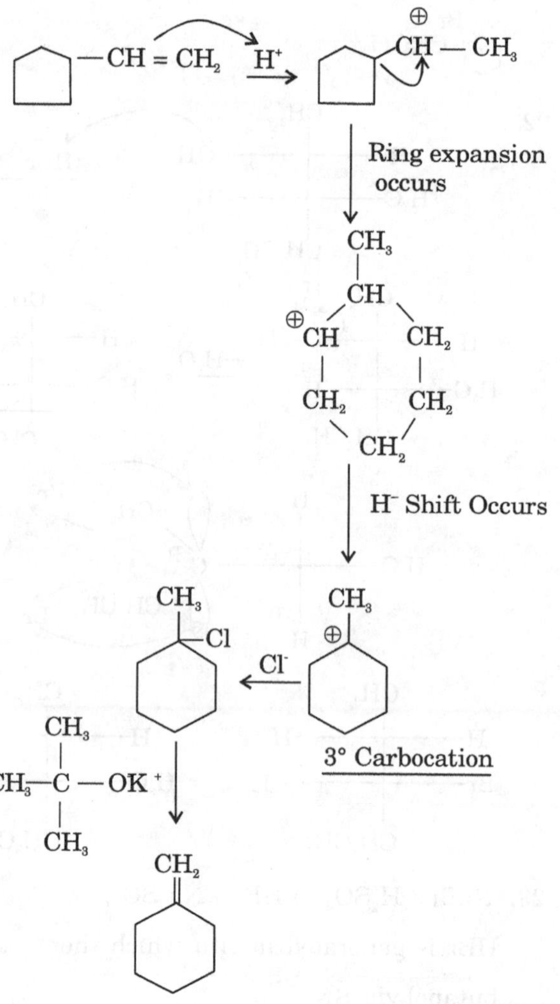

(Hoffmann's elimination product is formed)

28. Only unsaturated compounds give this test. Benzene does not give test for unsaturation.

30. Br_2 adds to alkene following anti-orientation.

Cis alkene + anti addition → Racemic mixture

Trans alkene + anti addition → Meso Compound

31. $CH_3-CH_2-CH=CH_2+HBr \rightarrow$ ... (1)

$CH_3-CH_2-CH=CH_2+H^+ \xrightarrow{Slow} CH_3-CH_2-\overset{\oplus}{C}H-CH_3$ ... (2)

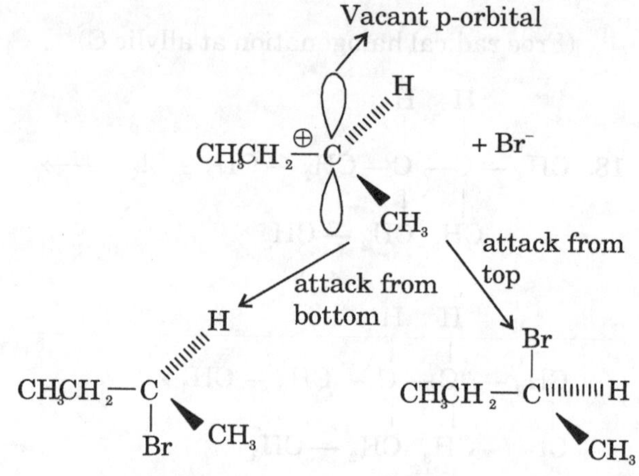

R - Configuration S - Configuration

32.

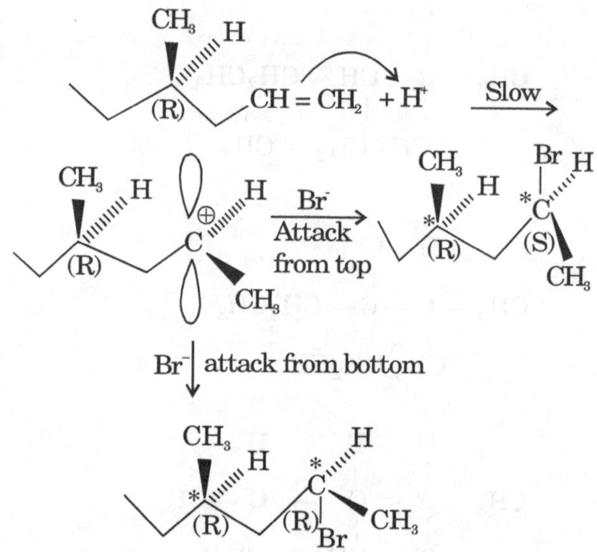

33. $\overset{S^+}{CH_3}-Br + AgF \longrightarrow CH_3-F + AgBr$

(Swarts reaction)

34. $CH_3-CH_2-CH_2-CH_3+Cl_2 \xrightarrow{hv}$

$CH_3-CH_2-CH_2-CH_2-Cl$

+

(±) $CH_3-CH_2-\underset{\underset{Cl}{|}}{CH}-CH_3$

→ These products are formed via free radical substitution.

During the formation of 2-chlorobutane, a 2° free radical is formed at which Cl then attacks to give the racemic mixture.

$$CH_3-CH_2-\dot{C}H-CH_3 \xrightarrow{Cl}$$

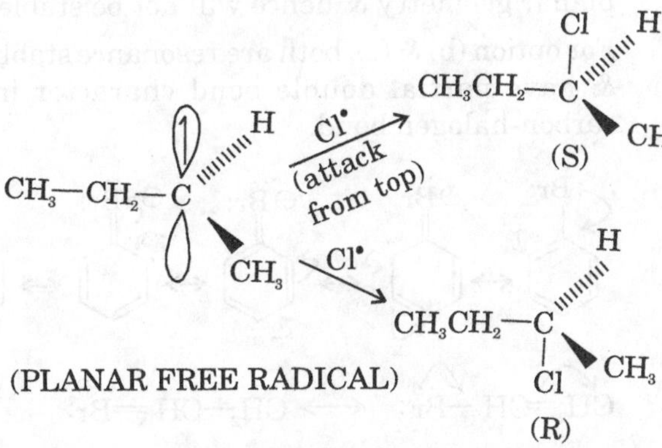

(PLANAR FREE RADICAL)

35. Relative rate of substitution of 3°, 2° & 1° hydrogens at 298 K towards Cl_2 is

3°H	2°H	1°H
5 :	3.8 :	1

$$CH_3-CH_2-CH_2-CH_3+Cl_2 \xrightarrow{hv} CH_3-CH_2-CH_2-CH_2-Cl$$

$6 \times 1 = 6$

(Considering probability & reactivity)

+

$$CH_3-CH_2-\underset{\displaystyle Cl}{\underset{|}{CH}}-CH_3$$

$4 \times 3.8 = 15.2$

$$\%\text{ age yield of 2-chlorobutane} = \frac{15.2}{21.2} \times 100$$

$$= 71.69\%$$

37. Borodine Hunsdiecker's reaction follows the following mechanism:-

$$R-\overset{O}{\overset{||}{C}}-OAg + Br_2 \longrightarrow R-\overset{O}{\overset{||}{C}}-O-Br + AgBr$$

(Hypobromite)

$$\downarrow$$

$$R\cdot\cdot\overset{O}{\overset{||}{C}}-\dot{O} + \dot{B}r$$

(Carboxyl free radical)

$$\dot{R} + CO_2$$

$$\dot{R} + \dot{B}r-O-\overset{O}{\overset{||}{C}}-R \longrightarrow R-Br + R-\overset{O}{\overset{||}{C}}-O^{\circ}$$

If an attempt is made to prepare 3° halide by this method, a 3° free radical is formed which is more inclined to undergo elimination & form an alkene, instead.

38. $CH_3CH_3 + I_2 \underset{}{\overset{hv}{\rightleftharpoons}} CH_3CH_2I + H-I$

$$2H-I + \underset{(conc.)}{2HNO_3} \longrightarrow I_2 + 2H_2O + 2NO_2$$

$$5HI + HIO_3 \rightarrow I_2 + H_2O$$

$$2HI + HgO \rightarrow I_2 + HgI_2 + H_2O$$

To check the reversibility of the reaction, H—I must be destroyed.

40. $2KI + H_2SO_4 \rightarrow 2KHSO_4 + 2HI$

$$2HI + H_2SO_4 \rightarrow H_2O + I_2 + SO_2 \uparrow$$

(Oxidising agent)

41.

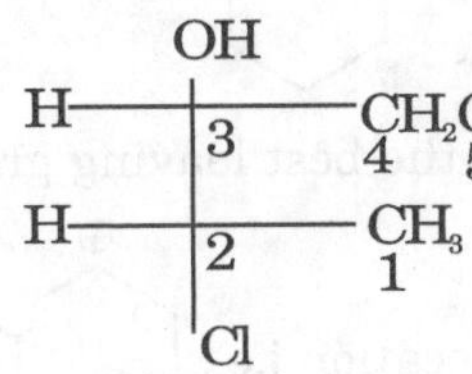

At C — 2

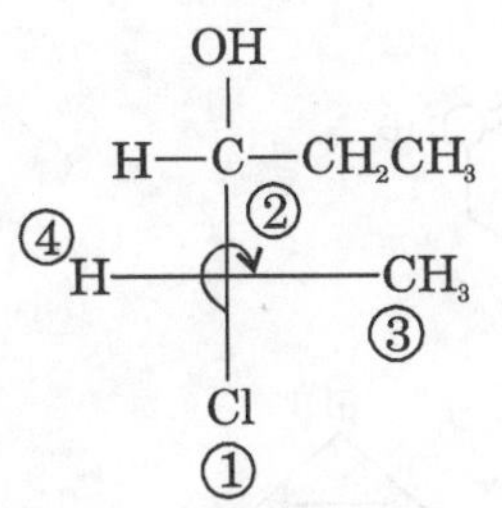

2S

At C — 3

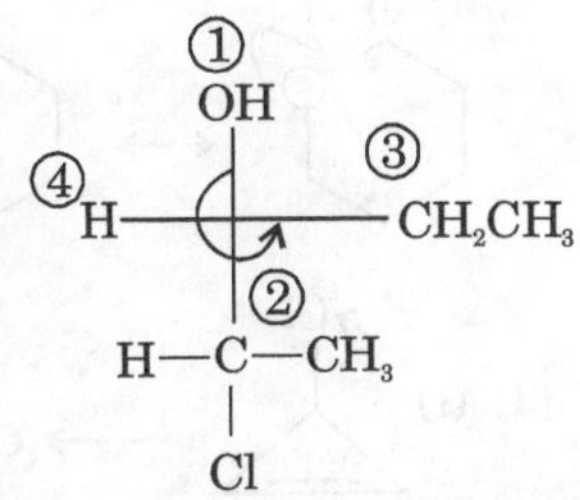

3R

So, the reactant is (2S, 3R)-2-chloro-pentan-3-ol. SN^2 occurs here with NaI & resultant product should be (2R, 3R)-2-iodopentan-3-ol (inversion of configuration)

In option 3-

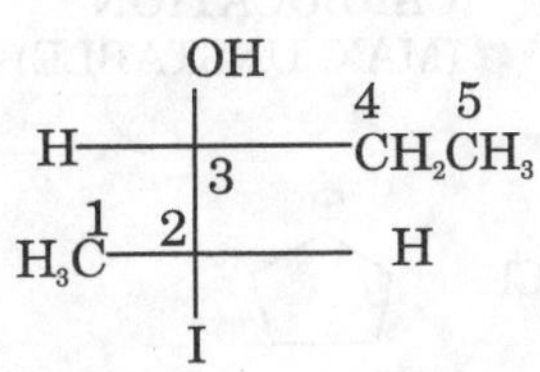

At C — 2

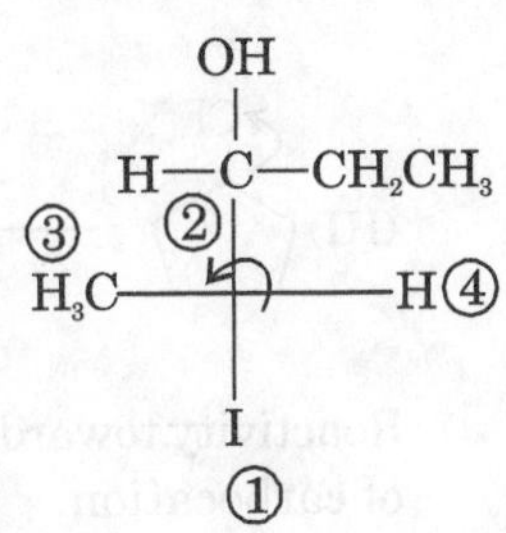

2R

At C — 3

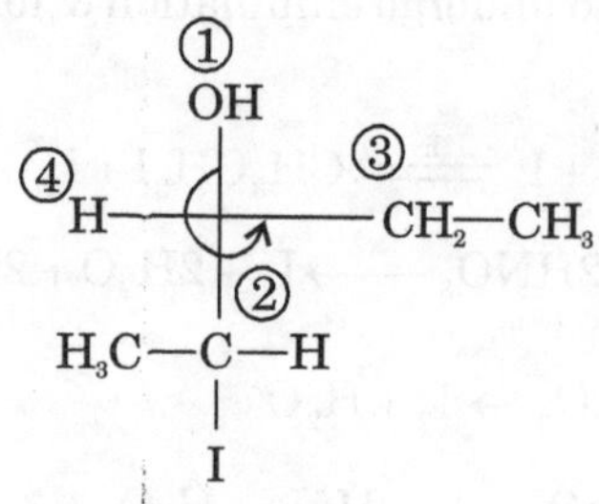

3R

So, option 3 is (2R, 3R)-2-iodopentan-3-ol.

42. For SN^2 reaction

Rate of reaction ∝ [Alkyl halide][Nucleophile]

43.

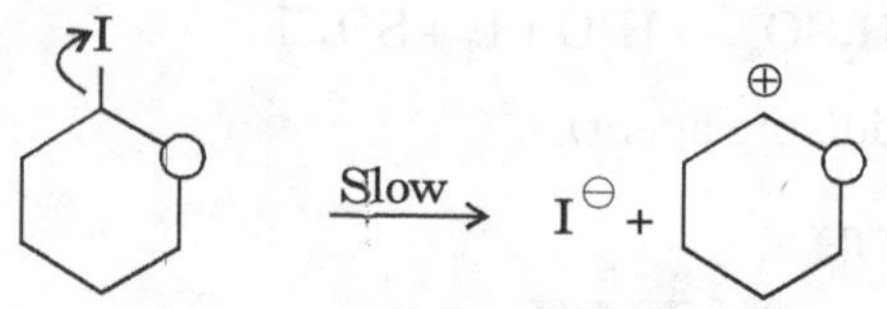

Among halide ions, I^- is the best leaving group.

Also, the resultant Carbocation i.e., 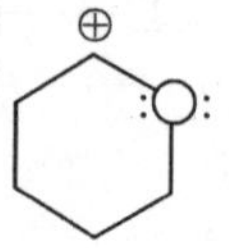

is stabilised by resonance.

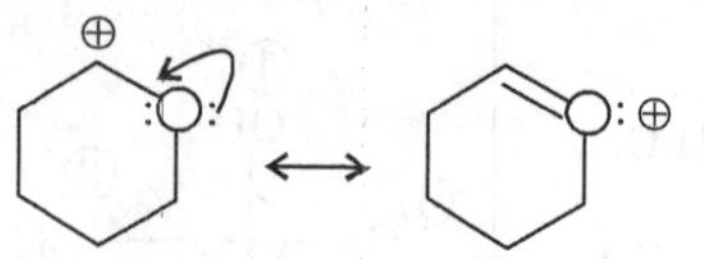

44. (I)

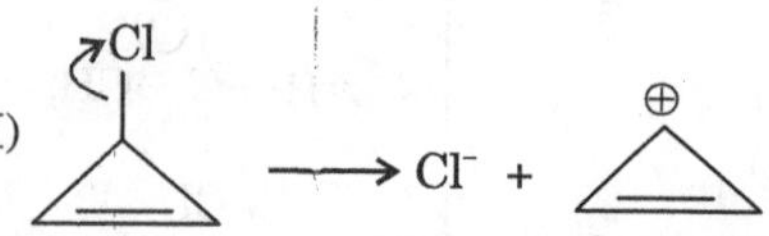

Aromatic Carbocation (Max. Stable)

(II)

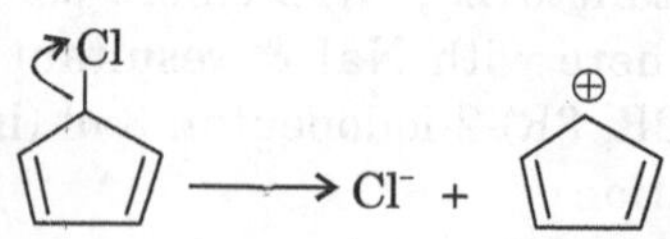

ANTI - AROMATIC CARBOCATION (MAX. UNSTABLE)

(III)

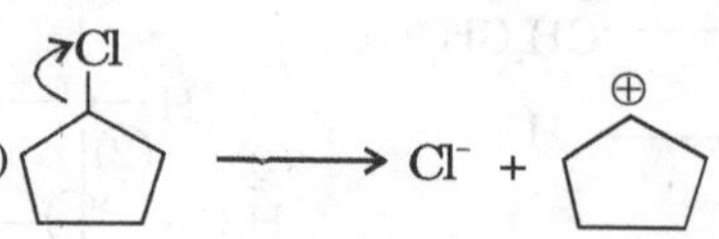

(2°Carbocation)

Reactivity towards SN^1 is governed by the stability of carbocation.

And stability follows the order- I > III > II

45.

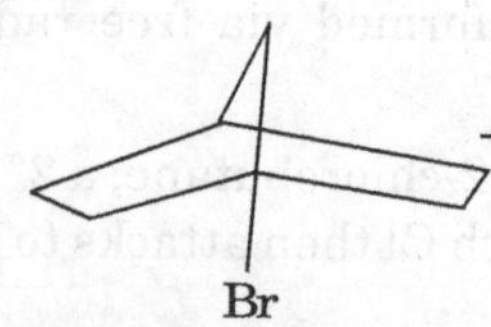

→ It is a bicyclocompound with halide at bridge head location.

SN^2 cannot occur because its a 3° halide. SN^1 cannot occur because carbocation will not attain planar geometry & hence will not be stable.

For option (b) & (c), both are resonance stablished & have partial double bond character in the carbon-halogen bond.

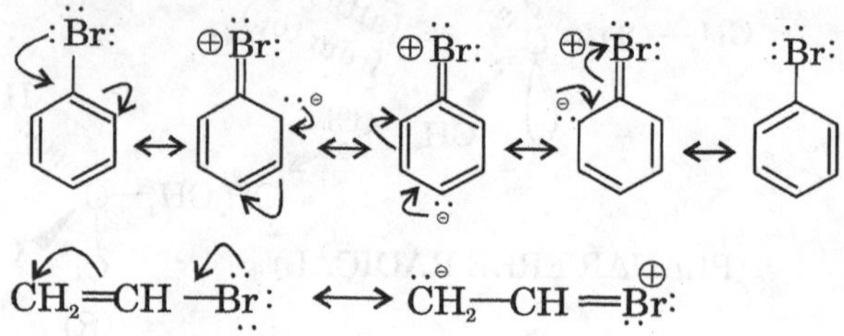

46. For option (a)

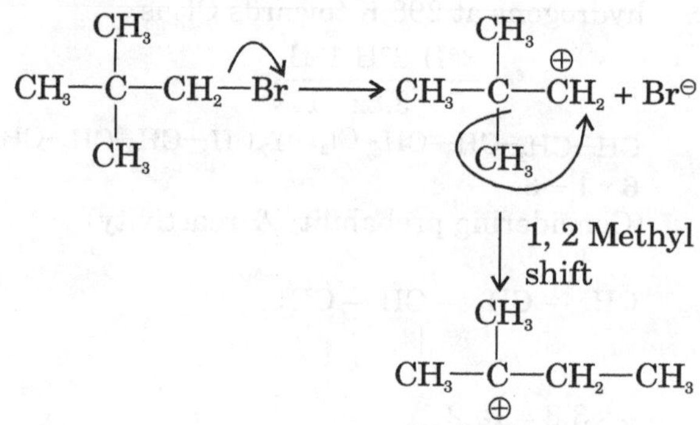

(3° Carbocation)

For option (b)

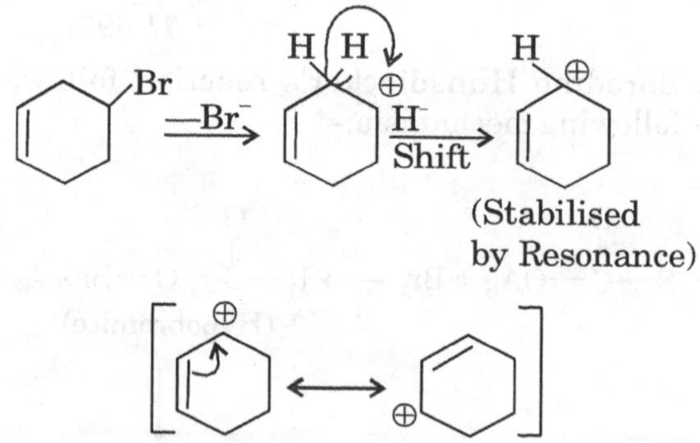

For option (c)

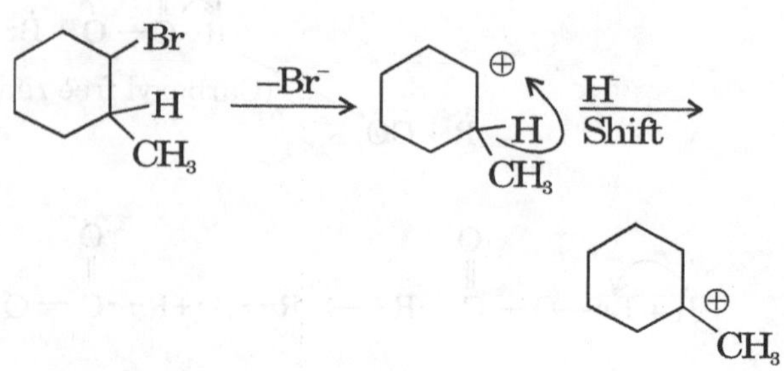

47. Inversion of configuration will occur at the C bearing the leaving group.

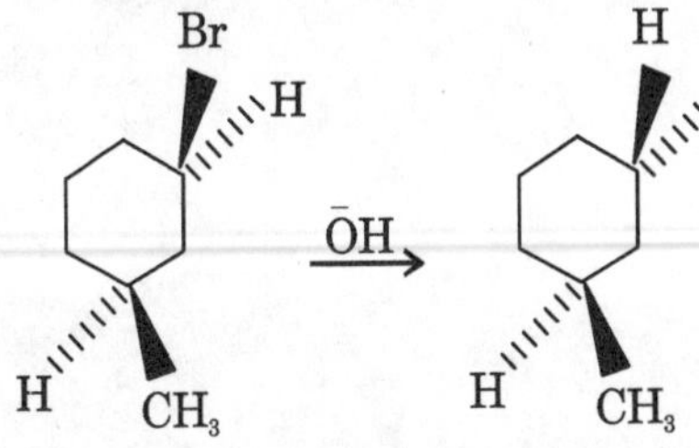

(1S, 3S) – Trans-3 - methyl cyclohexanol

48. Wrt option (d),
3° halides do not undergo SN^2 reactions owing to steric hindrance.

49. $>C=O$ exerts -I effect & stabilises the transitions state of SN^2. So, Bromide labelled as 'a' is most reactive towards SN^2 followed by 'c' & 'b'.

50. Presence of Carbonyl group at α – carbon is one of the most suitable substrate for SN^2 reaction. The transition state gets stabilised by p-orbital of $>C=O$ group.

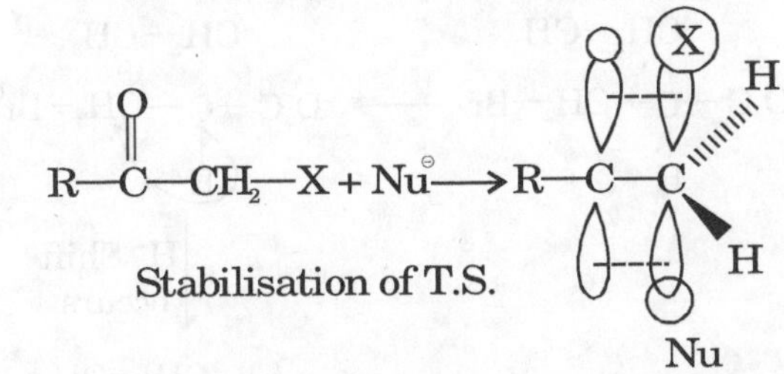

Stabilisation of T.S.

51. Br^- is a better leaving group than Cl^-. Also, in option (c), maximum stable carbocation is formed.

$$CH_3-\ddot{O}-CH_2-Br \longrightarrow \overset{\ominus}{Br} + CH_3-\ddot{O}-\overset{\oplus}{C}H_2$$

$$CH_3-\ddot{O}-\overset{\oplus}{C}H_2 \longleftrightarrow CH_3-\overset{\oplus}{O}=CH_2$$

(Octet of C gets completed)

52. SN^2 reaction occurs. 3° halides do not undergo SN^2 due to steric hindrance.

53. option (a),

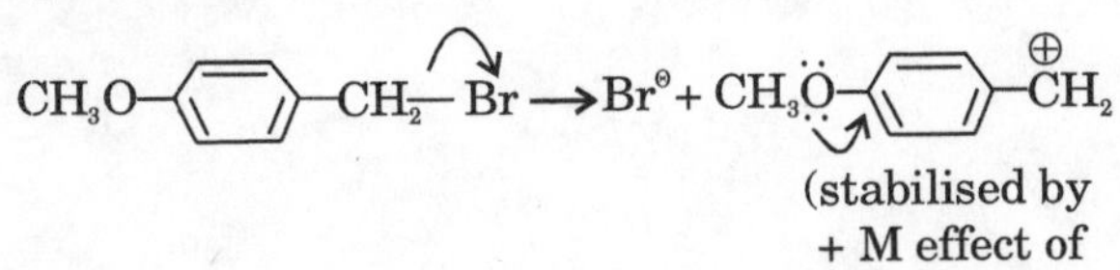

(stabilised by + M effect of p- OCH_3 gp.)

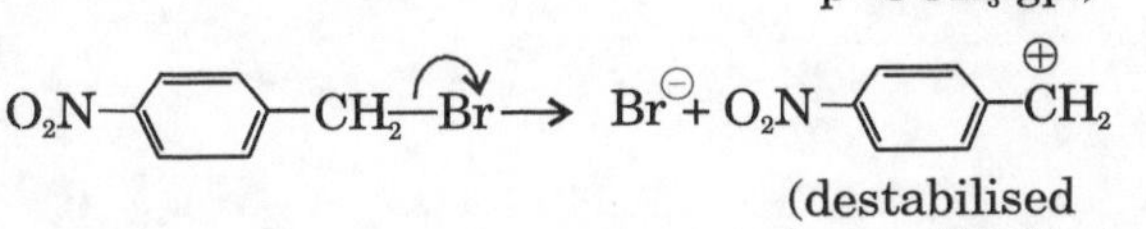

(destabilised by — M effect of —NO_2group)

option b,

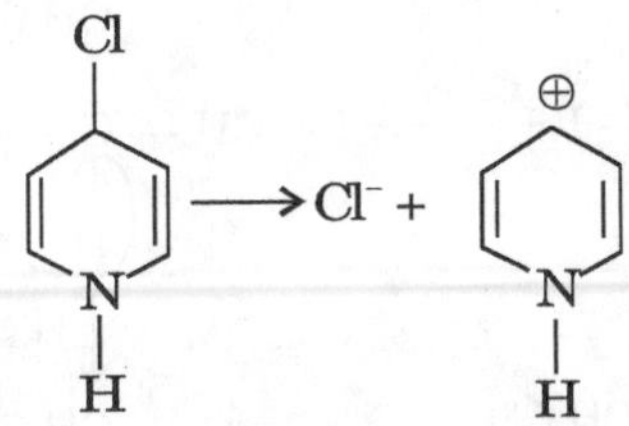

(Aromatic Carbocation highly stable)

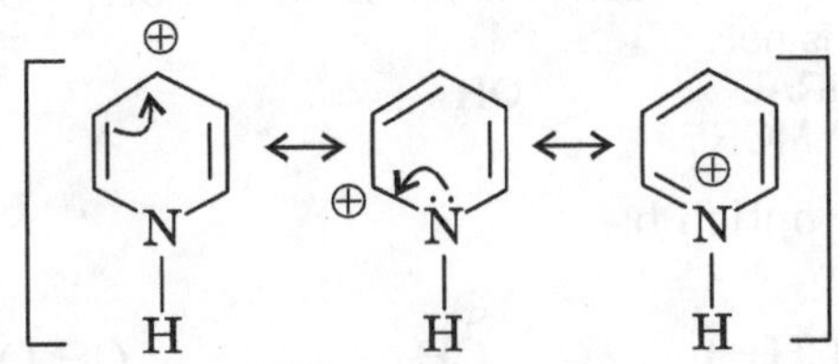

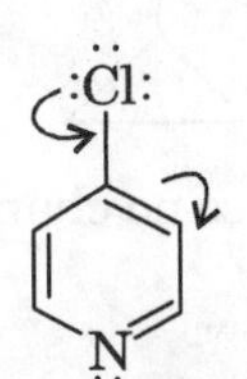

(there is already partial double bond character in the C—Cl bond, so it is tough to break)

Also,

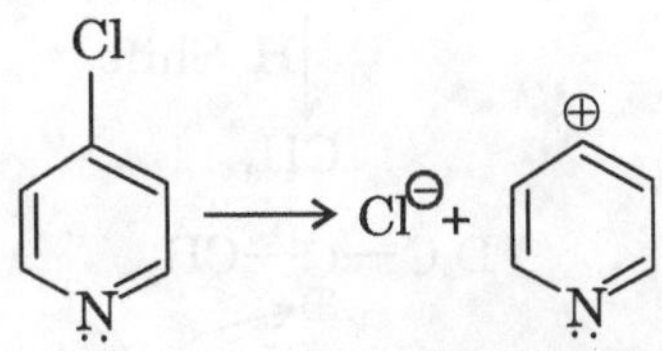

(NOT Stabilised by Resonance)

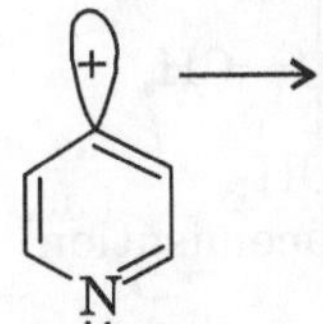

→ VACANT ORBITAL LIES IN THE PLANE OF RING, SO IT IS NOT STABILISED BY π electrons.

option (c),

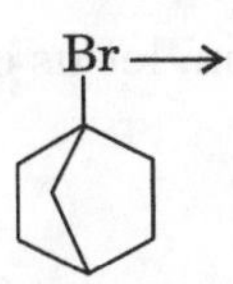

Br → Here, halide is at bridge head location so, carbocation is highly unstable. Hence, unreactive toward SN^1.

wrt option (d),

$$CH_2=CH-\ddot{C}l: \longleftrightarrow \overset{\ominus}{C}H_2-CH=\overset{\oplus}{C}l:$$

(VINYL CHLORIDE)

There is partial double bond character in the C—Cl bond. So, unreactive towards both SN^1 & SN^2.

54. For option (a):-

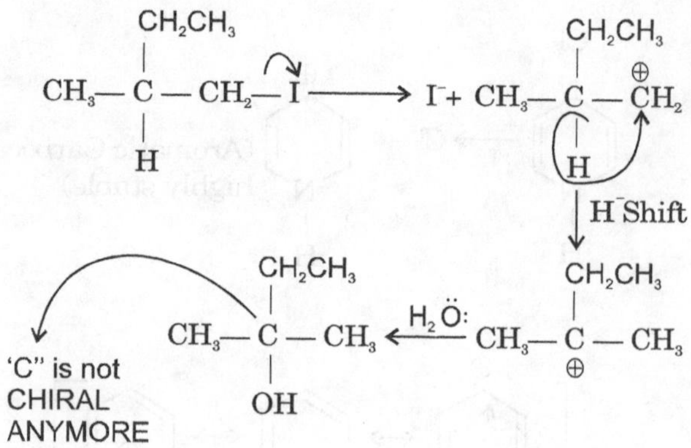

For option b:-

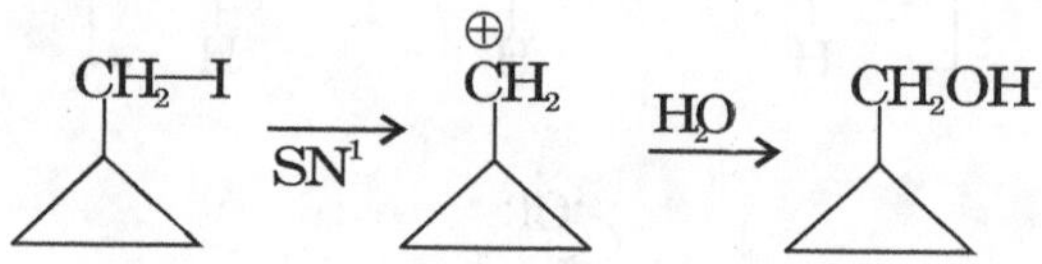

(No Chiral C, so no chance of racemisation)

For option c,

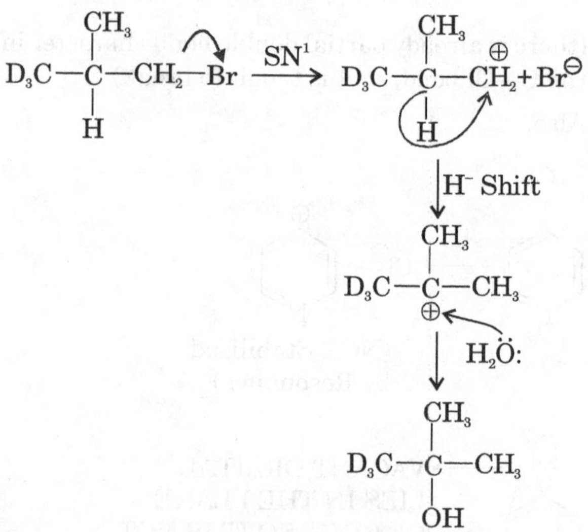

(No chiral C, no racemisation)

For option d,

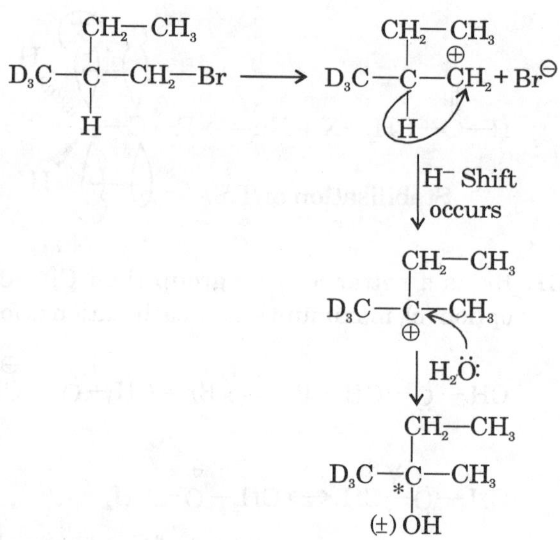

The Carbon marked '*' is chiral, so racemisation occurs.

55. To understand partial racemisation, let us consider the following reaction-

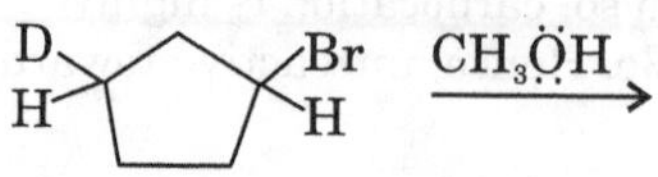

Step 1

Formation of a Carbocation

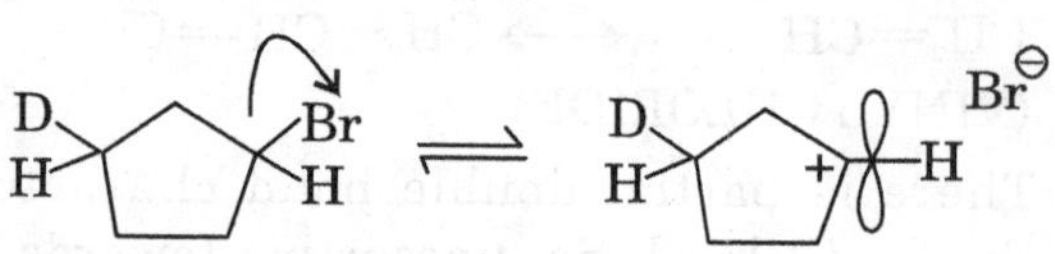

Step 2

Nucleophiolic attack

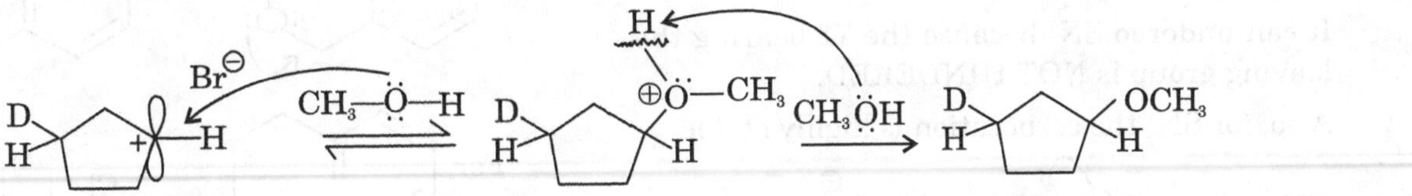

Front side is hindered by the leaving group

Cis form (40% Retention of Configuration)

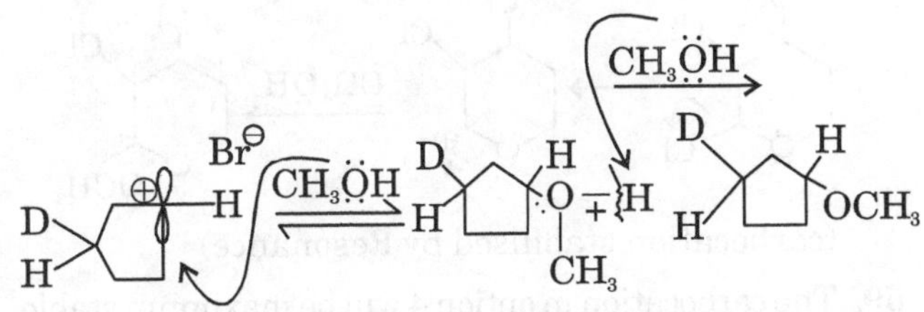

trans (60% inversion of configuration)

56. Wrt substrate 1 –

(1) Allyl halides are even more reactive than corresponding alkyl halides for SN^2.

(2) For eg:- allyl bromide is more reactive than propyl bromide for SN^2.

(3) It can be explained on the basis of strong -I of $>C=O$ group accompanied by allylic deloc-alisation of electrons in the Transition state.

(4) This process lower the energy of T.S. & hence increases the rate of reaction.

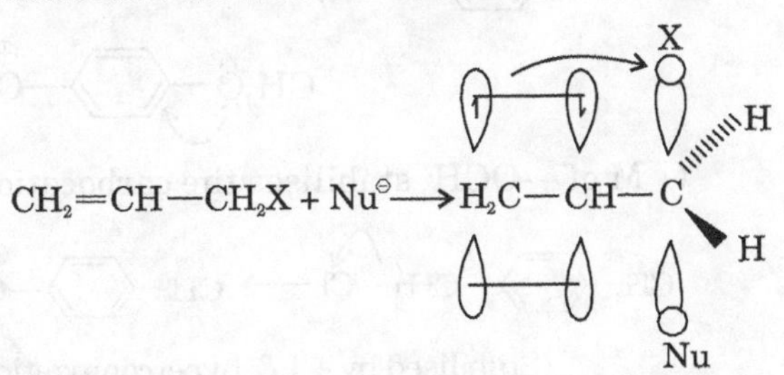

Same, stands valid for benzyl halide. Both, allyl & benzyl halides can undergo SN^2.

Both (allyl halide & benzyl halide) undergo SN^1 reactions also owing to stabilities of their carbocations.

$$CH_2=CH-CH_2-Cl \xrightarrow{SN^1} CH_2=CH-\overset{\oplus}{C}H_2 + Cl^-$$

(Allyl Chloride)

$$CH_2=CH-\overset{\oplus}{C}H_2 \longleftrightarrow \overset{\oplus}{C}H_2-CH=CH_2$$

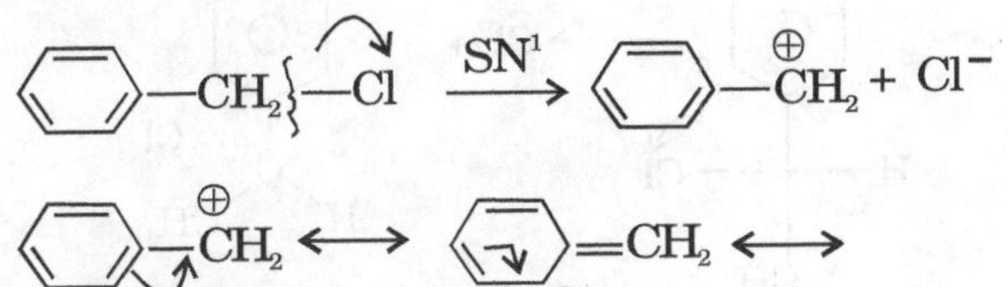

(BENZYLIC CARBOCATION)

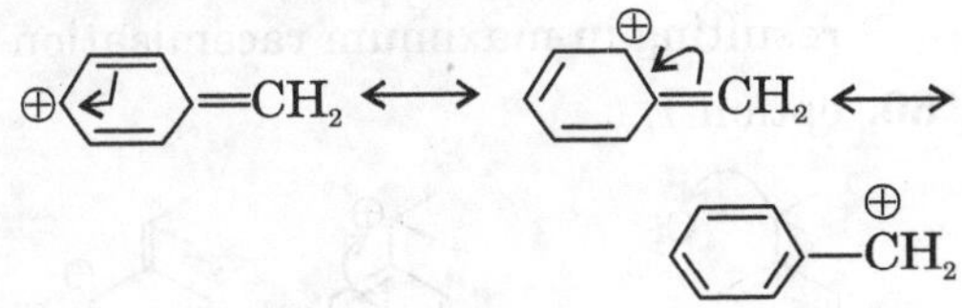

For 2nd Substrate

$$R-\overset{O}{\overset{\|}{C}}-CH_2-Cl$$

is highly reactive towards SN^2 (α-carbonyl compound) because of strong- I shown by $>C=O$ gp. Also, the p-orbital of carbonyl group are parellel to the p- orbital of C bearing the leaving group, thus stablishing the T.S.

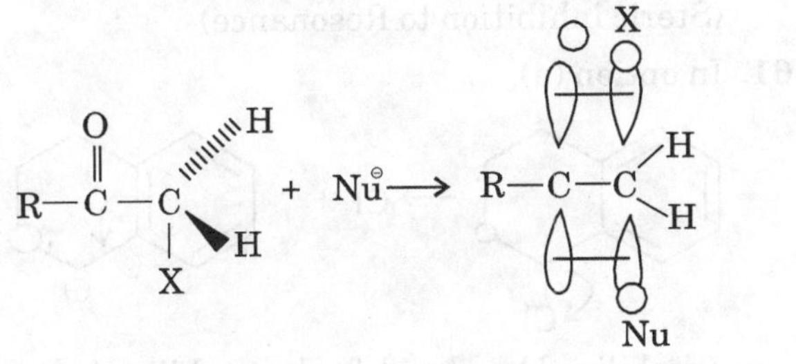

For 3rd Substrate

$CH_3—O—CH_2—Cl$

It can undergo SN^2 because the 'C' bearing the leaving group is NOT HINDERED.

Also, for SN^1 the carbocation is highly stable.

$$CH_3—O—CH_2—Cl \longrightarrow CH_3O\overset{\oplus}{C}H_2 + Cl^-$$

$$[CH_3—\ddot{O}—\overset{\oplus}{C}H_2 \longleftrightarrow CH_3—\overset{\oplus}{O}=CH_2]$$

57. The reaction follows SN^1 mechanism.

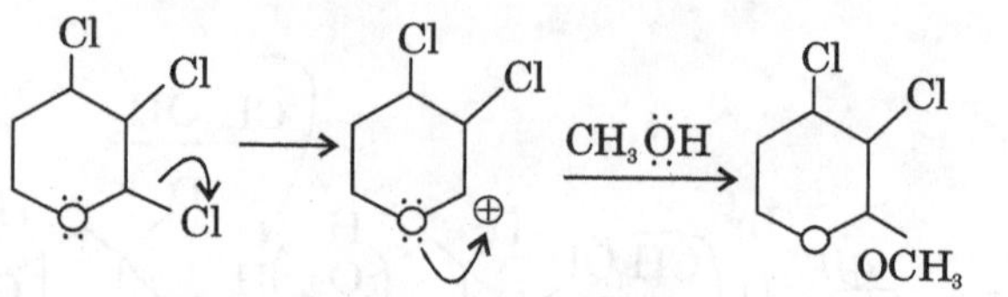

(carbocation stabilised by Resonance)

59. The carbocation in option 4 will be maximum stable.

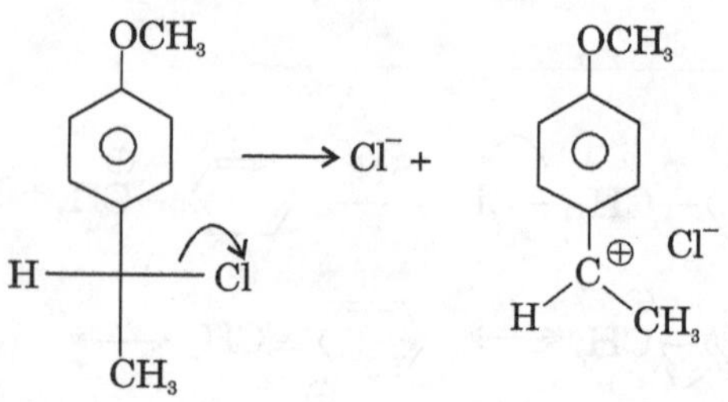

Since, carbocation is maximum stabilised, the halide ion will leave the carbocation readily resulting in maximum racemisation.

60. option 1,

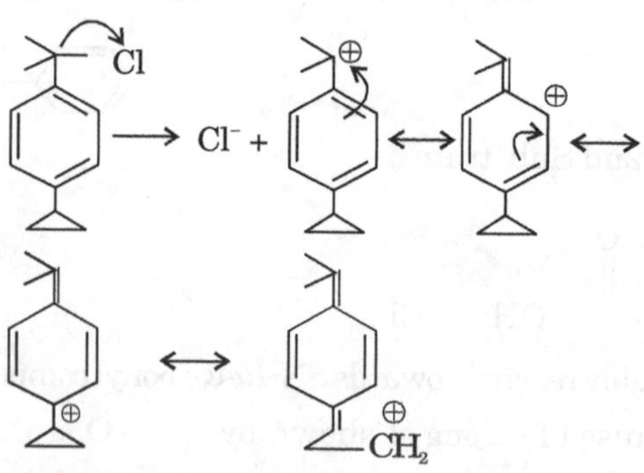

(stabilised by dancing resonance)

option 3,

Dancing resonance hampered due to SIR.

(Steric inhibition to Resonance)

61. In option (a),

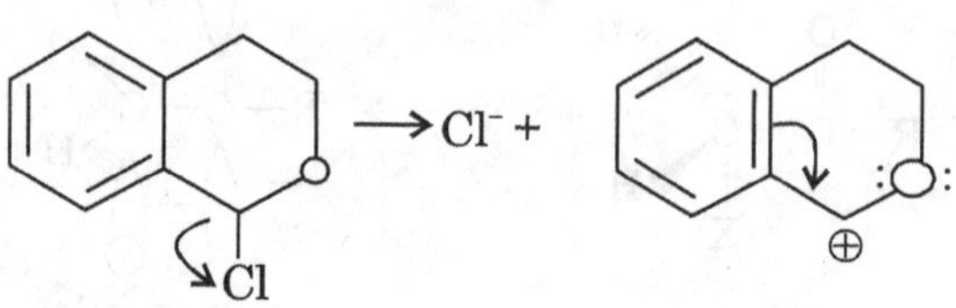

(Stabilised by π bond & also stabilised by lone pair of O)

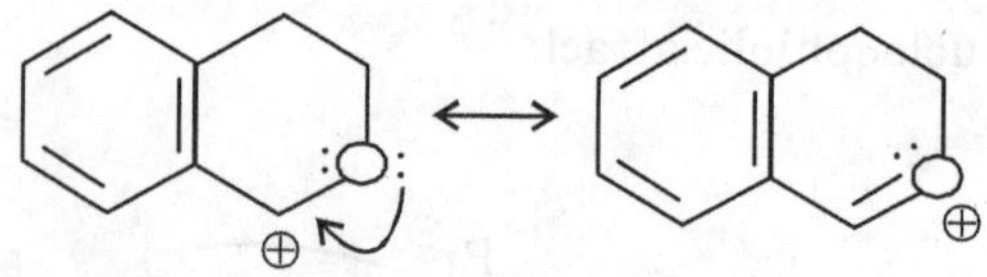

For,

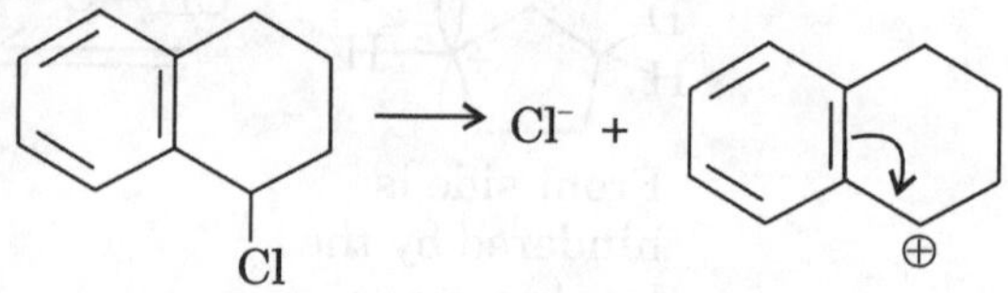

(Stabilised only by π bond)

For option (b),

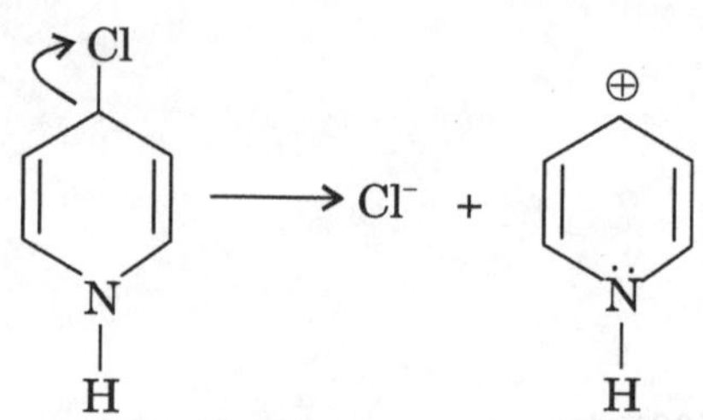

(AROMATIC)

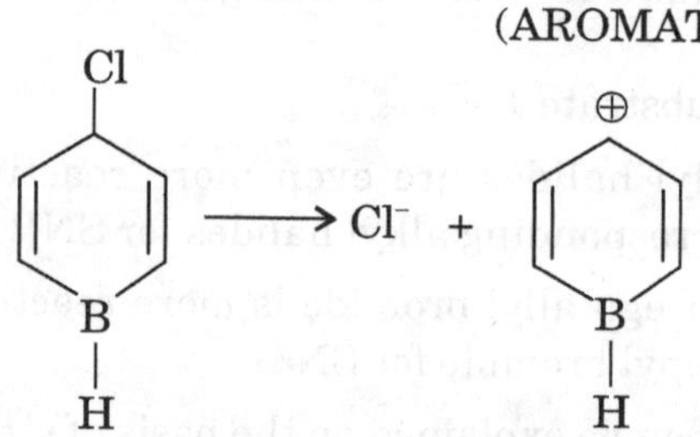

(ANTI - AROMATIC)

Stability:- AROMATIC > ANTI AROMATIC

For option (c),

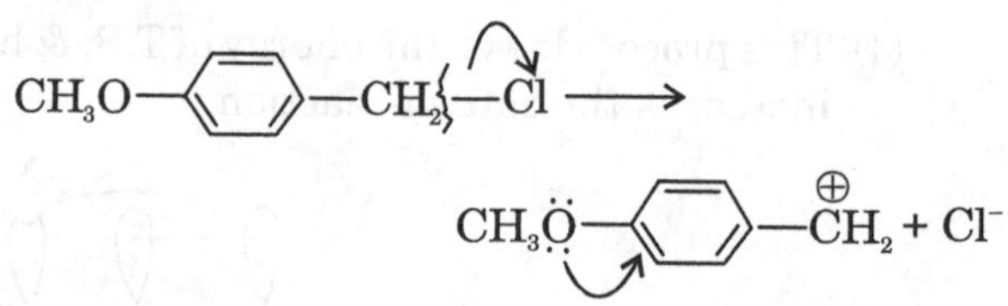

(+ M of —OCH_3 stabilises the carbocation more)

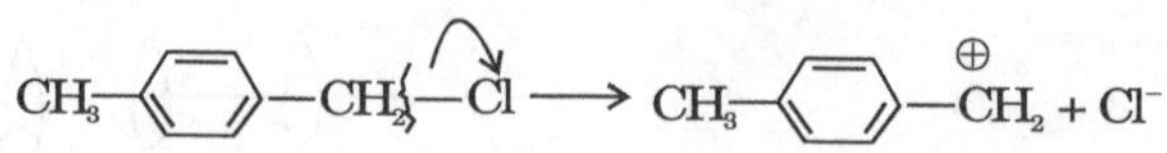

(Stabilised by + I & hyperconjugation)

Elimination Reactions

(E_1, E_2 & E_{1Cb})

62.

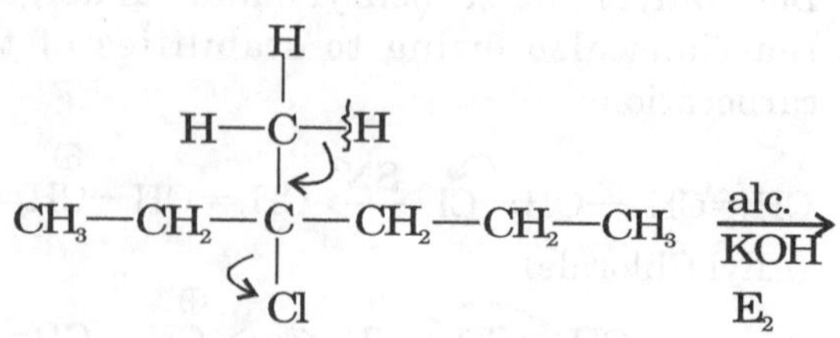

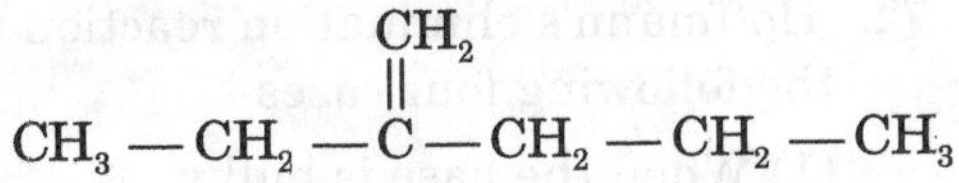

(neither geometrical nor optical, possible)

+

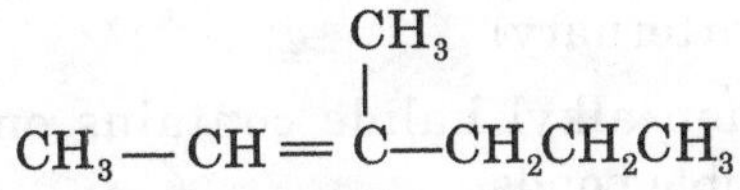

(Cis & trans)

+

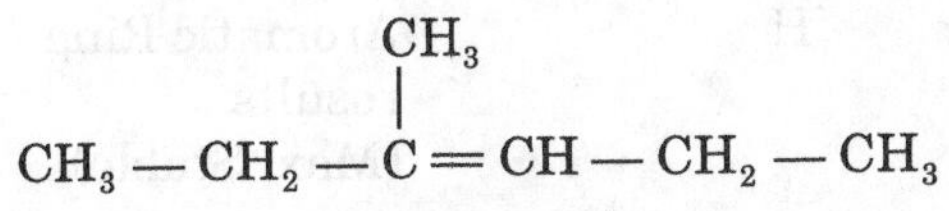

(Cis & Trans)

63.

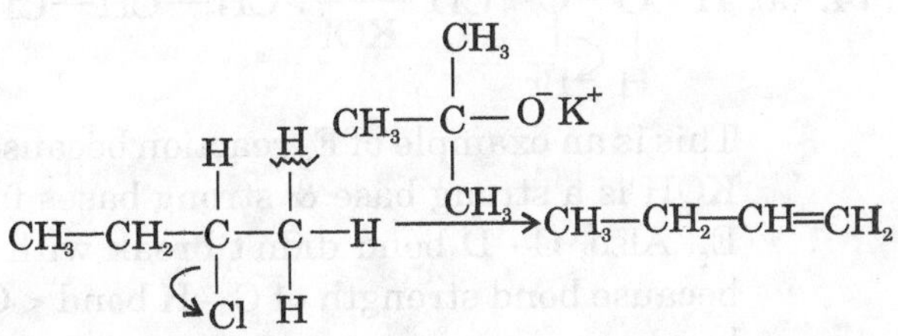

ter-butoxide is a bulky base (& a strong base). E_2 mechanism is favoured & Hoffmann's product is the major product.

64. Neopentyl halide cannot undergo E_2 elimination because it lacks β-hydrogen.

No 'H' attached with this C.

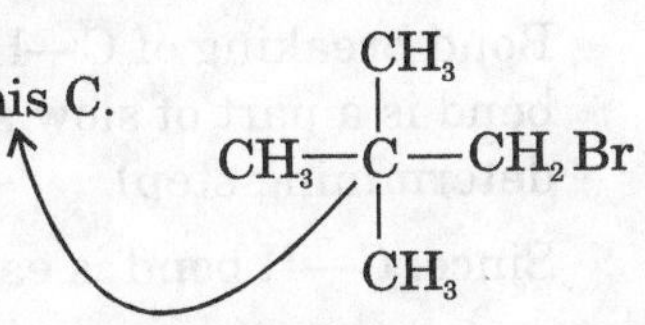

65. This reaction is an example of $E_{1\ cb}$ mechanism which occurs via carbanion formation. Poor leaving group favours $E_{1\ cb}$.

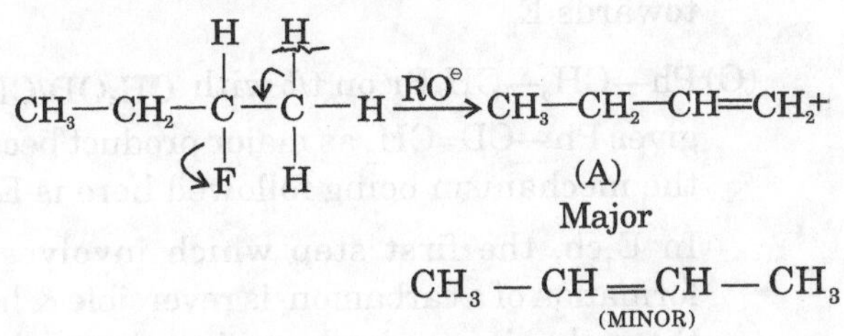

→ Hoffman's product is the major product (i.e. but-1-ene)

66. Stability of carbanion & presence of a poor leaving group (i.e., F^- ion) is the key here to solve this problem. The reaction occurs via E_{1cb} & Hoffmann's elimination rule is followed.

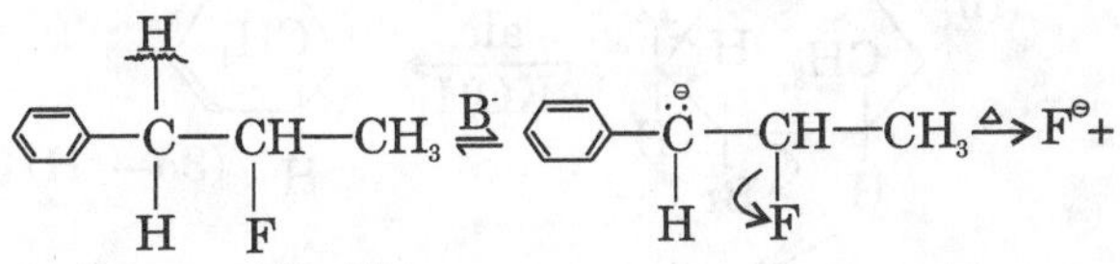

(Most acidic H is deprotonated)

67. For E_1, reactivity follows the order-3° halide > 2° halide > 1° halide (Based upon the stabilities of respective carbocations)

For E_2, reactivity follows the order-3° halide > 2° halide > 1° halide

(Based upon the stabilities of alkenes formed)

Also For E_2, reactivity follows the order-

Alkyl iodide > alkyl bromide > alkyl chloride > alkyl fluoride

(Based upon the leaving ability of halides ions which follows the order: $I^- > Br^- > Cl^- > F^-$)

68.

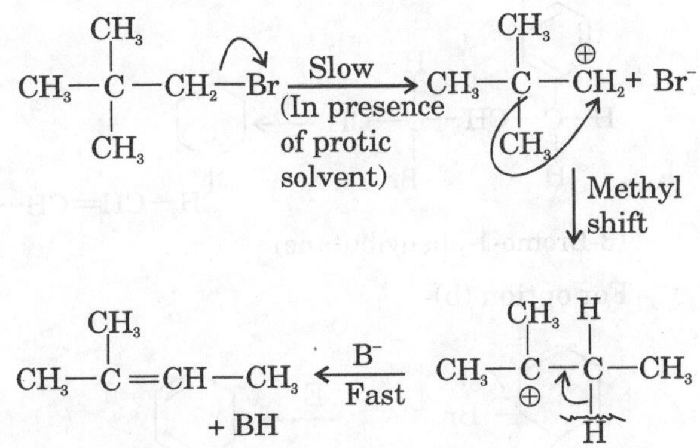

69. In molecule 1, an aromatic ring will be formed (max. stable)

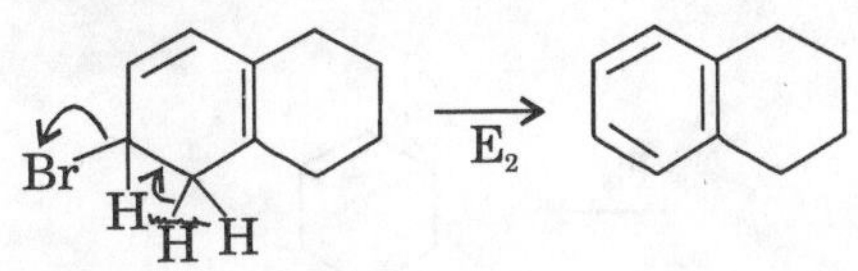

In molecule 3,

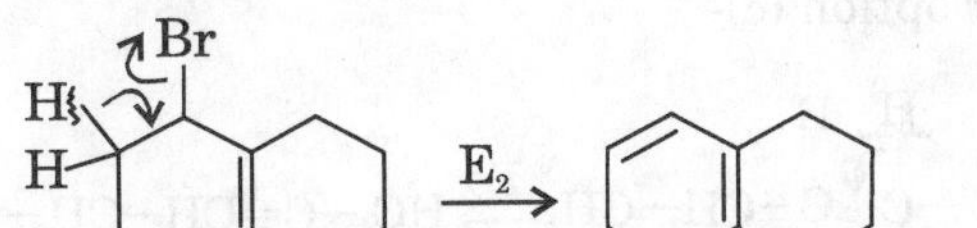

π bond - π bond Conjugation results

70. (a)

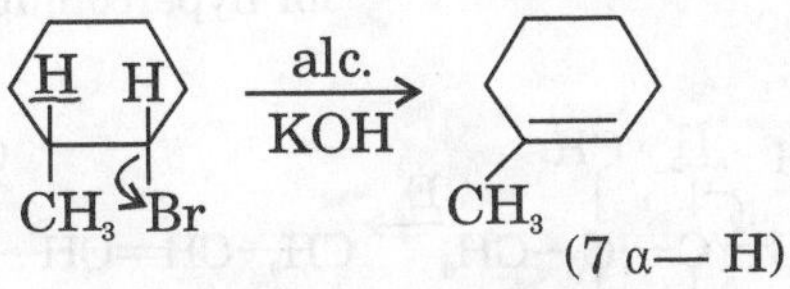

Elimination occurs with anti-periplanar orientation.

(b) 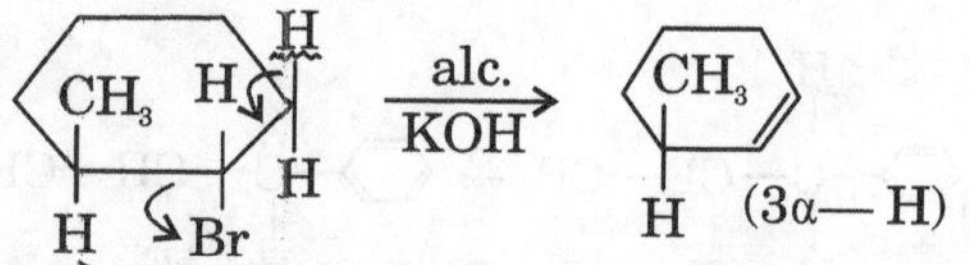

This 'H' is in syn periplanar Orientation

(c) 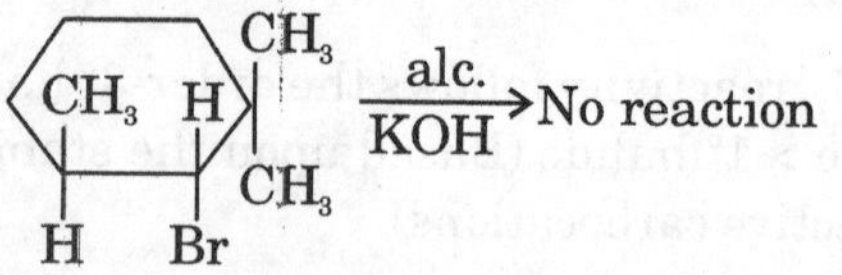

Non-availibility of Anti H wrt Br.

71. 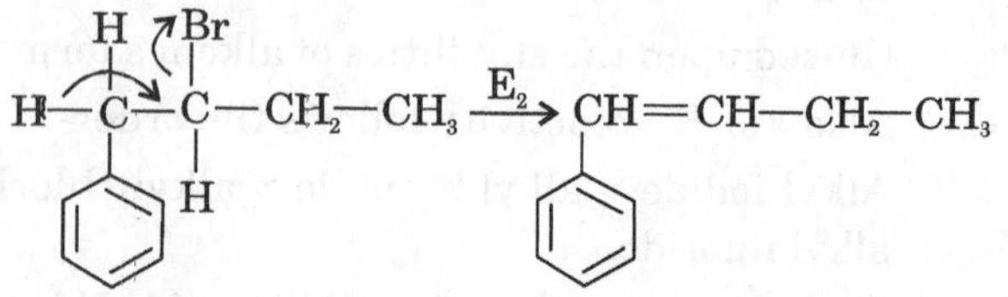

(2 - Bromo - 1 - phenyl butane) (π - π Conjugation) more stable alkene

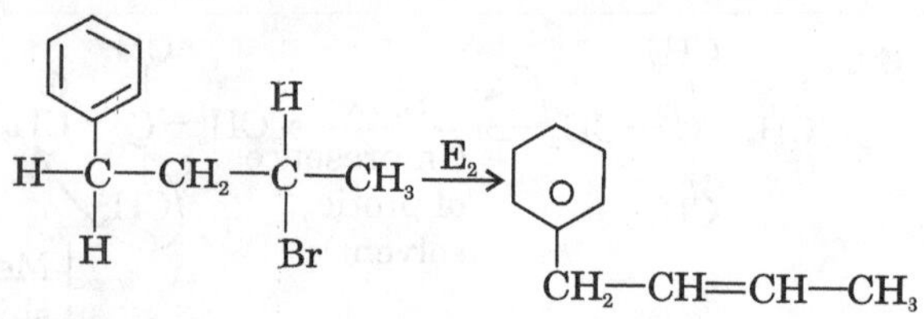

(3-Bromo-1-phenylbutane)

For option (b)-

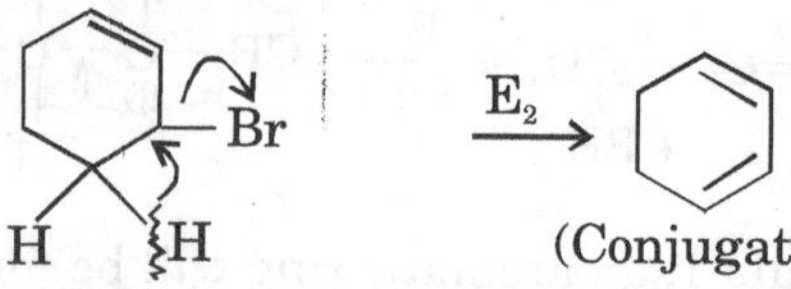

3 - Bromo cyclohexene (Conjugated diene) more stable

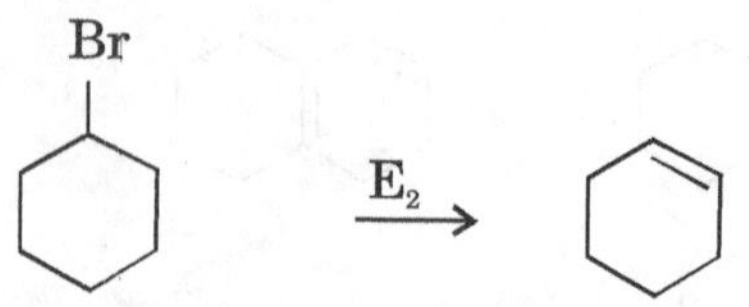

For option (c)-

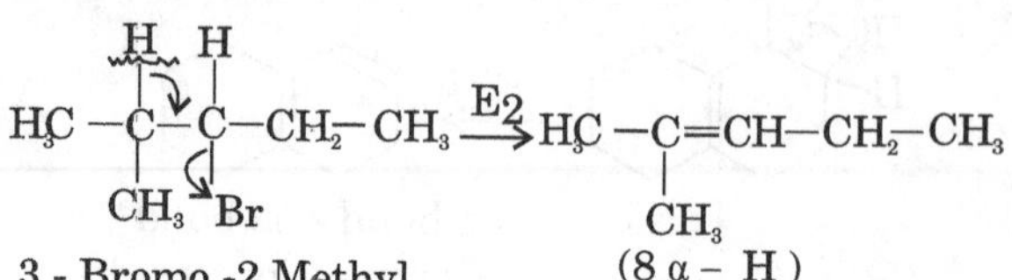

3 - Bromo -2 Methyl pentane (8 α - H) for hyperconjugation

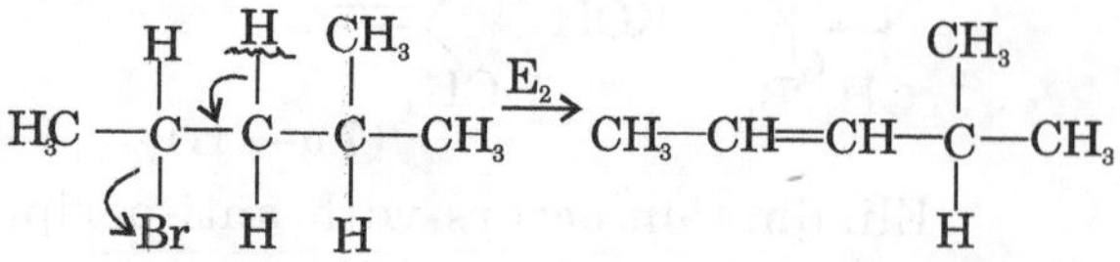

2 - Bromo - 4 - Methyl pentane (4 α - H)

72. Hoffmann's elimination reaction takes place in the following four cases-

(1) When the base is bulky

(2) When leaving group is poor eg. F^-, $\overset{\oplus}{N}R_3$, $\overset{\oplus}{S}R_2$

(3) Steric hindrance at β-carbon (eg. if Y–C is quarternary)

(4) When alkyl halide contains one or more double bonds.

73. 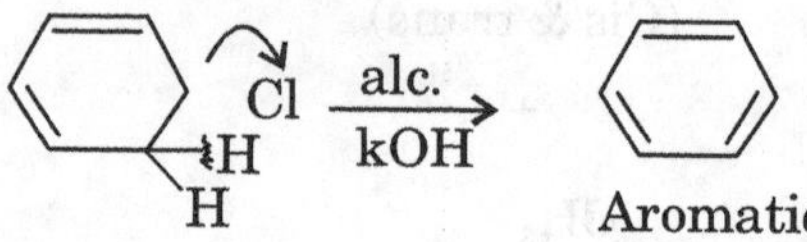

Aromatic Ring results (Max. Stable)

74. (a) 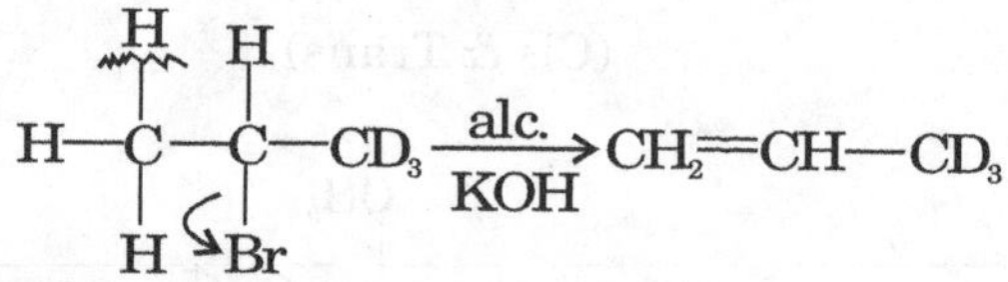

This is an example of E_2 reaction because alc. KOH is a strong base & strong bases favors E_2. Also, C—D bond didn't break with ease because bond strength of C—H bond < C—D bond.

(b) Reactivity of

$$Ph-\underset{Br}{\underset{|}{CH}}-CH_3 \;\&\; Ph-\underset{Br}{\underset{|}{CH}}-CD_3$$

for E_2 will be different.

Bond breaking of C—H/C—D bond & C—Br bond is a part of slow step (which is rate determining step)

Since, C—H bond is easy to cleave,

$\therefore Ph-\underset{Br}{\underset{|}{CH}}-CH_3$ is more reactive towards E_2.

(C) Ph—CH_2—CH_2Br on t/t with $CH_3OD/CH_3O^{\ominus}$ gives Ph—CD=CH_2 as major product because the mechanism being followed here is E_1cb. In E_1cb, the first step which involves the formation of a carbanion, is reversible & hence the carbanion, picks deuterium from solvent.

(D) Ph—CH_2—CH_2Br & Ph—CD_2—CH_2Br react with same rate for 'E_1 reaction'. In E_1 reaction, the slowest step involves the cleavage of C—Br bond, which is present in both. Breaking of C—H/C—D bond is part of fast step (which is not rate determining step)

75. (1) $CH_3-\underset{\underset{Cl}{|}}{CH}-CH_2-CH_2-CH_3$

$\xrightarrow[KOH]{alc.} CH_3-CH=CH-CH_2-CH_3$ +
Major P
(Cis + Trans)

$CH_2=CH-CH_2-CH_2-CH_3$

So, total 3 alkanes are possible.

(2) $CH_3-CH_2-\underset{\underset{Cl}{|}}{CH}-CH_2-CH_3 \xrightarrow[KOH]{alc.}$

$CH_3-CH=CH-CH_2-CH_3$
(Cis + TRANS)

(3) $CH_3-CH_2-CH_2-Cl \xrightarrow[KOH]{alc.} CH_3-CH=CH_2$
(Only one alkene is possible)

76. For molecule 1,

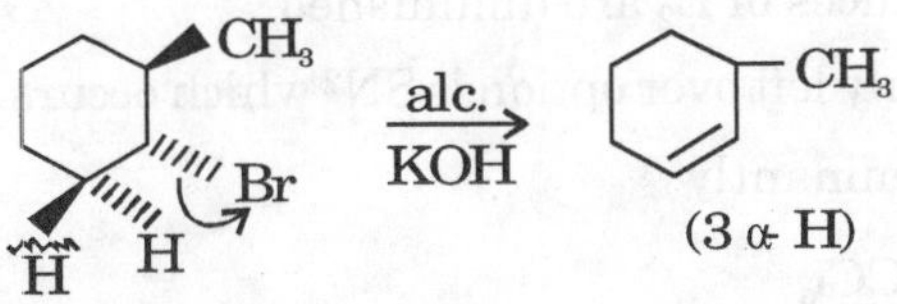

The 'H+' removed will have anti-orientation Br^-
For Molecule- 2

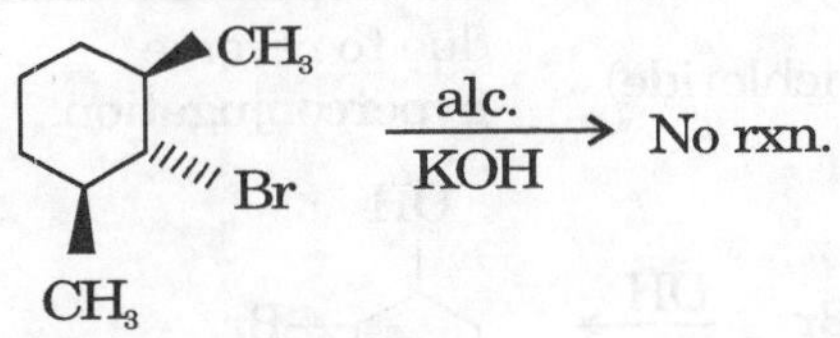

None of the H's on β — C is/are anti-periplanar.

For molecule- 3

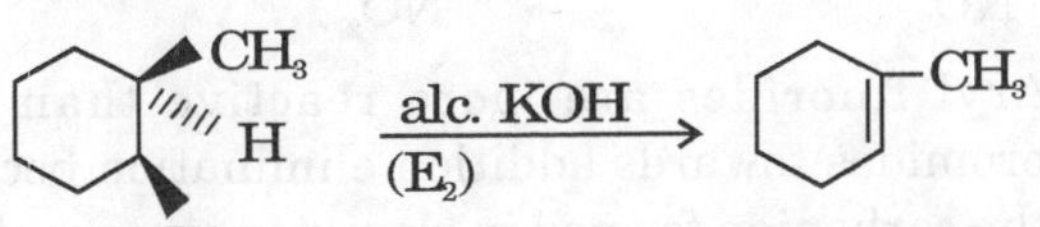

(Major product)
(7α - H)

Max, stable alkene will be formed by molecule 3, So reactivity towards E_2 follow the order-3>1>2

77. $CH_3-\underset{\underset{CH_3}{|}}{\overset{\overset{CH_3}{|}}{C}}-Br \xrightarrow{CH_3O^-Na^+} CH_3-\underset{\underset{CH_2}{\|}}{\overset{\overset{CH_3}{|}}{C}} + CH_3OH + NaBr$

(Major Product)

3° halides on reaction with anionic lewis base (strong base) undergoes E_2 predominantly.

78. For option 1, its a 1° alkyl halide. 1° halides, in general are reluctant to undergo elimination because alkenes formed are not very stable.

So, major product is formed via SN^2.

For option 2,

Its a 2° alkyl halide & with it, strong base like alkoxide prefers to perform E_2 mainly & a minor product is formed by SN^2.

For option 3-

Nucleophiles that are less basic than $\bar{O}H$ react with both 1° & 2° alkyl halides to give product of nucleophilic substitution in high yield.

Now, $\bar{C}N$ is a weaker base than $\bar{O}H$ because,

Acidic strength

$HCN > H_2O$

(pKa = 9.1) (pKa = 15.7)

79. 2° halides on reacting with a weaker nucleophile (like H_2O) undergo SN^1 mainly.

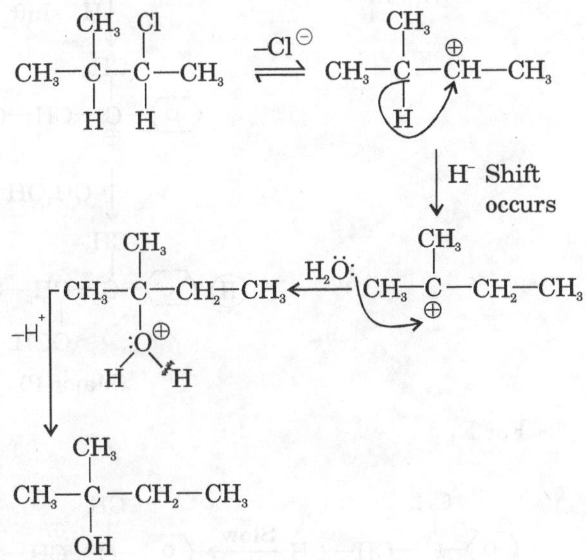

80. Isopropyl bromide is a secondary halide.

$CH_3-\underset{\underset{Br}{|}}{CH}-CH_3$

With 2° halides, weak basicity of nucleophiles favours substitution. In general, the nucleophiles which are less basic than $\bar{O}H$ give more substitution products rather than elimination.

Option 3 & 4 are hindered nucleophiles & bulky base favoring more elimination.

Out of option 1 & 2, $CH_3O^{\ominus}$ is more basic than $CH_3S^{\ominus}$. So, it will favor elimination more, in comparison to $CH_3S^{\ominus}$.

$CH_3S^{\ominus}$ is least basic. So, substitution product will dominate. Hence, substitution/elimination ratio is highest

81. For SN^1

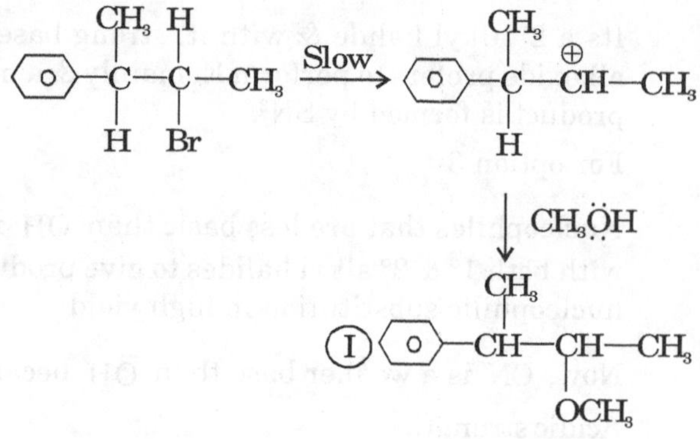

(Minor P)

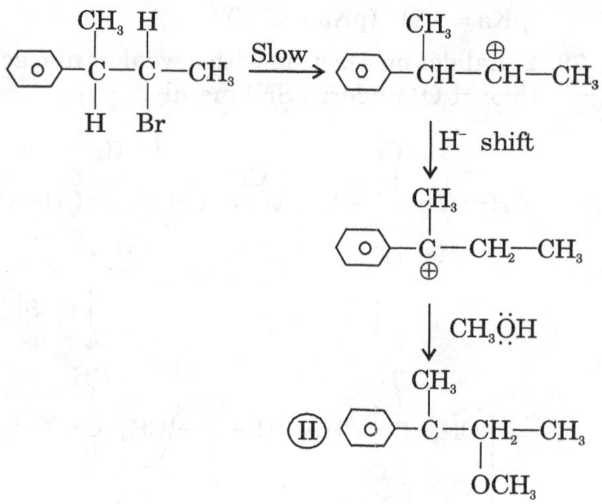

(Major P)

For E_1

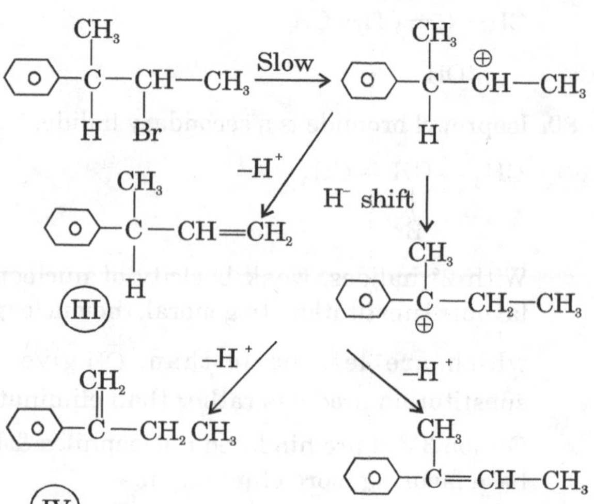

(Cis + TRANS)

(V) (VI)

82. (a) option is an alkyl fluoride (2° halide with ethoxide, a strong base). So, elimination is favored by Hoffmann's elimination (via E_1 cb)

(b) option is an alkyl bromide (2° halide) with a strong base (stronger than $\bar{O}H$); so elimination is favored via E_2 & Saytzeff's product is the major product.

(c) option is a 3° halide with bulky base. E_2 is favored & Hoffman's Product is the major product.

83. In option (a) ; its a 1° halide with little β-branching, weak nucleophile like 'alcohol' will tend to support SN^1 via hydride shift followed by nucleophillic attack.

In option (b), its a 3° halide with a strong base ($\bar{O}H$) favoring E_2 reaction.

Option (c) is a 1° halide which can neither undergo SN^1 nor E^1. Also; $(C_2H_5)_3$ N is not a strong base, so chances of E_2 are diminished.

The only left over option is SN^2 which occurs here, predominantly.

84.

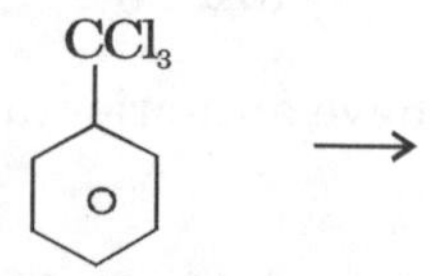

(Benzotrichloride)

It is meta directing for electrophillic attack due to reverse hyperconjugation.

85.

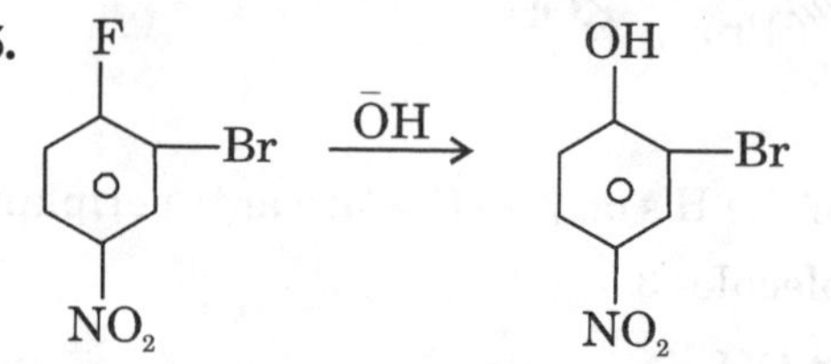

Aryl fluorides are more reactive than aryl bromides towards addition elimination because the carbanion formed in slow step is more stable in fluorides than bromides.

86. In the presence of light, free radical substitution occurs at benzylic C.

In the presence of lewis acid (as anhydrous $AlCl_3$), electrophillic aromatic substitution occurs & para product is major.

87. Aryl SN^2 involves the formation of carbanion. EWG's (electron withdrawing groups) will stabilise the carbanions & favour aryl SN^2.

88. Elimination addition (benzyne) mechanism involves loses of proton from a position which is ortho to halogen (i.e., most acidic H).

In option (d), i.e., 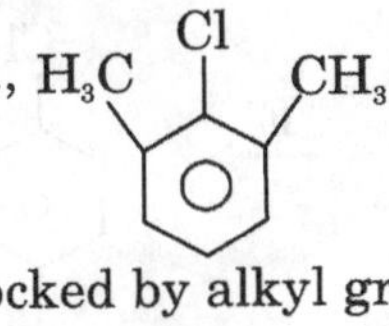, both the ortho positions are blocked by alkyl groups.

89. In the presence of $Na\overset{+}{\bar{N}}H_2$, aryl halide will undergo benzyne mechanism to form nucleophillic substitution product. Also, $\bar{N}H_2$ will act like a base & cause elimination to form an alkene.

90. In option (c), $-NO_2$ group is pushed out of plane of the ring due to repulsions by two adjacent methyl groups. Hence, the carbanion formed will not be stabilised by -M of nitro.

91. 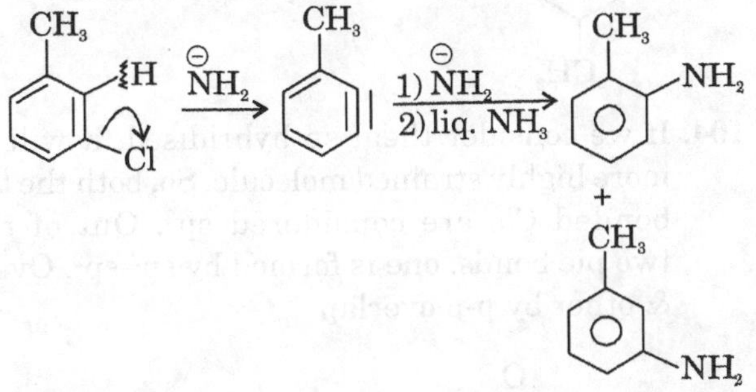

Also,

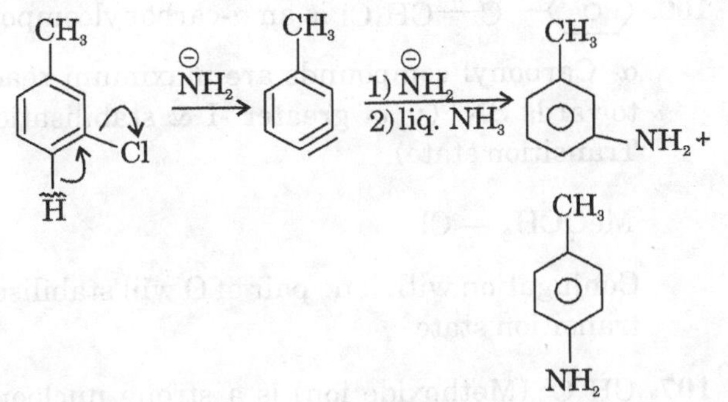

92. 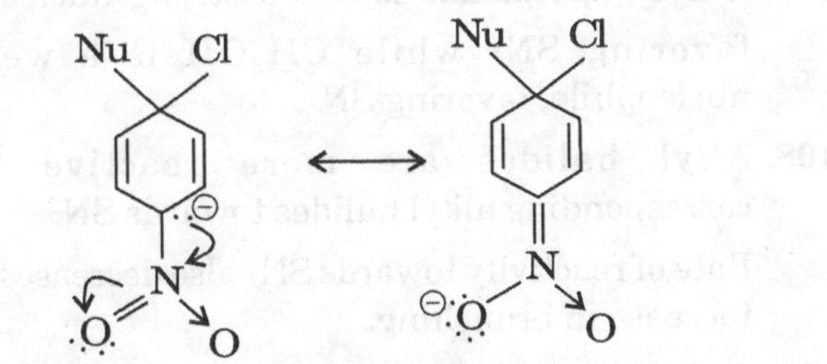

Carbanion stabilised by -M and – I of nitro.

93. 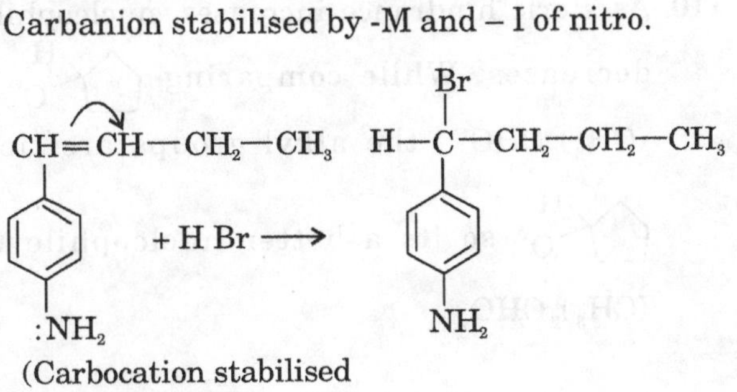

(Carbocation stabilised by + M of NH_2)

94. 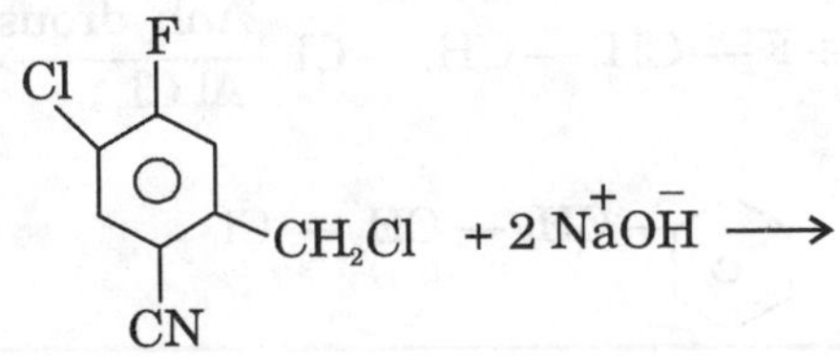

— CH_2Cl undergoes nucleophilic substitution. Also, –'CN' is present at para wrt F, so will stabilize the carbanion. Hence, 'F' gets substituted by –'OH' (by addition elimination)

95. —I of halogens will stabilize the carbanion.

96. Reaction (a) follows addition- elimination via formation of a carbanion (which is stabilised by —M & —I of NO_2)

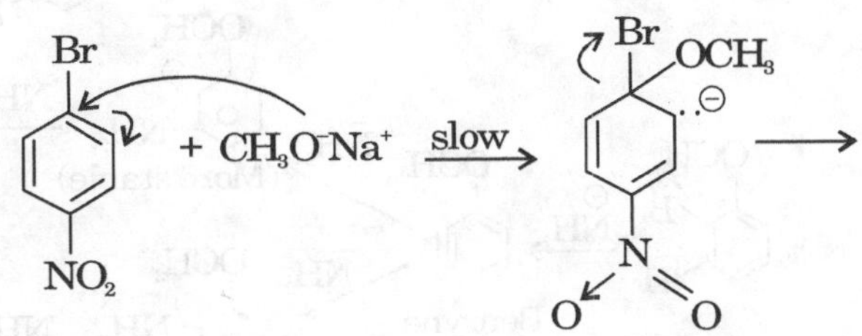

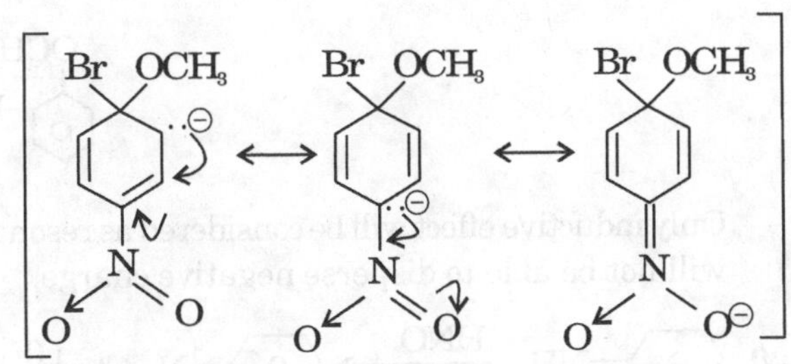

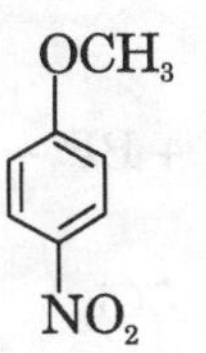

Reaction (b) follows S_N2

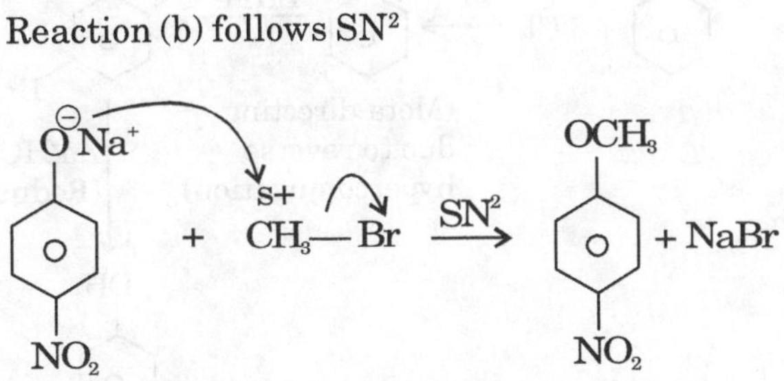

Reaction (c) does not occur because aryl halides do not undergo nucleophillic substitution easily because of partial double bond character.

97. 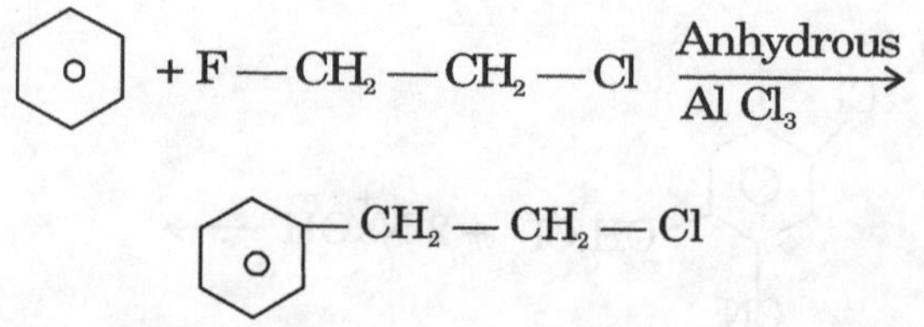

98. In option (d), benzyne mechanism cannot operate because there no 'H' available at 'ortho' to halogen.

Also, addition elimination cannot occur because the carbanion is not stabilised because of Electron donating groups.

99. 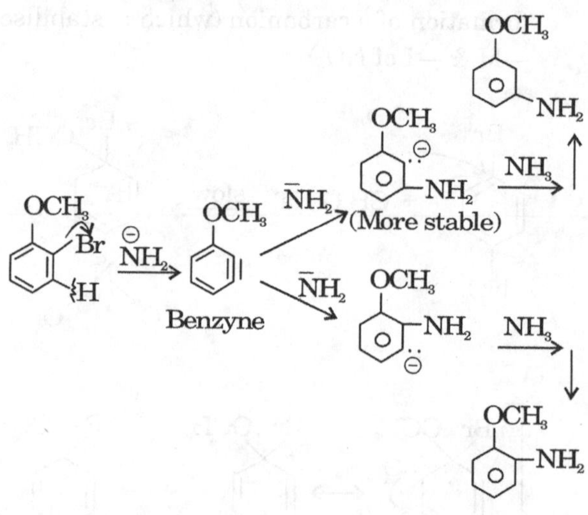

Only inductive effect will be considered as resonance will not be able to disperse negative charge.

100. 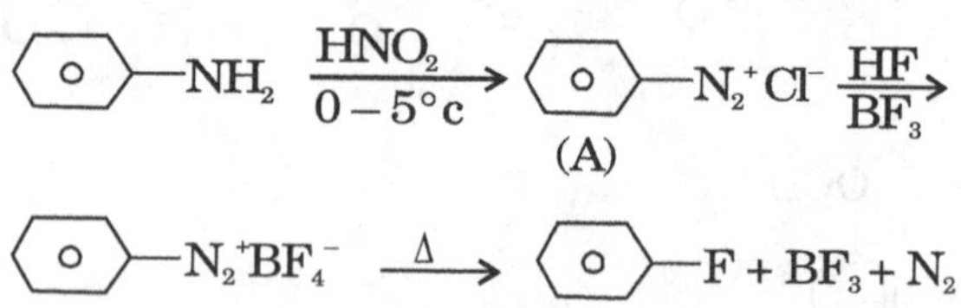

101. 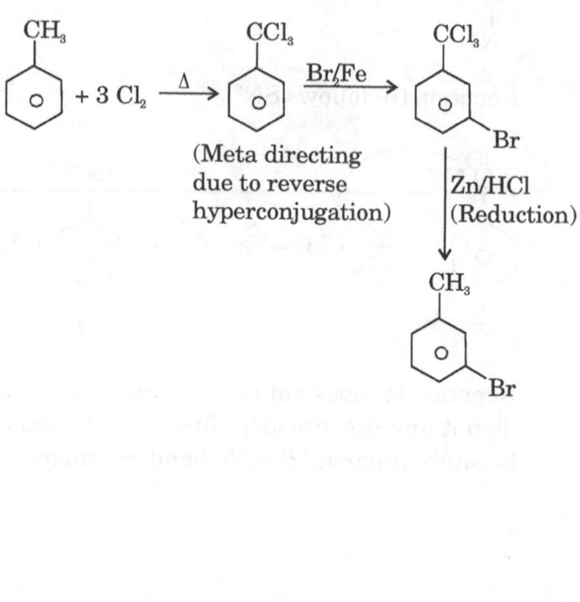

103. 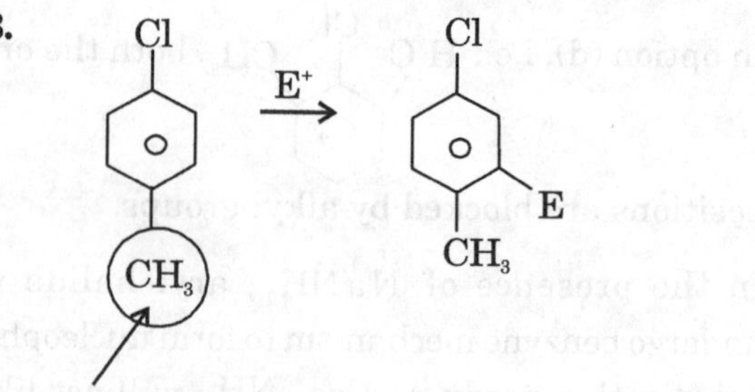

More activating group.
(O, p directing due to hyperconjugation)

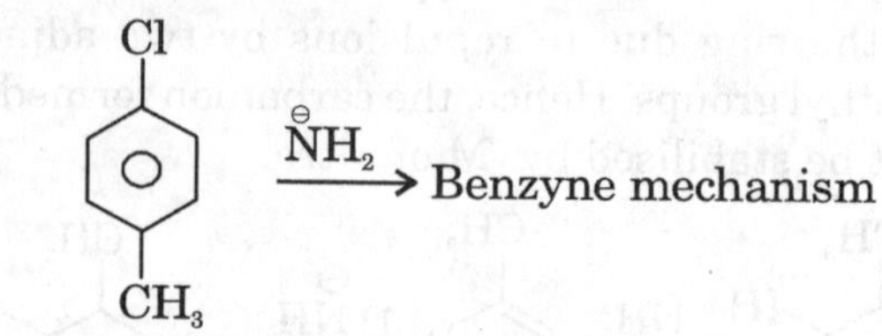

104. If we consider them sp hybridised, it will be a more highly strained molecule. So, both the triple bonded C's are considered sp^2. Out of these two pie bonds, one is formed by sp^2-sp^2. Overlap & other by p-p overlap.

106. 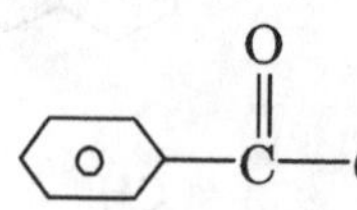 is an α-carbonylcompound.

α- Carbonyl compounds are maximum reactive towards SN^2 (∵ of greater -I & stabilisation of Transition state)

$Me\ddot{O}CH_2 - Cl$

Conjugation with lone pair of O will stabilise the transition state.

107. $CH_3O^{\ominus}$ (Methoxide ion) is a strong nucleophile favoring SN^2 while CH_3OH is a weaker nucleophile, favoring SN^1.

108. Allyl halides are more reactive than corresponding alkyl halides towards SN^2.

Rate of reactivity towards SN^2 also decreases with increase in branching.

110. As steric hindrance increases, nucleophilicity decreases. While comparing 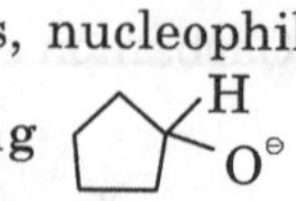 and $(CH_3)_2CHO^{\ominus}$, the alkyl groups are tied in 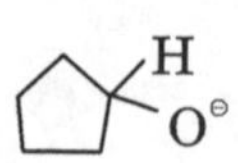 so its a better nucleophile than $(CH_3)_2CHO^{\ominus}$.

113. Reactivity is directly proportional to the stability of product formed.

(1) 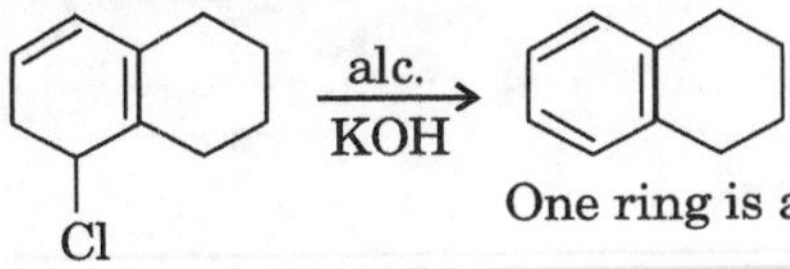

One ring is aromatic

(2) 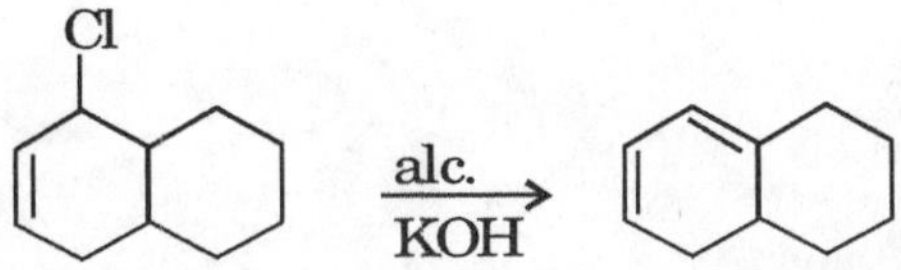

Conjugated diene is formed

(3) 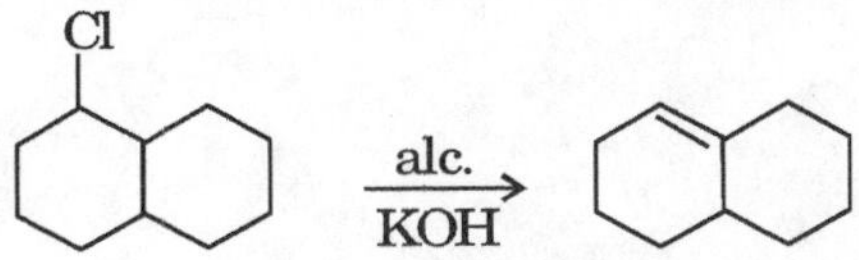

Isolated alkene is formed

114. Addition elimination occurs.

115. It's a case of alkyl fluoride & F^- is a poor leaving group. So, elimination will occur via E_1cb mechanism & Hoffmann's product will be the major product.

116. Wrt option 3, carbocation formed is max. stable.
– Resonance stabilised & also, it is away from $>C=O$ (Electron withdrawing group)

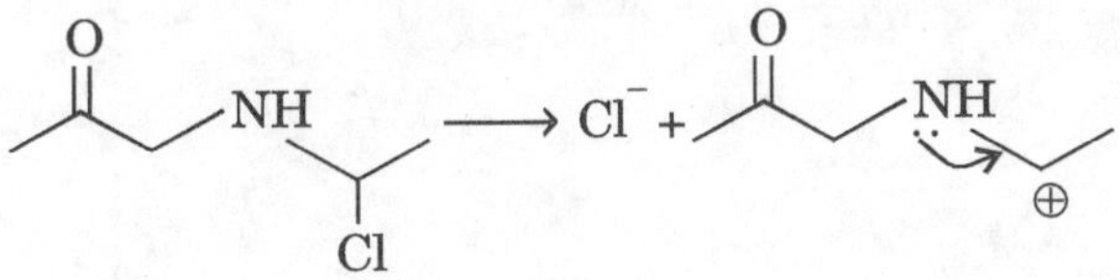

117. Presence of $-NO_2$ group will favour addition elimination reaction in Aryl halide. Also, Aryl fluorides are more reactive than aryl chlorides towards addition elimination. So, F^- gets substituted as follows-

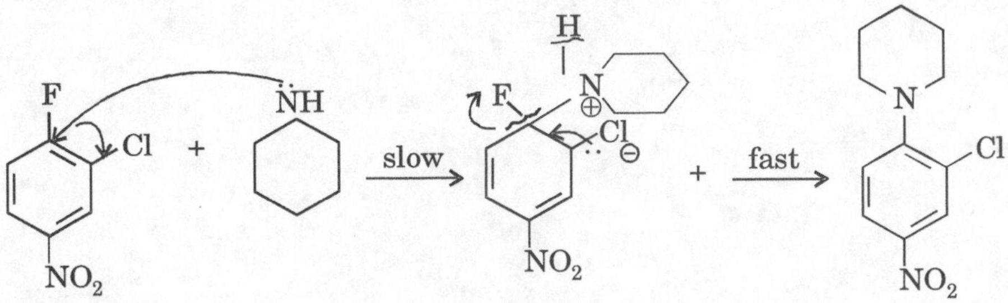

11

CHAPTER

Alcohols, Phenols and Ethers

Alcohols, Phenols & Ethers

1. Which of the following statements is /are true for glycerol?

(1) Its IUPAC name is propane – 1,2,3-triol

(2) It is a monohydric alcohol

(3) It is a trihydric alcohol

(4) It has one 2° alcoholic & one primary alcoholic group.

(a) 1, 2,& 4 but not 3 (b) 2 & 3 but not 1 & 4

(c) 1, 3 & 4 but not 2 (d) 1 & 3 but not 2 & 4

2. Which one of the following is ethyl methyl carbinol

(a) C_2H_5OH (b) CH_3OH

(c) $(CH_3)_2CHOH$ (d) $CH_3CH_2CH(OH)CH_3$

3. Which one of the following is named 'acid' but lacks 'COOH' group?

(a) Phthalic acid (b) Carbonic acid

(c) Picric acid (d) Phenyl acetic acid

4. Identify the mismatch

(a) Absolute alcohol – 100 % pure ethanol

(b) Wood spirit – Methanol

(c) Power alcohol – Ethanol & Petrol

(d) Rubbing alcohol – n–propyl alcohol

5. 1, 2, 3 – trihydroxy benzene is also known as–

(a) Pyrogallol (b) Phloroglucinol

(c) Resorcinol (d) Quinol

6. Ethers can act as–

(a) Lewis acid (b) lewis base

(c) Bronsted acid (d) amphiprotic species

7. Neopentyl alcohol is

(a) a primary alcohol (b) a secondary alcohol

(c) a tertiary alcohol (d) None of these

8. What is correct about ethylene glycol?

(a) It is a dihydric alcohol

(b) It is a vicinal diol

(c) It is a trihydric alcohol.

(d) Both a & b

9. The correct IUPAC name for isopropyl alcohol is

(a) Hexan – 2 – ol

(b) Butan – 2 – ol

(c) 3– methyl butan – 2 – ol

(d) Propan – 2 – ol

10. Which one of the following is a 3° allylic alcohol?

(a) $CH_2 = CH - OH$

(b) $CH_2 = CH - CH_2 - OH$

(c) $CH_2 = CH - C(CH_3)(OH) - CH_3$

(d) $CH_2 = CH - CH(CH_3) - OH$

11. Which of the following isomerism can be exhibited by methoxy methane ?

(a) Chain isomerism (b) Position isomerism
(c) Metamerism (d) None of these

12. 1 – methoxy propane & 1 – ethoxy ethane are –

(a) Functional isomers
(b) Position isomers
(c) Metamers
(d) Tautomers

Methods of Preparation of Alcohols

13. $CH_3-\underset{\underset{CH_3}{|}}{CH}-CH_2-NH_2 \xrightarrow[+HCl]{NaNO_2(aq)}$

The major product in the above reaction is –

(a) $CH_3-\underset{\underset{CH_3}{|}}{CH}-CH_2OH$

(b) $CH_3-\overset{\overset{CH_3}{|}}{\underset{\underset{CH_3}{|}}{C}}-OH$

(c) $CH_3-\overset{\overset{CH_3}{|}}{\underset{\underset{CH_3}{|}}{C}}-Cl$

(d) All of these

14. A 1° alcohol can be formed by reacting CH_3MgI with –

(a) ethyl acetate (b) epoxy ethane
(c) ethane nitrile (d) acetone

15. Which of the following reactions will yield 2 – Propanol?

(I) $CH_2=CH-CH_3 \xrightarrow{H_3O^+}$

(II) $CH_3CHO \xrightarrow[2)H_3O^+]{1)CH_3MgI}$

(III) $HCHO \xrightarrow[2)H_3O^+]{1)C_2H_5MgI}$

(IV) $CH_3-CH=CH_2 \xrightarrow[alk.KMnO_4]{cold}$

(a) both I & II (b) both II & III
(c) both II & IV (d) both I & III

16. The number of moles of sodium used for reacting with the final products (A) & (B) respectively are

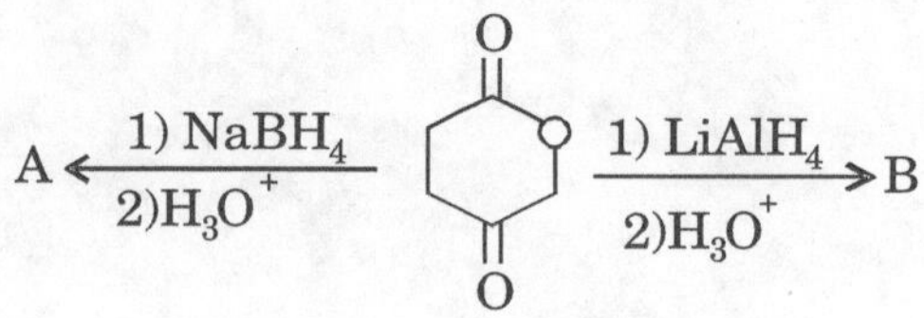

(a) 3,3 (b) 1,3
(c) 3,1 (d) 1,1

17. Consider the following three molecules

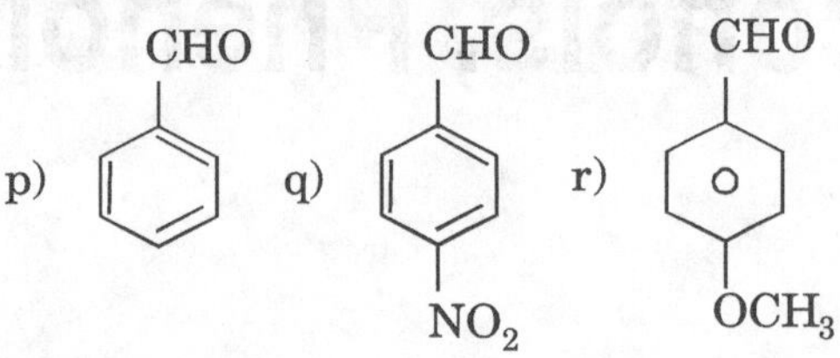

Correct order of reactivity of these molecules towards $NaBH_4$ is

(a) q > p > r (b) r > p > q
(c) r > q > p (d) p > q > r

18. Consider the following reaction–

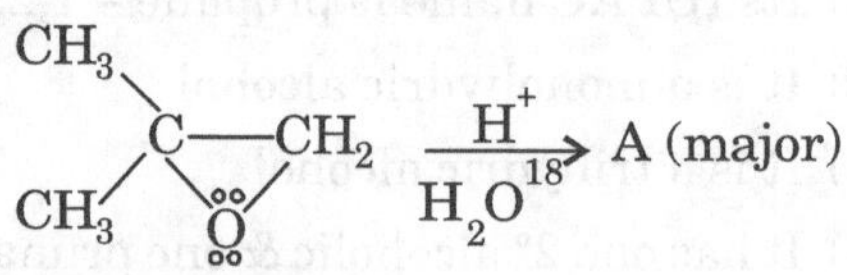

Then 'A' is

(a) $(CH_3)_2C(OH)-CH_2\overset{18}{O}H$

(b) $(CH_3)_3C-\overset{18}{O}H$

(c) $(CH_3)_2C(\overset{18}{O}H)-CH_2OH$

(d) $(CH_3)_2CH-CH_2-\overset{18}{O}H$

19. Consider the following reaction–

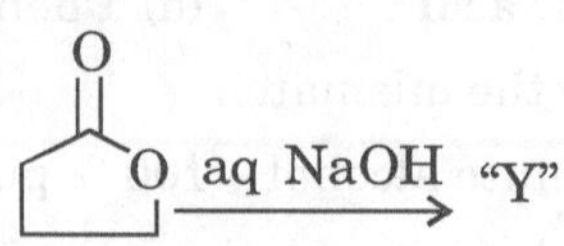

The product 'Y' in the above reaction is

(a) 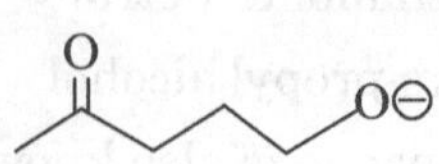 (b) 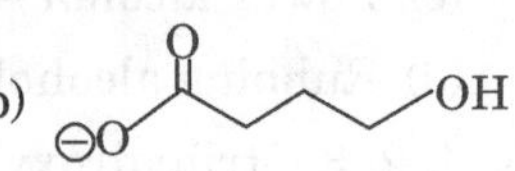

(c) 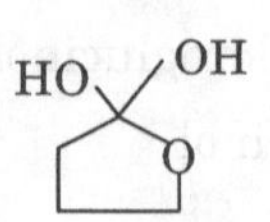 (d) 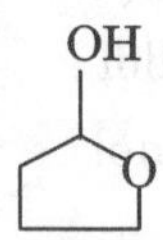

20. Identify 'X' in the following reaction –

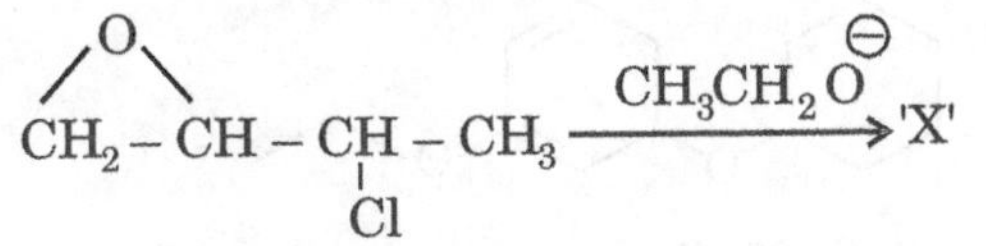

(a) 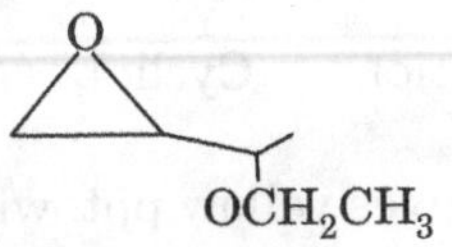 (b) 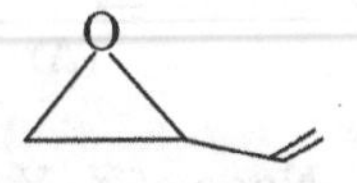

(c) 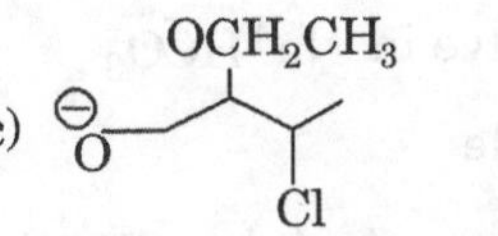 (d) 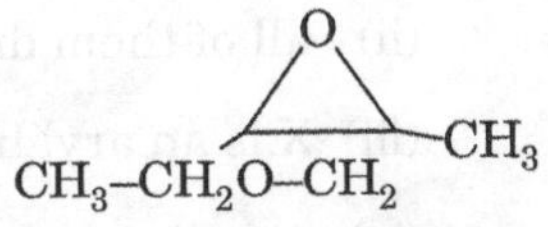

21. The enzyme which converts glucose to ethylalcohol is

(a) Zymase (b) Invertase

(c) Maltose (d) diastase

22. Which of the following enzyme converts maltose to glucose

(a) Invertase (b) Zymase

(c) Maltase (d) Diastase

23. Ethyl alcohol containing 9.5% methyl alcohol & 0.5% pyridine is called

(a) Spirit (b) Denatured spirit

(c) Rectified spirit (d) Absolute alcohol

24. Which of the following pairs can be used as a starting material to prepare phenyl-2-pentanol?

(a) 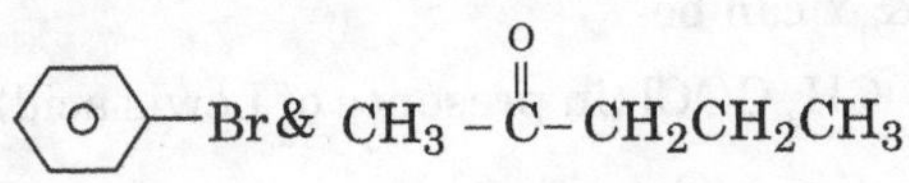

(b) 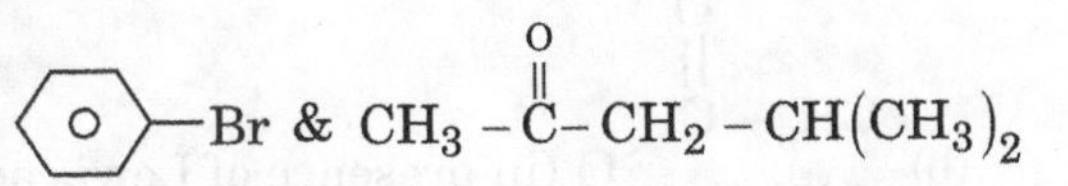

(c) 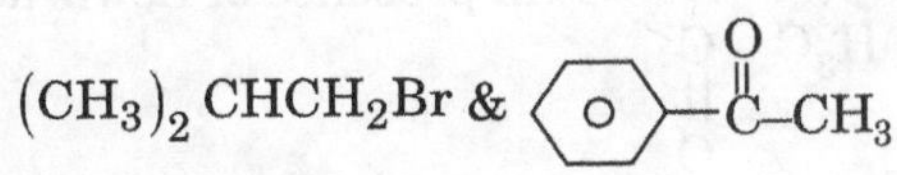

(d) None of these

25. Consider the reaction given below–

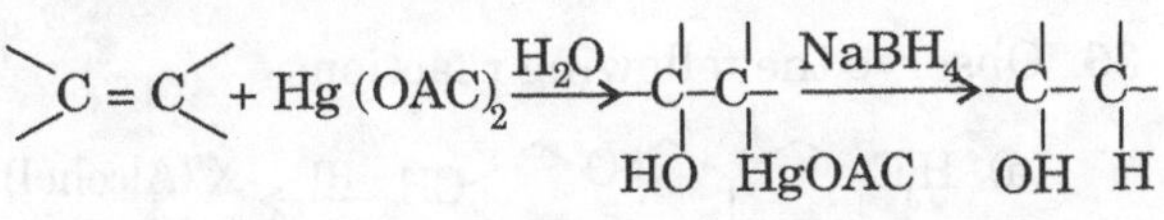

Select the correct statement (s)wrt reaction given

(1) It is called oxymercuration – demercuration

(2) Attack by water occurs giving product by markownikoffs orientation

(3) This reaction does not involve any rearrangements

(4) Oxymercuration involves electrophilic attack on the double bond by +vely charged mercury species.

(a) Only 1 is correct

(b) Only 2 & 3 are correct

(c) Only 1 & 4 are correct

(d) all are correct

26. Which of the following reactions result in the formation of 2–methyl–2–butanol?

(a) 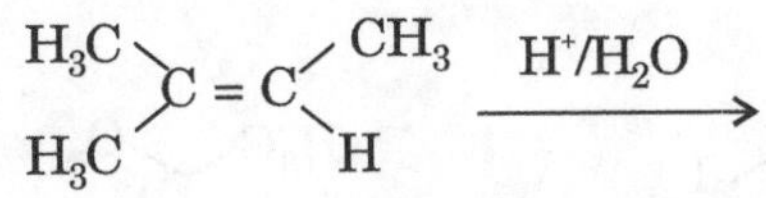

(b) 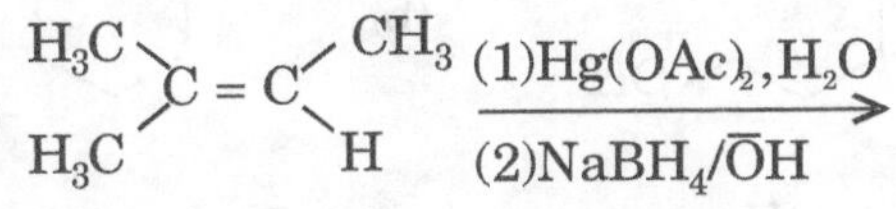

(c) 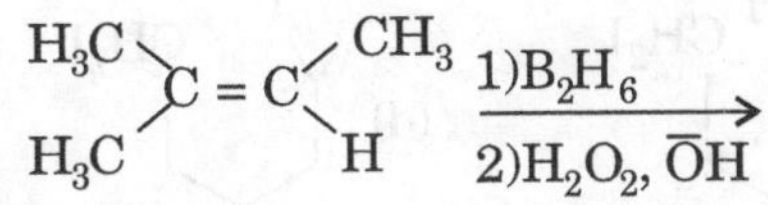

(d) Both a & b

27. What is true about Hydroboration –Oxidation ?

(a) Hydroboration involes the use of BH_3, which is a strong electrophile

(b) There is formation of a four membered cyclic transition state.

(c) There is syn addition of H & OH with anti markovnikov's Orientation

(d) All the statements are correct.

28. Which is correct wrt following reaction sequence

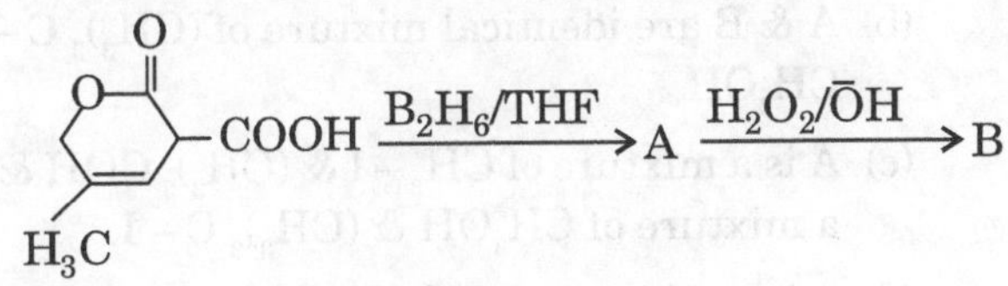

(a) A is 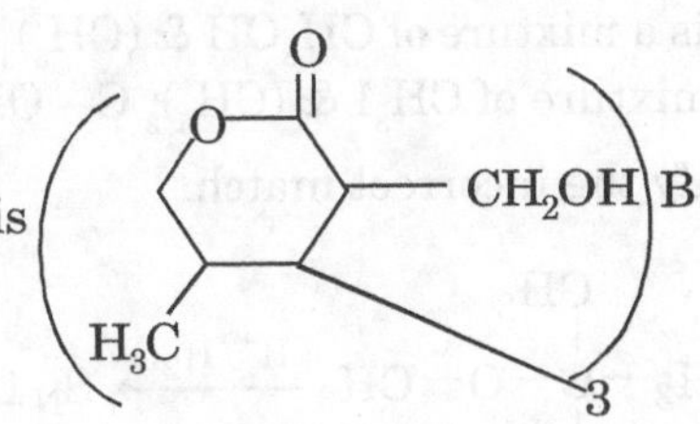

(b) A is 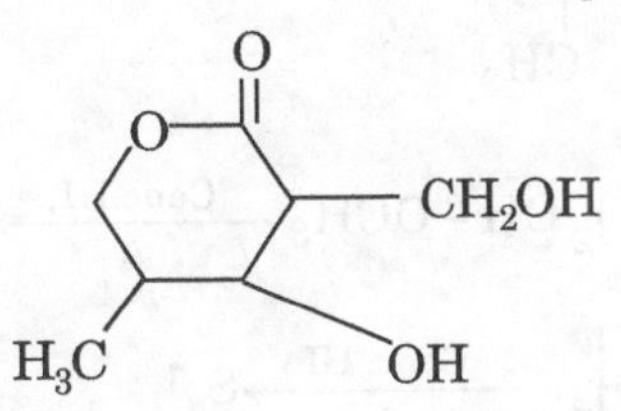

(c) B is 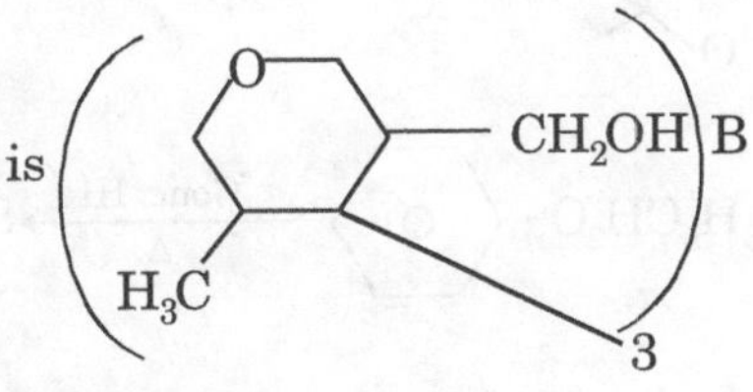

(d) None of these

Chemical Properties of Ether

29. Identify the final major product in the following reaction-

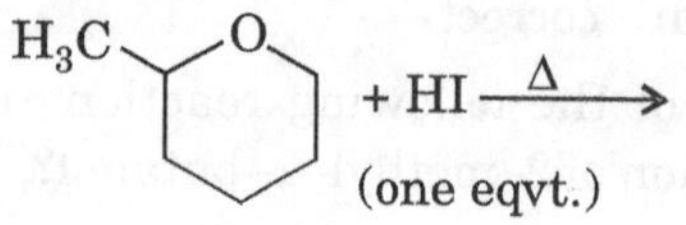

(a) 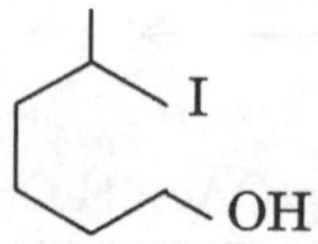 (b) 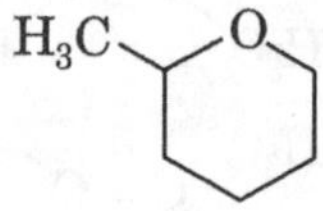

(c) 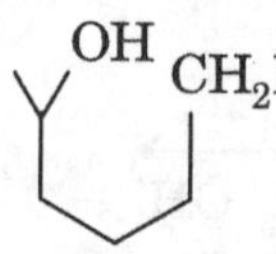 (d) 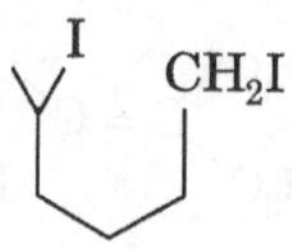

30. Identify the correct statement (s) wrt the following reaction-

$(CH_3)_3\ COCH_3$ (ether)

Conc. HI ↙ B (mixture); Anhyd. HI ↘ A (mixture)

(a) A & B are identical mixture of CH_3I & $(CH_3)_3$ COH

(b) A & B are identical mixture of $(CH_3)_3$ C – I & CH_3OH

(c) A is a mixture of CH_3 – I & $(CH_3)_3$ COH & B is a mixture of CH_3OH & $(CH_3)_3$ C – I.

(d) A is a mixture of CH_3OH & $(CH_3)_3$ C – I & B is a mixture of CH_3I & $(CH_3)_3$ C – OH.

31. Identify the incorrect match.

(a) $CH_3-\underset{CH_3}{\overset{CH_3}{C}}-O-CH_3 \xrightarrow{H^+/H_2O} S_N1$

(b) $(CH_3)_2CH-OCH_3 \xrightarrow[\Delta]{\text{Conc.HI,}} S_N2$

(c) 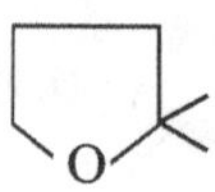 $\xrightarrow[\Delta]{\text{Conc. HI}} S_N1$

(d) $C_6H_5CH_2O$– 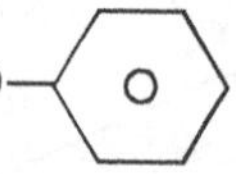 $\xrightarrow[\Delta]{\text{Conc. HI}} S_N2$

32. For the following reaction, what is correct?

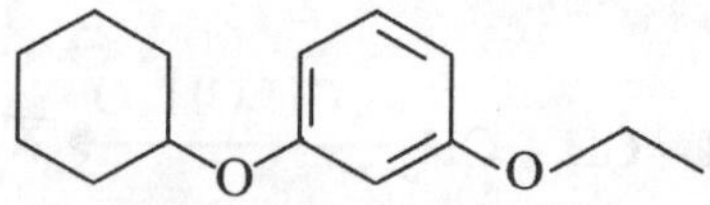

$\xrightarrow{\text{HI, 373 K}}$ X (Aromatic) + Y (Cyclic) + Z (Acyclic)

(i) None of X, Y, Z gives yellow ppt. with $IO^{\ominus}$

(ii) all of them dissolve in $Na^+H\overline{C}O_3$

(iii) X is an aryl halide

(iv) Acyclic product on attack by $\overline{O}H$ gives 'W' which gives positive holoform test.

(a) both iii & iv (b) only iv

(c) both i & iv (d) both i & iii

33. Which of the following can form coordinate complexes with Lewis acids?

(a) BF_3 (b) $AlCl_3$

(c) R–MgX (d) All of these

34. Diethyl ether reacts with PCl_5 to form

(a) ethanol & ethyl chloride

(b) ethyl chloride + H_3PO_3

(c) ethyl chloride + $POCl_3$

(d) ethyl chloride + H_3PO_2

35. Ethers can react with X & Y to form esters. Then X & Y can be-

(a) CH_3 COCl (in presence of Lewis acid)

(b) 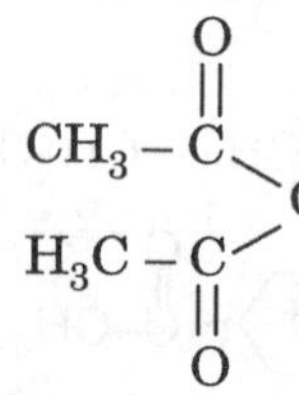 (in presence of Lewis acid)

(c) dil. H_2SO_4

(d) Both a & b

36. Observe the following reactions-

(a) 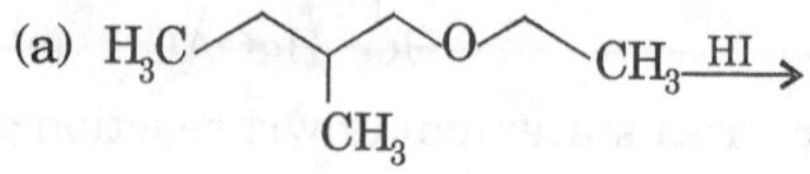 $\xrightarrow{HI}$ X (Alcohol) + Y (Alkyl halide)

(b) 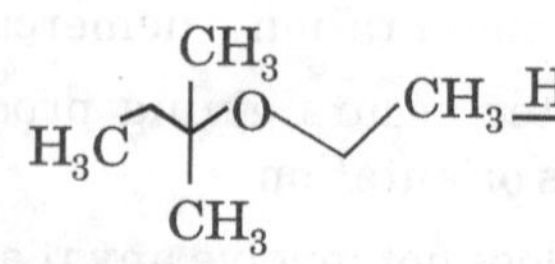 $\xrightarrow{HI}$ W (alcohol) + S (alkyl halide)

(c) $X \xrightarrow{R_1} S$

(d) $Y \xrightarrow{R_2} W$

The reagents R_1 & R_2 can be, respectively

(a) NaI/acetone, aq. $AgNO_3$

(b) aq. KOH, HI

(c) aq. $AgNO_3$, NaI/acetone

(d) HI, aq. KOH

37. The acidic hydrolysis of ether (X) shown below is fastest, when

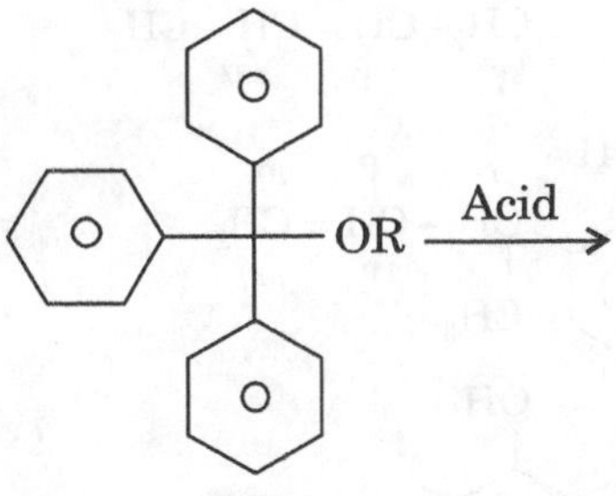

(X)

(a) one phenyl group is replaced by a methyl group

(b) one phenyl group is replaced by a para-methoxy phenyl group.

(c) two phenyl groups are replaced by two para-methoxy phenyl groups.

(d) No structural change is made to X.

38. Reagent (s) which can be used to bring about the following transformation is (are)-

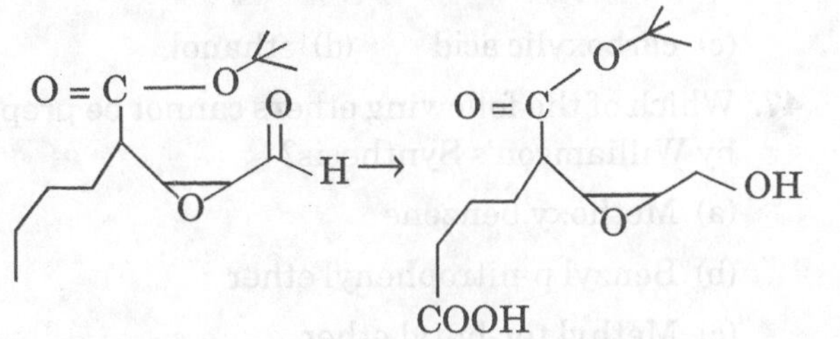

(a) $LiAlH_4$ in $(C_2H_5)_2O$ (b) BH_3 in THF

(c) $NaBH_4$ in C_2H_5OH (d) Raney Ni/H_2 in THF

39. Select the correct reaction.

(a) $CH_3-CH_2-O-CH_2-CH_3 \xrightarrow[h\nu]{Cl_2(\text{excess})} CCl_3-CCl_2-O-CCl_2-CCl_3$
Perchlorodiethyl ether

(b) $R-CH_2-O-CH_2-R+O_2 \xrightarrow{\text{light}} R-CH(O-OH)-OCH_2-R$ (peroxide)

(c) $R-O-R+\text{conc.}H_2SO_4 \xrightarrow{\Delta} ROH+RHSO_4$

(d) All are correct.

40. Select the incorrect statement (s).

(a) Etheral peroxides are explosive in nature

(b) Testing of ethers (from peroxides) is done by washing ether with a solution of Fe^{2+} salt followed by addition of KCNS.

(c) The peroxide from ether can be removed either by treating it with KI soln. or $FeSO_4$ where peroxide is reduced to ether & I^- ion is oxidised to I_2 molecule.

(d) None of these is INCORRECT

41. Consider the reaction given below-

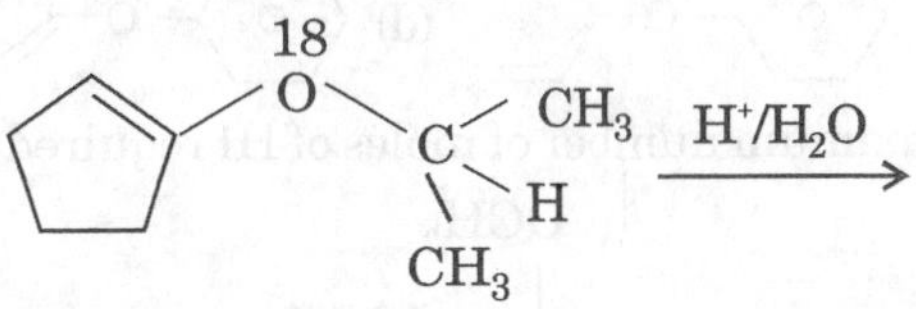

Products formed are-

(a) 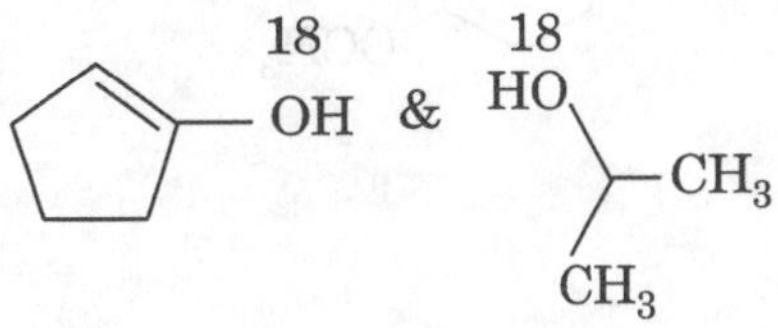

(b) 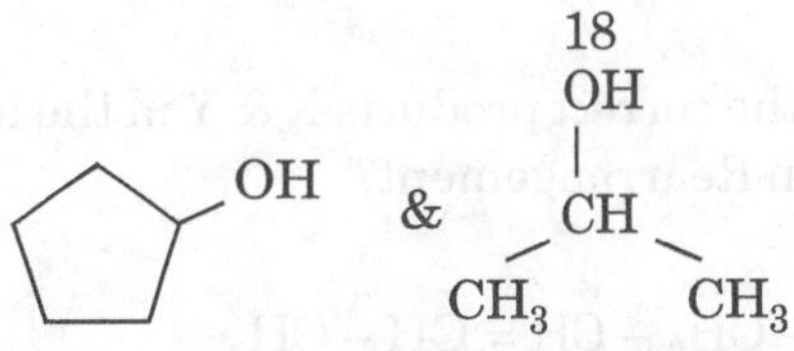

(c) 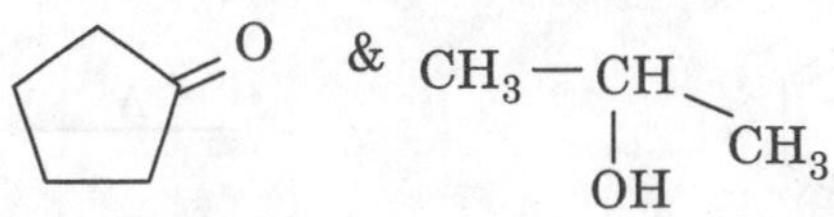

(d) 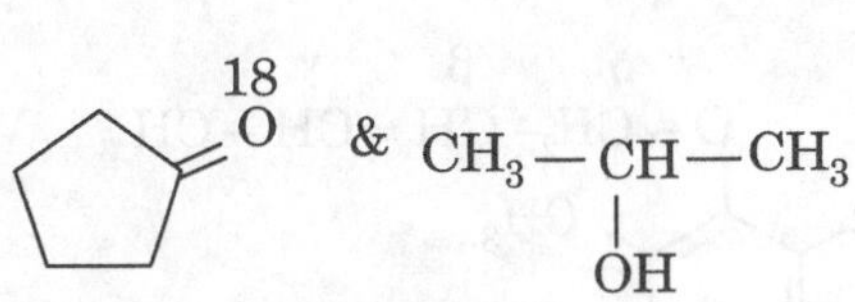

42. Consider the reaction given below-

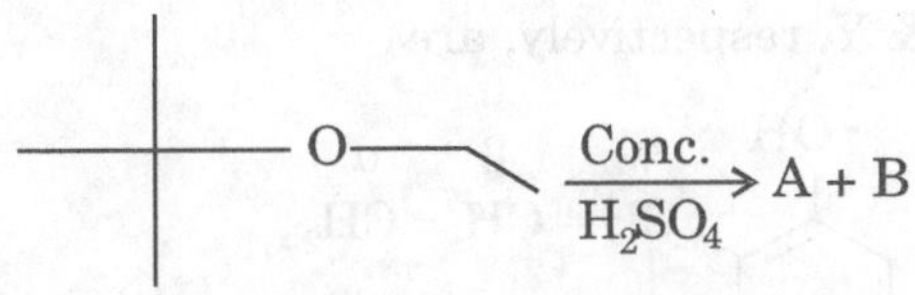

Out of the above main products, B is called grain alcohol. which one is NOT TRUE?

(1) B gives yellow ppt. with NaOH, Cl_2.

(2) A gives isobutyl alcohol in hydroboration oxidation.

(3) A on hydration with H^+, H_2O gives another compound with which Cu, Δ gives back A.

(4) A is a 3° alcohol.

(a) both 1 & 4

(b) 1 only

(c) 1, 2, 3 & 4

(d) both 2 & 4

43. Which of the following ethers can be cleaved by HI?

(a) 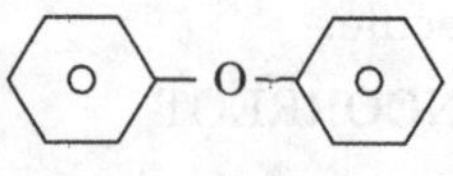 (b) 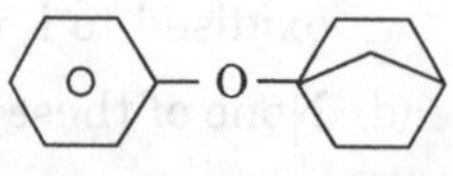

(c) 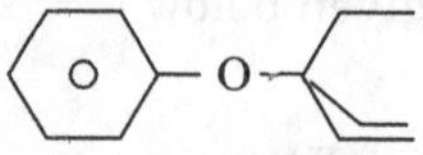 (d) 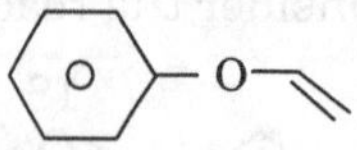

44. Maximum number of moles of HI required to react with 1 mole of 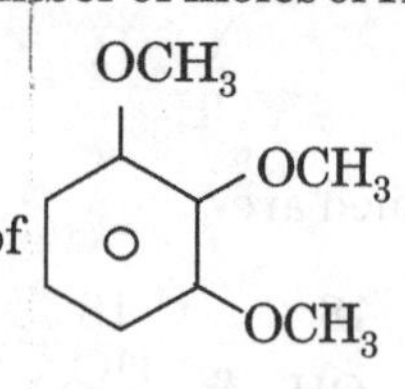 are-

(a) 3

(b) 6

(c) 9

(d) 5

45. Select the correct products X & Y in the following 'Claisen Rearrangement?'

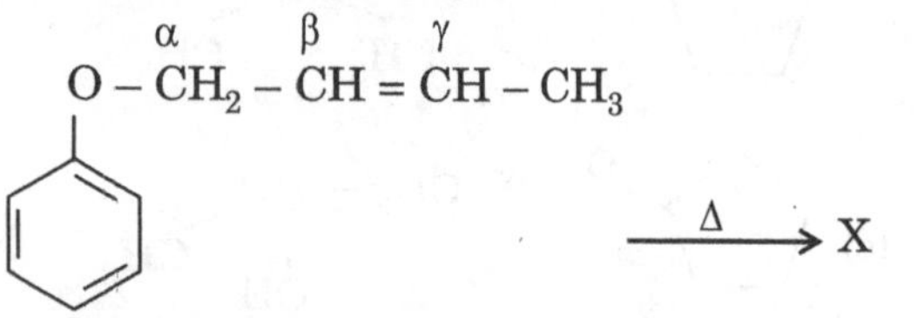

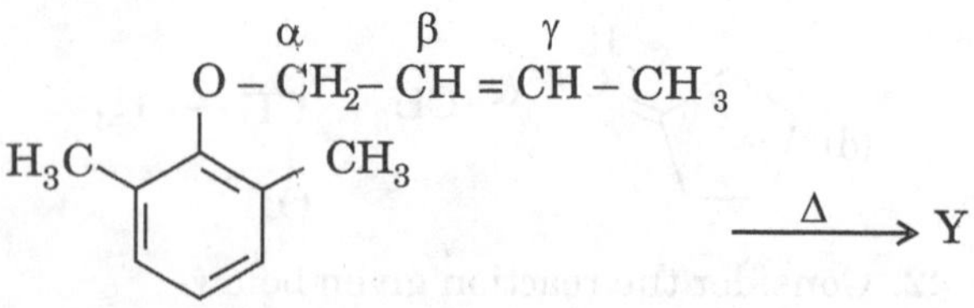

X & Y, respectively, are

(a) 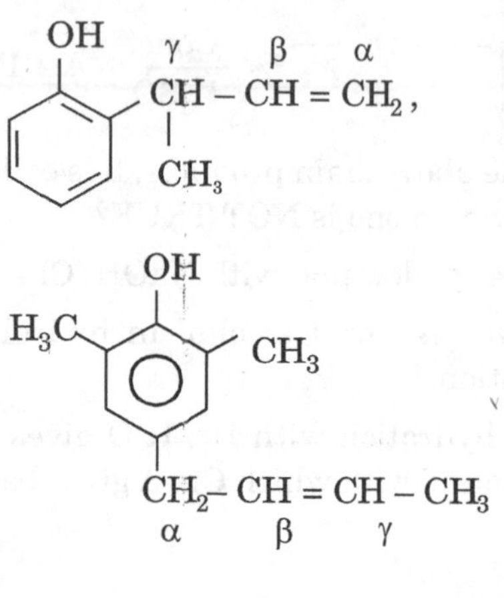

(b) 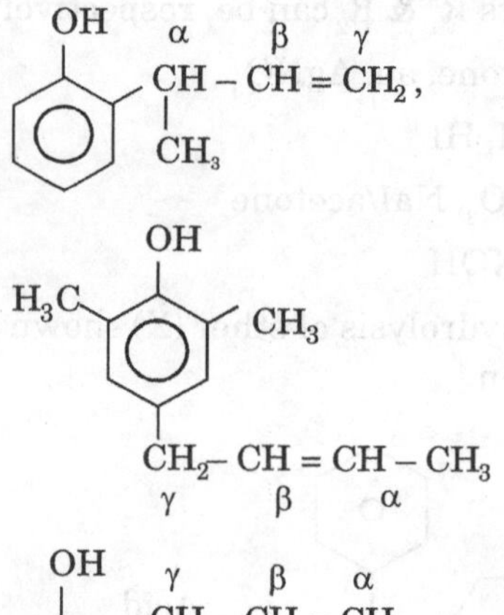

(c) 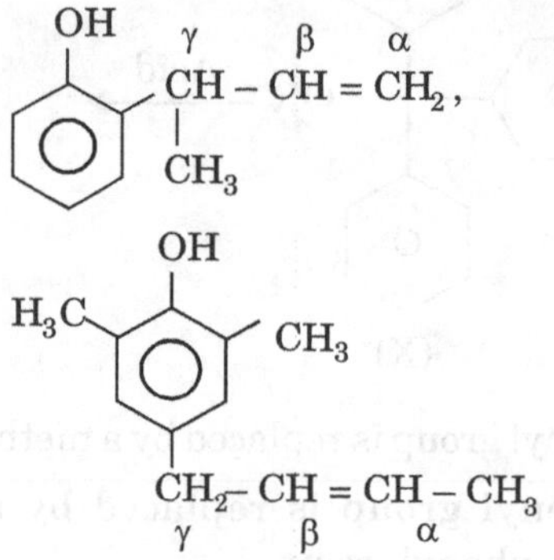

(d) None of these

Methods of Preparation of Ethers

46. The product obtained when sodium ethoxide & ethyl chloride are reacted is-

(a) ethoxyethane (b) ethyl alcohol

(c) carboxylic acid (d) ethanol

47. Which of the following ethers cannot be prepared by Williamson's Synthesis?

(a) Methoxy benzene

(b) Benzyl p-nitrophenyl ether

(c) Methyl ter-butyl ether

(d) Ditertiary butyl ether

48. Wich of the following results in the formation of ANISOLE?

(a) 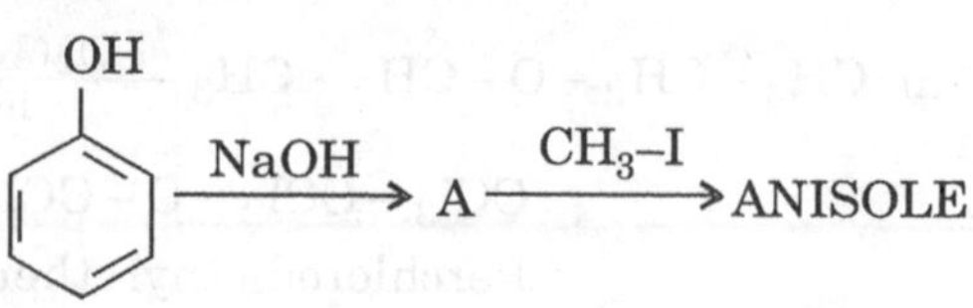

(b) $2C_6H_5OH + (CH_3)SO_4 \xrightarrow{NaOH}$ ANISOLE

(c) 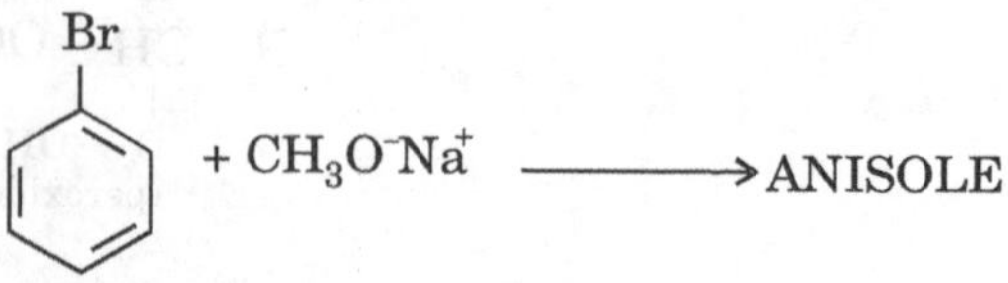

(d) Both a & b

49. Consider the following reaction-

$$RCH_2OH + CH_2N_2 \xrightarrow{HBF_4} RCH_2OCH_3 + N_2 \uparrow$$

Which of the following statements is/are true wrt reaction given above?

(a) It follows S_N2 mechanism.

(b) N_2 is the leaving group here.

(c) alcohol acts as a nucleophile.

(d) All are true.

50. Select the correct name of the reaction given below-

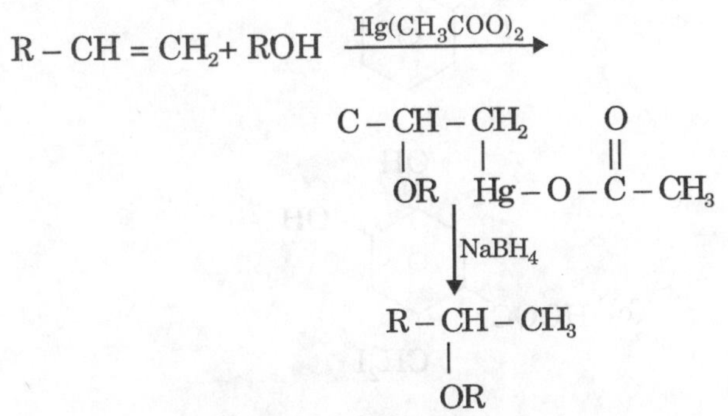

(a) Oxymercuration demercuration

(b) Alkoxymercuration demercuration

(c) Hydroboration oxidation

(d) None of these

51. Which of the following methods will give ether as major product?

(a) $CH_3-CH_2OH \xrightarrow[170°C]{Conc.H_2SO_4}$

(b) $2CH_3CH_2OH \xrightarrow[140°C]{Conc.H_2SO_4}$

(c) $CH_3OCH_2Cl + CH_3MgI \xrightarrow[ether]{dry}$

(d) Both (b) & (c)

52. Which of the following ethers cannot be prepared by Williamson's synthesis?

(1) R_3COCR_3

(2) ArOAr

(3) R – CH = CHOCH = CHR′

(4) $C_6H_5CH_2OC_2H_5$

(a) 1, 4 but not 2 & 3

(b) 1, 2, 3 but not 4

(c) 2 & 3 but not 1 & 4

(d) 2 & 4 but not 1 & 3

53. Which of the following is an approximate set of reactants for the preparation of 1-Methoxy -4 - nitro benzene?

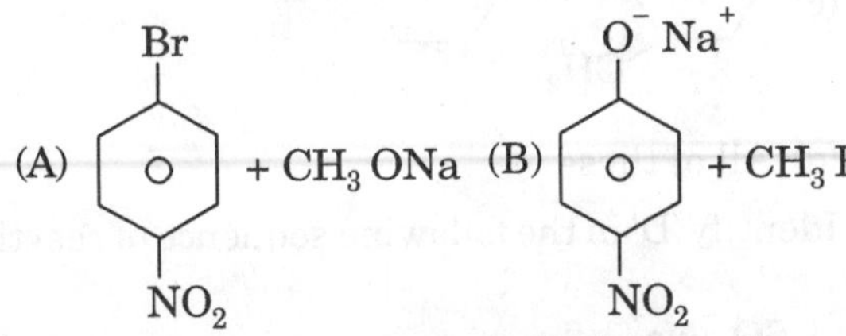

(a) A only (b) B only

(c) both A & B (d) Neither A nor B

54. Ease of dehydration of alcohols to ethers follows the order-

(a) 3° > 2° > 1° (b) 1° > 2° > 3°

(c) 2° > 1° > 3° (d) 2° > 3° > 1°

55. Consider the following two reactions-

$$2CH_3CH_2Br + \underset{(dry)}{Ag_2O} \longrightarrow X$$

$$CH_3CH_2Br + \underset{(moist)}{Ag_2O} \longrightarrow Y$$

X & Y in the above reactions are-

(a) CH_3CH_2OH, CH_3CH_2OH

(b) $CH_3CH_2OCH_2CH_3$, CH_3CH_2OH

(c) $CH_3CH_2OCH_2CH_2CH_3$, $CH_3CH_2OCH_3$

(d) Both a & c

56. What is 'Y' in the following reaction sequence?

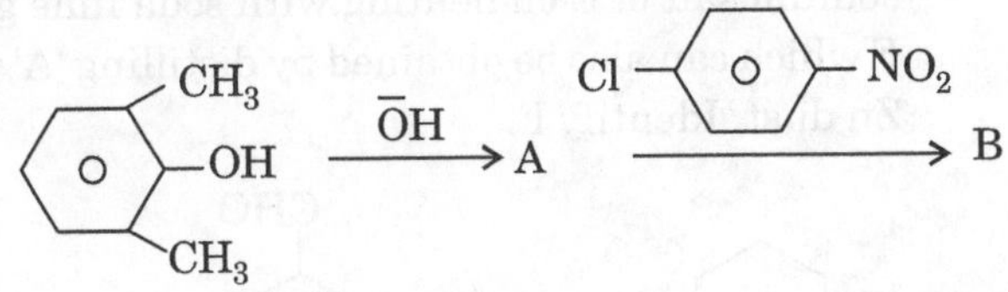

(a)

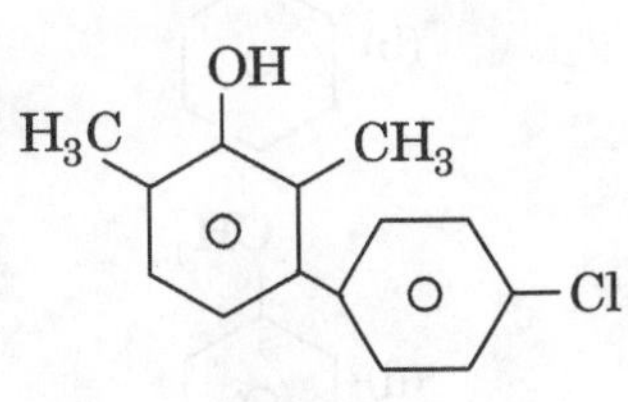

(b)

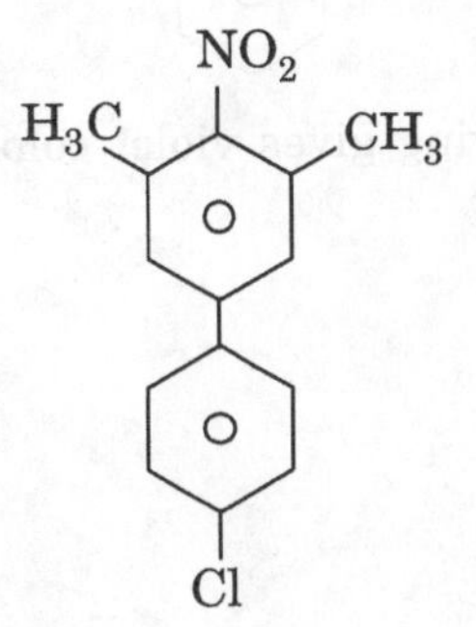

(c) 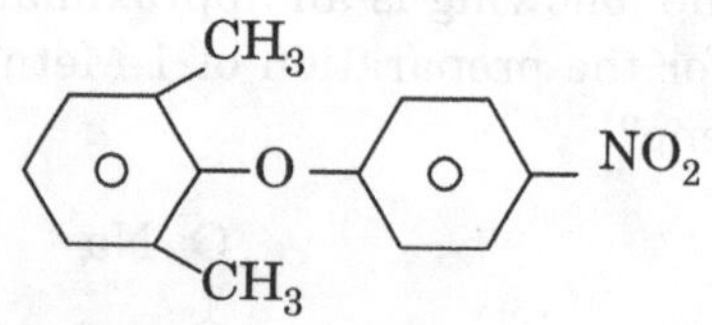

(d) All of these

57. Identify 'D' in the following sequence of reactions.

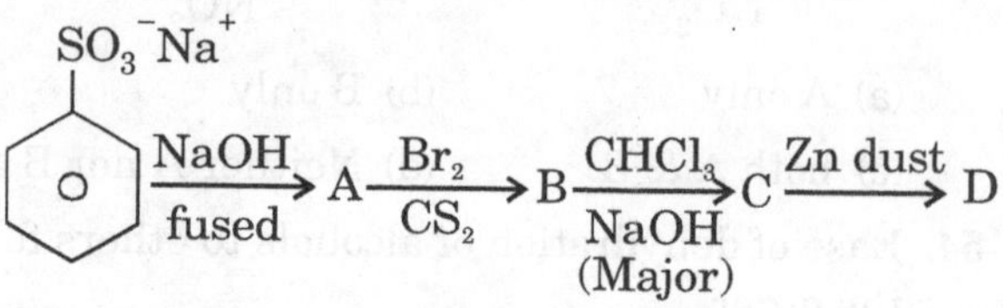

(a) 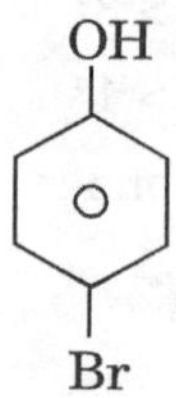 + HCHO (b) 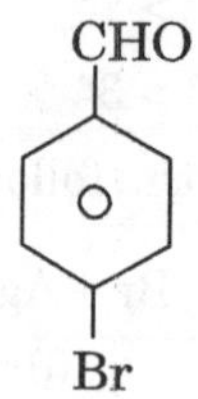

(c) 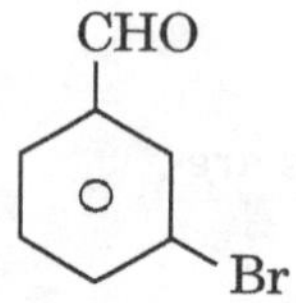 (d) 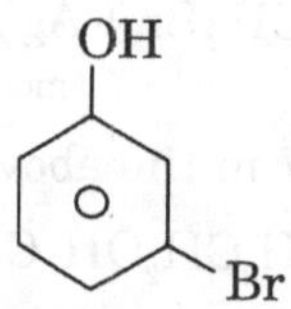

58. An organic compound 'A' on treatment with $CHCl_3$ & KOH gives B and C. B & C in turn give same compound 'D' when distilled with Zn dust. Oxidation of D yields 'E' of formula $C_7H_6O_2$. The sodium salt of E on heating with soda lime gives F which can also be obtained by distilling 'A' with Zn dust. Identify F.

(a) 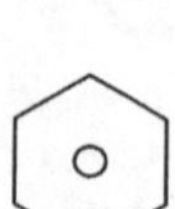 (b) 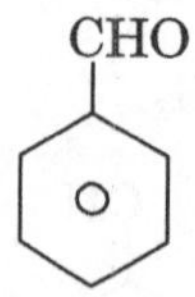

(c) 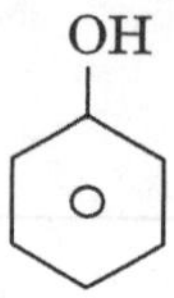 (d) 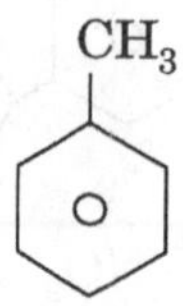

59. Which of the following gives violet colour with phenol?

(a) $NaHCO_3$

(b) Na_2CO_3

(c) $ZnCl_2$

(d) $FeCl_3$

60. The product 'X' of the following reaction can be-

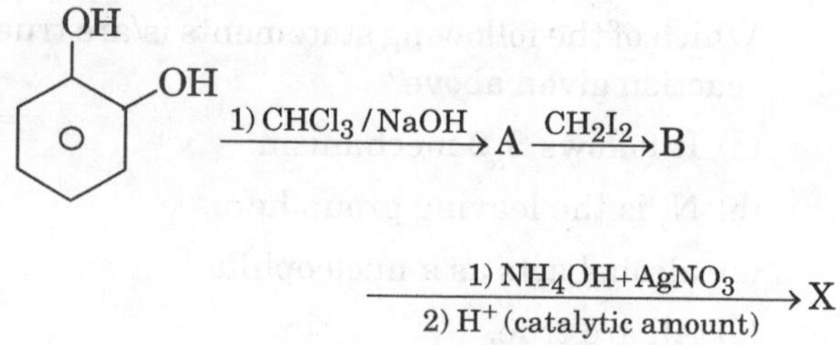

(a) 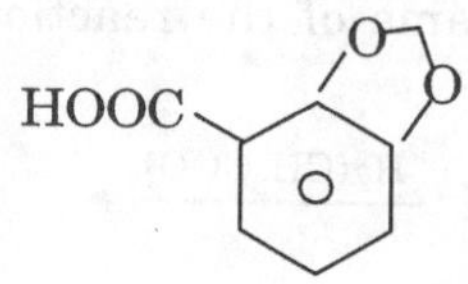

(b) 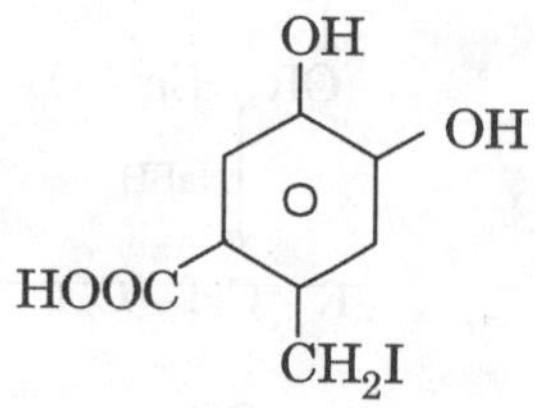

(c) 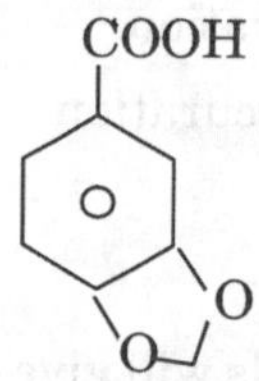

(d) Both a & c

61. The correct statement regarding the following reaction is-

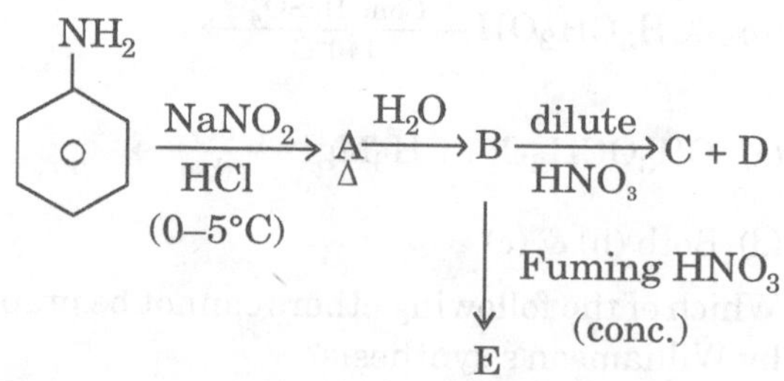

If C can form intramolecular hydrogen bonding & D can form intermolecular hydrogen bonding, the identify the correct order of acidic strength-

(a) E > D > C > B

(b) B > D > C > E

(c) C > D > B > E

(d) B > C > D > E

62. Select the correct reaction(s)-

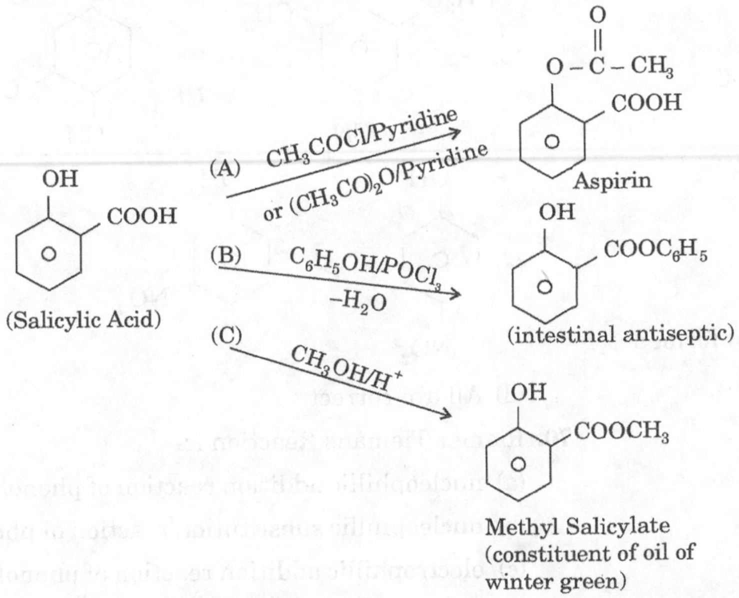

(a) only A is correct
(b) only B & C are correct
(c) only A & C are correct
(d) All are correct.

63. Select the correct statement about coupling reaction of phenol.

(1) It is an electrophilic substitution reaction of phenol.

(2) In coupling, benzene diazonium ion acts as an electrophile (with +ve charge resting on terminal N)

(3) Coupling of phenol is favored in optimum basic pH.

(4) Coupling of phenol is a nucleophilic substitution reaction.

(a) only 1 is correct
(b) only 1, 2 & 3 are correct
(c) only 2, 3 & 4 are correct
(d) All are correct

64. Yield of alkylated product of phenol is-

(a) high because ring is highly activated by + R of – OH group.

(b) high because ring is deactivated by +R of –OH group.

(c) very low because of co-ordination of $AlCl_3$ with oxygen atom of phenol forming $Ph-\overset{\oplus}{O}(H)-\overset{\ominus}{Al}Cl_3$ because of which ring is deactivated.

(d) very low because it is a nucleophilic substitution reaction.

65. Select the INCORRECT REACTION.

(a) 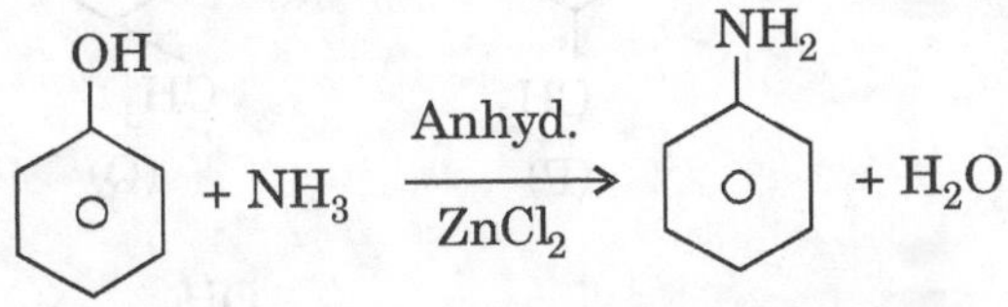

(b) 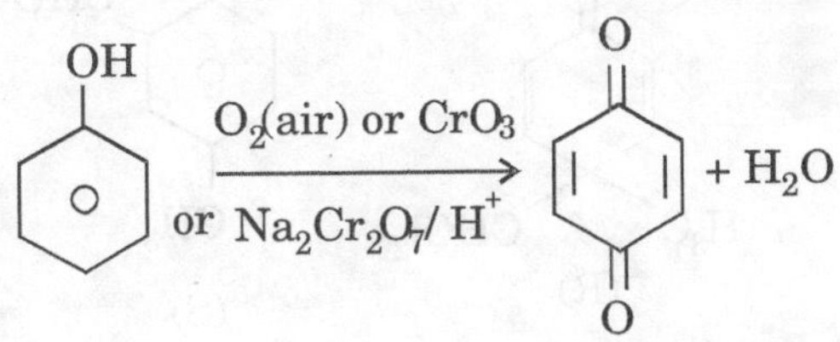

p-benzoquinone

(c) 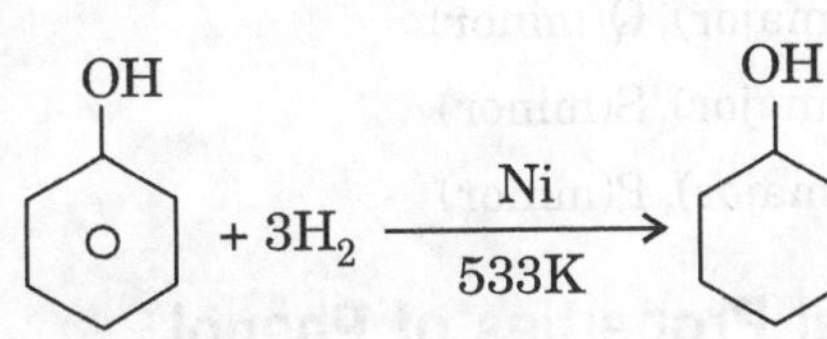

(d) None of these

66. Which of the following reacts with phenol to form phenolphthalein?

(a) Phthalic acid
(b) Isophthalic acid
(c) Phthalic anhydride
(d) Isophthalic anhydride

67. Identify X in following reaction-

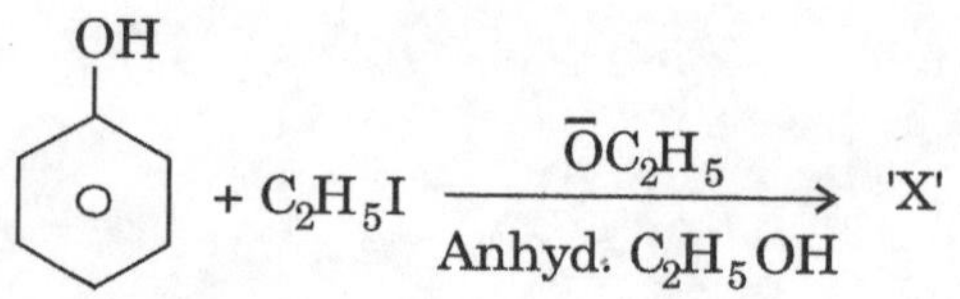

(a) $C_6H_5OC_2H_5$
(b) $C_2H_5OC_2H_5$
(c) $C_6H_5OC_6H_5$
(d) C_6H_5I

68. In the following reaction, the product(s) formed is (are)-

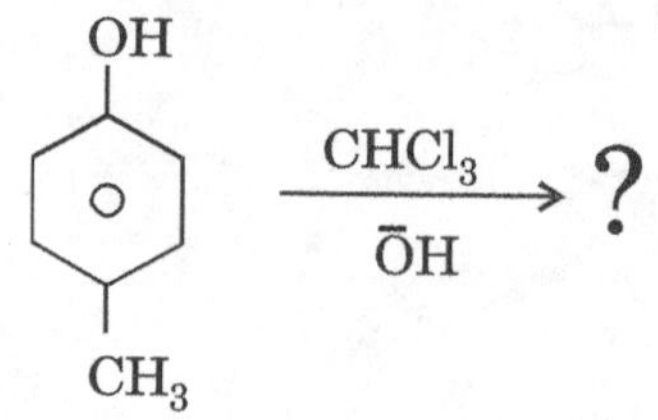

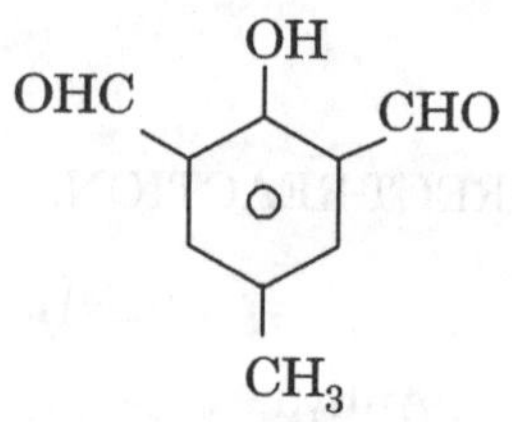
(P)

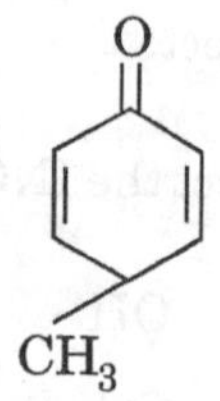
(Q)

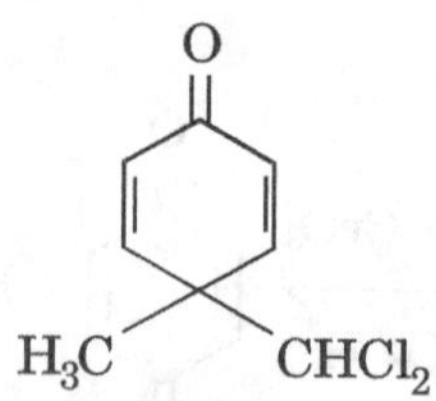
(R)

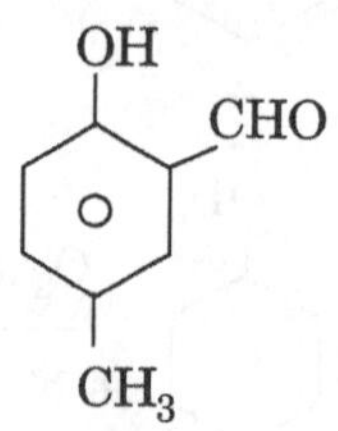
(S)

(a) R(minor), S(major)
(b) P(major), Q(minor)
(c) R(major), S(minor)
(d) S(major), P(minor)

Chemical Properties of Phenol

69. Which one is correct order of acidic strength?

(a) 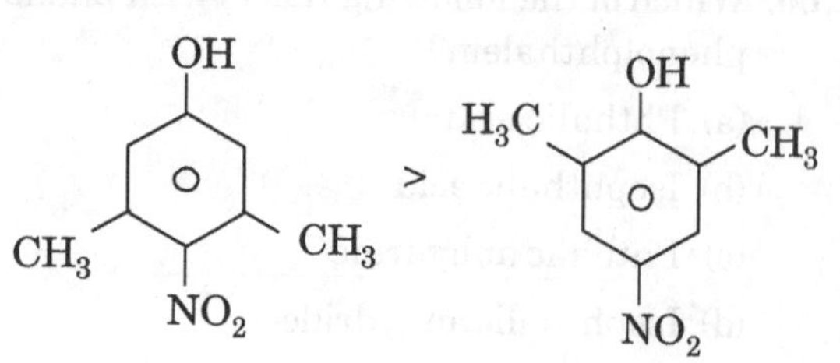

(b) 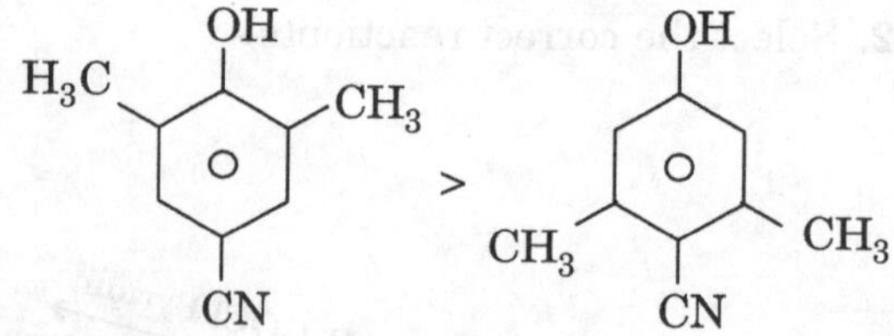

(c) 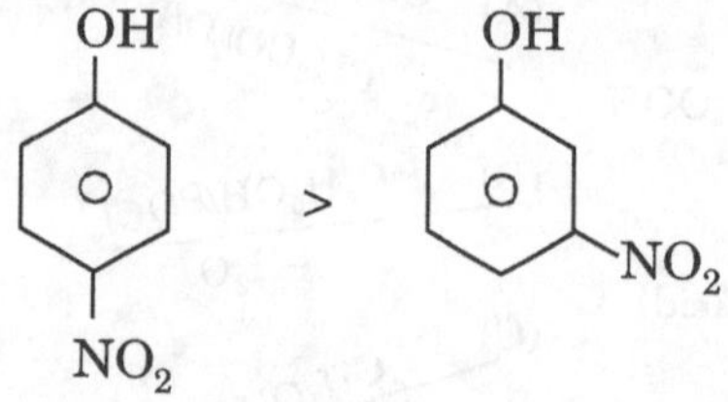

(d) All are correct

70. Riemer Tiemans Reaction is-
(a) nucleophillic addition reaction of phenol.
(b) nucleophillic substitution reaction of phenol
(c) electrophillic addition reaction of phenol
(d) electrophillic substitution reaction of phenol.

71. Which of the following is correct about major product?

(a) 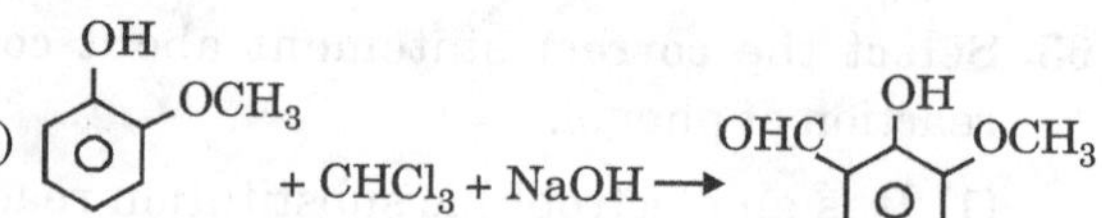

(b) 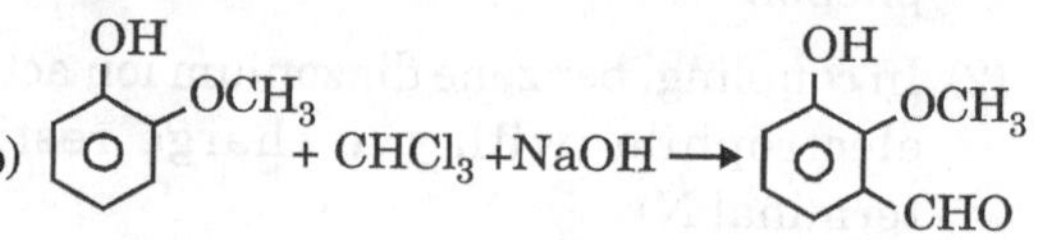

(c) 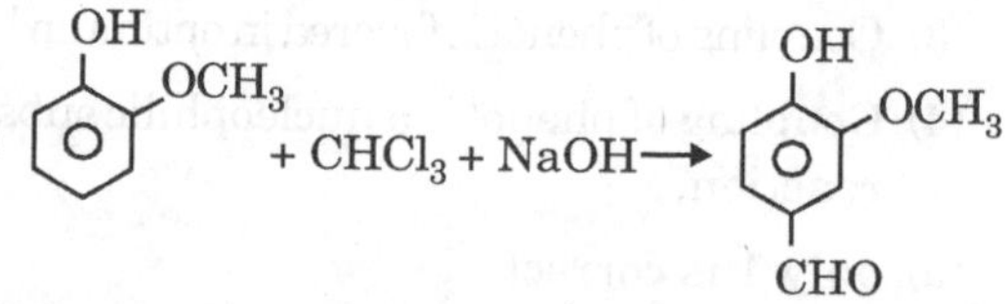

(d) Equimolar amount of a & c

72. Riemar Tiemann's formylation & Riemer Tiemann's carboxylation reactions are given as follows. Sum of 'X' & 'Y' is-

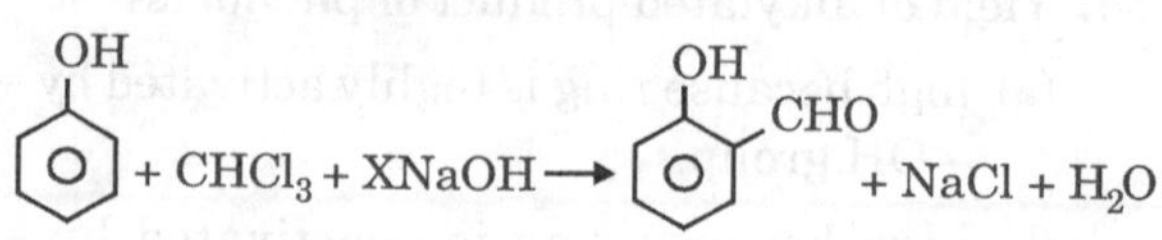

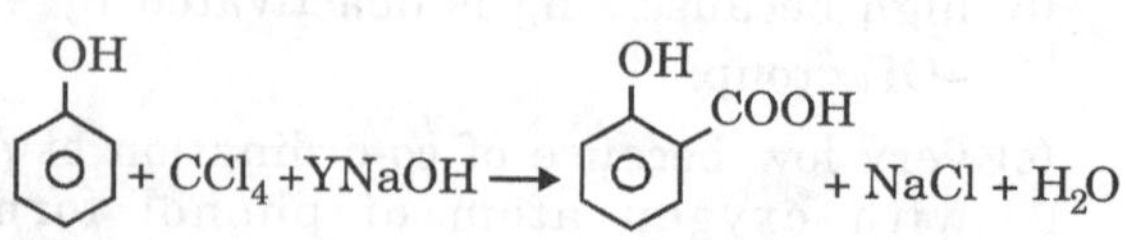

(a) 5
(b) 9
(c) 7
(d) 6

73. Identify the final product 'Z' in the following reaction sequence-

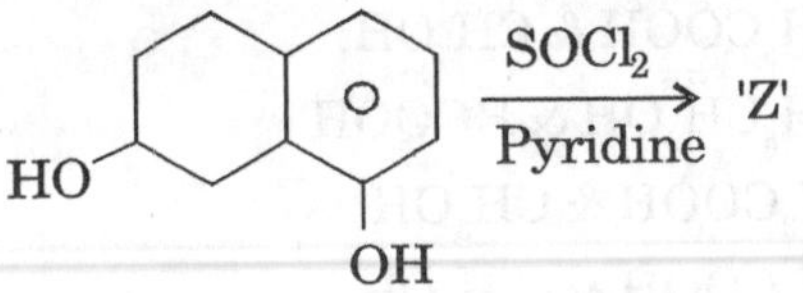

(a) 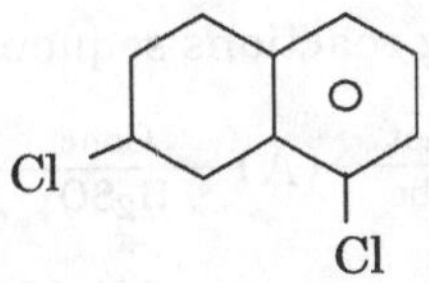 (b) 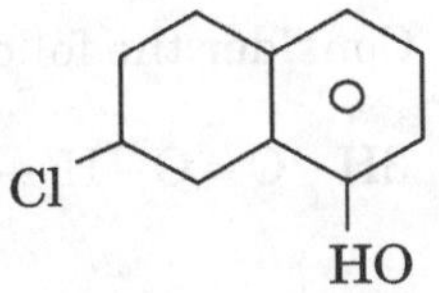

(c) 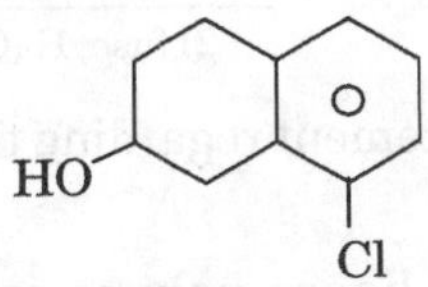 (d) All of these

74. Select correct statement about 'Fries Rearrangement'?

(1) It involves the rearrangement of phenyl esters like phenyl acetate (in the presence of lewis acids as Anhyd.$AlCl_3$) into hydroxy ketones.

(2) It is an example of electrophillic substitution reaction.

(3) $ArOCOCH_3$ will be less reactive than $ArOCOC_6H_5$ for this reaction.

(4) $ArOCOCH_3$ will be more reactive than $ArOCOC_6H_5$ for this reaction.

(a) only 1 & 2 are correct.

(b) only 2 & 3 are correct.

(c) only 1, 2 & 3 are correct.

(d) All are correct

75. Which of the following molecules will NOT undergo FRIES REARRANGEMENT?

(a) 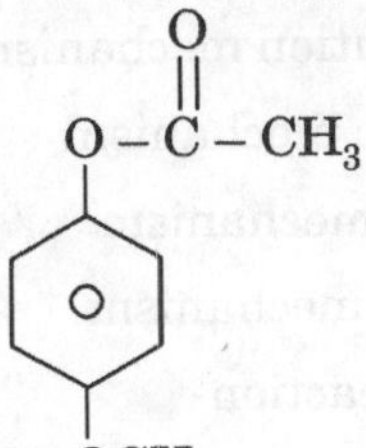 (b) 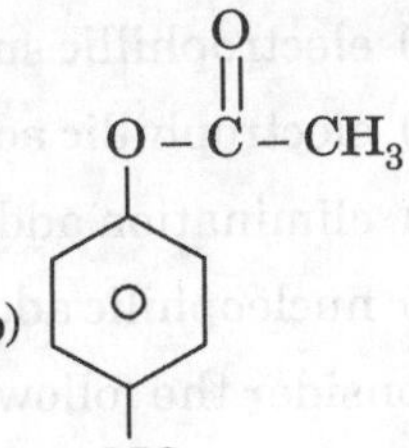

(c) 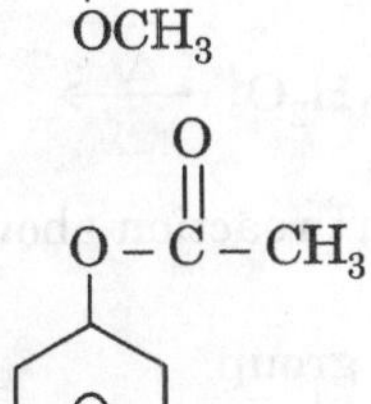 (d) All of these

76. Identify the final product 'B' in the following sequence of reactions.

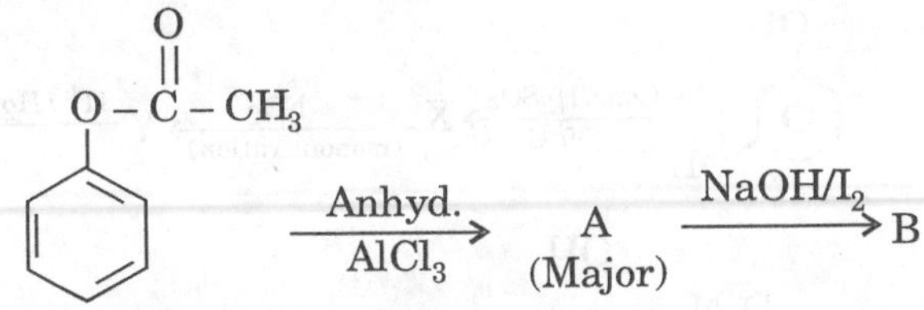

(a) 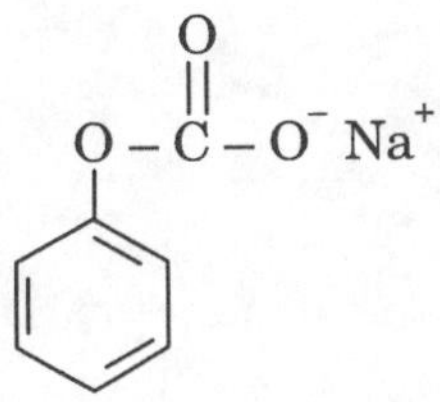 (b) 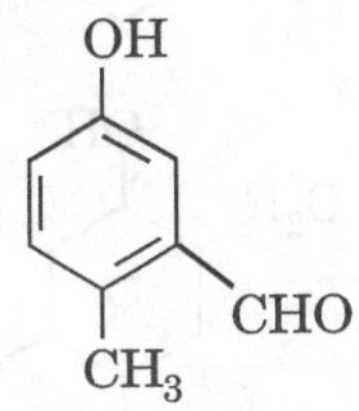

(c) 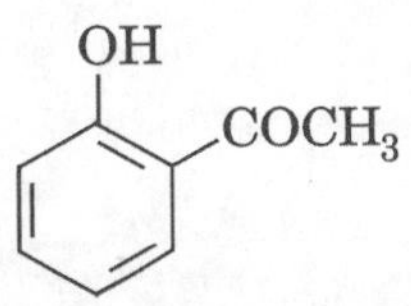 (d) 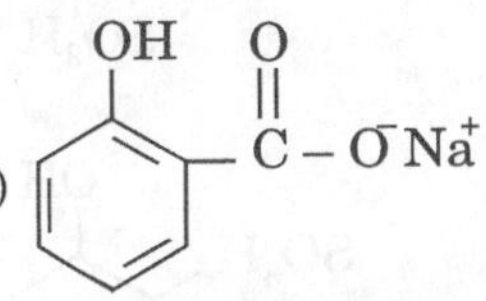

77. Which of the following is/are INCORRECTLY named?

(a) 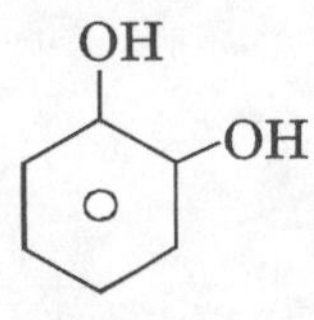 – Catechol

(b) 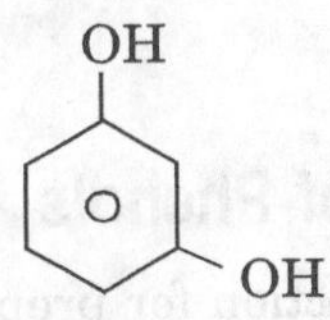 – Resorcinol

(c) 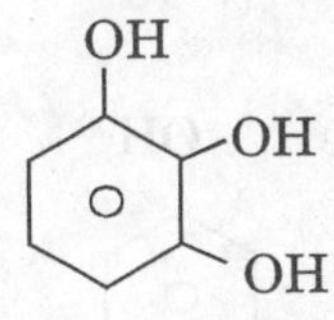 – Pyrogallol

(d) None of these

78. Phloroglucinol is subjected to Schotten Baumann's reaction for a long time. Then, its molar mass increases by-

(a) 210 gm (b) 312 gm

(c) 315 gm (d) 292 gm

79. Which of the following will increase the acidity of phenol?

(a) dil. HCl

(b) Conc. CH_3COOH

(c) Conc. H_2SO_4

(d) All of these

80. Identify the final product 'Z' in the following reaction sequence-

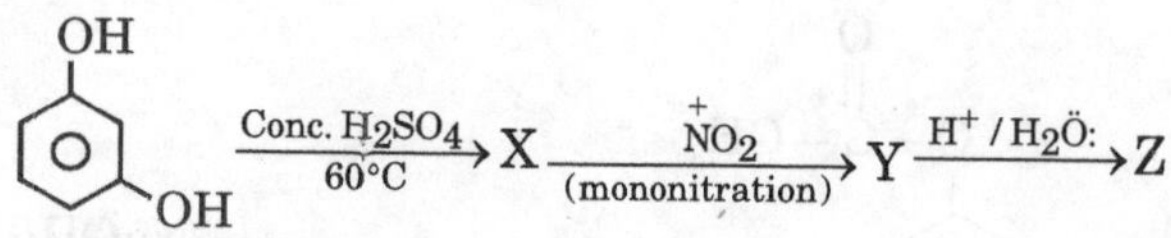

(a)

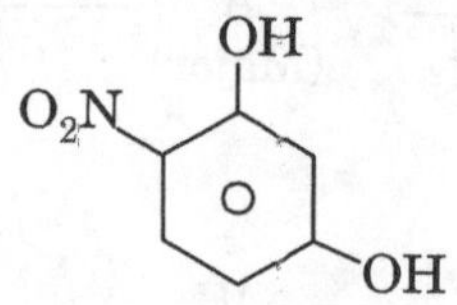

(b)

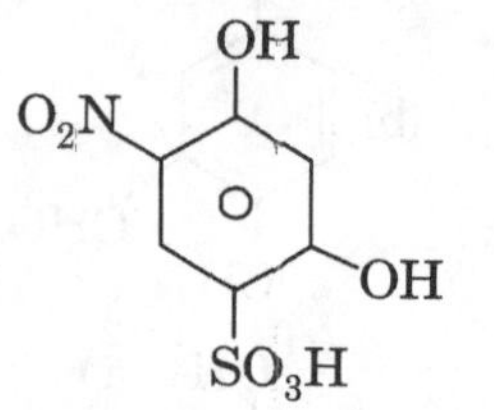

(c)

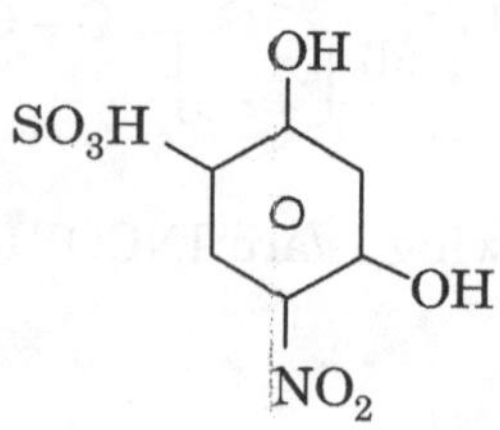

(d)

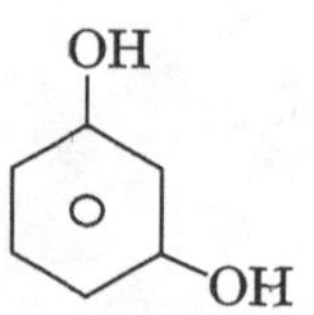

Methods of Preparation of Phenols

81. Consider the following reaction for preparation of phenol-

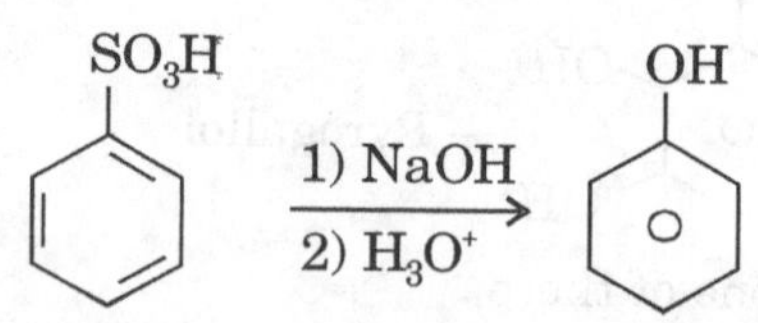

Select the correct statement (s) regarding above reaction-

(a) It proceeds by addition-elimination mech-anism of nucleophilic aromatic substitution.

(b) It proceeds by elimination-addition mech-anism of nucleophilic aromatic substitution.

(c) Hydroxide replaces the sulphite ion (SO_3^{2-}).

(d) Both a & c are correct.

82. The products of acidic hydrolysis of phenyl acetate are-

(a) C_6H_5COOH & CH_3OH

(b) $C_6H_5CH_2OH$ & $HCOOH$

(c) CH_3COOH & CH_3OH

(d) CH_3COOH & C_6H_5OH

83. Consider the following reactions sequence-

$$3H-C\equiv C-H \xrightarrow[\text{Fe tube}]{\text{Red hot}} (A) \xrightarrow[H_2SO_4]{\text{Conc.}} (B) \xrightarrow[\text{2) fuse, } H_3O^+]{\text{1) NaOH}} (C)$$

Identify the correct statement regarding the above sequence of reaction-

(A) 'A' is obtained by linear polymerisation of ethyne.

(B) Formation of 'B' from 'A' involves arenium ion as an intermediate.

(C) The product 'C' is a stronger acid than water.

(D) The product 'A' will decolourise pink colour of Baeyer's reagent.

(a) A, B & C but not D

(b) A, B & D but not C

(c) B & C but not A & D

(d) B & D but not A & C

84. Base promoted hydrolysis of chlorobenzene, shown below, proceeds via-

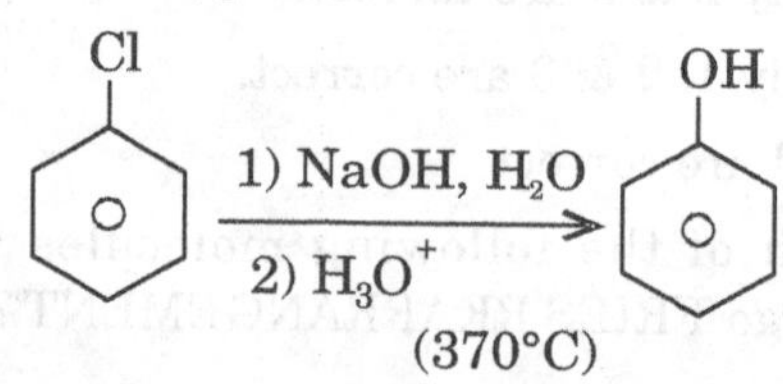

(a) electrophillic substitution mechanism

(b) electrophillic addition mechanism

(c) elimination addition mechanism

(d) nucleophilic addition mechanism

85. Consider the following reaction-

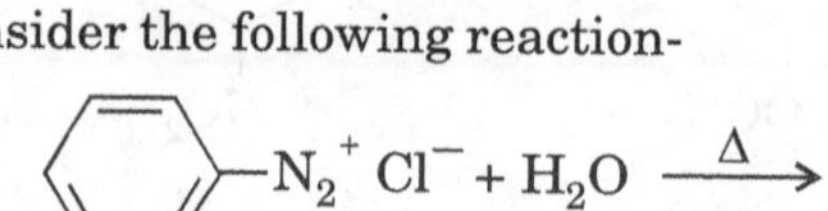

The correct statement wrt reaction above is-

(a) $\ddot{N}\equiv\ddot{N}$ is the leaving group.

(b) Phenol is formed

(c) It involves formation of phenyl cation

(d) All are correct

86. Select the correct statement (s).

(a) Phenyl shift occurs when phenol is formed from cumene.

(b) Cumene can be formed when propene reacts with benzene in the presence of protonic acid.

(c) Another name for cumene is isopropyl benzene

(d) All are correct.

87. Phenol is final product by which of the following reactions?

(a) 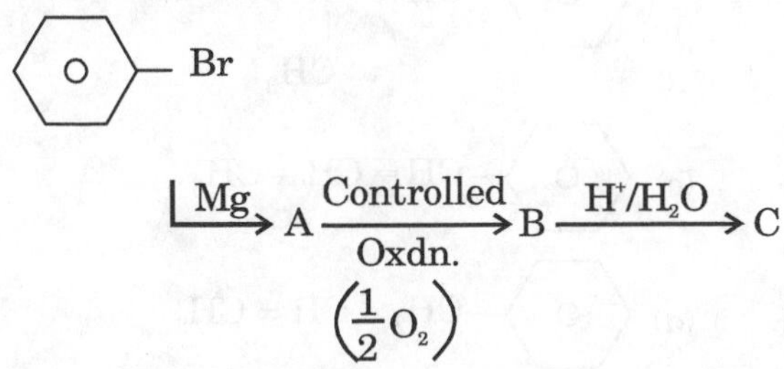

(b) 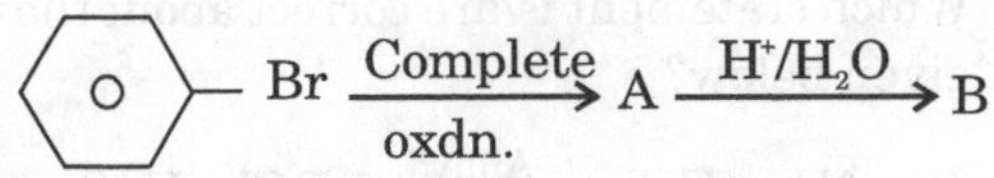

(c) 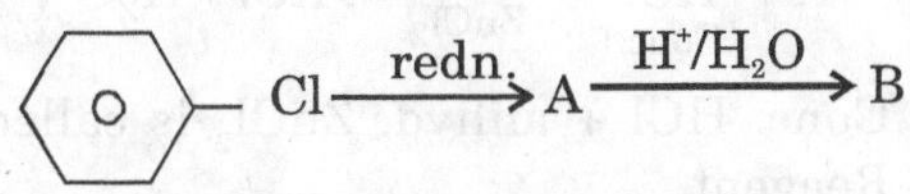

(d) All have phenol as final product.

Chemical Properties of Alcohol

88. Consider the following reaction-

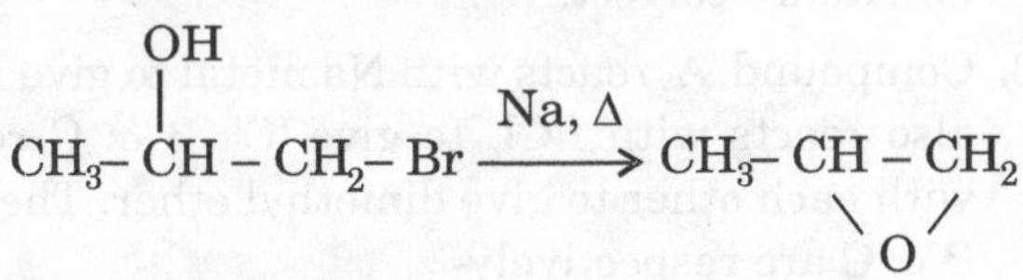

The reaction can be described as-

(a) Acid base reaction followed by intramolecular S_N1.

(b) Acid base reaction followed by intramolecular S_N2.

(c) E_2 reaction followed by addition reaction to a double bond.

(d) SN^2 followed by intramolecular S_N1.

89. 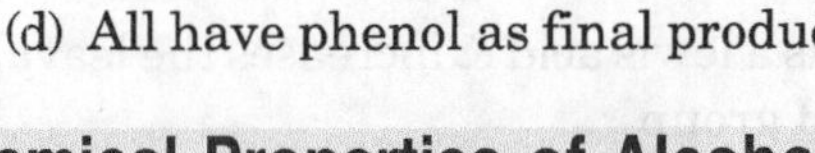 on reaction with one mole of CH_3MgBr gives-

(a) 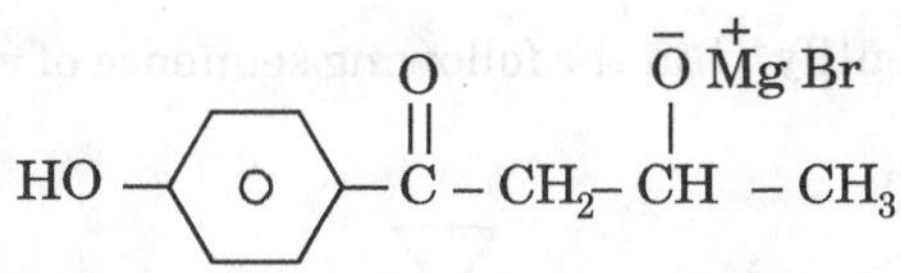

(b) 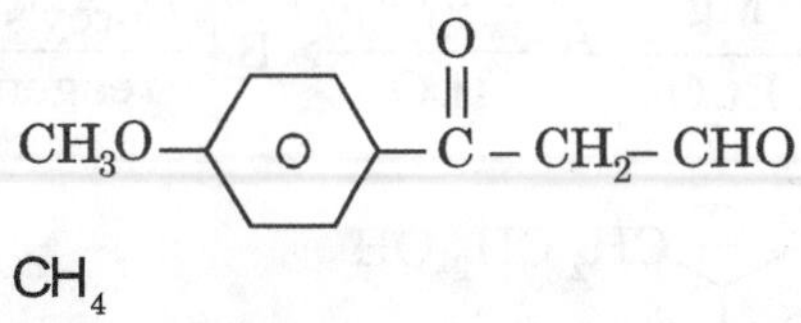

(c) CH_4

(d) None of these

90. Which alcohol is most reactive towards acid catalysed dehydration?

(a) 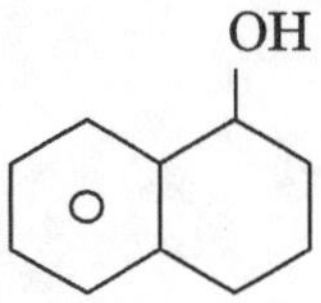

(b) 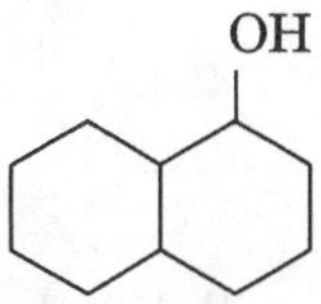

(c) 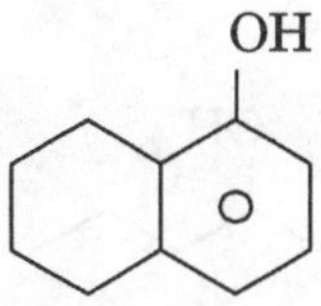

(d) 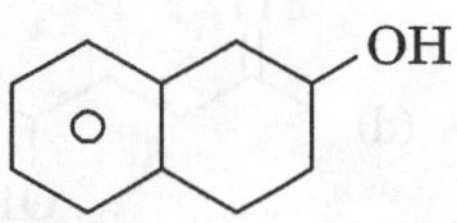

91. Identify 'X' in the following reaction-

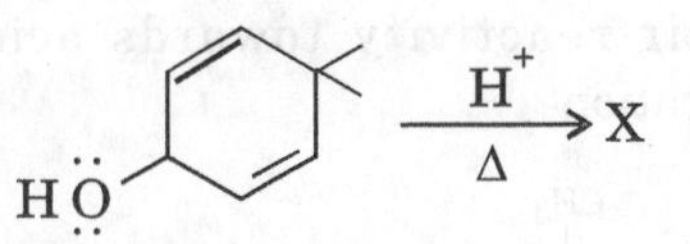

(a) 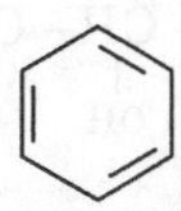

(b) 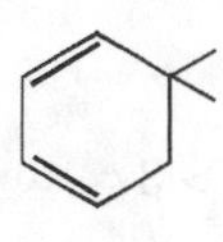

(c) 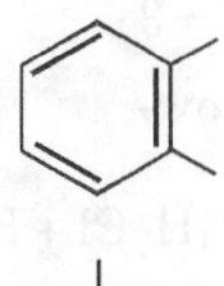

(d) 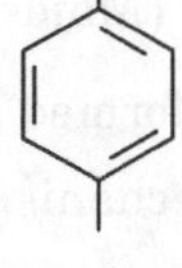

92. Identify 'C' in the following sequence of reaction-

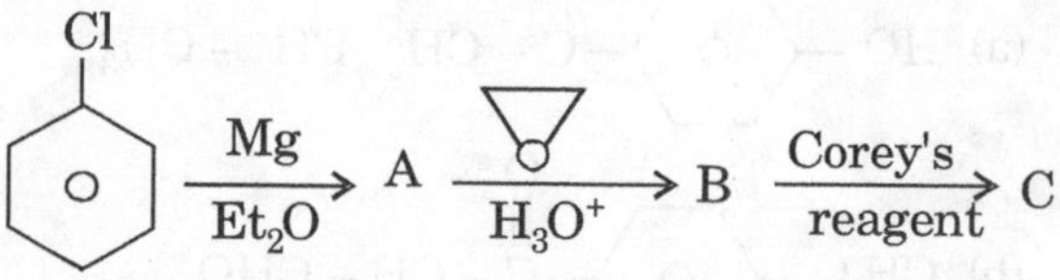

(a) 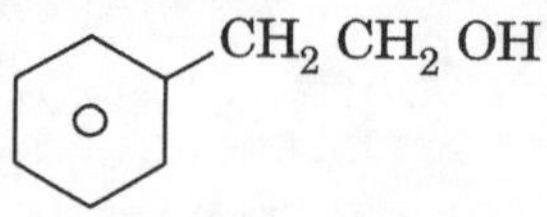

(b) 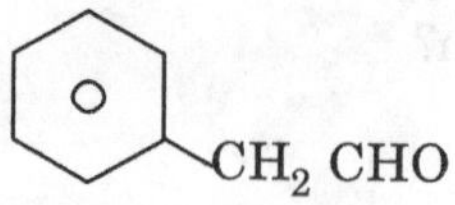

(c) 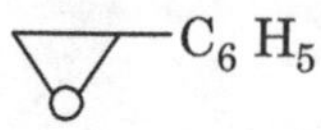

(d) 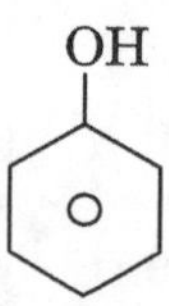

93. Which one of the following will dehydrate most easily in basic conditions?

(a) 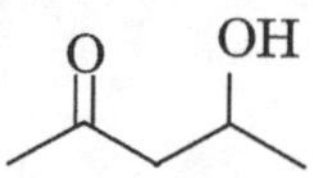
(b) 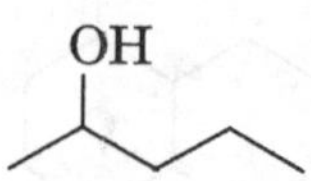
(c) 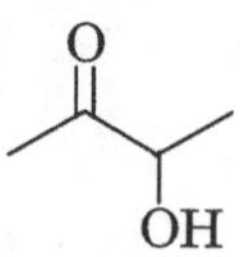
(d) 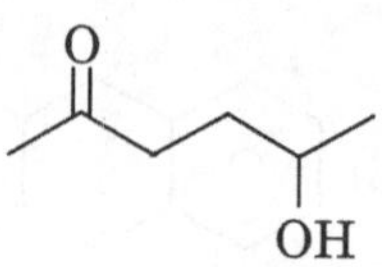

94. Arrange the following alcohols in decreasing order of their reactivity towards acid catalysed dehydration-

(1) $CH_3-C(CH_3)_2-OH$ (2) $CH_3-CH(OH)-CH_3$

(3) $CH_3-CH(CH_3)-CH_2OH$

(a) 1 > 2 > 3 (b) 2 > 1 > 3

(b) 3 > 2 > 1 (c) 1 > 2 = 3

95. Consider the reaction given below-

$$CH_3CH_2CH_2OH + HCl \longrightarrow \underset{(\text{Major P})}{C_3H_7Cl} + H_2O$$

Major P in the above reaction is formed by-

(a) S_N1 mechanism (b) S_N2 mechanism

(c) S_{N_i} mechanism (s) E_1 mechanism

96. Identify the major product 'Z' in the following reaction-

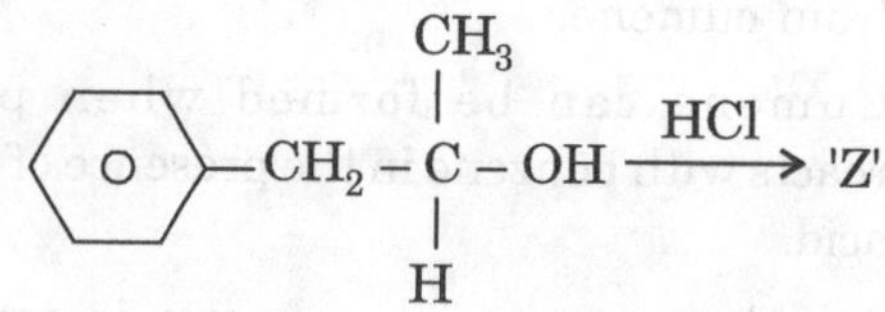

(a) 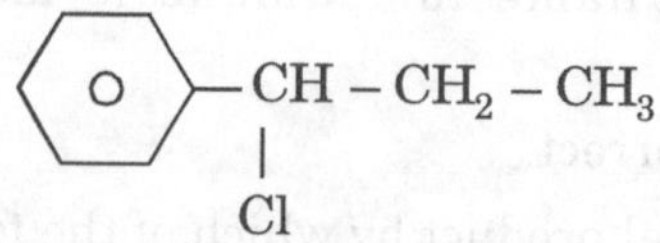

(b) 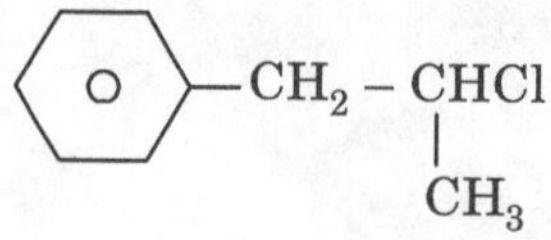

(c) 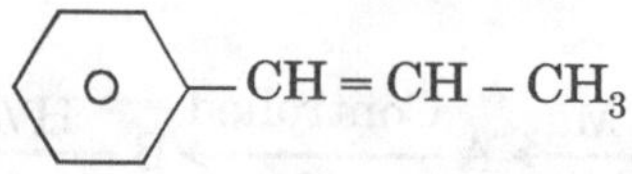

(d) 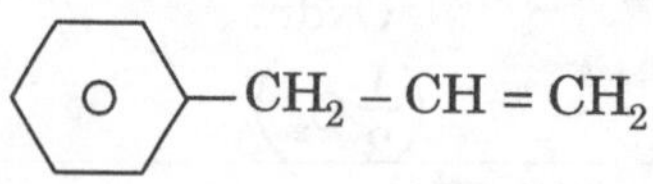

97. Which statement is/are correct about the reaction given below?

$$R-OH + \underset{(\text{Conc.})}{HCl} \xrightarrow[ZnCl_2]{\text{Anhyd.}} RCl + H_2O$$

(a) Conc. HCl + anhyd. $ZnCl_2$ is called Lucas Reagent.

(b) $ZnCl_2$ is a lewis acid & increases the leavability of –OH group

(c) $HO-\overset{\ominus}{Zn}Cl_2$ is the leaving group here.

(d) All are correct.

98. Compound 'A' reacts with Na metal to give B. 'A' also reacts with PCl_5 to give 'C'. B & C reacts with each other to give dimethyl ether. Then, A, B & C are respectively-

(a) CH_3OH, CH_3ONa, CH_3COCl

(b) CH_3OH, CH_4, CH_3Cl

(c) CH_3OH, CH_3ONa, CH_3Cl

(d) CH_3Cl, CH_4, CH_3OH

99. Order of reactivity of alcohols towards K metal follows the order-

(a) 1° > 2° > 3° (b) 3° > 2° > 1°

(c) 2° > 1° > 3° (d) 1° = 2° > 3°

100. When a mixture of PCl_3 & PCl_5 is heated with ethyl alcohol, a total of 4 moles of ethyl chloride are formed. Mole ratio of PCl_3 & PCl_5 in the mixture is-

(a) 3 : 1 (b) 1 : 1

(c) 1 : 3 (d) 2 : 1

101. Consider the following reaction & identify 'X'.

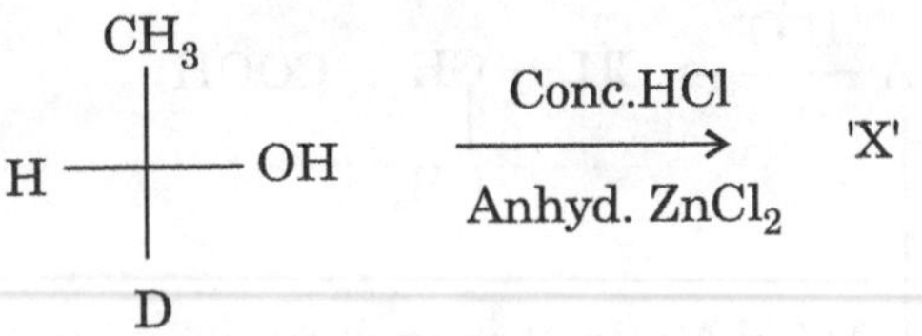

(a) 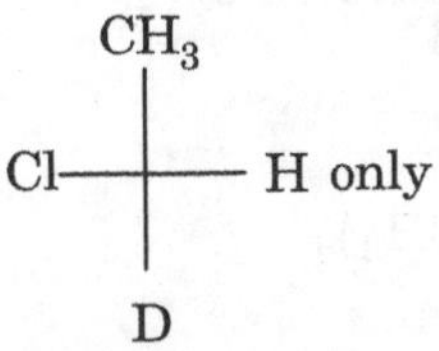 only

(b) 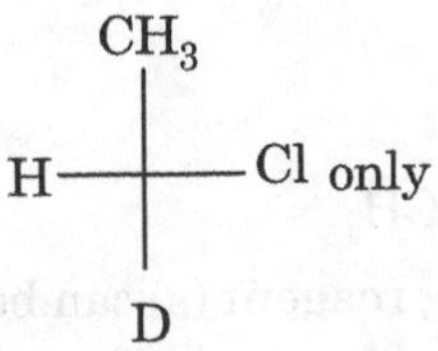 only

(c) Equimolar mixture of both a & b

(d) $CH_2 = CH - D$

102. An organic compound X on treatment with PCC in dichloromethane gives compound Y. Compound Y reacts with I_2 & alkali to give triiodomethane. The Compound 'X' is-

(a) CH_3CH_2OH (b) CH_3CHO

(c) CH_3COCH_3 (d) CH_3COOH

103. Which of the following reaction will give an alkyl halide?

(a) $CH_3CH_2OH + HCl \longrightarrow$

(b) $CH_3CH_2OH + HCl \xrightarrow[ZnCl_2]{Anhyd.}$

(c) $CH_3-\underset{CH_3}{\overset{CH_3}{C}}-OH + HCl \xrightarrow[(conc.)]{}$

(d) Both b & c

104. Which of the following is NOT the product of acid catalysed dehydration of-

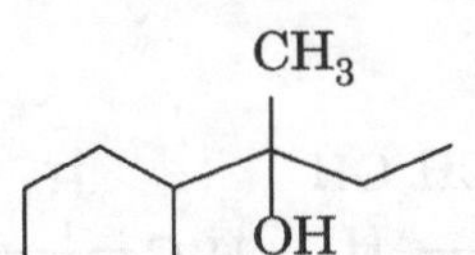

(a) 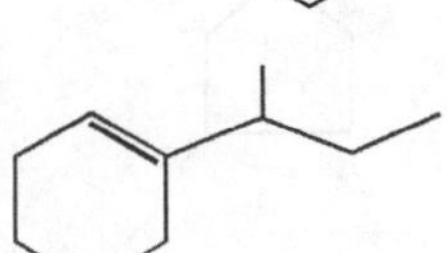

(b) 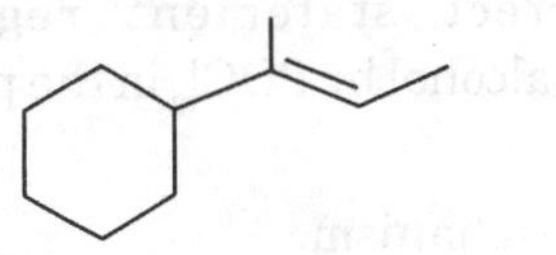

(c) 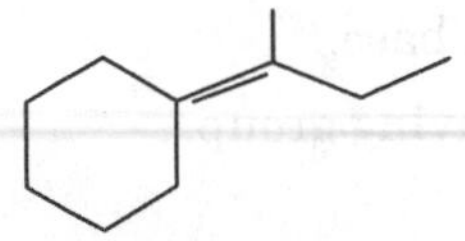

(d) 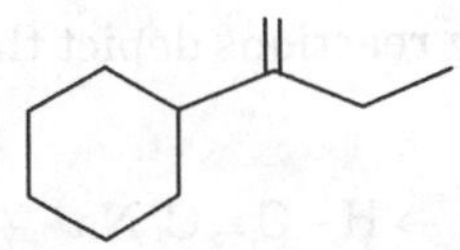

105. Which combination of acid & alcohol will give the best yield of an ester?

(a) $HCOOH + CH_3OH$

(b) $CH_3COOH + CH_3OH$

(c) $CH_3COOH + C_2H_5OH$

(d) $HCOOH + CH_3CH_2OH$

106. Which of the following ion is/are formed in the following reaction?

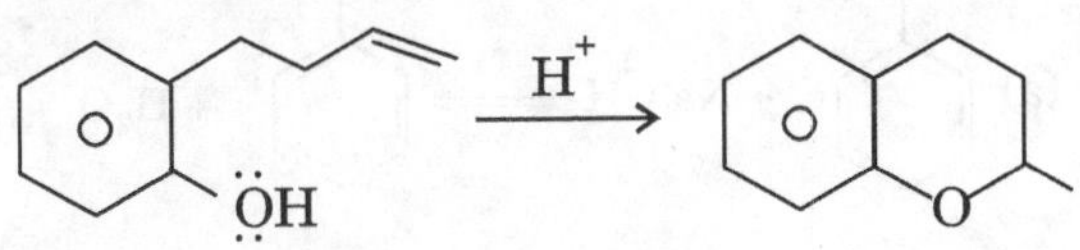

(a) 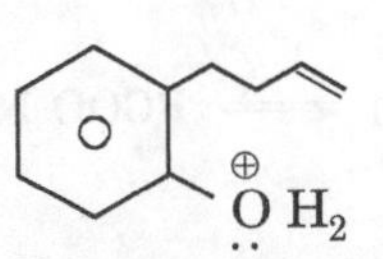

(b) 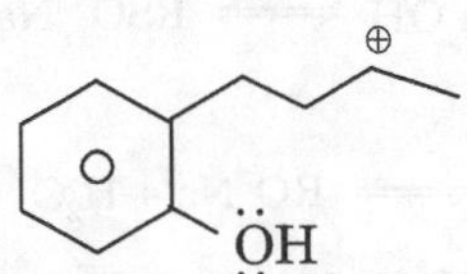

(c) 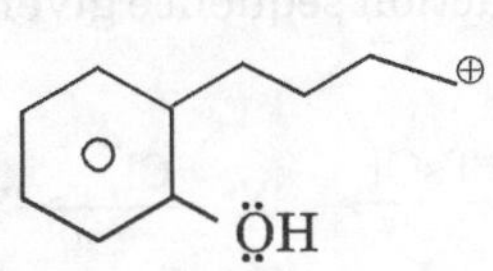

(d) All of these

107. What is the structure of ($C_4H_{10}O$) which can give +ve haloform test & can evolve H_2 gas with $LiAlH_4$?

(a) $CH_3 - O - CH_3$

(b) $CH_3 - \underset{CH_3}{\underset{|}{CH}} - CH_2OH$

(c) $CH_3 - \underset{OH}{\underset{|}{CH}} - CH_2CH_3$

(d) $CH_3 - CH_2 - O - CH_2CH_3$

108. Select the correct statement regarding dehydration of an alcohol by $POCl_3$ in the presence of Pyridine.

(a) It follows E_2 mechanism.

(b) Pyridine acts as a base.

(c) $PCl_2O_2^-$ is the leaving group.

(d) All are correct.

109. Which of the following reactions depict the acidic nature?

(a) $H-C\equiv C-H+Na \rightarrow H-C\equiv C^-Na^+ + \frac{1}{2}H_2 \uparrow$

(b) $NH_3+Na \rightarrow NaNH_2 + \frac{1}{2}H_2 \uparrow$

(c) $R-OH+Na \rightarrow RO^-Na^+ \frac{1}{2}H_2 \uparrow$

(d) All the reactions depict acidic nature

110. In which of the following, equilibrium predominantly lies to left hand side?

(a) 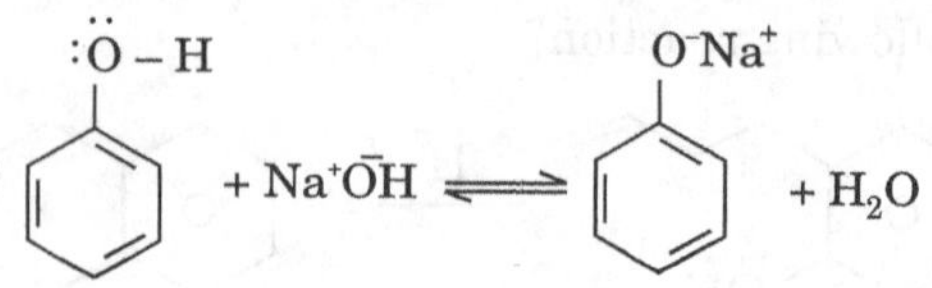

(b) $R-\overset{O}{\overset{||}{C}}-\ddot{O}-H + Na^+\bar{O}H \rightleftharpoons RCOO^-Na^+ + H_2O$

(c) $R-\overset{O}{\overset{||}{\underset{\underset{O}{||}}{S}}}-\ddot{O}-H + Na^+\bar{O}H \rightleftharpoons RSO_3^-Na^+ + H_2O$

(d) $R\ddot{O}-H + Na^+\bar{O}H \rightleftharpoons RO^-Na^+ + H_2O$

111. What is 'Y' in the reaction sequence given below?

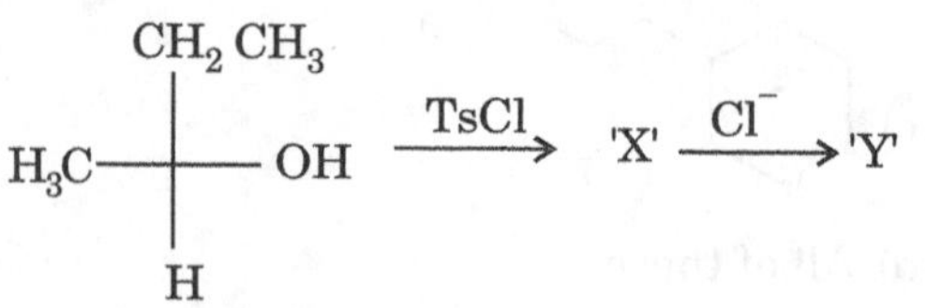

(a) 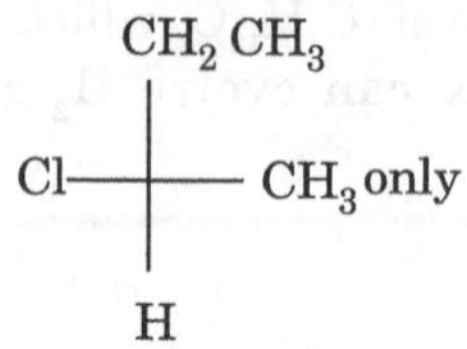

(b) 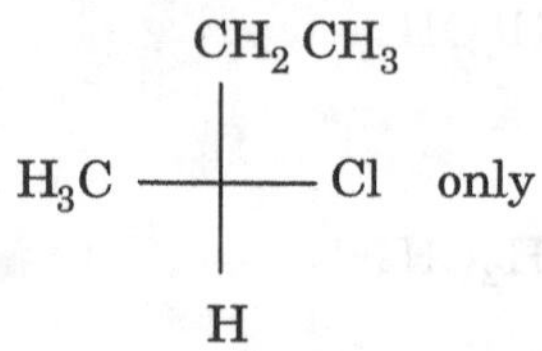

(c) Equimolar mixture of 1 & 2

(d) None of these

112. Identify 'B' in the following reaction map-

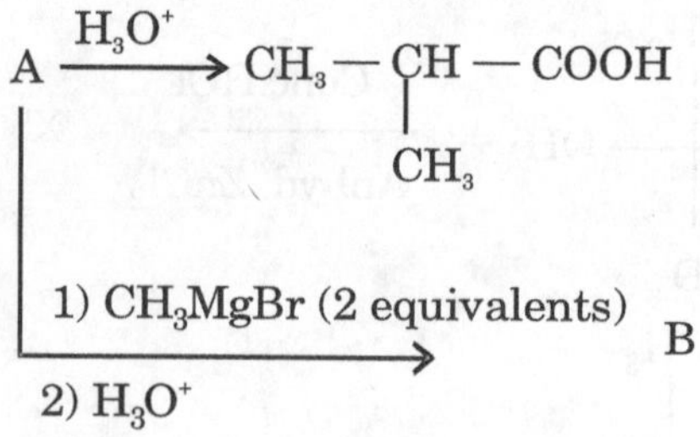

(a) $(CH_3)_2CH-C(CH_3)_2$ with OH on the C

(b) $(CH_3)_2CH-CH_3$

(c) $(CH_3)_2CHCOCH_3$

(d) $(CH_3)_2CHCOCH_2-CH_3$

113. Which of the following reagent (s) can be used to carry out the following conversion?

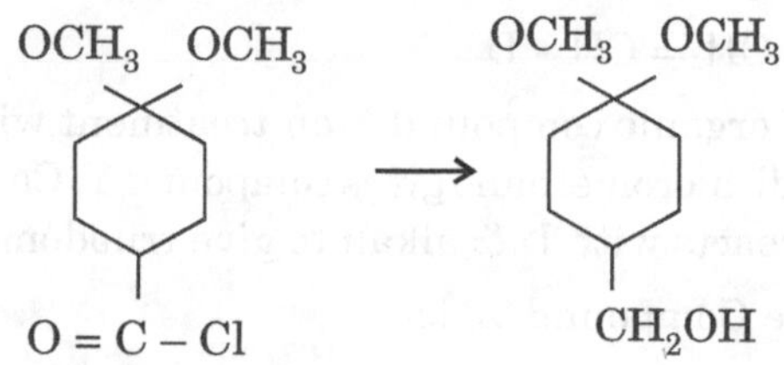

(a) $NaBH_4$ | H_3O^+

(b) (i) $LiAlH_4$ (ii) H_3O^+

(c) B_2H_6 | H_3O^+

(d) Both a & b

114. An optically active alcohol A($C_8H_{16}O$) on strong oxidation gives B. 'A' on heating with acid (dehydration) gives C(C_8H_{14}) as major product. 'C' on ozonolysis produces D (C_5H_8O) and $CH_3-\underset{\underset{O}{||}}{C}-CH_3$. 'D' on reduction with $LiAlH_4$ gave 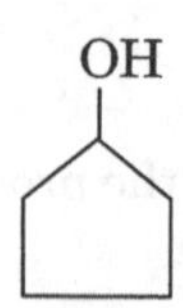 Then A, B, C & D could be, respectively

(a) 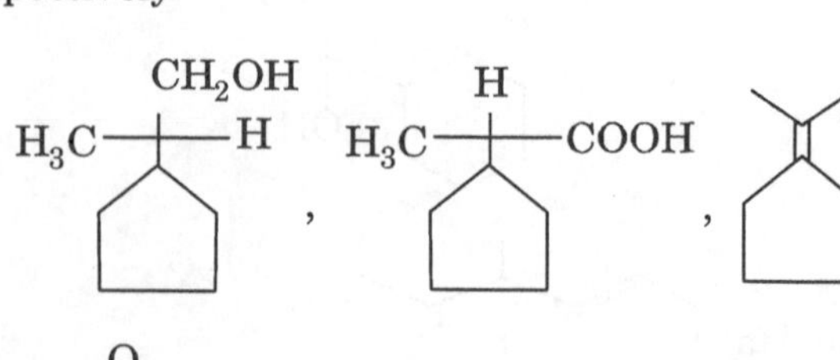

& 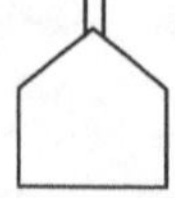

(b) 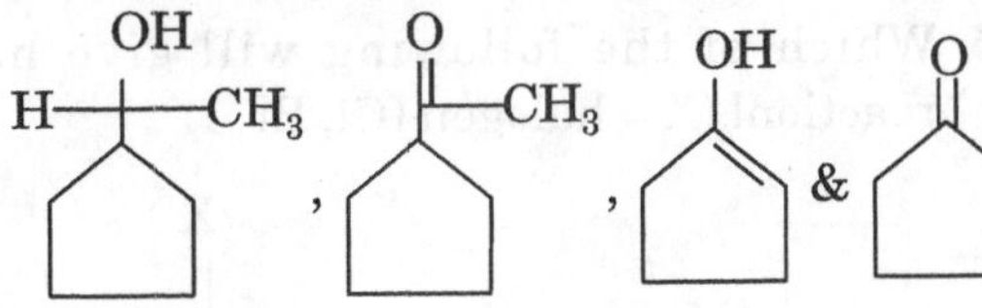

(c) 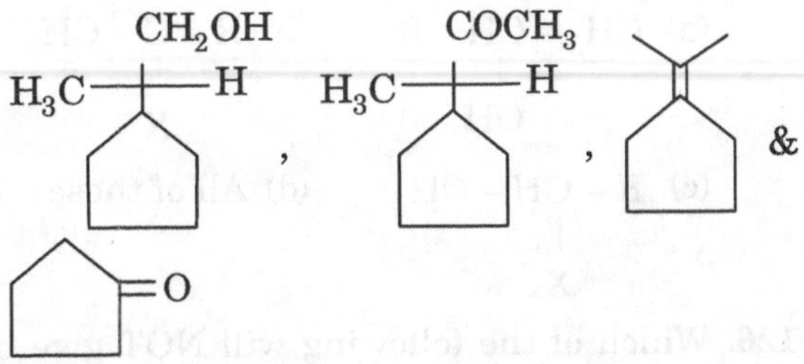

(d) None of these

115. Which of the following is the correct order of reactivity towards acid catalysed dehydration?

(a) $CH_2 = CH - CH(OH) - CH_3 > CH_3 - CH_2 - CH(OH) - CH_3 > CH_2 = CH - OH$

(b) 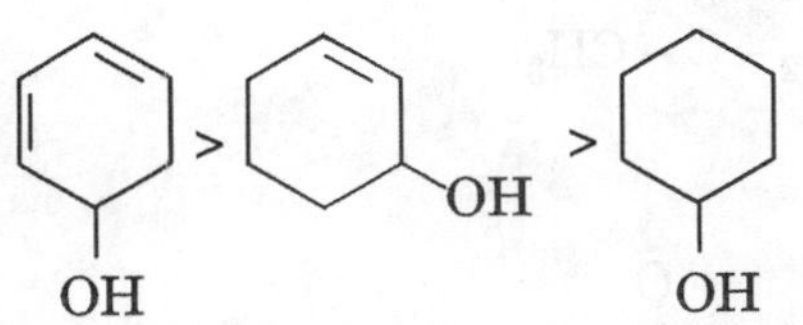

(c) $(CH_3)_3C - OH > CH_3 - CH(OH) - CH_3 > CH_3 - CH_2OH$

(d) All are correct.

116. Select the correct statement.

(a) Esters can undergo both acidic & basic hydrolysis.

(b) Acidic hydrolysis of esters is reversible but basic hydrolysis is irreversible

(c) Carboxylic acid and an alcohol is formed in acidic hydrolysis of esters whereas carboxylate ion & an alcohol is formed in basic hydrolysis of esters.

(d) All are correct.

117. Which of the following is/are correct?

(a) 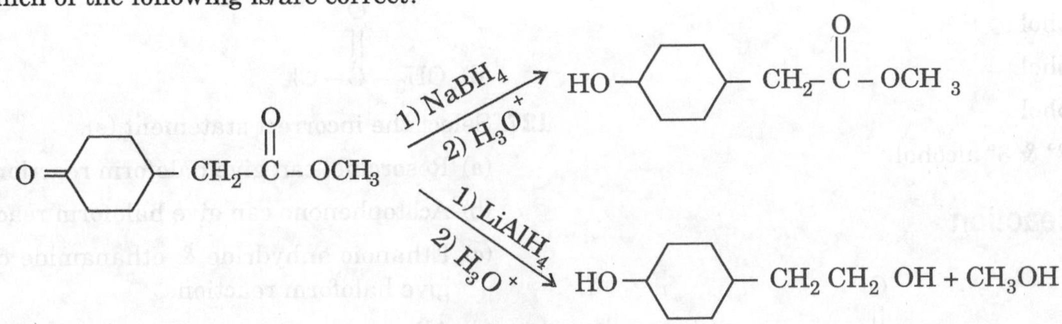

(b) $CH_3 - CH = CH - CH_2 - CH_3 \xrightarrow[2)\ H_3O^+]{1)\ LiAlH_4} CH_3CH_2CH_2CH_2CH_3$

(c) $C_6H_5 - CH = CH - CHO \xrightarrow[2)\ H_3O^+]{1)\ LiAlH_4} C_6H_5CH_2CH_2CH_2OH$

(d) Both a & c are correct

118. Identify the INCORRECT reaction.

(a) $CH_3CH_2OH \xrightarrow[300°C,\ -H_2]{Cu} CH_3CHO$

(b) $CH_3 - CH(CH_3) - OH \xrightarrow[-H_2]{Cu/300°C} CH_3 - \overset{O}{\overset{\|}{C}} - CH_3$

(c) $CH_3 - C(CH_3)_2 - OH \xrightarrow[-H_2O]{Cu/300°C} CH_3 - C(CH_3) = CH_2$

(d) None of these

119. Which of the following reagent selectively oxidises 1° allylic & benzylic alcohols to aldehydes & 2° allylic & benzylic alcohols to Ketones?

(a) H_2CrO_4 (b) MnO_2
(c) PCC (d) PDC

120. Which of the following reagent (s) is/are best suited to cause acid catalysed dehydration of an alcohol?

(a) Conc. H_2SO_4 (b) Conc. HCl
(c) Conc. HNO_3 (d) All of these

121. Consider the following reaction-

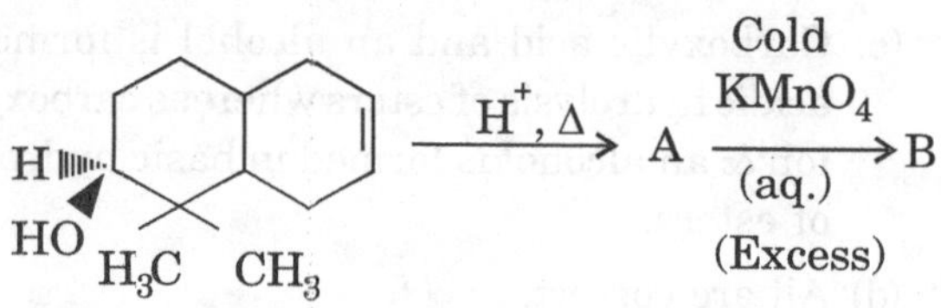

The number of hydroxyl group in final product 'B' are-

(a) 2 (b) 3
(c) 5 (d) 4

122. Which of the following results in 'blood red' coloration in Victor Meyer's test?

(a) 1° alcohol
(b) 2° alcohol
(c) 3° alcohol
(d) Both 2° & 3° alcohol

Haloform Reaction

123. Beginning from $CH_3-\overset{O}{\overset{\|}{C}}-H$ which steps are required to form haloform?

(a) Oxidation, halogenation, basic hydrolysis
(b) Only basic hydrolysis
(c) halogenation & basic hydrolysis only
(d) None of these

124. Beginning from CH_3CH_2OH, which of the following steps are required to form haloform?

(a) Only basic hydrolysis
(b) Oxidation, halogenation & then basic hydrolysis
(c) Oxidation & basic hydrolysis only.
(d) halogenation & basic hydrolysis only.

125. Which of the following will give haloform reaction! (X = halogen (Cl, Br, I)

(a) $CH_3-\underset{OH}{\underset{|}{CH}}-R$ (b) $R-\overset{X}{\overset{|}{\underset{X}{\underset{|}{C}}}}-CH_3$

(c) $R-\underset{X}{\underset{|}{CH}}-CH_3$ (d) All of these

126. Which of the following will NOT give haloform reaction?

(a) $CH_3-\overset{O}{\overset{\|}{C}}-CH_2-\overset{O}{\overset{\|}{C}}-CH_3$

(b) $\underset{Cl}{\underset{|}{CH_2}}-\overset{O}{\overset{\|}{C}}-CH_3$

(c) $CHCl_2-\overset{O}{\overset{\|}{C}}-CH_3$

(d) $CH_3-\overset{O}{\overset{\|}{C}}-Cl$

127. Select the incorrect statement (s).

(a) Resorcinol can give haloform reaction.
(b) Acetophenone can give haloform reaction.
(c) Ethanoic anhydride & ethanamide can also give haloform reaction.
(d) All are correct.

Brain Teasers

128. With reference to the scheme given, which of the given statement(s) about T, U, V & W is/are correct?

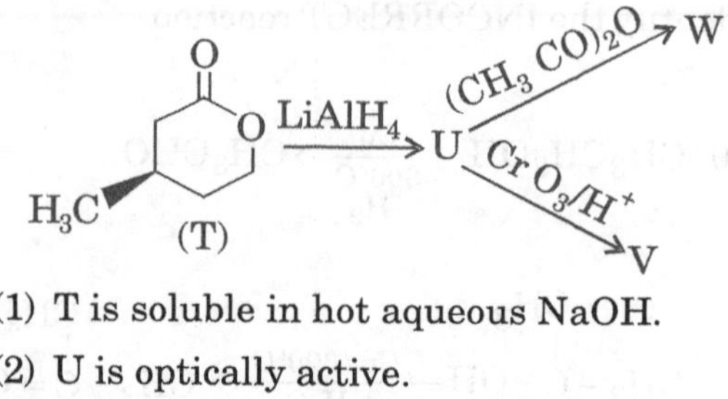

(1) T is soluble in hot aqueous NaOH.
(2) U is optically active.
(3) Molecular formula of W is $C_{10}H_{18}O_4$.

(4) V gives effervescence on treatment with aq. $NaHCO_3$.

(a) Only 1, 3 & 4 are correct.
(b) Only 1, 2, 3 are correct.
(c) Only 3 & 4 are correct.
(d) Only 1 & 3 are correct.

129. Among the following reactions, which will give salicylic acid (after acidification)?

(a) 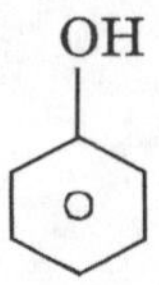 $+ CHCl_3 + NaOH \longrightarrow$

(b) 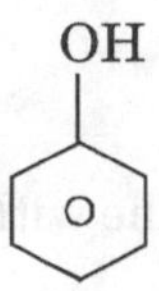 $+ CCl_4 + NaOH \longrightarrow$

(c) 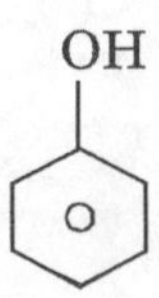 $+ CO_2 + NaOH \longrightarrow$

(d) Both b & c

130. Consider the following reaction-

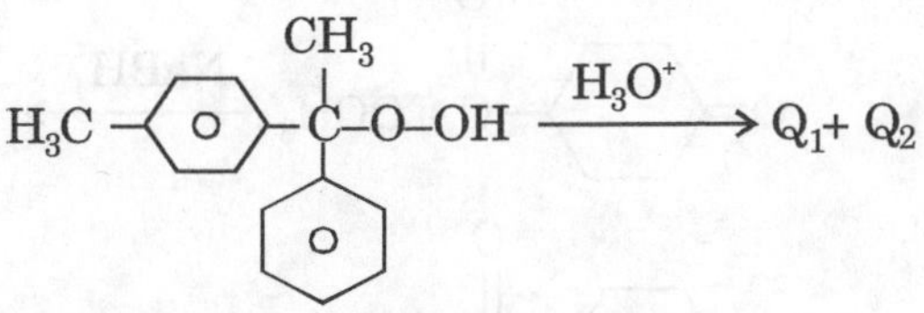

($Q_2 + FeCl_3 \rightarrow$ violet colour)

$Q_1 + NaOH/I_2 \rightarrow Q_3 + Q_4$ (yellow ppt.)

Select the correct statement wrt the reaction given above

(a) Q_3 on reaction with Ag gives acetylene.
(b) Q_4 on reaction with sodalime gives benzene.
(c) Q_1 can react with 2, 4 - DNP.
(d) All of these are correct.

131. Select the correct order of acidic strength

(1) 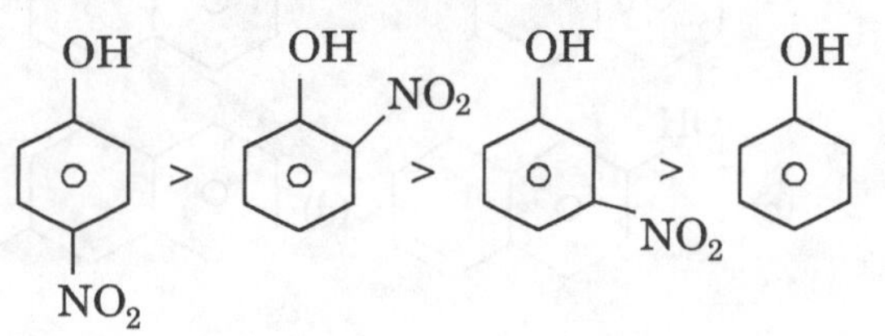

(2) 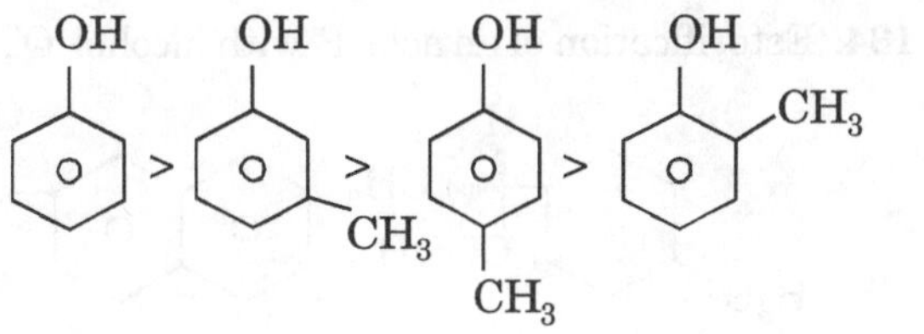

(3) 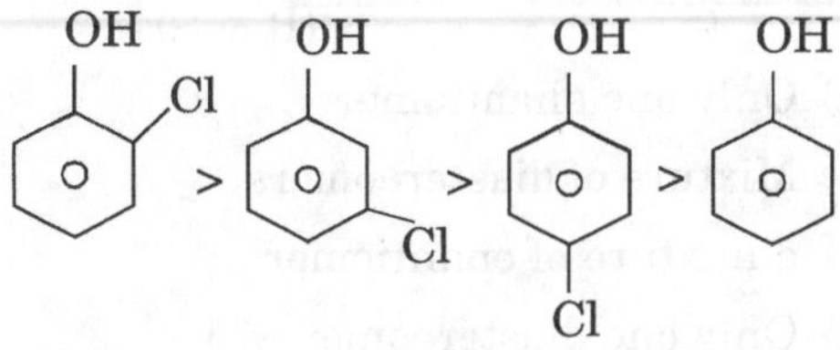

(4) 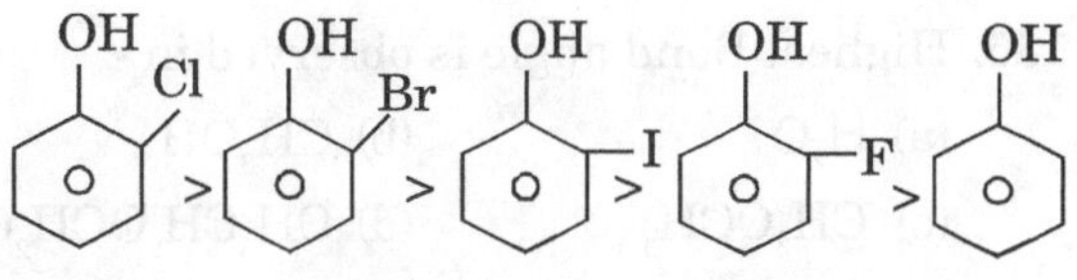

(5) 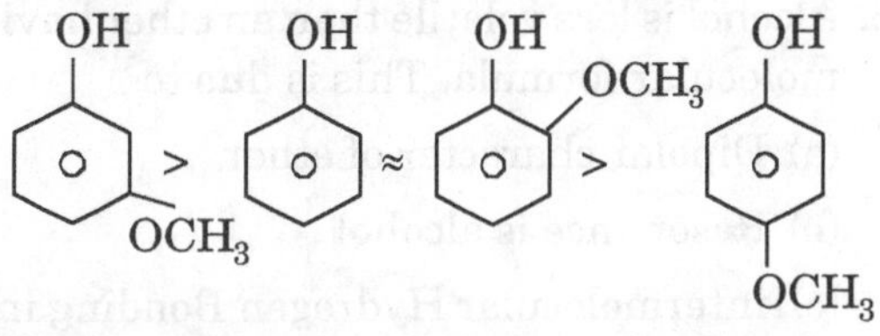

(a) Only 1, 2 & 3 are correct
(b) Only 1, 2 & 4 are correct
(c) Only 3 is correct
(d) All are correct.

132. Which of the following will NOT give effervescence with carbonates and Bicarbonates?

(a) 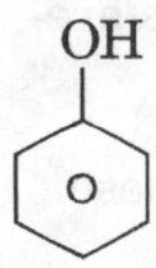 (b) 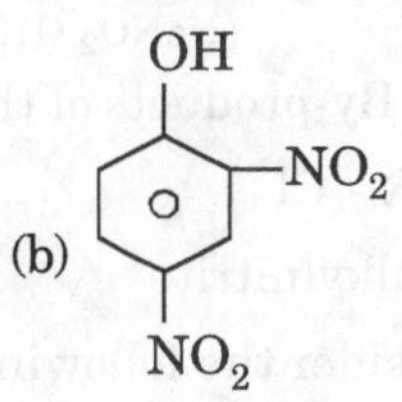

(c) 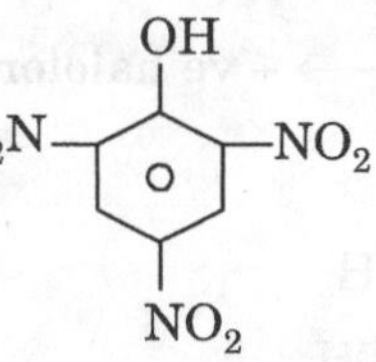 (d) Both b & c

133. Maximum number of moles of HI required to react with 1 mole of 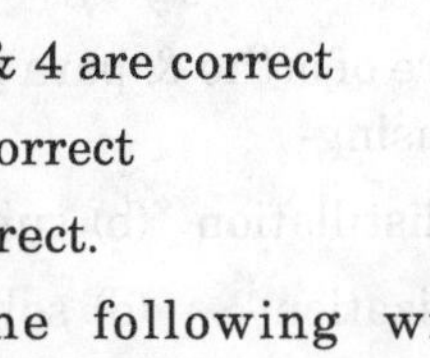 is/are-

(a) 3
(b) 6
(c) 11
(d) 7

134. Esterification of an acid 'P' with alcohol 'Q', will give

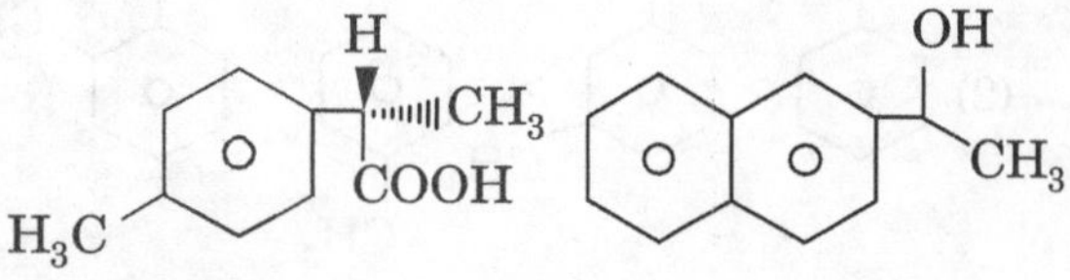

(S) – P (R & S) – Q

(a) Only one enantiomer

(b) Mixture of diastereomers

(c) a mixture of enantiomer

(d) Only one diastereomer

135. Highest Bond angle is observed in -

(a) H_2O (b) CH_3OH

(c) CH_3OCH_3 (d) $CH_3CH_2OCH_2CH_3$

136. Alcohol is less volatile than an ether having same molecular formula. This is due to-

(a) Dipolar character of ether

(b) Resonance is alcohol

(c) intermolecular Hydrogen Bonding in alcohol

(d) intermolecular Hydrogen Bonding in ether

137. 1 : 1 mixture of ortho & para nitrophenols can be separated using-

(a) steam distillation (b) sublimation

(c) crystallization (d) solvent extraction

138. $R-NH_2 + \underset{(NaNO_2/HCl)}{HNO_2} \longrightarrow$

The By-products of this reaction is/are-

(a) R – Cl (b) alkene

(c) alkylnitrite (d) All of these

139. Consider the following reaction-

$$(A) \xrightarrow[Pb(AcO)_4]{HIO_4 \text{ or}} B \longrightarrow +\text{ve haloform.}$$

(A) may be-

(a) $(CH_3CH_2CHOH)_2CH_2$

(b) $CH_3CHOHCHOHCH_3$

(c) $CH_3CHOHCOCHOHCH_3$

(d) Both b & c

140. $CH_3-CH=CH-CH(OH)-CH_3 \xrightarrow[\text{Reagent}]{\text{Jones}} X$

Product 'X' is -

(a) $CH_3CH_2CH_2CH(OH)CH_3$

(b) $CH_3CH{=}CHCOCH_3$

(c) Both a & b are correct

(d) $CH_3CH_2CH_2COCH_3$

141. Consider the following conversion-

$$CH_3-\underset{OH}{CH}-CH_2-CH=CH-CH_2-\underset{OH}{CH}-C_6H_5$$

$$\longrightarrow CH_3-\underset{OH}{CH}-CH_2-CH=CH-CH_2-\underset{C_6H_5}{\overset{O}{\overset{||}{C}}}$$

The Reagent which can be used for above conversion is-

(a) PCC

(b) $KMnO_4/\overline{O}H$

(c) MnO_2

(d) dil.HNO_3

142. Product of reaction of diazomethane with phenol is-

(a) anisole + oxygen

(b) anisole + nitrogen

(c) benzene + nitrogen

(d) benzene + oxygen

143. The product formed in the following reaction is –

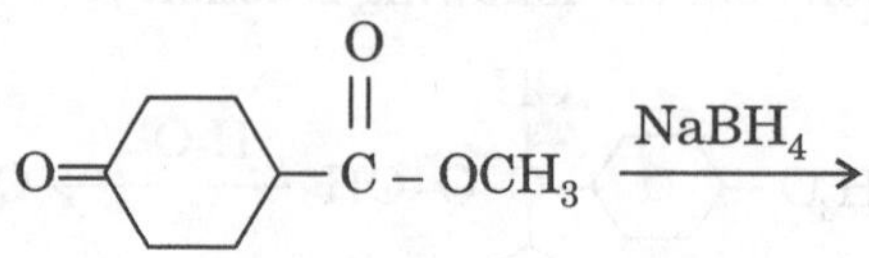

(a) 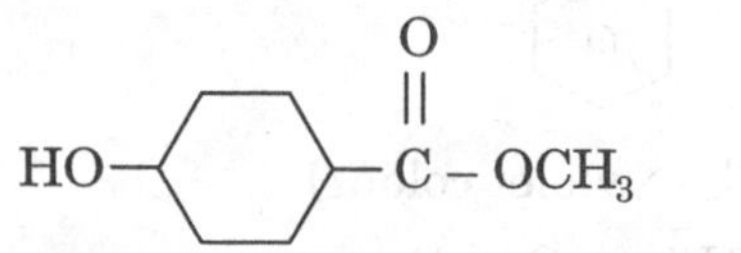

(b) 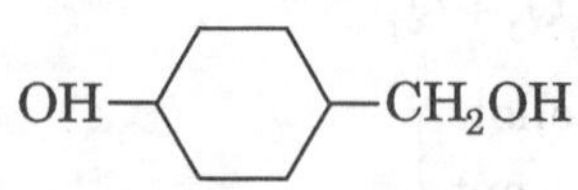

(c) 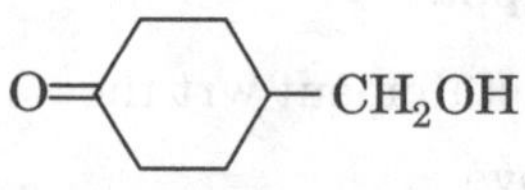

(d) None of these

144. Which one of the following is maximum reactive towards acid catalysed dehydration ?

(a) 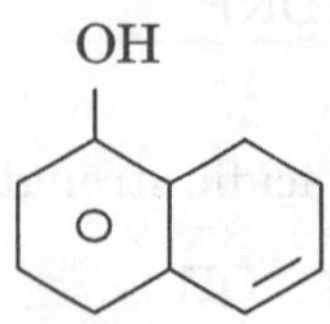

(b) 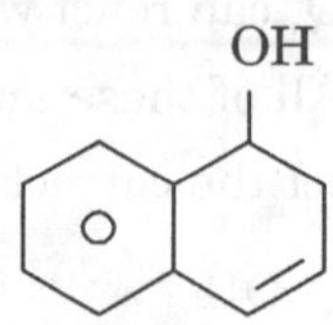

(c) 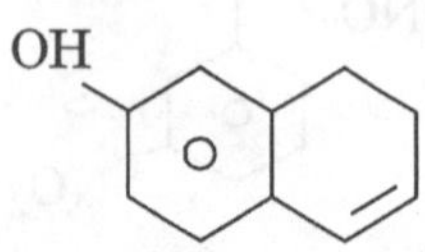

(d) 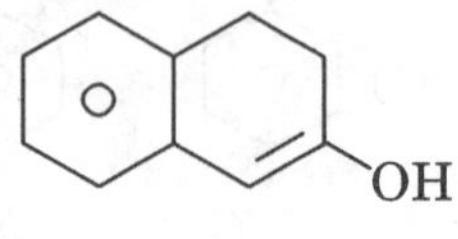

145. Consider the following reaction –

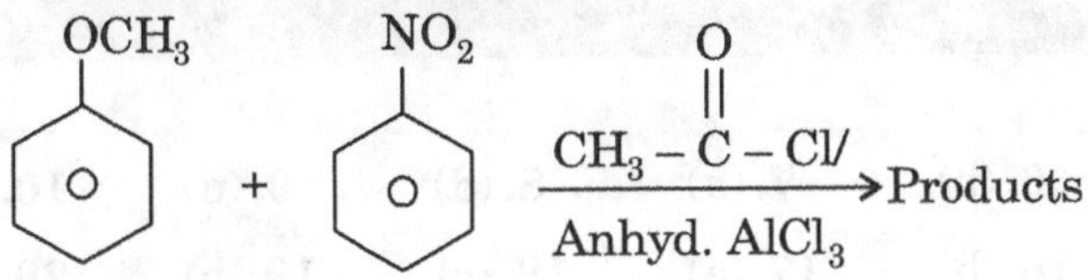

Possible products is/are

(a) 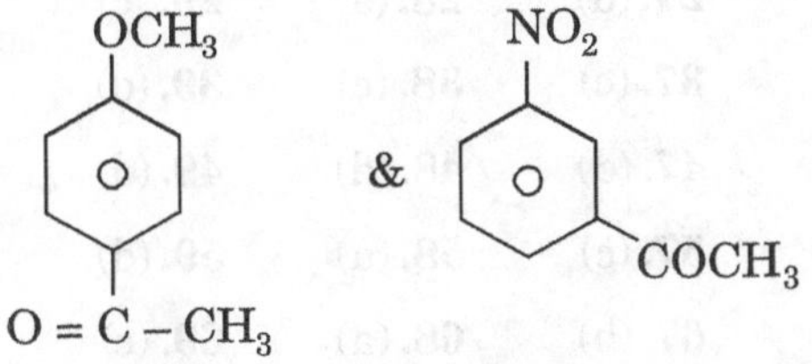

(b) 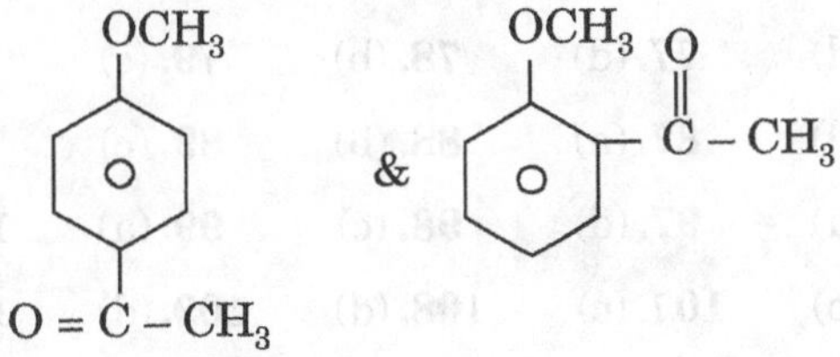

(c) Only 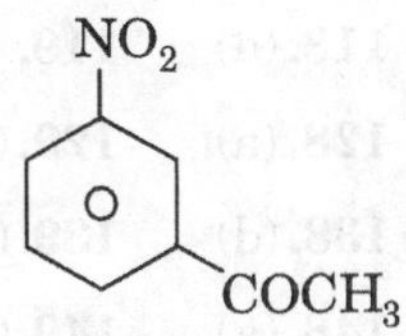

(d) Only 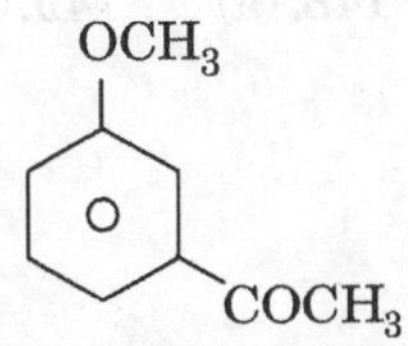

146. Which of the following will give a silver mirror with tollen's reagent ?

(a) CH_3CHO (b) C_6H_5CHO

(c) $CH_3-\overset{O}{\overset{||}{C}}-CH_2OH$ (d) All of these

147. Which of the following can give immediate turbidity with Lucas Reagent ?

(a) 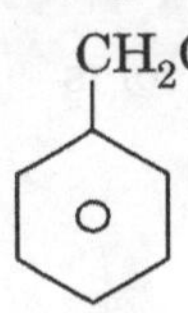

(b) $CH_2=CH-CH_2-OH$

(c) 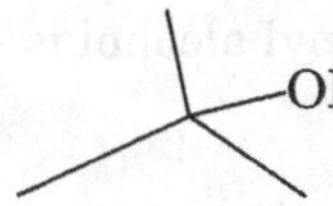

(d) All of these

148. The compound which on reduction with $LiAlH_4$ gives two different alcohols is –

(a) CH_3COOCH_3 (b) $CH_3COOC_2H_5$

(c) CH_3COCH_3 (d) CH_3CH_2CHO

149. HBr reacts with $CH_2=CH-OCH_3$ under anhydrous conditions at room temperature to give–

(a) CH_3CHO & CH_3Br (b) $BrCH_2CHO$ & CH_3OH

(c) $BrCH_2CH_2OCH_3$ (d) $CH_3-\underset{Br}{\underset{|}{CH}}-OCH_3$

150. The final product in the following reactions is –

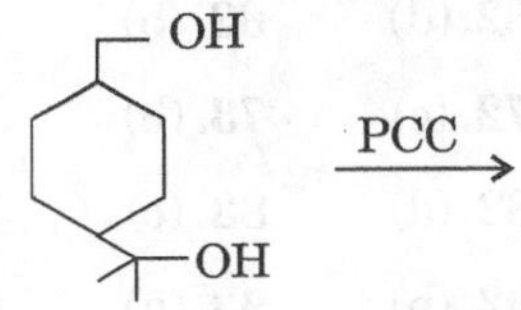

(a) 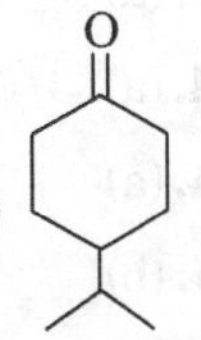 (b) 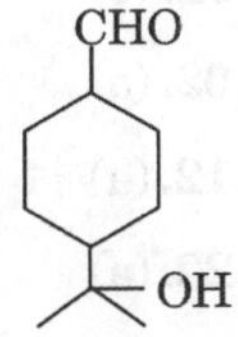

(c) 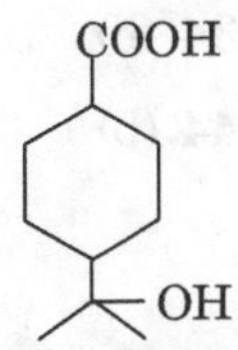 (d) 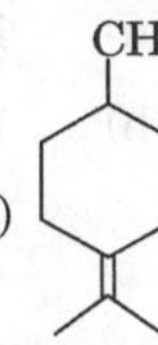

151. Give the products of the following reaction –

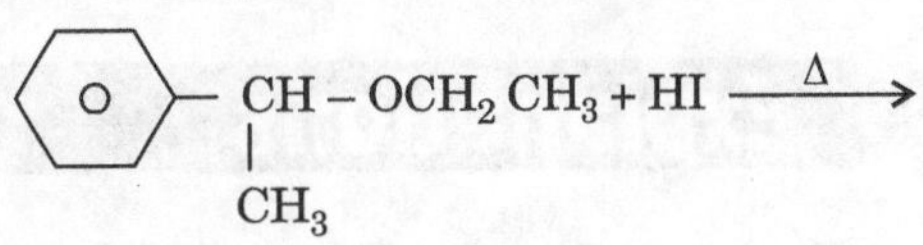

(a) 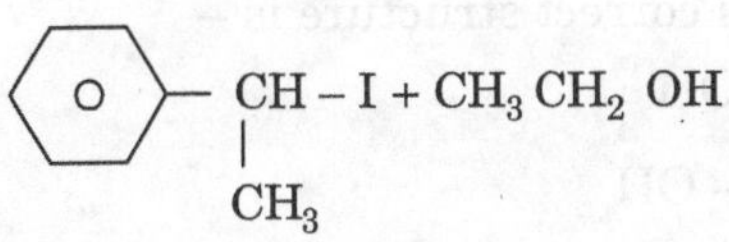

(b) $CH_3CH_2I + CH_3CH_2OH +$ 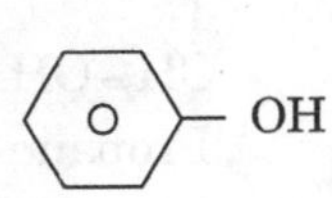

(c) 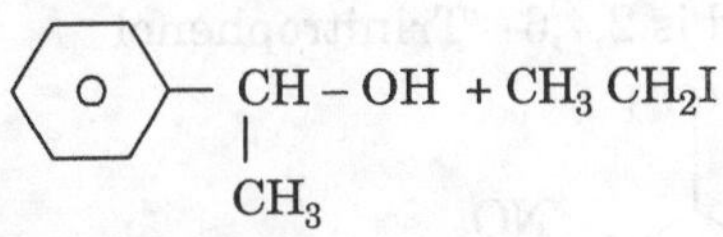

(d) None of these

Answers

1. (c)	**2.** (d)	**3.** (c)	**4.** (d)	**5.** (a)	**6.** (b)	**7.** (a)	**8.** (d)	**9.** (d)	**10.** (c)
11. (d)	**12.** (c)	**13.** (b)	**14.** (b)	**15.** (a)	**16.** (b)	**17.** (a)	**18.** (c)	**19.** (b)	**20.** (d)
21. (a)	**22.** (c)	**23.** (b)	**24.** (a)	**25.** (d)	**26.** (d)	**27.** (d)	**28.** (a)	**29.** (c)	**30.** (c)
31. (d)	**32.** (b)	**33.** (d)	**34.** (c)	**35.** (d)	**36.** (d)	**37.** (c)	**38.** (c)	**39.** (d)	**40.** (d)
41. (d)	**42.** (a)	**43.** (c)	**44.** (a)	**45.** (a)	**46.** (a)	**47.** (d)	**48.** (d)	**49.** (d)	**50.** (b)
51. (d)	**52.** (b)	**53.** (c)	**54.** (b)	**55.** (b)	**56.** (c)	**57.** (c)	**58.** (a)	**59.** (d)	**60.** (d)
61. (a)	**62.** (d)	**63.** (b)	**64.** (c)	**65.** (d)	**66.** (c)	**67.** (b)	**68.** (a)	**69.** (c)	**70.** (d)
71. (c)	**72.** (c)	**73.** (b)	**74.** (c)	**75.** (b)	**76.** (d)	**77.** (d)	**78.** (b)	**79.** (c)	**80.** (a)
81. (d)	**82.** (d)	**83.** (c)	**84.** (c)	**85.** (d)	**86.** (d)	**87.** (a)	**88.** (b)	**89.** (c)	**90.** (a)
91. (c)	**92.** (b)	**93.** (a)	**94.** (a)	**95.** (b)	**96.** (a)	**97.** (d)	**98.** (c)	**99.** (a)	**100.** (b)
101. (a)	**102.** (a)	**103.** (d)	**104.** (a)	**105.** (a)	**106.** (b)	**107.** (c)	**108.** (d)	**109.** (d)	**110.** (d)
111. (a)	**112.** (a)	**113.** (d)	**114.** (a)	**115.** (d)	**116.** (d)	**117.** (d)	**118.** (d)	**119.** (b)	**120.** (a)
121. (d)	**122.** (a)	**123.** (c)	**124.** (b)	**125.** (d)	**126.** (d)	**127.** (c)	**128.** (a)	**129.** (d)	**130.** (d)
131. (d)	**132.** (a)	**133.** (b)	**134.** (b)	**135.** (d)	**136.** (c)	**137.** (a)	**138.** (d)	**139.** (d)	**140.** (b)
141. (c)	**142.** (b)	**143.** (a)	**144.** (b)	**145.** (b)	**146.** (d)	**147.** (d)	**148.** (a)	**149.** (d)	**150.** (b)
151. (a)									

Explanations

1. Glycerol's correct structure is –

$$\begin{array}{l} CH_2{-}OH \\ | \\ CH{-}OH \\ | \\ CH_2{-}OH \end{array}$$

Propane-1,2,3-triol

3. Picric acid is 2,4,6 – Trinitrophenol

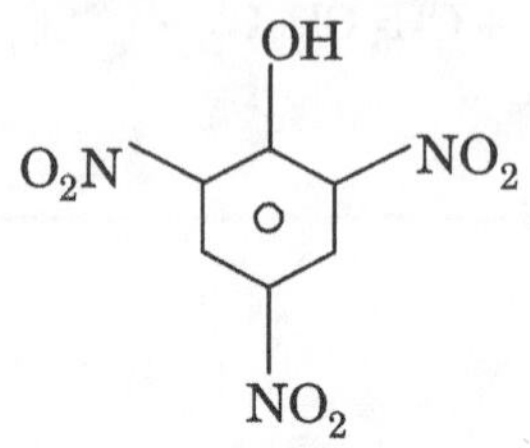

6. General formula of ethers is R–Ö–R 'O' has two lone pairs resting on it & so it can act as lewis base.

7.
$$CH_3-\underset{\displaystyle CH_3}{\overset{\displaystyle CH_3}{\underset{|}{\overset{|}{C}}}}-CH_2\,OH$$

(Neopentyl alcohol, 1° alcohol)

8. Correct formula for ethylene glycol is

$$\begin{array}{l} CH_2{-}OH \\ | \\ CH_2-OH \end{array}$$

9. Correct formula for isopropyl alcohol is

$$CH_3 - \underset{\displaystyle CH_3}{\underset{|}{CH}} - OH$$

IUPAC Name:– Propan – 2 – ol

12. $CH_3O{-}CH_2{-}CH_2{-}CH_3$ & $CH_3CH_2OCH_2CH_3$ (1-methoxy propane) (1-ethoxy ethane) are metamers

13. The reaction occurs via carbocation formation.

Mechanism is as follows

(1) $NaNO_2 + HCl \rightarrow HNO_2 + NaCl$

(2) 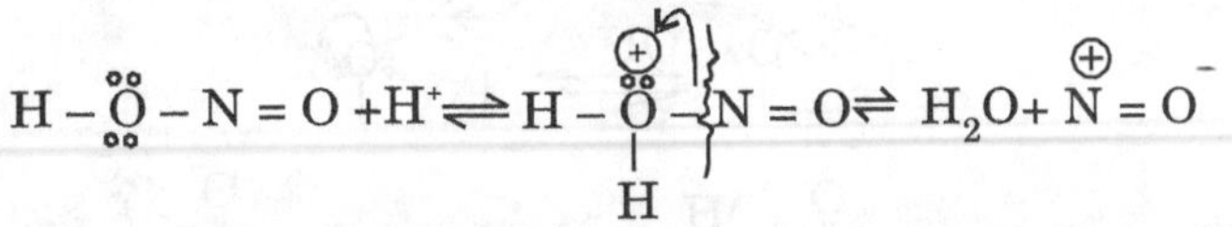

(3) 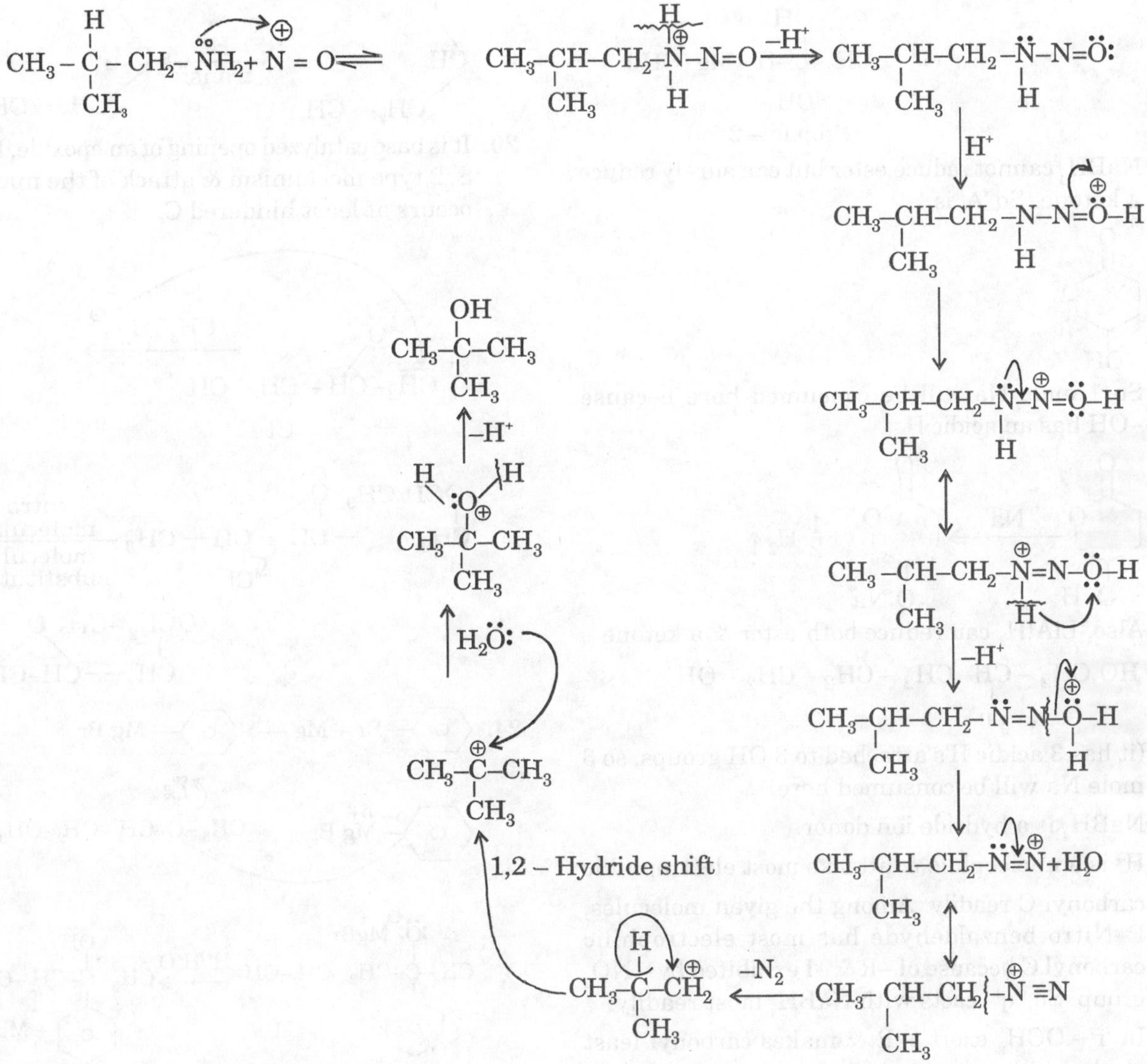

14. 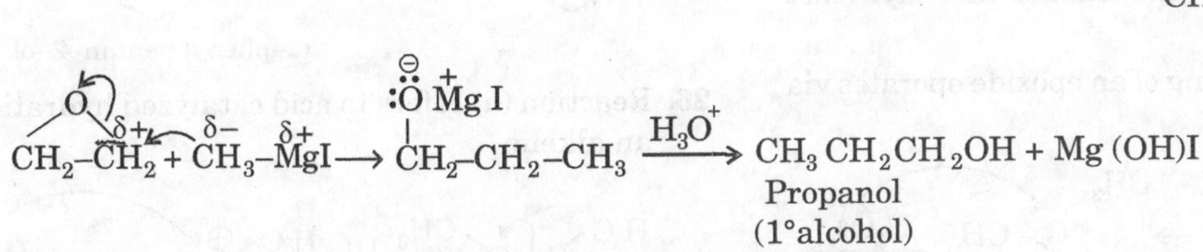

15. Reaction 1 represents acid catalysed hydration of an alkene.

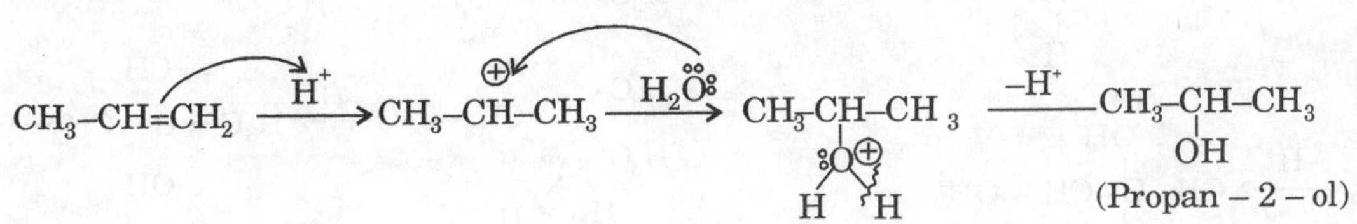

Reaction II involves attack of Grignard's reagent on ethanal.

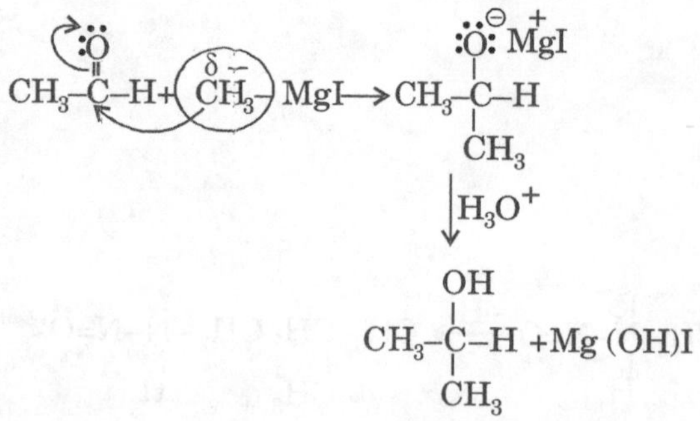

(Propan – 2–ol)

16. $NaBH_4$ cannot reduce ester but can surely reduce a ketone. So 'A' is

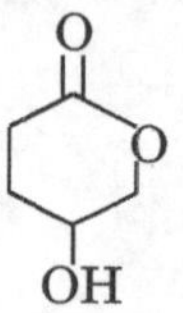

So 1 mole Na will be consumed here because –OH has an acidic H

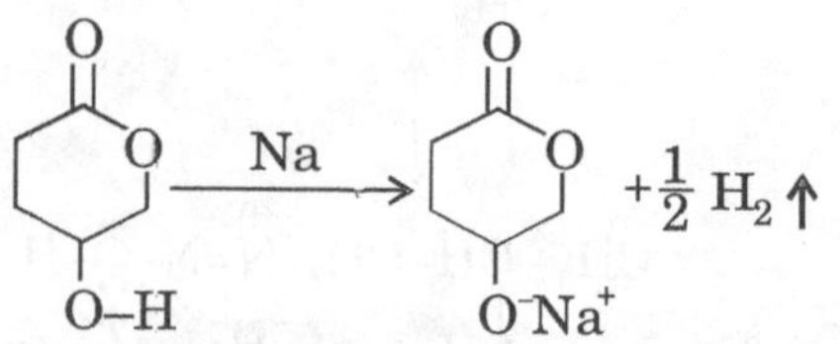

Also, $LiAlH_4$ can reduce both ester & a ketone

$HO\,CH_2 - \underset{|}{CH}(OH) - CH_2 - CH_2 - CH_2 - OH$

(it has 3 acidic H's attached to 3 OH groups, so 3 mole Na will be consumed here)

17. $NaBH_4$ is a hydride ion donor.

H^- is a nucleophile & attacks most electrophillic carbonyl C readily. Among the given molecules, P–Nitro benzaldehyde has most electrophilic carbonyl C because of –R & –I exhibited by – NO_2 group. So, 'q' reacts with $NaBH_4$ most readily.

In 'r' –OCH_3 exert + R & makes carbonyl least electrophillic

18. Acid catalyzed opening of an epoxide operates via S_N1 type

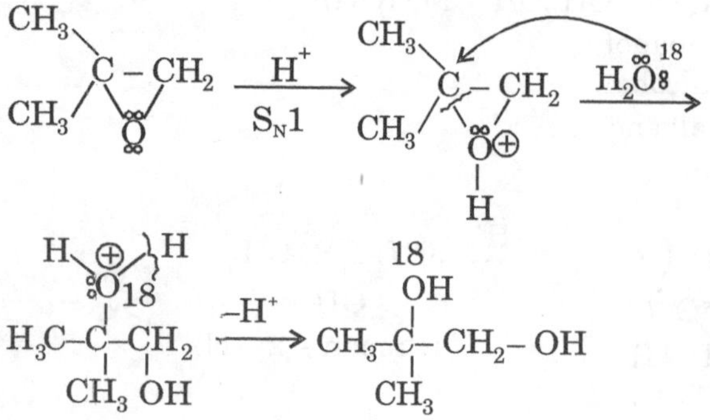

19. The reaction is an example of base catalyzed hydrolysis of an ester

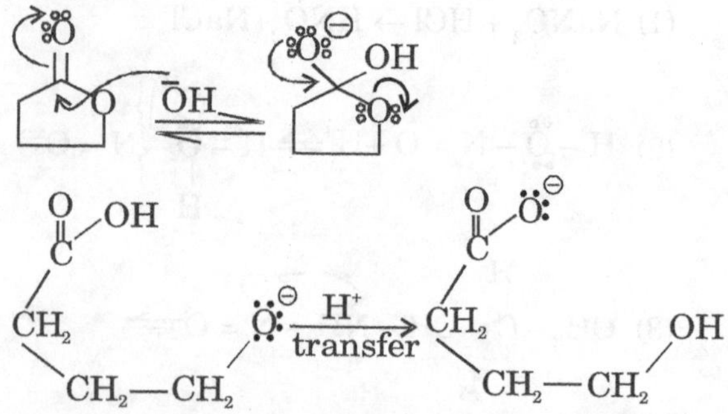

20. It is base catalyzed opening of an epoxide. It follows S_N2 type mechanism & attack of the nucleophile occurs at least hindered C.

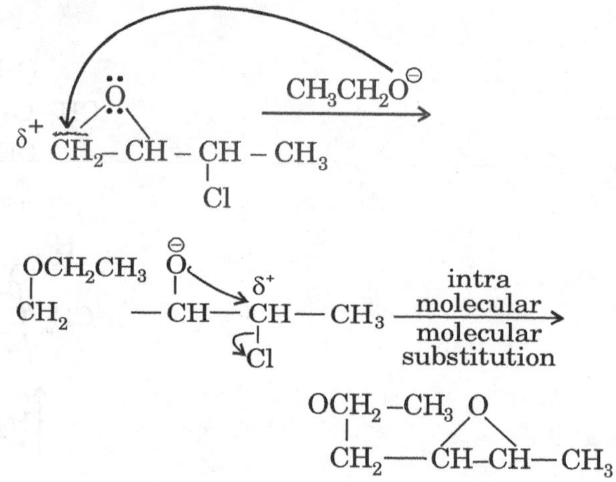

24.

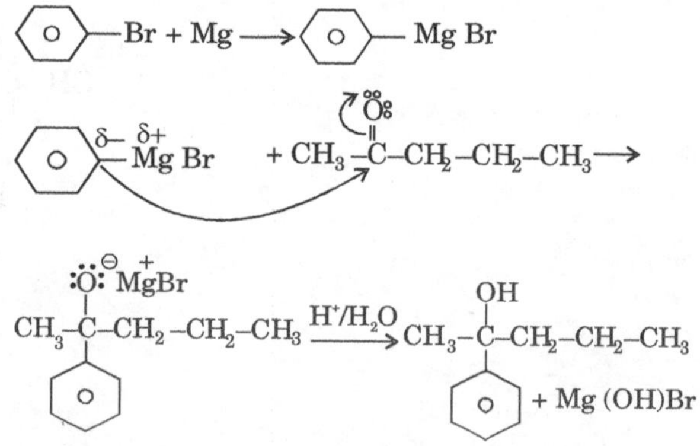

(2–phenyl pentan–2–ol)

26. Reaction (a) refers to acid catalyzed hydration of an alkene

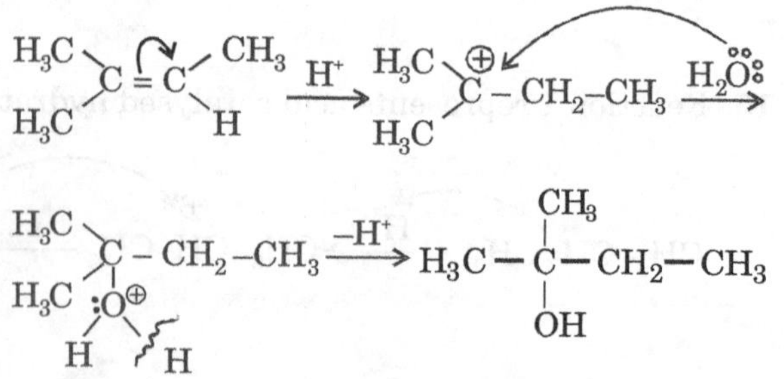

Reaction 2 is oxymercuration demercuration

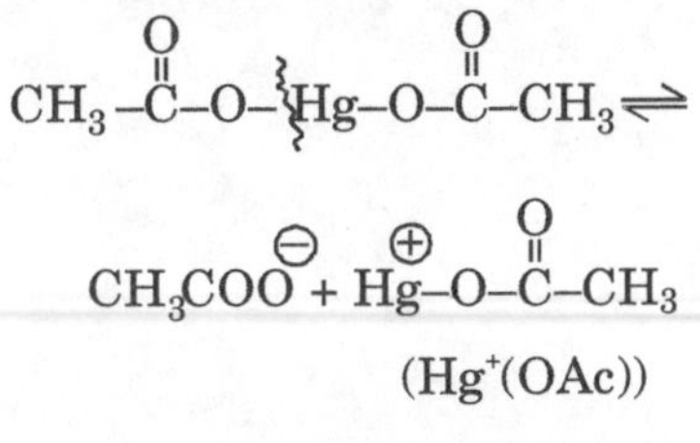

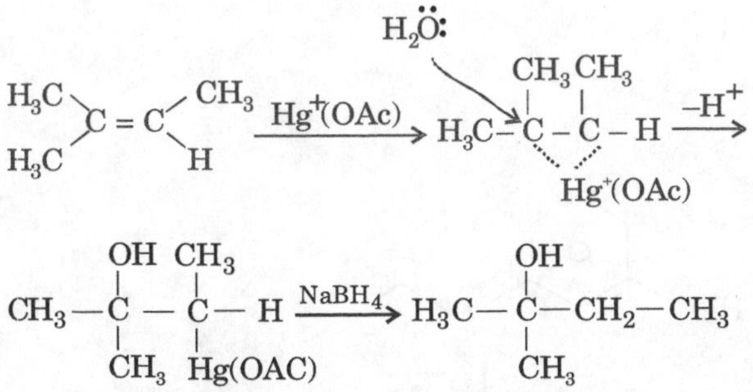

28. B_2H_6/THF besides reacting at C = C bond also reduces – COOH to $-CH_2OH$

29. 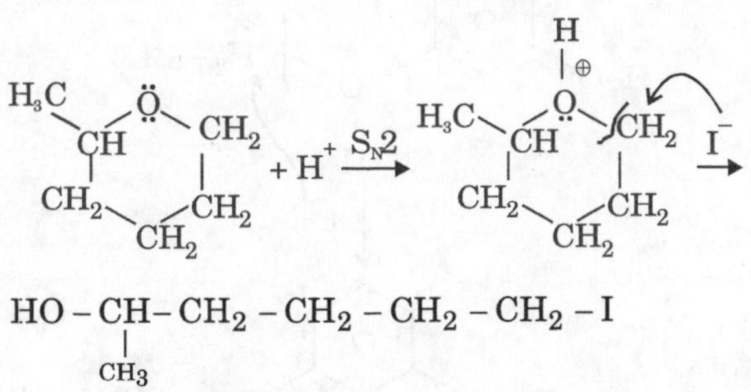

30. 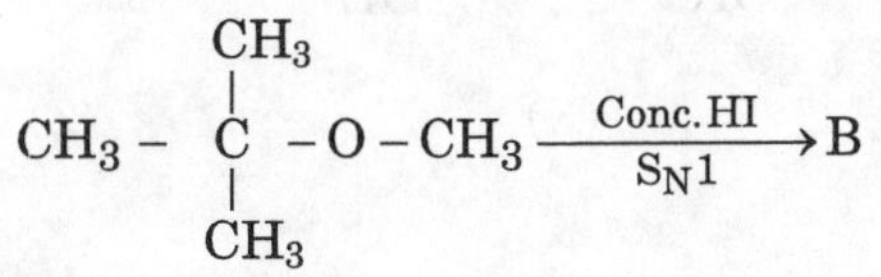

<u>Mechanism</u>

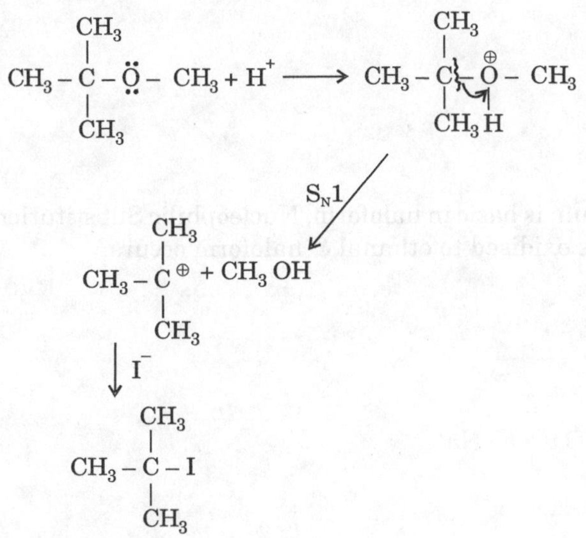

So, Mixture B has 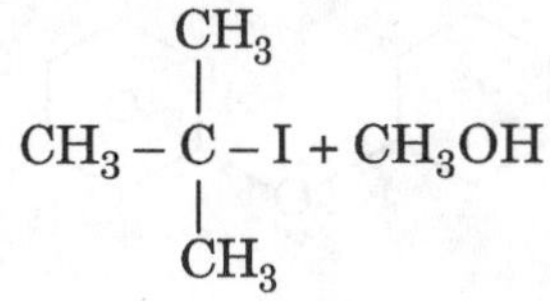

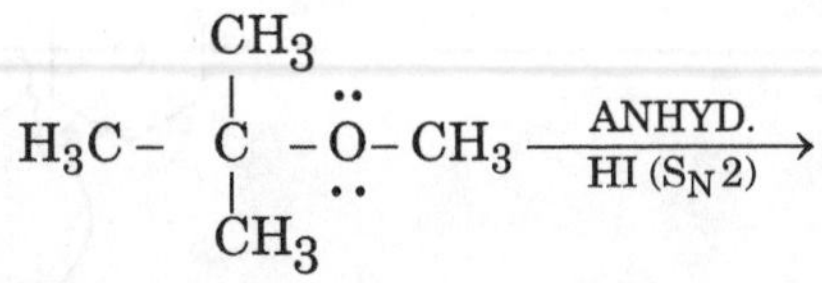

<u>Mechanism</u>

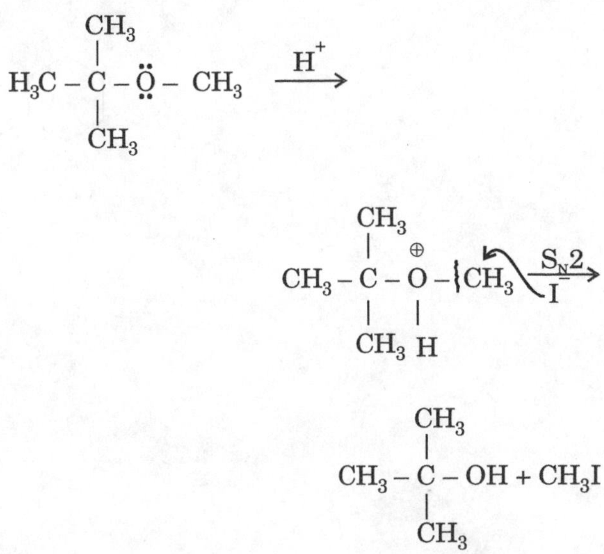

(Mixture A)

31. Wrt option (d)

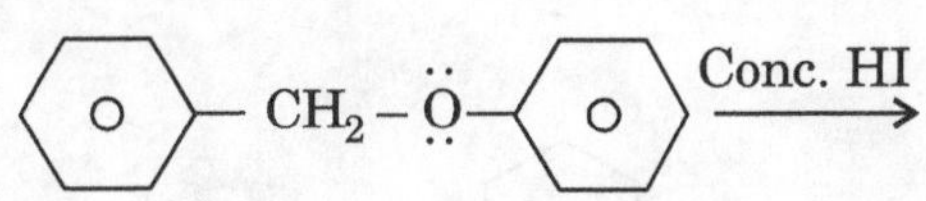

Mechanism

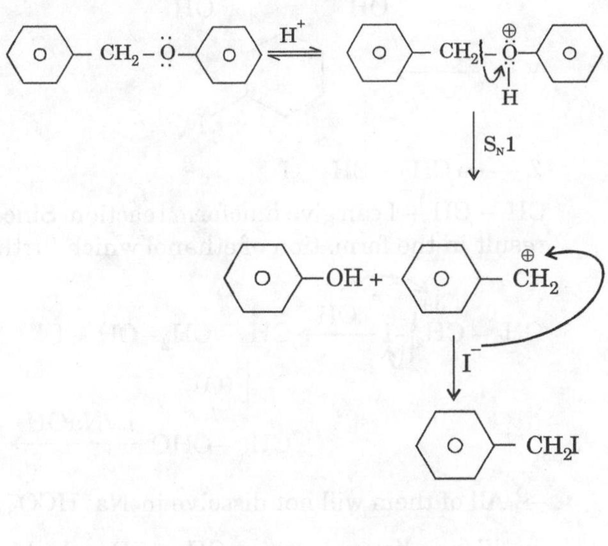

32.

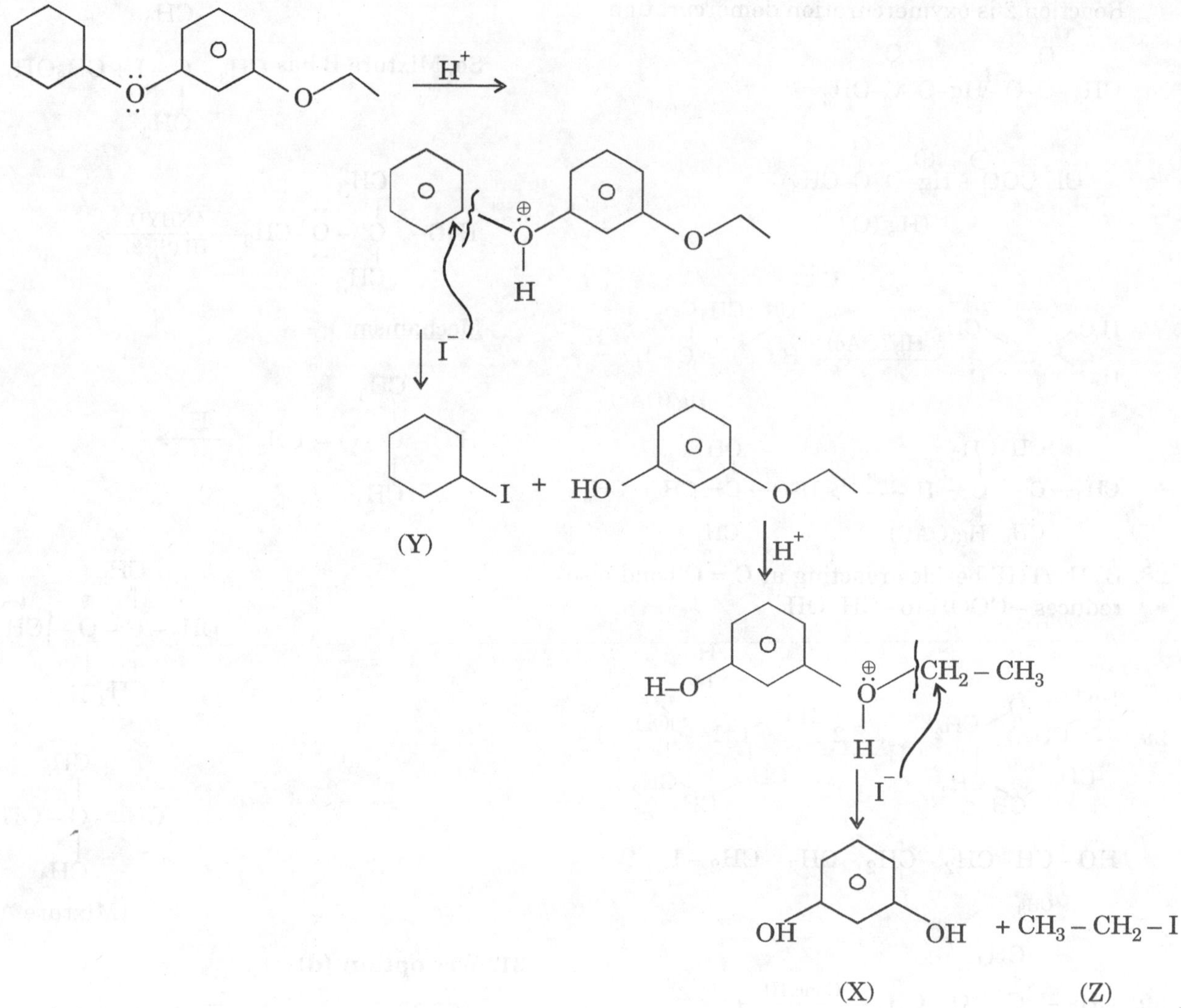

So,

X $\longrightarrow$ 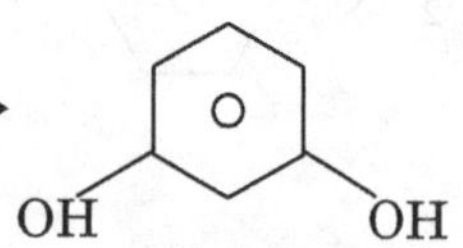

Y $\longrightarrow$ 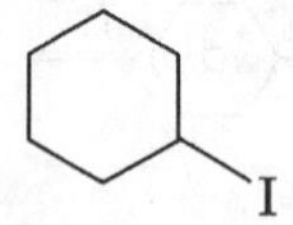

Z $\longrightarrow CH_3-CH_2-I$

CH_3-CH_2-I can give haloform reaction. Since medium is basic in haloform, Nucleophilic Substitution can result in the formation of ethanol which further gets oxidised to ethanal & haloform occurs.

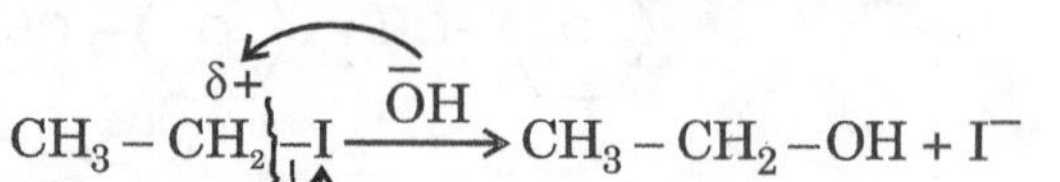

$$CH_3-\overset{\delta+}{CH_2}-I \xrightarrow{\bar{O}H} CH_3-CH_2-OH + I^-$$

$$\downarrow (O)$$

$$CH_3-CHO \xrightarrow{I_2/NaOH} CHI_3 + HCOO^-Na^+$$

→ All of them will not dissolve in $Na^+HCO_3^-$.

→ 'Z' (acyclic product) i.e. CH_3-CH_2-I which gives haloform test.

33. All given options are lewis acids.

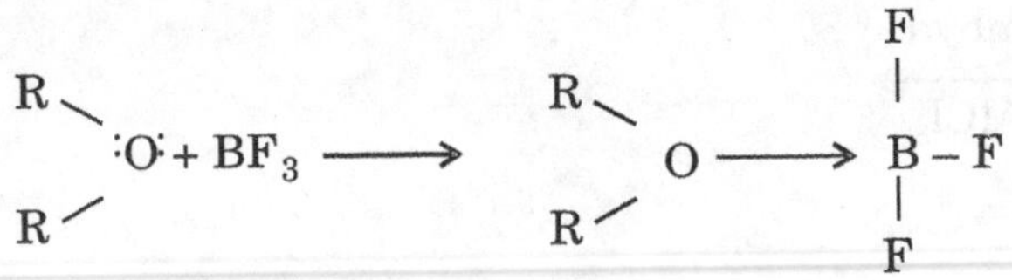

Boron trifluoride etherate (complex)

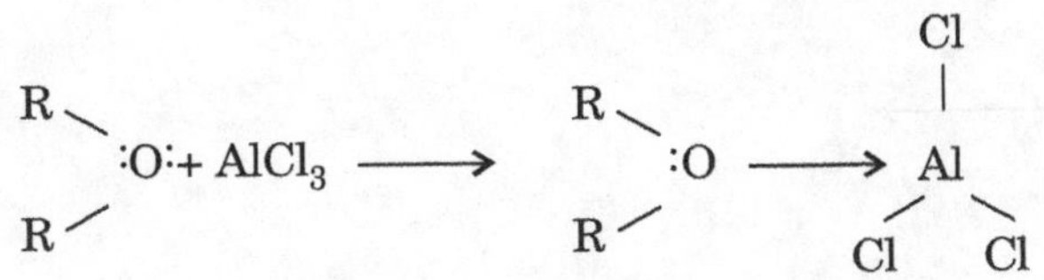

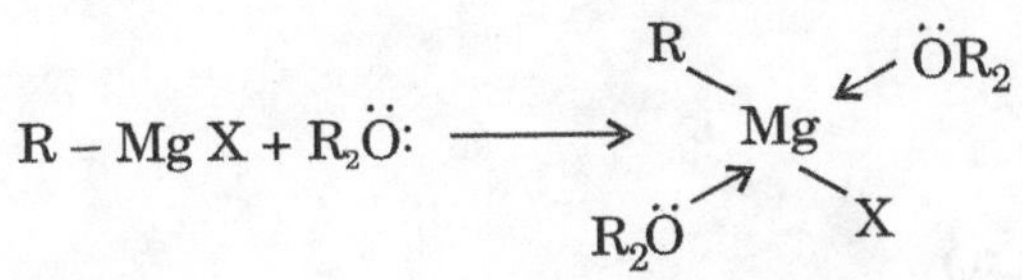

etherate

34. 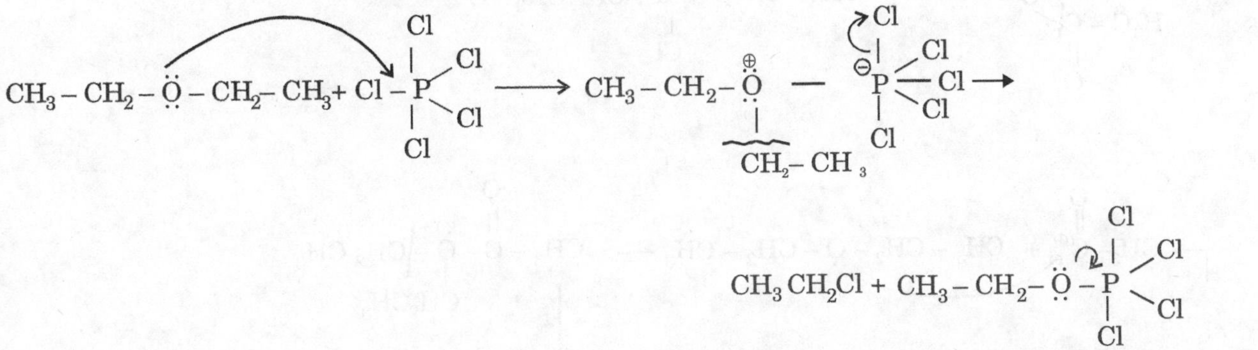

(P = O pπ–dπ bond is strong)

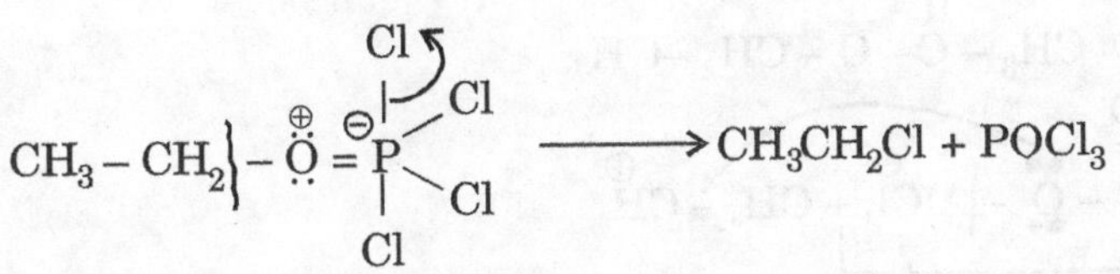

35. $CH_3-CH_2-O-CH_2-CH_3+CH_3-\overset{O}{\overset{\|}{C}}-Cl\xrightarrow[AlCl_3]{Anhyd.}$

(1) $CH_3-\overset{O}{\overset{\|}{C}}-Cl+AlCl_3\longrightarrow CH_3-\overset{O}{\overset{\|}{C}}\oplus+AlCl_4^-$

(2) 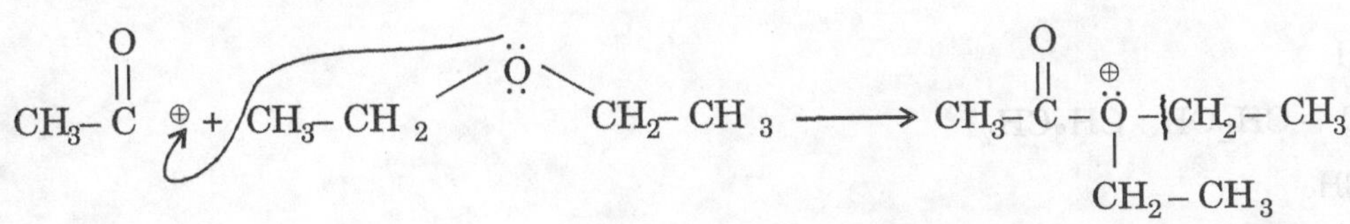

$\xrightarrow{AlCl_4^-} CH_3-\overset{O}{\overset{\|}{C}}-OCH_2CH_3+CH_3CH_2Cl+AlCl_3$

(3)

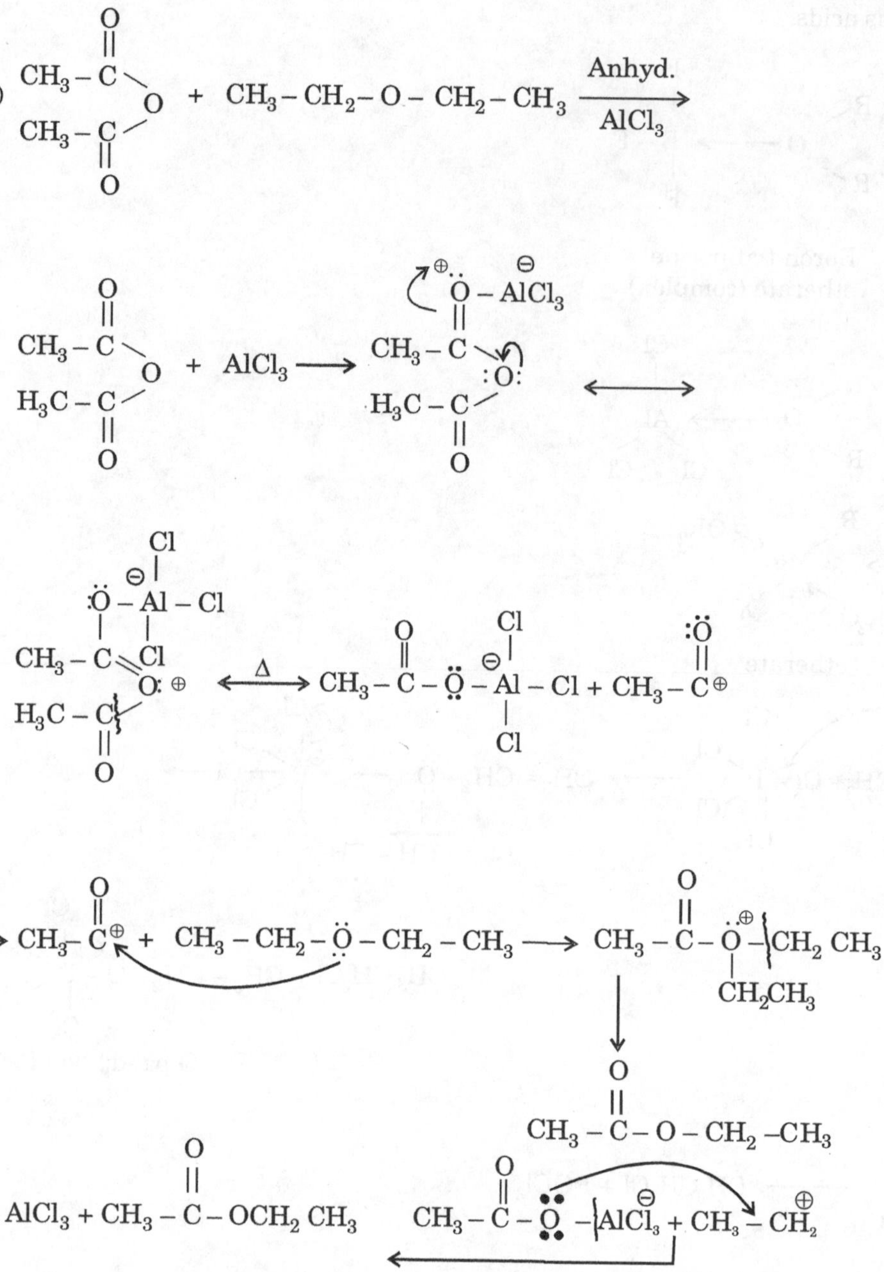

36.

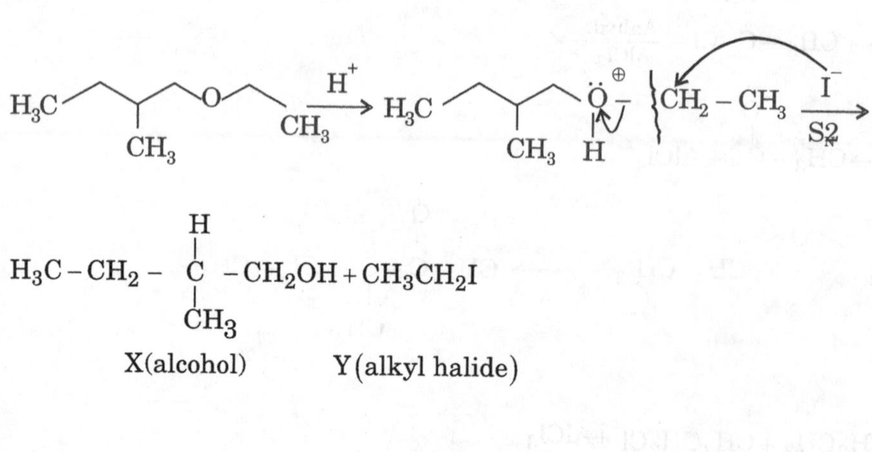

Wrt b option

$$H_3C-CH_2-\underset{CH_3}{\overset{CH_3}{C}}-O-CH_2-CH_3 \xrightarrow{HI}$$

$$H_3C-CH_2-\underset{CH_3}{\overset{CH_3}{C}}-\underset{H}{\overset{\oplus}{O}}-CH_2-CH_3 \xrightarrow[I^-]{S_N1} \underset{(W)}{CH_3\,CH_2\,OH} + \underset{(S)}{CH_3-CH_2-\underset{CH_3}{\overset{CH_3}{C}}-I}$$

$$\rightarrow X \xrightarrow{R_1} S$$

$$\underset{(X)}{H_3C-CH_2-\underset{CH_3}{\overset{H}{C}}-CH_2OH} \xrightarrow[S_N1]{HI} \underset{(S)}{CH_3-CH_2-\underset{CH_3}{\overset{CH_3}{C}}-I}$$

$$\rightarrow Y \xrightarrow{R_2} W$$

$$\underset{(Y)}{CH_3CH_2I} \xrightarrow{aq.KOH} \underset{(W)}{CH_3CH_2OH}$$

37. 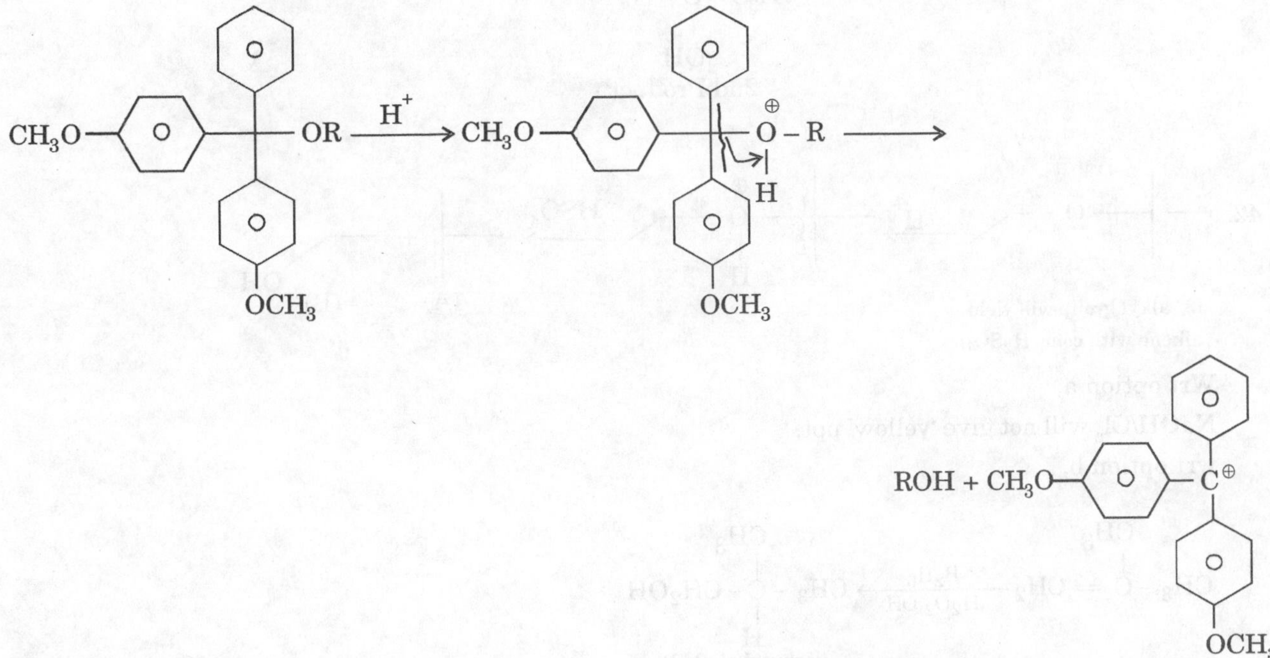

Presence of $-OCH_3$ groups at para-positions will help stabilise the carbocation.

40. Ether, Oxidises $Fe^{2+} \rightarrow Fe^{3+} \xrightarrow{CNS^{\ominus}} Fe(CNS)_3$
(with peroxide) Red colour

41.

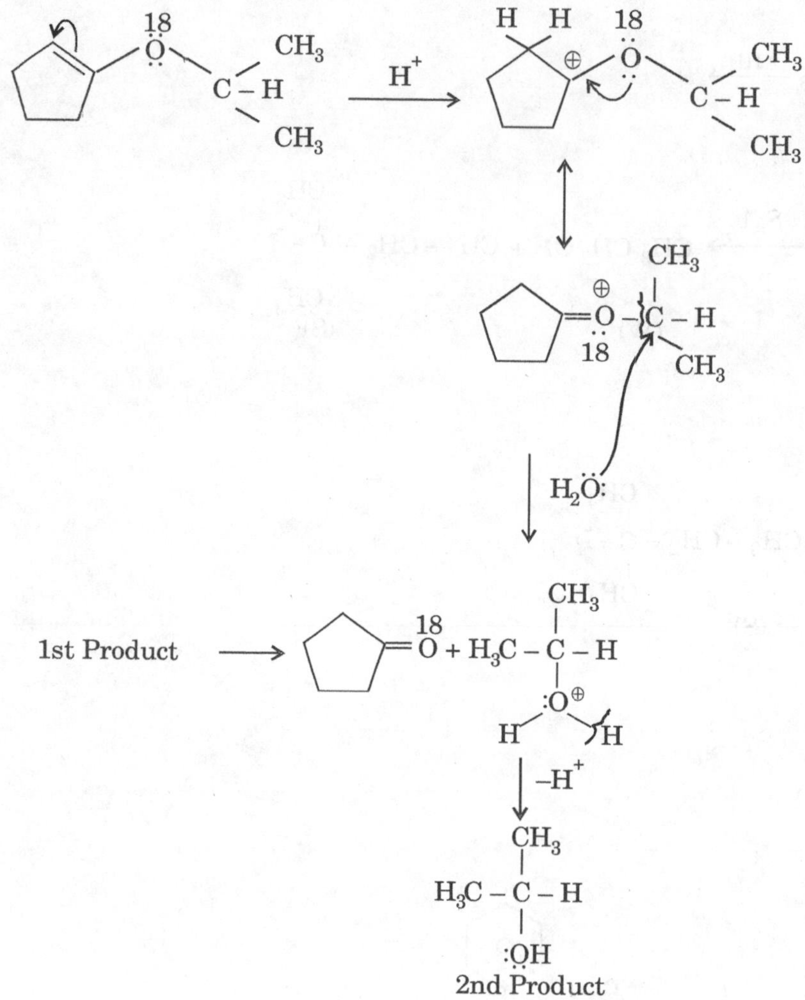

42.

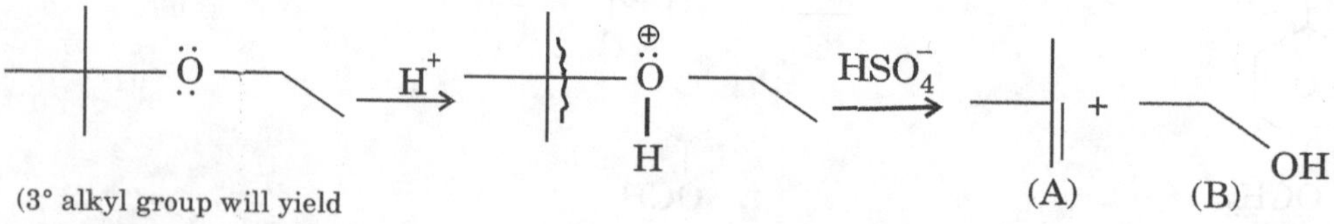

(3° alkyl group will yield alkene with conc. H_2SO_4)

Wrt option a,

$NaOH/Cl_2$ will not give 'yellow' ppt.

wrt option b,

$$CH_3-\overset{\overset{CH_3}{|}}{C}=CH_2 \xrightarrow[H_2O_2,\bar{O}H]{B_2H_6} CH_3-\underset{\underset{H}{|}}{\overset{\overset{CH_3}{|}}{C}}-CH_2OH$$

(isobutyl alcohol)

Wrt option c,

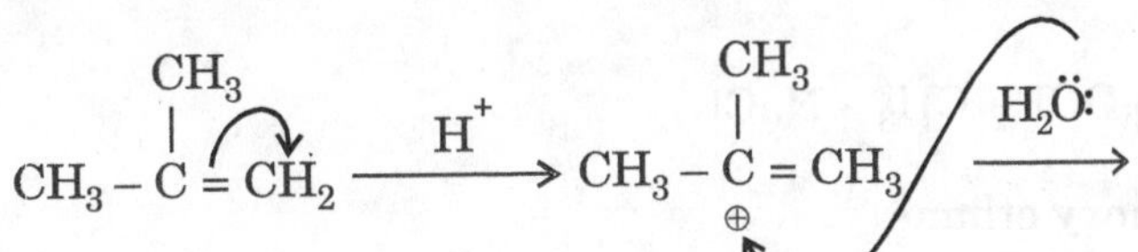

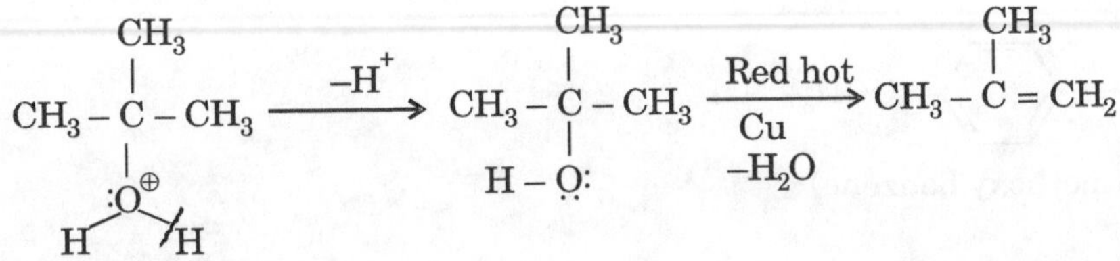

wrt option d,

'A' is not a 3° alcohol. It is an alkene.

44.

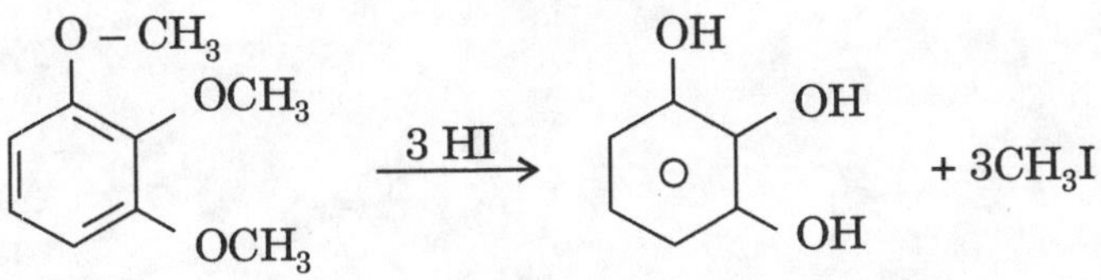

45.

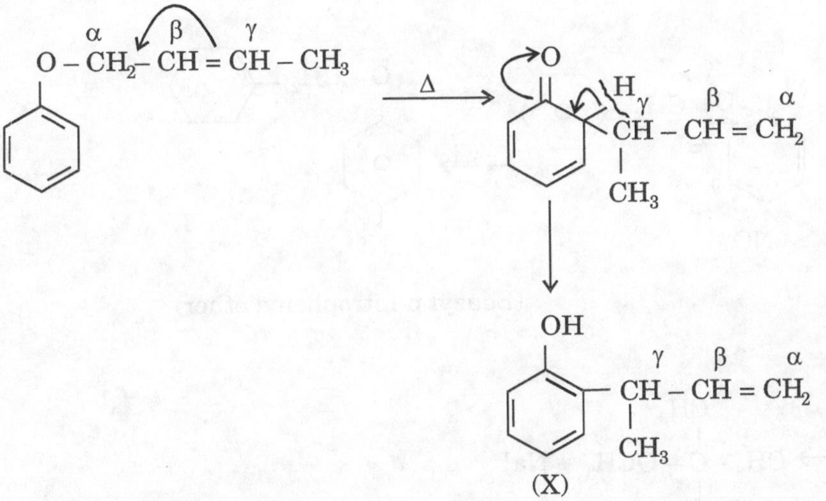

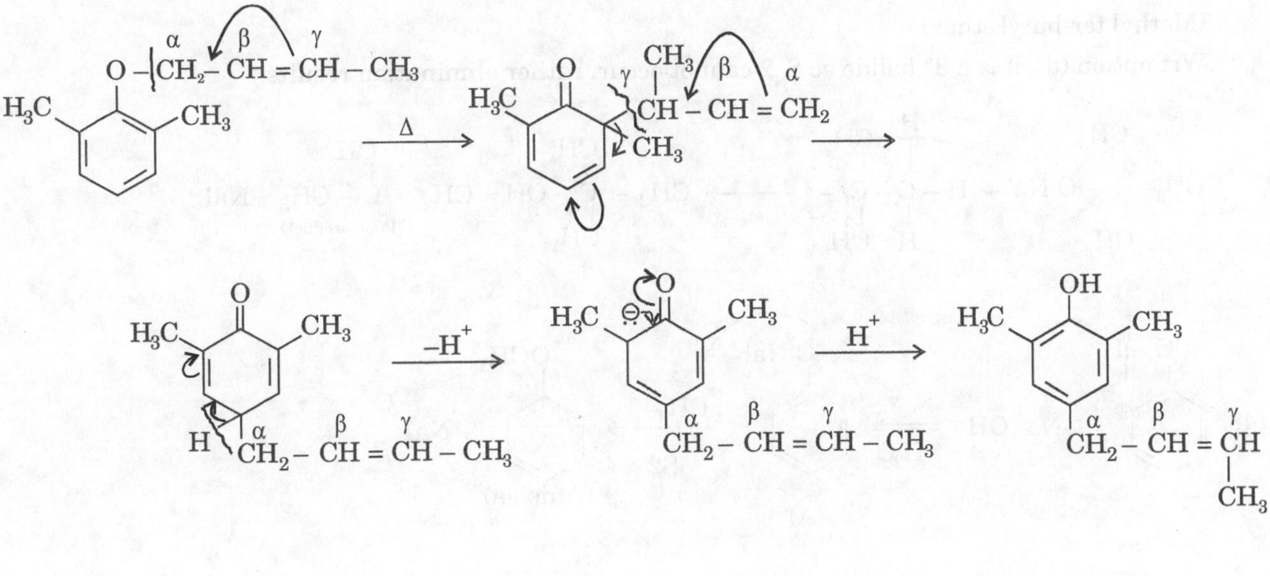

46. $C_2H_5O^- Na^+ + CH_3 - \overset{\delta+}{C}H_2 - Cl \xrightarrow{S_N2} C_2H_5OCH_2\,CH_3 + NaCl$

(Williamson's synthesis) (ethoxy ethane)

47. Wrt option (a),

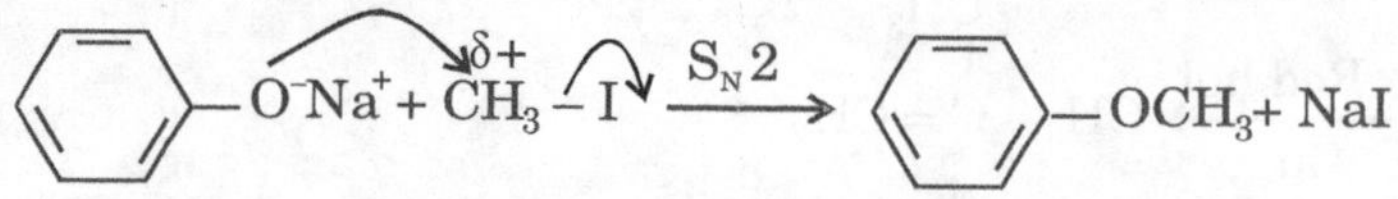

(methoxy benzene)

Wrt option (b),

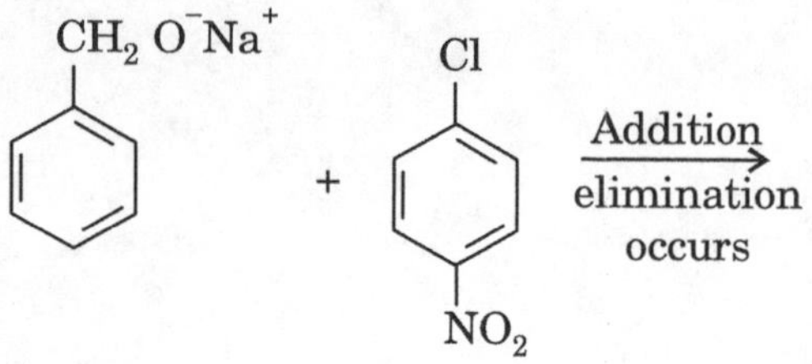

Mechanism

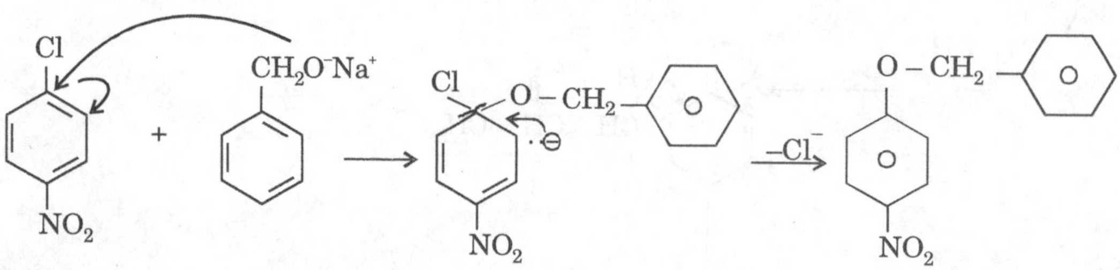

(Benzyl p-nitrophenyl ether)

Wrt option (c),

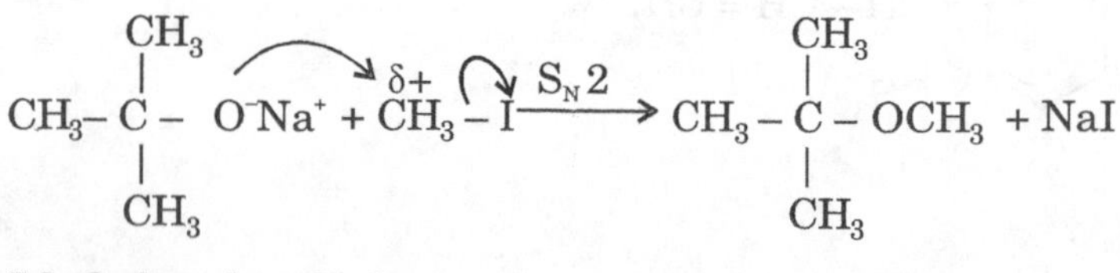

(Methyl ter-butyl ether)

Wrt option (d), it is a 3° halide so S_N2 cannot occur. rather elimination results.

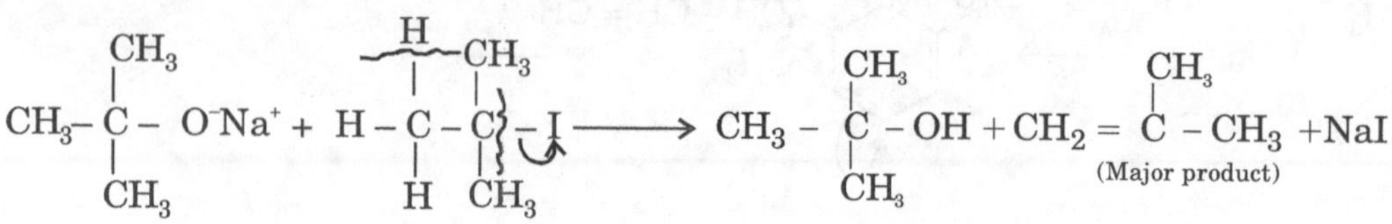

48.

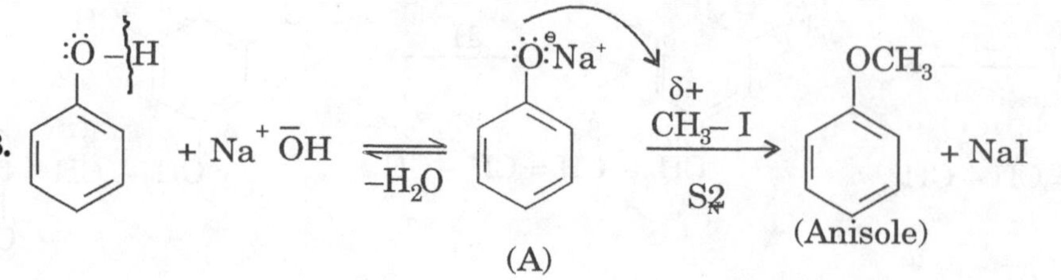

Wrt (b) option,

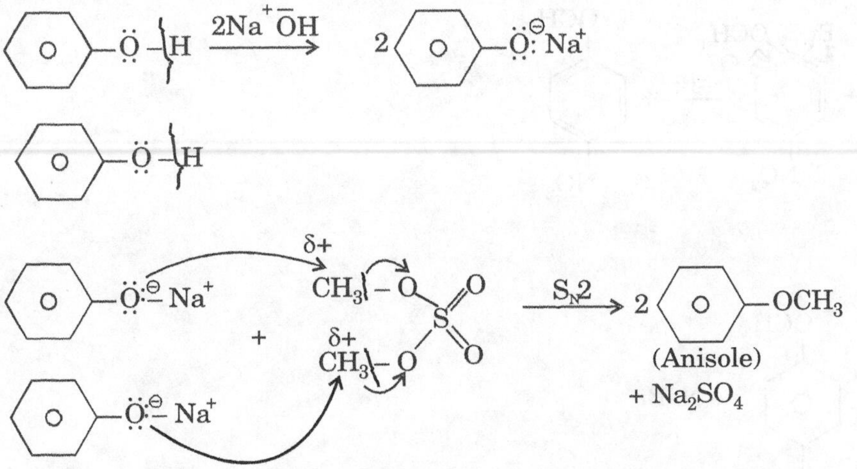

Wrt (c) option, S_N2 cannot occurs in Aryl halides.

49. (1) $\overset{..\ominus}{CH_2}-\overset{\oplus}{N}\equiv N \xrightarrow{HBF_4} CH_3-\overset{\oplus}{N}\equiv N$

(2)

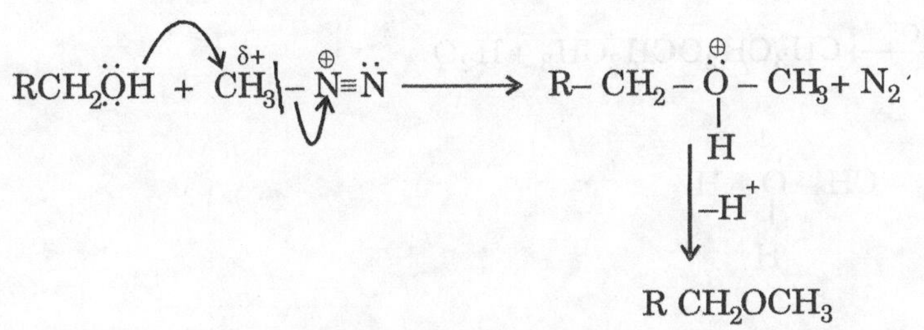

51. Wrt option (b), $CH_3CH_2OH + HO-CH_2-CH_3 \xrightarrow[140°C]{Conc.H_2SO_4} CH_3CH_2OCH_2CH_3$

Wrt option (c), $CH_3O-\overset{\delta+}{CH_2}-Cl \xrightarrow[S_N2]{\overset{\delta-}{CH_3}-MgI} CH_3OCH_2CH_3 + Mg(Cl)I$

52. Wrt 1

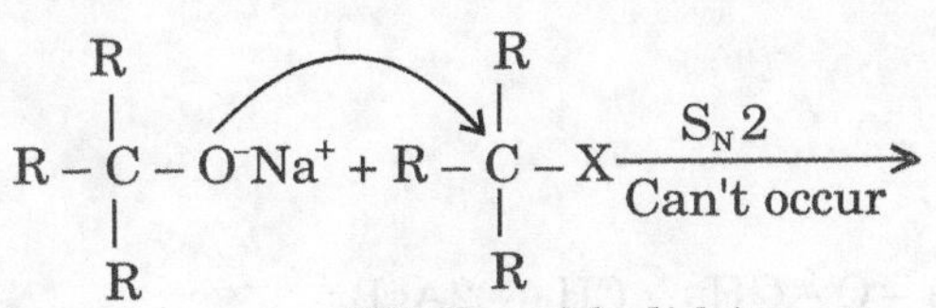

(Hindered halide)

Wrt 2

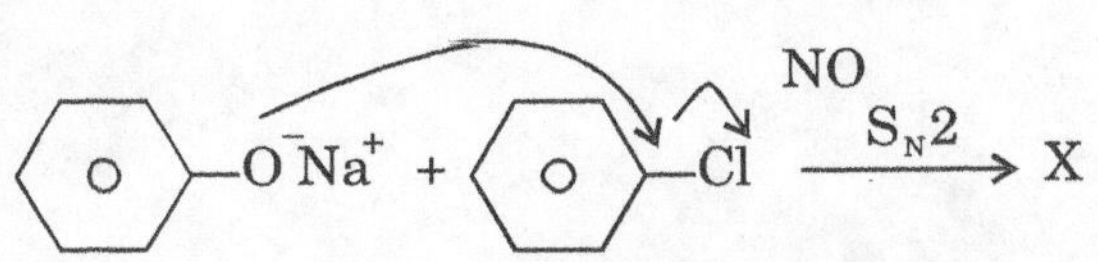

(Partial double bond character in C—Cl bond)

Wrt 3

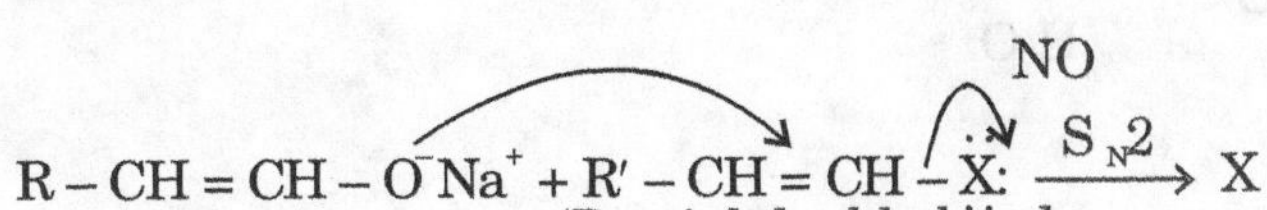

(Partial double bond character in C — X bond)

53. Wrt A, Aryl S_N2 (addition elimination) can occur-

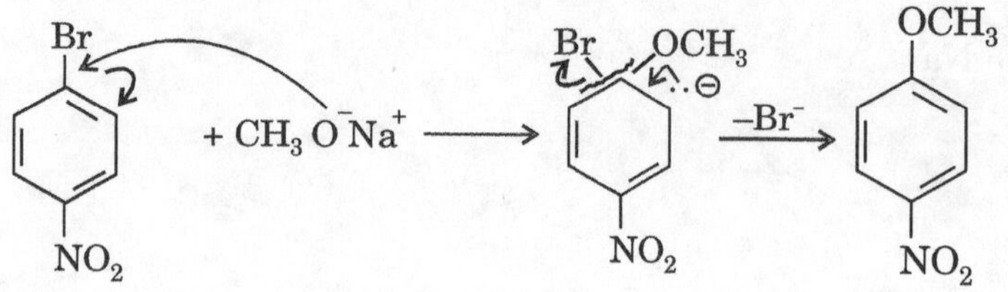

Wrt B,

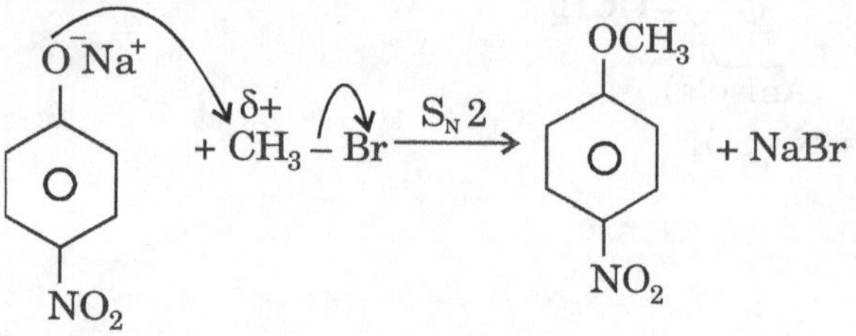

54. The reaction follows SN^2 mechanism.

$$CH_3CH_2OH + HOCH_2CH_3 \xrightarrow[140°C]{Conc.H_2SO_4} CH_3CH_2OCH_2CH_3 + H_2O$$

(1) $CH_3 - CH_2 - \ddot{O} - H + H^+ \rightleftharpoons CH_3 - CH_2 - \overset{\oplus}{\ddot{O}}(H) - H$ (from $H_2SO)_4$

(2) $CH_3 - \overset{\delta+}{CH_2} - \overset{\oplus}{O}(H) - H + CH_3 - CH_2 - \ddot{O}H \overset{S_N2}{\rightleftharpoons} CH_3 - CH_2 - \overset{\oplus}{\ddot{O}}(H) - CH_2 - CH_3 + H_2O$

$\xrightarrow{-H^+} CH_3 - CH_2 - \ddot{O} - CH_2 - CH_3$

1° alcohols will undergo SN^2 fastest to yield ethers.

55. With dry Ag_2O, oxide ion acts as nucleophile.

$$CH_3CH_2 - Br + O^{2-} + CH_3CH_2 - Br \overset{S_N2}{\rightleftharpoons} CH_3 - CH_2 - O - CH_2 - CH_3 + 2AgBr$$

(from Ag_2O)

Wth moist Ag_2O (AgOH), $\bar{O}H$ acts as a nucleophile.

$$CH_3 - CH_2 - Br + \bar{O}H \longrightarrow CH_3CH_2OH + AgBr$$

56. (1) 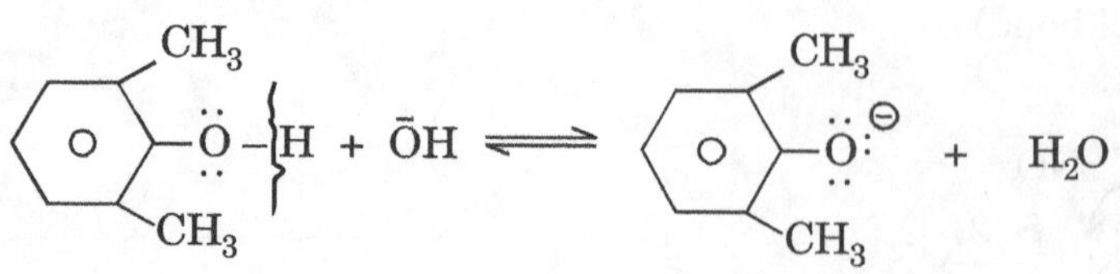

(2)
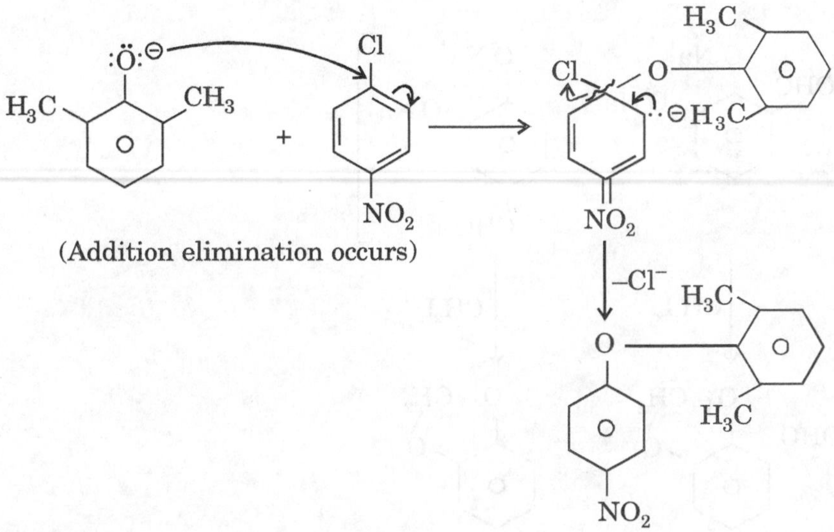

(Addition elimination occurs)

57.
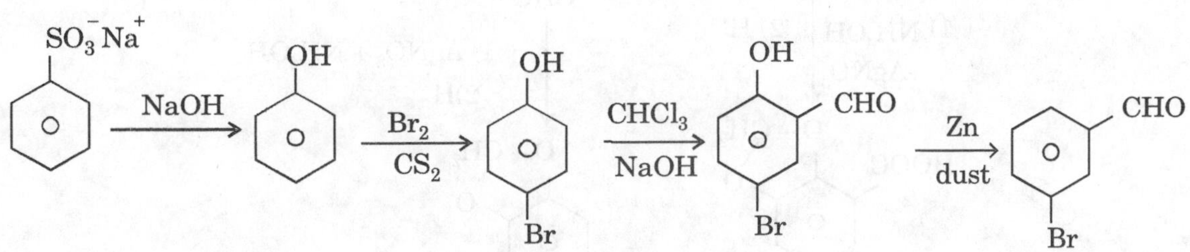

58.
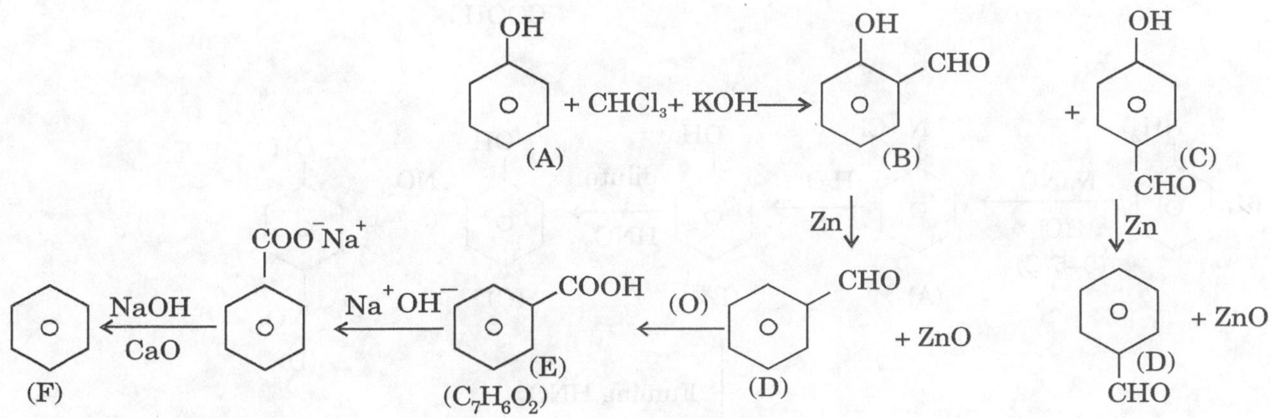

Benzene can also be obtained by heating 'A' (phenol) with Zn dust.

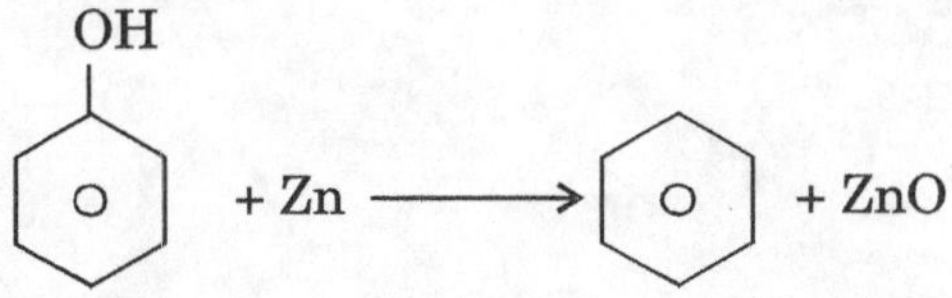

59.

(Voilet coloured complex)

60. 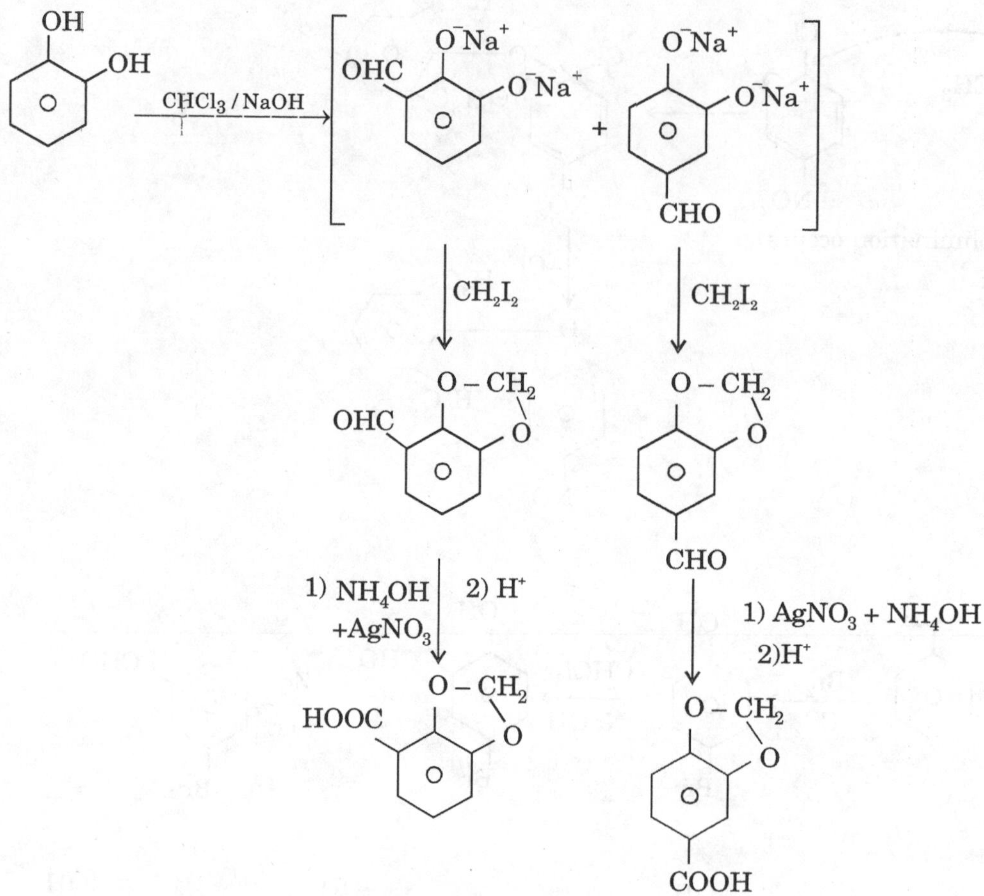

61. 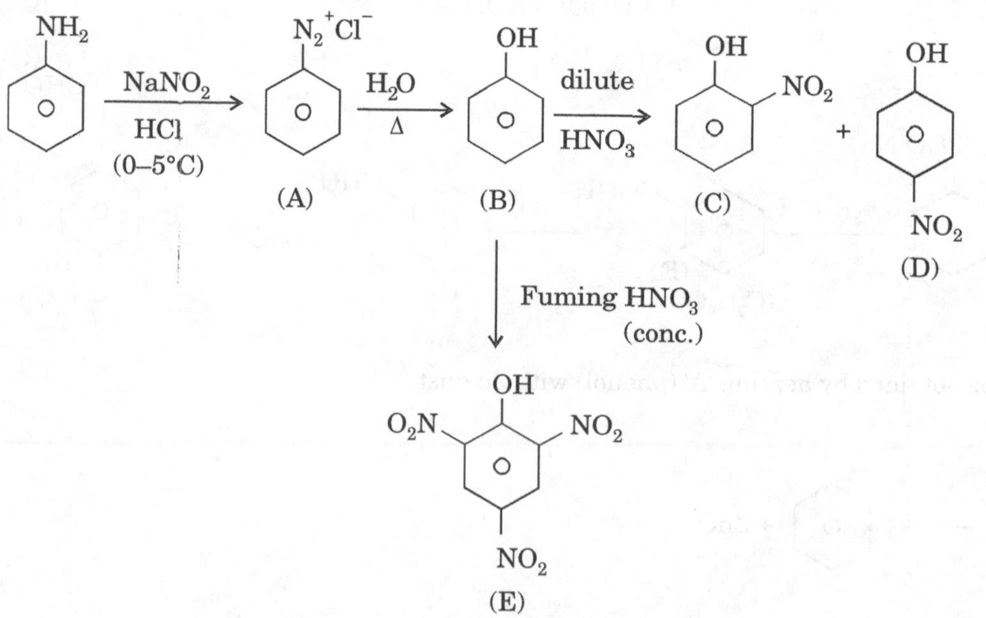

Presence of electron withdrawing groups increase the acidic strength of phenols.
So, acidic strength follows the order-
E > D > C > B

63. Its mechanism is as follows

Reaction

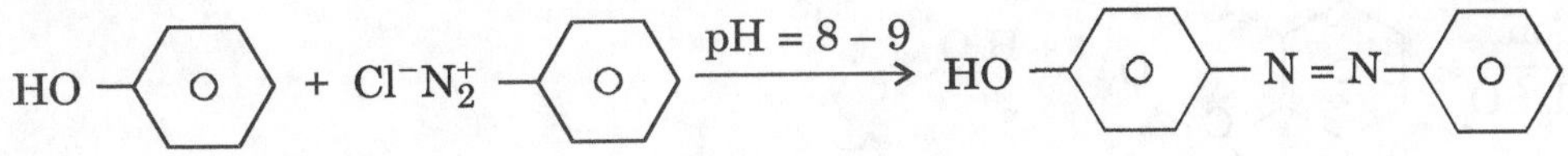

Mechanism: Since medium is basic-

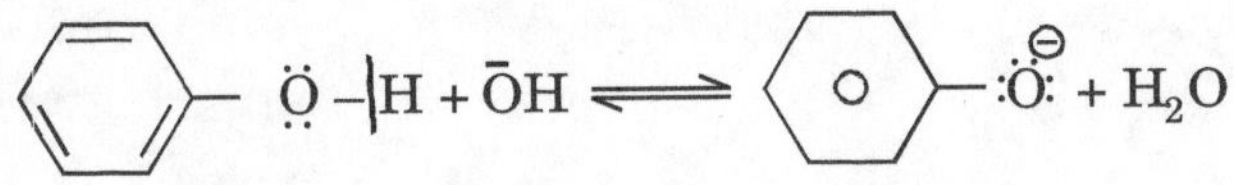

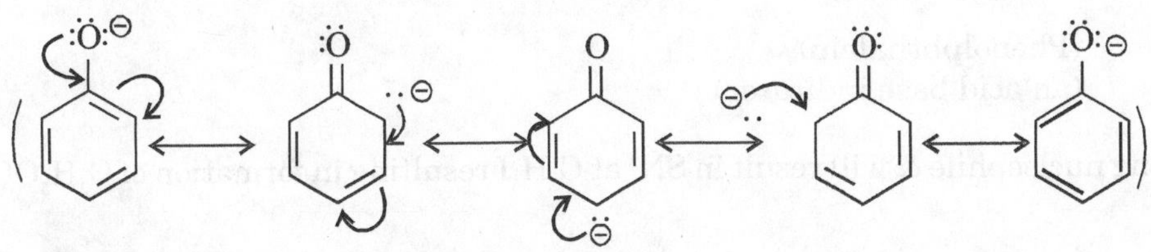

Major product is obtained at para-position.

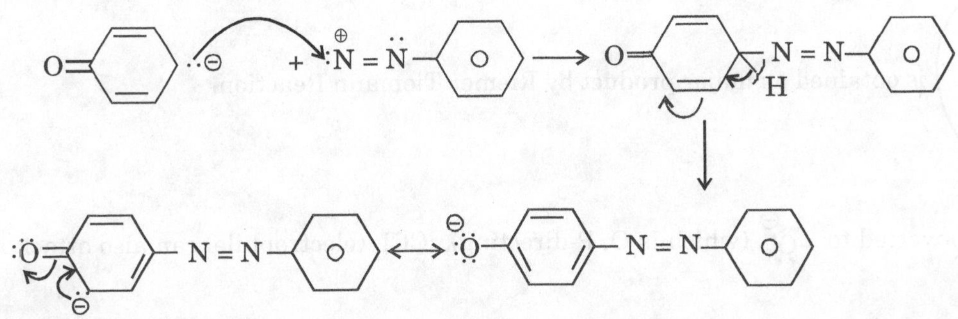

Benzene diazonium ion is a weak electrophile. In order to enhance the reaction rate, basic medium converts phenol to phenoxide so that the Ring becomes more e^- rich (ring is activated).

Also, it is an electrophilic substitution reaction in which benzene diazonium ion (an electrophile) substitutes H^+ (another electrophile)

64.

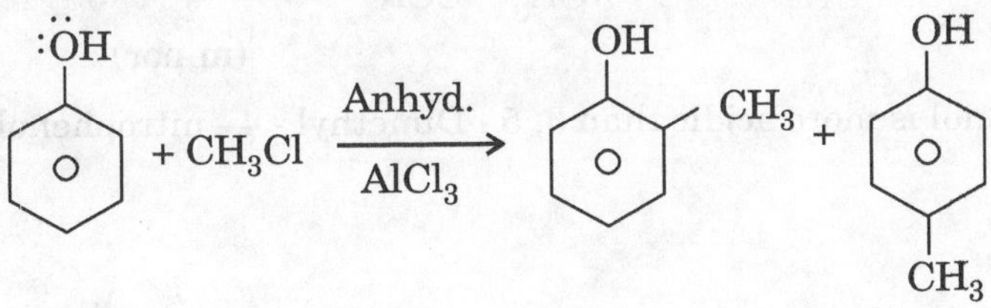

(VERY POOR YIELD)

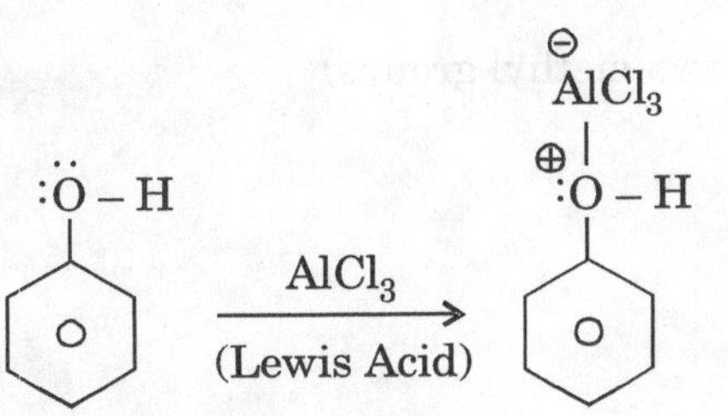

(O bearing +ve charge now deactivates the Ring)

66. 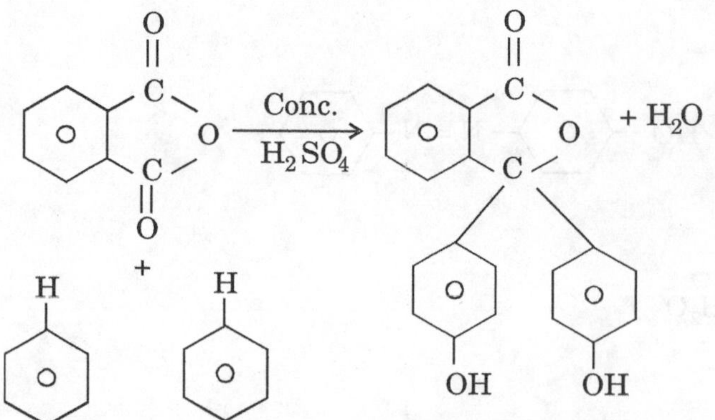
(Phenolphthalein)
(an acid base indicator)

67. $C_2H_5O^{\ominus}$ is itself a very strong nucleophile & will result in SN^2 at C_2H_5I resulting in formation of $C_2H_5OC_2H_5$.

$$CH_2O_5^{\ominus} \quad + \quad CH_3-CH_2-I \longrightarrow C_2H_5OCH_2CH_3 + I^-$$

68. 'S' 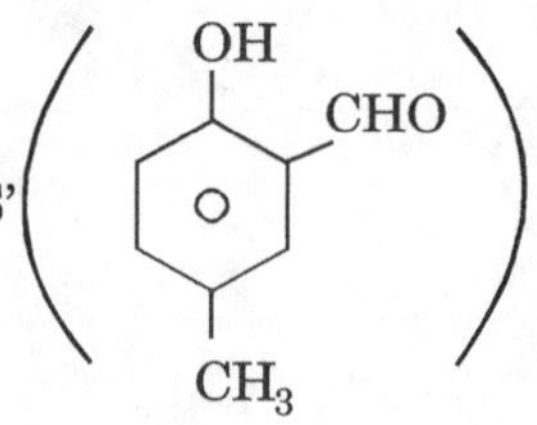 is obtained as major product by Riemer Tiemann Reaction.

Since –OH group is converted to $-\ddot{O}^{\ominus}$ (which is O, P-directing), $:CCl_2$ (electrophile) can also attack at P-position.

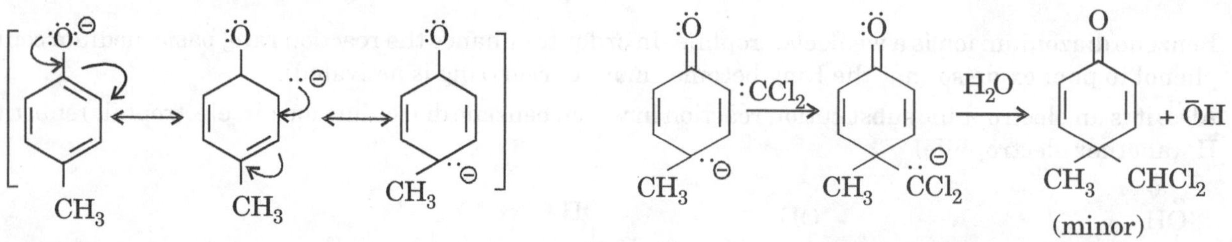
(minor)

69. Wrt option (a) 1, 2, 6 - Dimethyl - 4 - nitrophenol is more acidic than 3, 5 - Dimethyl - 4 - nitrophenol.

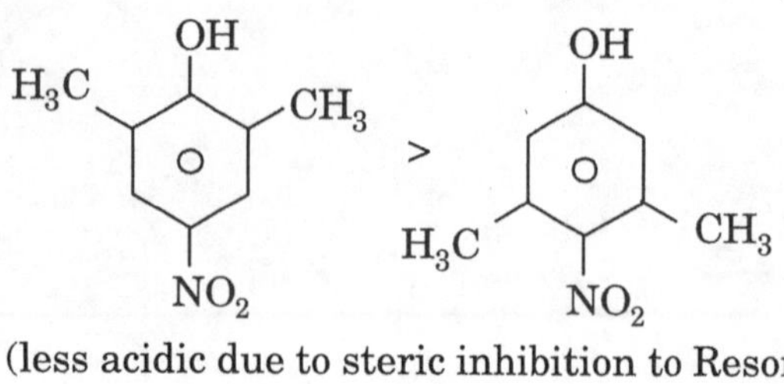
(less acidic due to steric inhibition to Resonance' due to adjacent two methyl groups)

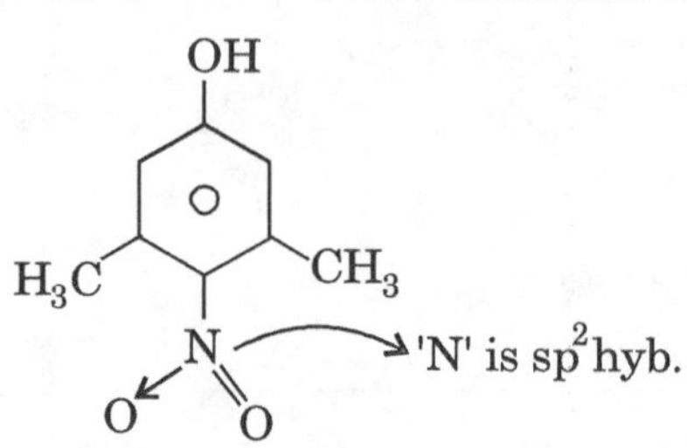
(it is flared and has triagonal planar geometry, will suffer repulsions from two methyl groups)

Wrt option b-3, 5 - Dimethyl - 4 - cyanophenol is more acidic than isomeric 2, 6 - Dimethyl - 4 - cyanophenol.

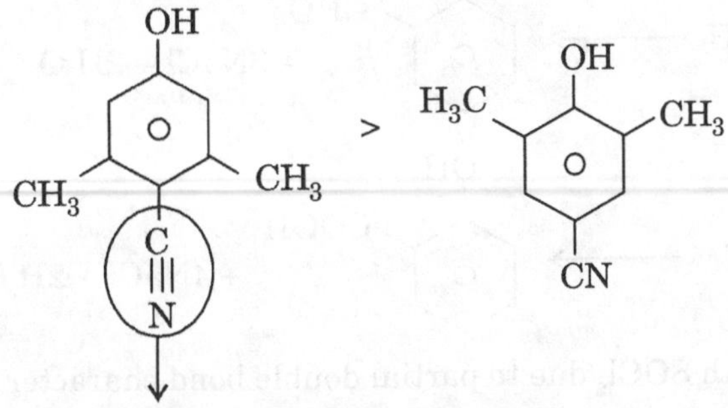

'C' in CN is sp hybridised imparting linear geometry NO 'STERIC INHIBITION TO RESONANCE' is observed because CN is not flared & cannot suffer significant repulsions from methyl groups.

Wrt option c, – NO_2 at para will exert – M & – I thus making paranitrophenol more acidic.

– M will be insignificant at meta position

70. Mechanism of Riemer Tiemanns reaction is as follows-

(1) 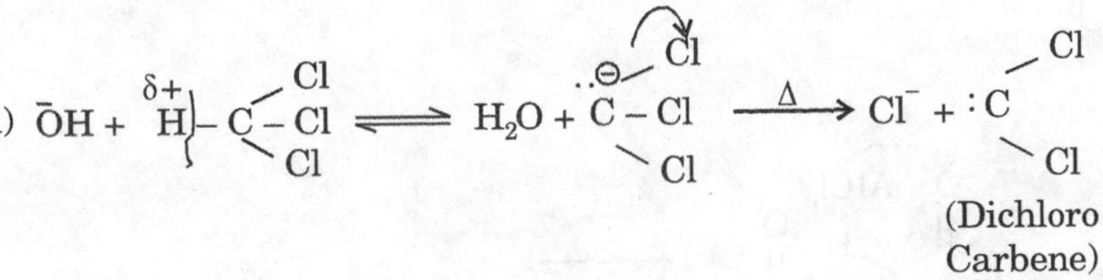

(2) 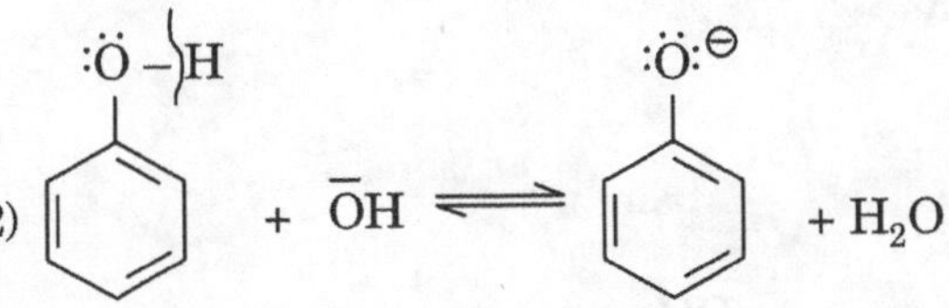

(3) 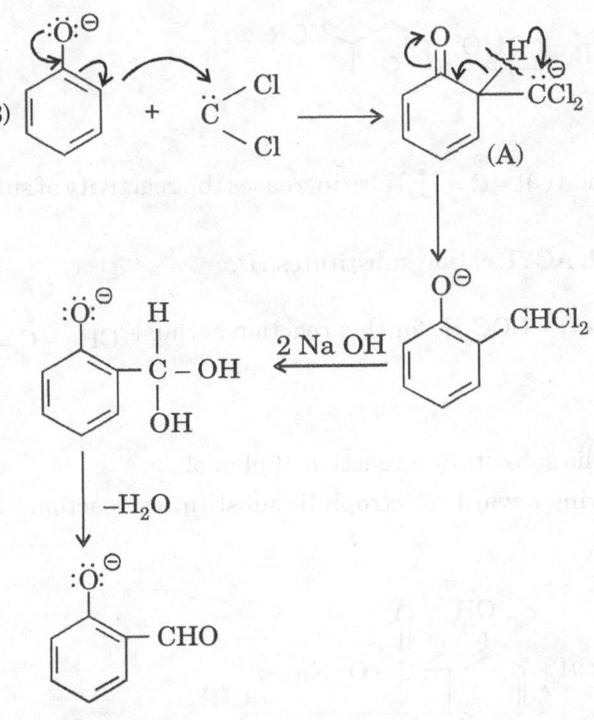

It is evident from molecule marked 'A', that dichlorocarbene (an electrophile) substitutes H^+, So it is an electrophilic substitution reaction.

72. 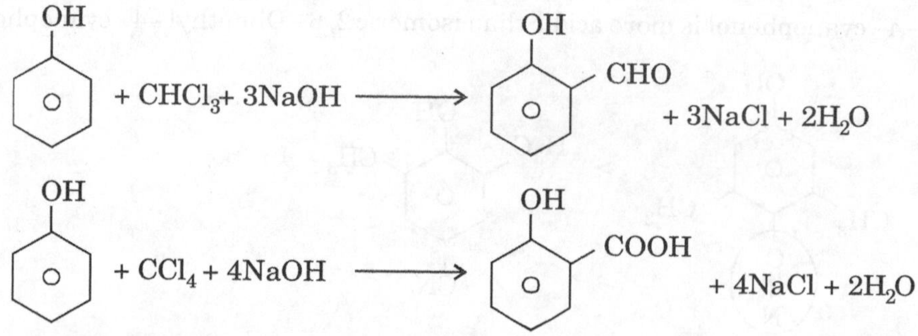

73. Phenols will not react with $SOCl_2$ due to partial double bond character in C – O bond.

74. Mechanism of Fries Rearrangement

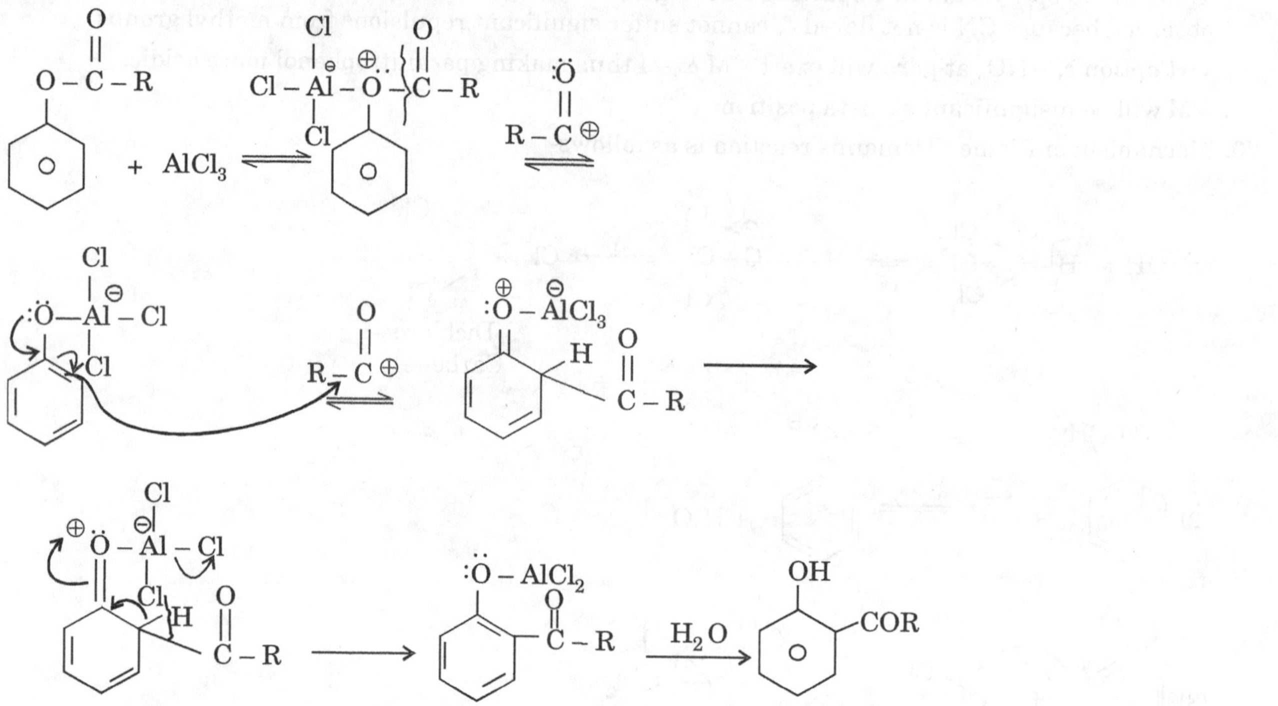

ANY factor which increases the stability of acyl cation ($R - \overset{\oplus}{C} = \ddot{O}:$) also increases the reactivity of substrate for this reaction.

It is an electrophilic substitution reaction in which ACYL cation substitutes H^+.

So, Ar – O – $COCH_3$ will be less reactive than Ar – O – COC_6H_5 for this reaction because $CH_3 - \overset{\oplus}{C} = \ddot{O}:$ is less stable than $C_6H_5 - \overset{\oplus}{C} = \ddot{O}:$.

75. Fries Rearrangement is an example of electrophillic substitution reaction of phenol.
Electron withdrawing groups will deactivate the ring towards electrophilic substitution reaction.

76. 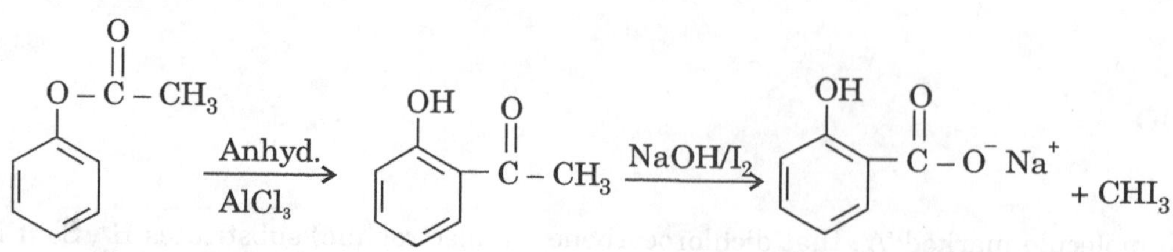

78. 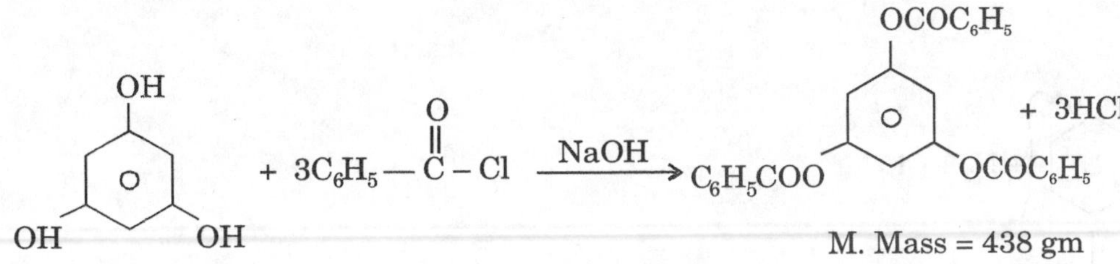

M. Mass = 126 gm

M. Mass = 438 gm

Increase in molar mass = 438 – 126 = 312 gm

79. 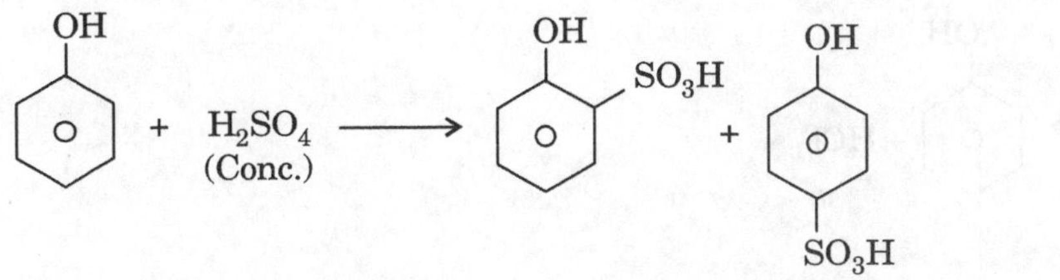

Once – SO_3H is introduced O – ring, its acidic strength will increase in comparison to phenol.

80. 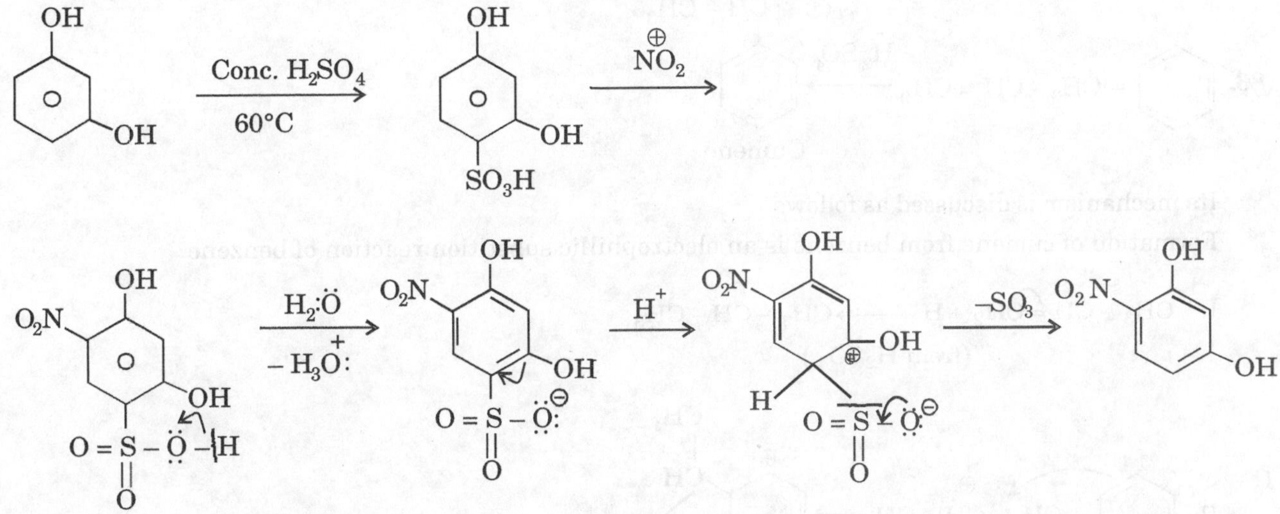

82. 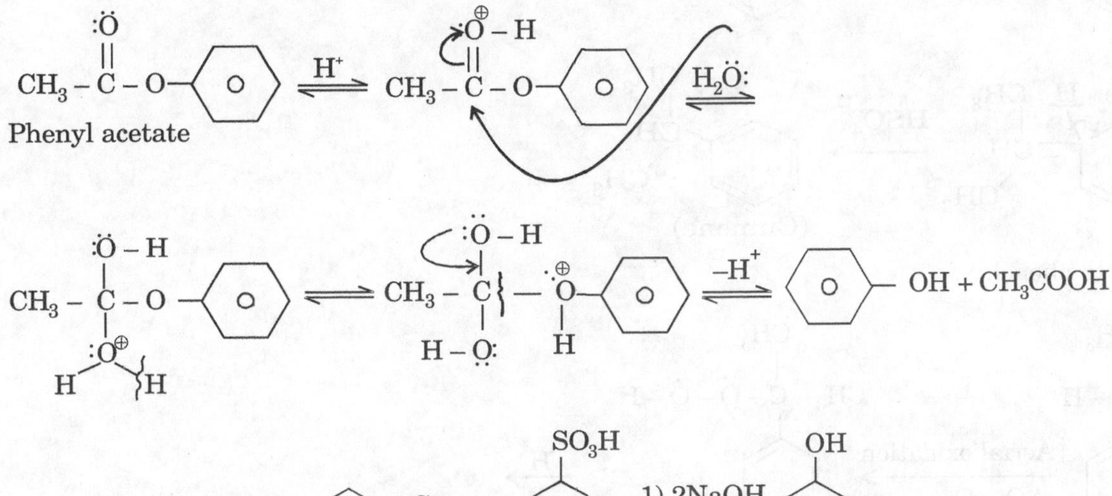

83. 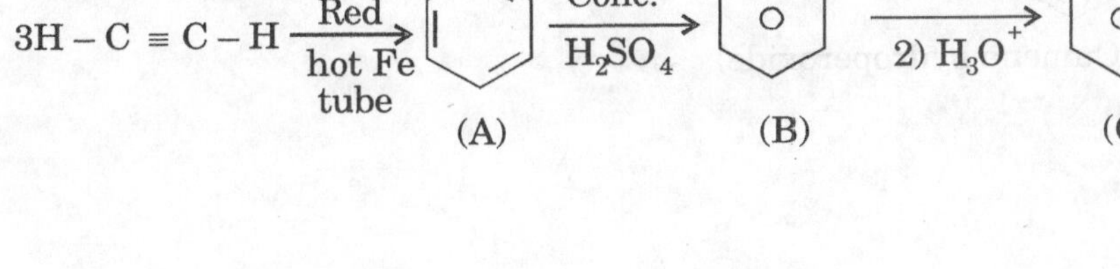

85.

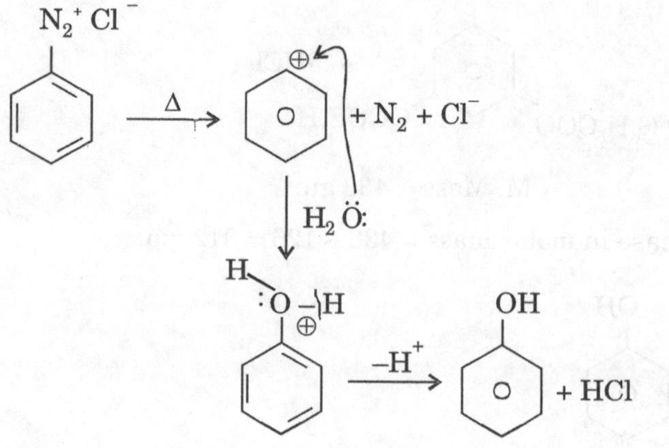

86.

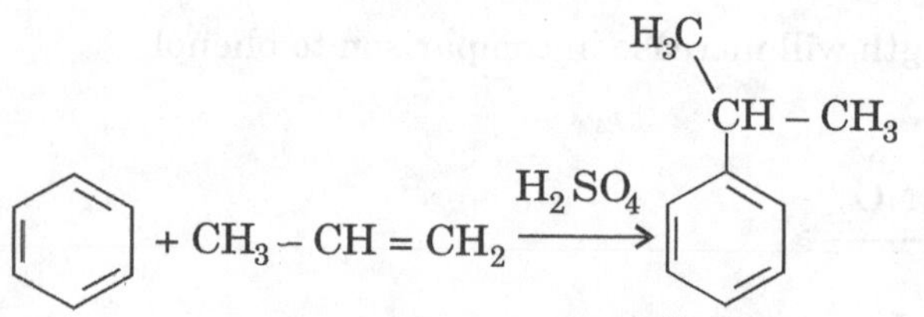

Cumene

Its mechanism is discussed as follows-

Formation of cumene from benzene is an electrophillic substition reaction of benzene.

I. $CH_3 - CH = CH_2 + H^+ \longrightarrow CH_3 - \overset{\oplus}{C}H - CH_3$
(from H_2SO_4)

II.

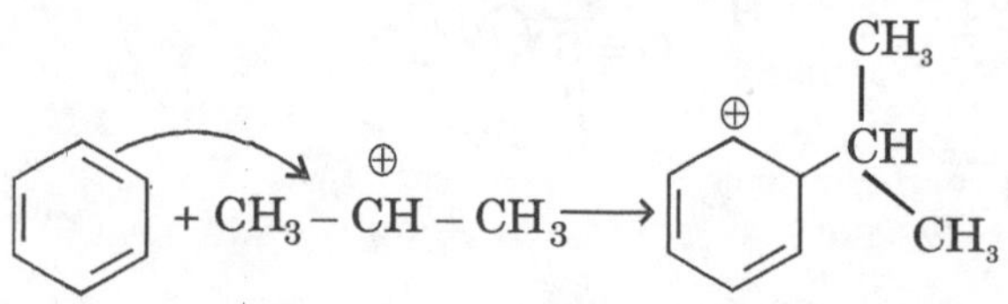

III.

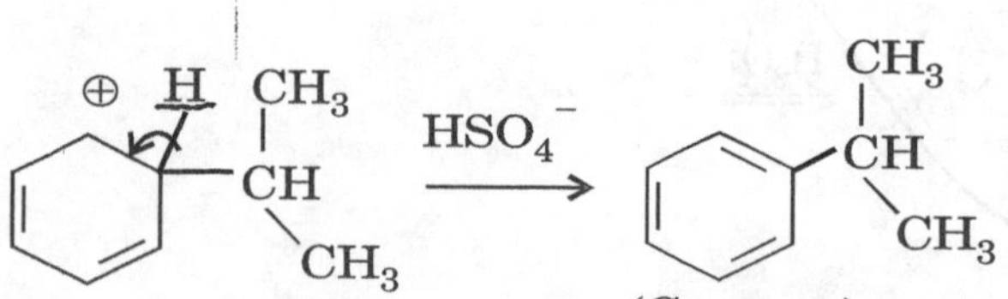

(Cumene)

Cumene to phenol.

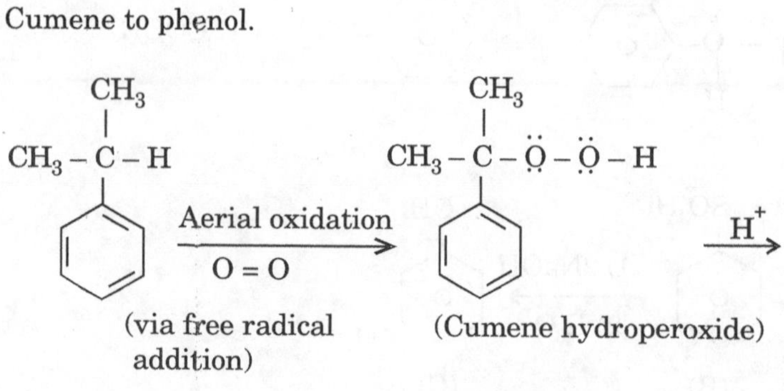

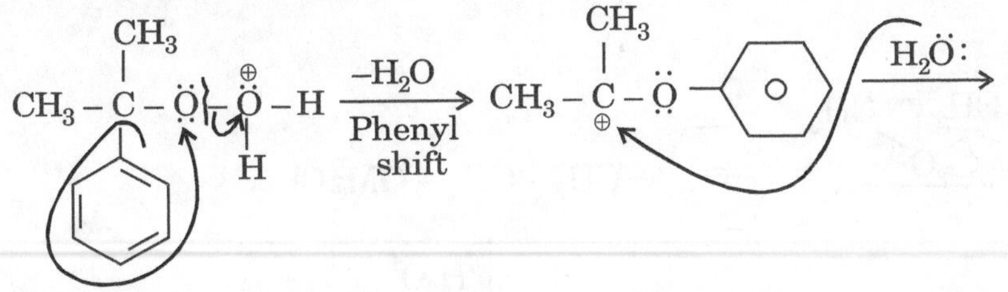

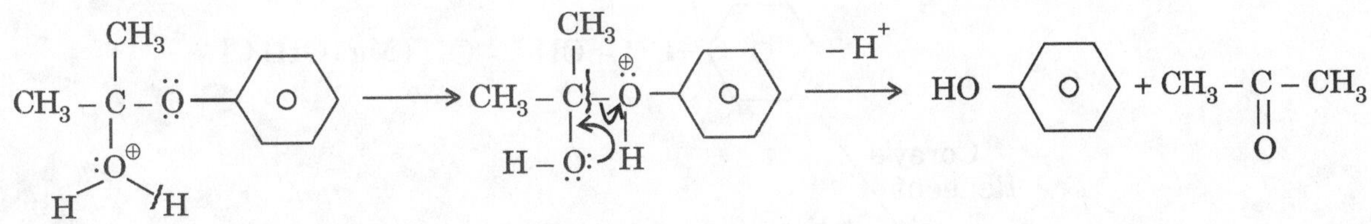

87.

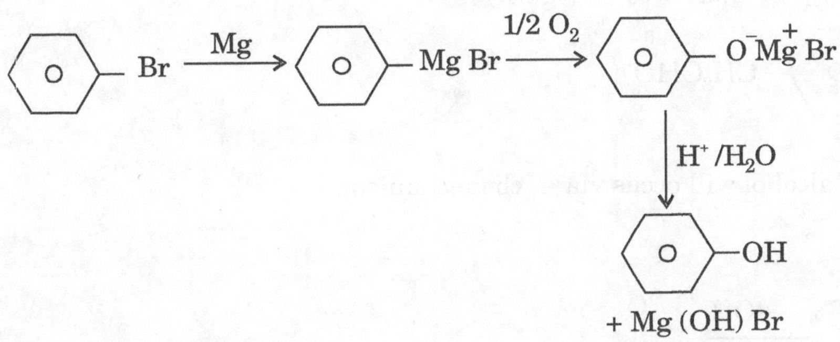

88. Reaction with Na will occur since alcohol has an acidic H.

$$Na \xrightarrow{\Delta} Na^+ + e^-$$
(hot)

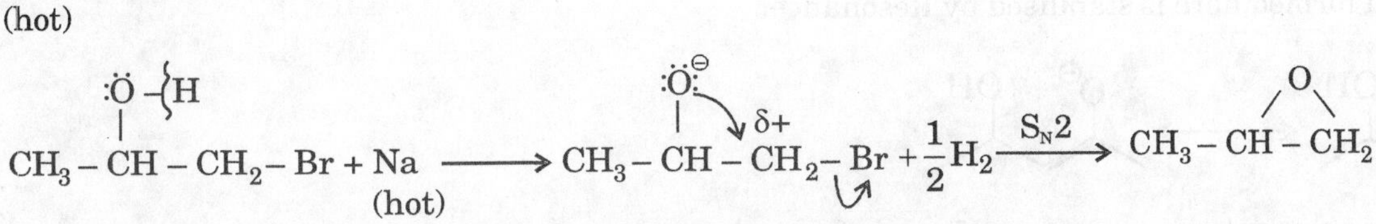

89. Grignard's reagent will act like bronsted base & pull acidic H (with –OH)

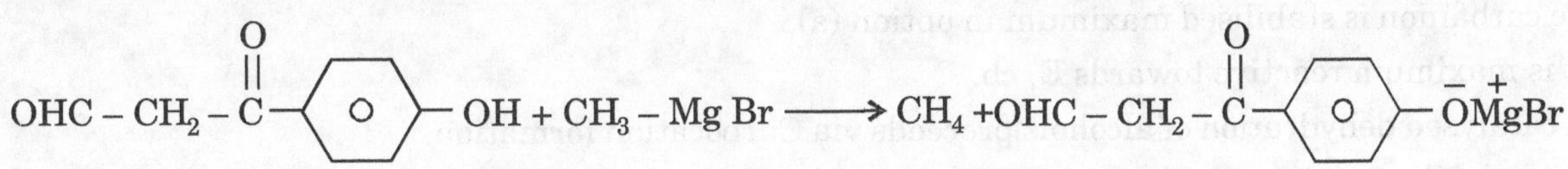

90.

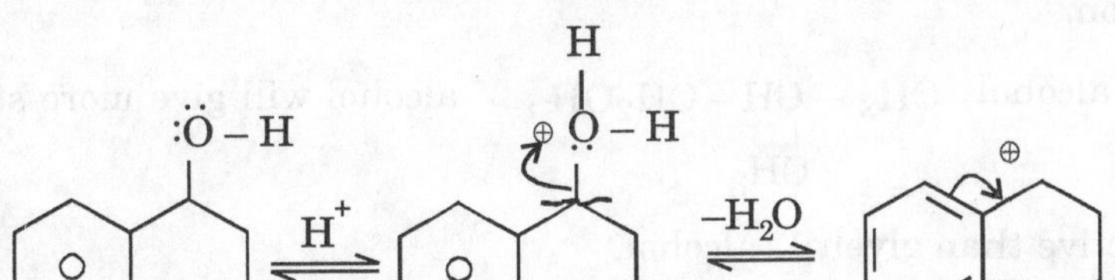

(Carbocation is stabilised by resonance)

91.

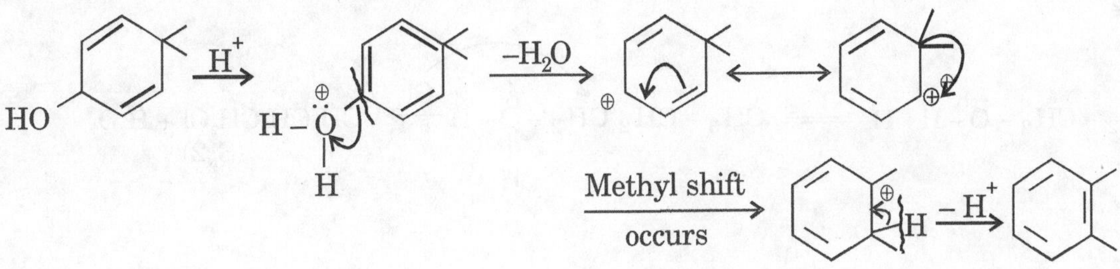

92. 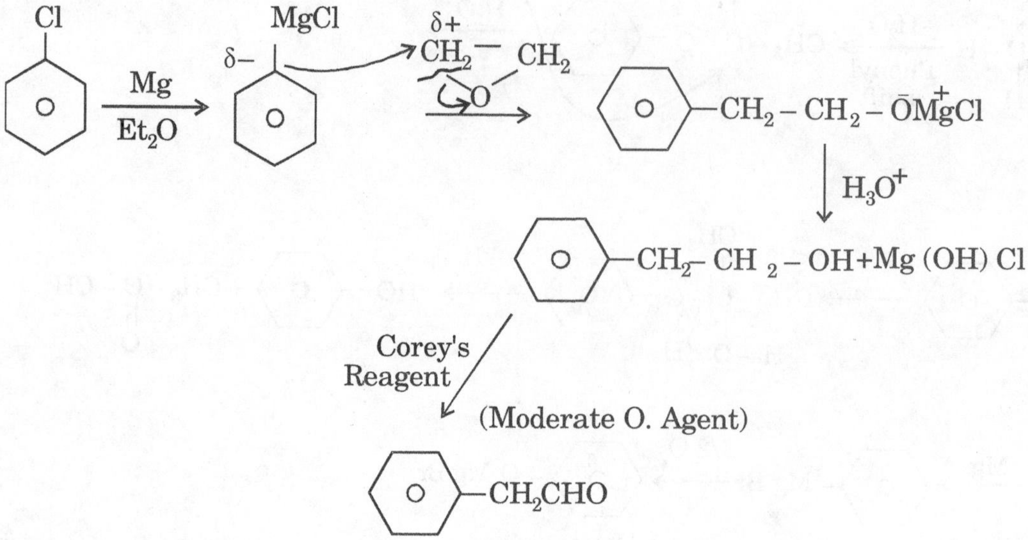

93. In basic conditions, dehydration of alcohol will occus via $\in_1$ cb mechanism.
option (a),

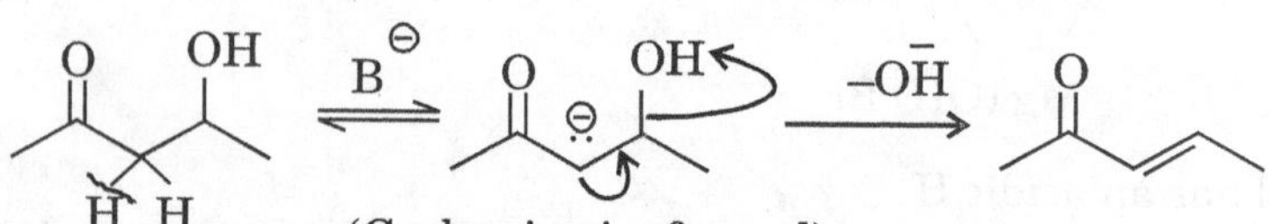

(Carbanion is formed)

Carbanion formed here is stabilised by Resonance.

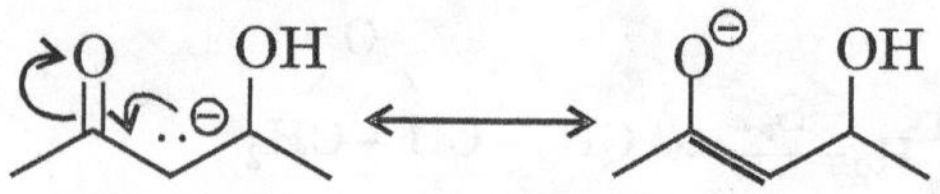

Also, $\bar{O}H$ is a poor leaving group, so E_1 cb is favored.
Since carbanion is stabilised maximum in option (a),
So it is maximum reactive towards E_1 cb.

94. Acid catalysed dehydration of alcohols proceeds via Carbocation formation.
3° alcohol will give max. stable Carbocation.

Among 2° alcohol $CH_3-\underset{\large OH}{\underset{|}{CH}}-CH_3$ & 1° alcohol $CH_3-\underset{\large CH_3}{\underset{|}{CH}}-CH_2OH$, 2° alcohol will give more stable Carbocation in first go. So, it is more reactive than given 1° alcohol.

95. 1° alcohols react with halogen acids via SN^2.
$CH_3CH_2CH_2OH + HCl \rightarrow$
<u>Mechanism</u>

$$CH_3-CH_2-CH_2-\ddot{O}-H + H^+ \rightleftharpoons CH_3-CH_2\,CH_2-\overset{\oplus}{\ddot{O}}(H)-H \xrightarrow{Cl^-} CH_3CH_2CH_2Cl + H_2O \quad (S_N2)$$

96. 2° & 3° alcohols react with halogen acids via S_N1.

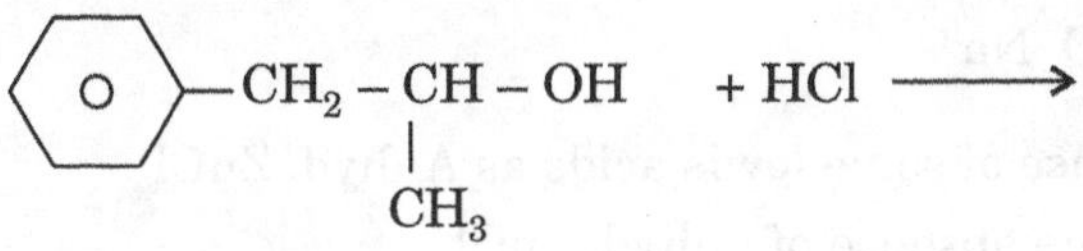

Mechanism

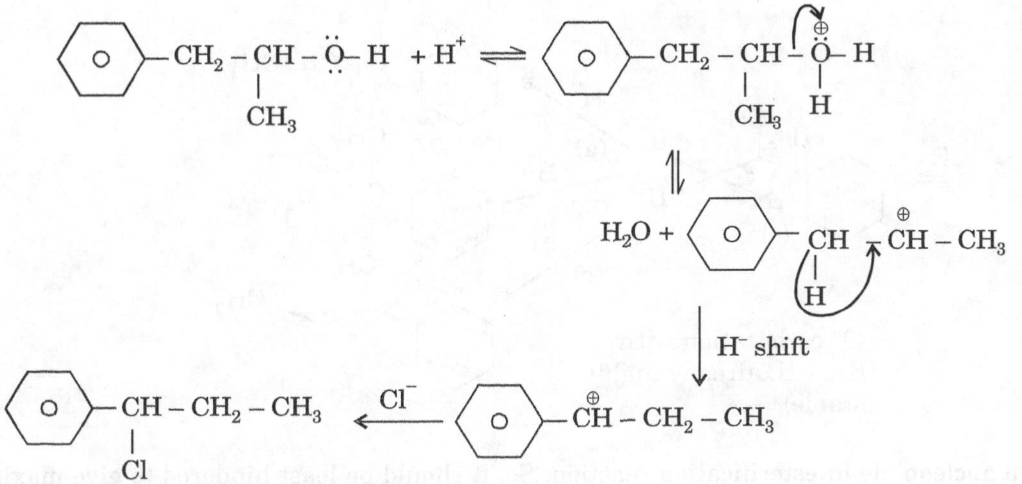

97. $ROH + \underset{(Conc.)}{HCl} \xrightarrow[ZnCl_2]{Anhyd.} RCl + H_2O$

Mechanism

$$R-\underset{\substack{|\\H}}{\ddot{O}}: + \underset{(Lewis\ acid)}{ZnCl_2} \longrightarrow R-\underset{\substack{|\\H}}{\overset{\oplus}{O}}-\overset{\ominus}{Z}nCl_2 \longrightarrow R^{\oplus} + HO-\overset{\ominus}{Z}nCl_2 \xrightarrow{Cl^-} RCl$$

$$HO-\overset{\ominus}{Z}nCl_2 \xrightarrow{H^+} H_2O + ZnCl_2$$

98. $\underset{(A)}{CH_3O-H} + \underset{(hot)}{Na} \longrightarrow \underset{(B)}{CH_3O^-Na^+} + \frac{1}{2}H_2\uparrow$

$$CH_3OH + PCl_5 \longrightarrow \underset{(C)}{CH_3Cl} + POCl_3$$

$$\underset{(B)}{CH_3O^-Na^+} + \underset{(C)}{CH_3-Cl} \xrightarrow{S_N2} CH_3OCH_3 + NaCl$$

99. Reaction with Na or K metal depicts the acidic nature of alcohols.

Since, Acidic strength $\propto \frac{1}{+I_{effect}}$, the correct order of acidic strength is 1° > 2° > 3°. So, 1° alcohol is maximum reactive towards Na or K.

100. $3\ ROH + PCl_3 \longrightarrow 3RCl + H_3PO_3$ ...(1)

$ROH + PCl_5 \longrightarrow RCl + POCl_3 + HCl$ ...(2)

It is evident from given reactions, if 4 moles of RCl are formed then PCl_3 & PCl_5 will be used in 1 : 1 molar ratio.

101. Lucas reagent reacts with 1°alcohols via SN^2. So, only 'INVERSION OF CONFIGURATION' occurs.

102. $CH_3CH_2OH \xrightarrow{PCC} CH_3CHO \xrightarrow[NaOH]{I_2} CHI_3 + HCOO^-Na^+$

103. The reactions of 1° & 2° alcohols with HCl require the use of some lewis acids as Anhyd. $ZnCl_2$. Tertiary alcohols react readily with conc. HCl even in the absence of anhyd. $ZnCl_2$.

104. 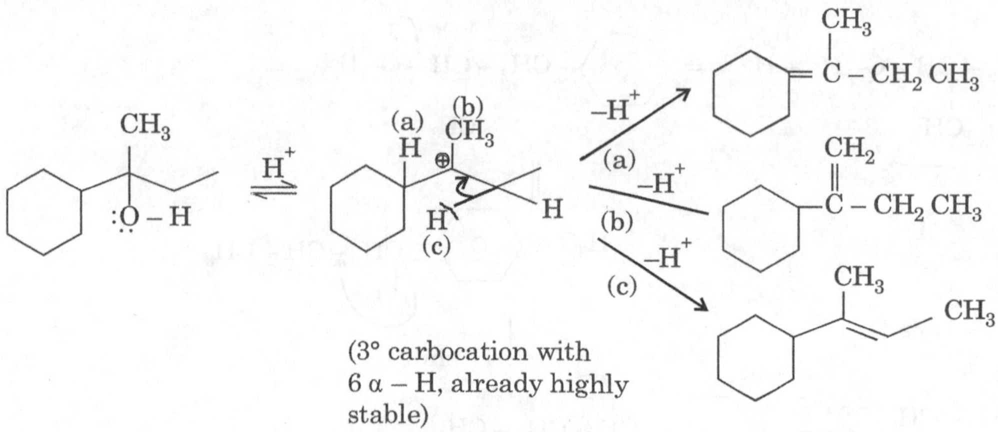

105. Alcohol acts as a nucleophile in esterification reaction. So, it should be least hindered to give maximum yield of an ester. Also, acid should have smallest alkyl group / H to offer least hindrance to attacking nucleophile.

106. 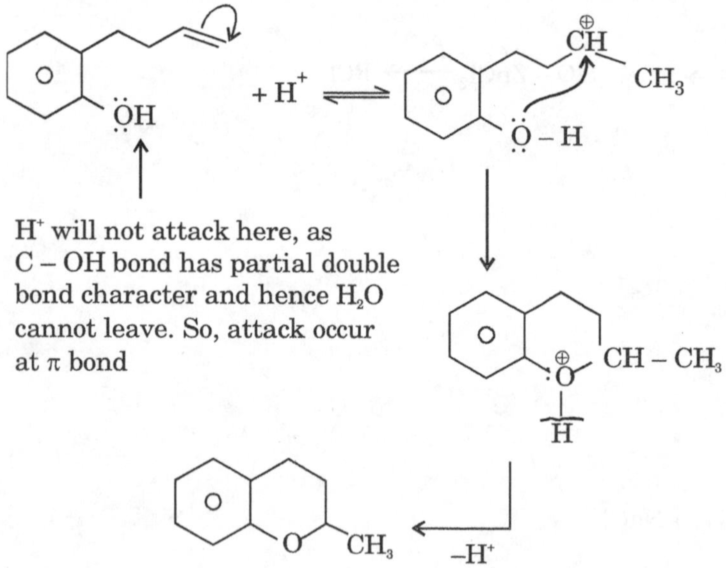

107. Option (c) has $CH_3-\underset{\large OH}{\underset{|}{CH}}-$ group, so it will give +ve haloform test.

Also, $LiAlH_4$ will react with alcohol & H^- ion

will tend to act like a base because it cannot substitute $\overline{O}H$ ($\because$ it's a poor leaving group)

$$CH_3-\underset{:\ddot{O}-H}{\underset{|}{CH}}-CH_2-CH_3 \xrightarrow[\text{(from } LiAlH_4)]{H^-} CH_3-\underset{:\ddot{O}:^{\ominus}}{\underset{|}{CH}}-CH_2CH_3 + H_2\uparrow$$

108. Suggested mechanism is as follows-

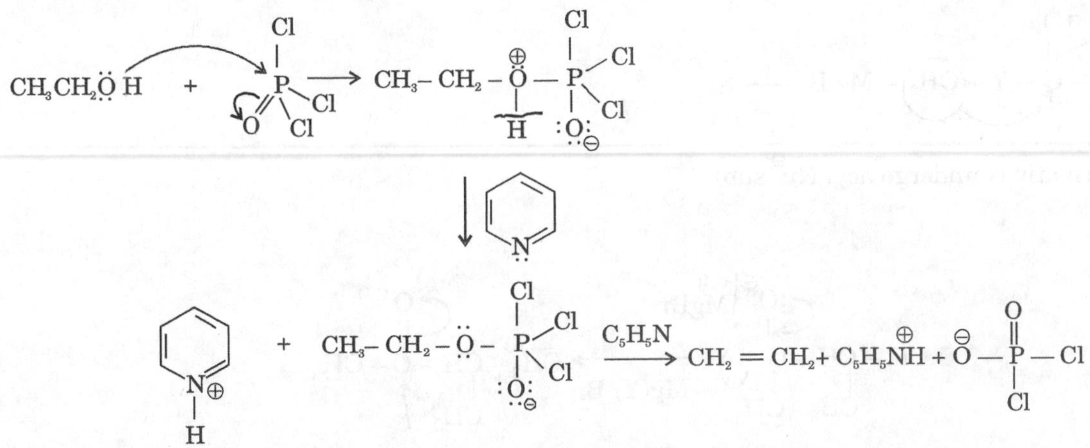

110. In (d) option, H_2O is more acidic than an alcohol. So, equilibrium will lie to the left hand side.

111.

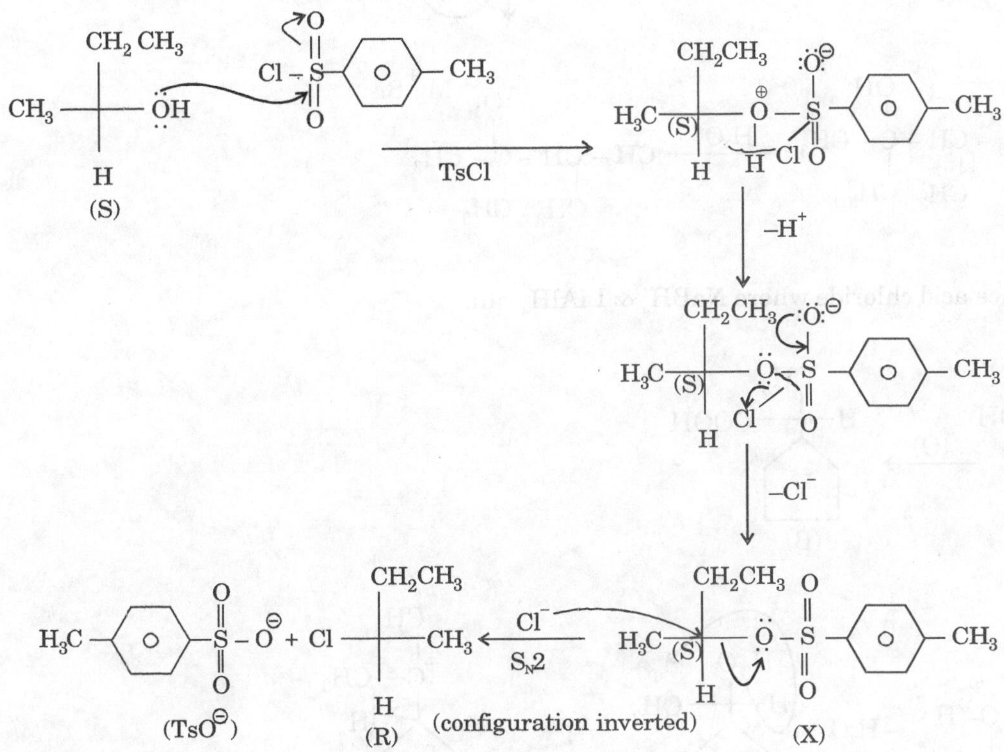

112. Since an acid $CH_3-\underset{\displaystyle CH_3}{\underset{|}{CH}}-COOH$ is formed by hydrolysis of 'A', ∴ 'A' must be an ester or some other acid derivative which has $CH_3-\underset{\displaystyle CH_3}{\underset{|}{CH}}-\overset{\displaystyle O}{\overset{\|}{C}}-Y$.

'Y' could be –Cl, –OR, $-O-\overset{\displaystyle O}{\overset{\|}{C}}-R$.

'A' undergoes reaction with Grignards reagent, which means-

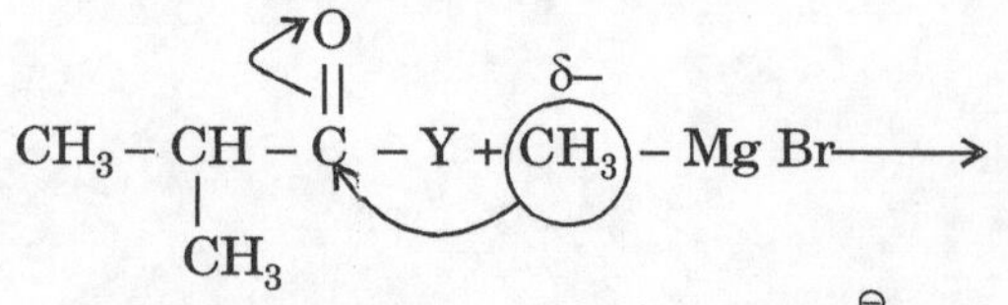

(Acid derivatives undergo acyl $Nu^{\ominus}$ sub).

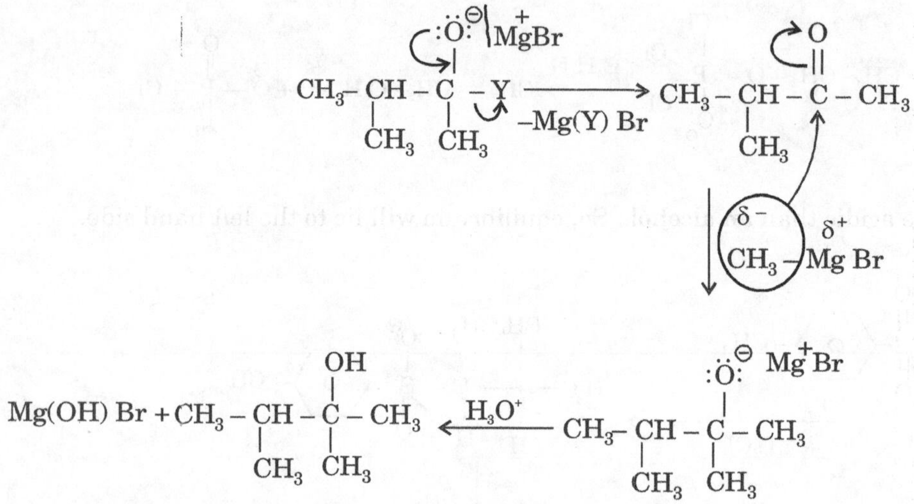

113. B_2H_6 can not reduce acid chloride where $NaBH_4$ & $LiAlH_4$ can.

114.

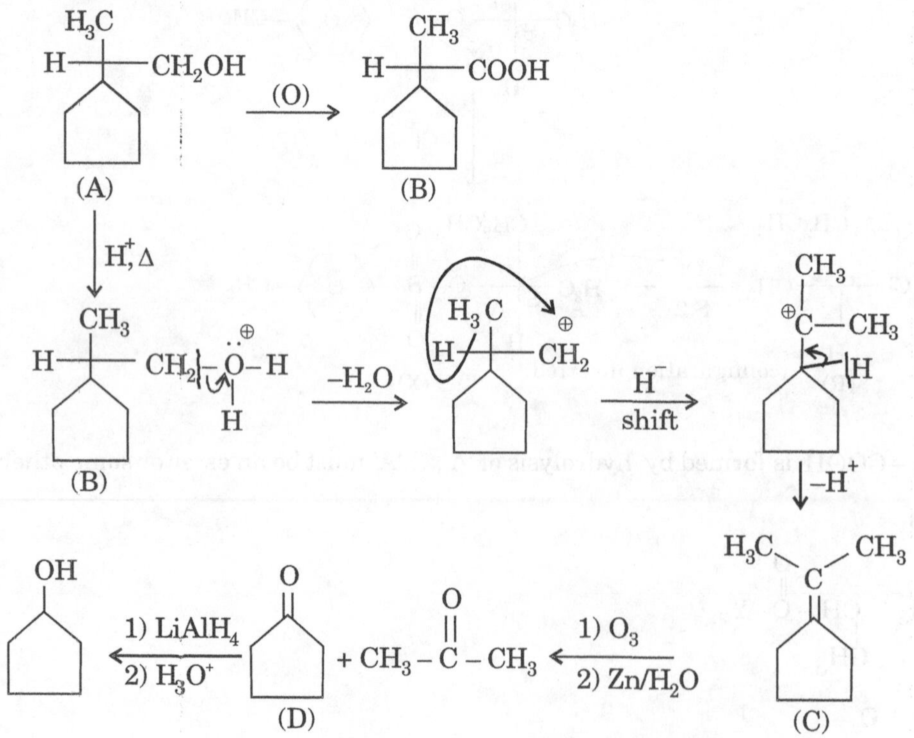

115. Stability of Carbocation is the major concern. Also, in allyl alcohol product will be a conjugated diene.

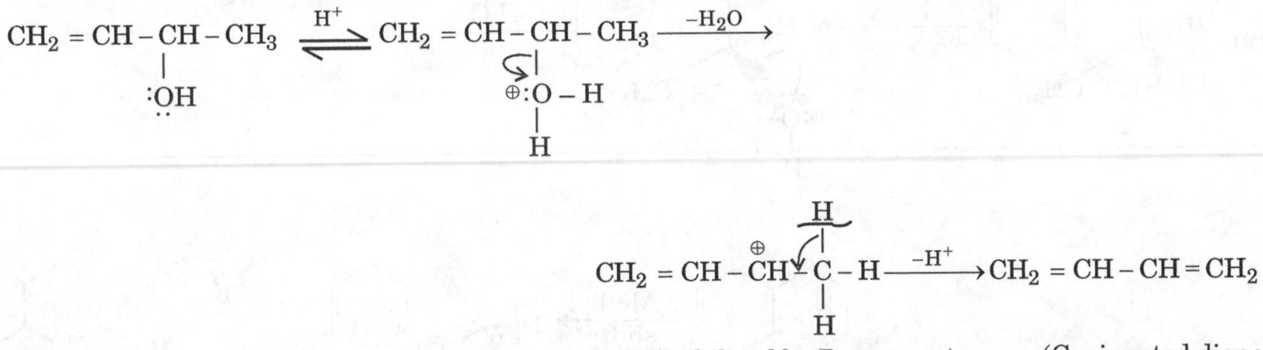

116. Acidic hydrolysis of an ester

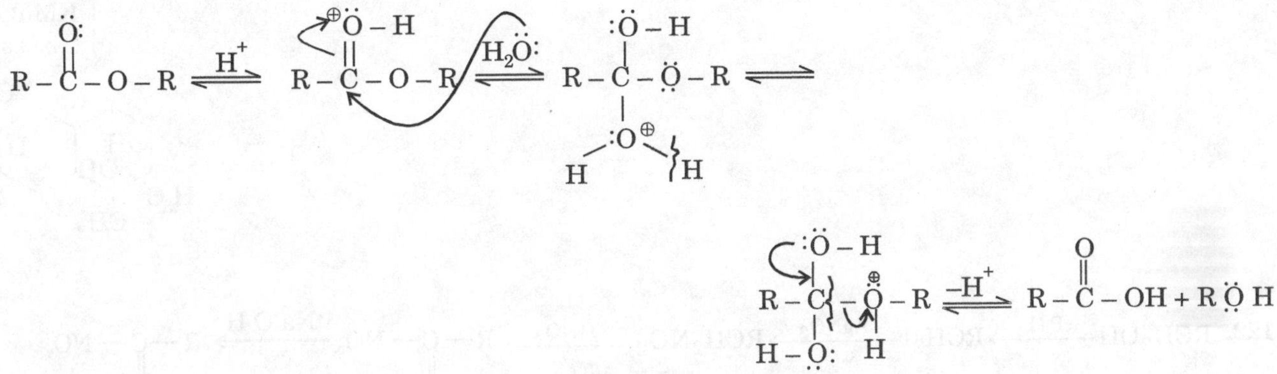

Basic hydrolysis of an ester

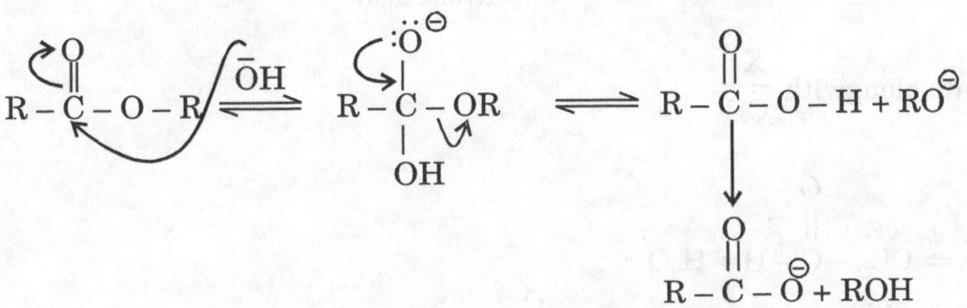

(irreversible, because stable carboxylate ion is formed)

117. (1) $NaBH_4$ cannot reduce ester & will reduce only ketone
Also, $LiAlH_4$ will reduce both ester & ketone

(2) $LiAlH_4$ cannot reduce isolated double bond
∵ H^- gets repelled by π electron cloud.

(3) In β – aryl – α, β – unsaturated aldehyde, the e^- density in alkene region is reduced & H^- ion manages to attack i.e. reducing alkene & aldehyde.

120. Acid catalysed dehydration of alcohols proceeds via Carbocation formation. Cl^-, being a good $Nu^{\ominus}$ can attack carbocation & form alkyl halide rather than acting as base & causing elimination. Conc. HNO_3 is a strong oxidising agent which can oxidise alcohol.

121.

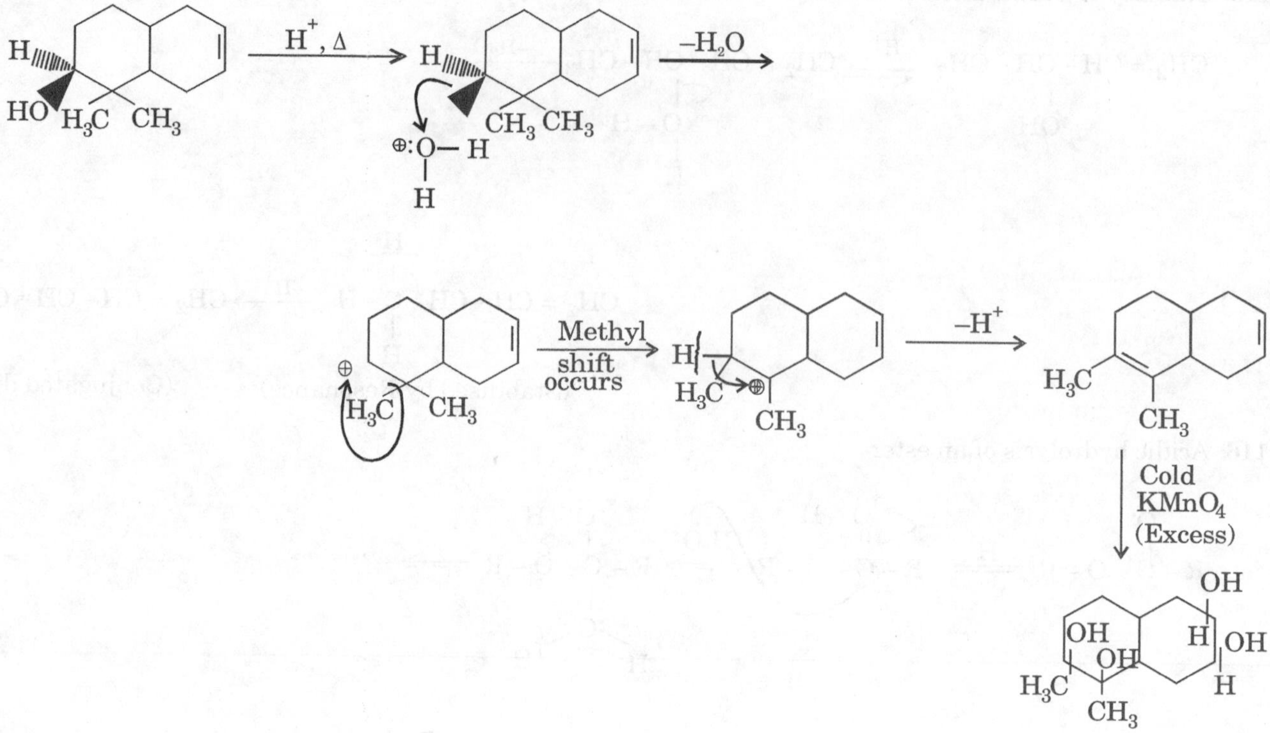

122.

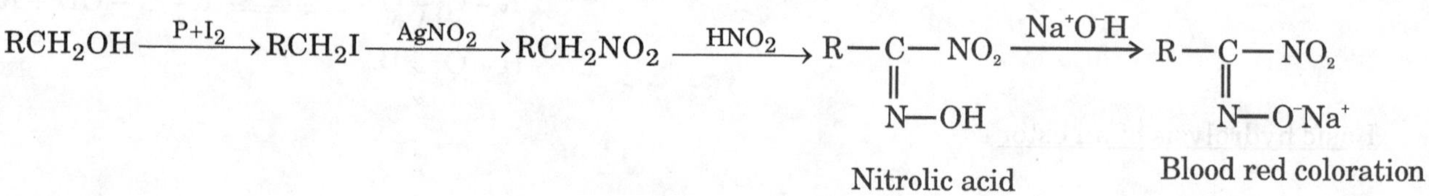

123. Haloform involves the substrate alongwith $\frac{X_2}{\bar{O}H}$.

(i)

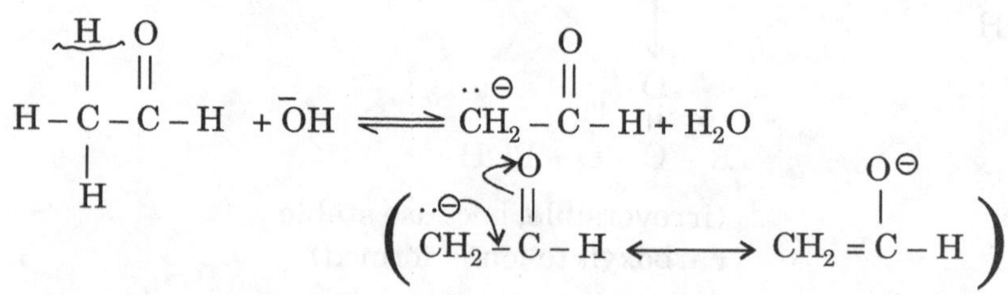

(ii)

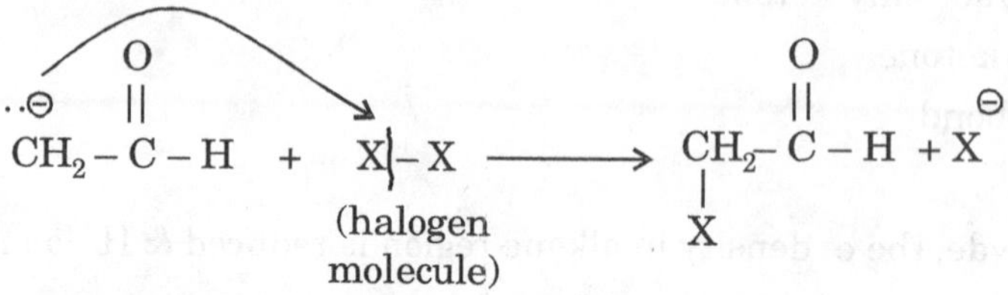

(iii)

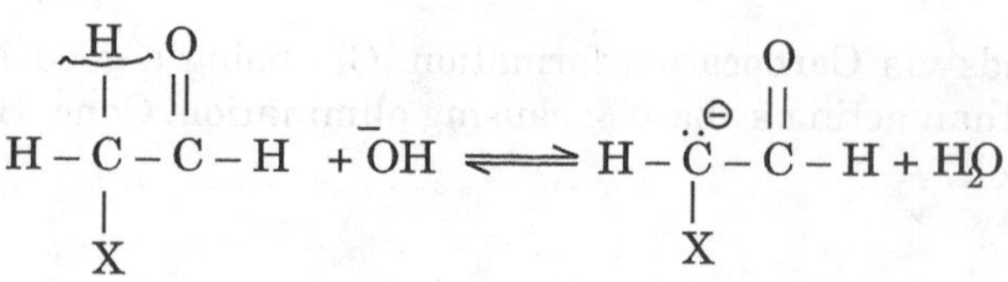

(iv) 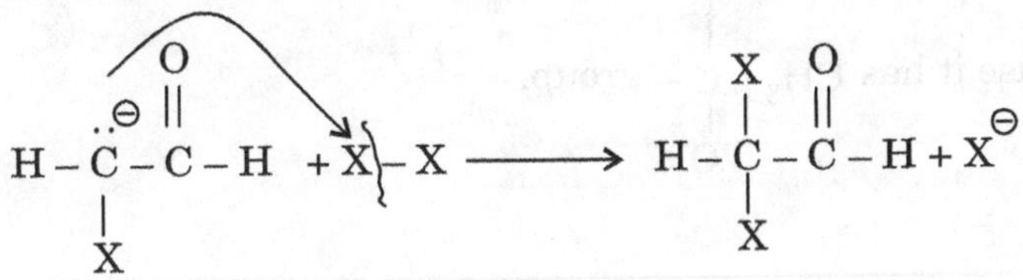

(v) 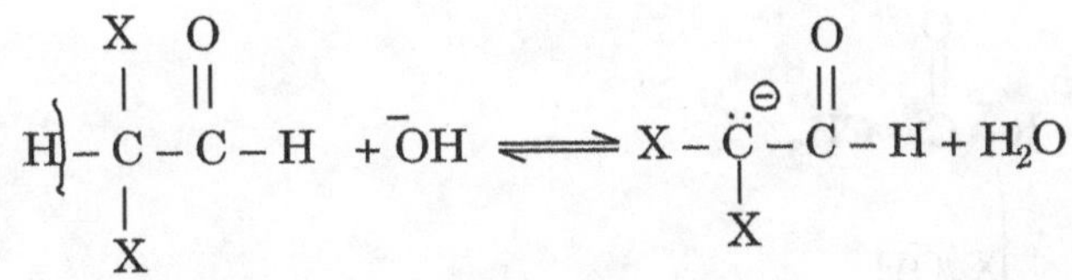

(vi) 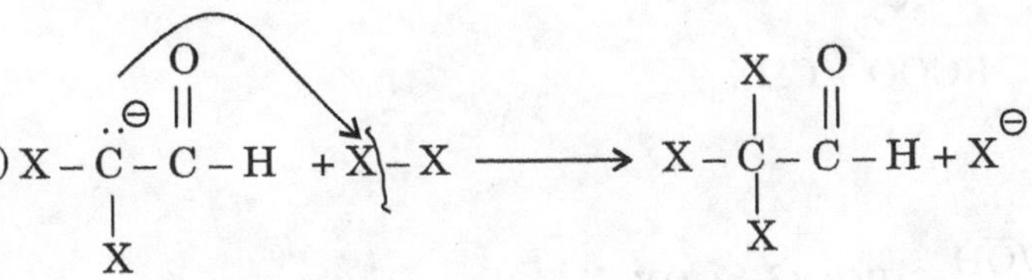

These all steps from (i) to (vi) come under the category of halogenation. Now, basic hydrolysis is carried out.

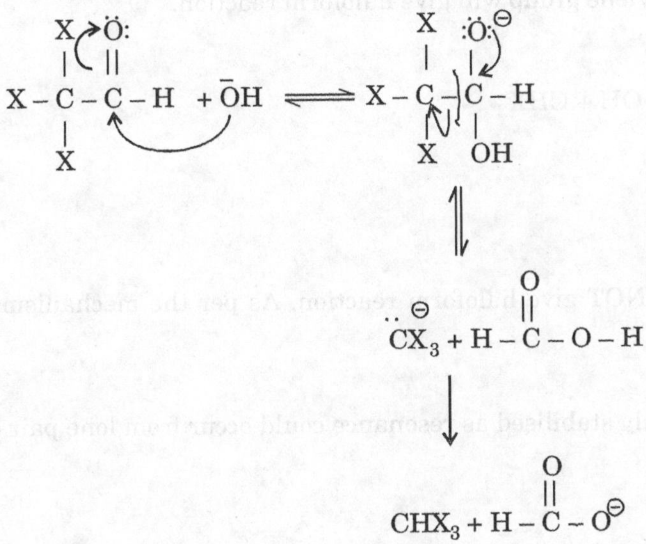

124. $NaOH + X_2 \longrightarrow NaX + NaXO + H_2O$

(NaX + NaXO) wil act as O-Agent

$$CH_3-CH_2OH \xrightarrow{(O)} CH_3-\overset{O}{\overset{\|}{C}}-H$$

Followed by oxidation, halogenation & hydrolysis will occur as described in the previous question.

125. Option a will give haloform reaction because it has $CH_3-\underset{OH}{\overset{H}{C}}-$ group.

Wrt option b

$$R-\underset{X}{\overset{X}{C}}-CH_3 \xrightarrow{\overline{O}H} R-\underset{OH}{\overset{OH}{C}}-CH_3 \xrightarrow{-H_2O} R-\overset{O}{\overset{\|}{C}}-CH_3 \xrightarrow{X_2/\overline{O}H} R\overset{\ominus}{COO} + CHX_3$$

wrt. option c

$$R-\underset{X}{CH}-CH_3 \xrightarrow{\overline{O}H} R-\underset{OH}{CH}-CH_3 \xrightarrow{X_2/\overline{O}H} RCO\overset{\ominus}{O} + CHX_3$$

126. Wrt. option a

1, 3-dicarbonyl compounds having active methylene group will give haloform reaction.

$$CH_3-\overset{O}{\overset{\|}{C}}-\underset{H}{\overset{H}{C}}-\overset{O}{\overset{\|}{C}}-CH_3 \xrightarrow[2)\ H_3O^+]{1)\ X_2/\overline{O}H} 2\ CH_3COOH + CHX_3$$

Option b & c will give haloform.

Option 'd' has $CH_3-\overset{O}{\overset{\|}{C}}-$ group. but will still NOT give haloform reaction. As per the mechanism, the conjugate base of $CH_3-\overset{O}{\overset{\|}{C}}-Cl$ will not be highly stabilised as resonance could occur from lone pair of Cl also.

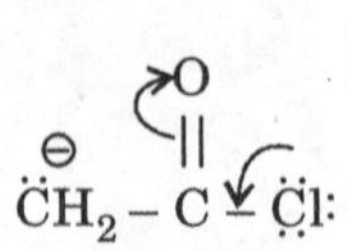

Also, $CH_3-\overset{O}{\overset{\|}{C}}-Cl$ will be reactive towards Nucleophilic acyl substitution also.

127. Wrt. option a

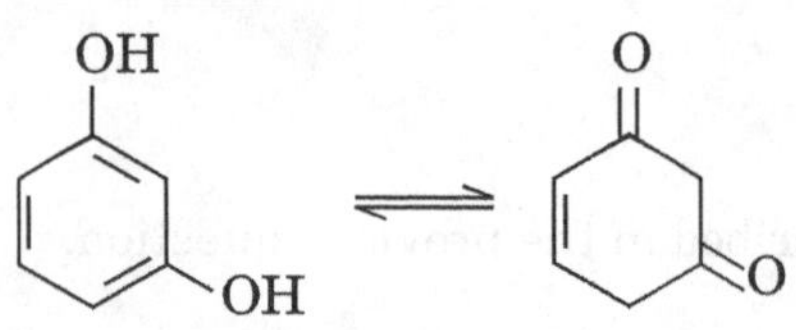

Now,

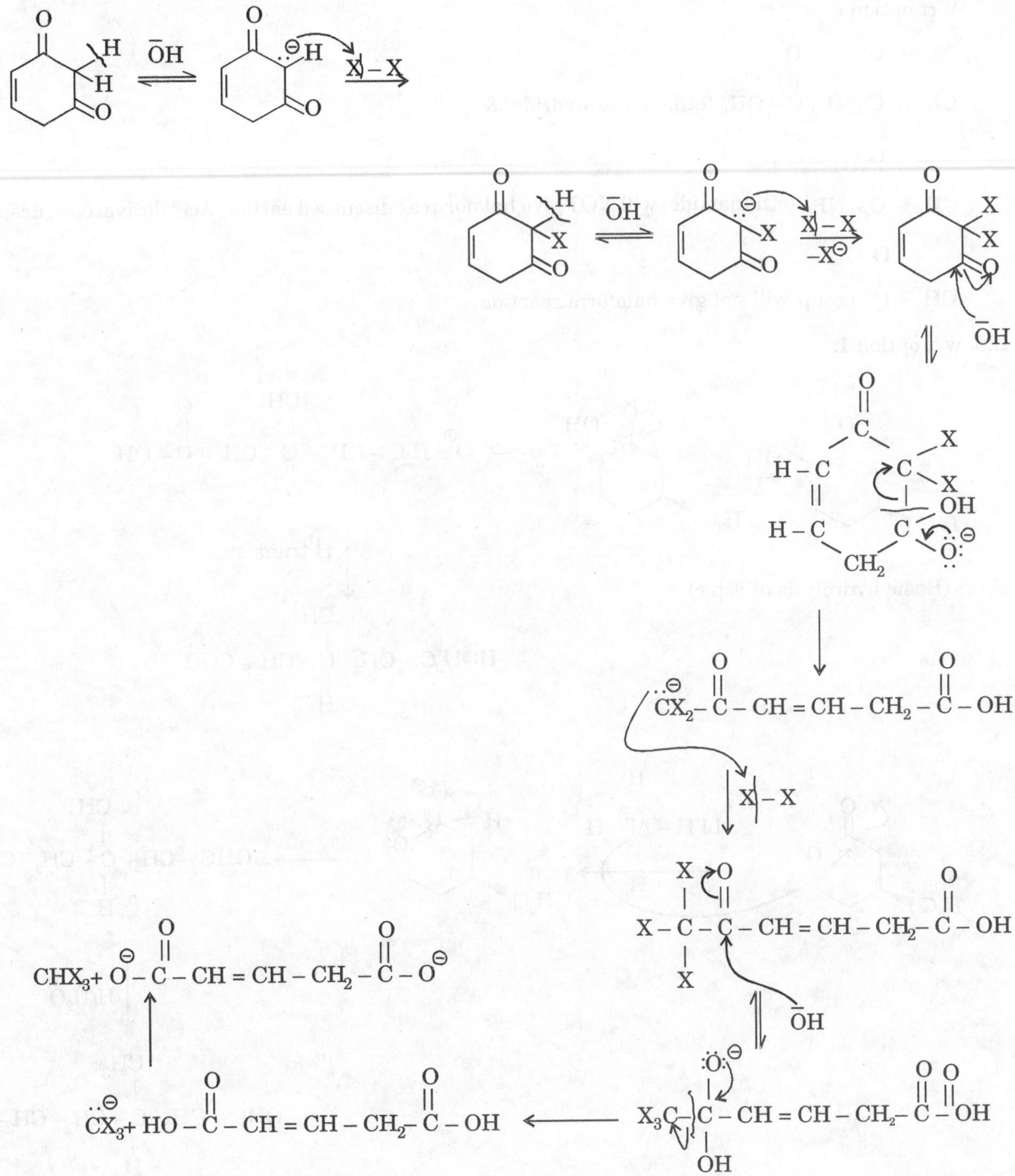

Wrt. option b

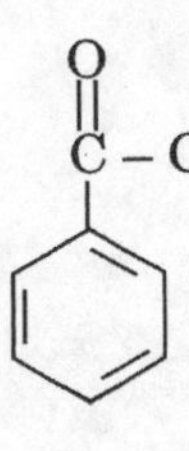

(Acetophenone), will give haloform reaction because it has $CH_3-\overset{O}{\overset{||}{C}}-$ gp

Wrt option c

$CH_3-\overset{\overset{\large O}{||}}{C}-O-\overset{\overset{\large O}{||}}{C}-CH_3$ (ethanoic anhydride) &

$CH_3-\overset{\overset{\large O}{||}}{C}-NH_2$ (ethanamide) will NOT give haloform as discussed earlier, Acid derivatives, despite having

$CH_3-\overset{\overset{\large O}{||}}{C}-$ group will not give haloform reaction.

128. wrt option 1,

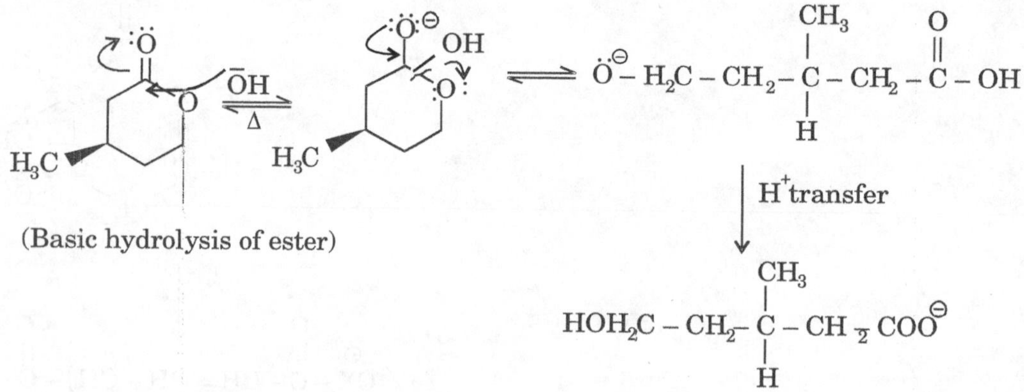

(Basic hydrolysis of ester)

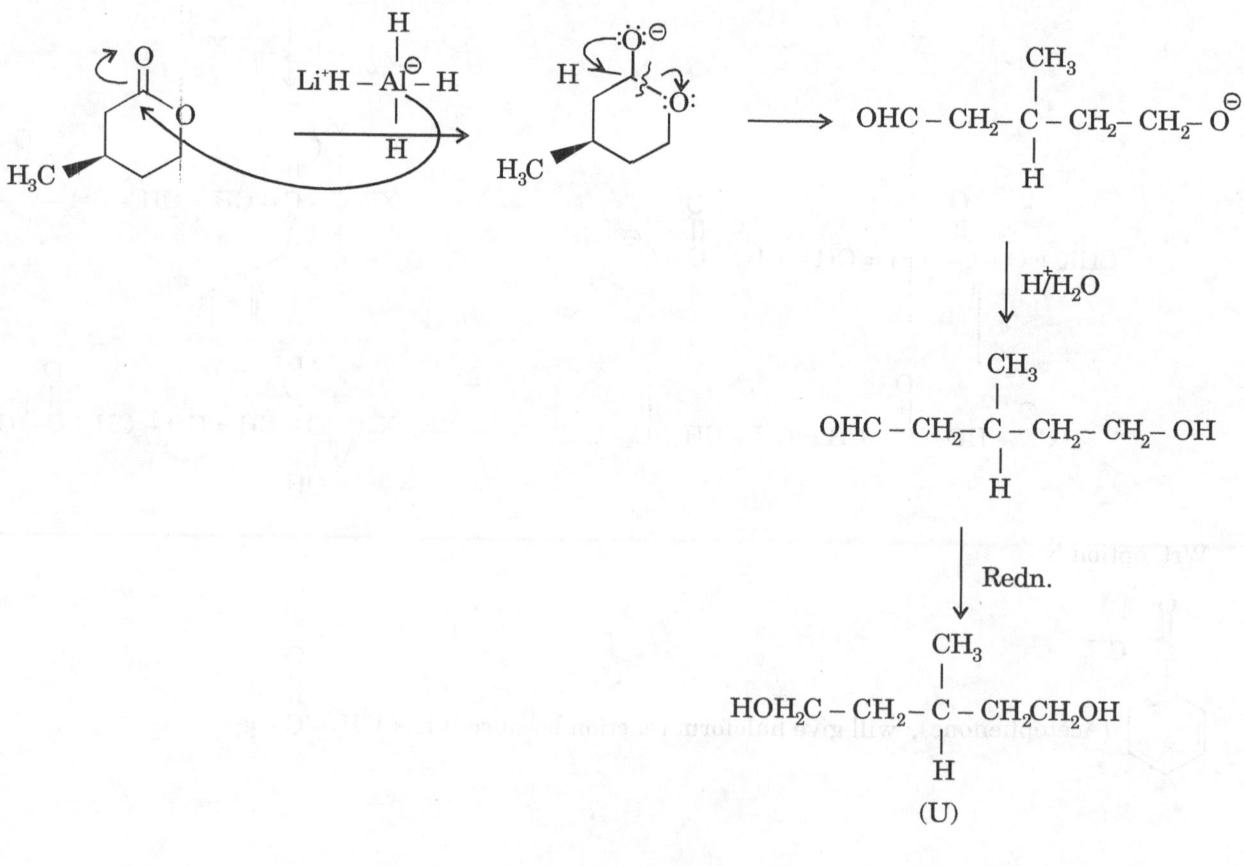

(U)

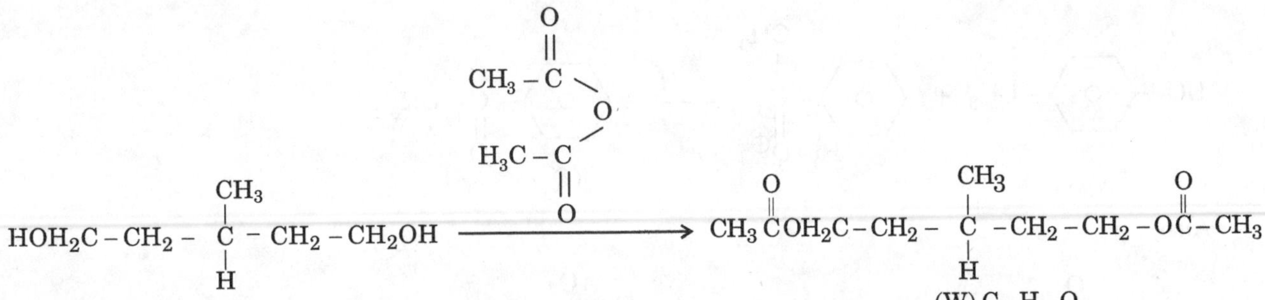

(U) (W) $C_{10}H_{18}O_4$

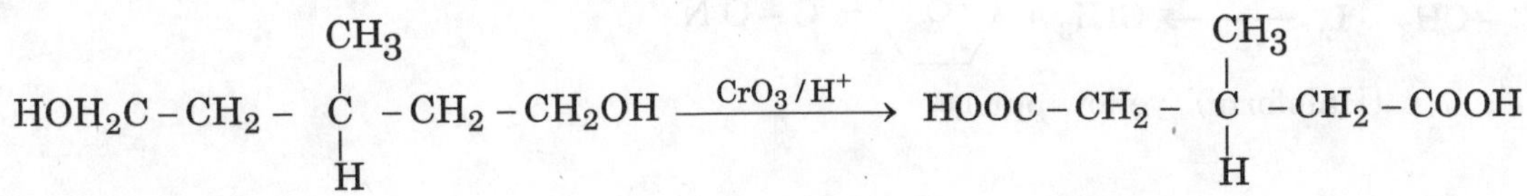

(V)

Since 'V' is Carboxylic acid, it gives effervescence with aq. $NaHCO_3$.

129. 2nd Reaction is Riemer Tiemann's Carboxylation. 3rd Reaction is Kolbe's reaction. Both will give salicylic acid (after acidification)

130.

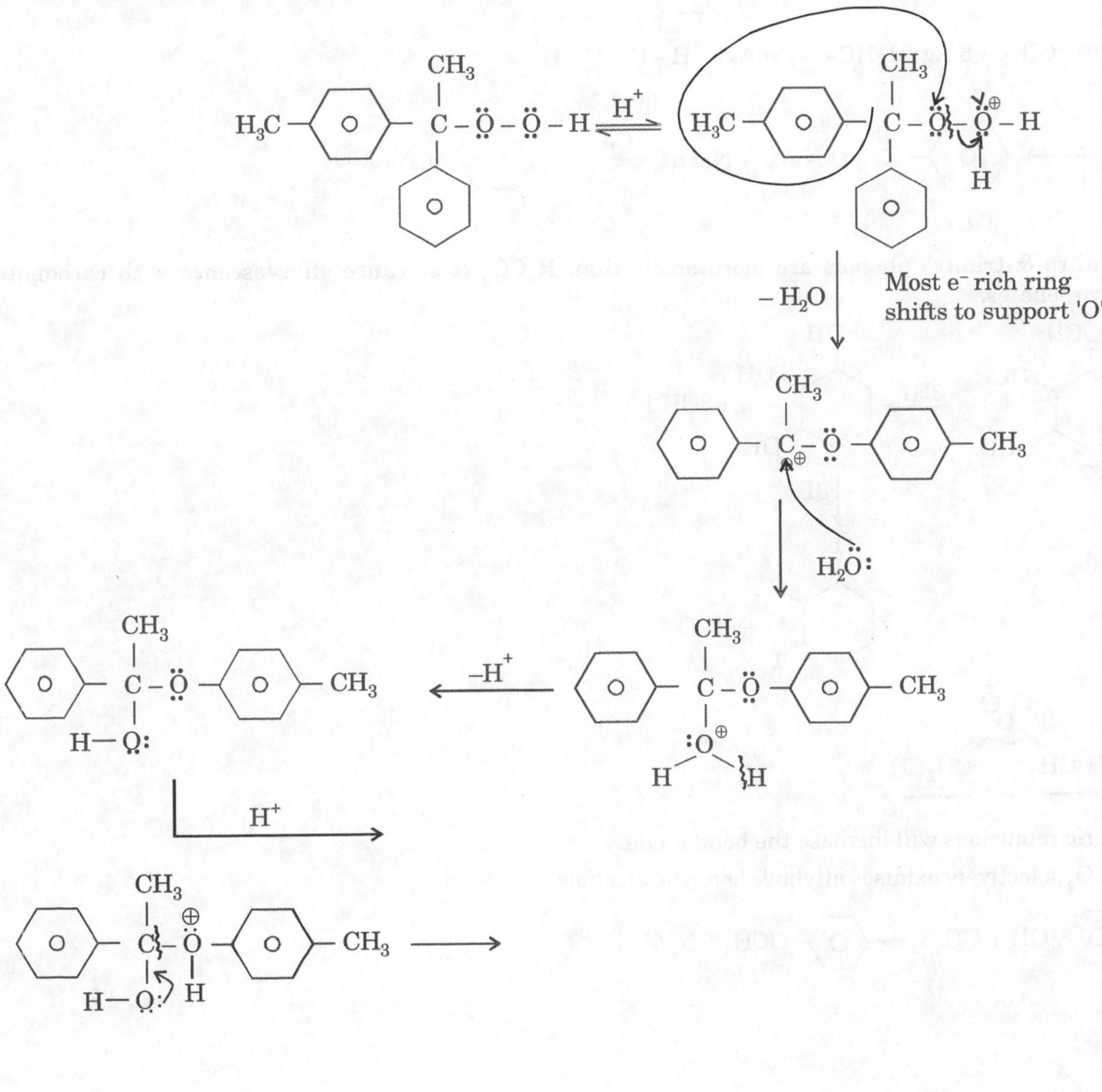

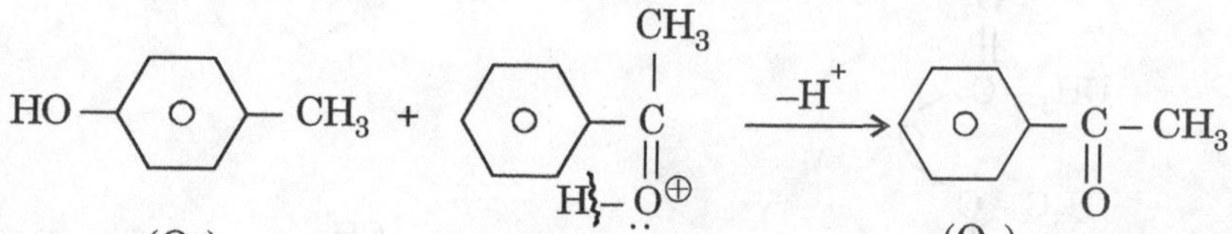

(Q2) (Q1)

Also,

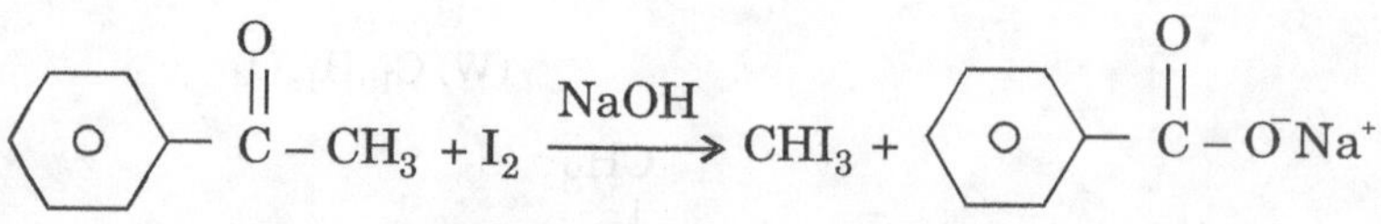

(Q1) (Haloform) (yellow ppt.)

$Q_3 \longrightarrow CHI_3$

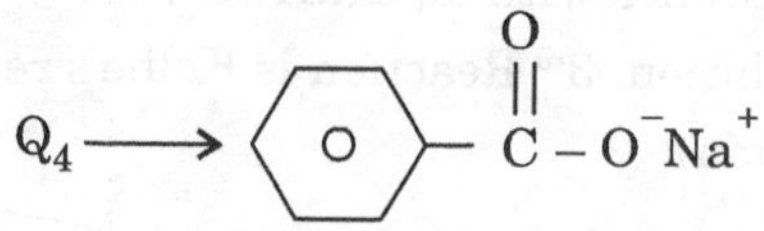

Now, $CHI_3 + 6\,Ag + I_3HC \longrightarrow 6AgI + H-C\equiv C-H$

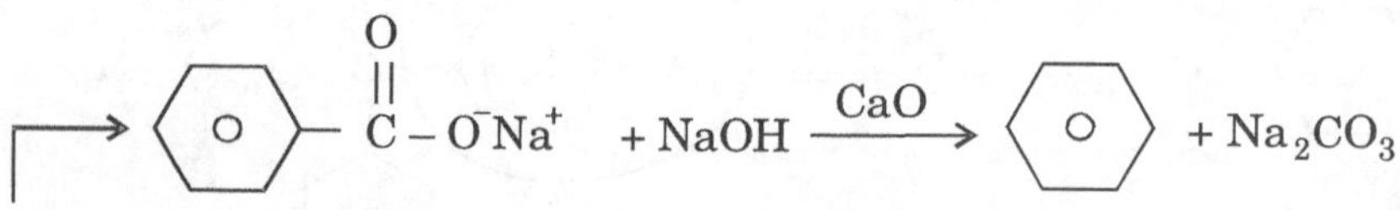

(Q4)

132. Dinitro & trinitro phenols are more acidic than H_2CO_3 & so cause effervescence with carbonates & bicarbonates.

133.

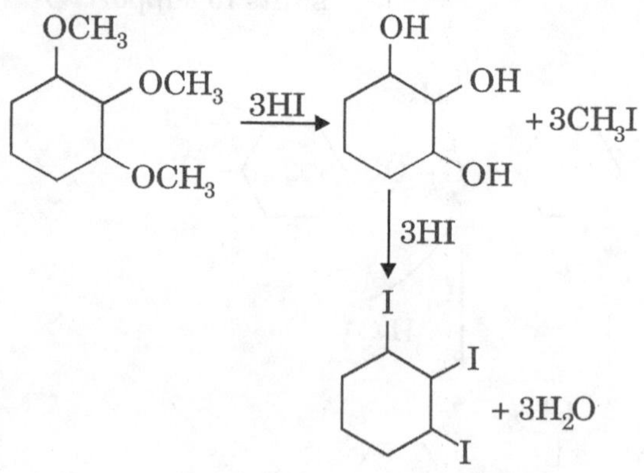

135.

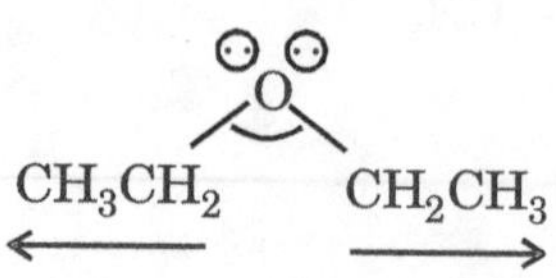

Steric repulsions will increase the bond angle.

141. MnO_2 selectively oxidises allylic & benzylic alcohols.

142.

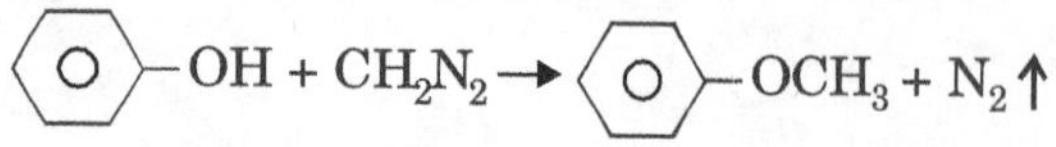

143. $NaBH_4$ will reduce ketone & not Ester.

144. Carbocation formed in option (b) is maximum stable.

145. Electrophilic aromatic substitution occurs at anisole 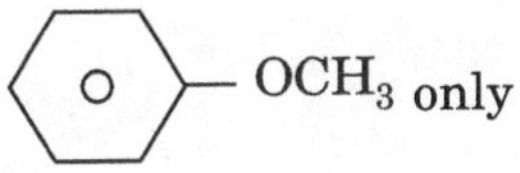

Nitrobenzene is highly deactivated.

146. All aldehydes (aliphatic and aromatic) & α–hydroxy ketone will give tollen's reagent test.

147. All the given molecules will form stable carbocations so will give immediate turbidity with Lucas reagent.

148. (1) $CH_3COOCH_3 \xrightarrow[2)H_3O^+]{1)LiAlH_4} CH_3CH_2OH + CH_3OH$

(2) $CH_3COOC_2H_5 \xrightarrow[2)H_3O^+]{1)LiAlH_4} CH_3CH_2OH + C_2H_5OH$

(3) $CH_3COCH_3 \xrightarrow[2)H_3O^+]{1)LiAlH_4} CH_3-CH(OH)-CH_3$

(4) $CH_3CH_2CHO \xrightarrow[2)H_3O^+]{1)LiAlH_4} CH_3-CH_2-CH_2-OH$

149. Cleavage of ether cannot occur at room temperature with halogen acid. So attack occurs at the pie bond.

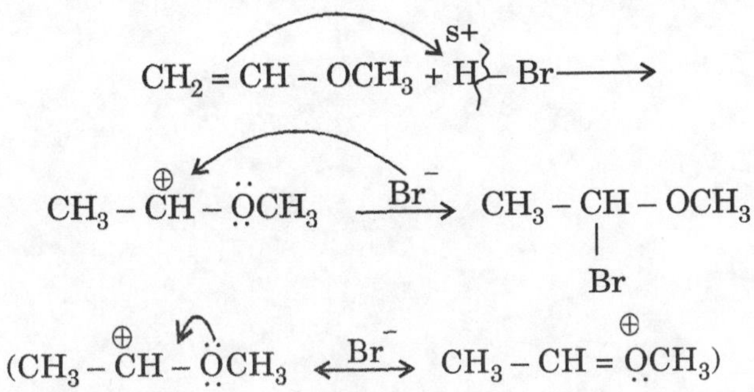

150. PCC will oxidise 2° alcohol to ketone. It cannot oxidise 3° alcohol

151. Since a stable carbocation can be formed here, that cleavage of ether will occur via SN.

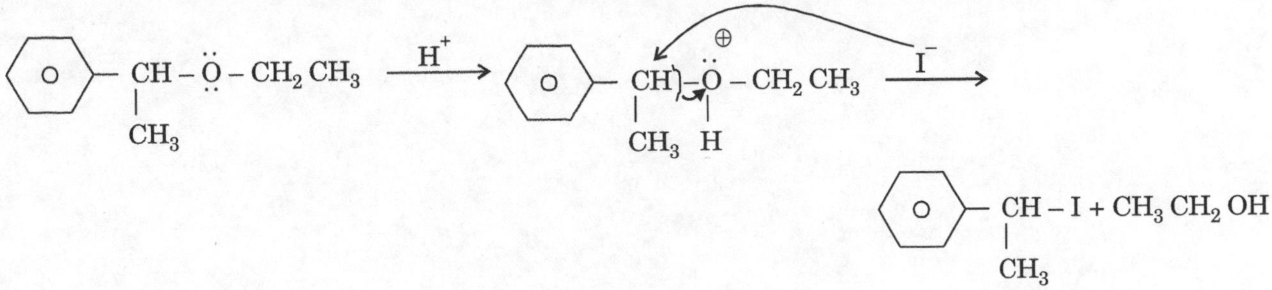

CHAPTER 12

Aldehydes, Ketones and Carboxylic Acid

Preparation of Aldehydes & Ketones

1. Stephen's reaction is used to convert

(a) aldehydes to ketones

(b) ketones to alcohols

(c) aldehydes to carboxylic acids

(d) Cyanides to aldehydes.

2. Select the incorrect match.

REACTION	Name of Reaction
(a) $RCOCl + H_2 \xrightarrow[BaSO_4]{Pd} RCHO + HCl$	Rosenmund's reduction
(b) 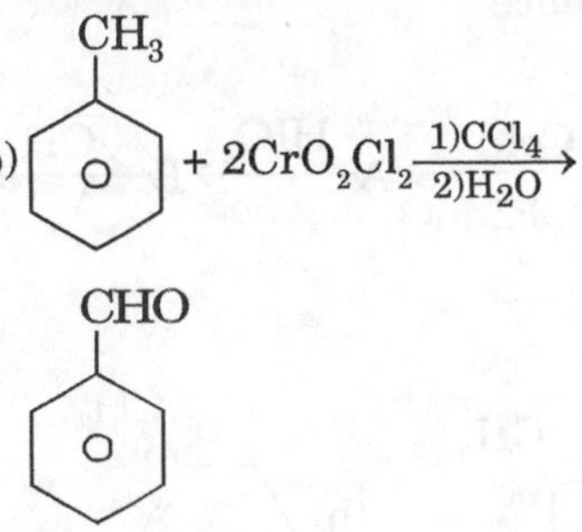	Etard's reaction
(c) $CH_3 - CH = CH_2 + H_2O + PdCl_2 \xrightarrow{CuCl_2} CH_3 - \underset{\underset{O}{\parallel}}{C} - CH_3 + Pd + 2HCl$	Wacker's process

(d) None of these

3. What is true about Gattermann's aldehyde synthesis?

(a) It is an electrophilic substitution reaction.

(b) It involves the use of lewis acid as anhyd. $AlCl_3$.

(c) It involves the formation of an imine.

(d) All are correct.

4. Select the wrong statement about Gattermann Koch reaction.

(a) It involves formylation of benzene.

(b) It is an electrophilic substitution reaction

(c) Formyl carbocation is the attacking electrophile.

(d) It is a nucleophilic substitution reaction

5. Select the major product in the following reaction

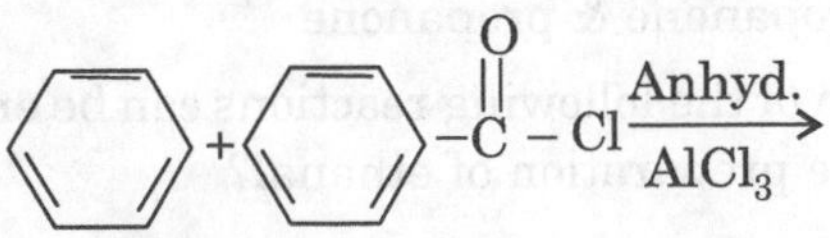

(a) Acetophenone

(b) Benzophenone

(c) Acetaldehyde

(d) Acetone

6. Select 'Z' in the following reaction:

$$H - C \equiv C - H \xrightarrow{CH_3MgBr} X \xrightarrow[H_3O^+]{CO_2\,/} Y \xrightarrow[H_2SO_4]{HgSO_4\,/} Z$$

(a) $OHC - CH_2 - COOH$

(b) $OHC - CH_2 - CHO$

(c) $CH_2(COOH)_2$

(d) $CH_3 - CH_2 - CHO$

7. Which one of the following is oxidised to prepare butan – 2 – one?

(a) 1 – propanol (b) 2 – propanol

(c) 2 – butanol (d) isopropyl alcohol

8. Consider the following reaction:

$$CH_3-CH_2-CH_2-CH_2MgBr + H_2C\underset{O}{-}CH_2 \longrightarrow A \xrightarrow{H_3O^+} B \xrightarrow[CH_2Cl_2]{PCC} C$$

The final product 'C' in the above reaction is –

(a) hexanone

(b) 2 – methyl pentan – 3 – one

(c) Pentan – 2 – one

(d) hexanal

9. Identify A & B, respectively, in the following reactions:

$$\text{Propyne} \xrightarrow{HgSO_4,\ dil.\ H_2SO_4} A$$

$$\text{Propyne} \xrightarrow[2) H_2O_2, \bar{O}H]{1) BH_3, THF} B$$

(a) Propanal & propanone

(b) Propanone & propanal

(c) Propanone & propane

(d) Propanone & propanone

10. Which of the following reactions can be employed for the preparation of ethanal?

(a) $CH_3-C\equiv N \xrightarrow[2) H_3O^+]{1) DIBAL-H}$

(b) $CH_3-C\equiv N \xrightarrow[2) H_3O^+]{1) SnCl_2 + HCl}$

(c) $CH_3-C\equiv N \xrightarrow[2) H_3O^+]{1) Pd/BaSO_4 + H_2}$

(d) All of these

11. Which of the following is NOT suitable for the preparation of an aldehyde?

(a) $CH_3-CH=CH-CH_2-CN \xrightarrow[2) H_2O]{1) DIBAL-H} CH_3-CH=CH-CH_2CHO$

(b) $CH_3-\overset{O}{\overset{\|}{C}}-OC_2H_5 \xrightarrow[(2)\ H_2O]{(1)\ DIBAL-H} CH_3CHO + C_2H_5OH$

(c) $C_6H_5CH_3 \xrightarrow[(CH_3CO)_2O]{CrO_3} A \xrightarrow{H_3O^+} C_6H_5CHO$

(d) 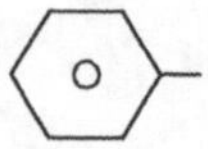 $-CH_3 \xrightarrow[\text{(excess) } h\nu]{Cl_2} A \xrightarrow[375\ k]{H_2O} C_6H_5CHO$

12. Ethyl acetate $\xrightarrow[2)\ H_3O^+]{1) CH_3MgBr\ (1\ mole)}$ A

The Product 'A' Can –

(1) give iodoform test

(2) further react with $CH_3MgBr\,|\,H_3O^+$ to give test – butanol.

(3) also be obtained by ozonolysis of 2, 3 – dimethyl 2 – butene.

The correct statement (s) is | are –

(a) 1 only

(b) 1, 2 & 3 only

(c) 1 & 3 but not 2

(d) 1 & 2 but not 3

Chemical Properties of Aldehydes & Ketones

13. The correct order of following molecules towards nucleophilic addition is –

(a) $HCHO > CH_3COCH_3 > PhCOCH_3 > PhCOPh$

(b) $PhCOCH_3 > CH_3COCH_3 > HCHO > PhCOPh$

(c) $CH_3COCH_3 > HCHO > PhCOCH_3 > PhCOPh$

(d) $HCHO > CH_3COCH_3 = PhCOCH_3 > PhCOPh$

14. Identify the final product 'C' in the following reaction sequence –

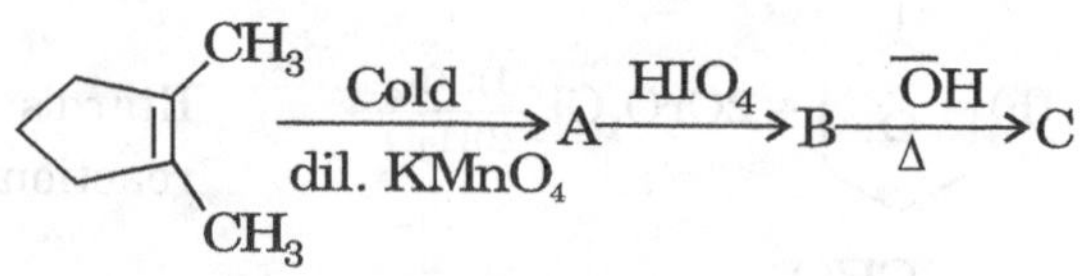

(a) 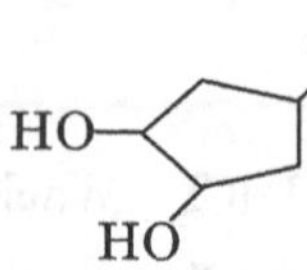

(b) 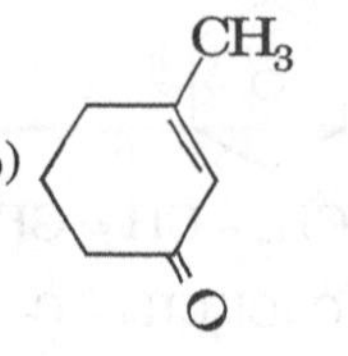

(c) 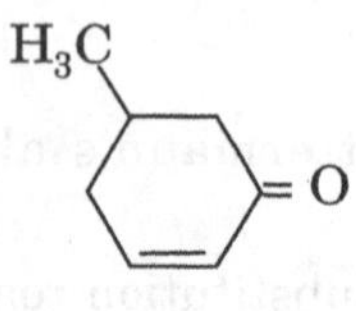

(d) 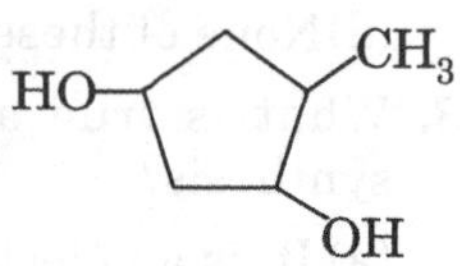

15. P–Cresol reacts with $CHCl_3$ in alkaline medium to give a compound A, which adds HCN to form a compound B. The latter on acidic hydrolysis gives a chiral carboxylic acid. The Structure of acid is

(a) 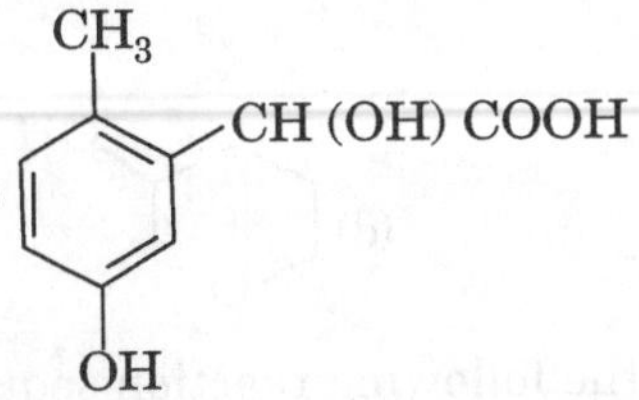

(b) 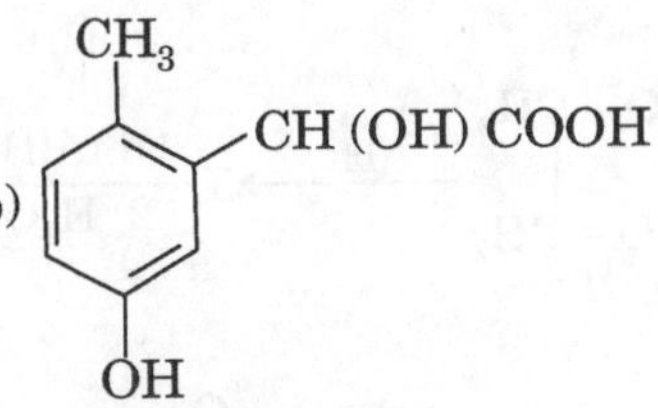

(c) 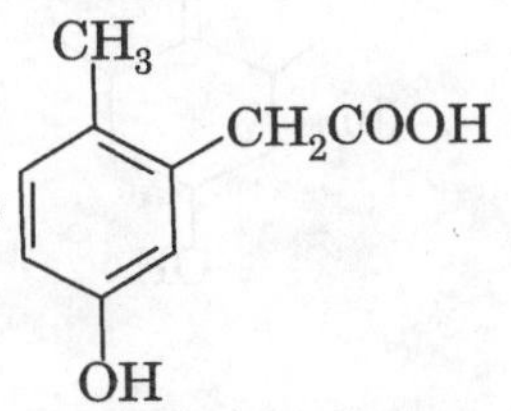

(d) 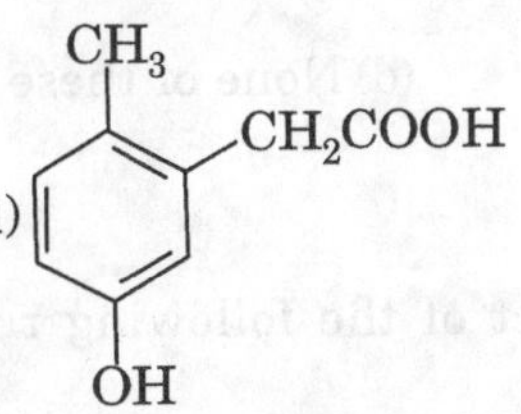

16. Consider the following reactions –

$$CH_3-CH_2-\underset{\underset{H}{|}}{C}=\boxed{O+H_2}\ NNH\,CONH_2 \xrightarrow{H^+}$$

$$H_2O + \underset{(A)}{CH_3-CH_2-CH=NNHCONH_2}$$

$$CH_3-CH_2-\underset{\underset{H}{|}}{C}=\boxed{O+H_2}\ NCONHNH_2 \xrightarrow{H^+}$$

$$H_2O + \underset{(B)}{CH_3-CH_2-CH=N\,CONHNH_2}$$

Out of two products (A & B) listed above, the correct 'Semi – Carbazone' is –

(a) A

(b) B

(c) either A or B

(d) None of these

17. Identify X, Y & Z in the following reaction sequence –

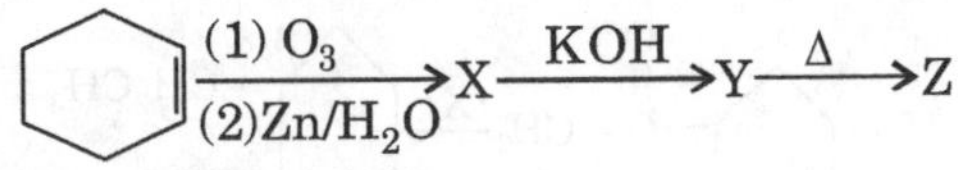

(a) $OHC-(CH_2)_4-CHO$;

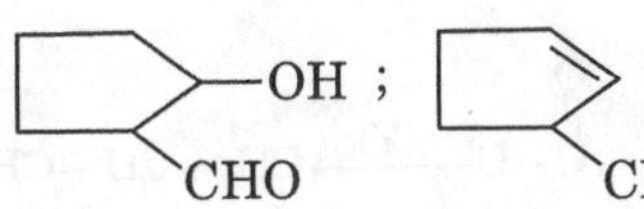

(b) $HO-\overset{\overset{O}{||}}{C}-(CH_2)_4-CHO$;

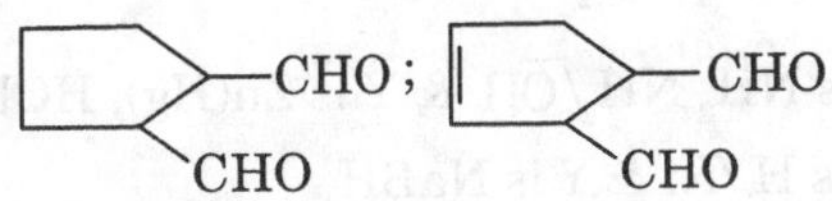

(c) $HO-\overset{\overset{O}{||}}{C}-(CH_2)_4-COOH$;

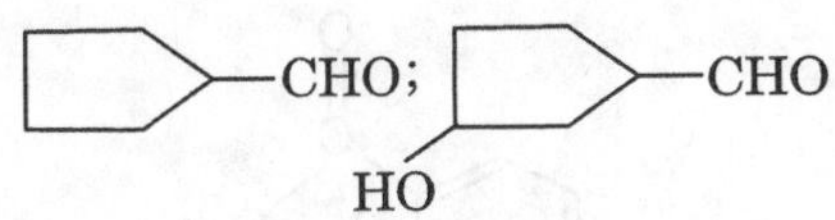

(d) $OHC-(CH_2)_4-CHO$;

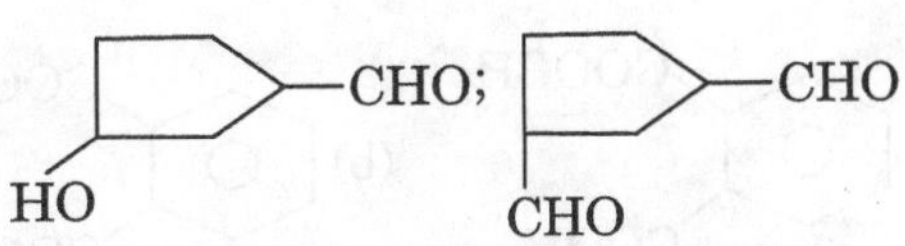

18. Identify 'A' in the following reaction –

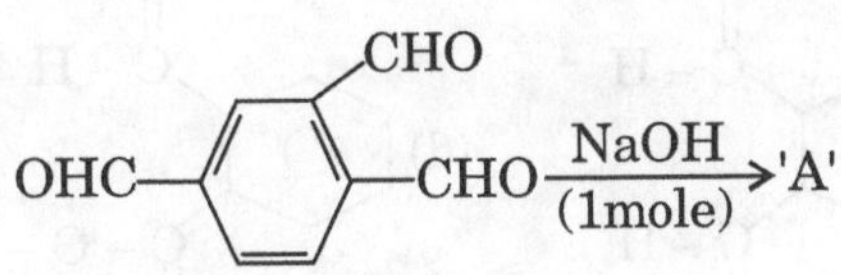

(a) 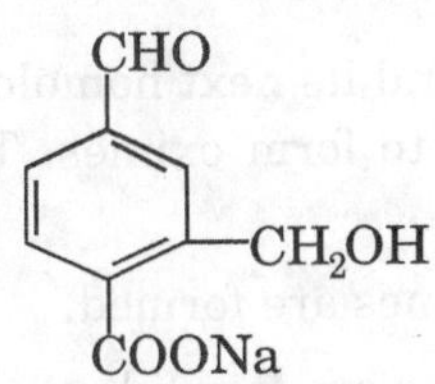

(b) 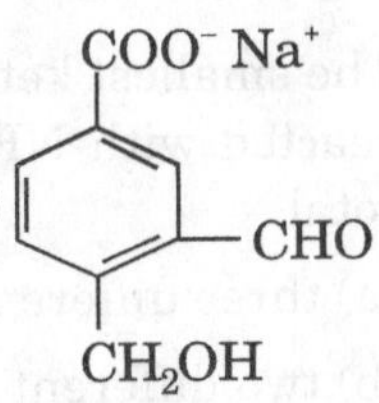

(c) 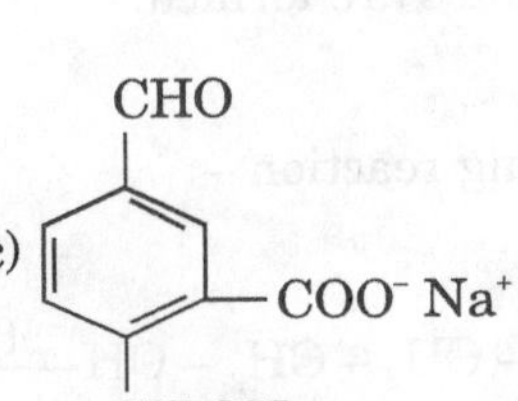

(d) 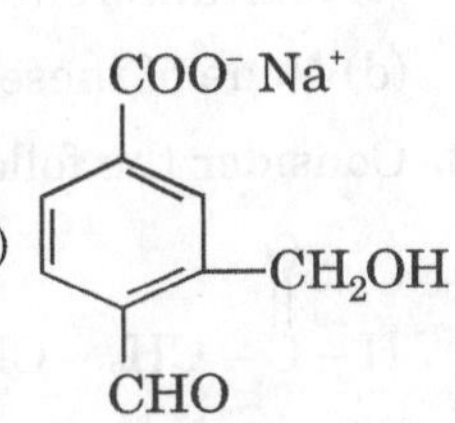

19. Most appropriate reagents for the following transformations are –

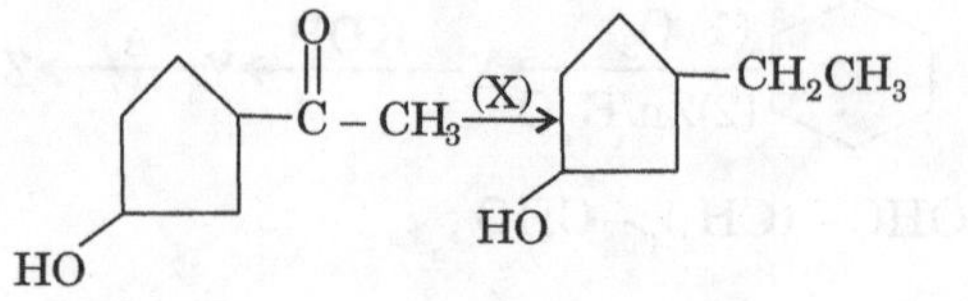

$$CH_3-\underset{Br}{CH}-CH_2-\overset{O}{\overset{\|}{C}}-H \xrightarrow{(Y)} CH_3-\underset{Br}{CH}-CH_2-CH_3$$

(a) X is Zn(Hg), HCl & Y is $NH_2NH_2/\overline{O}H$

(b) X is $NH_2NH_2/\overline{O}H$ & Y is $NaBH_4$

(c) X is $NH_2NH_2/\overline{O}H$ & Y is Zn(Hg), HCl

(d) X is H_2/Ni & Y is $NaBH_4$

20. Which of the following reactants on reaction with conc. NaOH followed by acidification gives the following lactone as the only product?

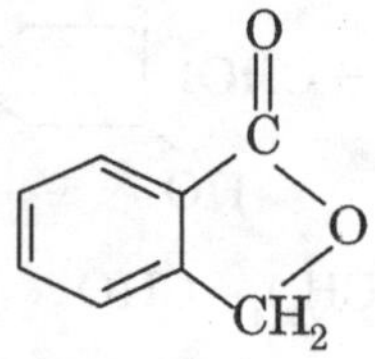

(a) 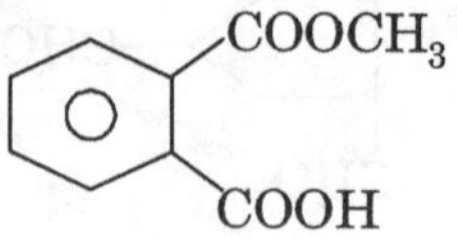 (b) 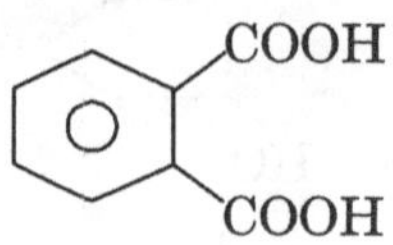

(c) 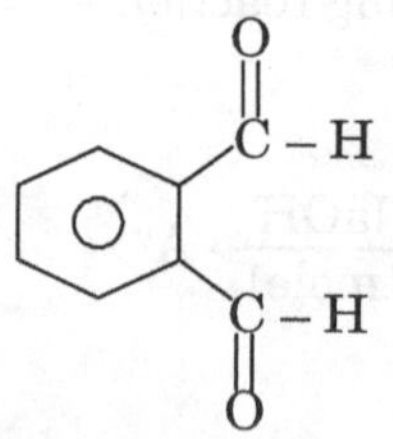 (d) 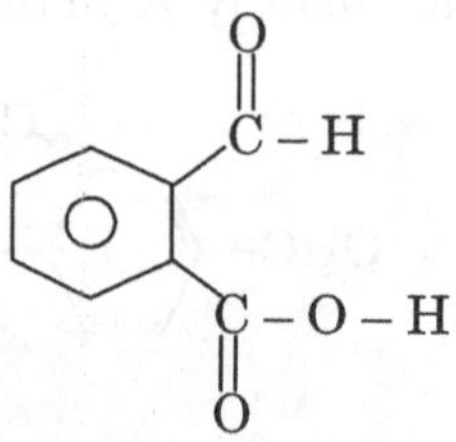

21. The smallest ketone and its next homologue are reacted with NH_2OH to form oximes. Then, in total –

(a) three different oximes are formed.

(b) two different oximes are formed.

(c) four different oximes are formed.

(d) None of these

22. Consider the following reaction –

$$H-\overset{O}{\overset{\|}{C}}-CH_2-CH_2-CH_2-CH_2-OH \xrightarrow{H^+} 'A'$$

'A' in the above reaction is –

(a) 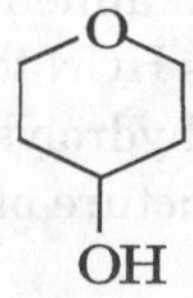 (b) 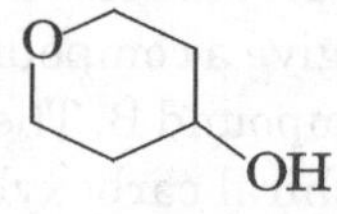

(c) 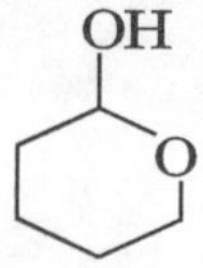 (d) 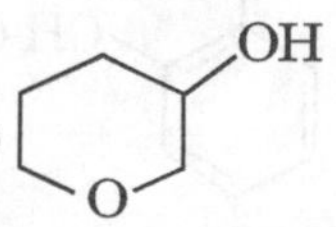

23. Identify 'Z' in the following reaction sequence –

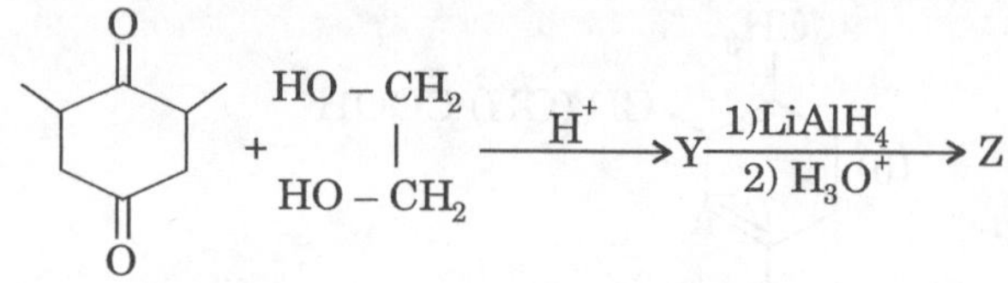

(a) 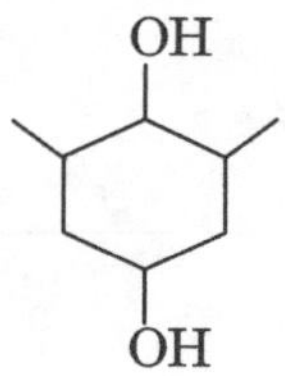 (b) 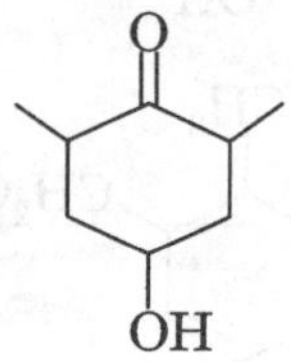

(c) 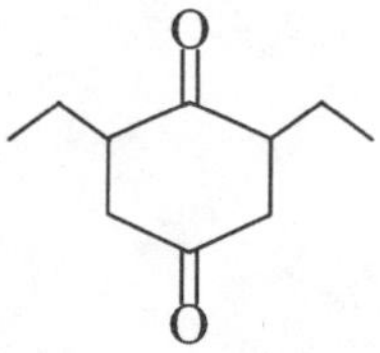 (d) None of these

24. The correct product of the following reaction is –

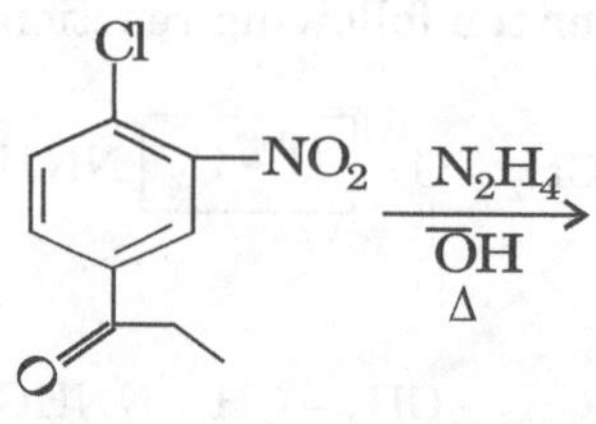

(a) 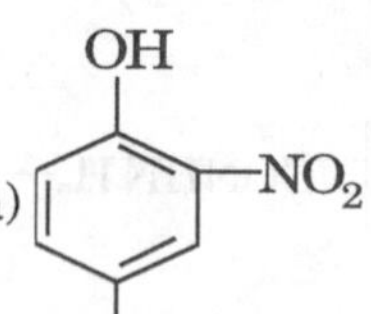 (b) 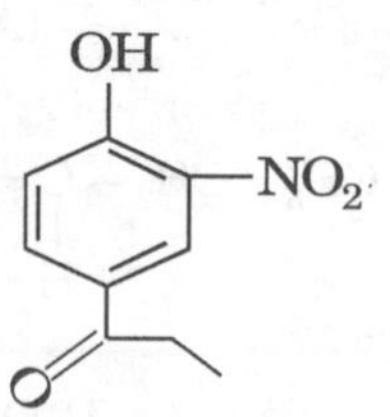

(c) 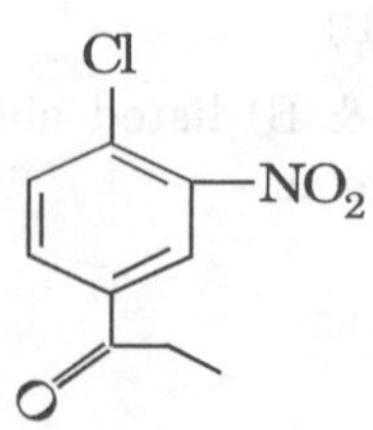 (d) 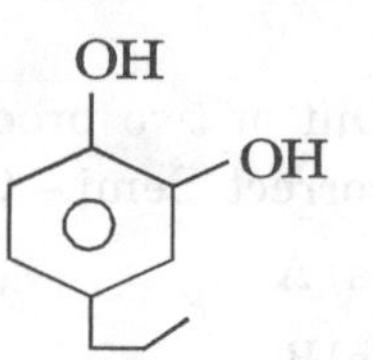

25. Identify the final product in the following sequence of reactions –

$$CH_3-CH_2-\overset{O}{\overset{\|}{C}}-CH_2-CH_2-\overset{O}{\overset{\|}{C}}-H \xrightarrow[\substack{CH_2-OH\\ |\\ CH_2-OH}]{\overset{+}{H}} A \xrightarrow[H_3\overset{+}{O}]{CH_3MgBr} B$$

(a) 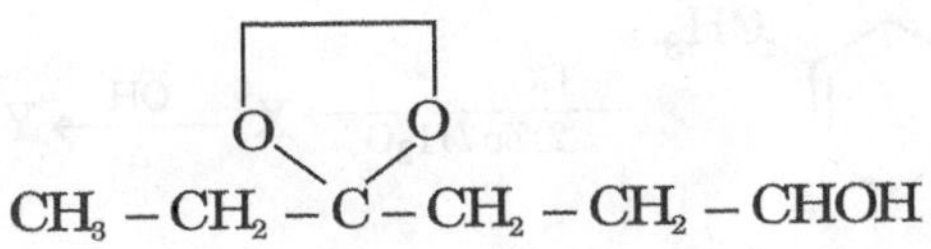

(b) $CH_3-CH_2-\underset{OH}{\overset{H}{\overset{|}{\underset{|}{C}}}}-CH_2CH_2CHO$

(c) $CH_3-CH_2-\underset{CH_3}{\overset{OH}{\overset{|}{\underset{|}{C}}}}-CH_2-CH_2-CHO$

(d) None of these

26. Positive Tollen's test is given by

(a) $CH_3-\overset{O}{\overset{\|}{C}}-H$ (b) 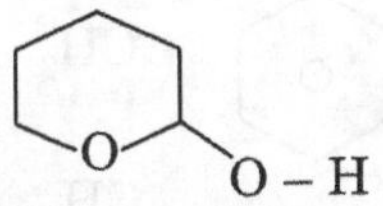

(c) 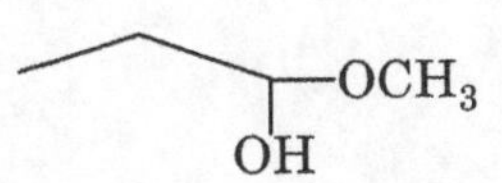 (d) All of these

27. 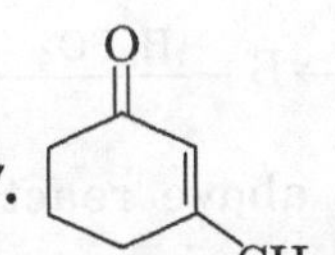 is the final product obtained when one of the following is reacted with base;

(a) $CH_3-\overset{O}{\overset{\|}{C}}-(CH_2)_3-\overset{O}{\overset{\|}{C}}-CH_3$

(b) $H_3C-CH_2-CH_2-\overset{O}{\overset{\|}{C}}-CH_2-\overset{O}{\overset{\|}{C}}-CH_3$

(c) $H_3C-\overset{O}{\overset{\|}{C}}-(CH_2)_3-\overset{O}{\overset{\|}{C}}-CH_2-CH_3$

(d) $CH_3-\overset{O}{\overset{\|}{C}}-CH_2-CH=CH-\overset{O}{\overset{\|}{C}}-\underset{CH_3}{\underset{|}{CH_2}}$

28. 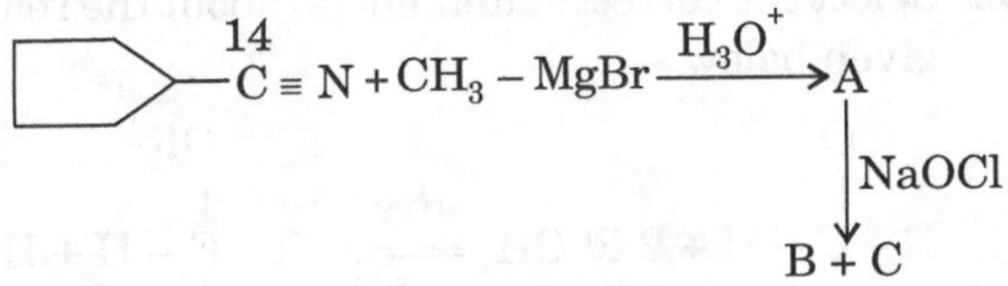

Products (B) & (C), respectively are –

(a) $\overset{14}{C}HCl_3$; 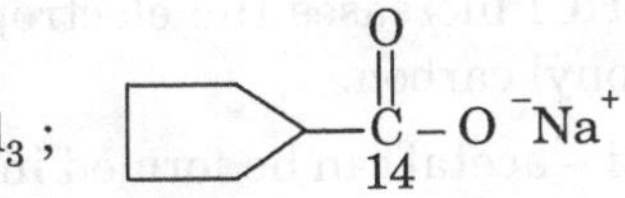

(b) $\overset{14}{C}HCl_3$; 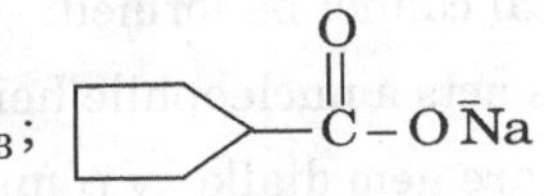

(c) $CHCl_3$; 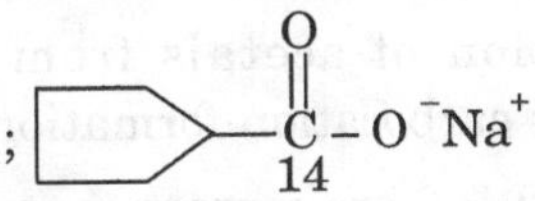

(d) None of these

29. Identify the final product 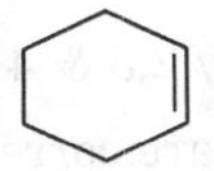 $\xrightarrow[(2)\ H_2O]{(1)\ O_3} A \xrightarrow[\Delta]{Ba(OH)_2} B \xrightarrow[\bar{O}H]{N_2H_4} C$

(a) Cyclopentanone

(b) Cyclopentane

(c) Cyclopentanal

(d) Cyclopentane carboxylic acid

30. Which of the following will give diastereomers?

(a) $CH_3-\overset{O}{\overset{\|}{C}}-H + HCN \xrightarrow{\bar{O}H}$

(b) $CH_3-\overset{O}{\overset{\|}{C}}-CH_3 + HCN \xrightarrow{\bar{O}H}$

(c) 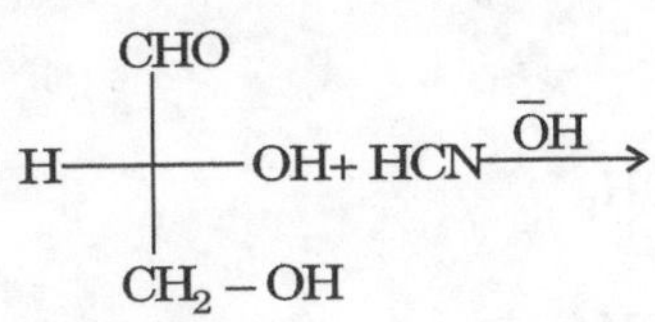

(d) Both a & b

31. Which of the following can give positive test with fehling's solution?

(a) 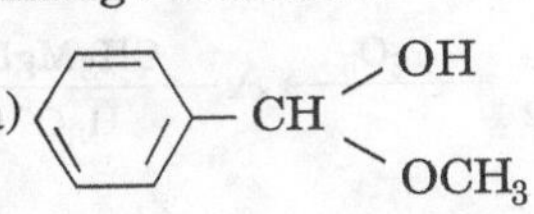

(b) 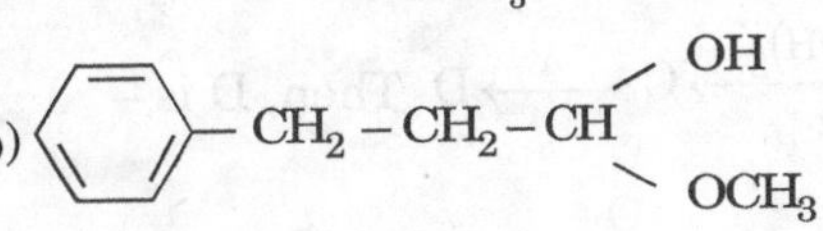

(c) 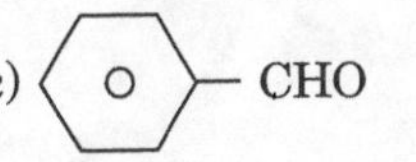

(d) All of these

32. Select the correct statement (s) about the reaction given below –

$$R-\overset{\overset{\displaystyle O}{||}}{C}-H + 2\,R'\,OH \underset{HCl}{\overset{dry}{\rightleftharpoons}} R-\underset{\underset{\displaystyle OR'}{|}}{\overset{\overset{\displaystyle OR'}{|}}{C}}-H + H_2O$$

1. Dry HCl increases the electrophilicity of the carbonyl carbon.
2. Hemi – acetal can be formed in basic medium but acetal cannot be formed
3. Alcohols acts a nucleophile here.
4. Acetals are gem dialkoxy compounds.
5. Formation of acetals from hemi-acetals involves carbocation formation.

(a) only 1, 2 & 3 are correct

(b) only 1, 2 & 4 are correct

(c) only 2,3 & 4 are correct

(d) all are correct.

33. The major product obtained in the following reaction is –

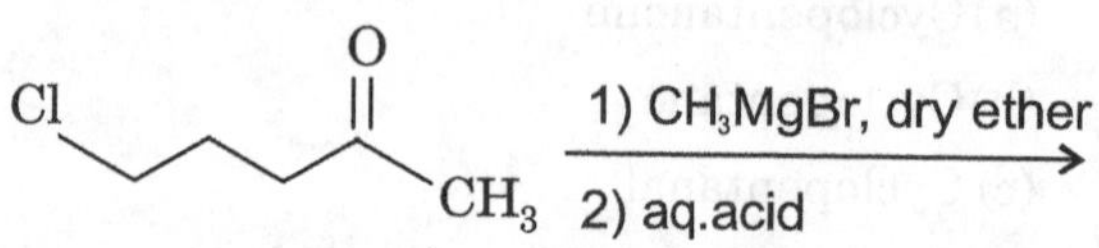

(a) 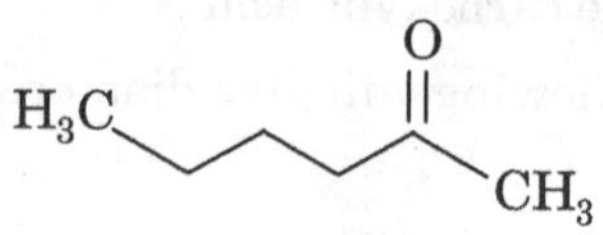

(b) 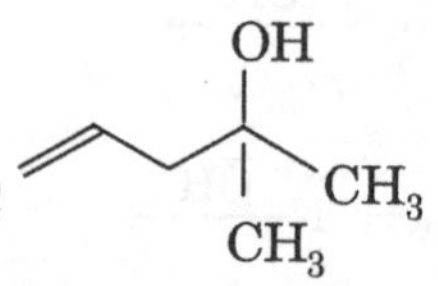

(c) 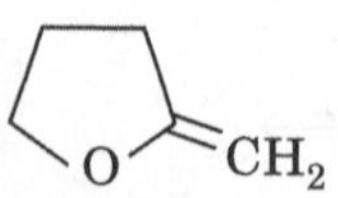

(d) 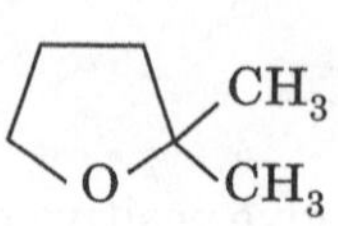

34. 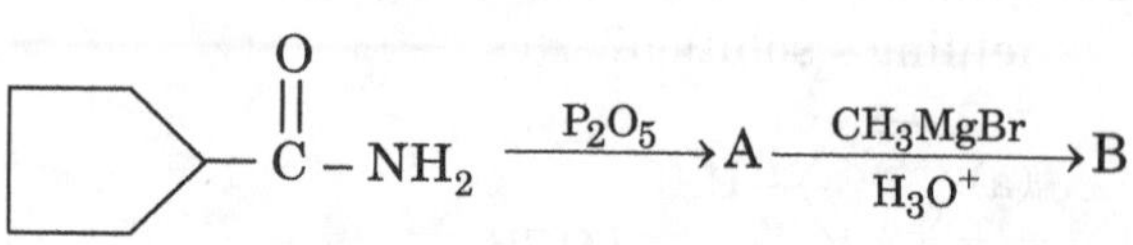

$\xrightarrow[I_2]{Ca(OH)_2}$ C $\xrightarrow{\Delta}$ D Then, D is –

(a) 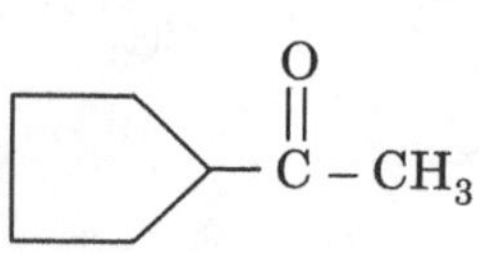

(b) 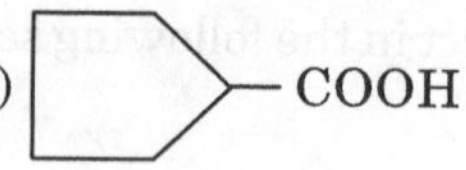

(c) 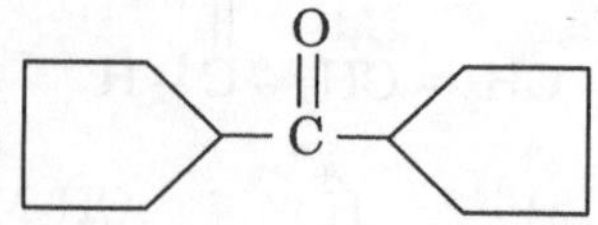

(d) 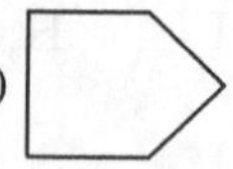

35. 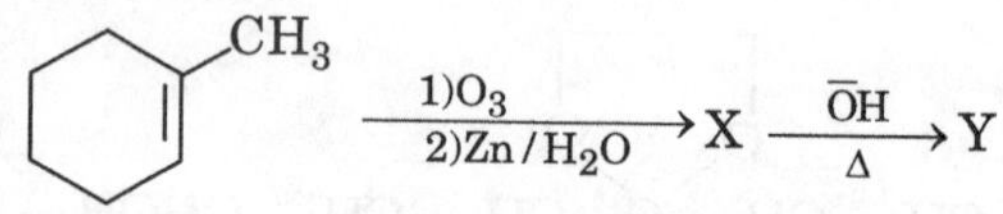

Product 'Y' in the above reaction is –

(a) 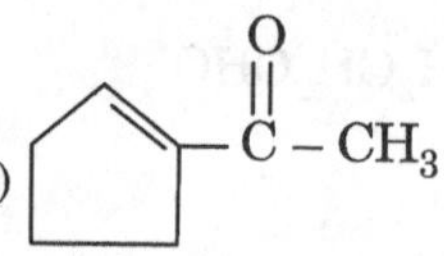

(b) 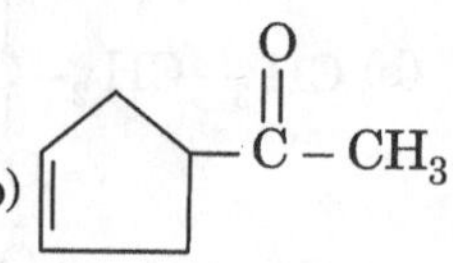

(c) 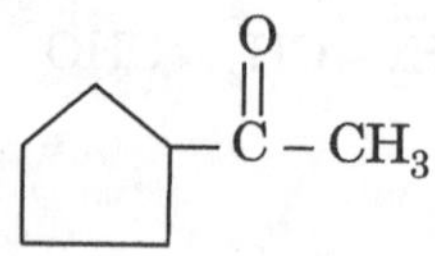

(d) None of these

36. 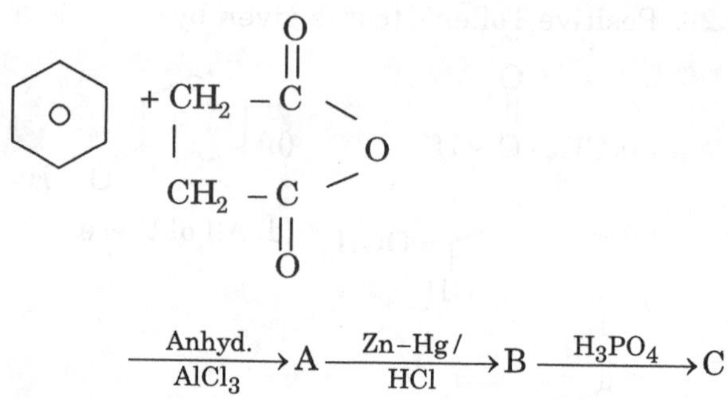

The final product 'C' in the above reaction sequence is –

(a) 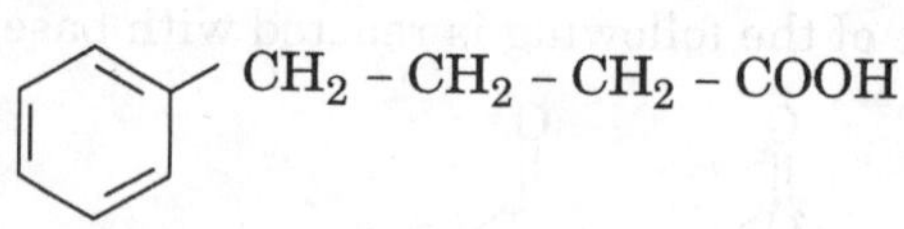

(b) 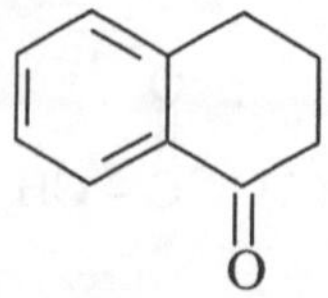

(c) 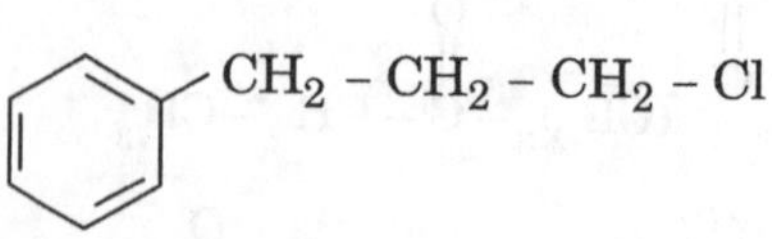

(d) None of these

37. 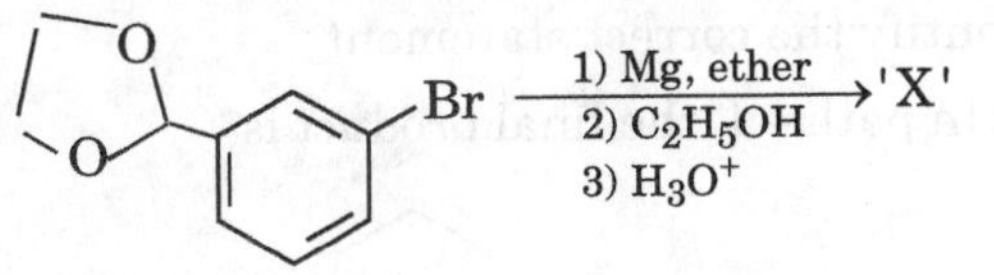

'X' in the above reaction is –

(a) 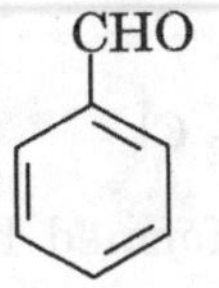

(b) 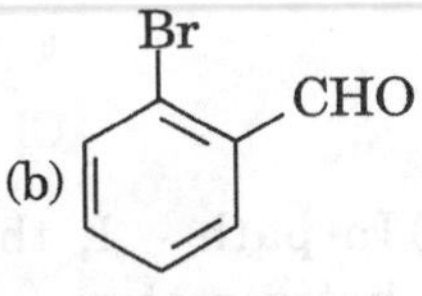

(c) 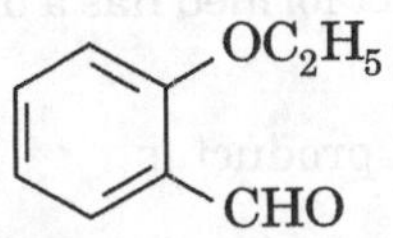

(d) 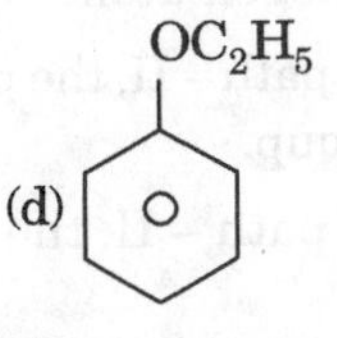

38. Identify 'B' in the following sequence of reactions

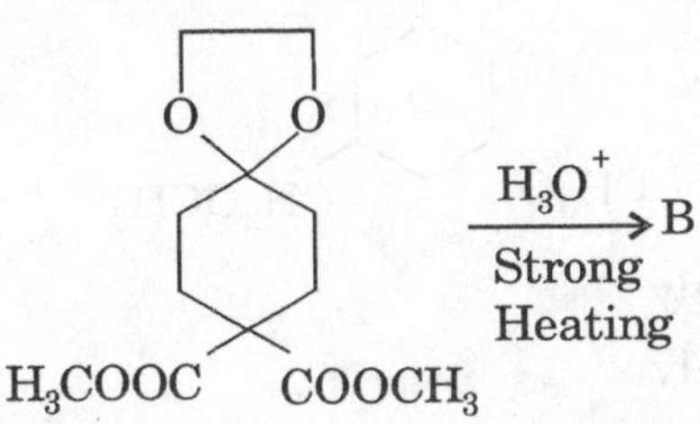

(a) 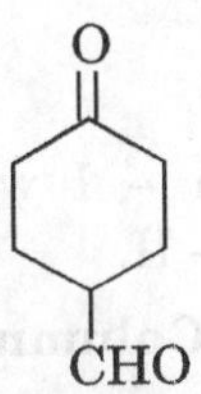

(b) 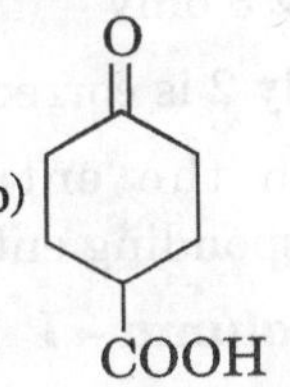

(c) 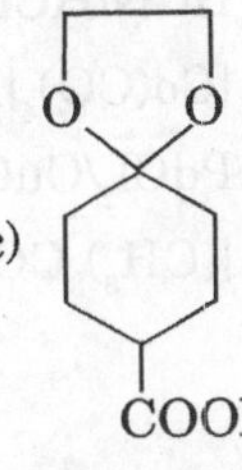

(d) All of these

39. Identify 'A' in the following reaction

$$H-\overset{O}{\overset{\|}{C}}-CH_2-CH_2-\overset{O}{\overset{\|}{C}}-OEt \xrightarrow[\substack{2)\ LiAlH_4,\ H_3O^+ \\ 3)\ H_3O^+}]{1)\ CH_2OH-CH_2OH\ /\ H^+} \text{'A'}$$

(a) $\underset{OH}{\underset{|}{CH_2}}-CH_2-CH_2-CHO$

(b) $\underset{CH_2}{\overset{CHO}{|}}-CH_2-\underset{CH_2}{\overset{CHO}{|}}$

(c) $HOH_2C-CH_2-CH_2-COOH$

(d) $CH_2O-CH_2-CH_2-COOH$

40. 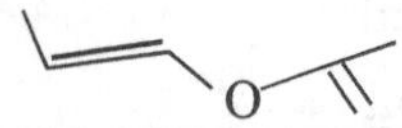 $\xrightarrow{H_3O^+} A + B$

Compounds A & B can be distinguished by

(a) 2, 4 – DNP (b) Fehling's solution

(c) $NaHSO_3$ (d) All of these

41. Consider the following reaction

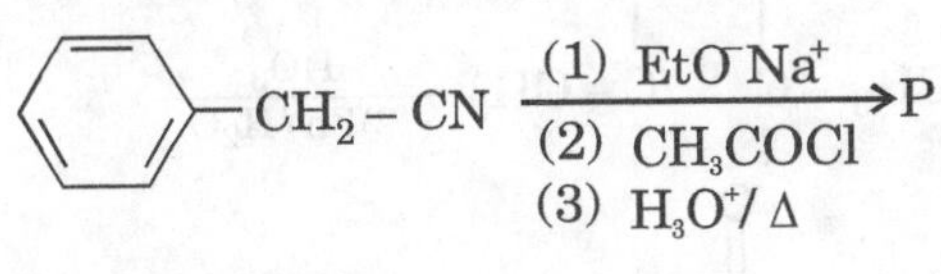

The product P is –

(a) 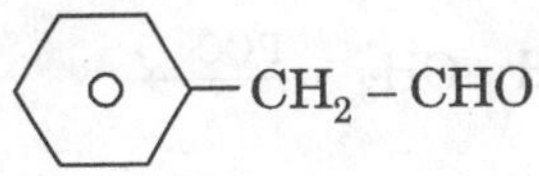

(b) 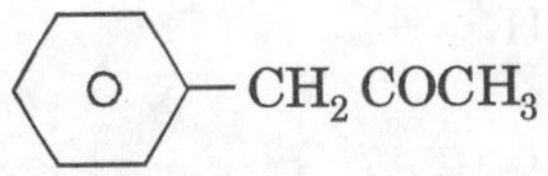

(c) 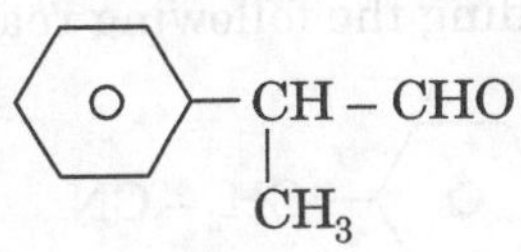

(d) 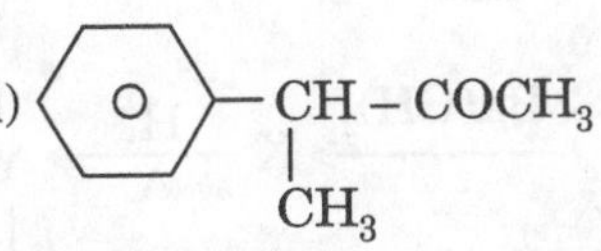

42. 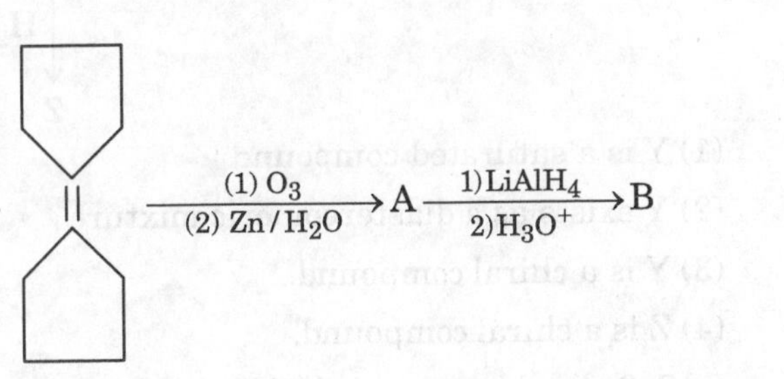

Which of the following statement is incorrect wrt above sequence?

(a) Compound 'A' is same which is obtained by heating calcium adipate.

(b) B give blue colour with (a) $P_4 + I_2$ (b) $AgNO_2$ (c) HNO_2 (d) $Na^+\overline{O}H$

(c) Formation of C involves rearrangement of carbocation

(d) D on halogenation gives only one Monochlorinated product.

43. 1 – Methyl cyclohexa –1,3-diene on ozonolysis in the presence of Zn/H_2O yields –
(a) 6 – oxoheptanal
(b) 4 – oxopentanal & glyoxal
(c) 2 – oxopentanal & glyoxal
(d) 3 – hydroxy pentanal & glycolic acid.

44. Which of the following reactions can be used to prepare ketones?

(a) $CH_3-\underset{CH_3}{\overset{|}{C}}=\underset{CH_3}{\overset{|}{C}}-CH_3 \xrightarrow[2)Zn/H_2O]{1)O_3}$

(b) $2CH_3-\overset{O}{\overset{||}{C}}-Cl+(CH_3)_2Cd \rightarrow$

(c) $CH_3CH_2-\underset{OH}{\underset{|}{CH}}-CH_3 \xrightarrow{PCC}$

(d) All of these

45. What is true regarding the following reaction?

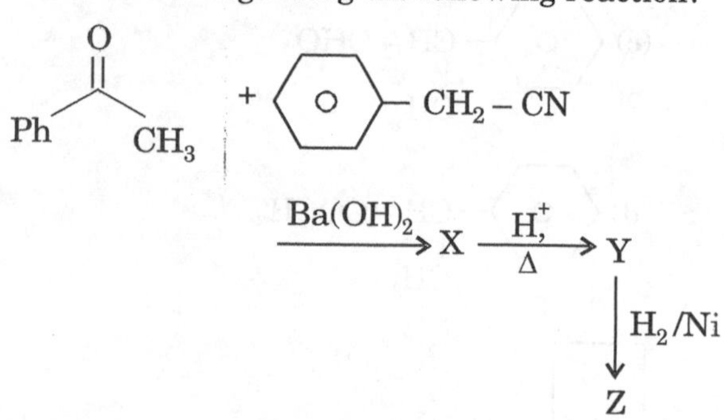

(1) Y is a saturated compound
(2) Y exists as a diastereomeric mixture
(3) Y is a chiral compound.
(4) Z is a chiral compound.
(a) 2, 3, 4 only (b) 1 & 4 only
(c) 2 & 4 only (d) All are correct

46. Consider the following reaction –

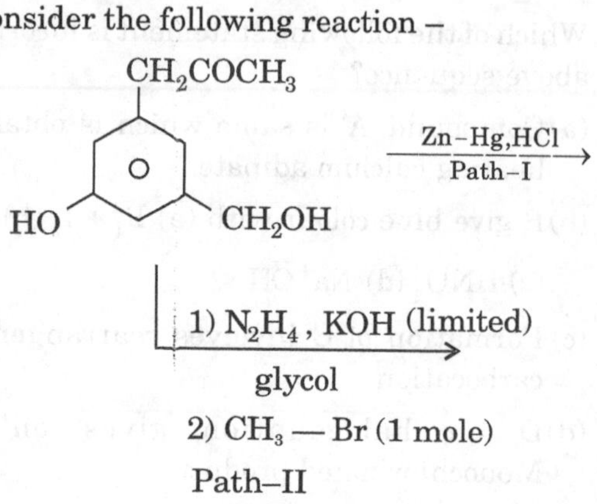

Identify the correct statement
(1) In path – I, the final product is

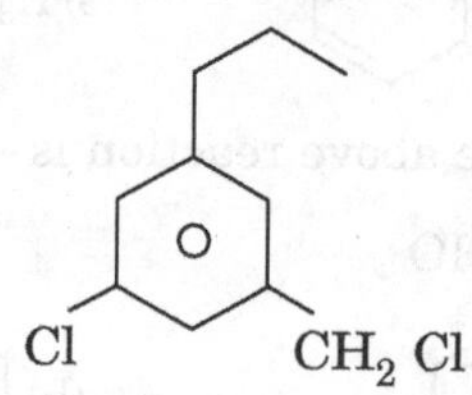

(2) In path – I, the product formed has one halogen atom.
(3) In path – II, the product formed has a one – OH group.
(4) In path – II, the final product is

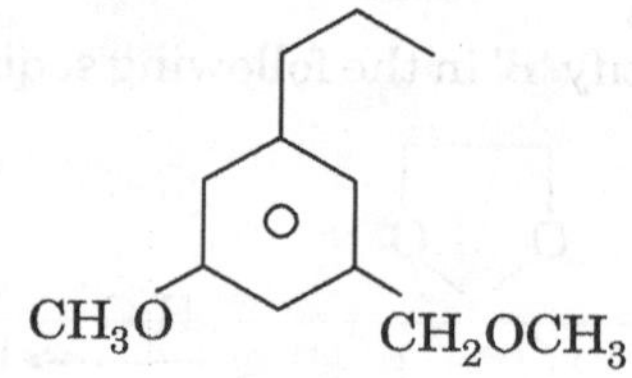

(a) 1 & 3 only
(b) 1 & 4 only
(c) 2 & 3 only
(d) only 2 is correct

47. Match the entry in column – I with its corresponding entry in column – II.

Column – I	Column – II
(A) Oppenauer oxidation	(i) $HCN/HCl, AlCl_3$
(B) Wacker's process	(ii) $[Co(CO)_4]_2$
(C) Hydroformylation	(iii) $PdCl_2/CuCl$
(D) Gattermann aldehyde synthesis	(iv) $[(CH_3)_3CO]_3Al$

(a) A – iv, B – iii, C – ii, D – i
(b) A – i, B – ii, C – iii, D – iv
(c) A – iv, B – i, C – iii, D – ii
(d) A – iii, B – iv, C – i, D – ii

48. In which one of the following all the compounds will give positive tollens test?

(a) 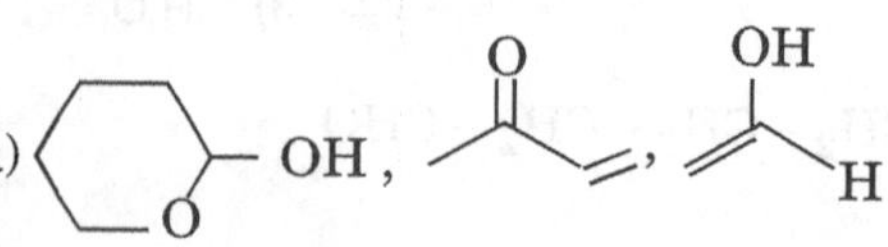

(b) 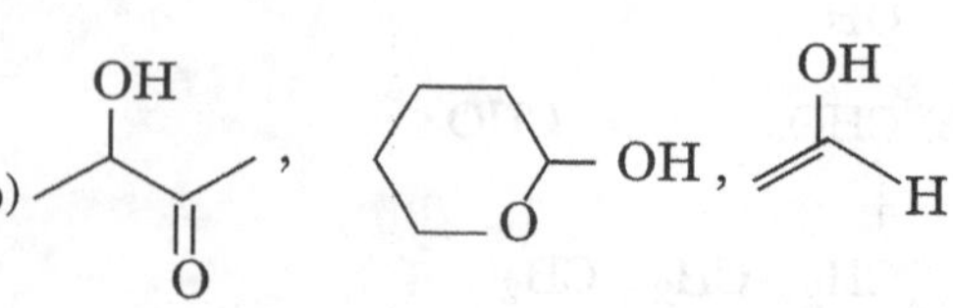

(c) 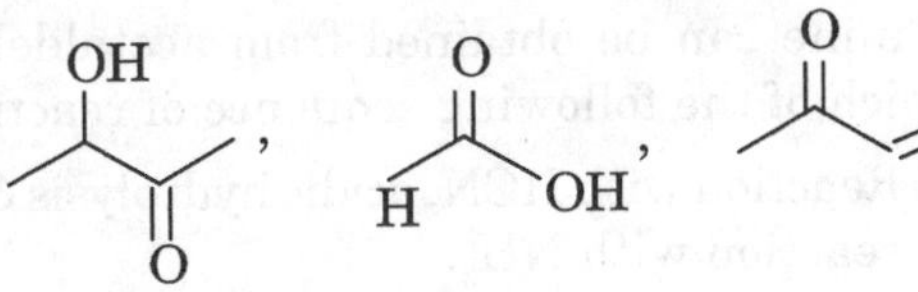

(d) 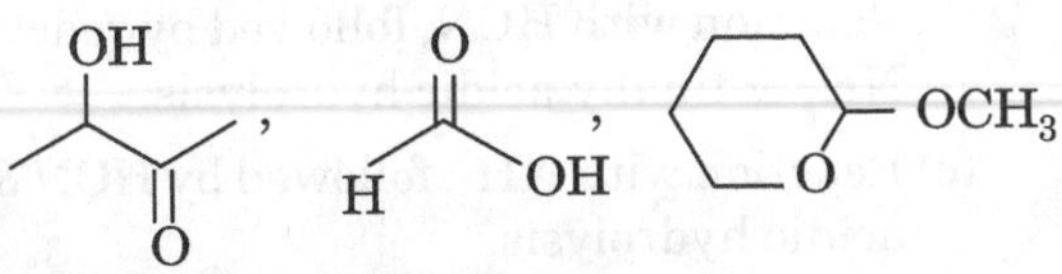

49. A carbonyl compound X gets oxidised to Y which gives positive tollens test. X, when treated with 2, 3, 5 – trihydroxy benzaldehyde in acidic medium forms Z. Z is then treated with Zn – Hg/HCl. The final product is –

(a) 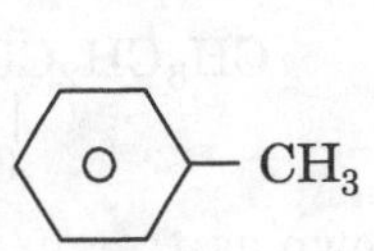 (b) 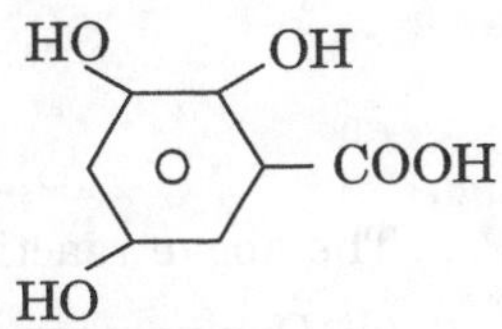

(c) CH_4 (d) HCOOH

50. Consider the following reaction –

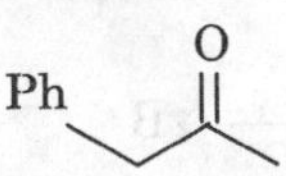 $+ Cl_2 \xrightarrow{Ca(OH)_2} Q + P$ (trihalogenated compound)

$Q \xrightarrow{\Delta} R \xrightarrow{HCN} S$

Select the incorrect statement regarding the above sequence of reactions.

(a) Product P has acidic H atom.

(b) R can react with Brady's reagent.

(c) R is a symmetrical ketone

(d) S is a racemic mixture.

51. A ketone (X) when reacted with C_2H_5 Mg Br (followed by hydrolysis), gave a product which on dehydration gives an alkene. The alkene on ozonolysis gave diethyl ketone & an acetaldehyde. The ketone (x) is –

(a) dimethyl ketone (b) diethyl ketone

(c) ethyl propyl ketone (d) ethyl methyl ketone.

52. Which of the following can undergo intramolecular Cannizaro's reaction?

(a) $Ph - \overset{O}{\overset{||}{C}} - CHO$ (b) $Ph - \overset{O}{\overset{||}{C}} - \underset{Br}{\underset{|}{CH}} - Br$

(c) 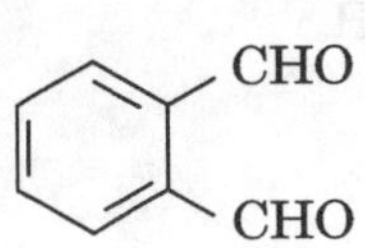 (d) All of these

53. Consider the following reaction & identify the final product 'B' in the reaction.

$$\begin{matrix} CHO \\ | \\ CHO \end{matrix} \xrightarrow[NaOH]{50\%\ Conc.} A \xrightarrow[\Delta]{H^+} B$$

(a) $CH_2 = CH - CO_2H$ (b) 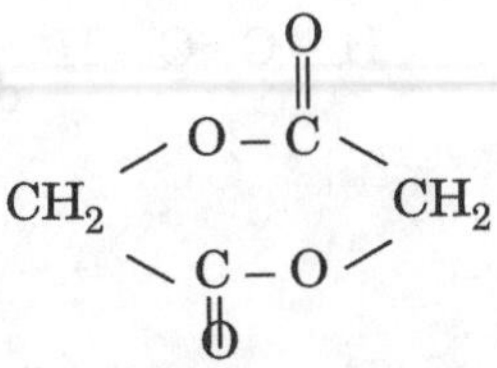

(c) 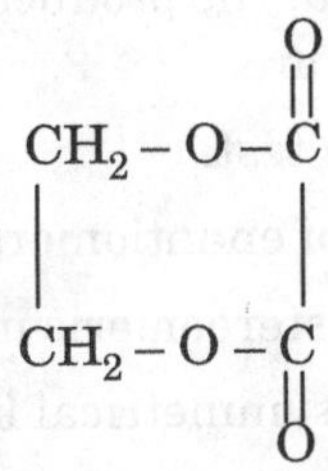 (d) $H_2C = C = O$

54. Identify 'Z' in the following reaction –

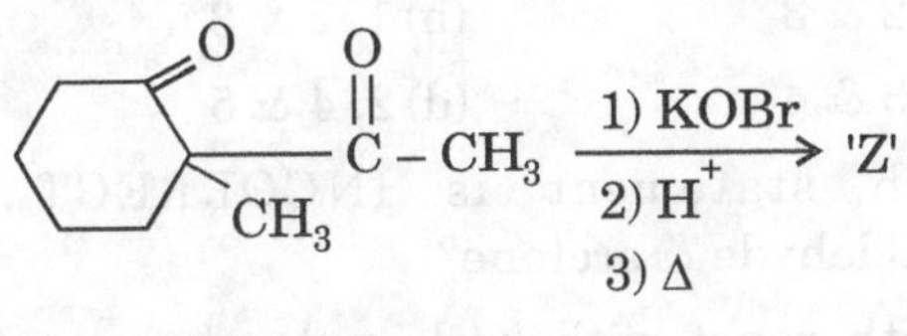

(a) 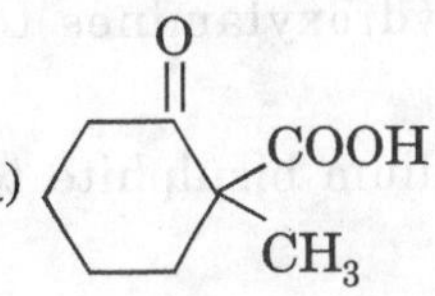 (b) 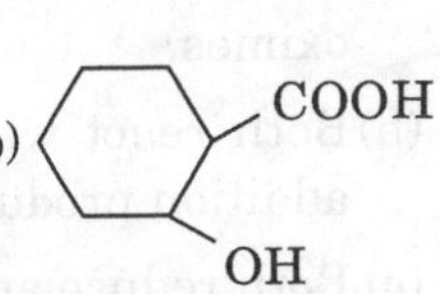

(c) 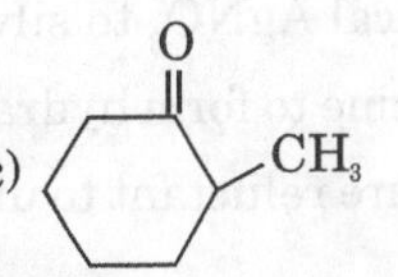 (d) 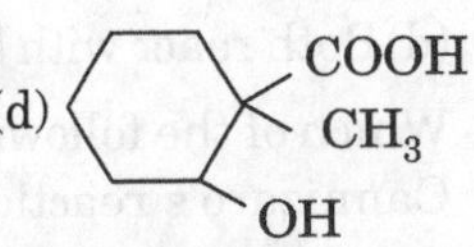

55. Ethanal forms 'X' total number of acetals (including stereoisomers) with glycerol. The value of X is

(a) 2 (b) 4

(c) 6 (d) 8

56. Select the correct option

$$CH_3 - \overset{O}{\overset{||}{C}} - H \xrightarrow[2) H_3O^+]{1) NaBD_4}$$

(a) $CH_3 - \overset{OD}{\overset{|}{\underset{D}{\underset{|}{C}}}} - H$ (b) $CH_3 - \overset{OH}{\overset{|}{\underset{D}{\underset{|}{C}}}} - H$

(c) $CH_3 - \overset{OD}{\overset{|}{\underset{H}{\underset{|}{C}}}} - H$ (d) $CH_3 - CH_2OH$

57. Consider the following reaction

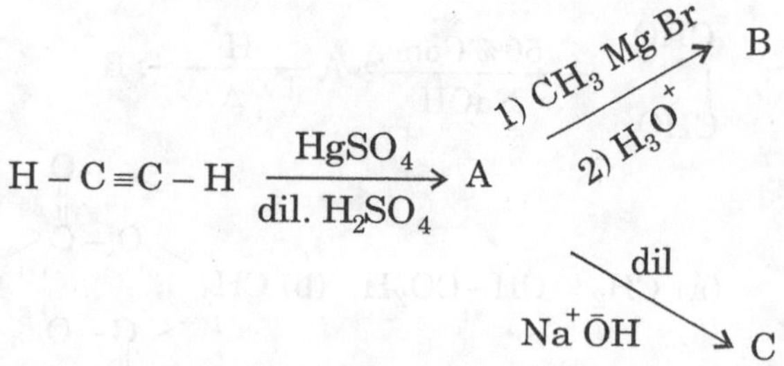

The correct statements about the products in the above sequence of reaction are

(1) B can give +ve iodoform test.

(2) C can exist in the form of enantiomers.

(3) C on heating gives a diastereomeric mixture.

(4) B on oxidation gives unsymmetrical ketone.

(5) B gives red colour in Victor – meyer's test.

(a) 1, 2 & 3 (b) 1, 2 & 3

(c) 2, 3 & 4 (d) 2, 4 & 5

58. Which statement is INCORRECT wrt Acetaldehyde & acetone?

(a) Both react with hydroxylamines to form oximes.

(b) Both react with sodium bisulphite to form addition products.

(c) Both reduce ammoniacal $AgNO_3$ to silver.

(d) Both react with hydrazine to form hydrazones.

59. Which of the following is/are reluctant to undergo Cannizaro's reaction?

(a) $Cl_3C-\overset{O}{\overset{||}{C}}-H$

(b) 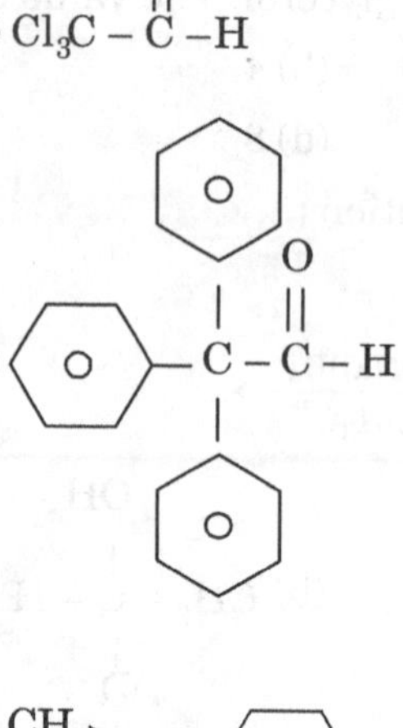

(c) 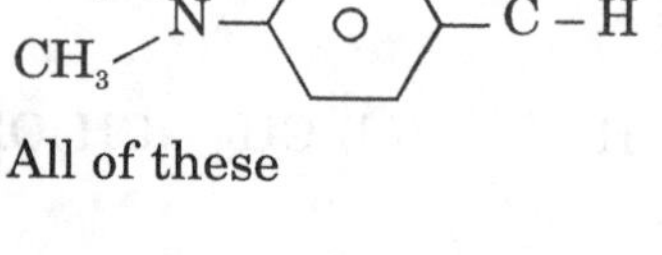

(d) All of these

60. Alanine can be obtained from acetaldehyde by which of the following sequence of reactions?

(a) Reaction with HCN, acidic hydrolysis & finally reaction with NH_3.

(b) Reaction with HCN, followed by reaction with NH_3 & finally acidic hydrolysis.

(c) Reaction with NH_3, followed by HCN & finally acidic hydrolysis.

(d) Reaction with $NaHSO_3$, followed by NH_3 & finally acidic hydrolysis.

Carboxylic Acids & its Derivatives

61. $CH_3-CH_2-CH=CH_2+CO+H_2O \xrightarrow{H^+} CH_3CH_2\underset{COOH}{\underset{|}{C}H}-CH_3$

The above reaction is known as

(a) Oxo process (b) Wacker's process

(c) Kolbe's reaction (d) Koch reaction

62. Consider the reaction

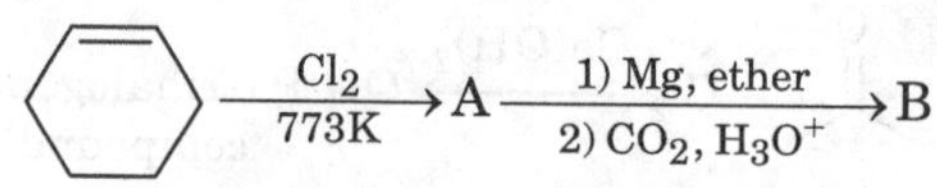

In the above reaction, product B is-

(a) 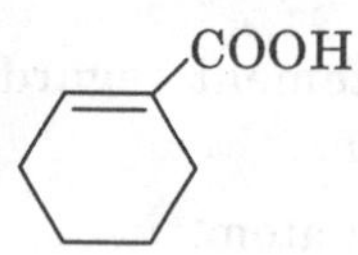 (b) 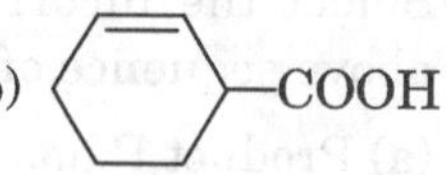

(c) 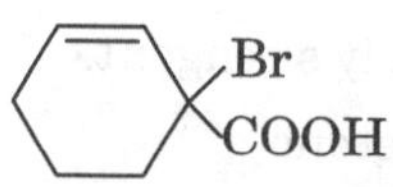 (d) 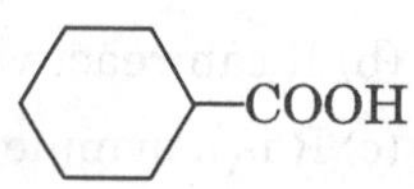

63. Consider the following sequence of reactions-

$R-CH_2-CH_2COOH$

$\xrightarrow[\text{Red P}]{Br_2} A \xrightarrow{KCN} B \xrightarrow[2)\ H_3O^+]{1)\ Li\ AlH_4} C$

The product 'C' is-

(a) $R-CH_2\underset{CONH_2}{\underset{|}{C}H}-CONH_2$

(b) $R-CH_2-\overset{CONH_2}{\overset{|}{C}H}-COOH$

(c) $R-CH_2-\underset{CH_2NH_2}{\underset{|}{C}H}-CH_2OH$

(d) $R-\underset{COOH}{\underset{|}{C}H}-CH-CH_2NH_2$

64. What are X & Y in the following reaction?

$$R-\overset{O}{\overset{\|}{C}}-O-\underset{CH_3}{\underset{|}{\overset{CH_3}{\overset{|}{C}}}}-CH_3 \xrightarrow{H^+/H_2O^{18}} X+Y$$

X & Y, respectively, are-

(a) $CH_3-\underset{CH_3}{\underset{|}{\overset{CH_3}{\overset{|}{C}}}}-O^{18}H,\quad R-COOH$

(b) $RCH_2O^{18}H, CH_3-CH_2-CH_2COOH$

(c) $CH_3-\underset{CH_3}{\underset{|}{\overset{CH_3}{\overset{|}{C}}}}-OH,\quad R-\overset{O}{\overset{\|}{C}}-O^{18}-H$

(d) $CH_3-\underset{CH_3}{\underset{|}{\overset{H}{\overset{|}{C}}}}-\overset{O}{\overset{\|}{C}}-OH\quad R-\overset{O}{\overset{\|}{C}}-\overset{18}{O}-H$

65. Which of the following will not give HVZ reaction?

(a) CH_3-CH_2-COOH

(b) $CH_3-\underset{CH_3}{\underset{|}{CH}}-COOH$

(c) $CH_3-\underset{CH_3}{\underset{|}{\overset{CH_3}{\overset{|}{C}}}}-COOH$

(d) All of these

66. In the following reaction, what is X?

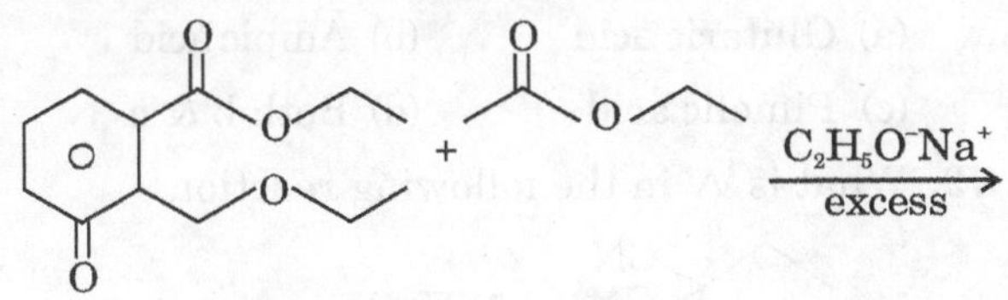

(a)

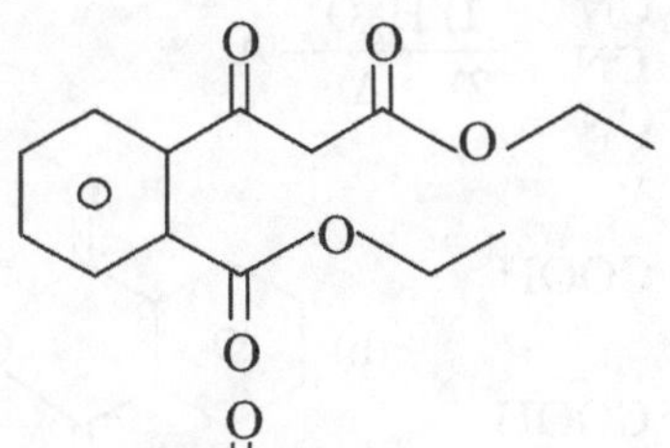

(b)

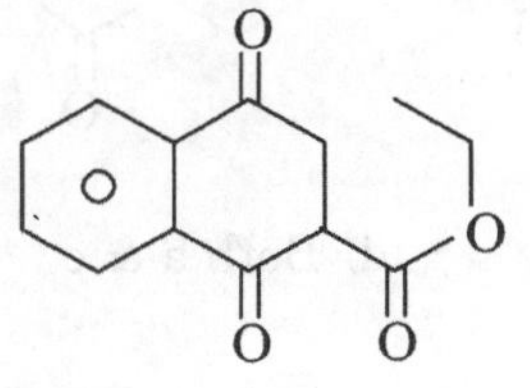

(c)

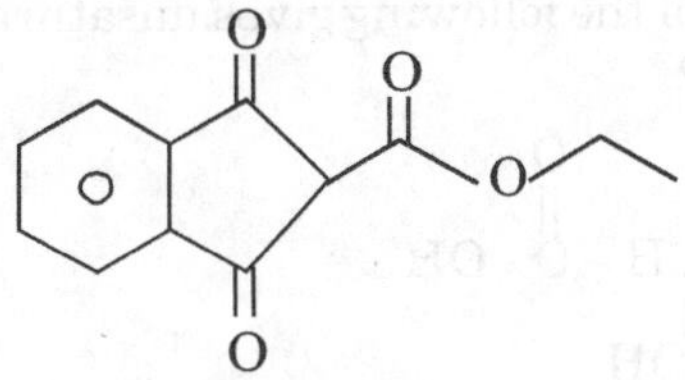

(d)

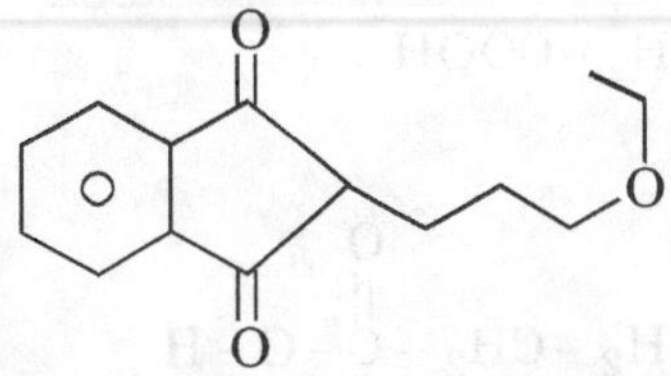

67. Identify the final product in the following reaction sequence.

$$H-\overset{O}{\overset{\|}{C}}-CH_2-CH_2-\overset{O}{\overset{\|}{C}}-O-H \xrightarrow[\text{2) } H_3O^+]{\text{1) } NaBH_4} A \xrightarrow[\text{(Catalytic amt.)}]{H^+} B$$

(a)

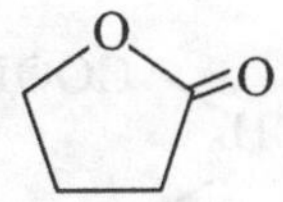

(b) $CH_2=CH-CH_2\,COOH$

(c) $CH_2=CH-CH_2\,CONH_2$

(d) $CH_3-CH=CH-COOH$

68. What is 'X' in the given reaction?

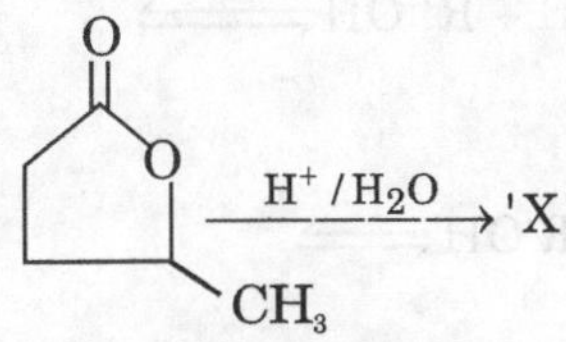

(a) $HOOC-CH_2-CH_2-\underset{OH}{\underset{|}{CH}}-CH_3$

(b) $CH_3-CH_2-CH_2-CH_2-COOH$

(c) $HO-CH_2-CH_2-CH_2-COOH$

(d) $CH_3-CH_2-\underset{OH}{\underset{|}{CH}}-CH_2-COOH$

69. The number of moles of CO_2 evolved in the following reaction is/are

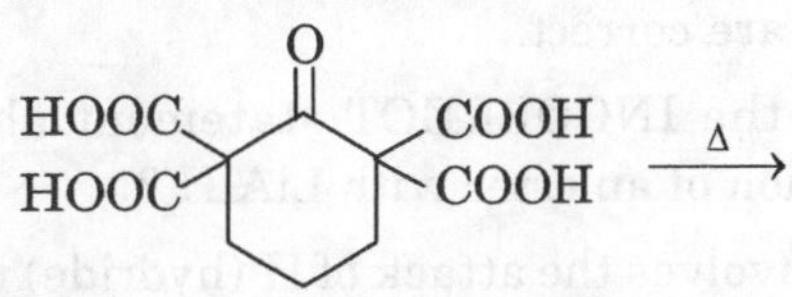

(a) 2 (b) 4

(c) 3 (d) 1

70. Which one of the following gives unsaturated acid an heating?

(a) $CH_3-\underset{OH}{\underset{|}{CH}}-\overset{O}{\overset{||}{C}}-OH$

(b) $\underset{OH}{\underset{|}{CH_2}}-CH_2-COOH$

(c) $\underset{OH}{\underset{|}{CH_2}}-CH_2-CH_2-\overset{O}{\overset{||}{C}}-O-H$

(d) All of these

71. Which one of the following will NOT yield a cyclic compound on heating?

(a) $\begin{matrix} CH_2-COOH \\ | \\ CH_2-COOH \end{matrix}$ (b) $CH_2\begin{matrix} \diagup CH_2-COOH \\ \diagdown CH_2-COOH \end{matrix}$

(c) 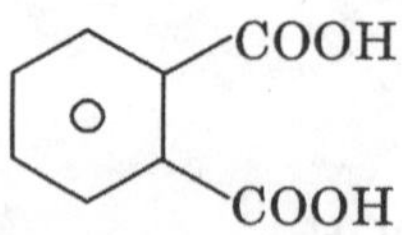

(d) $CH_2\begin{matrix} \diagup COOH \\ \diagdown COOH \end{matrix}$

72. Which of the following reactions will result in the formation of an ester?

(a) $R-\overset{O}{\overset{||}{C}}-O-H+R'OH \overset{H^+}{\rightleftharpoons}$

(b) $R-\overset{O}{\overset{||}{C}}-Cl+R'OH \rightleftharpoons$

(c) $R-\overset{O}{\overset{||}{C}}-O-H+CH_2N_2 \longrightarrow$

(d) All of these

73. Which of the following statement is/are correct about hydrolysis of an ester?

(a) Basic hydrolysis of ester is called saponification.

(b) Basic hydrolysis of an ester is irreversible owing to the formation of stable carboxylate ion.

(c) The product of basic hydrolysis of an ester and basic hydrolysis of an amide is carboxylate ion.

(d) All are correct.

74. Select the INCORRECT statement about the reduction of an ester with $LiAlH_4$?

(a) It involves the attack of H^-(hydride) ion.

(b) An aldehyde is formed during the reduction process.

(c) Reduction of an ester with $LiAlH_4$ results in the formation of Carboxylic acid & an alcohol.

(d) Both (a) & (b) are incorrect.

(Check out its complete mechanism in EXPLANATIONS')

75. Which of the following will result in the formation of formic acid & a primary amine?

(a) $R-C\equiv N \xrightarrow{H^+/H_2O}$

(b) $R-N^+\equiv \ddot{C}^{\ominus} \xrightarrow[H_2O]{\bar{O}H/}$

(c) $R-\overset{\oplus}{N}\equiv \ddot{C}^{\ominus} \xrightarrow{H^+/H_2O}$

(d) All of these

(Check out complete explanations & mechanisms)

76. Consider the following reaction-

$$R-\overset{O}{\overset{||}{C}}-\ddot{\underset{..}{O}}-H+SOCl_2 \longrightarrow RCOCl+SO_2+Cl^-$$

Now, select the correct statement(s)

(a) Either oxygen atom of acid can attack sulfur.

(b) Chlorosulfite is formed during the reaction.

(c) $SOCl_2$ is called sulfuryl chloride

(d) Both (a) & (b) are correct.

77. The final product of the following reaction is –

$$R-\overset{O}{\overset{||}{C}}-O-H \xrightarrow{2R'-Li} A \xrightarrow{H_3O^+} B \xrightarrow{\Delta} C$$

(a) Aldehyde (b) Ketone

(c) acid chloride (d) anhydride

78. Which of the following dicarboxylic acids on heating undergo decarboxylation & dehydration, both?

(a) Glutaric acid (b) Adipic acid

(c) Pimelic acid (d) Both b & c

79. What is 'A' in the following reaction

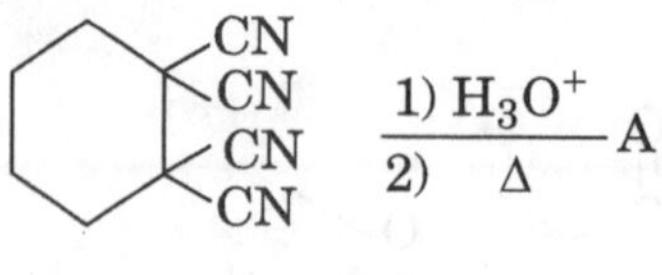

(a) 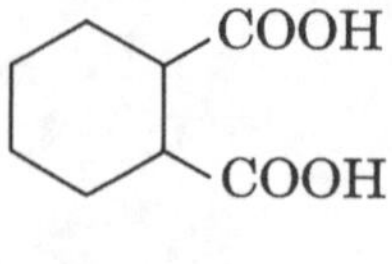

(b) 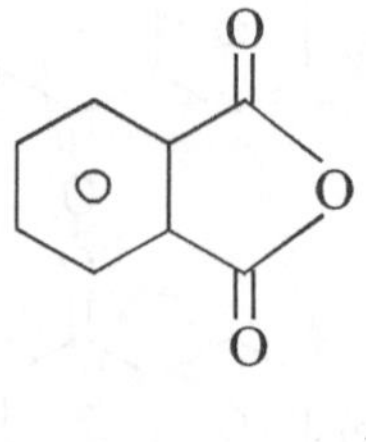

(c) 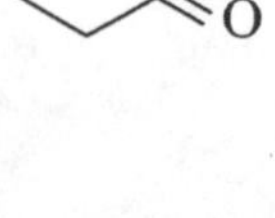

(d) Both a & c

80. Identify the correct statement(s)

(a) Ka_1, of Maleic acid is greater than that of fumaric acid but Ka_2 of fumaric acid is greater than that of maleic acid.

(b) Fumaric acid does not form an anhydride.

(c) Phthalic acid is stronger acid than isophthalic or terephthalic acid.

(d) All statements are correct.

81. Which one of the following is NOT soluble in $NaHCO_3$ solution?

(a) 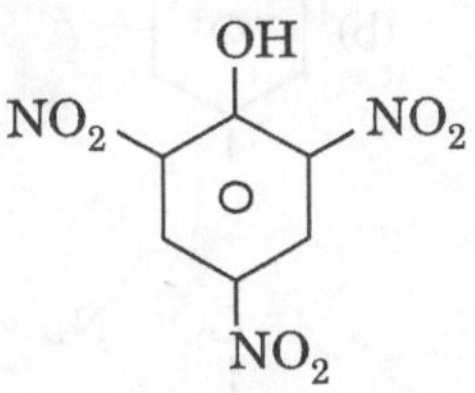

(b) 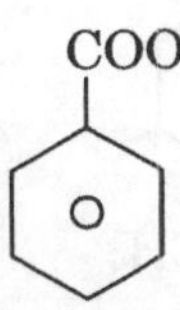

(c 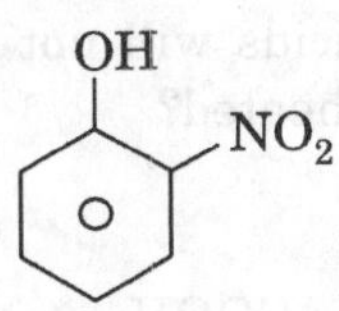

(d) 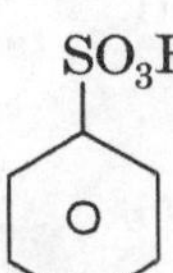

82. Which of the following isomeric tetracarboxylic acids will form 2 isomeric monoanhydrides?

(a) 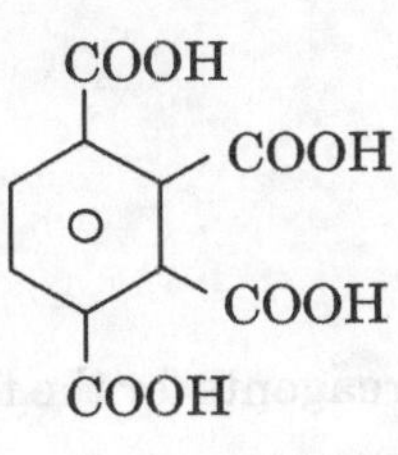

(b) 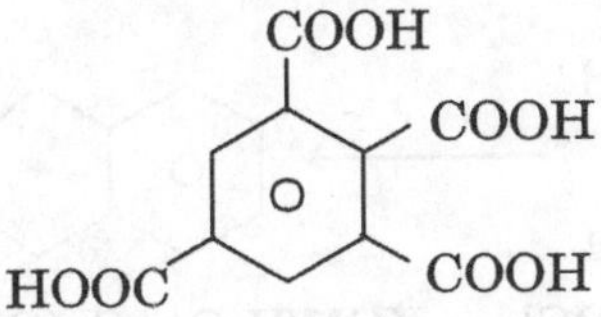

(c) 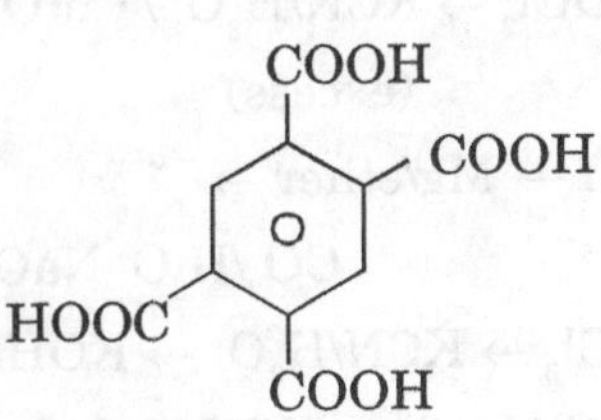

(d) Both b & c

83. Which of the following can form 'Di-ANYDRIDE'?

(a) 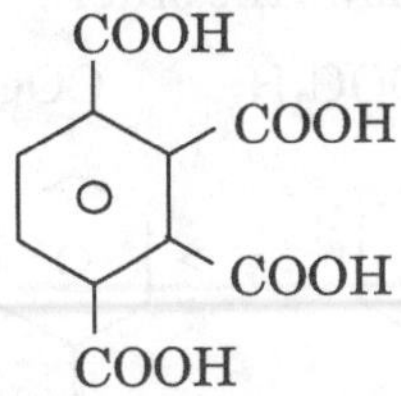

(b) 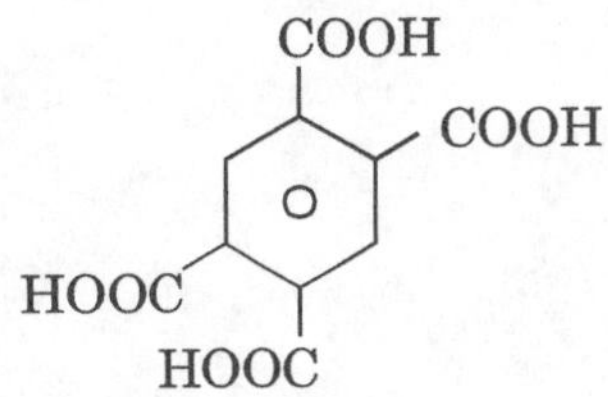

(c) 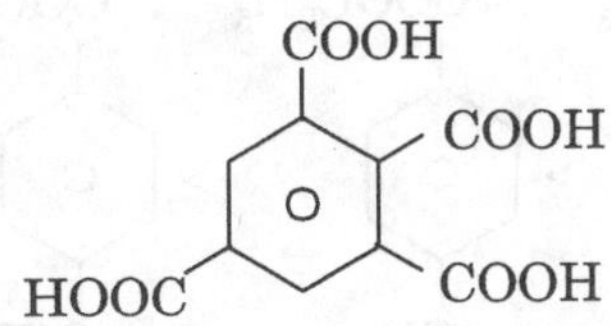

(d) Both a & b

84. Identify 'C' in the following reaction sequence

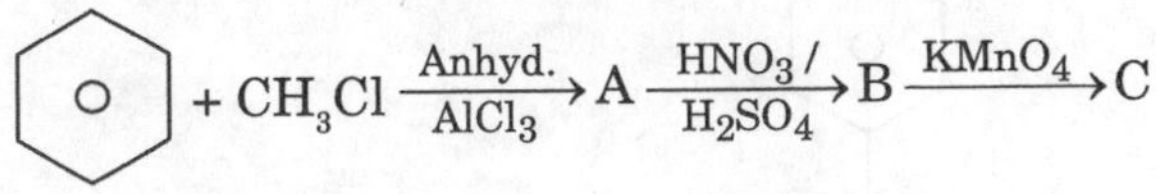

(a) 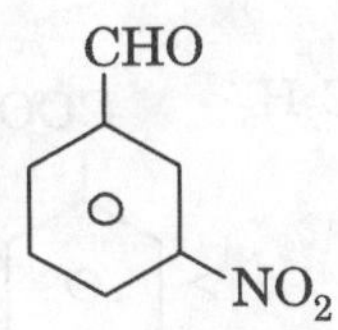

(b) 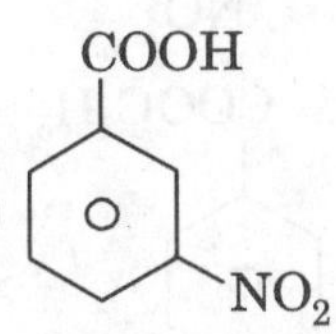

(c) 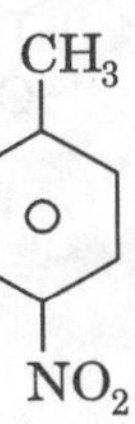

(d) 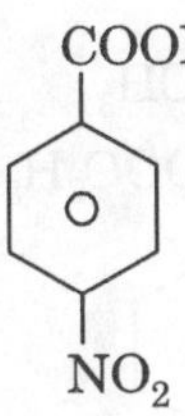

85. Select the correct statement(s).

(a) Oximes are less acidic than hydroxyl amines.

(b) 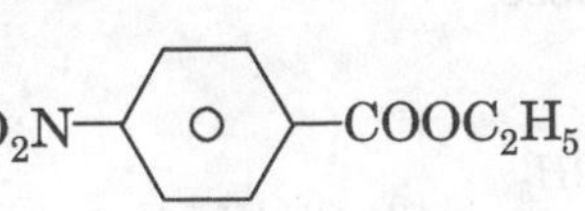 is more reactive than 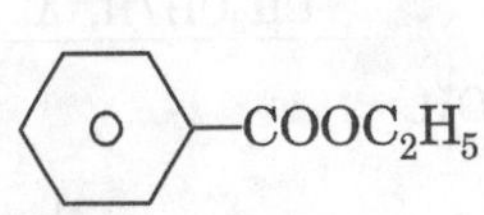 towards basic hydrolysis

(c) Benzoyl chloride is less reactive than acetyl chloride for Nucleophilic acyl substitution.

(d) All are correct.

86. The reactivity of following esters towards base catalysed hydrolysis follows the order-

(a) 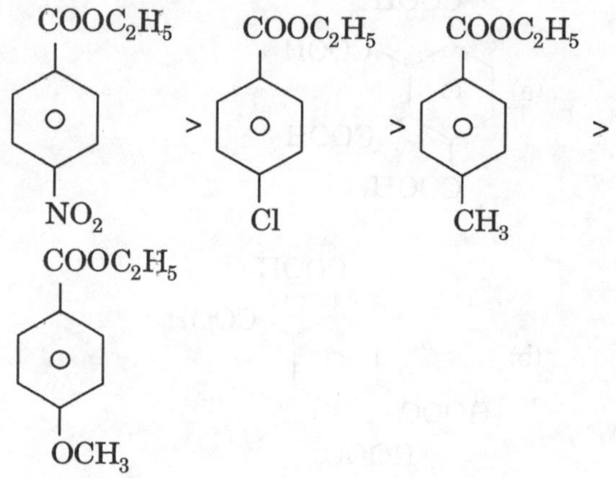

(b) 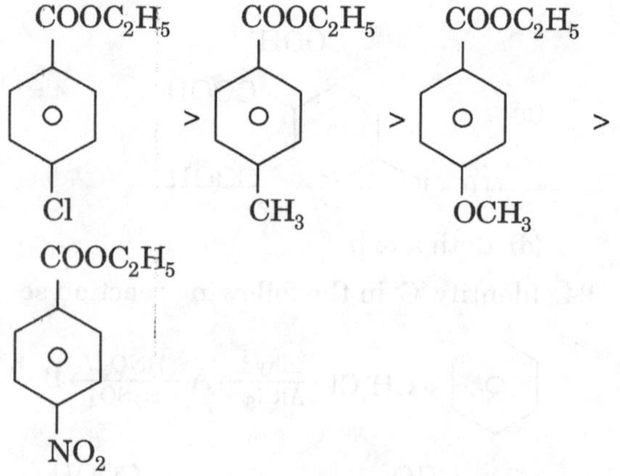

(c) 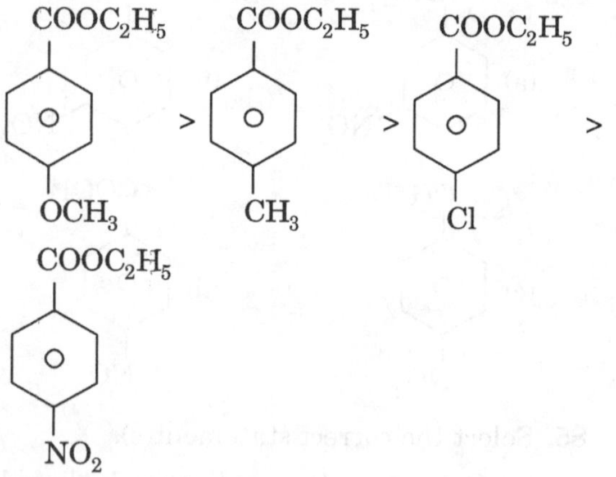

(d) None of these

87. 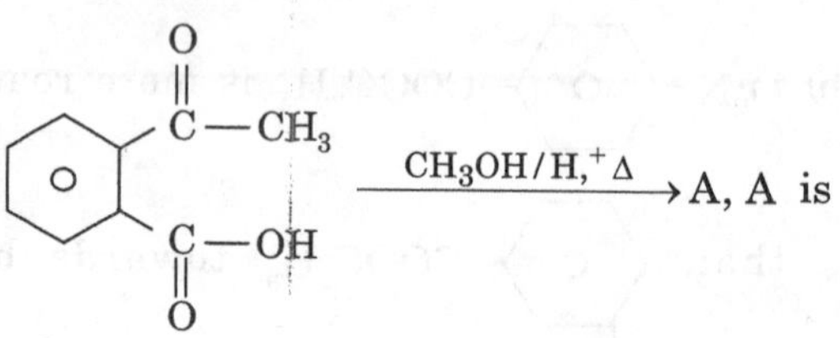

(a) 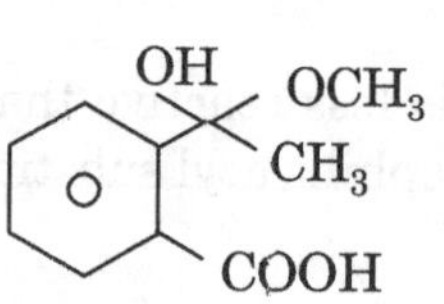 (b) 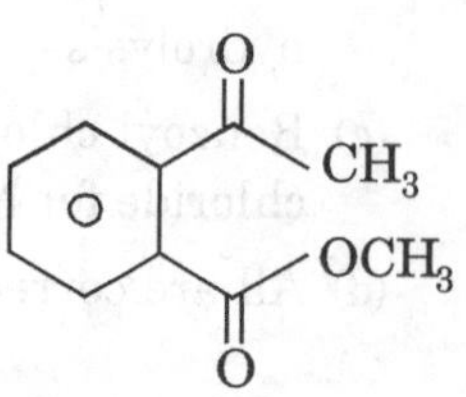

(c) 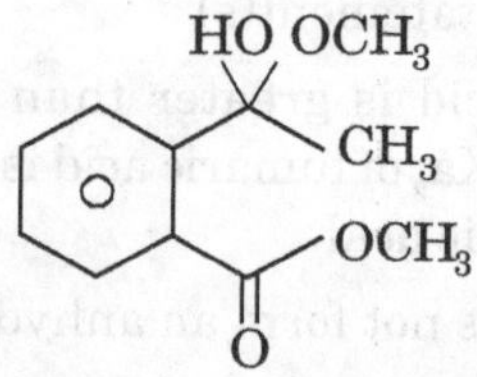 (d) 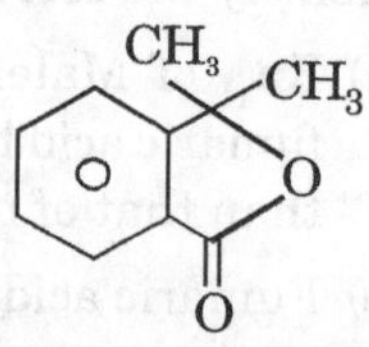

88. Which of the following undergoes soda lime decarboxylation at the fastest rate?

(a) 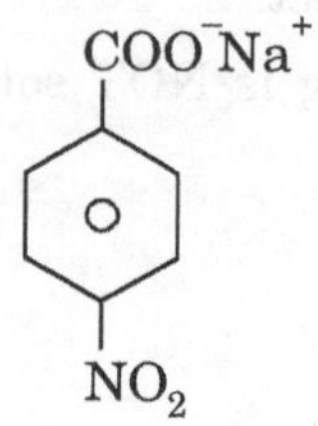 (b) 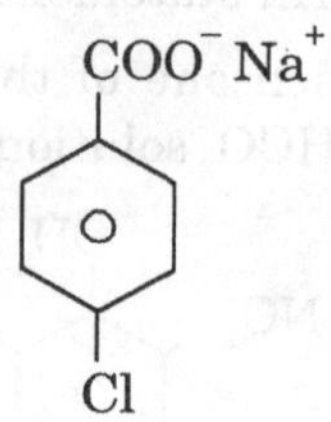

(c) 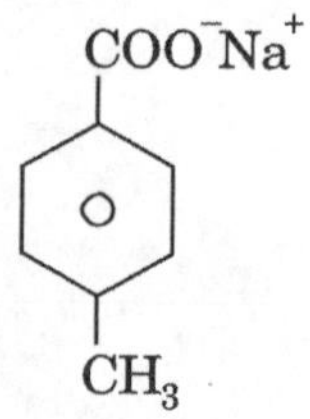 (d) 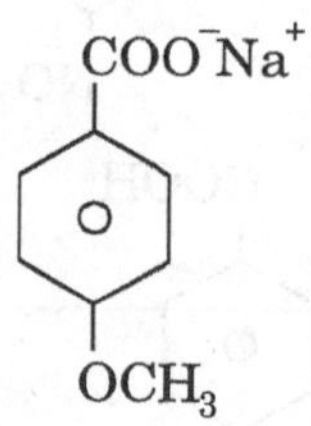

89. Which of the following acids will not undergo decarboxylation on being heated?

(a) $CH_3-CH_2-\overset{O}{\overset{||}{C}}-CH_2-COOH$

(b) $CH_3-\overset{O}{\overset{||}{C}}-CH_2-COOH$

(c) 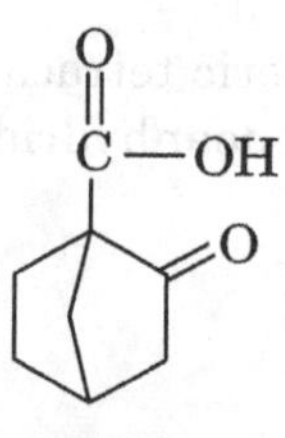

(d) All of these

90. The correct sequence of reagents for the following conversion, is-

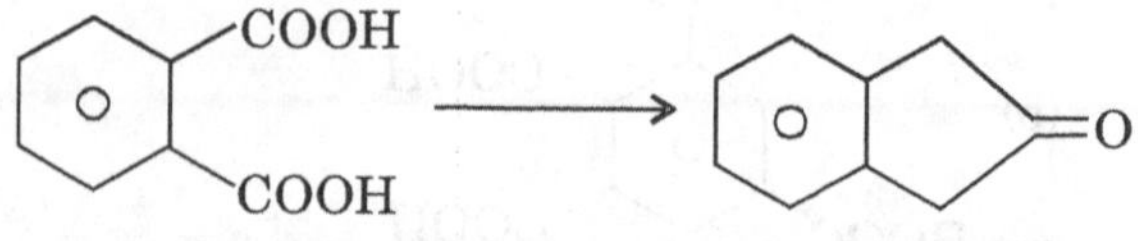

(a) $LiAlH_4 \rightarrow SOCl_2 \rightarrow KCN/H_3O^+ / Ca(OH)_2/\Delta$ (excess)

(b) $LiAlH_4 \rightarrow HI \rightarrow Mg/ether \rightarrow CO_2/H_3O^+ \; NaOH/CaO\Delta$

(c) $LiAlH_4 \rightarrow PCl_3 \rightarrow KCN/H_3O^+ \rightarrow KOH/CaO, \Delta$

(d) $LiAlH_4 \rightarrow HCl/ZnCl_2 \rightarrow KCN/H_3O^+ \rightarrow CaO, \Delta$

91. Identify the final product of the following reaction-

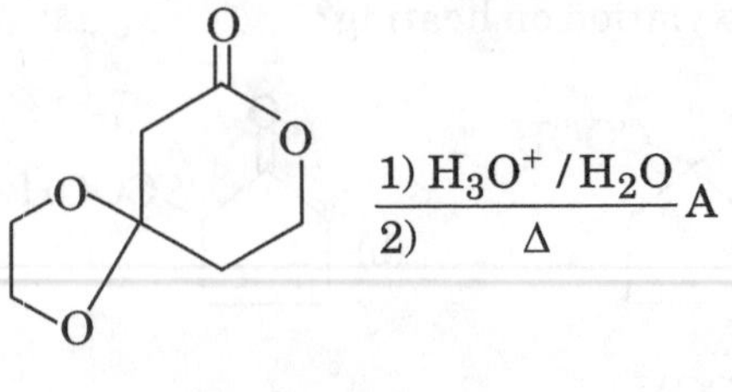

(a) $CH_3-\overset{O}{\overset{||}{C}}-CH_2CH_2\ OH$

(b) $HOOC-CH_2-\overset{O}{\overset{||}{C}}-CH_2-CH_2\ OH$

(c) $\underset{CH_2}{\overset{CONH_2}{|}}\ -\ \overset{O}{\overset{||}{C}}-CH_2-CONH_2$

(d) None of these

92. Consider the following three reduction reactions

$$R-\overset{O}{\overset{||}{C}}-Cl \xrightarrow[2)\ H_3O^+]{1)\ LiAlH_4} X, (RCO)_2O \xrightarrow[2)\ H_3O^+]{1)\ LiAlH_4} Y,$$

$$R-\overset{O}{\overset{||}{C}}-O-R \xrightarrow[2)\ H_3O^+]{1)\ LiAlH_4} Z$$

Now, X, Y & Z respectively, are –

(a) Aldehyde, aldehyde, Ketone

(b) Aldehyde, aldehyde, aldehyde

(c) Ketone, Carboxylic acid, alcohol

(d) alcohol, alcohol, alcohol

93. Arrange the following acid derivatives in the decreasing order of their reactivities towards acyl nucleophilic substitution-

(a) Acid chloride > Acid anhydride > Ester > Acid amide

(b) Acid anhydride > Acid chloride > Ester > acid amide

(c) Ester > acid amide > acid anhydride > acid chloride

(d) None of these

94. Select the correct order of acidic strength.

(a) $O_2N-CH_2-COOH > Cl-CH_2-COOH > CH_3-COOH$

(b) Oxalic acid > Malonic acid > Formic acid

(c) $H-C\equiv C-CH_2-COOH > CH_2=CH-CH_2-COOH > CH_3-CH_2-CH_2-COOH$

(d) All are correct

95. 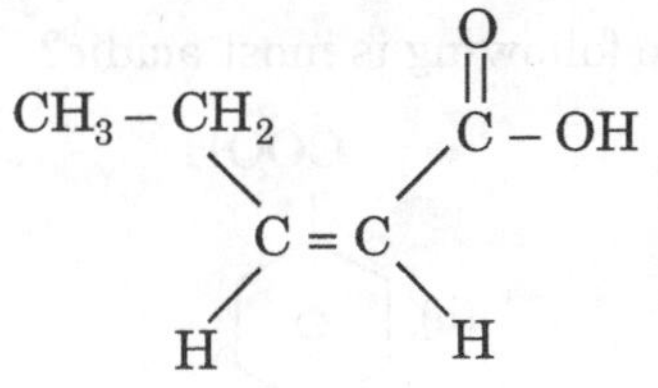 is more acidic than

(Cis form)

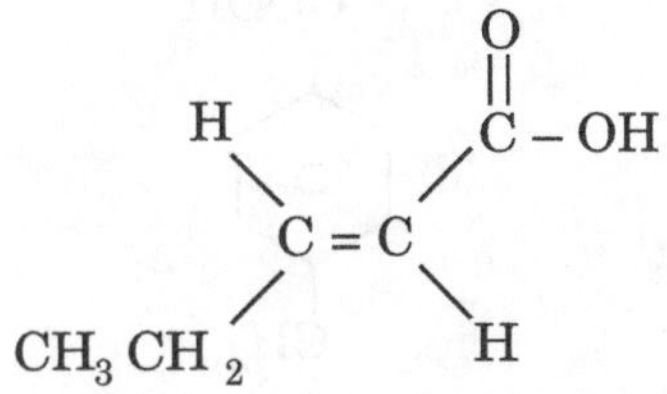 because-

(Trans form)

(a) –I effect of vinylic C's more in trans than in Cis.

(b) –I effect of vinylic C's is more in Cis than in trans.

(c) Due to steric repulsions in Cis form, +M of VINYL towards - COOH gets hampered i.e. co-planarity of C = C with – COOH is lost.

(d) All of these

96. Identify compound Y in the following reaction –

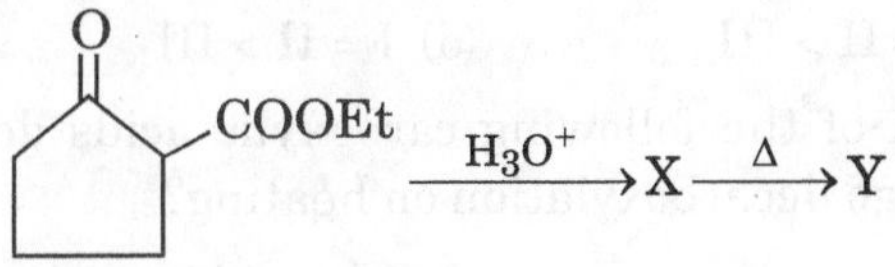

The compound Y is

(a) 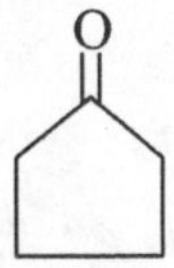 (c) 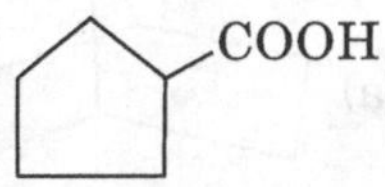

(c) 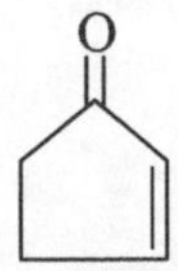 (d) 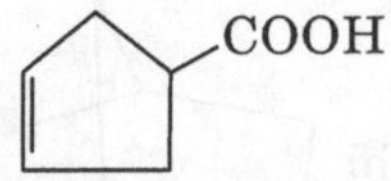

97. With reference to the scheme given, which of the given Statement(s) about T, U, V & W is/are IN correct?

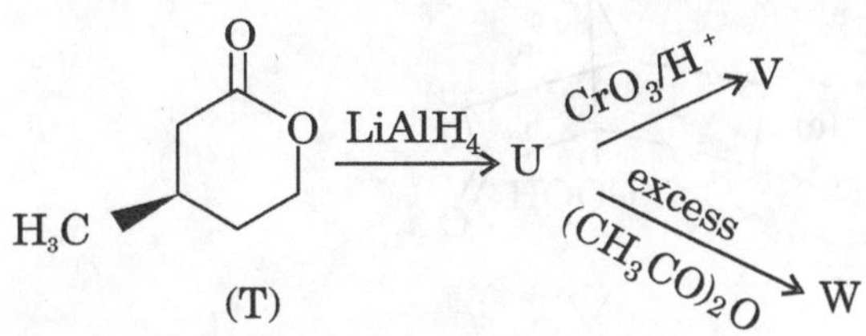

(T)

(a) T is soluble in hot aq. NaOH

(b) U is optically active

(c) Molecular formula of W is $C_{10}H_{18}O_4$.

(d) V gives effervescence on treatment with aq. $NaHCO_3$.

98. Which one of the following is most acidic?

(a) 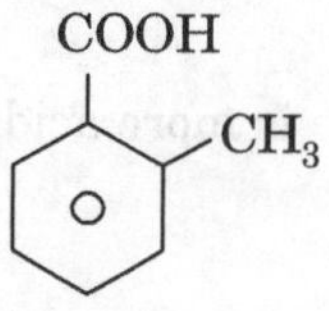

(b) 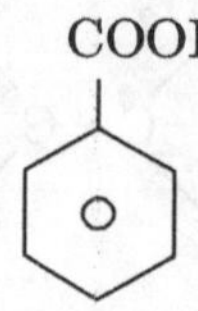

(c) 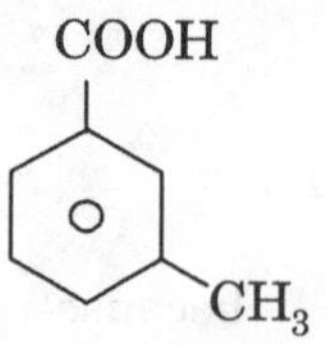

(d) 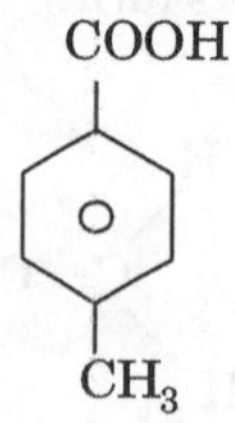

99. Arrange the following acids in the decreasing order of their acidic strengths-

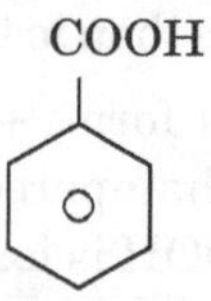
(I)

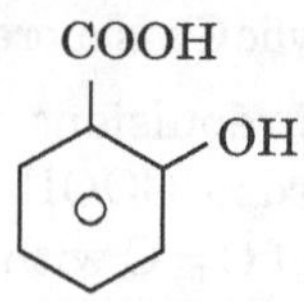
(II)

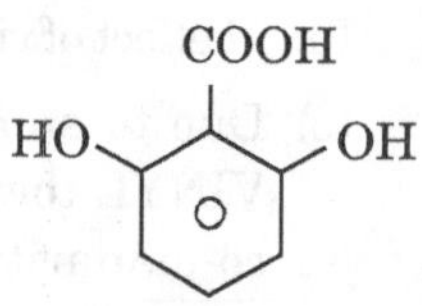
(III)

(a) III > II > I (b) II > I > III

(c) I > II > III (d) I = II > III

100. Which of the following carboxylic acids do not undergo decarboxylation on heating?

(a) 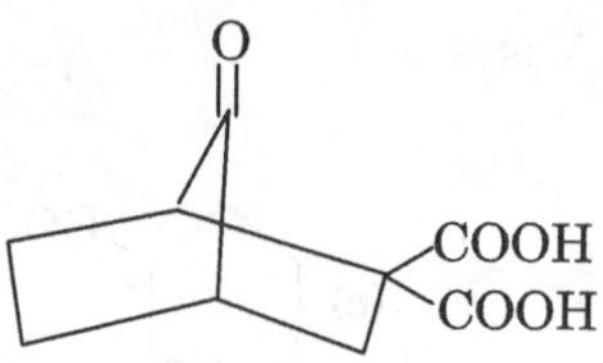

(b) 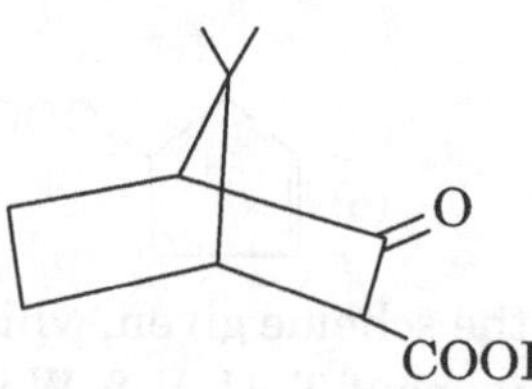

(c) 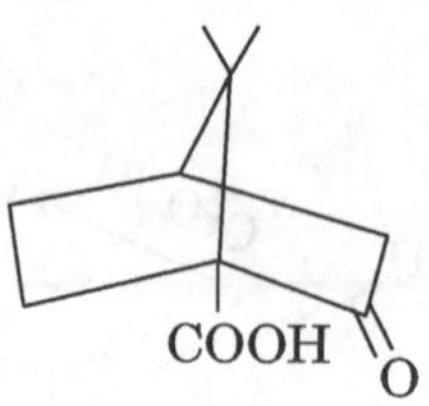

(d) 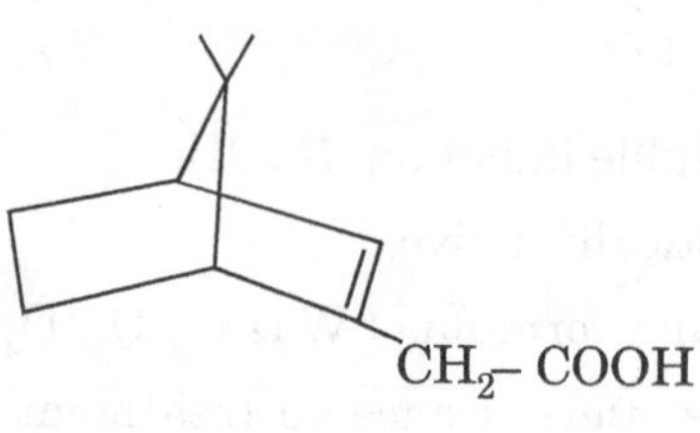

101. Which of the following acids undergo decarboxylation on heating?

(a) 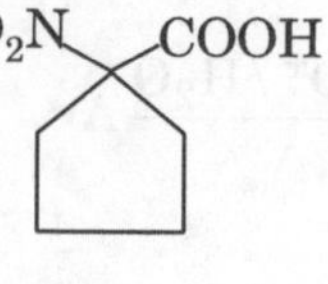

(b) 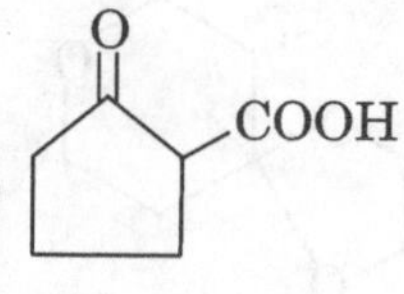

(c) 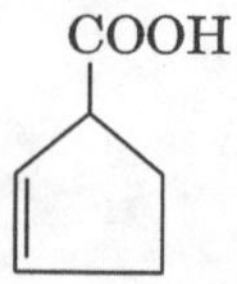

(d) All of these

102. Which of the following statement is/are correct about the reaction given below?

$$CH_3-\overset{O}{\overset{\|}{C}}-OC_2H_5 + CH_3-\overset{O}{\overset{\|}{C}}-OC_2H_5 \xrightleftharpoons{C_2H_5O^-Na^+}$$

(A) It involves the formation of a carbanion.

(B) It follow acyl nucleophilic substitution.

(C) It involves formation of a β-Keto ester.

(D) It is called claisen Ester condensation,

(E) Acetoacetic ester is formed in this reaction

(F) Acetoacetic ester has acidic protons between the two $>C=O$ groups & $EtO^{\ominus}$ converts acetoacetic ester into its conjugate base shifting the reaction to completion.

(a) Only A is correct

(b) A, B & C only are correct

(c) B, C, D & E are correct

(d) All are correct

103. Which of the following statement is/are correct about HVZ reaction?

(a) Carboxylic acids having α-H can undergo HVZ reaction

(b) It involves formation of a free radical

(c) It does not involve formation of an acid halide

(d) All are correct.

104. Which of the following compound react with hydroxylamine in dilute acidic solution?

(a) 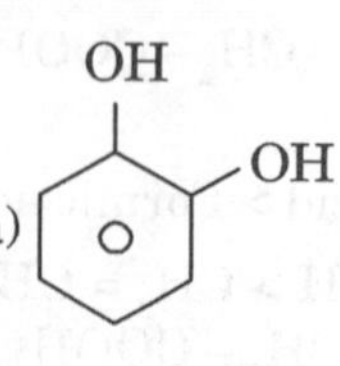

(b) 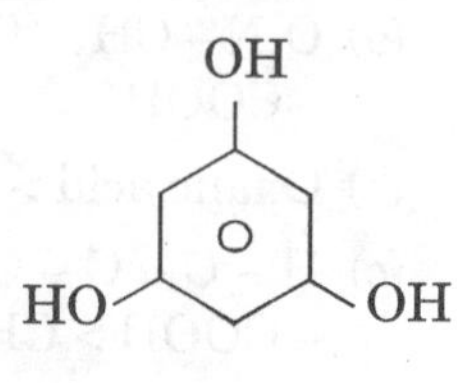

(c) 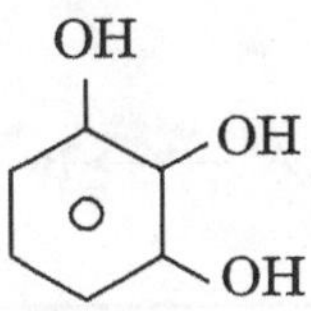 (d) 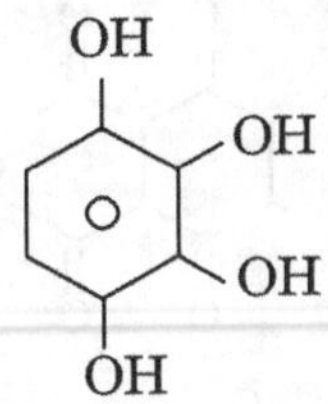

105. Consider the following reaction –

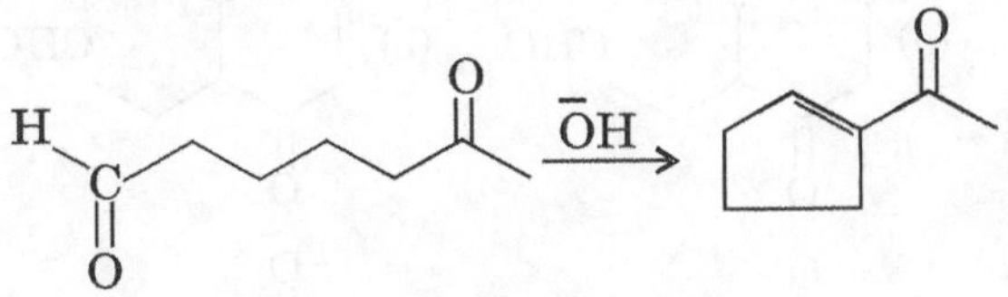

The above reaction involves –

(a) 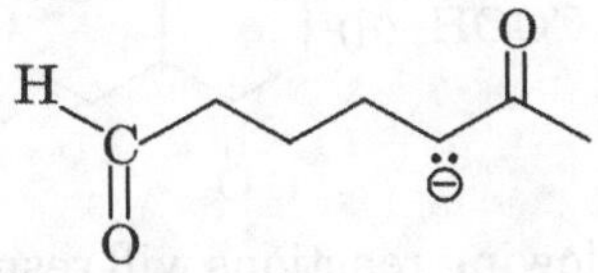

(b) 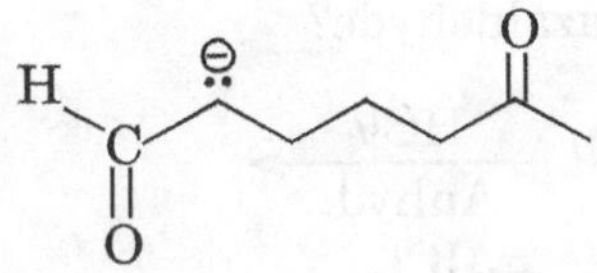

(c) 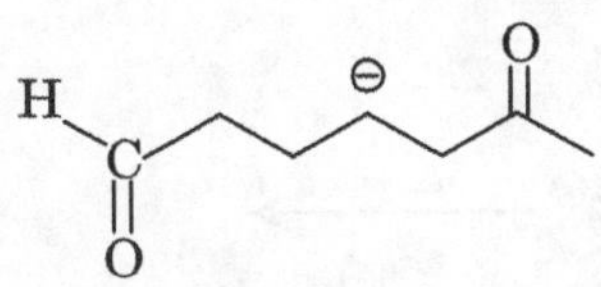

(d) None of these

106. Identify the correct products in the following reactions.

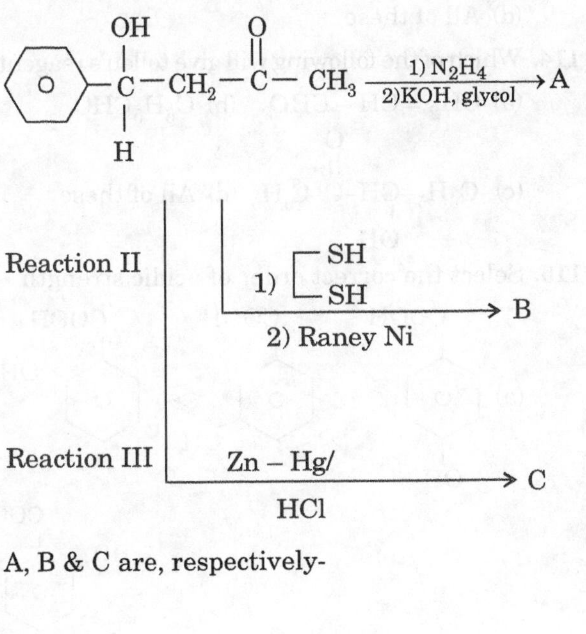

A, B & C are, respectively-

(a) 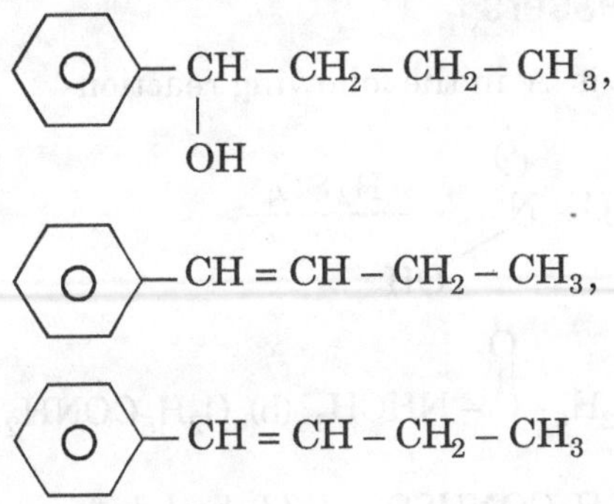

(b) 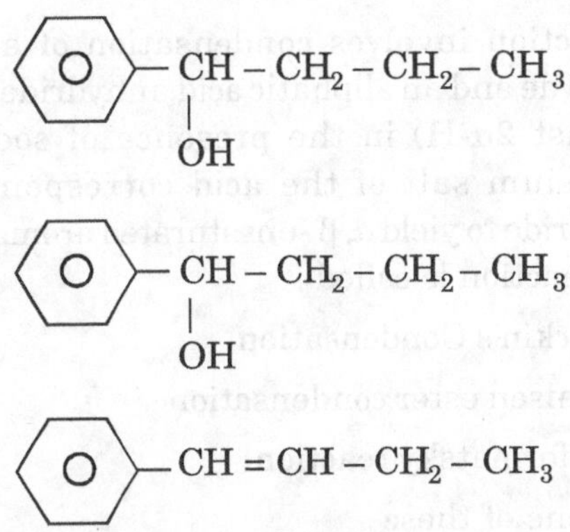

(c) 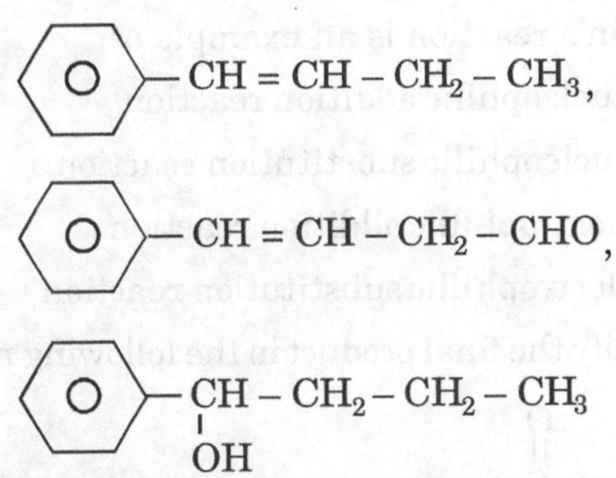

(d) None of these

107. Identify the final product of the following reaction

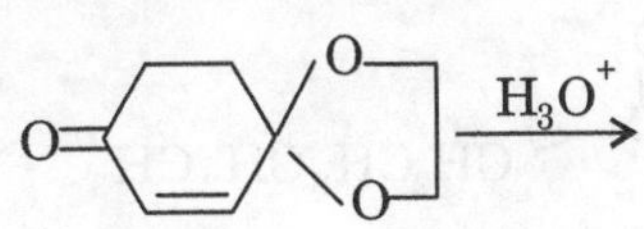

(a) 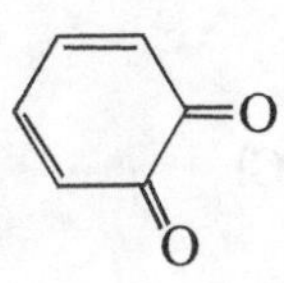 (b) 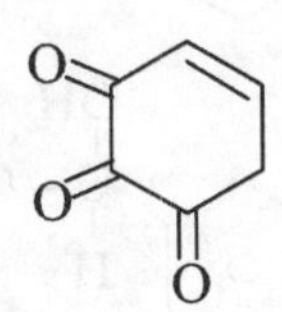

(c) 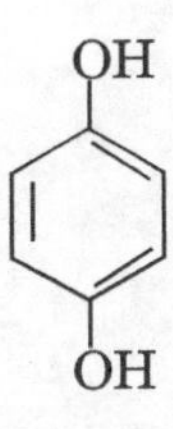 (d) 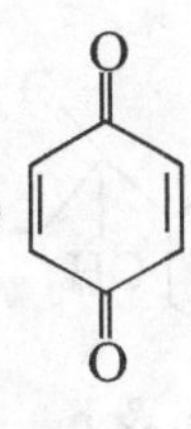

Brain Teasers

108. What is 'A' in the following reaction-

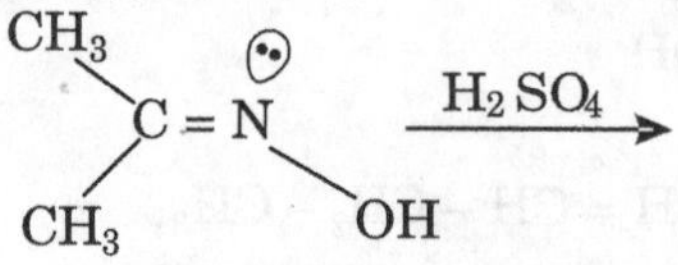

(a) $C_2H_5-\overset{O}{\overset{||}{C}}-NHCH_3$ (b) $C_2H_5CONH_2$

(c) $C_2H_5CONHSO_4$ (d) both b & c

109. A reaction involves condensation of aromatic aldehyde and an aliphatic acid anhydride (having at least 2α-H) in the presence of sodium or potassium salt of the acid corresponding to anhydride to yield α, β -unsaturated aromatic acid. The reaction is called-

(a) Perkin's Condensation

(b) Claisen ester condensation

(c) Reformatsky reaction

(d) None of these

110. Perkin's reaction is an example of

(a) Nucleophilic addition reaction

(b) Nucleophilic substitution reaction

(c) Electrophillic addition reaction

(d) Electrophillic substitution reaction

111. Identify the final product in the following reaction-

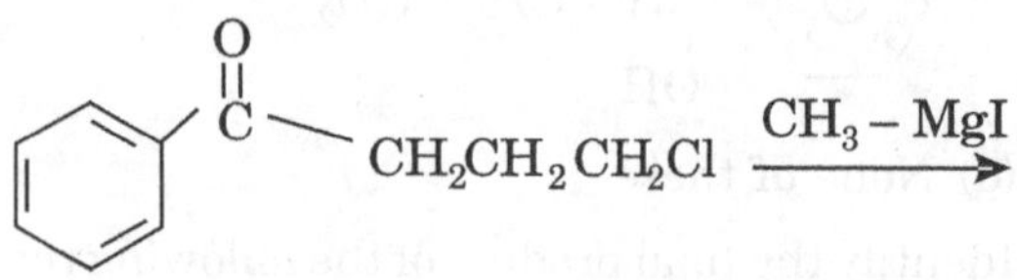

(a) 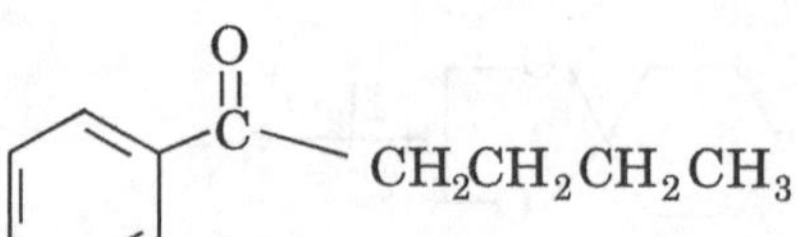

(b) 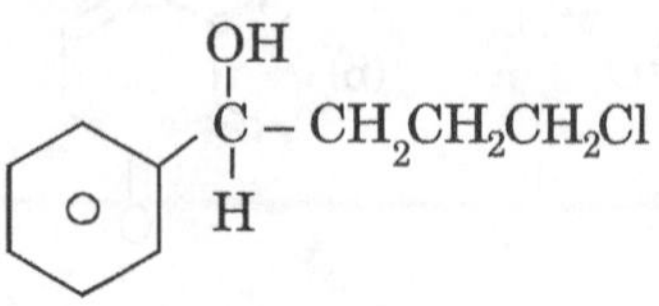

(c) 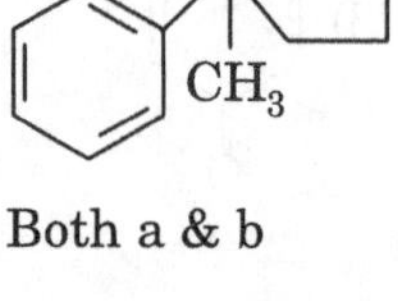

(d) Both a & b

112. Identify X in the following reaction-

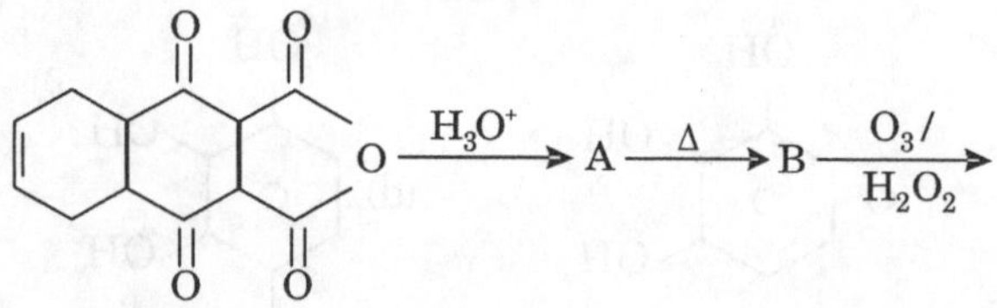

(a) 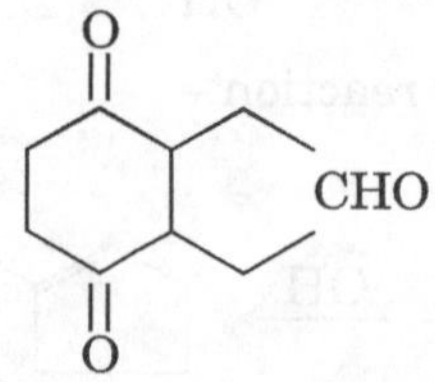 (b) 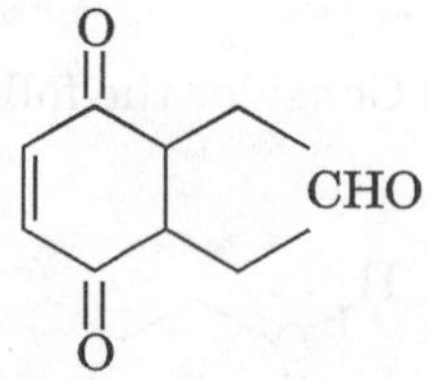

(c) 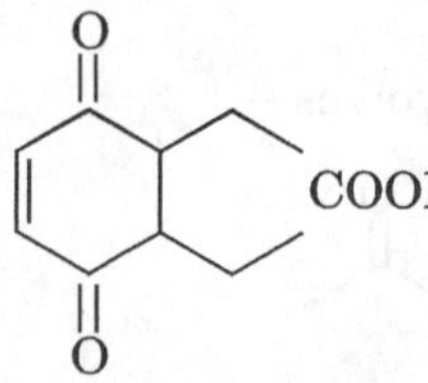 (d) 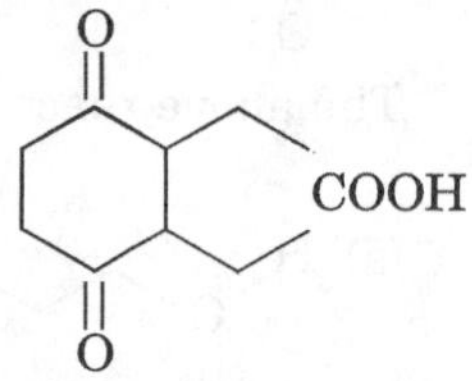

113. Which of the following reactions will result in the formation of benzaldehyde?

(a) 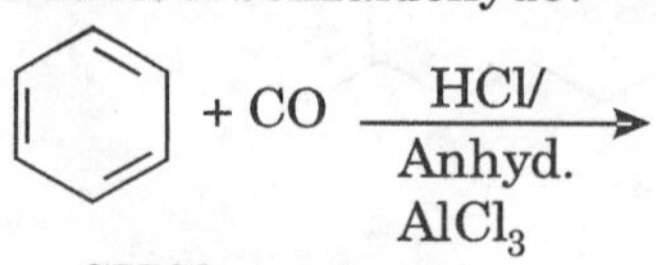

(b) 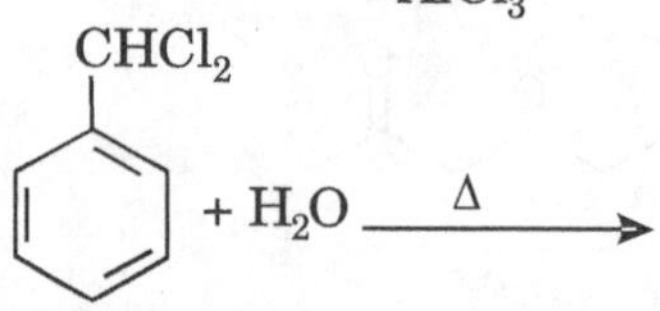

(c) 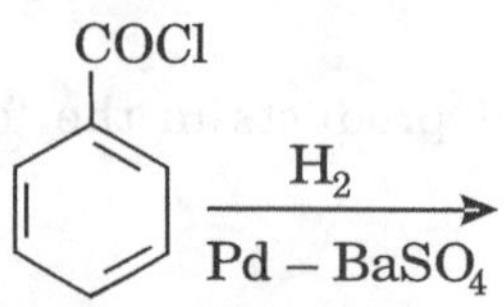

(d) All of these

114. Which of the following will give tollen's reagent test?

(a) $CH_2 = CH - CHO$ (b) C_6H_5CHO

(c) $C_6H_5-\underset{OH}{\underset{|}{CH}}-\overset{O}{\overset{||}{C}}-C_6H_5$ (d) All of these

115. Select the correct order of acidic strength

(a) 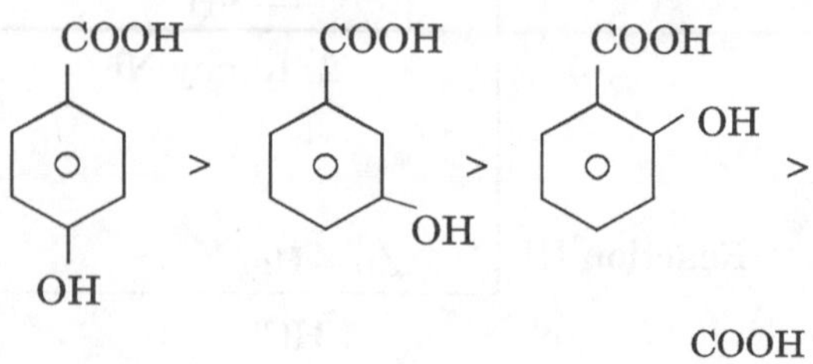

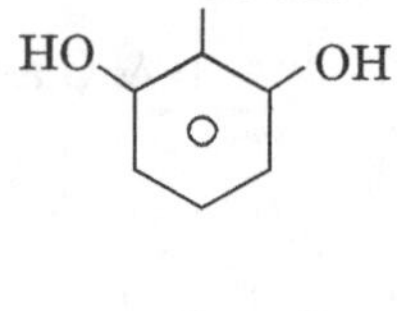

(b) 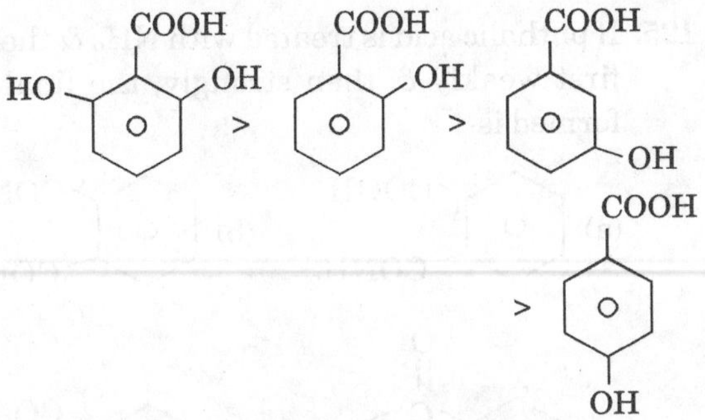

(c) 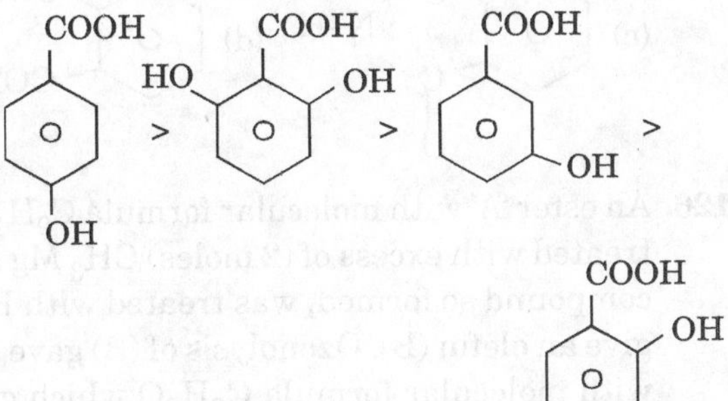

(d) None of these

116. Consider the following reaction-

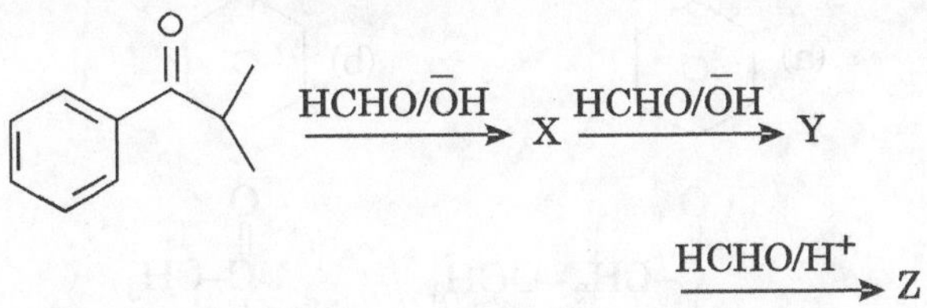

The major product in this reaction is-

(a) Aldol (b) Ketol

(c) Hemi-acetal (d) Acetal

117. In moderate concentration of the base, Cannizaro's reaction follow "X" order kinetics & in high Concentration of the base, it follows 'Y' order kinetics. Hence, X&Y, respectively, are-

(a) 1&2 (b) 2&3

(c) 3&4 (d) 4&5

118. Consider the following two dehydration steps of aldols-

(Reaction 1)

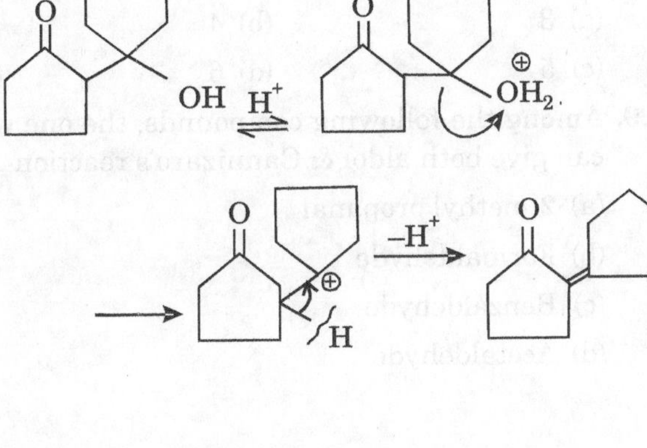

(Reaction 2)

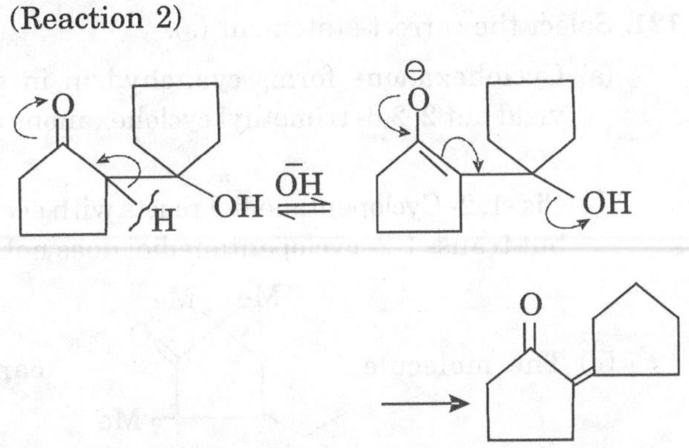

The Mechanisms followed in reaction 1 & reaction 2, respectively are-

(a) S_N1, E_1 (b) E_1, E_2

(c) S_N2, E_2 (d) E_1, E_1cb

119. Identify the mismatch-

Reactions	Name of Reaction
(a) 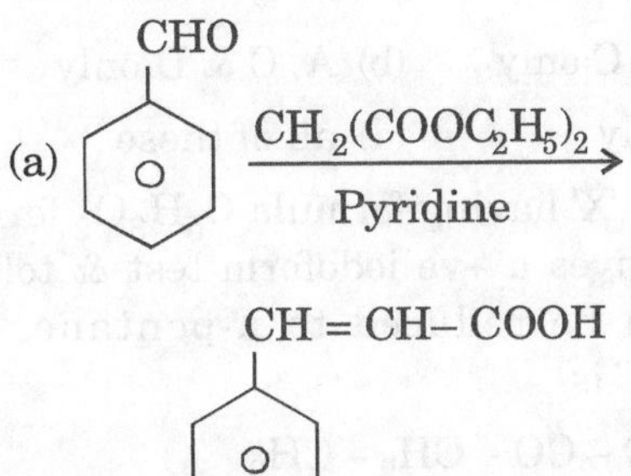	Knoevengel Reaction
(b) $>C=O + Br-\underset{\displaystyle R}{\underset{|}{CH}}-COOC_2H_5 \xrightarrow[H_2O]{Zn/\Delta}$	Reformatsky Reaction
(c) $R-\overset{\displaystyle O}{\overset{\|}{C}}-R' \xrightarrow{R''CO_3H} R-\overset{\displaystyle O}{\overset{\|}{C}}-OR' + R''\,COOH$	Baeyer villiger oxidation

(d) None of these

120. Consider the following reaction-

$$2CH_3CH_2COOC_2H_5 \xrightarrow{C_2H_5O^-Na^+} A \xrightarrow{H^+/H_2O} B \xrightarrow{\Delta} C + CO_2$$

'C' in the above reaction is-

(a) an aldehyde

(b) a ketone

(c) a carboxylic acid

(d) none of these

121. Select the correct statement (s).

(a) Cyclohexanone forms cyanohydrin in good yield but 2, 2,6- trimethyl cyclohexanone does not.

(b) Cis -1, 2- Cyclopentanediol reacts with acetone but trans- 1-2- cyclopentanediol does not.

(c) The molecule 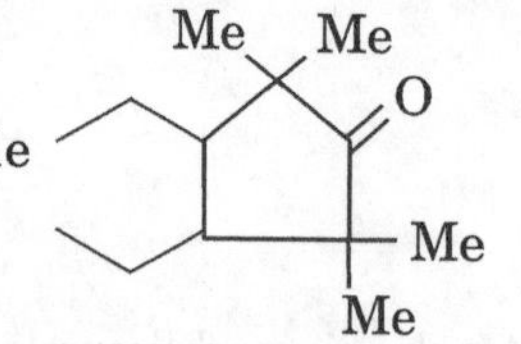 , cannot undergo aldol because it lacks α-H.

(d) All are correct

122. Which of the following will react with ammoniacal $AgNO_3$ Solution?

(A) HCOOH (B) RNHOH

(C) $CH_3-C\equiv C-H$ (D) $CH_3COCH(OH)CH_3$

(a) both A & C only (b) A, C & D only

(c) A & D only (d) all of these

123. A compound 'X' having formula $C_5H_8O_2$ forms a dioxime & gives a +ve iodoform test & tollen's test. It can be reduced to n-pentane. The compound 'X' is-

(a) $CH_3-CO-CO-CH_2-CH_3$

(b) $CH_3-CO-CH_2\,CH_2CHO$

(c) $CH_3-CO-CH(CH_3)-CHO$

(d) $(CH_3)_2-CO-CH_2CHO$

124. In the following sequence of reaction identify the final product.

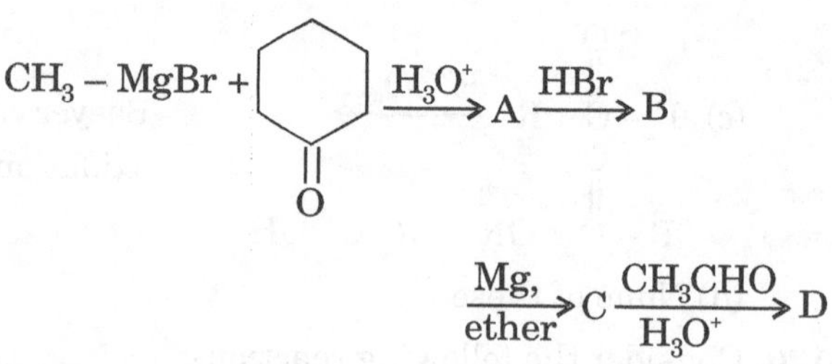

'D' is –

(a) 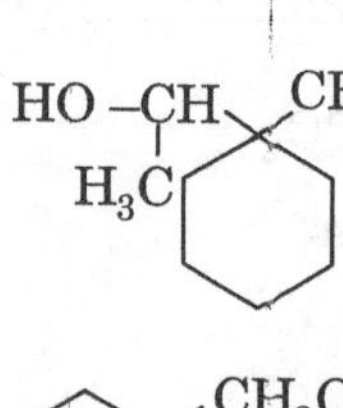 (b) 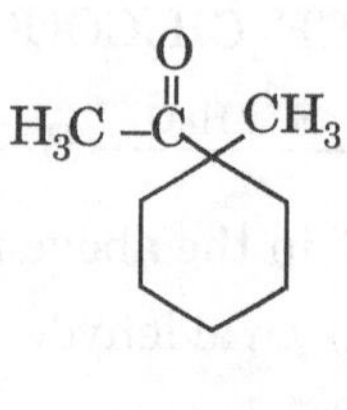

(c) 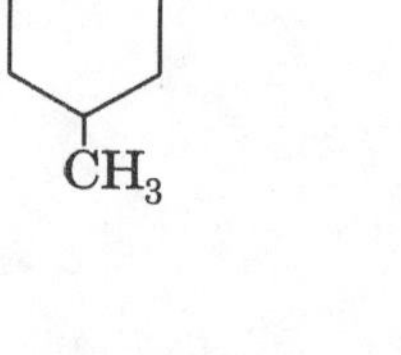 (d) All of these

125. If phthalic acid is treated with NH_3 & then heated first weakly & then strongly, the final product formed is-

(a) 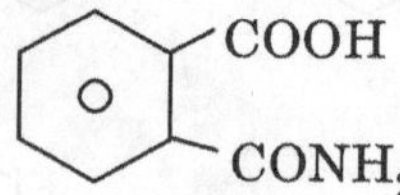 (b) 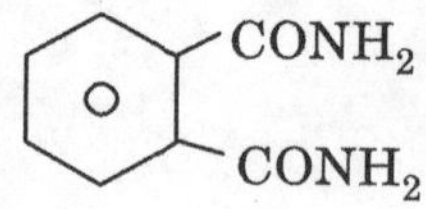

(c) 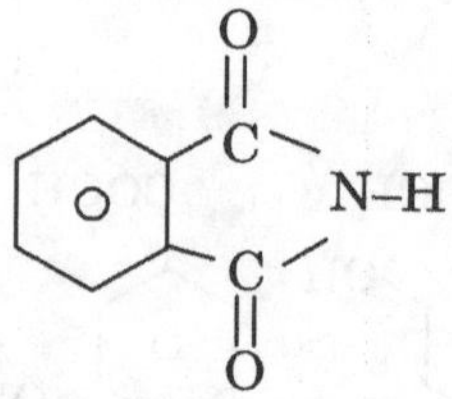 (d) 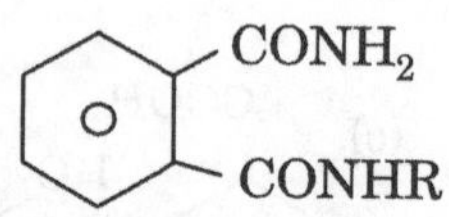

126. An ester 'A' with molecular formula $C_9H_{10}O_2$ was treated with excess of (2 moles) $CH_3\,Mg\,Br$ & the compound so formed, was treated with H_2SO_4 to give an olefin (B). Ozonolysis of (B) gave a ketone with molecular formula C_8H_8O which gives +ve iodoform test. The correct structure for 'A' is -

(a) 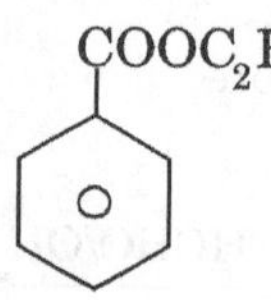 (b) 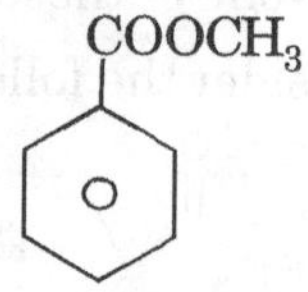

(c) 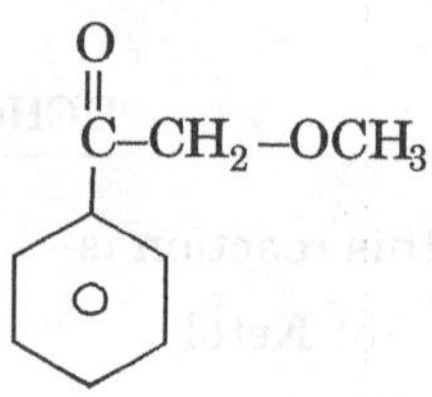 (d) 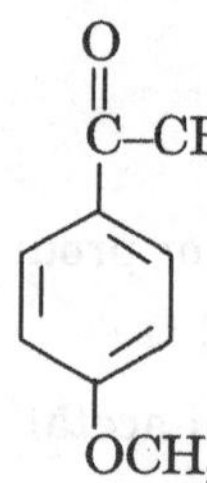

127. Formula of ketone 'X' is $C_6\,H_{12}O$ (having mol. mass = 100). How many of these will give racemic mixture with $NaBH_4$?

(a) 3 (b) 4

(c) 5 (d) 6

128. Acetone and butan-2-one undergo both self & cross aldol (ketol) which loses water to give α, β – unsaturated ketones. The number of isomeric α, β – unsaturated ketones formed is/are (excluding stereoisomers in products)

(a) 3 (b) 4

(c) 5 (d) 6

129. Among the following compounds, the one which can give both aldol & Cannizaro's reaction-

(a) 2-methyl propanal

(b) Formaldehyde

(c) Benzaldehyde

(d) Acetaldehyde

130. Propanal will react most readily with-

(a) $H_2N\text{-}NH_2$ (b) $H_2N\text{-}NHCONH_2$

(c) $Ph\text{-}NH\text{-}NH_2$ (d) $H_2N\text{-}OH$

131. Which of the following is/are reluctant to give Cannizaro's reaction?

(a) $Cl_3C\text{–}C(=O)\text{–}H$

(b) 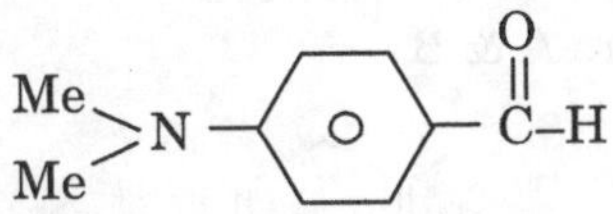

(c) HCHO

(d) Both a & b

132. 4 moles of NH_3 & 6 moles of HCHO react with each other to give -

(a) Diacetone ammonia

(b) Hexamethylenetetramine

(c) Urotropine

(d) Both b & c

133. The number of aldol reactions that occur in the given transformation is/are-

$CH_3CHO + 4HCHO \xrightarrow[\text{NaOH}]{\text{Conc.aq.}}$ 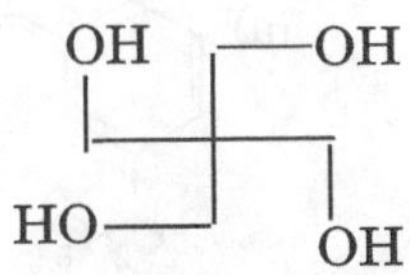

(a) 1 (b) 2

(c) 3 (d) 4

134. Consider the following reactions & Identify 'A' & 'B' respectively-

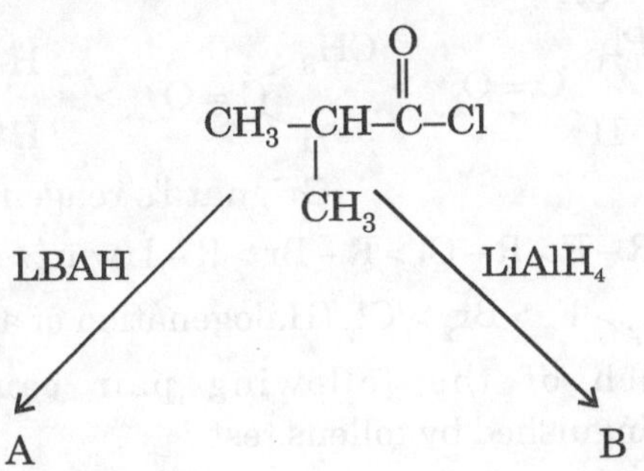

(LBAH is lithium tri-t-butoxyaluminium hydride) A & B, respectively, are-

(a) aldehyde, alcohol

(b) aldehyde, aldehyde

(c) alcohol, alcohol

(d) aldehyde, imine

135. Molecule 'X' ($Ph\text{-}CH = CHCOCH_3$) can be converted into molecules given in column-I by reactions given in column-II. Select the mismatch

Column-I	Column-II (Reagent/ Reaction)
(a) $Ph-CH = CH-CH(OH)-CH_3$	$\rightarrow$ MPV Reduction/ $LiAlH_4$
(b) $Ph-CH = CH\ COOH$	$\rightarrow I_2/NaOH$
(c) $Ph-CH=CH-CH_2-CH_3$	$\rightarrow$ Wolf kishner's reduction

(d) None of these

136. Which of the following reactions represent pinacol- pinacolone rearrangement?

(a) 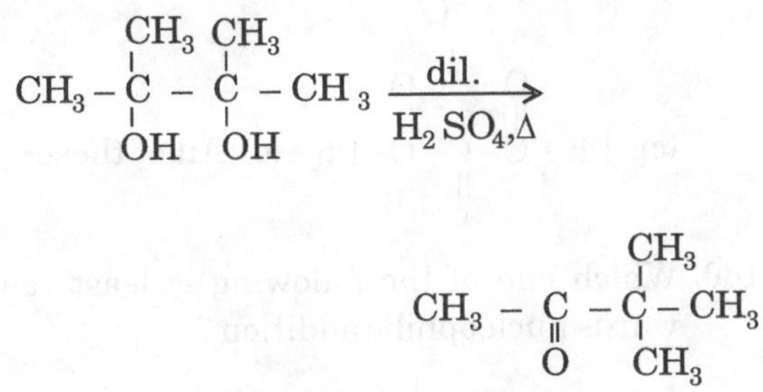

(b) 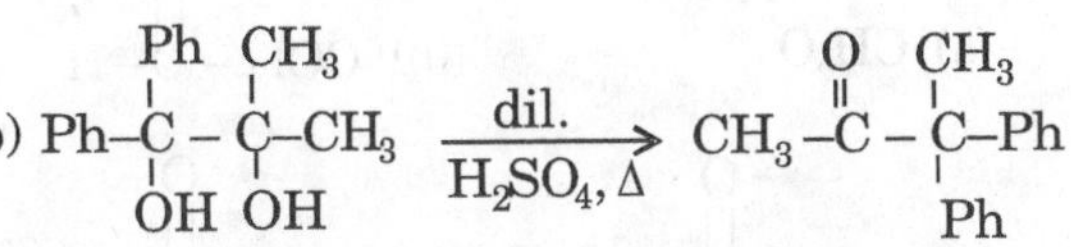

(c) 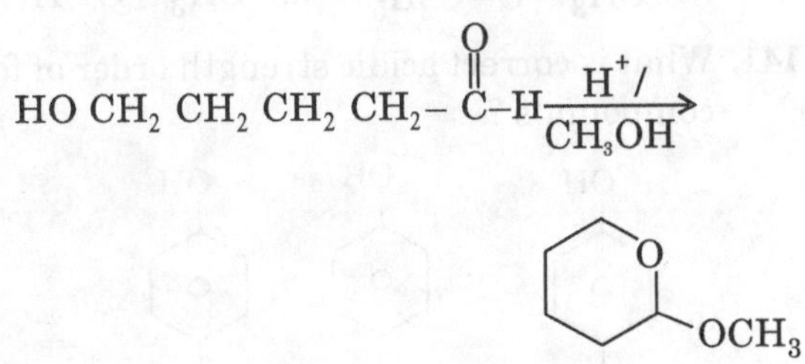

(d) Both a & b

137. The correct name of the following reaction is-

$$Ph-\overset{O}{\overset{\|}{C}}-CH_3 + CF_3\ CO_3H \rightarrow CH_3-\overset{O}{\overset{\|}{C}}-OPh + CF_3COOH$$

(a) Knovengeal reaction

(b) Beckmann's Rearrangement

(c) Favorskii rearrangement

(d) Baeyer Villiger's oxidation

138. Rank the following in order of increasing value of the equilibrium constant for hydration, $k_{hyd.}$

(1) 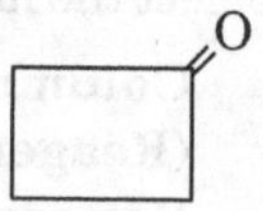 (2) 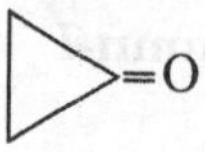

(3) $(CH_3)_3C-\overset{O}{\overset{||}{C}}-C(CH_3)_3$

(a) 3 > 2 > 1 (b) 2 > 1 > 3

(c) 3 > 1 > 2 (d) 2 > 3 > 1

139. Which of the following forms stable Hydrate?

(a) 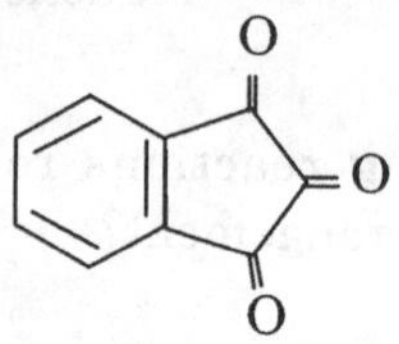 (b) $Cl_3C-\overset{O}{\overset{||}{C}}-H$

(c) $Ph-\overset{O}{\overset{||}{C}}-\underset{O}{\underset{||}{\overset{O}{\overset{||}{C}}}}-C-Ph$ (d) All of these

140. Which one of the following is least reactive to wards nucleophilic addition ?

(a) CH_2O (b) $CCl_3-\overset{O}{\overset{||}{C}}-H$

(c) $CH_3-\overset{O}{\overset{||}{C}}-C_2H_5$ (d) $CH_3-\overset{O}{\overset{||}{C}}-H$

141. What is correct acidic strength order of following compounds ?

(a) 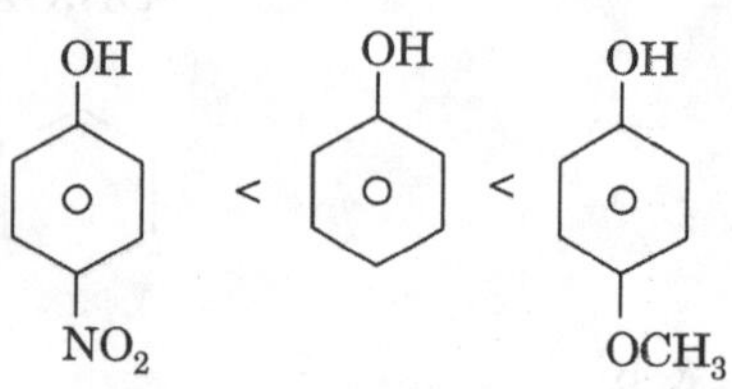

(b) 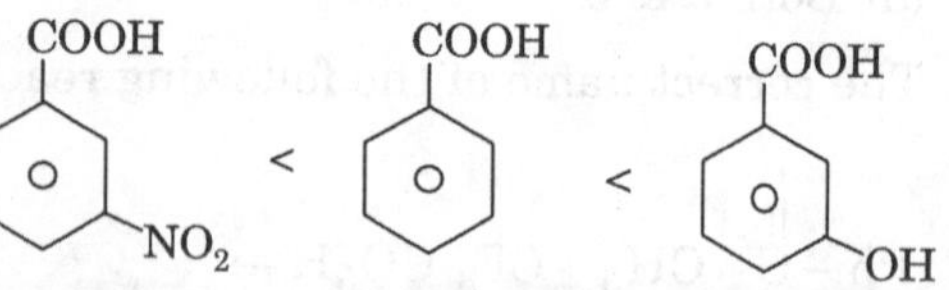

(c) 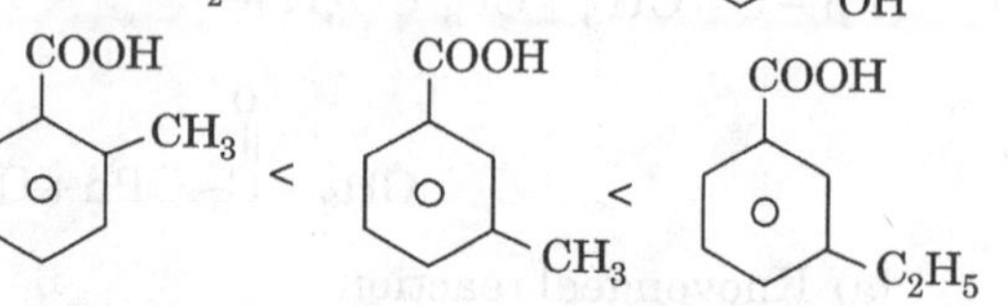

(d) 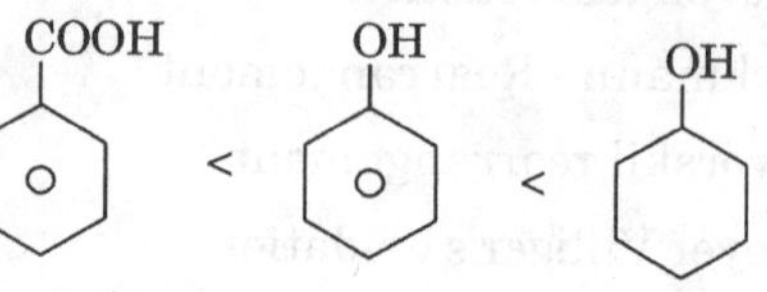

142. 2 isomers, A & **B**, both on ozonolysis give same products $\xrightarrow[2)\ Zn/H_2O]{1)\ O_3}$ 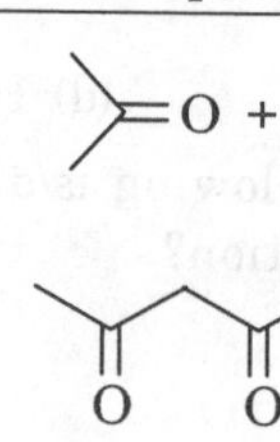 + HCHO

Identify isomers A & B –

(a) 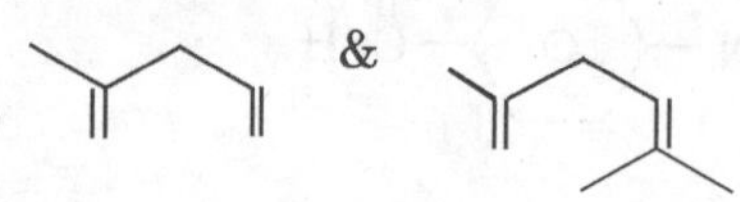

(b) 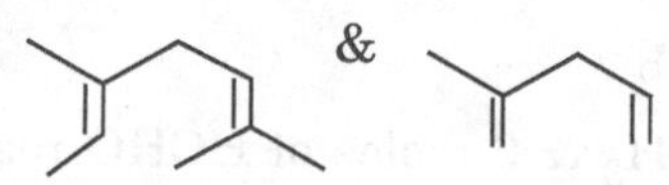

(c) 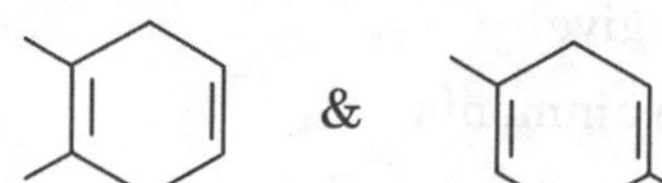

(d) 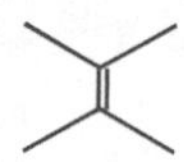 & $CH_2 = CH_2$

143. Which of the following is correct order of reactivity for –

(a) 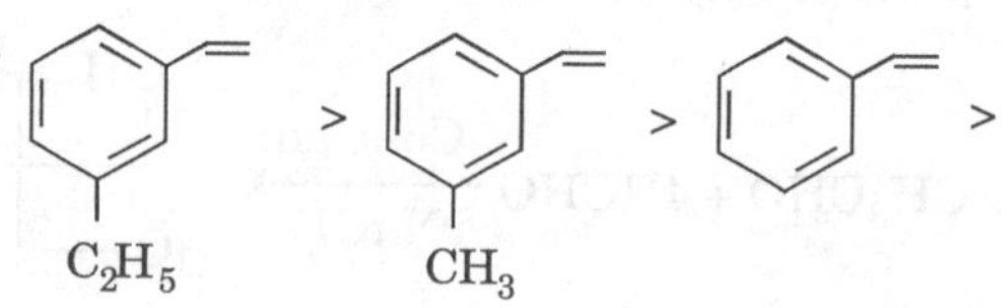

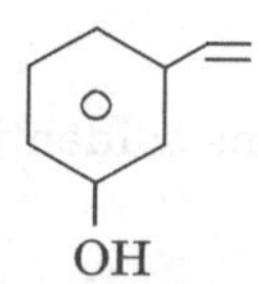 (Electrophilic addition reaction)

(b) Ph(H)C = O > CH_3(H)C = O > H(H)C = O

(Grignard's reagent)

(c) R – F > R – Cl > R – Br > R – I (wurtz reaction)

(d) $I_2 > F_2 > Br_2 > Cl_2$ (Halogenation of alkanes)

144. Which of the following pair cannot be distinguished by tollens test ?

(a) CH_3COCH_3, 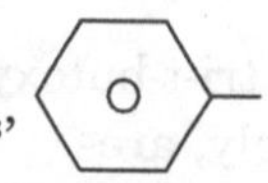 – CHO

(b) HCOOH, CH_3COCH_3

(c) CH_3CHO, 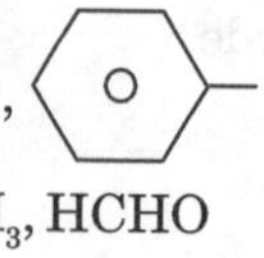 – CH_2CHO

(d) $PhCOCH_3$, HCHO

Answers

1. (d)	**2.** (d)	**3.** (d)	**4.** (d)	**5.** (b)	**6.** (a)	**7.** (c)	**8.** (d)	**9.** (b)	**10.** (d)
11. (d)	**12.** (b)	**13.** (a)	**14.** (b)	**15.** (b)	**16.** (a)	**17.** (a)	**18.** (a)	**19.** (c)	**20.** (c)
21. (a)	**22.** (c)	**23.** (d)	**24.** (a)	**25.** (c)	**26.** (d)	**27.** (a)	**28.** (c)	**29.** (b)	**30.** (c)
31. (b)	**32.** (d)	**33.** (d)	**34.** (c)	**35.** (a)	**36.** (b)	**37.** (a)	**38.** (b)	**39.** (a)	**40.** (b)
41. (b)	**42.** (c)	**43.** (b)	**44.** (d)	**45.** (c)	**46.** (c)	**47.** (a)	**48.** (b)	**49.** (c)	**50.** (d)
51. (b)	**52.** (d)	**53.** (b)	**54.** (c)	**55.** (c)	**56.** (b)	**57.** (a)	**58.** (c)	**59.** (d)	**60.** (b)
61. (d)	**62.** (b)	**63.** (c)	**64.** (a)	**65.** (c)	**66.** (c)	**67.** (a)	**68.** (a)	**69.** (b)	**70.** (b)
71. (d)	**72.** (d)	**73.** (d)	**74.** (c)	**75.** (c)	**76.** (d)	**77.** (b)	**78.** (d)	**79.** (b)	**80.** (d)
81. (c)	**82.** (a)	**83.** (d)	**84.** (d)	**85.** (d)	**86.** (a)	**87.** (d)	**88.** (a)	**89.** (c)	**90.** (a)
91. (a)	**92.** (d)	**93.** (a)	**94.** (d)	**95.** (c)	**96.** (a)	**97.** (b)	**98.** (a)	**99.** (a)	**100.** (c)
101. (d)	**102.** (d)	**103.** (a)	**104.** (b)	**105.** (a)	**106.** (b)	**107.** (c)	**108.** (a)	**109.** (a)	**110.** (a)
111. (c)	**112.** (d)	**113.** (d)	**114.** (d)	**115.** (b)	**116.** (d)	**117.** (c)	**118.** (d)	**119.** (d)	**120.** (b)
121. (d)	**122.** (d)	**123.** (b)	**124.** (a)	**125.** (c)	**126.** (a)	**127.** (c)	**128.** (d)	**129.** (a)	**130.** (a)
131. (d)	**132.** (d)	**133.** (c)	**134.** (a)	**135.** (d)	**136.** (d)	**137.** (d)	**138.** (b)	**139.** (d)	**140.** (c)
141. (c)	**142.** (a)	**143.** (a)	**144.** (c)						

Explanations

1. $R-C\equiv N \xrightarrow[HCl]{SnCl_2} R-CH=NH \xrightarrow{H_3O^+} RCHO + NH_3$

3. 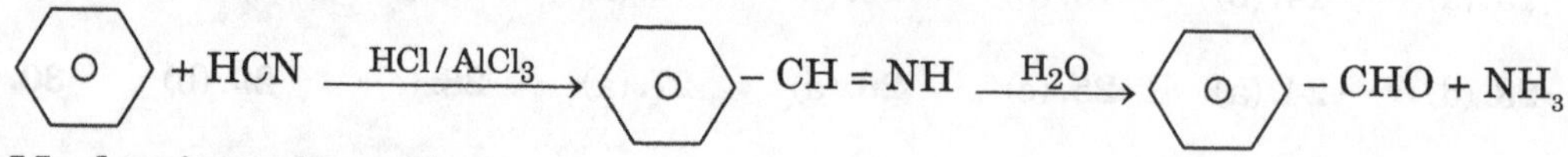

Mechanism of reaction

1. $H-\ddot{Cl}: + AlCl_3 \longrightarrow H^+ + AlCl_4^-$

2. $H-C\equiv \ddot{N} + H^+ \rightleftharpoons H-C\equiv \overset{\oplus}{N}-H \longleftrightarrow H-\overset{\oplus}{C}=N-H$

(electrophile is generated)

3. 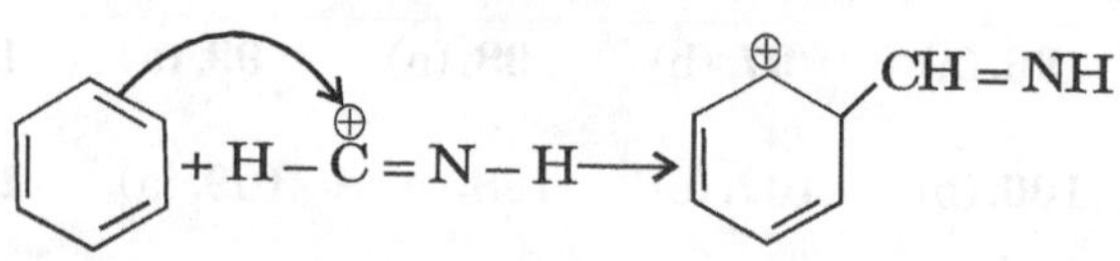

4. 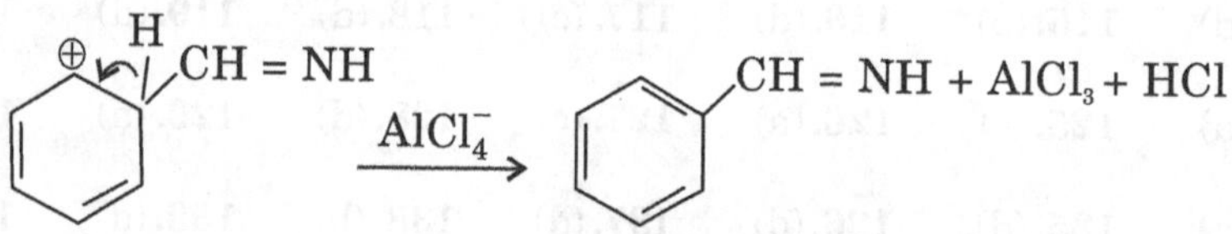

Benzaldimine

5. 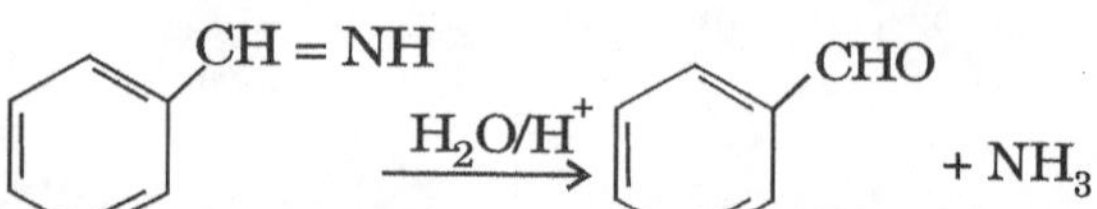

5. This reaction is an example of electrophillic substitution reaction of benzene.

(a) 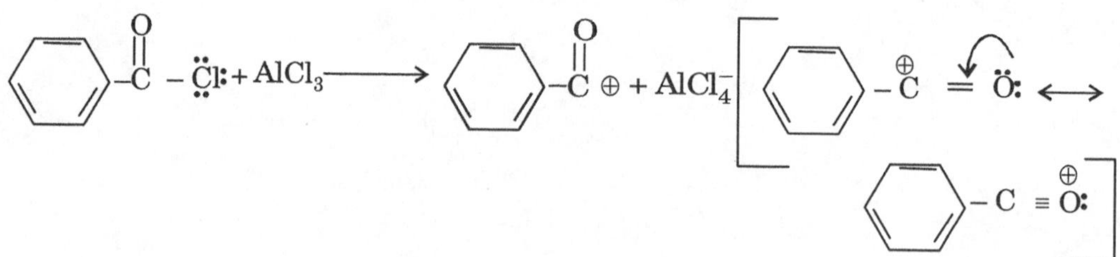

(b) 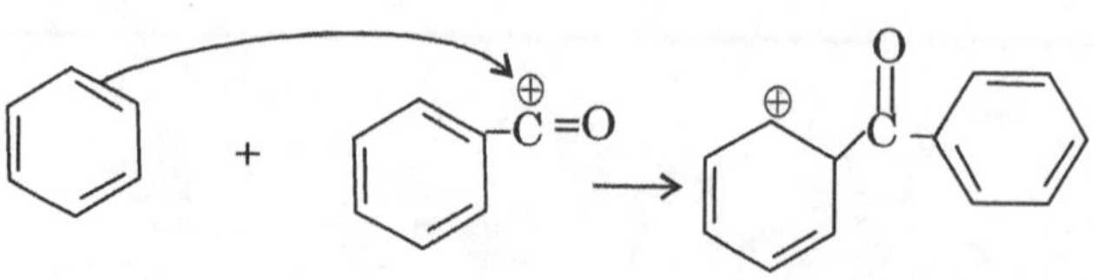

(c) 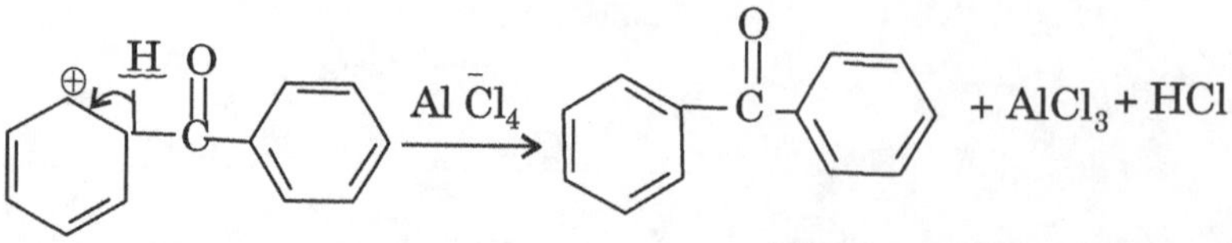

(BENZOPHENONE)

6. Mechanism

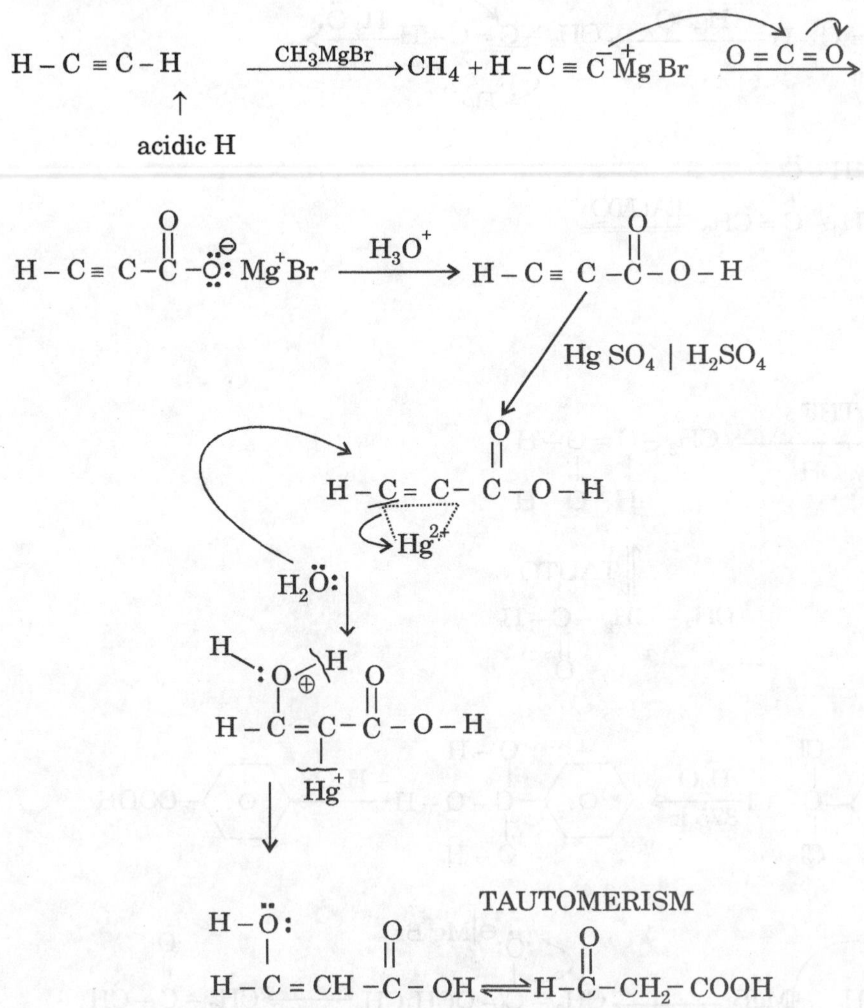

7. $$CH_3-\underset{\displaystyle OH}{\underset{|}{CH}}-CH_2-CH_3 \xrightarrow{PCC} CH_3-\underset{\displaystyle O}{\underset{||}{C}}-CH_2-CH_3$$

8.

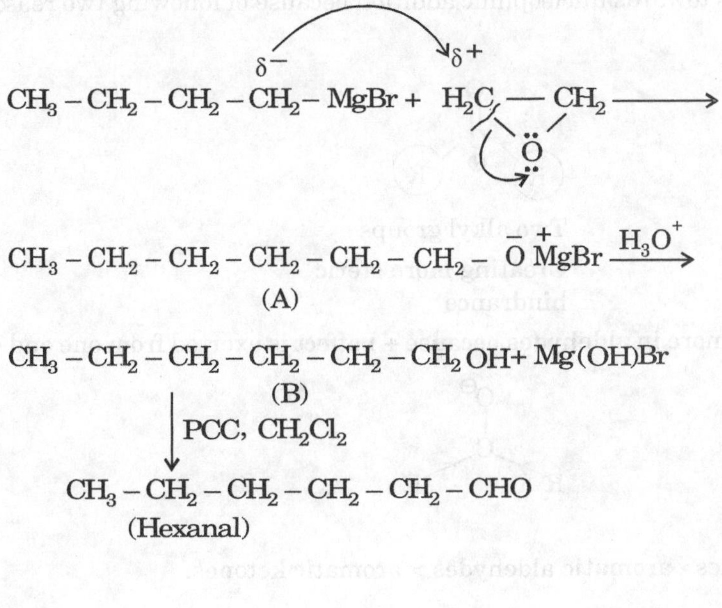

9. Kucherov's reaction 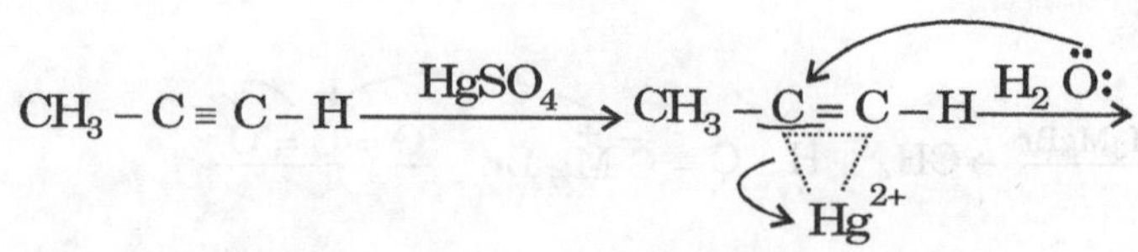

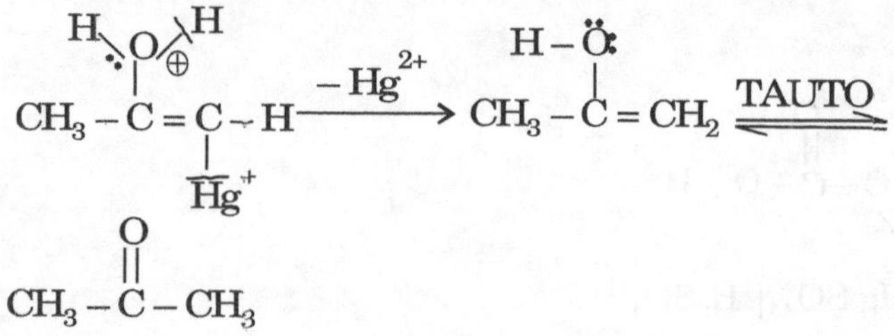

$$CH_3-C\equiv C-H \xrightarrow[2)\ H_2O_2,\ \bar{O}H]{1)\ BH_3,\ THF} CH_3-\underset{H}{\underset{|}{C}}=\underset{O-H}{\underset{|}{C}}-H$$

(Hydroboration – oxidation)

$$\Big\Updownarrow \text{TAUTO}$$

$$CH_3-CH_2-\underset{O}{\underset{||}{C}}-H$$

11. Wrt option (d)

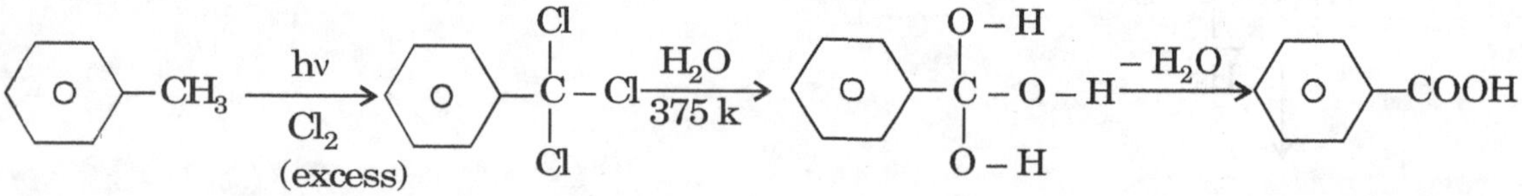

12. 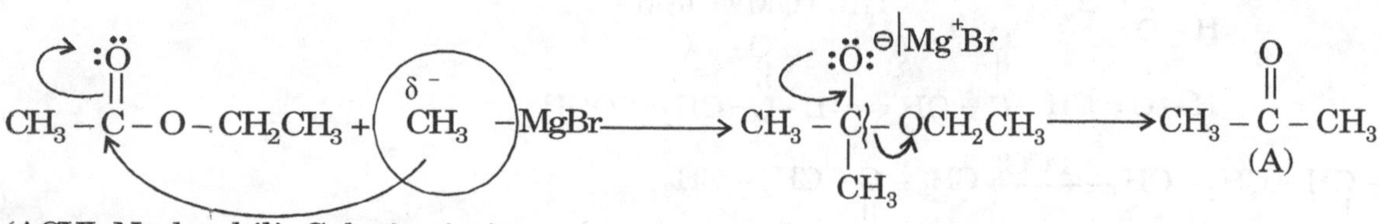

(ACYL Nucleophilic Substitution)

13. Aldehydes are more reactive than ketones towards nucleophilic addition because of following two reasons –

(a) Less steric hindrance in aldehydes.

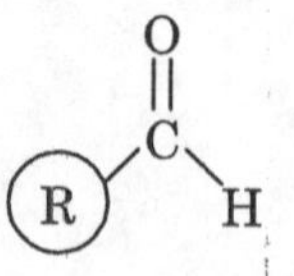

relatively less steric hindrance

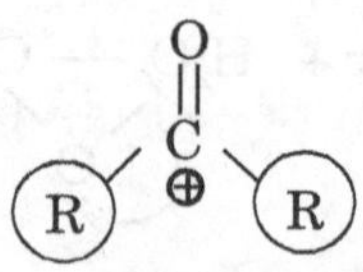

Two alkyl groups Creating more steric hindrance

(b) Electrophilicity of carbonyl carbon is more in aldehydes because + I effect is exerted from one end only.

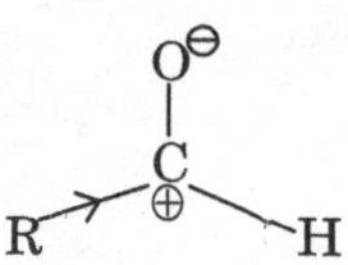

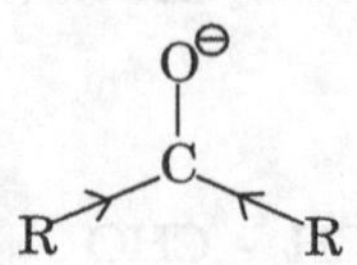

Reactivity towards Nu $^{\ominus}$ addition

Aliphatic aldehydes > aliphatic ketones> aromatic aldehydes > aromatic ketones.

14. 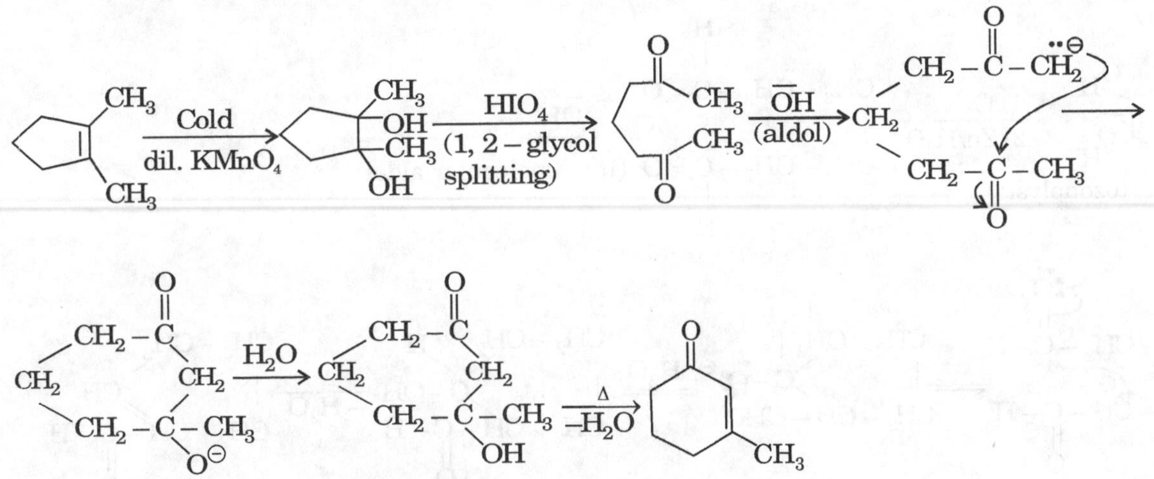

15. 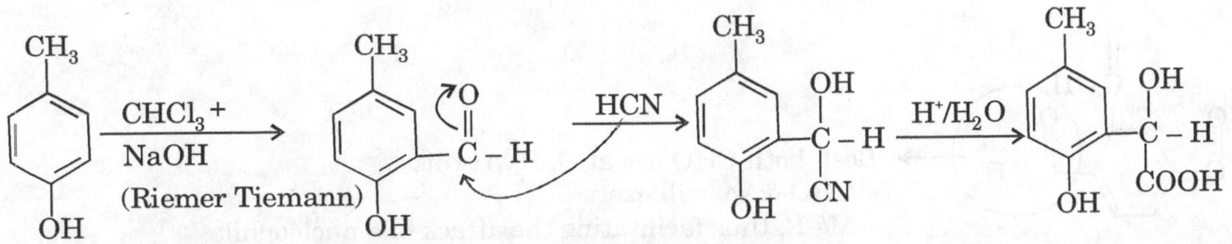

16. Semi – Carbazide is an ammonia derivative. It undergoes addition – elimination type of mechanism with carbonyl Compounds under optimum acidic conditions.

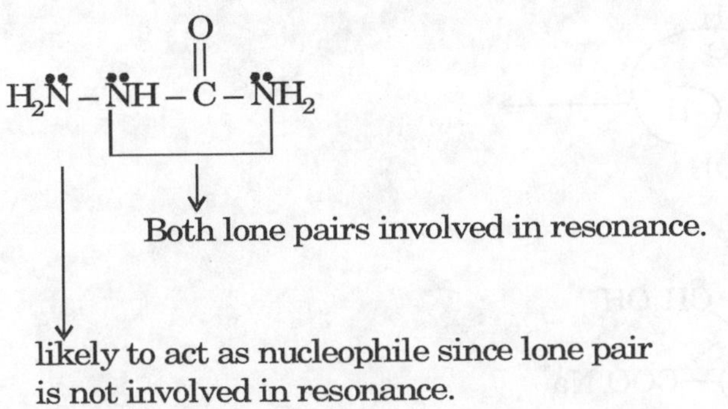

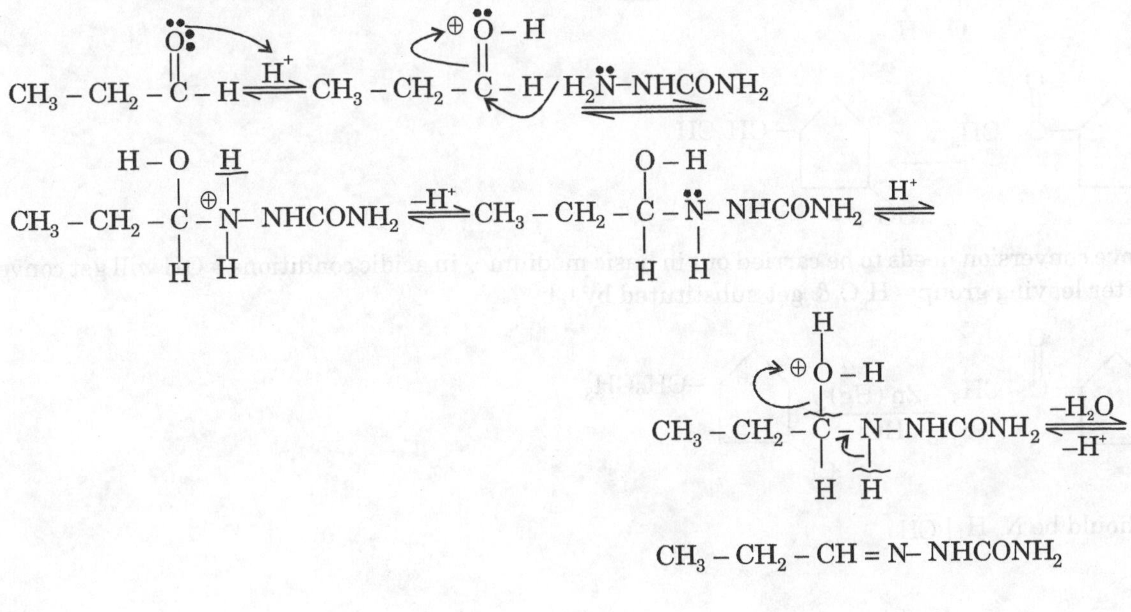

17. 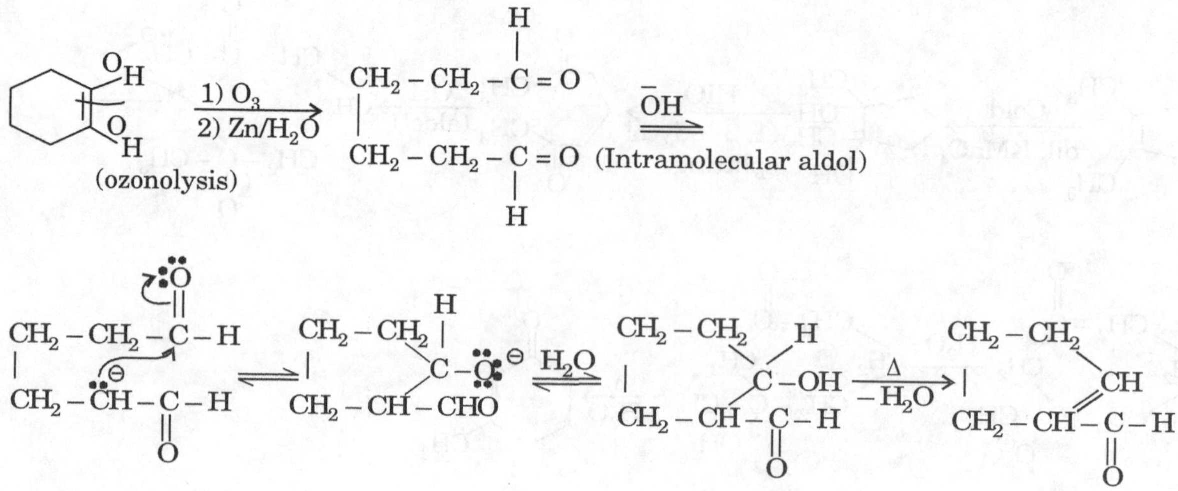

18. 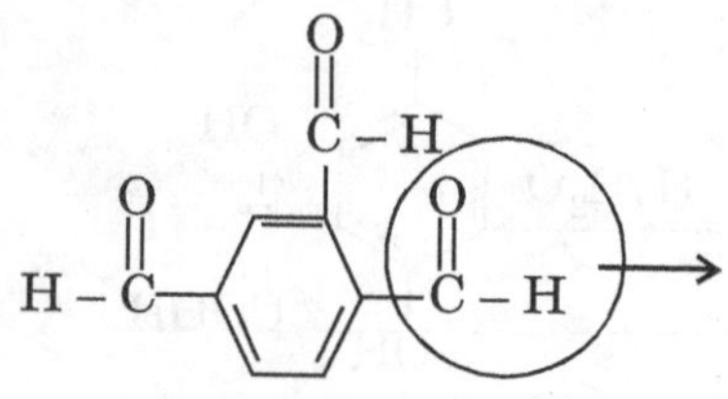

→ Rest, both-CHO are at O, P wrt this – CHO & so, will exert – M/–R, thus facilitating the attack of a nucleophile

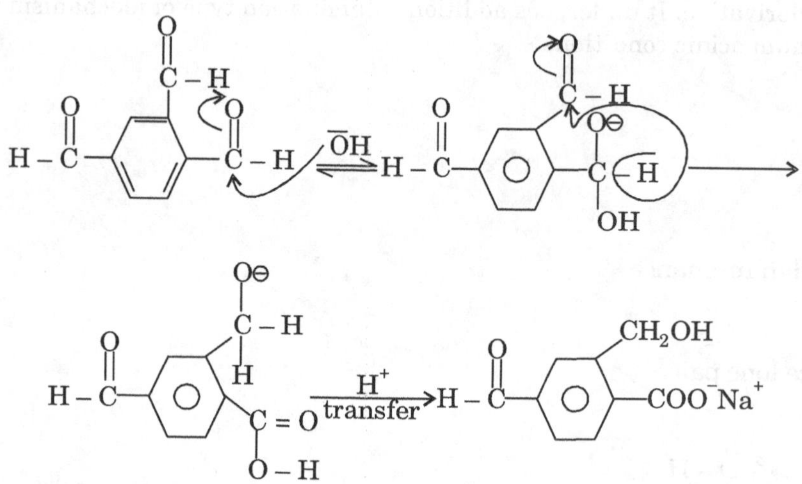

19.

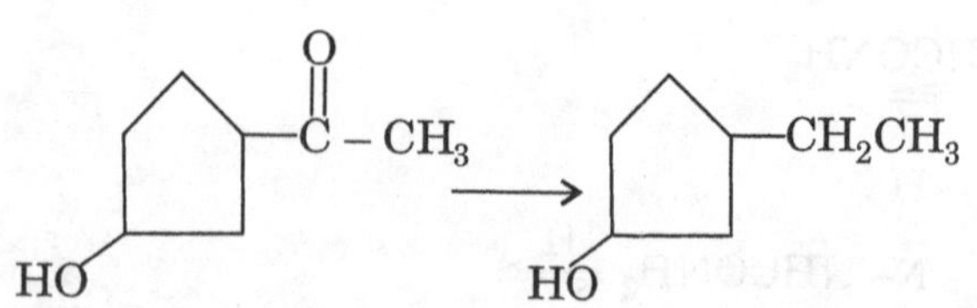

The above conversion needs to be carried out in basic medium ∵ in acidic conditions – OH will get converted to a better leaving group – H_2O & get substituted by Cl^-

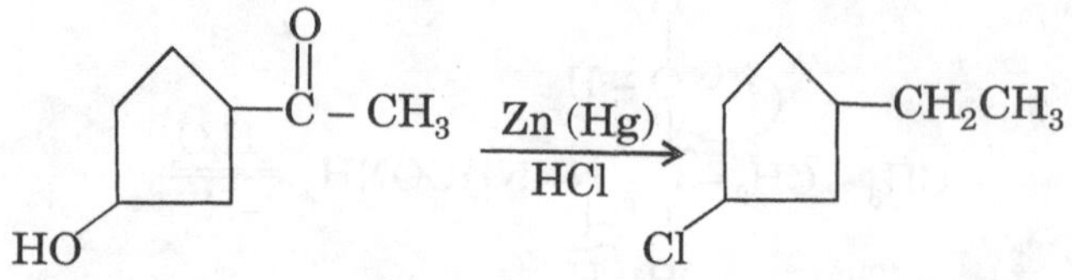

So, X should be $N_2H_4 \mid \overline{O}H$.

Also, for

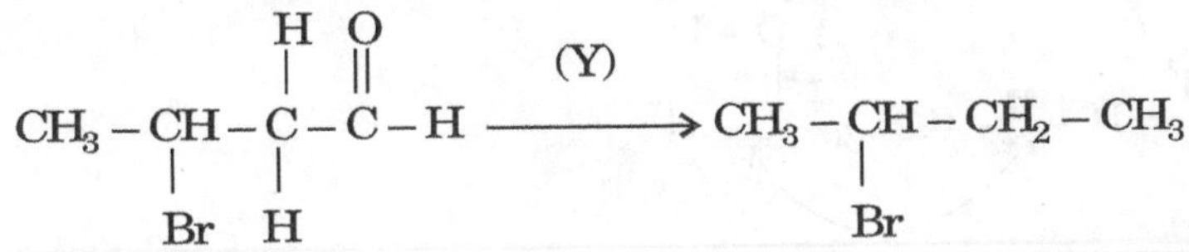

If the above conversion is carried in basic medium (Wolf Kishner's reduction), elimination reaction will occur.

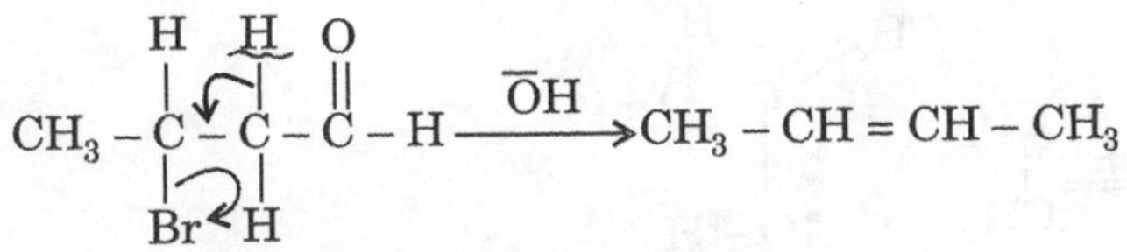

Hence, Y should be acidic medium i.e.

Clemmensen's reduction. (using Zn(Hg)HCl)

20.

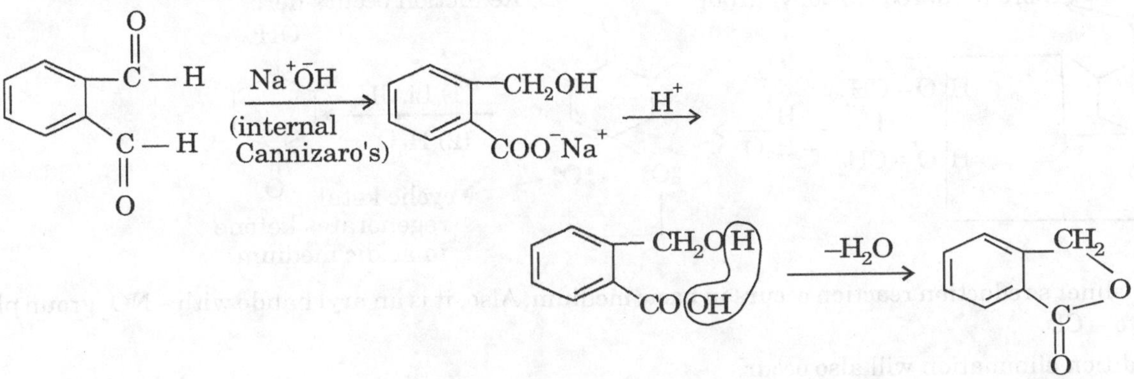

(intramolecular esterification in acidic medium) (Lactone)

21.

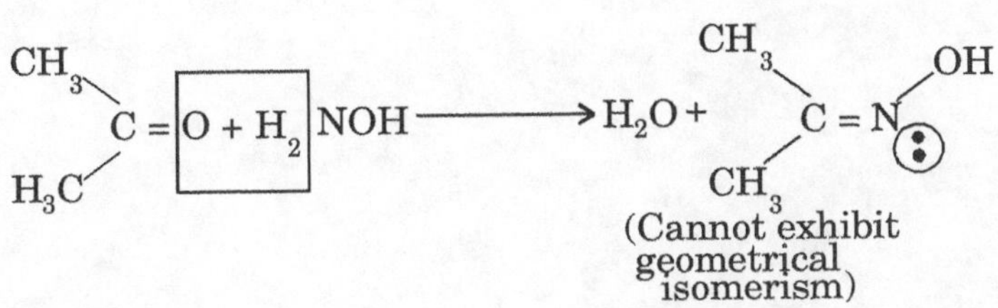

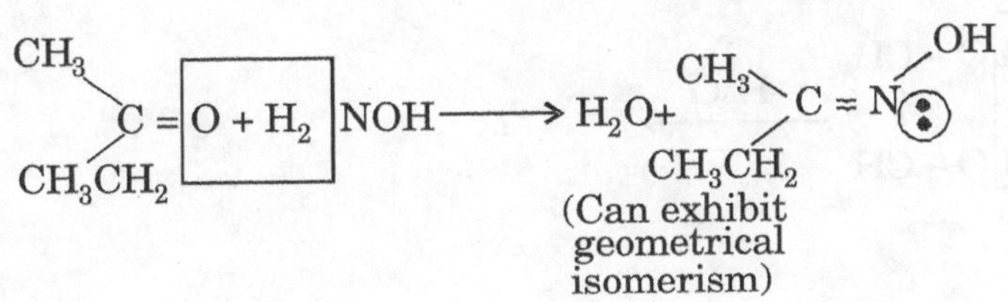

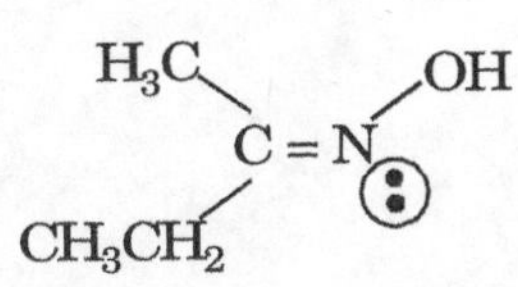

(Syn – methyl ethyl ketoxime)

or

Anti – ethyl methyl ketoxime

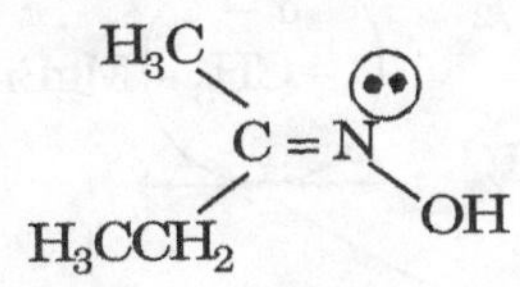

(Syn – ethyl methyl ketoxime)

or

Anti – methyl ethyl ketoxime

22. The given reaction is an example of intramolecular hemi – acetal formation.

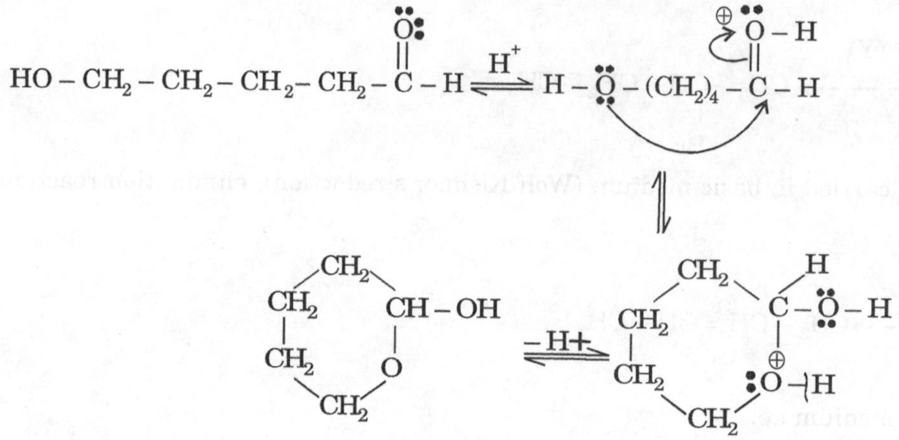

23.

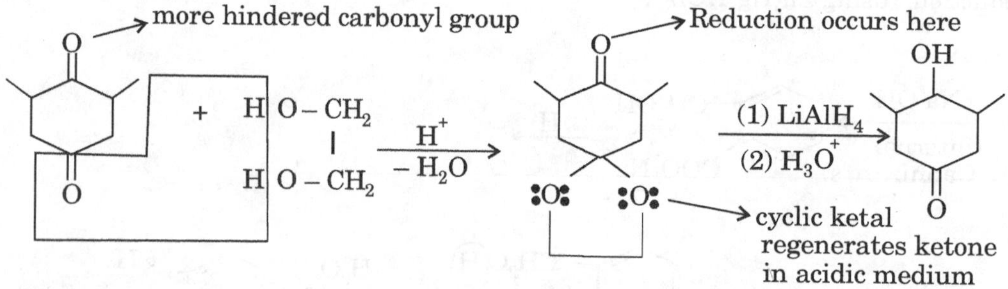

24. Wolf kishner's reduction reaction occurs in basic medium. Also, it is an aryl halide with $-NO_2$ group placed ortho to – Cl.

So, addition elimination will also occur.

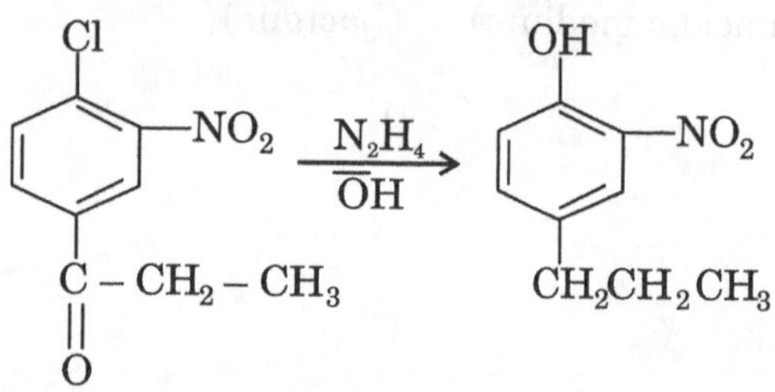

25.

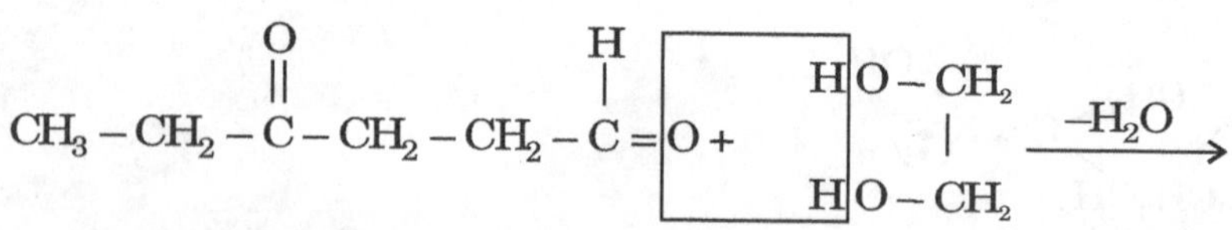

(Aldehydes are more reactive than ketones towards nucleophilic addition)

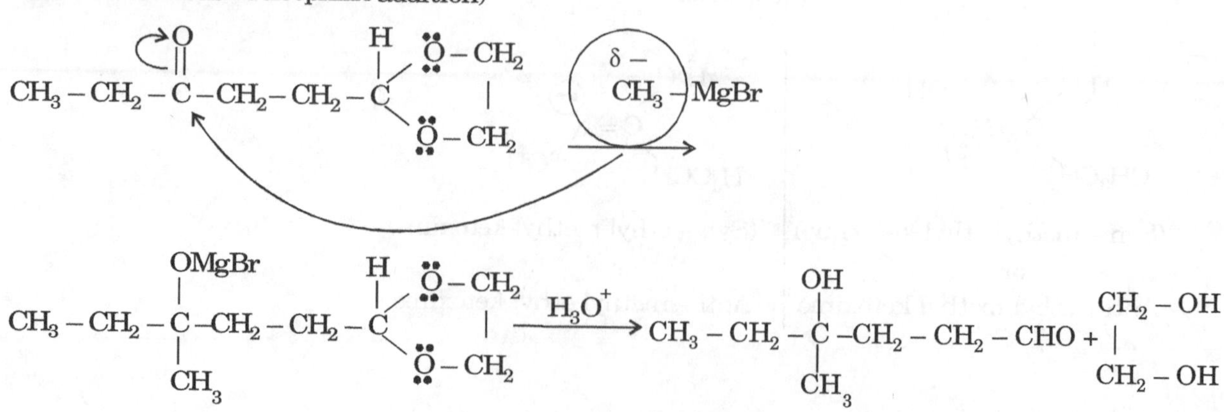

26. Aldehydes & hemi – acetals give +ve tollen's test. Tollens test involves basic medium.

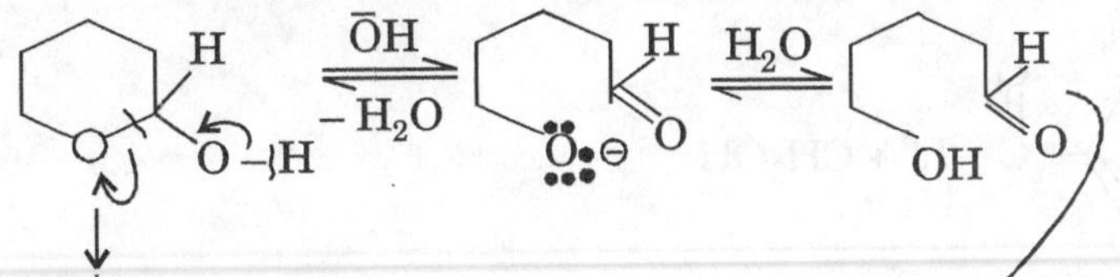

Cyclic hemi – acetal
Option 3 is also a hemi-acetal.

aldehydic group is generated which will give +ve tollen's test.

27. Perform retro aldol in the product Aldols are β – hydroxy aldehyde or β hydroxy ketones.

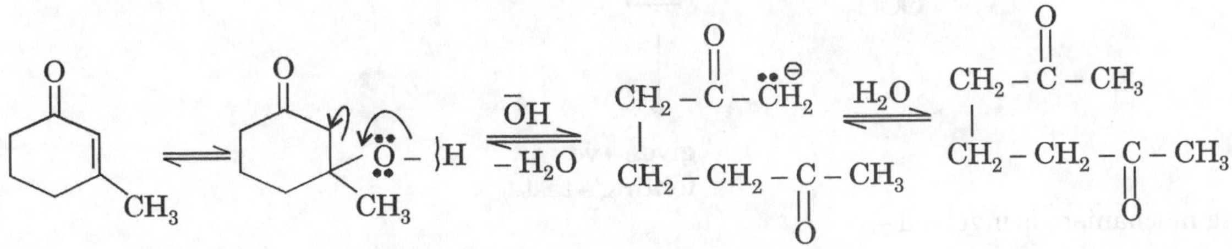

28.

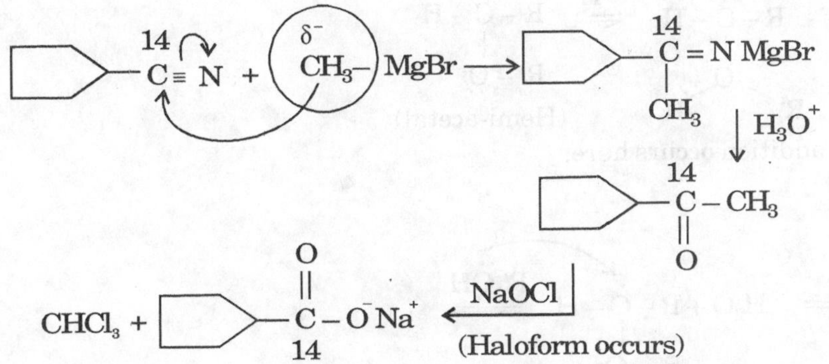

29.

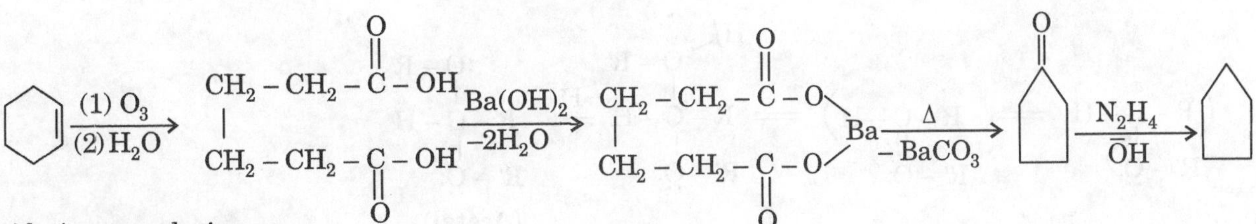

Oxidative ozonolysis occurs due to formation of H_2O_2 & in the absence of Zn)

30.

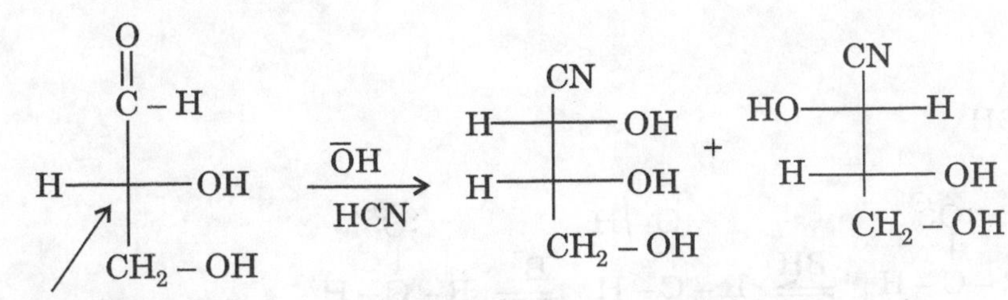

Pre–existing Chiral C

31. Fehlings solution has basic medium.

For option – (a)

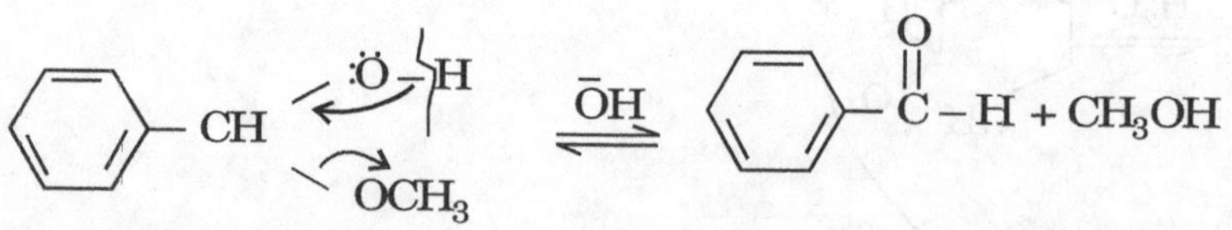

So, reaction is reversed & hemi – acetal again forms benzaldehyde. (which however does not give + ve fehling's test)

For option – (b)

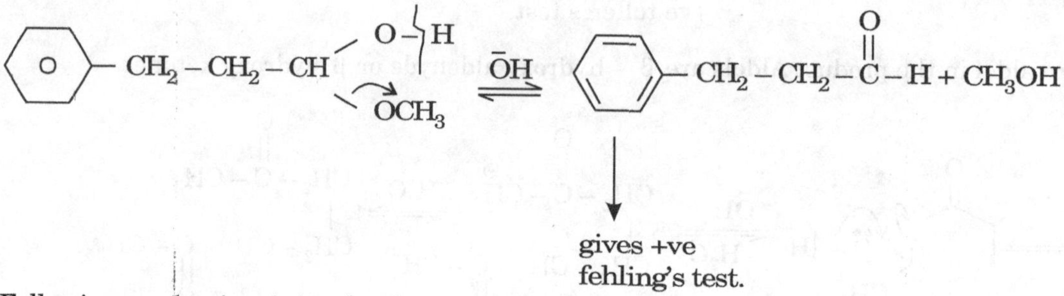

32. Following mechanism is involved –

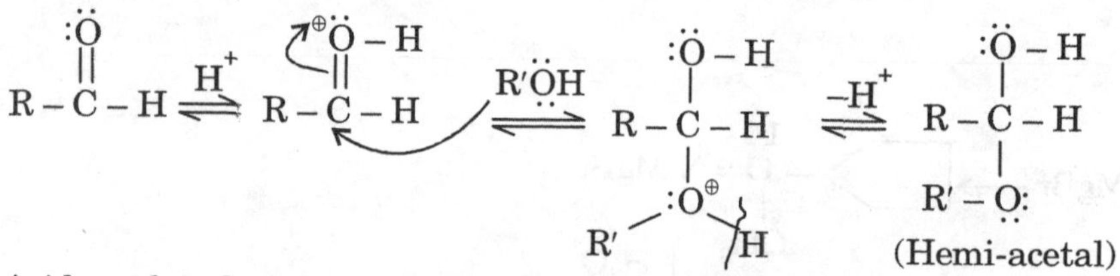

Acid catalysed nucleophilic (R'OH) addition occurs here.

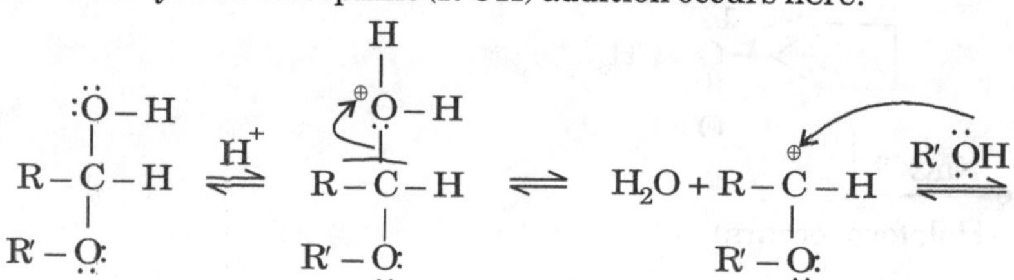

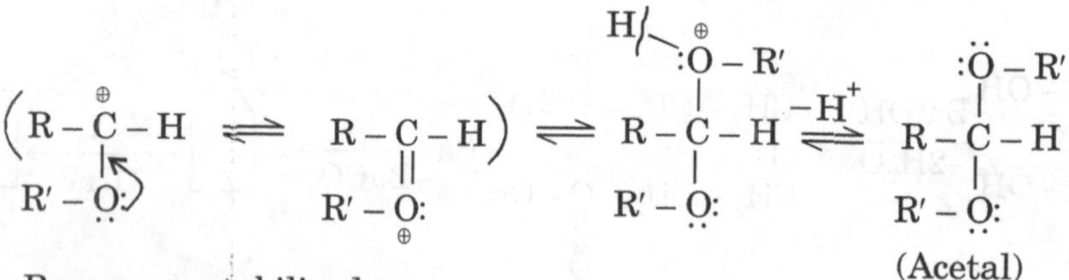

Resonance stabilised

If we attempt base catalysed reaction, then

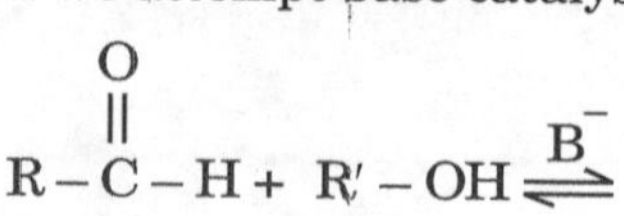

1. $R'-\ddot{O}-H + B^{-} \rightleftharpoons R'\ddot{O}^{\ominus} + BH$

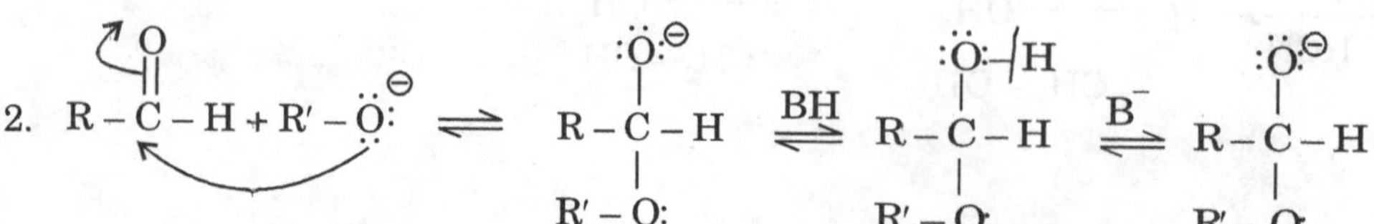

(Hemi-acetal) Now, nothing can happen further

Acidic medium had converted – OH to a good Leaving group ($-H_2O$), after which alcohol (nucleophile) attacked.

But, with base, $\bar{O}H$ can't leave & so, alcohol cannot attack. So, hemi – acetal can't be converted into acetal in basic medium.

33. 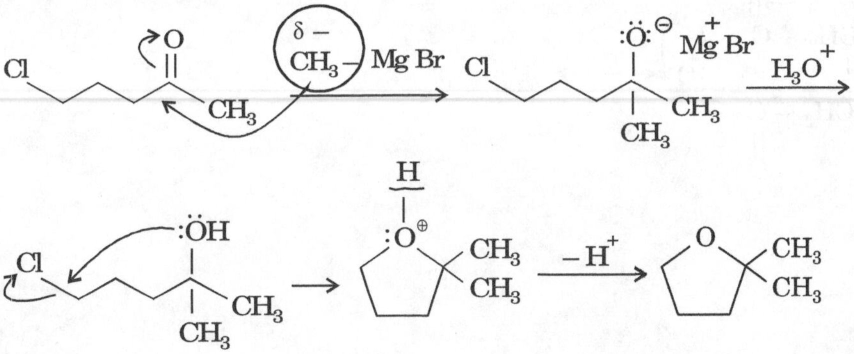

34. 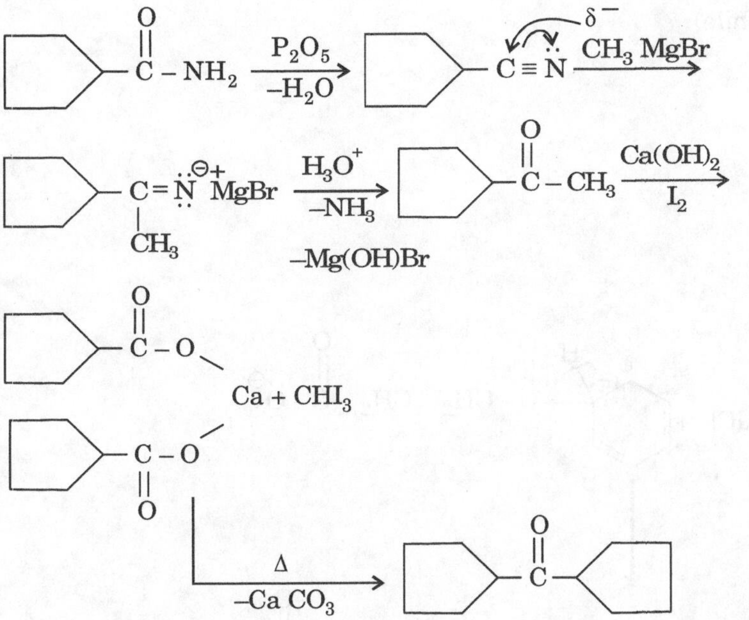

35. 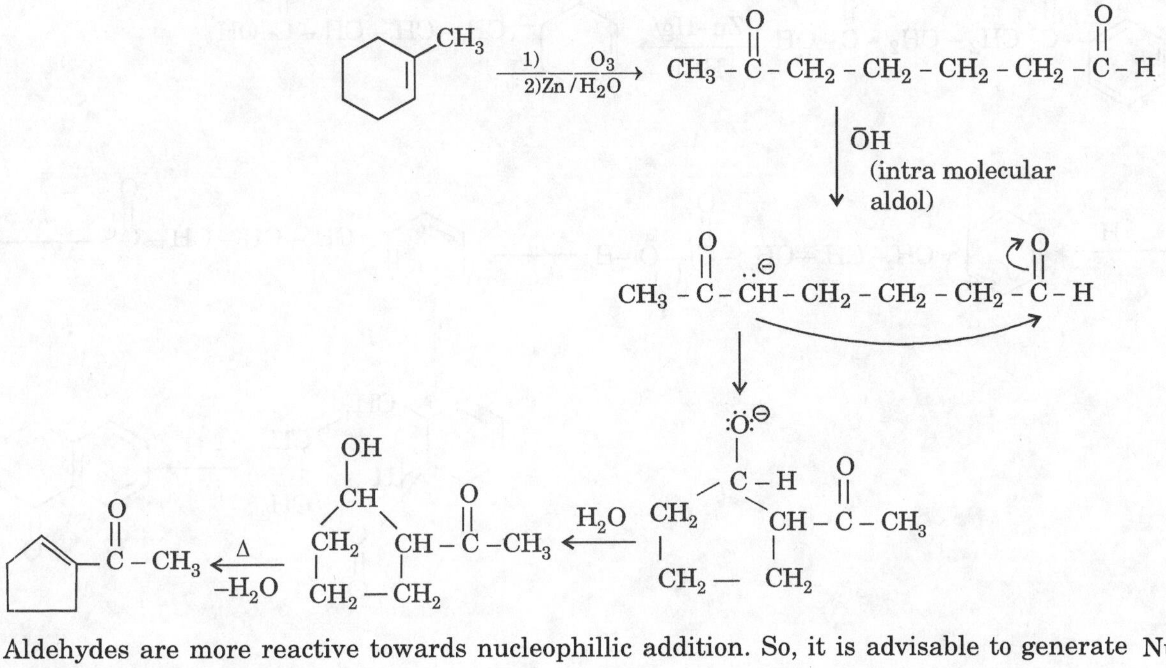

Aldehydes are more reactive towards nucleophillic addition. So, it is advisable to generate $Nu^{\ominus}$ from ketone & perform addition on an aldehyde

36. Benzene undergoes electrophilic substitution reaction with succinic anhydride.

I.

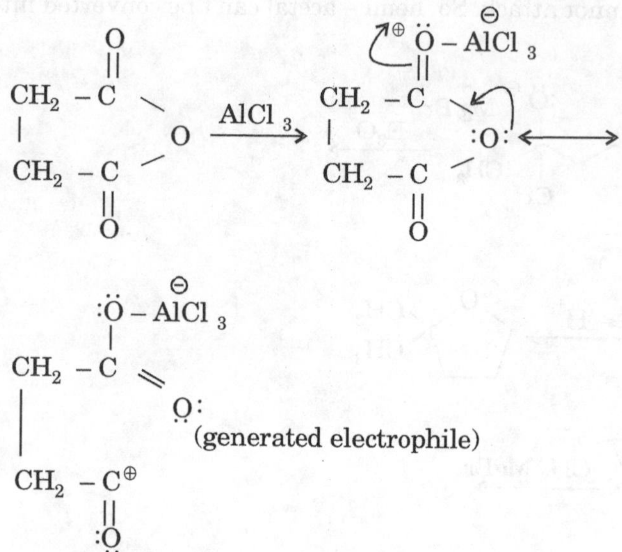

II. Attack on ring

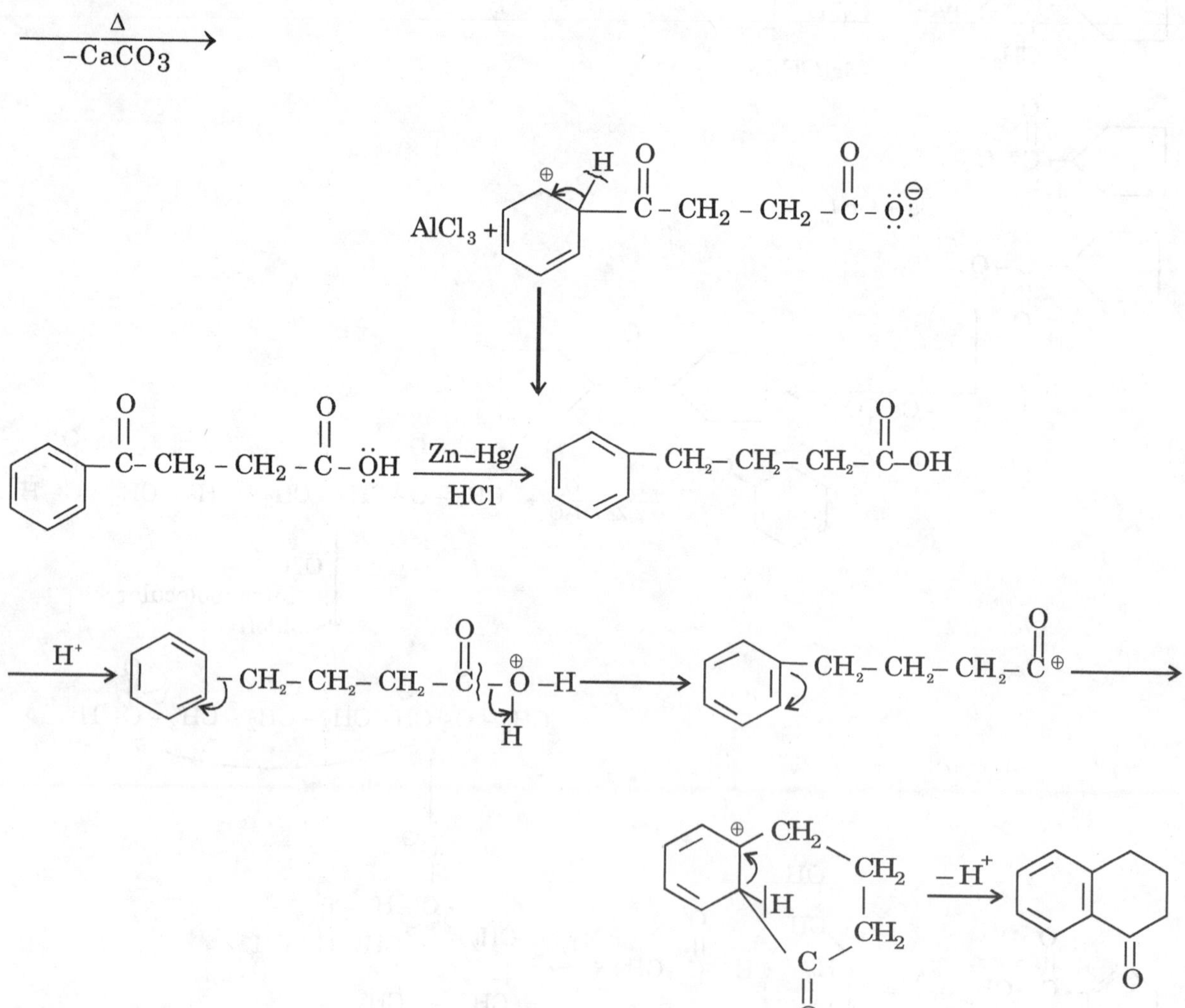

37. 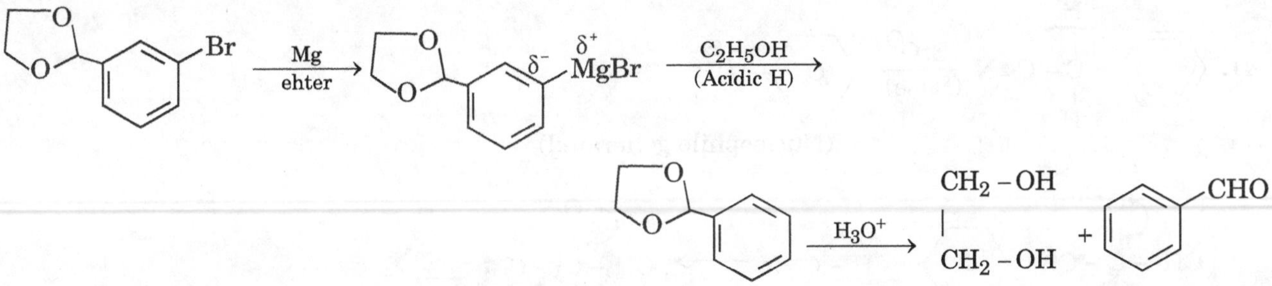

38. 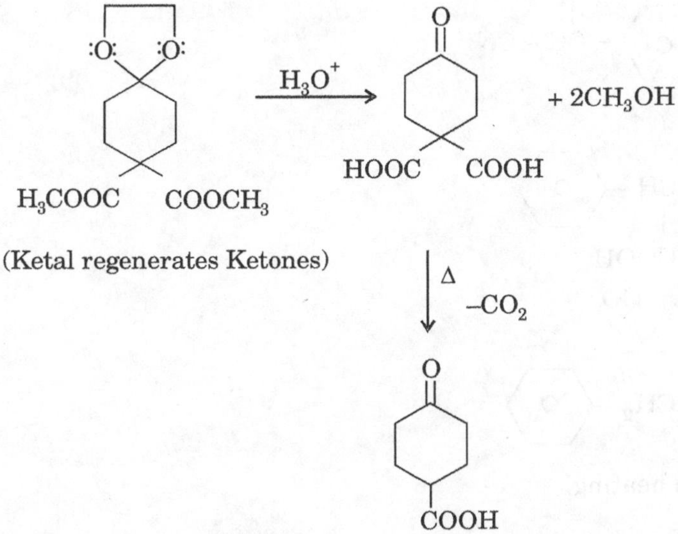

(Ketal regenerates Ketones)

39. 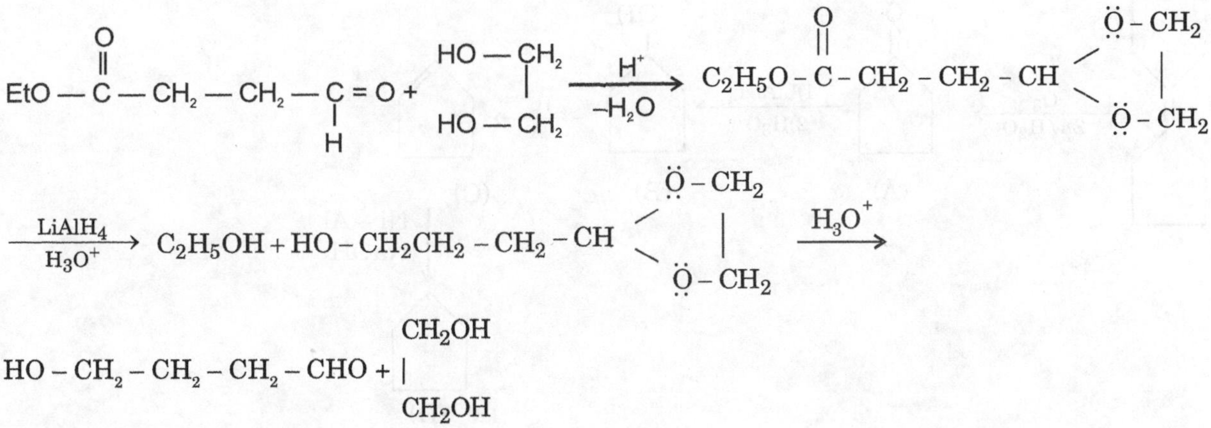

40. 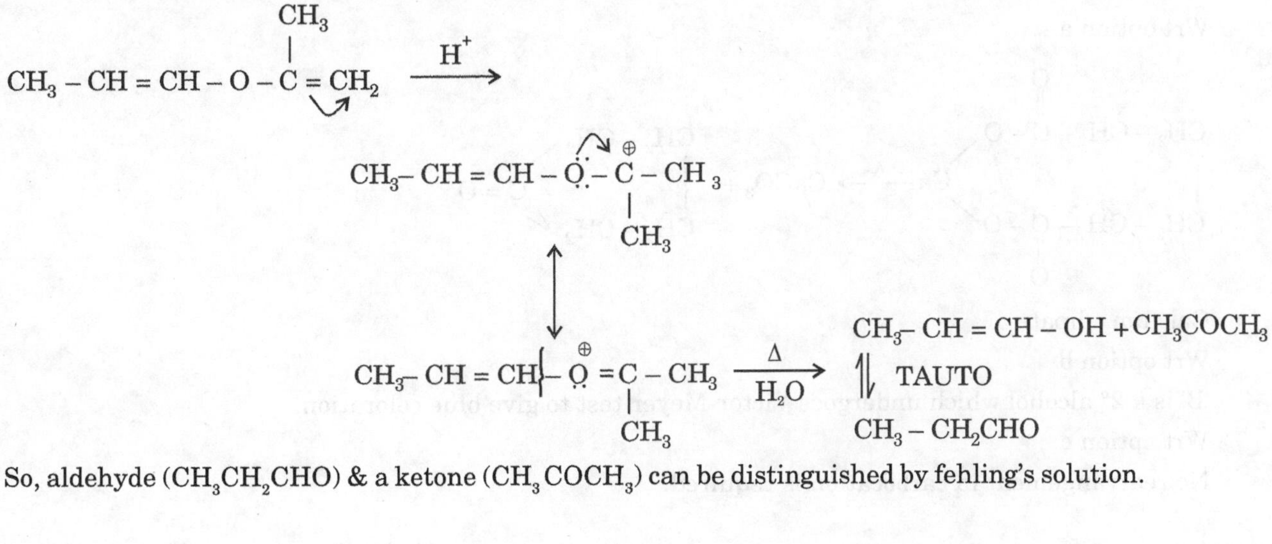

So, aldehyde (CH_3CH_2CHO) & a ketone (CH_3COCH_3) can be distinguished by fehling's solution.

41.

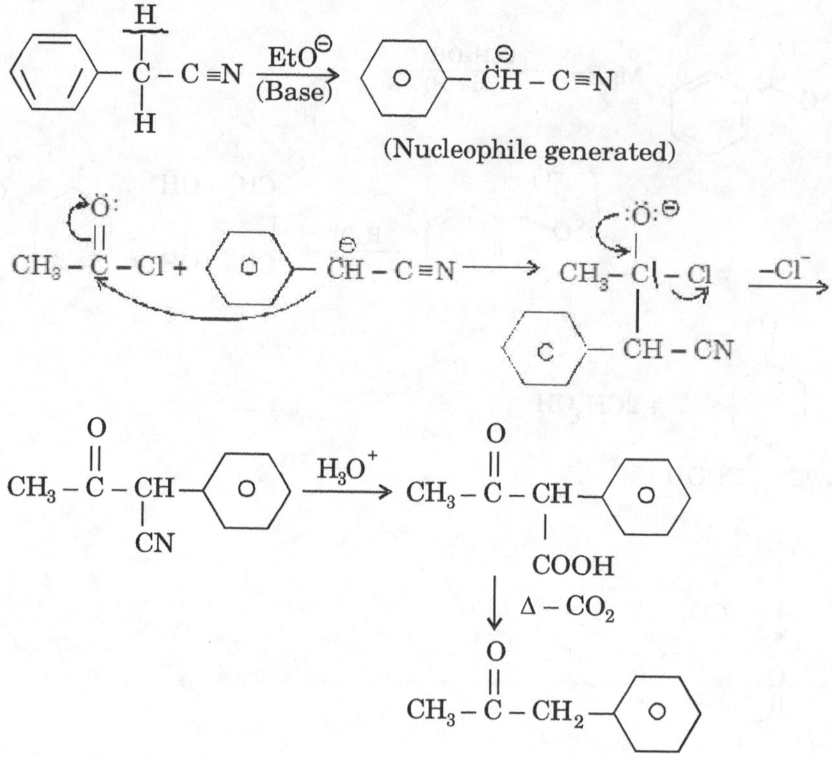

(β - keto acids undergo decarboxylation upon heating)

42.

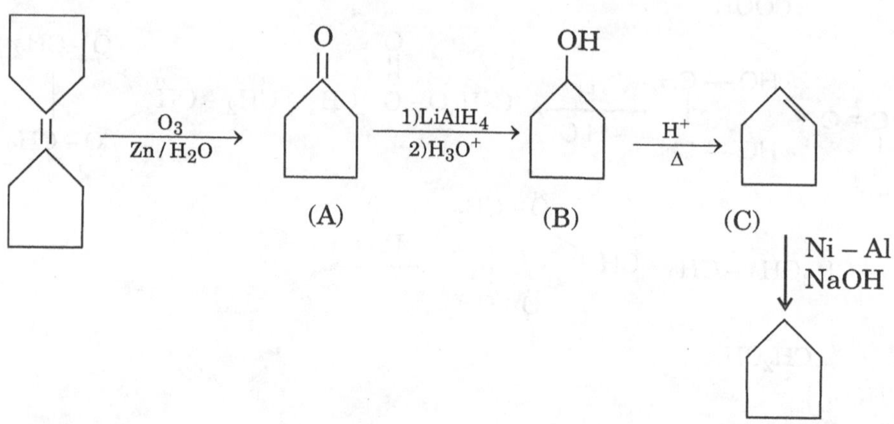

Wrt option a

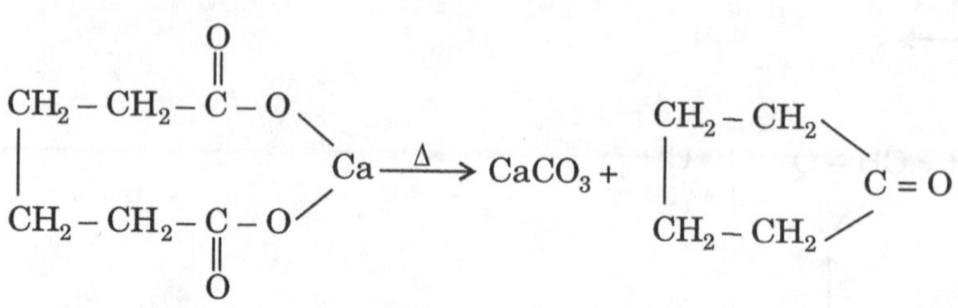

Calcium adipate

Wrt option b

'B' is a 2° alcohol which undergoes Victor-Meyer test to give blue coloration.

Wrt option c

No rearrangement in carbocation is required.

43. 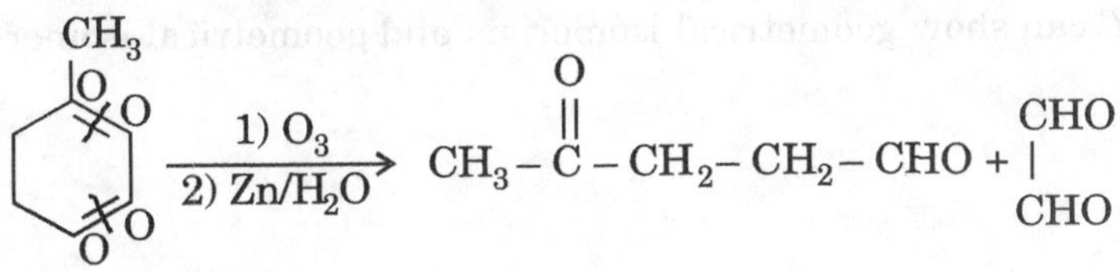

44. Wrt option a

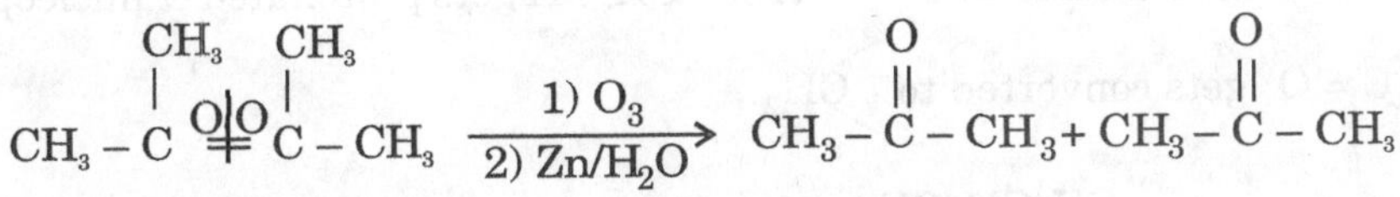

wrt option b

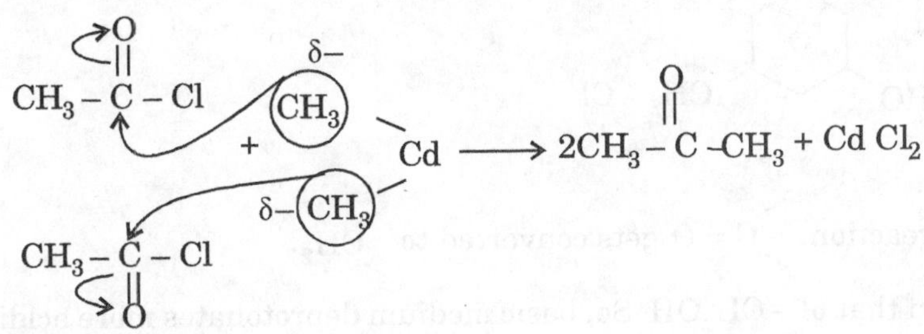

(Acyl Nuc. Sub.)

45. 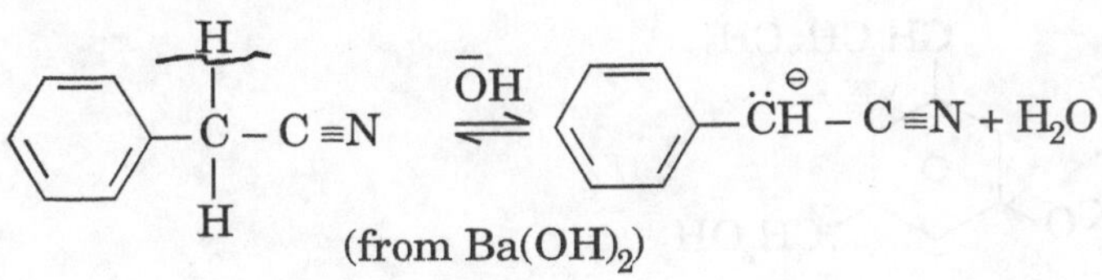

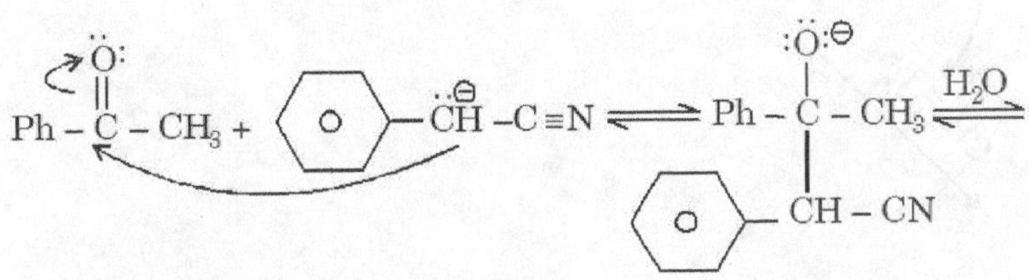

(Nucleophilic addition on ketone)

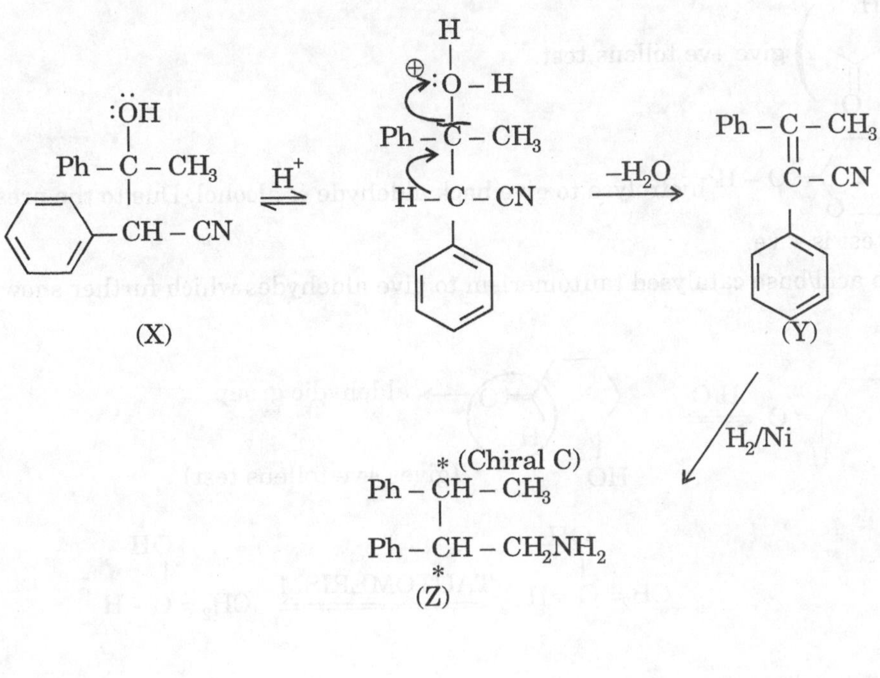

Now, 'Y' is NOT a saturated compound. 'Y' can show geometrical isomerism and geometrical isomers are diastereomers.

'Y' has No chiral C's.

'Z' has chiral C's.

46. Consider path – I

It is Clemmenson's reduction. Since, the medium is acidic – OH of – CH_2OH gets protonated & nucleophilic substitution results. Besides, $>C=O$ gets converted to $>CH_2$.

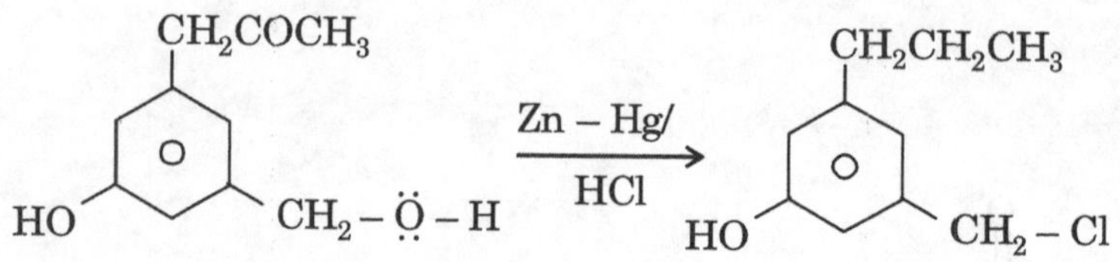

Consider path – II

Path – II is Wolf Kishner's reduction reaction. $>C=O$ gets converted to $>CH_2$.

Also, –OH of phenol is more acidic than that of – CH_2OH. So, basic medium deprotonates more acidic H & then nucleophilic substitution results.

(c) 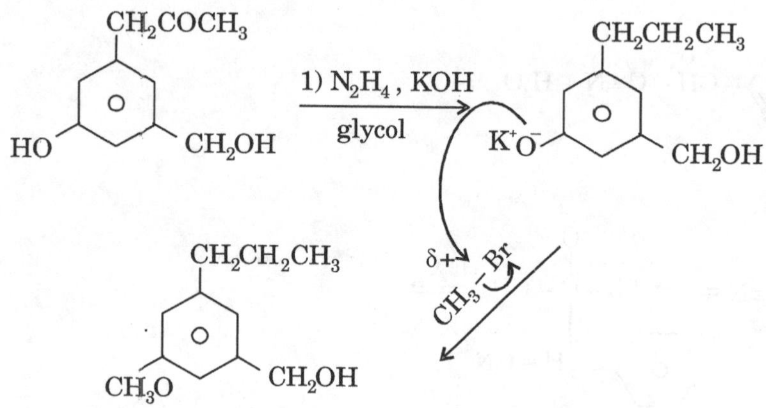

48. α – hydroxy ketones 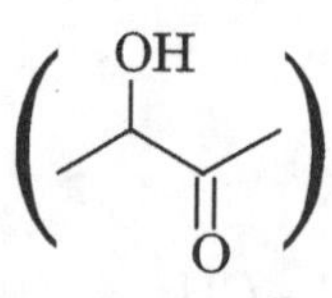 give +ve tollens test.

Also, hemi – acetals like 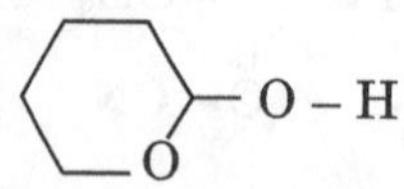 hydrolyse to give back aldehyde & alcohol. Due to the presence of aldehydic group, tollens test is + ve.

Also, vinyl alcohols undergo acid/base catalysed tautomerism to give aldehydes which further show + ve tollens test.

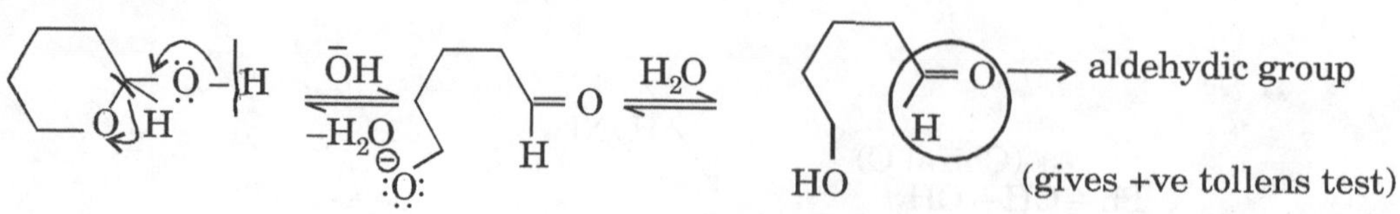

$$CH_2=\overset{OH}{\overset{|}{C}}-H \xrightleftharpoons{\text{TAUTOMERISM}} CH_2=\overset{OH}{\overset{|}{C}}-H$$

49. 'X' is HCHO. On getting oxidised, it gives Y(HCOOH) which gives tollen's test positive.

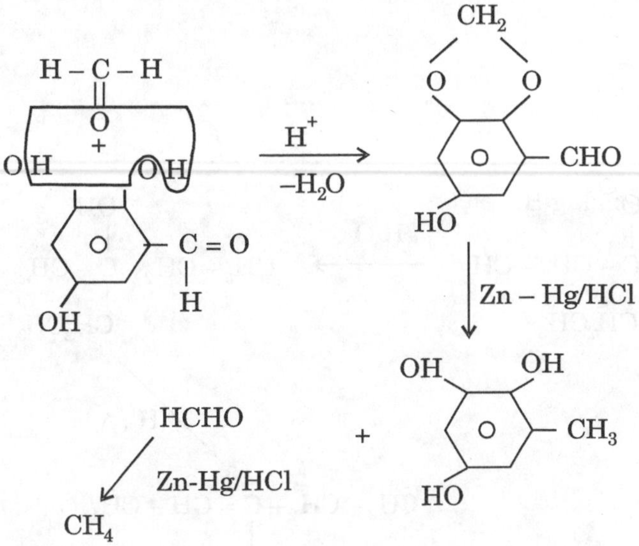

50. $Ph-CH_2-\overset{O}{\overset{||}{C}}-CH_3 + Cl_2 \xrightarrow{Ca(OH)_2} CHCl_3 + (Ph-CH_2-\overset{O}{\overset{||}{C}}-O)_2Ca \xrightarrow[-CaCO_3]{\Delta}$

(Haloform reaction)

$\underset{(P)}{CHCl_3} + \underset{(Q)}{(Ph-CH_2-\overset{O}{\overset{||}{C}}-O)_2Ca} \xrightarrow[-CaCO_3]{\Delta} \underset{(R)}{Ph-CH_2-\overset{O}{\overset{||}{C}}-CH_2-Ph}$

$\xrightarrow{HCN} \underset{(S)}{Ph-CH_2-\overset{OH}{\underset{CN}{C}}-CH_2-Ph}$

$H \rightarrow C(\rightarrow Cl)_3$ has an acidic H.

'R' is a symmetrical ketone.

'S' lacks a chiral C. So, no racemic mixture is formed.

51. Alkene $\xrightarrow[2)Zn/H_2O]{1)O_3} CH_3CH_2-\underset{CH_2CH_3}{C}=O + O=\underset{H}{C}-CH_3$

Alkene was $\longrightarrow CH_3CH_2-\underset{CH_2CH_3}{C}=CH-CH_3$

Alcohol was either

$CH_3-CH_2-\overset{OH}{\underset{CH_2-CH_3}{C}}-CH_2-CH_3$ OR $CH_3-CH_2-\overset{H}{\underset{CH_2CH_3}{C}}-\overset{OH}{\underset{H}{C}}-CH_3$

So, diethyl ketone could be the answer.

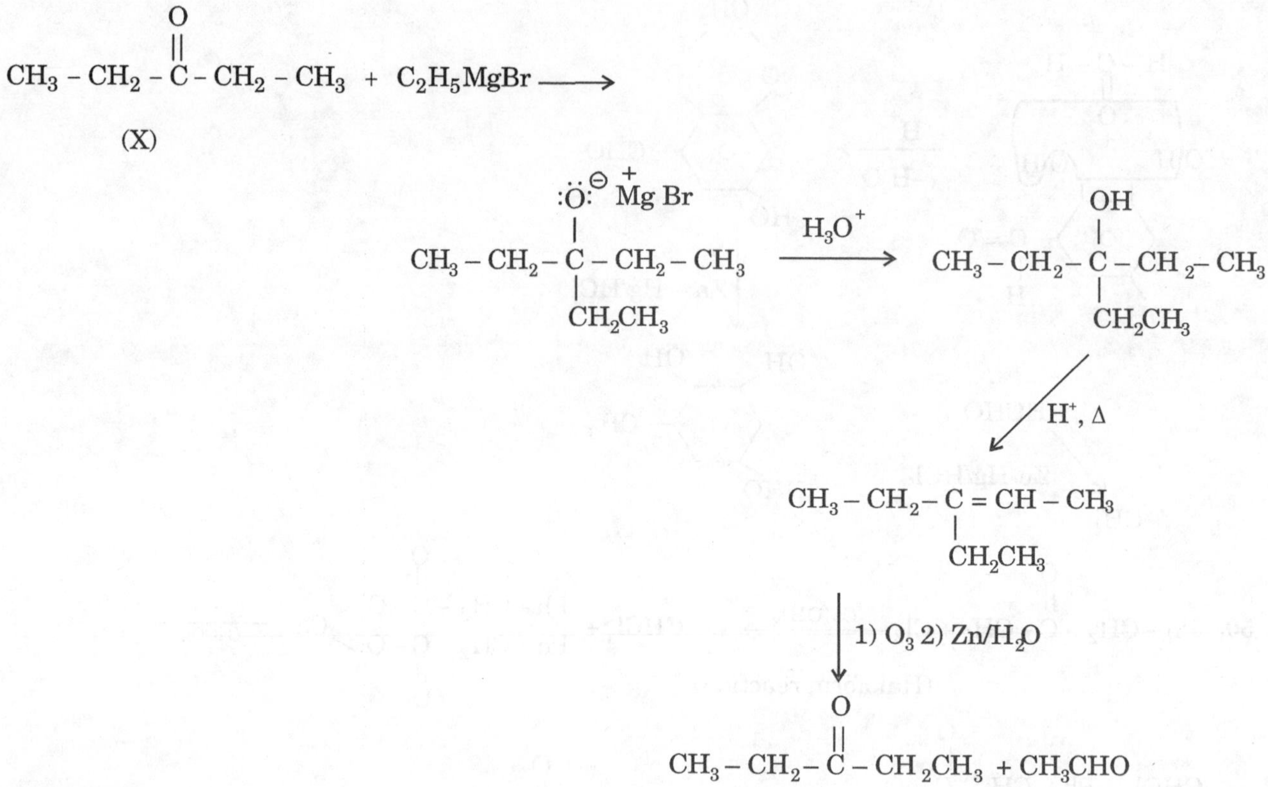

52. Wrt option a

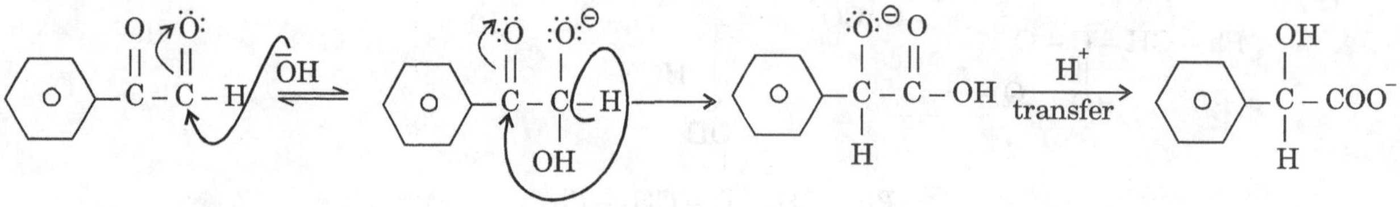

Wrt option b

In presence of a strong base, nucleophilic substitution occurs.

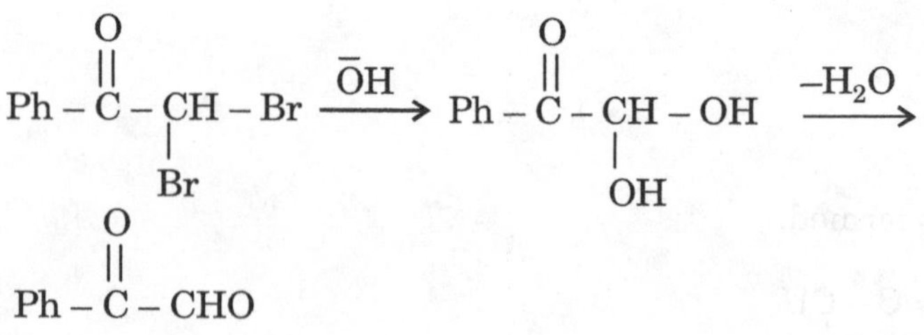

(Which can undergo internal Cannizaro)

Wrt option c

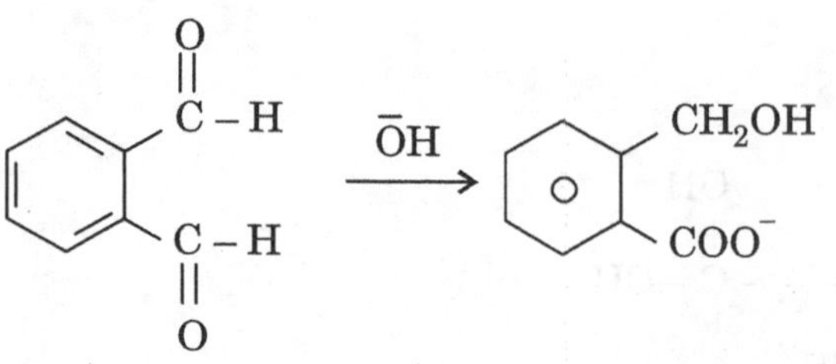

53. 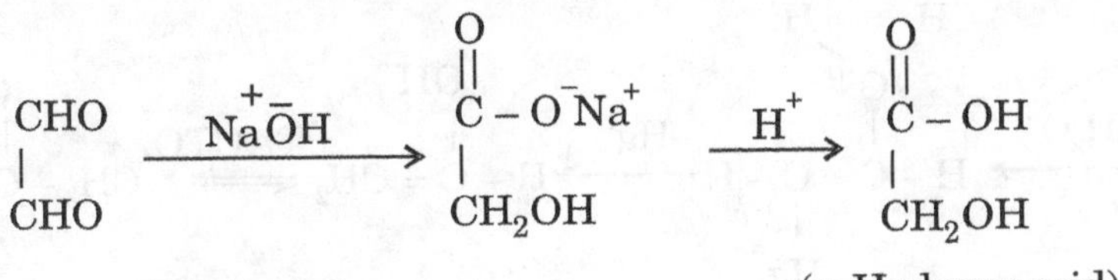

(Cannizaro's reaction) (α-Hydroxy acid)

α – Hydroxy acids on being heated undergo intermolecular esterification.

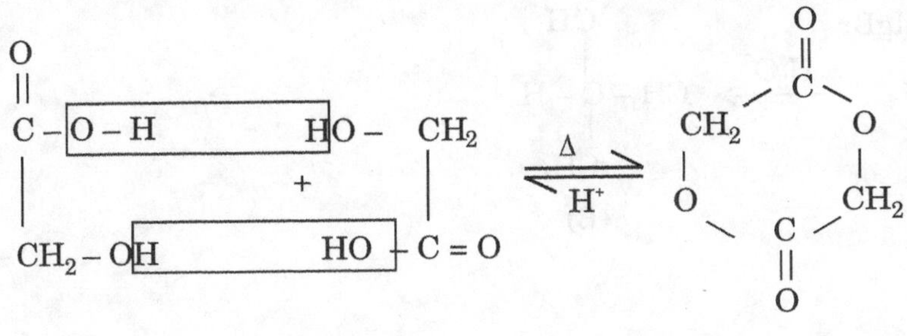

54. 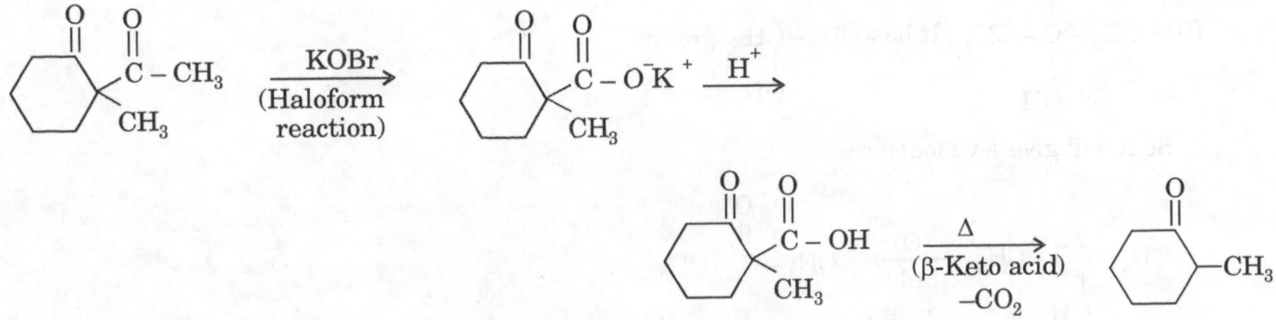

55. 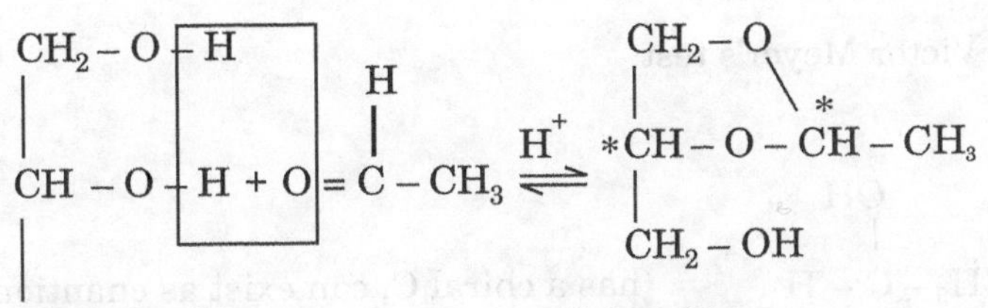

* – Chiral C's

(Two chiral C's)

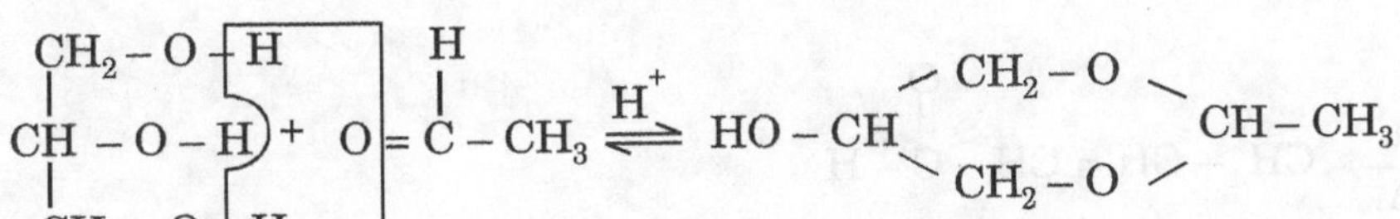

(Stereomers = 2)

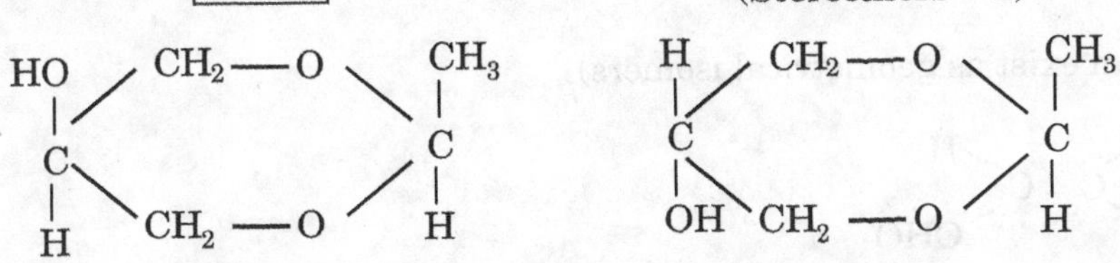

Cis form Trans form

56. $NaBD_4$ will give D^-

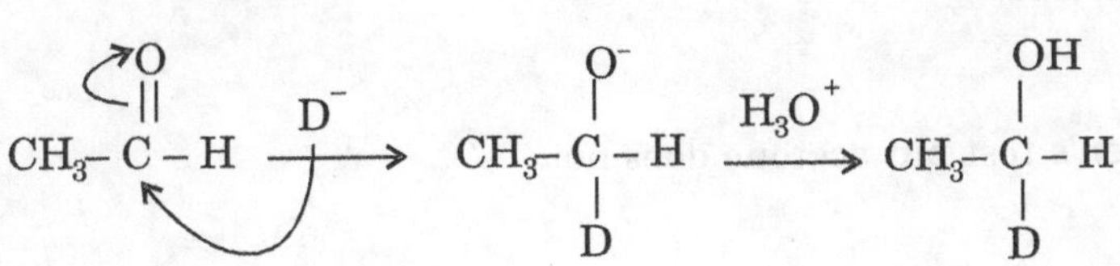

57.

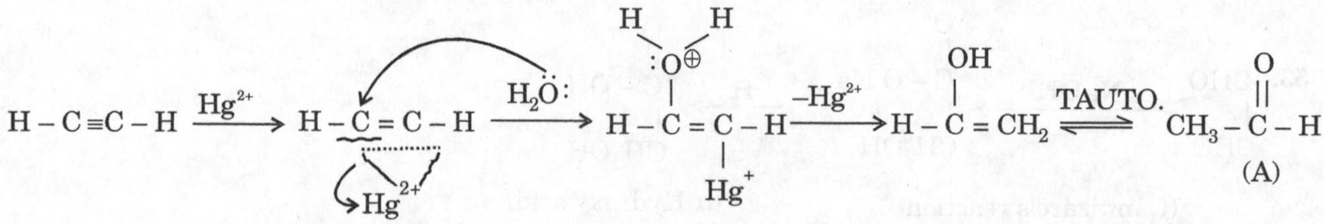

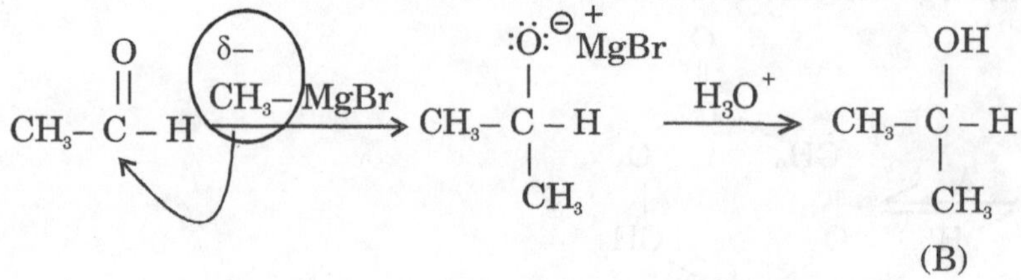

(B) is $CH_3-\underset{OH}{\overset{H}{C}}-CH_3$. It has $CH_3-\underset{OH}{CH}-$ group

So it will give + ve iodoform.

$$CH_3-\underset{OH}{CH}-CH_3 \xrightarrow[\text{Mild oxdn.,}]{(O)} CH_3-\overset{O}{\overset{\|}{C}}-CH_3 \text{ (Symmetrical Ketone)}$$

(B) is a 2° alcohol, will NOT give red color in Victor Meyer's test.

Also,

$$CH_3-\overset{O}{\overset{\|}{C}}-H + \underset{\text{(Alcohol occurs)}}{CH_3-\overset{O}{\overset{\|}{C}}-H} \xrightarrow[Na^+\bar{O}H]{\text{dil.}} CH_3-\overset{OH}{\overset{|}{\underset{*}{C}}}-H \quad (CH_2-\overset{O}{\overset{\|}{C}}-H \text{ on } C^*)$$

(has a chiral C, can exist as enantiomers)

$$\text{(C) } CH_3-\underset{H}{\overset{OH}{C}}-CH_2-\overset{O}{\overset{\|}{C}}-H \xrightarrow[\Delta]{H^+} CH_3-CH=CH-\overset{O}{\overset{\|}{C}}-H$$

(Can exist as geometrical isomers)

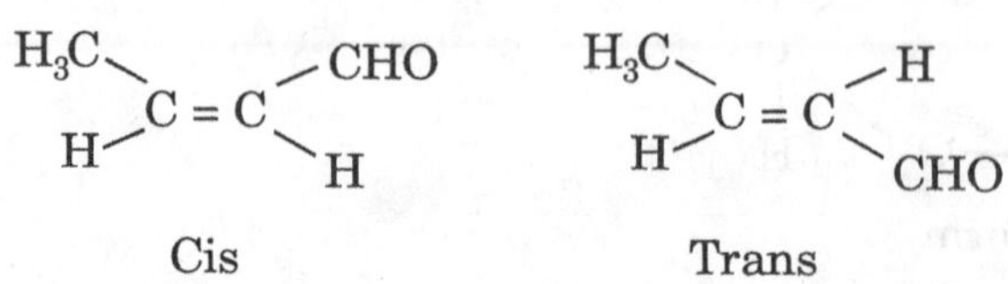

Cis Trans

Geometrical isomers are also diastereomers.

58. $CH_3-\overset{O}{\overset{\|}{C}}-H$ (acetaldehyde) gives + ve tollen's test but acetone does not.

59. Wrt option (a)

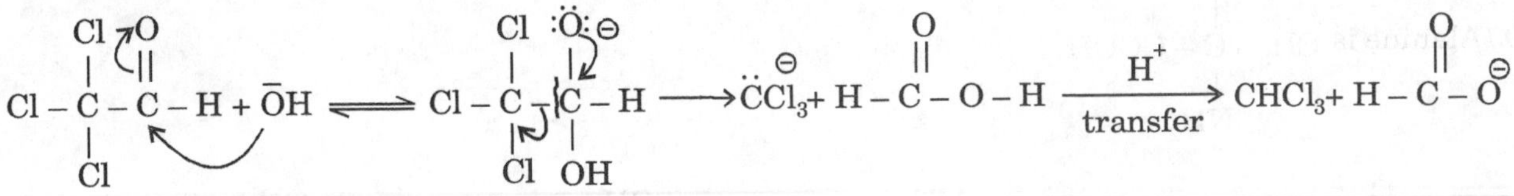

($\overset{\ominus}{\ddot{C}}Cl_3$ is a much better leaving group, so leaves readily)

Wrt option (b)

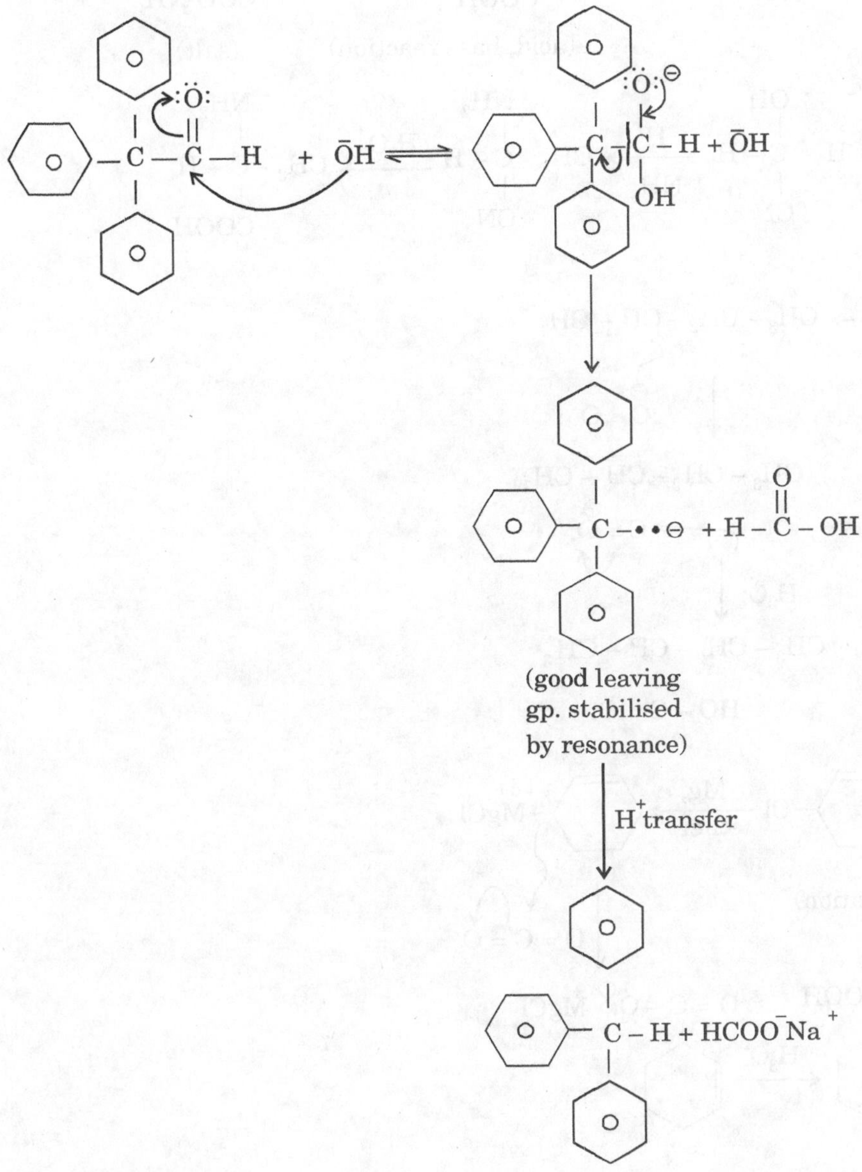

Wrt option – (c)

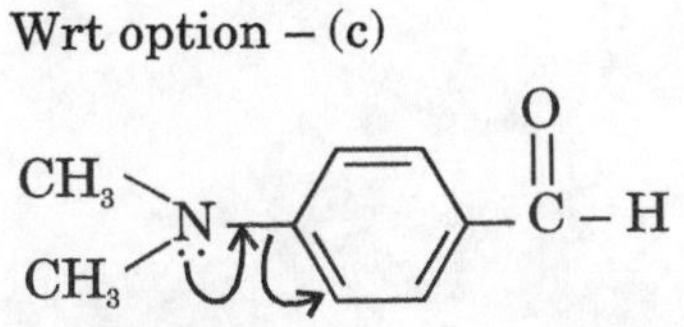

(strong e– donating tendency of $(CH_3)_2$ N decreases the electrophilicity of >C=O 'C' there by decreasing the probability of attack by a nucleophile)

60. Alanine is $CH_3-\underset{NH_2}{\overset{H}{C}}-COOH$

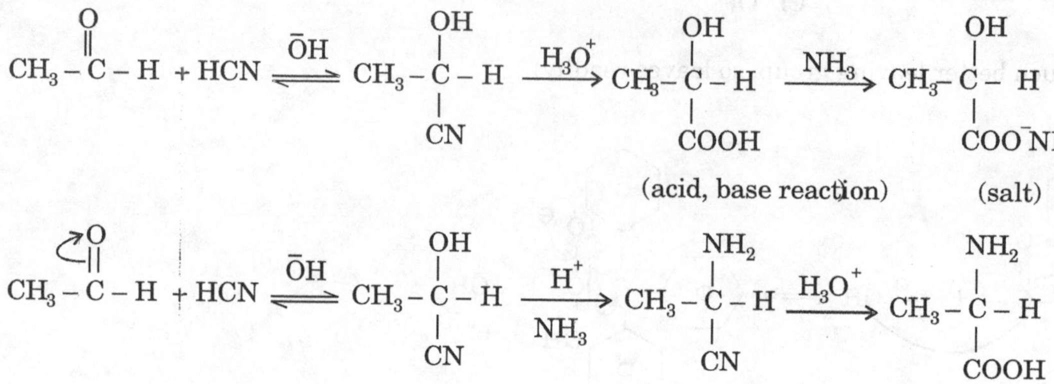

61.

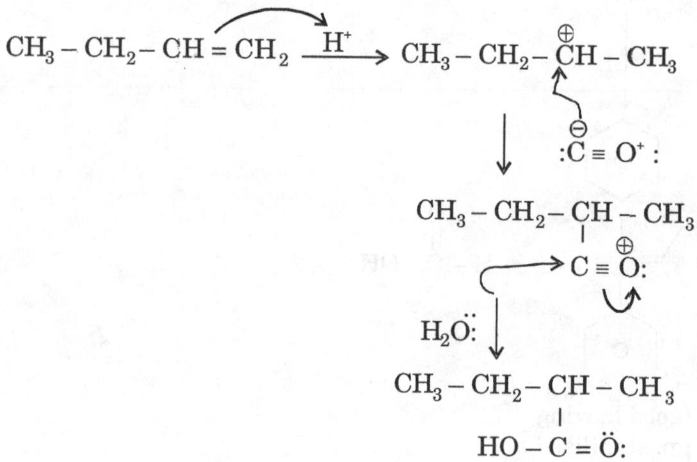

62.

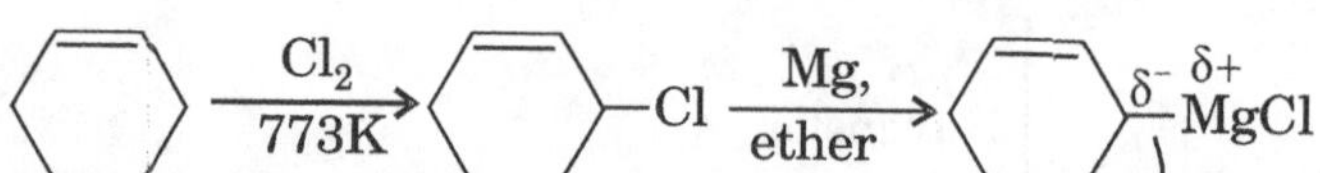

(high T favors allylic halogenation) via formation of free radical)

63.

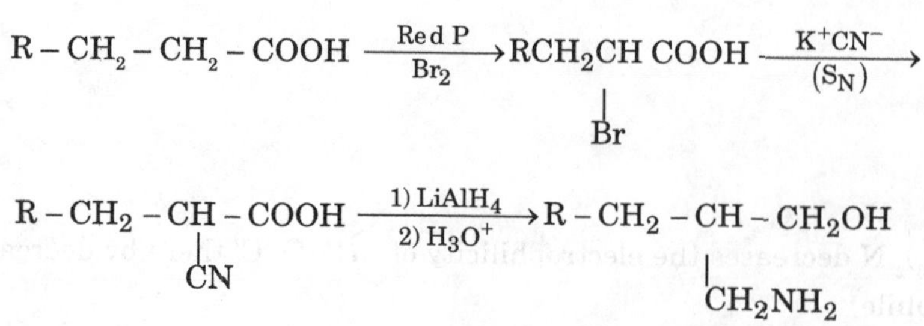

64. Due to greater stability of ter-butyl carbocation, mechanism of acidic hydrolysis followed is acyl S_N1.

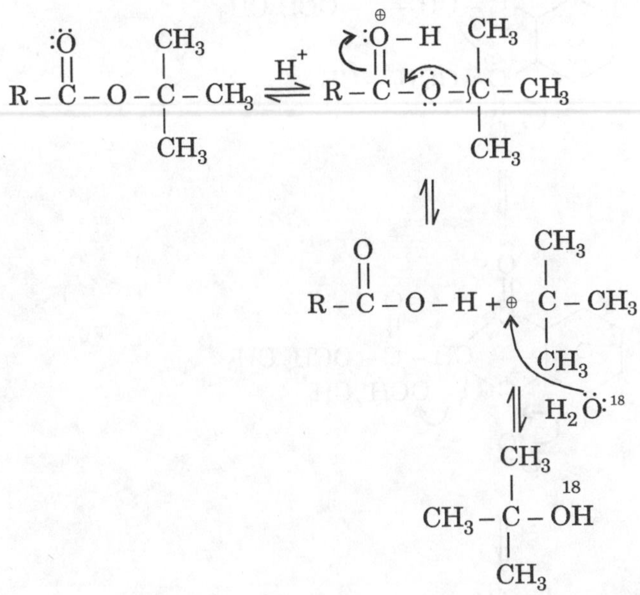

65. Option (c) lacks α – H. So, will not give HVZ Reaction.

66.

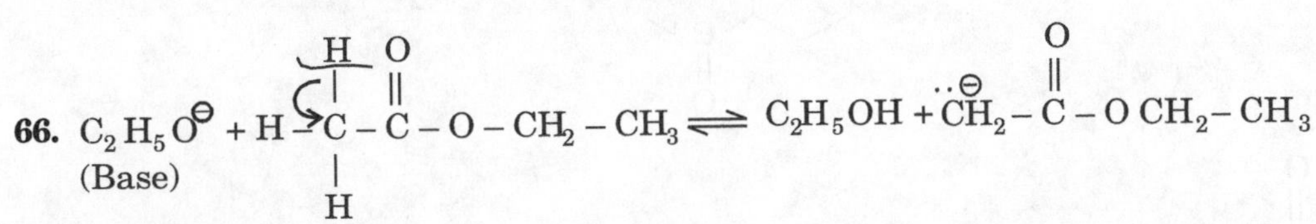

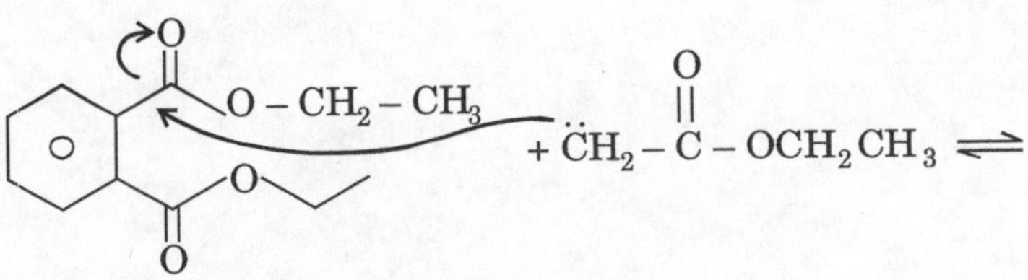

(Acyl $Nu^{\ominus}$ sub. on Ester)

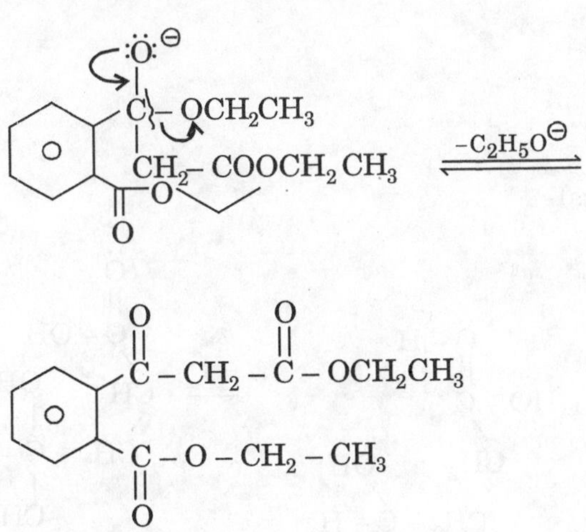

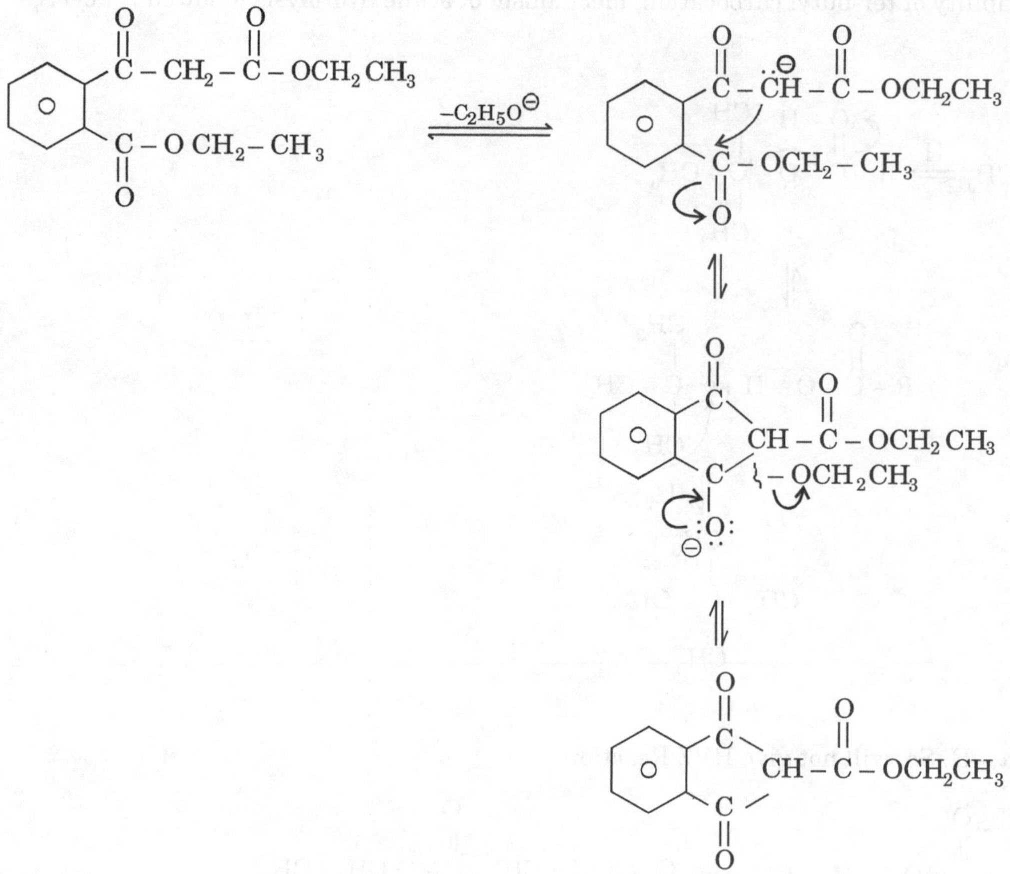

67.

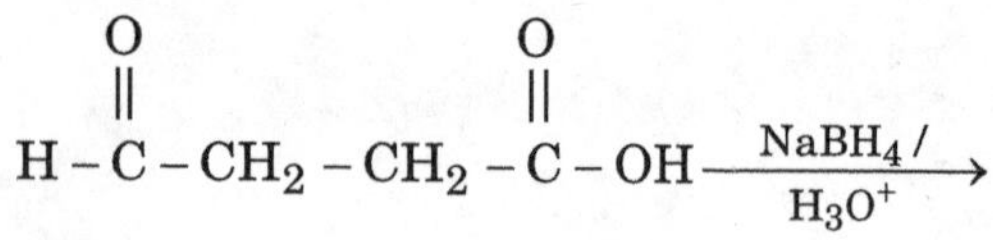

[$NaBH_4$ does not reduce C.acid)

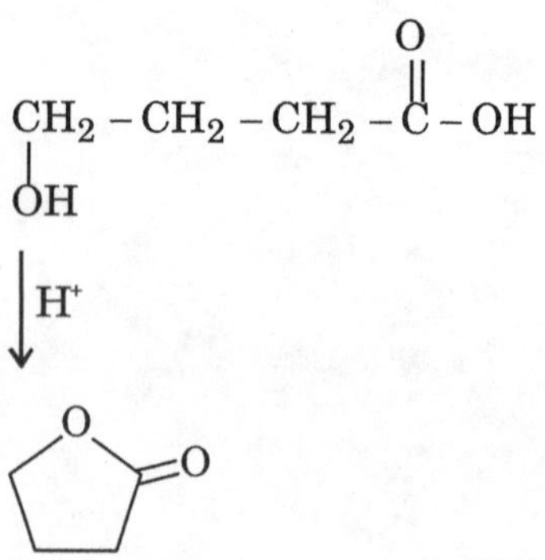

(Lactone formation i.e intramolecular esterification occurs)

68.

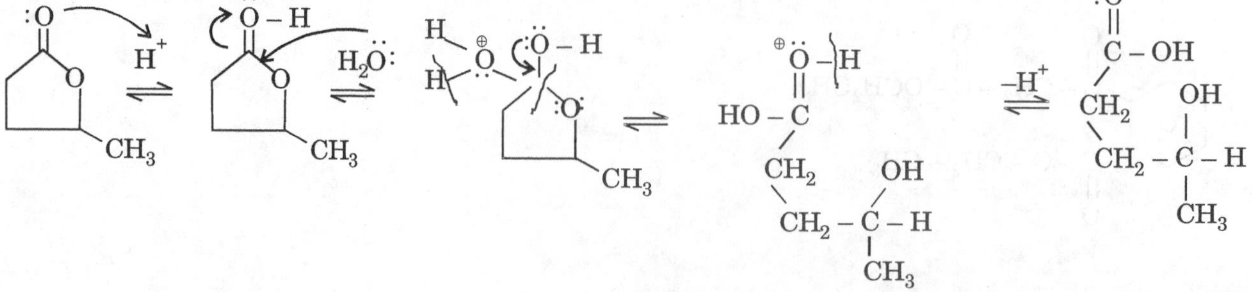

69. Gem dicarboxylic acids & β-Keto acids undergo decarboxylation upon heating.

70. α-hydroxy acids $\xrightarrow{\Delta}$ Intermolecular esterification

β-hydroxy acids $\xrightarrow[-H_2O]{\Delta}$ α, β - unsaturated acids

γ-hydroxy acids $\xrightarrow{\Delta}$ Intramolecular esterification.

71.

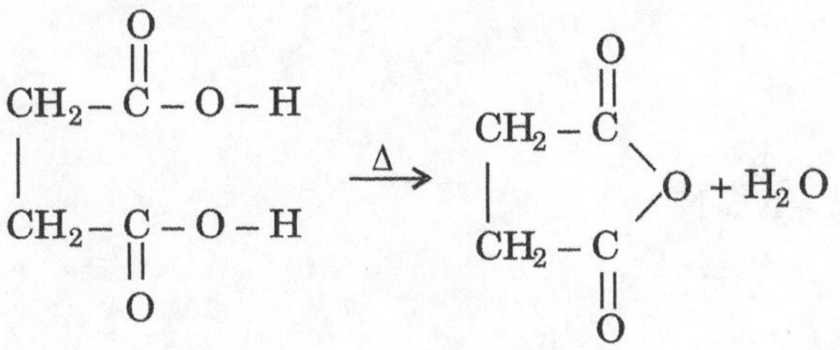

(Succinic acid)

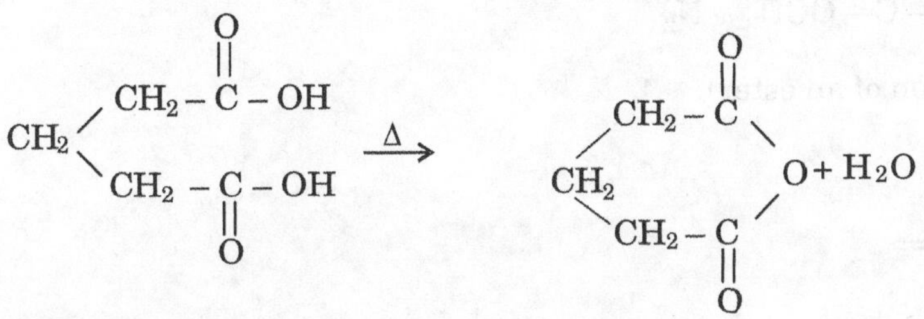

(Glutaric acid)

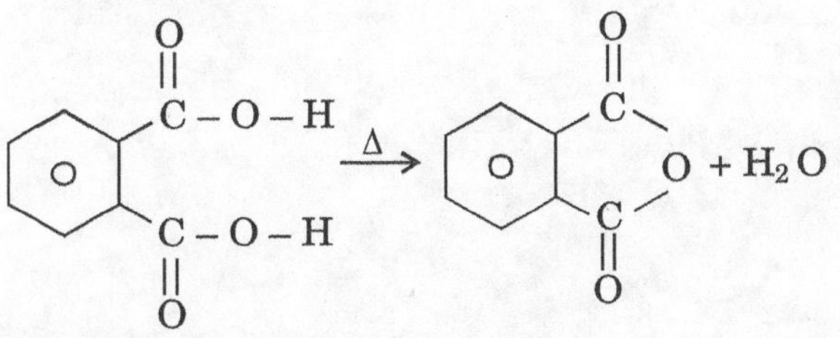

(Phthalic acid)

5 & 6 membered rings are stable

$$CH_2\begin{matrix} COOH \\ COOH \end{matrix} \xrightarrow{\Delta} CO_2 + CH_3COOH$$

Malonic acid.

72. Wrt option (a)

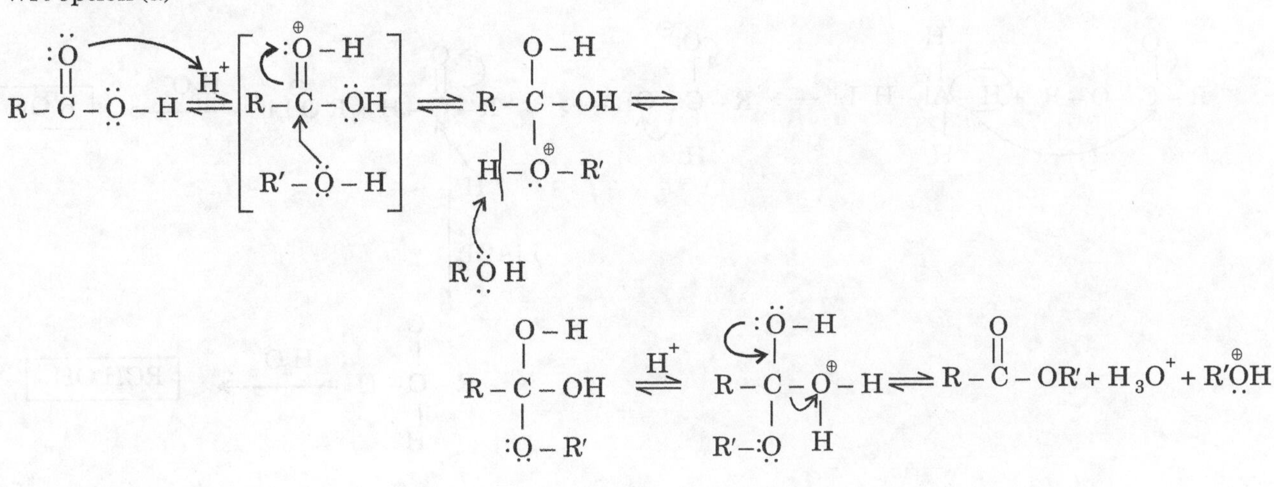

Wrt option (b),

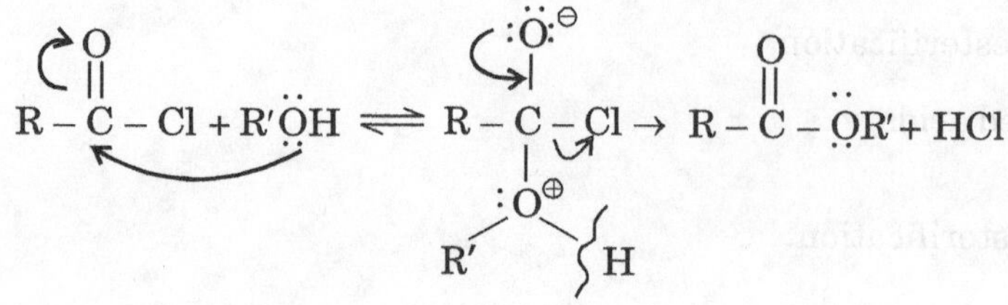

Wrt option (c)

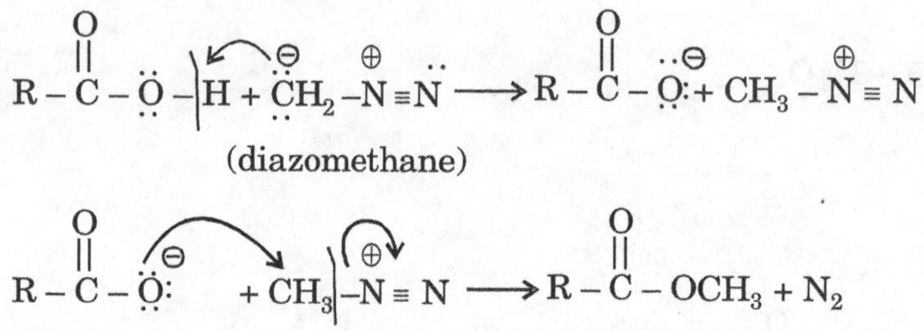

73. Basic hydrolysis of an ester (Saponification of an ester)

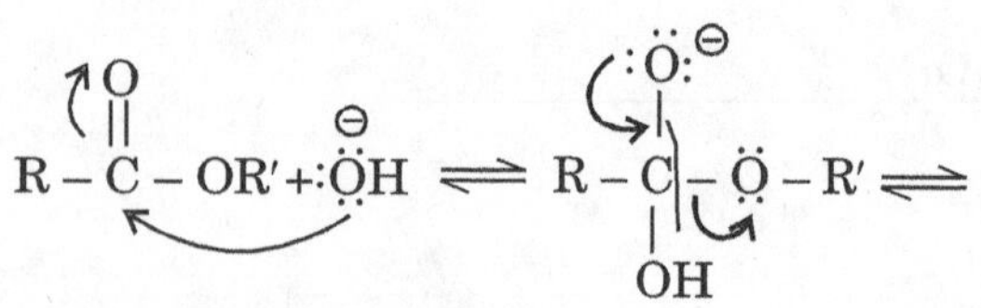

(Acyl Nucleophilic sub.)

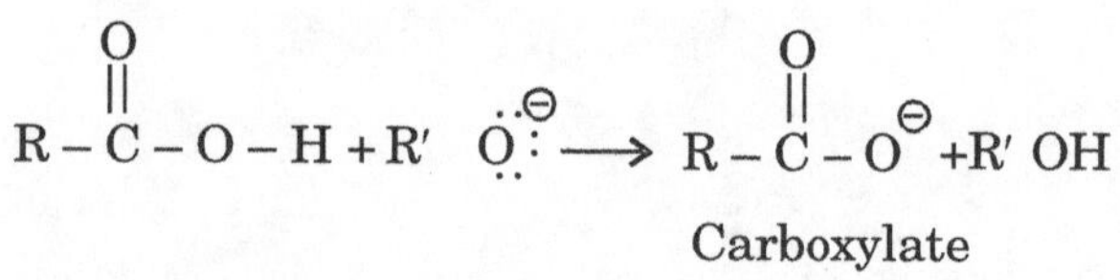

Basic hydrolysis of an amide

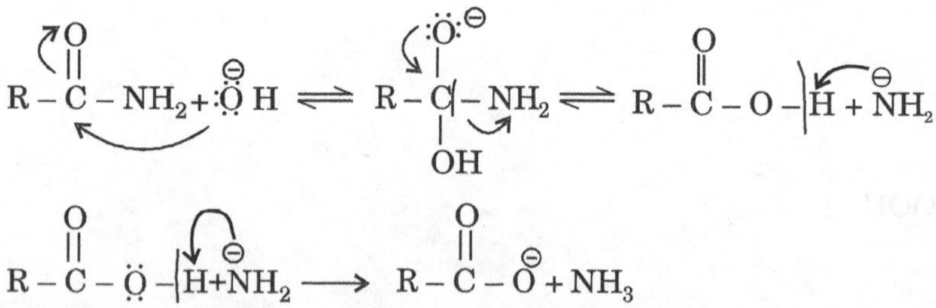

74. Mechanism of Reduction of an ester with $LiAlH_4$.

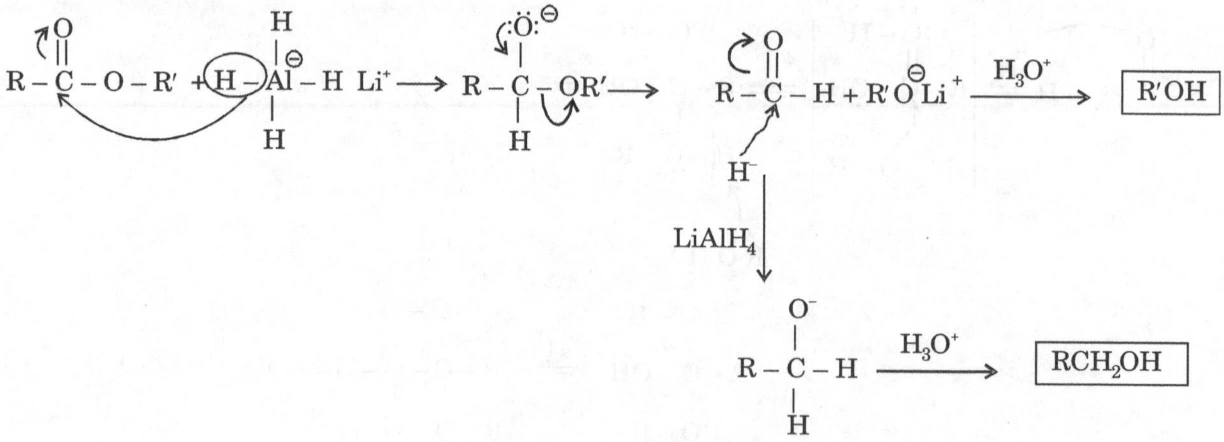

75. Complete hydrolysis of Alkyl Cyanides

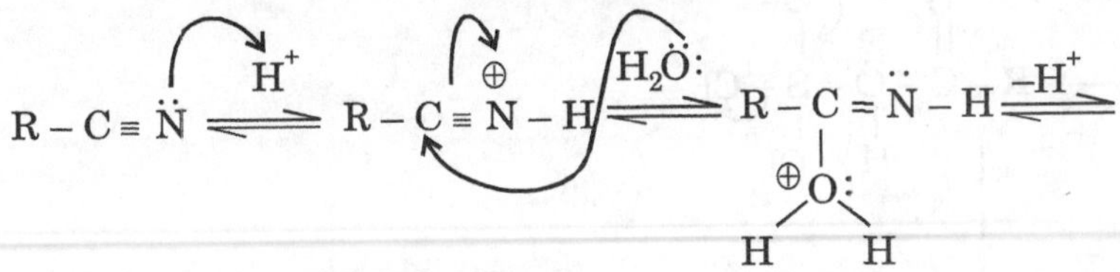

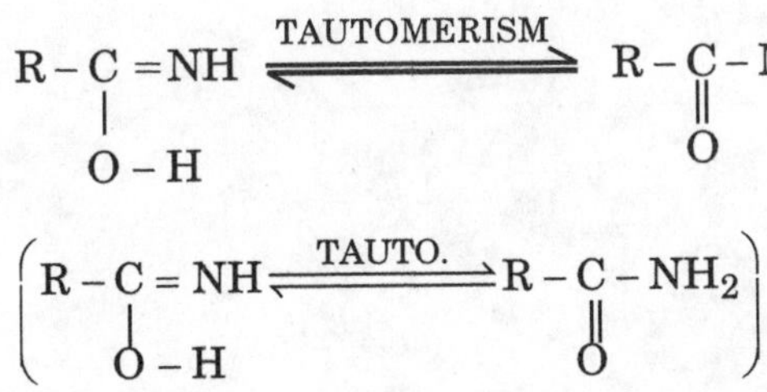

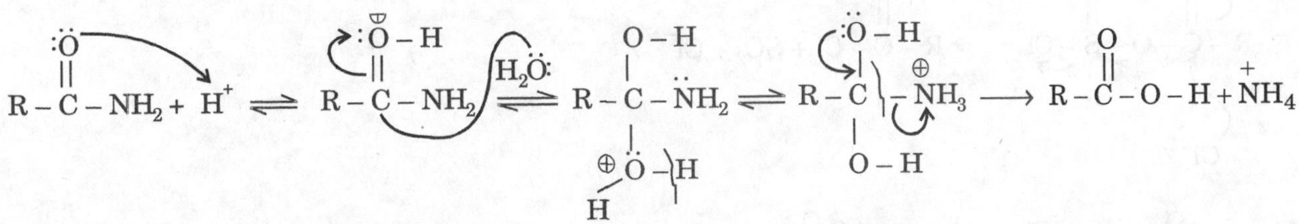

wrt option (b).

$R-\overset{\oplus}{N}\equiv\overset{..\ominus}{C}$ Cannot undergo $-\overline{O}H$ (basic) hydrolysis because $\overline{O}H$ cannot attack at N(which already has a complete octet) & will be repelled from – vely charged C.

Wrt option (c),

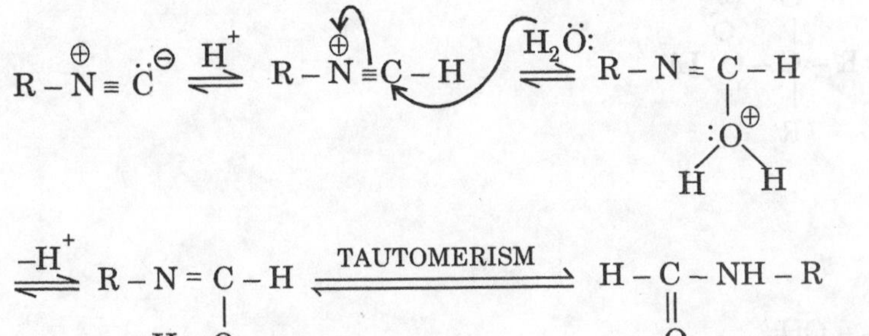

(substituted amide)

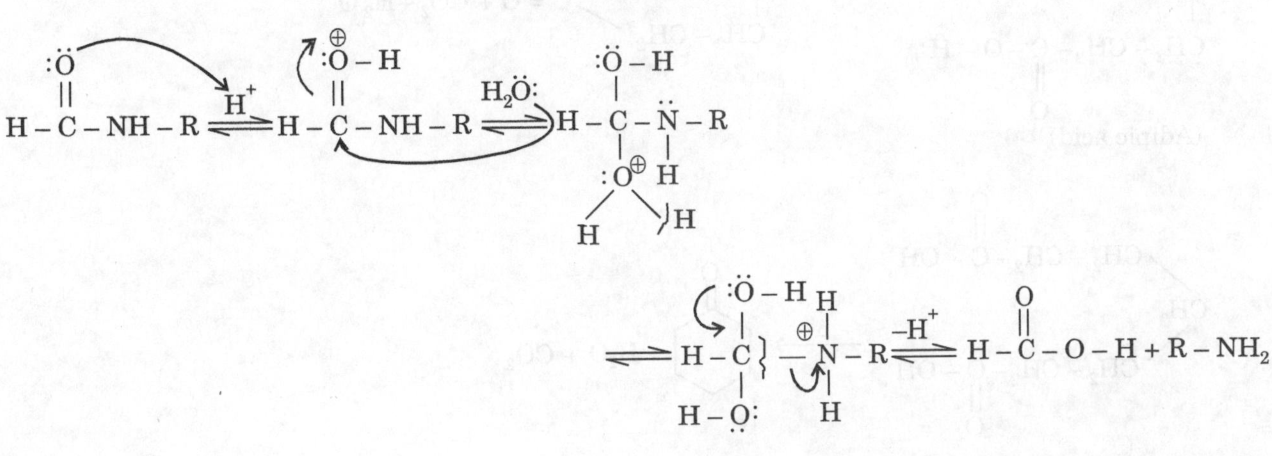

76. 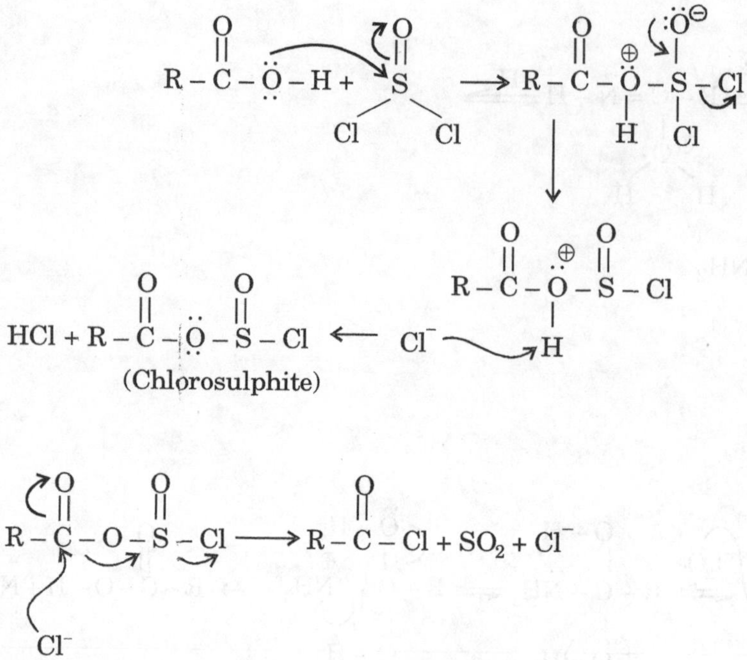

77. 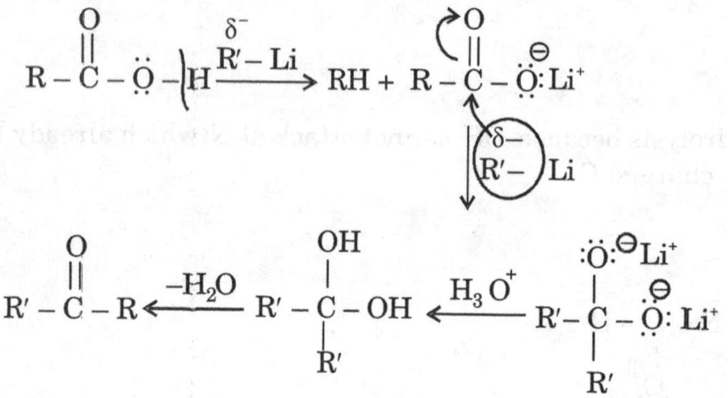

78. Adipic acid

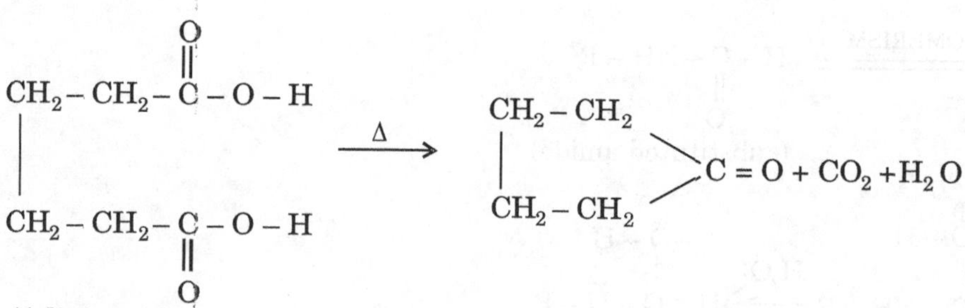

(Adipic acid)

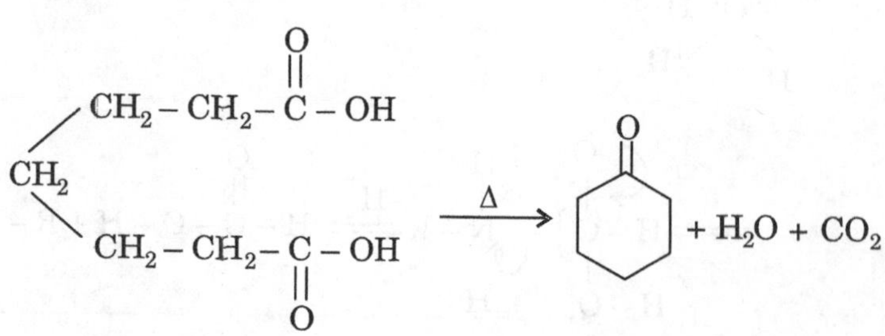

(Pimelic acid)

79.

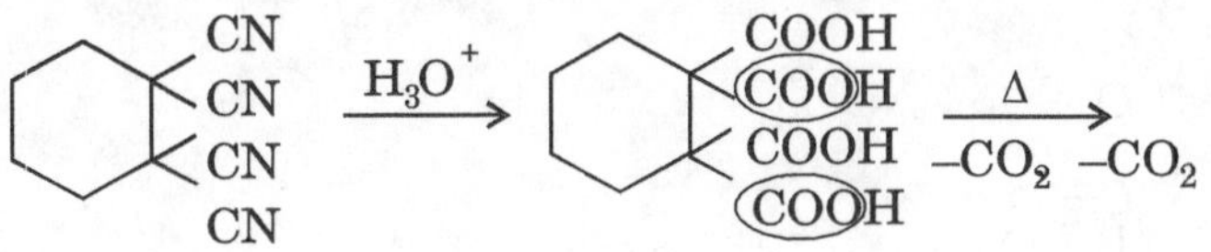

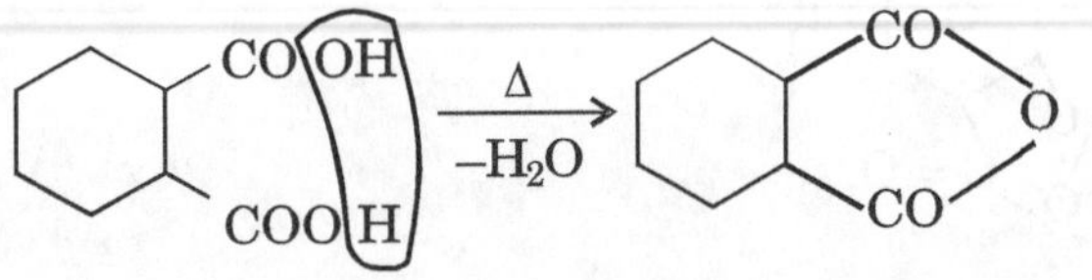

(gem dicarboxylic acids undergo decarboxylation when heated)

80.

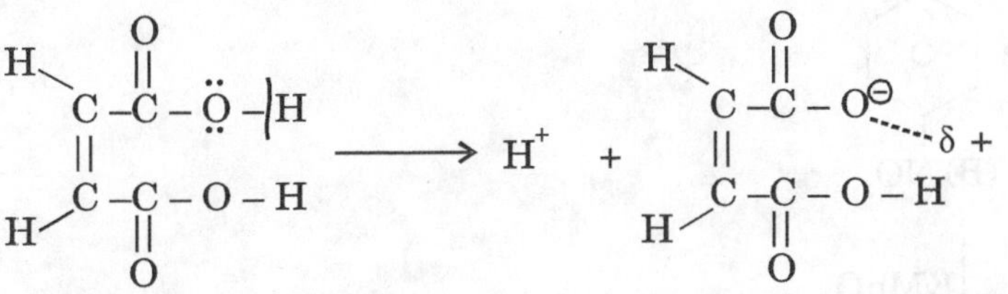

Conjugate base of maleic acid is stabilised by intramolecular H-bonding. So, Ka_1 is greater than Ka_1 of Fumaric acid (trans form). But Ka_2 of maleic acid is smaller because the H left is involved in intramolecular H–Bonding.

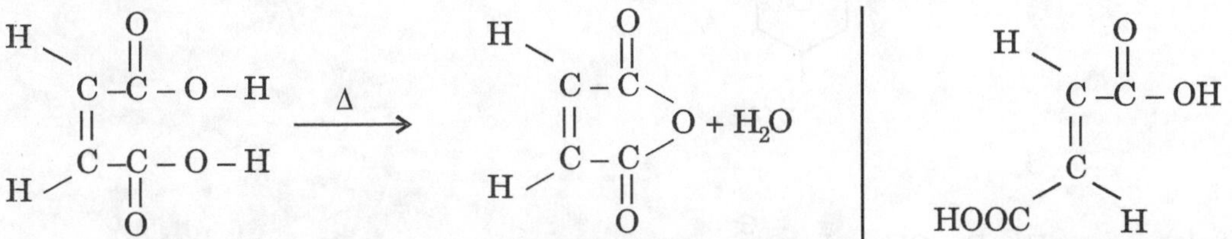

(Maleic acid) (Maleic anhydride) (Fumaric acid)

$\xrightarrow{\Delta}$ No anhydride formation because the two –COOH are oppositely oriented.

81. Acids, which are more acidic than carbonic acid will react with $NaHCO_3$.

82. Only 1, 2-dicarboxylic acids undergo dehydration on being heated.

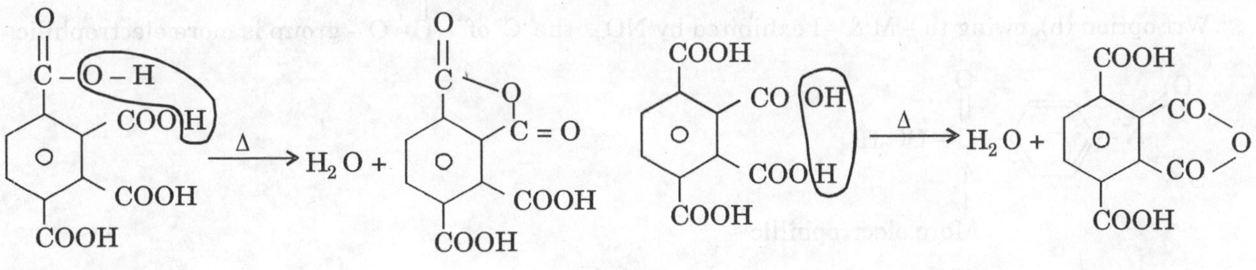

83. Wrt option (a)

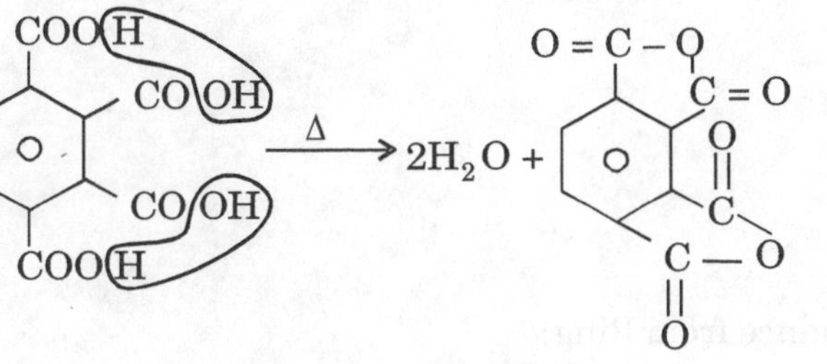

Wrt option (b)

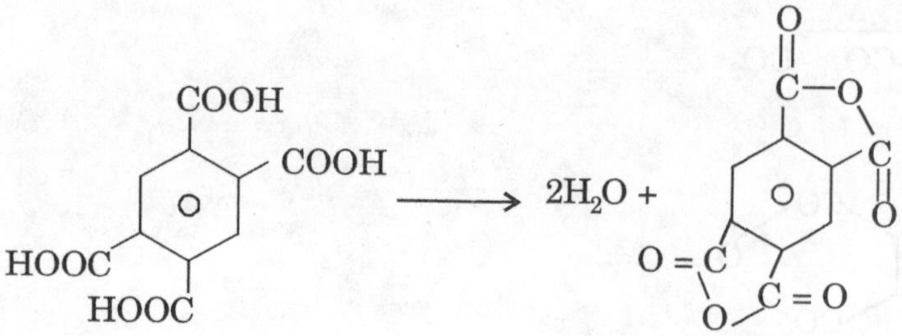

84.

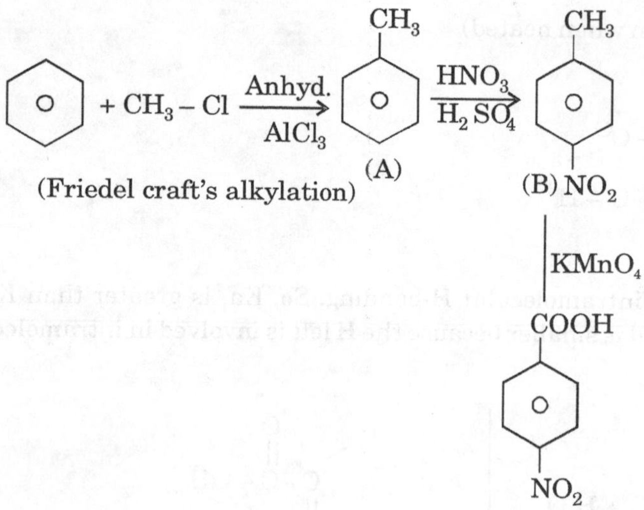

85. Wrt option (a),

$$R-CH=N-\ddot{O}-H \longrightarrow H^{+} + R-CH=N-\ddot{O}:^{\ominus}$$

$$[R-CH=N-\ddot{O}:^{\ominus} \leftrightarrow R-\overset{\ominus}{\ddot{C}H}-N=\ddot{O}:]$$

Oximes have an acidic H attached to O & also, it conjugate base is stabilised by resonance.

Wrt option (b), owing to – M & –I exhibited by NO_2, the 'C' of $-\overset{O}{\overset{\|}{C}}-O-$ group is more electrophilic.

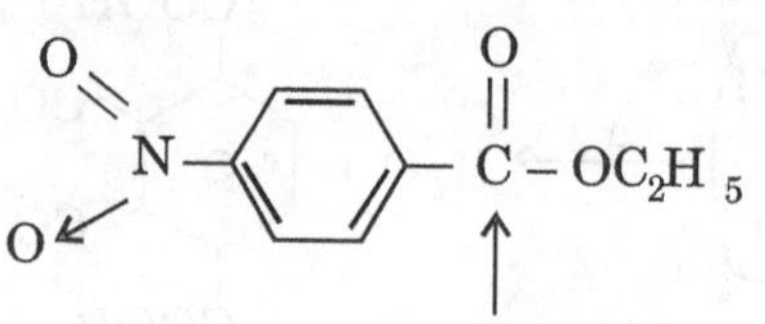

(More susceptible to attack by $\overline{O}H$)

Wrt option (c),

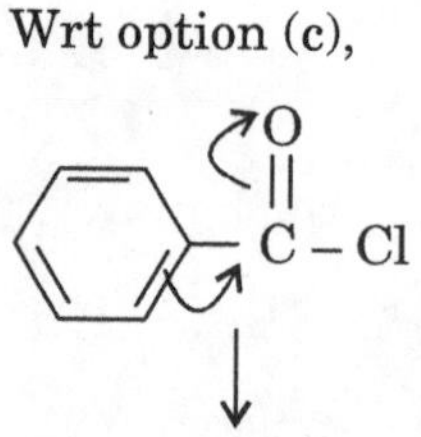

(electrophilicity of this C is compromised ∵ of resonance from Ring)

This is absent in Acetyl chloride (CH_3COCl)

86. Base catalysed hydrolysis of an ester is an example of Acyl Nucleophilic substitution.

Electron withdrawing groups increase the electrophilicity of carboxyl 'C' thereby increasing the rate of basic hydrolysis.

87. Ketones are more reactive than acid towards nucleophilic attack ∵ the electrophilicity of caboxyl C is reduced due to resonance

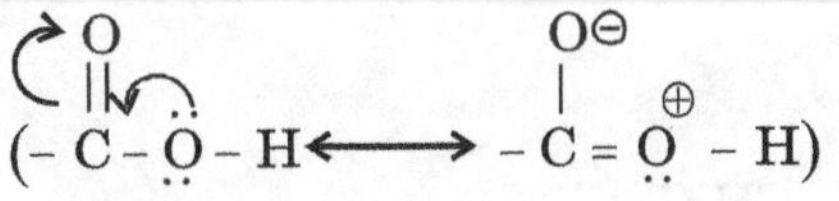

So,

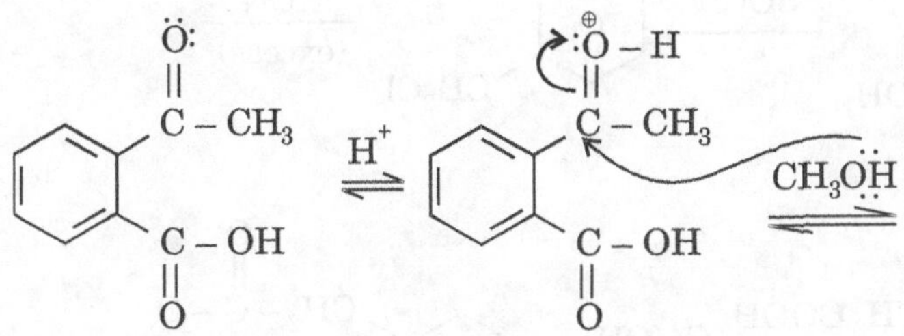

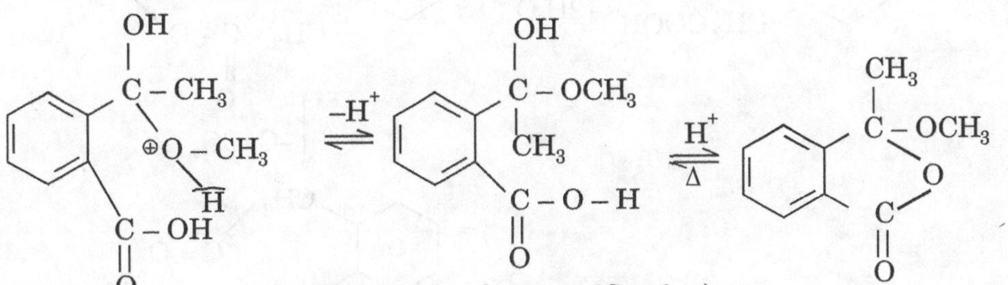

(intramolecular esterification)

88. Mechanism of soda lime decarboxylation

(1) $R-\overset{\overset{O}{||}}{C}-\ddot{O}-H + Na^{+}\bar{O}H \rightleftharpoons R-\overset{\overset{O}{||}}{C}-\ddot{O}:^{\ominus}\ Na^{+} + H_2O$

(2) $R-\overset{\overset{O}{||}}{C}-\ddot{O}:^{\ominus} \xrightarrow{\Delta} R-\overset{\overset{O}{||}}{C}-\ddot{O}:^{\ominus} \xrightarrow{\Delta} CO_2 + R^{\ominus}$

(3) $R^{\ominus} \xrightarrow{H_2O} RH + \bar{O}H$

So, the reaction involves formation of a carbanion, which is stabilised max. by $-NO_2$. ($-I$ of $-NO_2$).

89. <u>Mechanism</u>: β-Keto acids undergo decarboxylation via formation of a 6 membered cyclic transition state, followed by conversion of Keto into enol form.

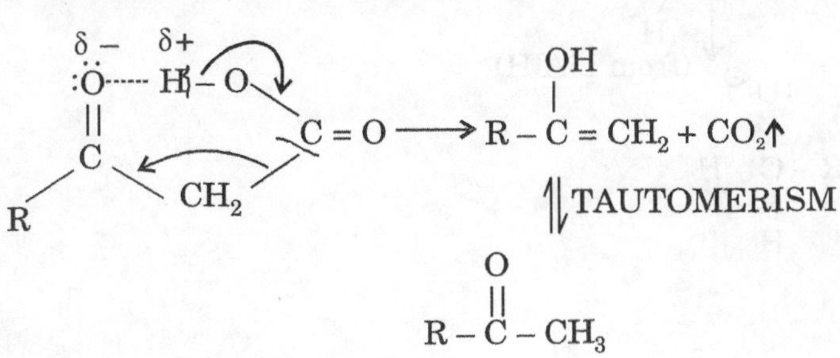

Wrt option (c), enol form cannot be formed because it will be a violation of BREDT'S RULE.

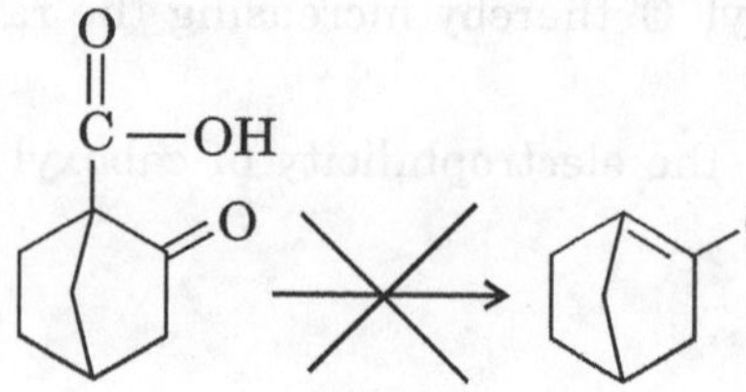

90. 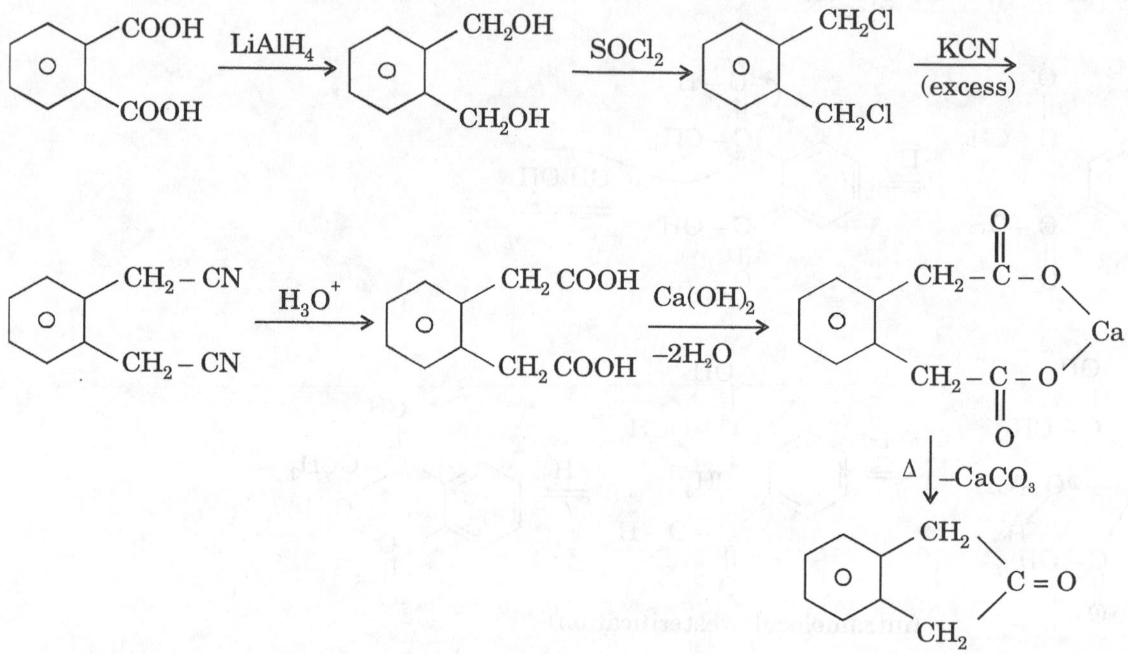

91. Hydrolysis of acetal & cyclic ester occurs to form β-Keto acid which upon heating undergoes decarboxylation.

$$HO-\overset{\overset{O}{\|}}{C}-CH_2-\overset{\overset{O}{\|}}{C}-CH_2-CH_2OH \xrightarrow{\Delta} CH_3-\overset{\overset{O}{\|}}{C}-CH_2-CH_2OH+CO_2\uparrow$$

92. All the three are acid derivatives & will undergo acyl nucleophilic substitution. A short mechanism is demonstrated.

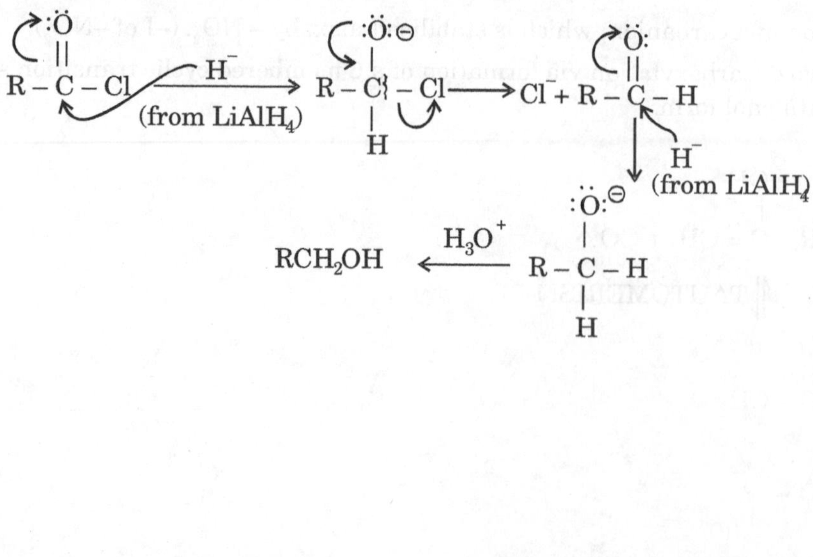

With anhydride

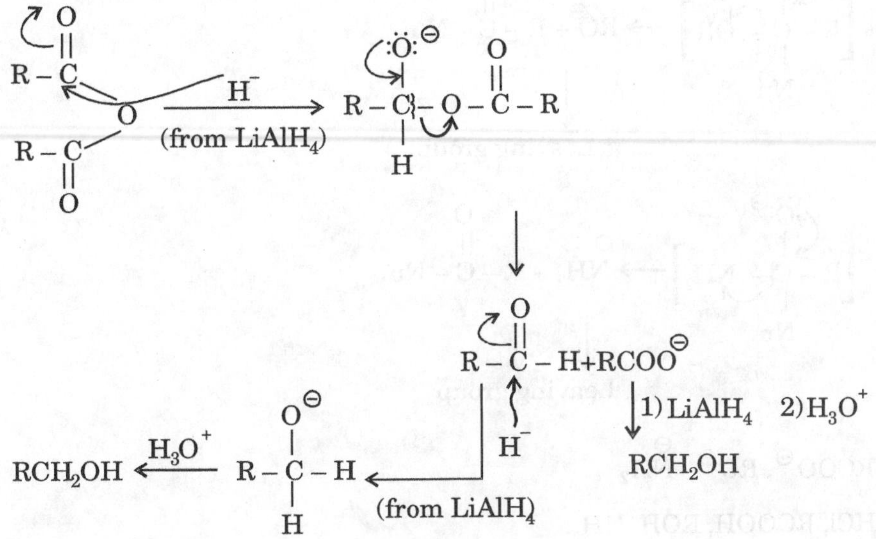

#

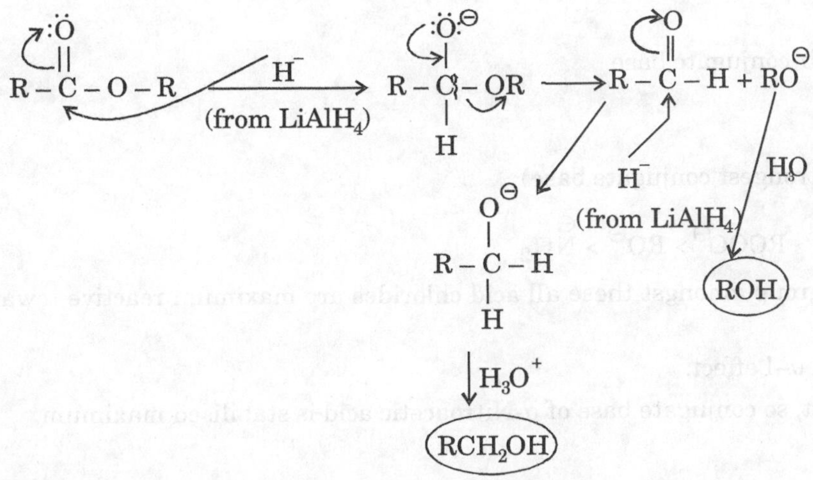

93. **Acid derivatives undergo acyl nucleophilic substitution reactions.**

(1)

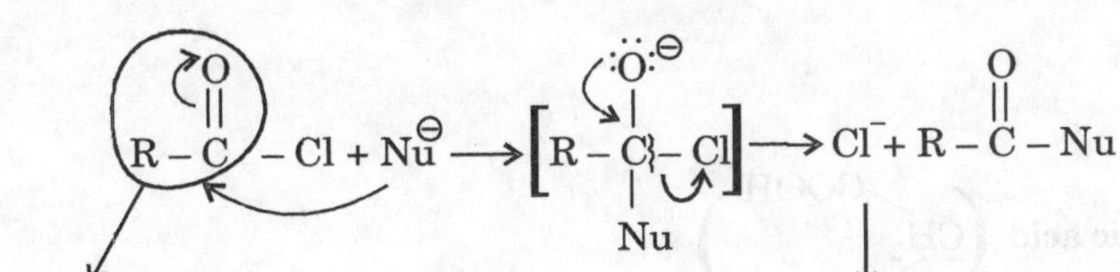

(2)

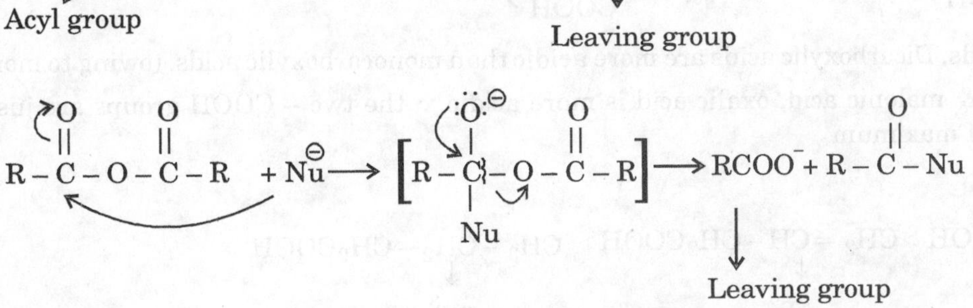

(3) 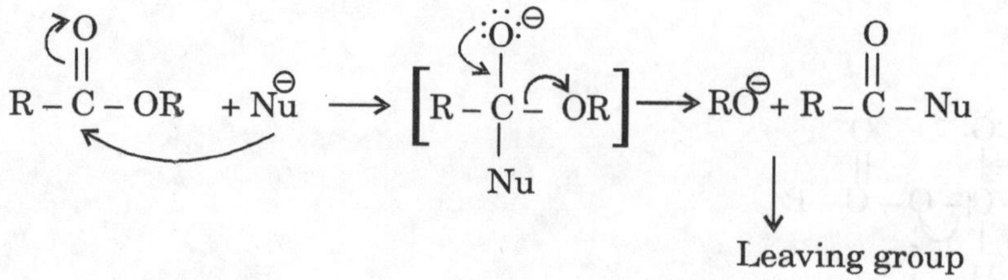

(4) 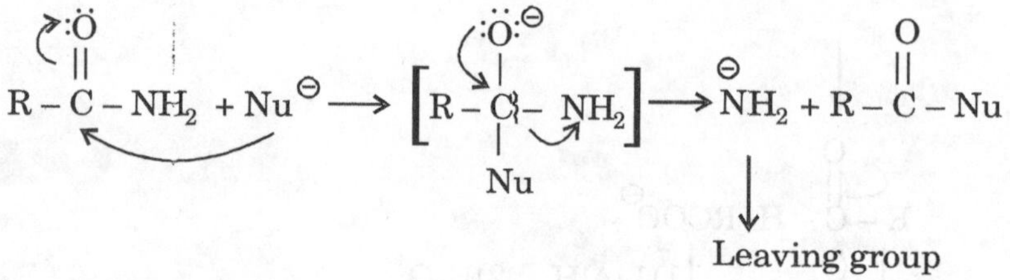

So, leaving groups are – Cl^-, $RCOO^{\ominus}$, $RO^{\ominus}$, $\overset{\ominus}{N}H_2$

Their Conjugate acids are – HCl, RCOOH, ROH, NH_3.

<u>Order of their acidic strength</u>

$HCl > RCOOH > ROH > NH_3$

Order of Basic strength of their conjugate base

$\overset{\ominus}{N}H_2 > RO^{\ominus} > RCOO^{\ominus} > \overset{\ominus}{Cl}$

(NH_3 is weakest acid, so has strongest conjugate base)

Order of leaving ability: – $Cl^- > RCOO^{\ominus} > RO^{\ominus} > \overset{\ominus}{N}H_2$

Since, Cl^- is the best leaving group amongst these all acid chlorides are maximum reactive towards acyl Nucleophilic substitution.

94. Wrt option (a), Acidic strength α–I effect.

– NO_2 exerts maximum-I effect, so conjugate base of α-Nitroacetic acid is stabilised maximum.

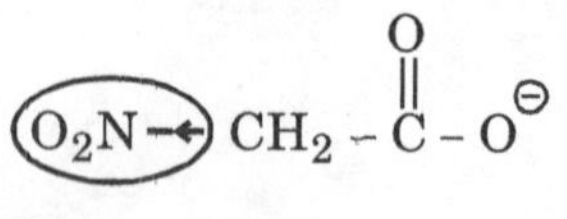

Max. – I effect

Wrt option (b)

Oxalic acid $\left(\begin{array}{l}COOH \\ | \\ COOH\end{array}\right)$ & Malonic acid $\left(CH_2 \begin{array}{l}\diagup COOH \\ \diagdown COOH\end{array}\right)$

are dicarboxylic acids. Dicarboxylic acids are more acidic than monocarboxylic acids. (owing to more EWG)

Out of Oxalic acid & malonic acid, oxalic acid is more acidic ∵ the two – COOH groups are just placed adjacent & exert – I maximum

Wrt. option (c),

$$\underset{\substack{\downarrow \\ \text{sp hybridised} \\ \text{(max. electro - ve)}}}{H-C\equiv C}-CH_2COOH > \underset{\substack{\downarrow \\ sp^2 \\ \text{(less electro - ve)}}}{CH_2=CH}-CH_2COOH > CH_3-\underset{\substack{\downarrow \\ sp^3}}{CH_2}-CH_2COOH$$

95. 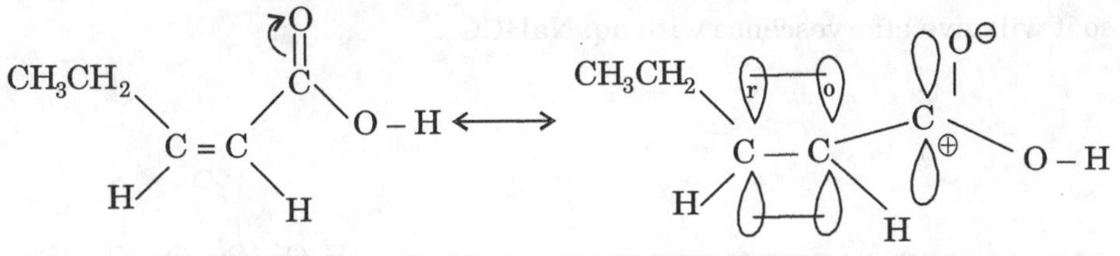

(Cis form)

Due to repulsions, planarity of these p-orbitals is lost due to which resonance occurrs from O of – OH creating +ve charge on O – H, making it more acidic.

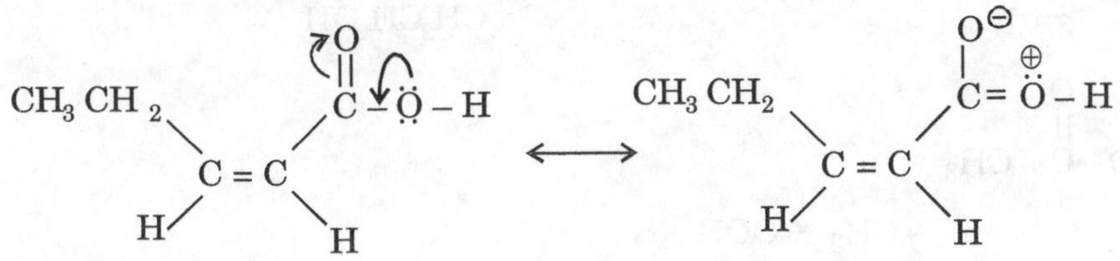

96. 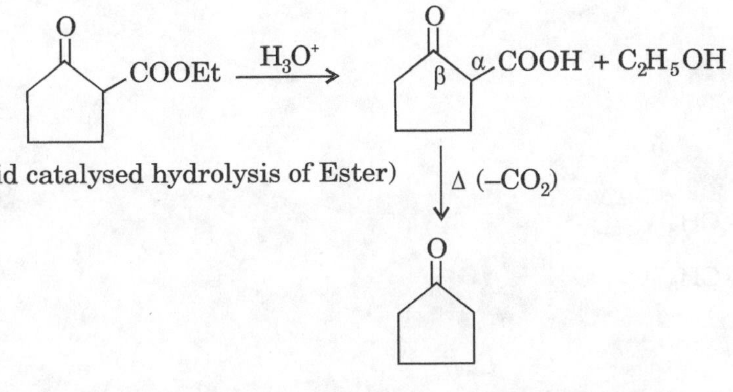

(Acid catalysed hydrolysis of Ester)

(β-Keto acids undergo decarboxylation on being heated)

97. 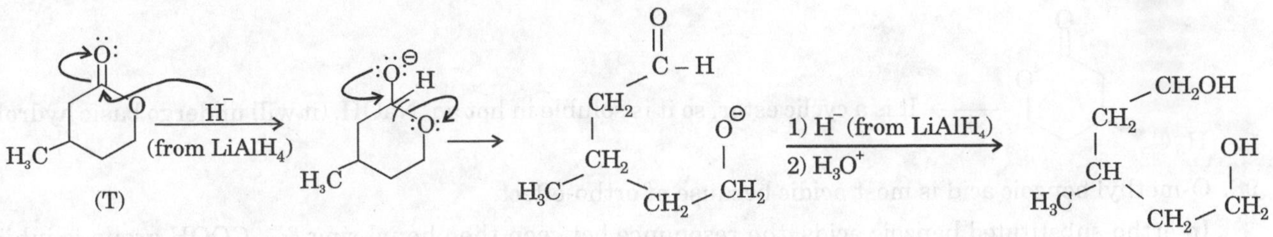

So, U is $H_3C-CH\begin{cases}CH_2-CH_2-OH\\CH_2-CH_2-OH\end{cases}$

↓

No Chiral C

Now, $U \xrightarrow{CrO_3/H^+}$

$$CH_3-CH\begin{cases}CH_2CH_2OH\\CH_2CH_2OH\end{cases} \xrightarrow[\text{(Oxidation)}]{CrO_3/H^+} CH_3-CH\begin{cases}CH_2COOH\\CH_2COOH\end{cases}$$

(V)

'V' is a dicarboxylic acid, so it will give effervescence with aq. $NaHCO_3$.

Also, U $\xrightarrow[\text{excess}]{(CH_3CO)_2O}$

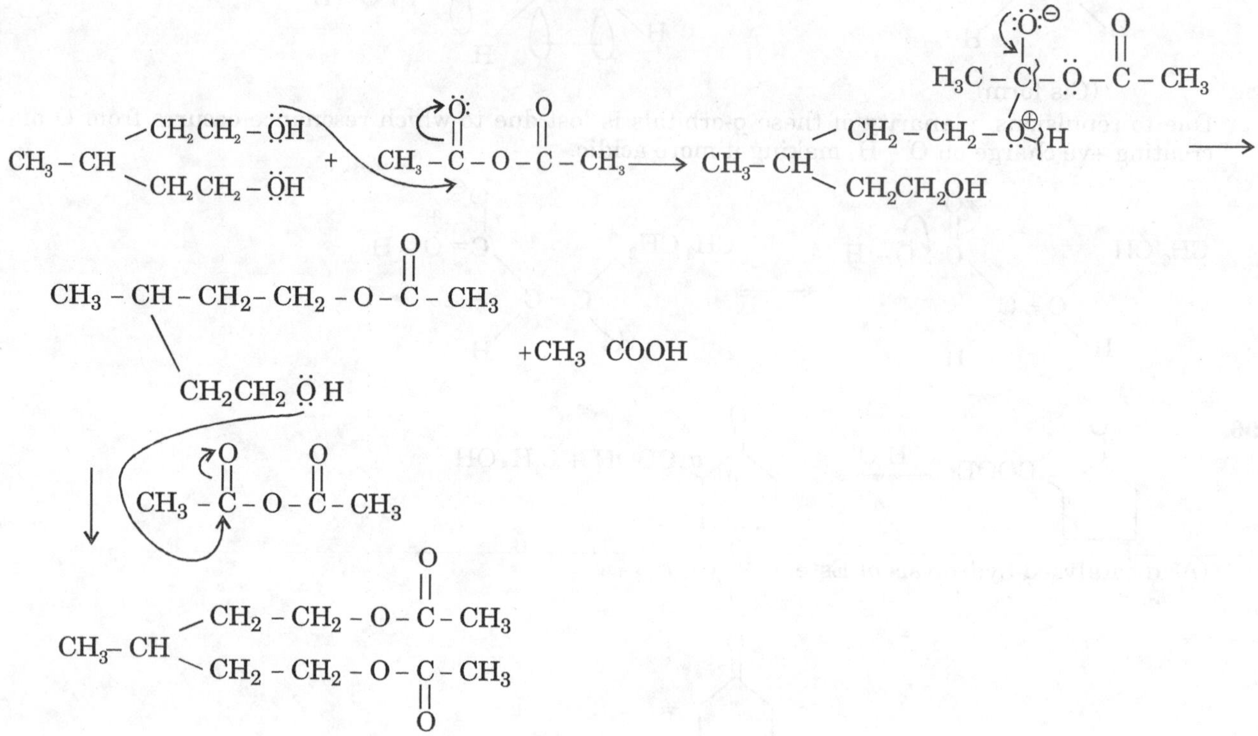

(W)

Wrt option (a)

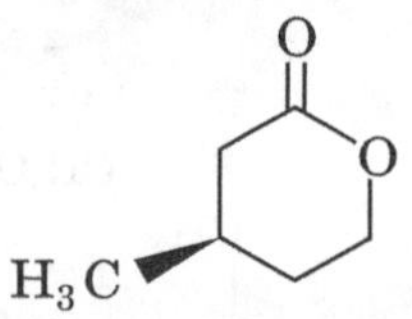

⟶ It is a cyclic ester, so it is soluble in hot aq. NaOH. (it will undergo basic hydrolysis)

98. O-methyl benzoic acid is most acidic because of ortho-effect.
In ortho-substituted benzoic acids, the resonance between the phenyl ring & – COOH group is inhibited due to loss of Co-planarity b/w the two groups due to steric repulsions.

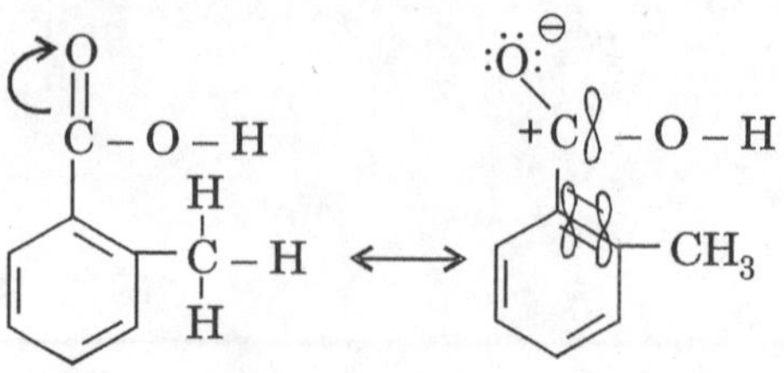

These p-orbitals do not remain in same plane. So, πe^- transfer cannot occur from p-orbital of ring to vacant p-orbital of C.

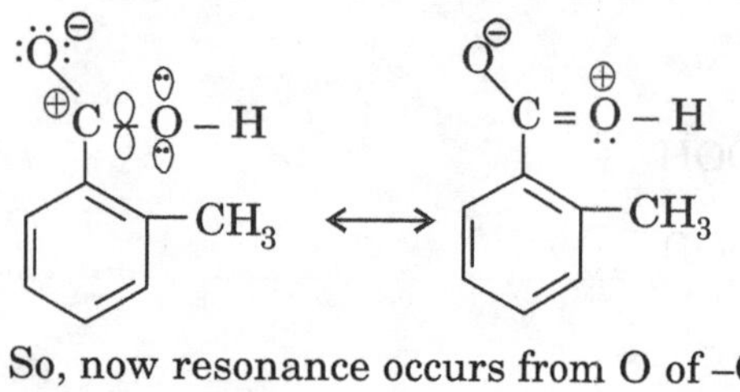

So, now resonance occurs from O of –OH creating +ve charge on O making H highly acidic.

99. In both II & III, ortho effect is pronounce. Also, in III, the conjugate base is highly stabilised by intramolecular H-bonding from 2 ends. So it is max. acidic.

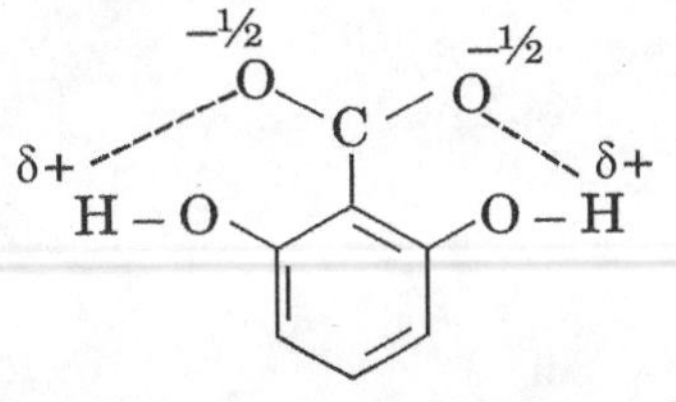

100. Enol form cannot be formed at bridge head location. It'll be a violation of BREDT'S Rule.

101. W.r.t option (a),

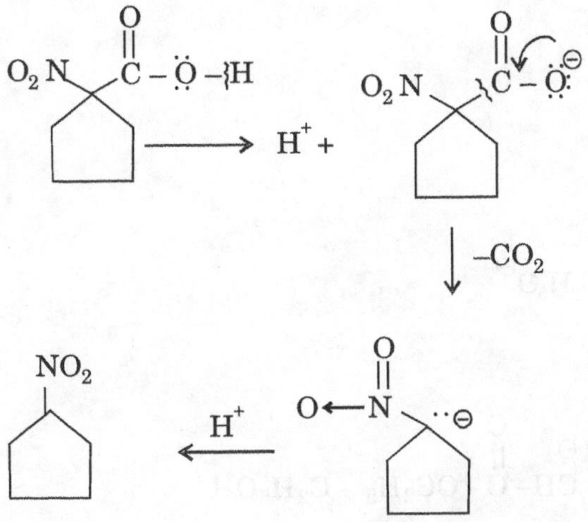

(stabilised by Resonance)

w.r.t option (b),

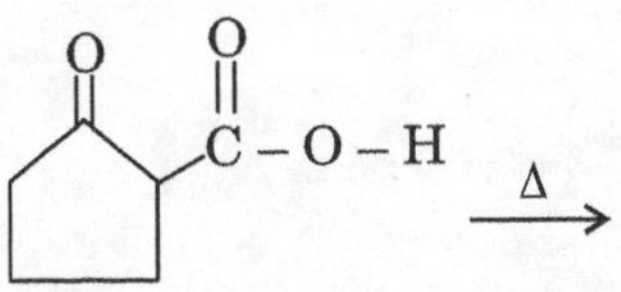

It can be explained either through formation of stable enolate ion or through formation of cyclic transition state.

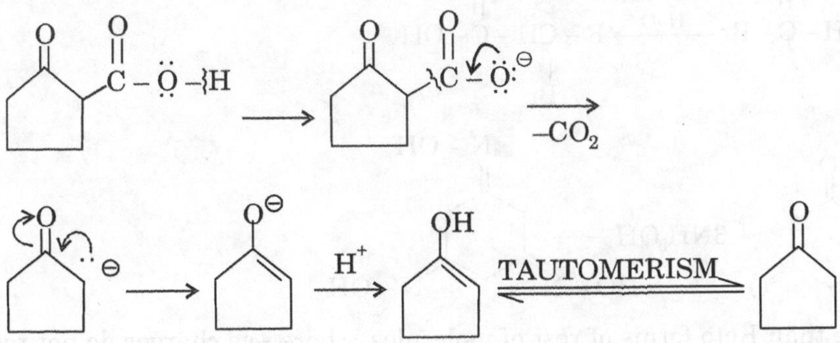

Wrt option (c)

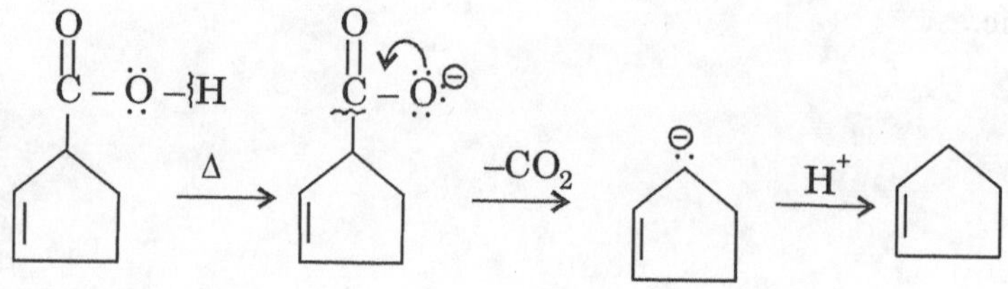

102.

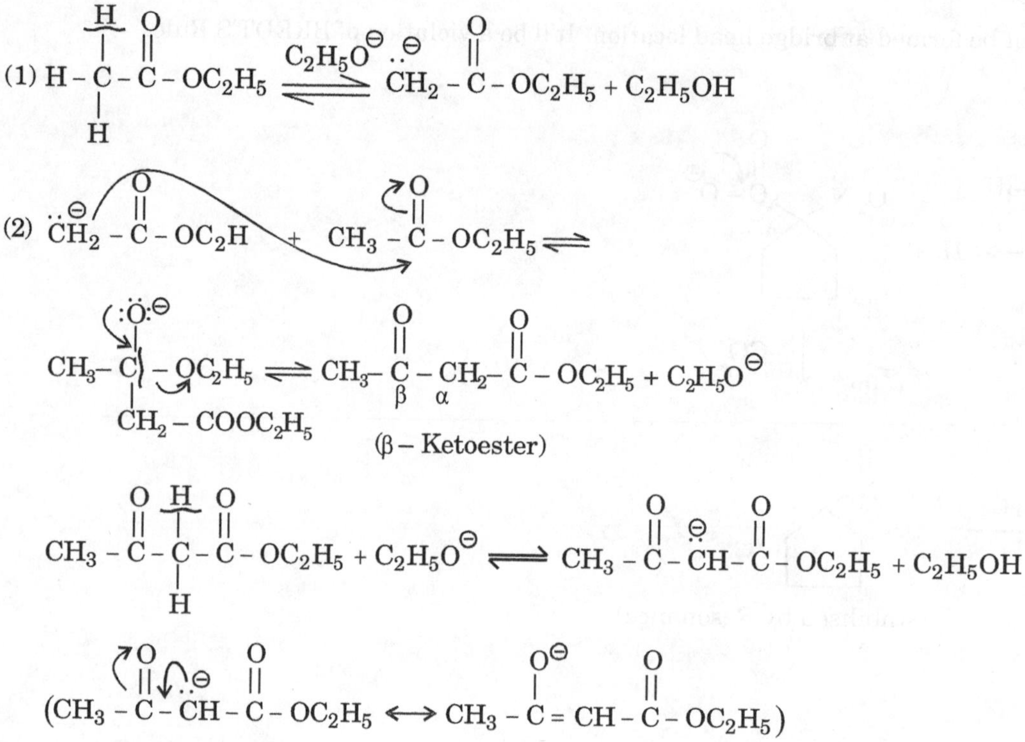

103.

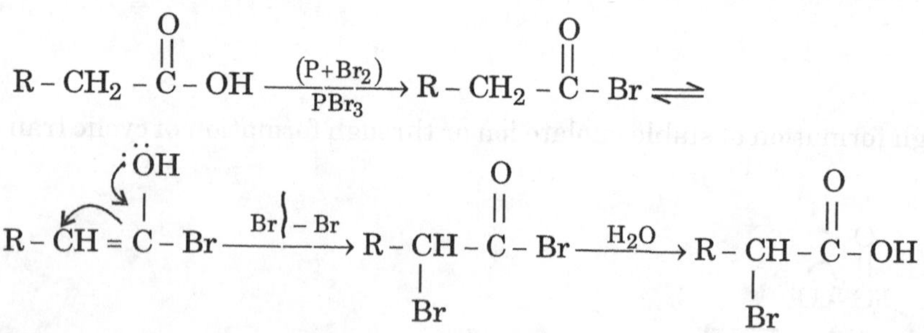

104.

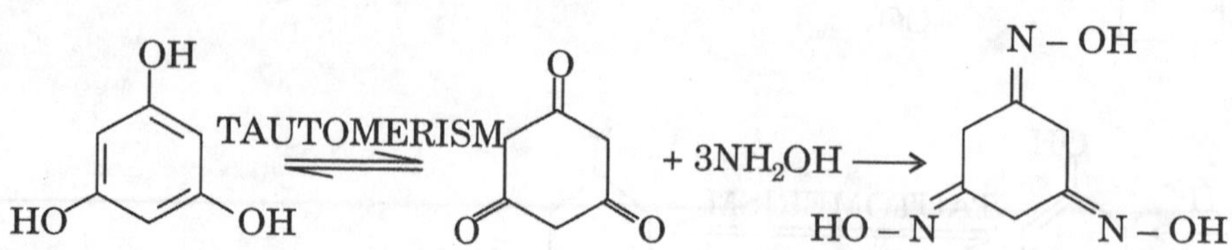

[its Keto form is relatively stable than Keto forms of rest of molecules ∵ here +ve charges do not rest on adjacent C's]

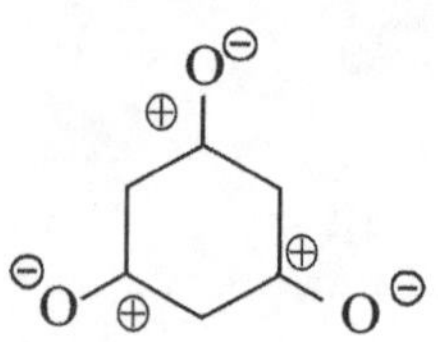

105. Since aldehydes are more reactive than Ketones towards nucleophilic addition, nucleophiles are made from Ketone end & attack occurs at an aldehyde i.e. intermolecular aldal.

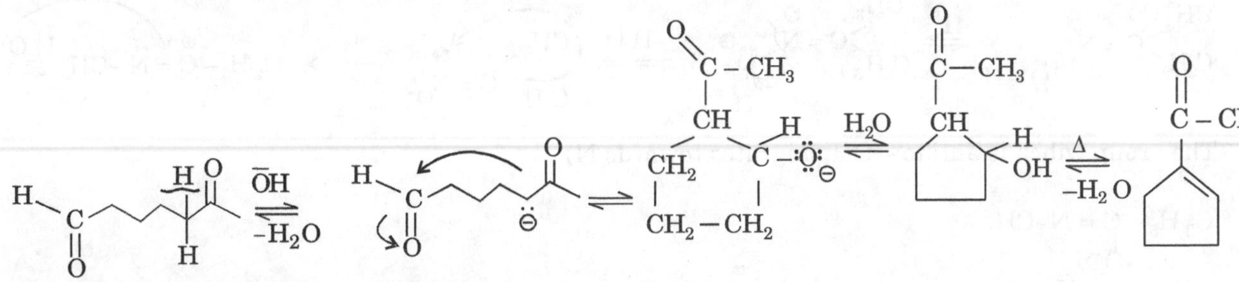

Also, 5 & 6 membered sings are stable.

106. Reaction I refers to Wolf Kishner's

Reduction reaction which occurs in basic medium

(1) 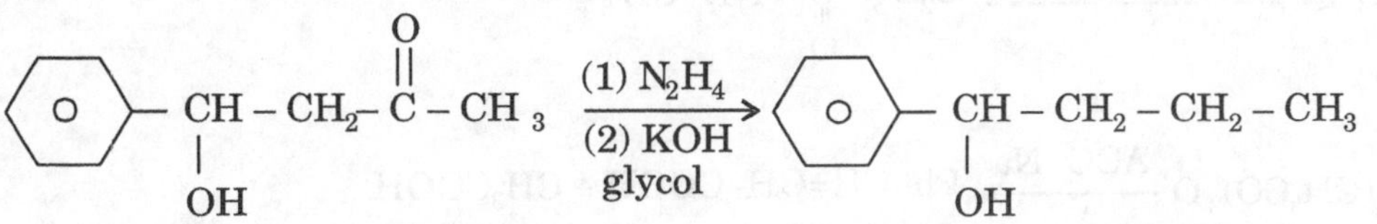

(2) 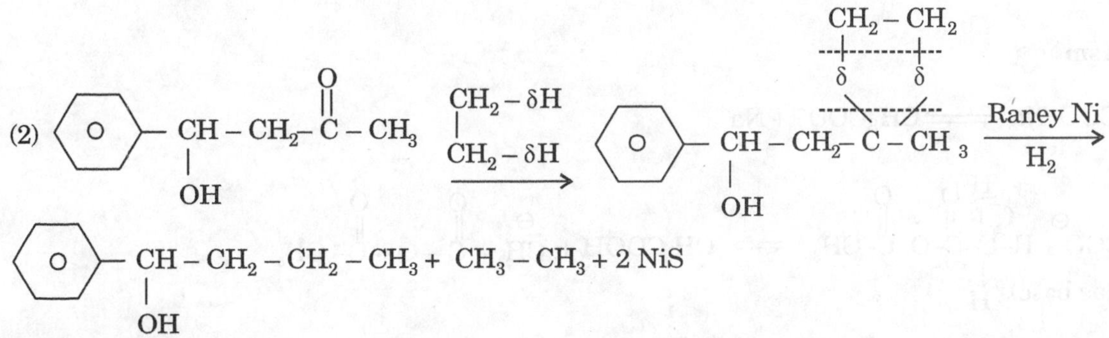

Wrt Reaction (c)-

It is Clemmenson's redn.

(in acidic medium)

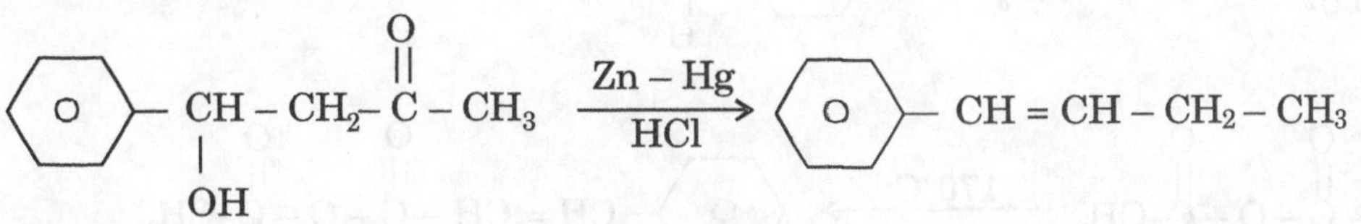

(acidic medium protonates –OH causing dehydration (elimination), besides converting >C = O to >CH$_2$ group)

107. 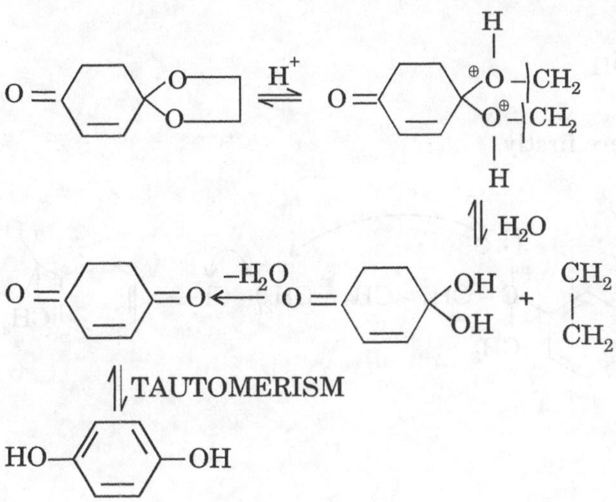

108. It is an example of Beckmann's Rearrangement

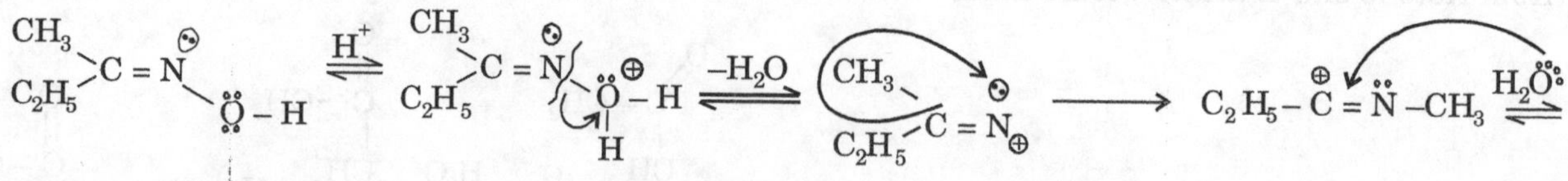

The group wihch is anti to – OH, migrates towards N)

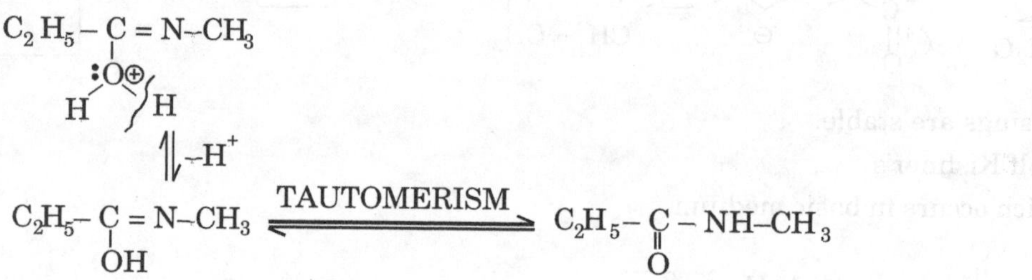

110. 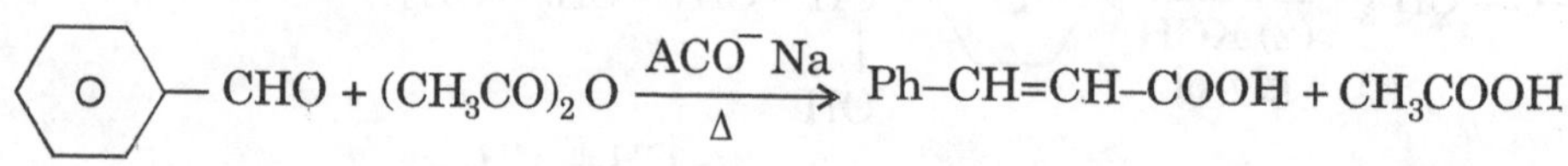

Mechanism

(a) $CH_3COO^-Na^+ \rightleftharpoons CH_3COO^- + Na^+$

(b) 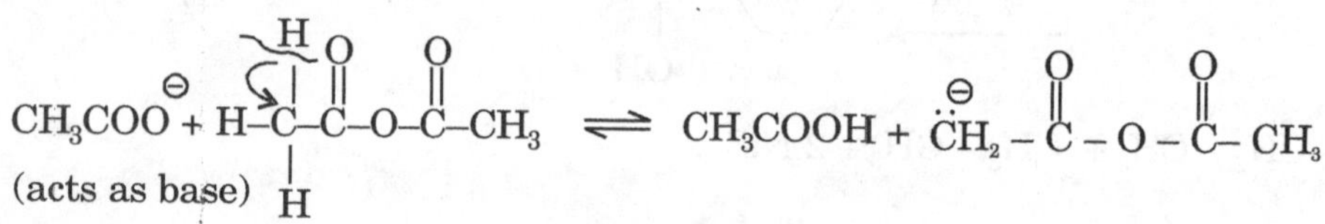

(c) 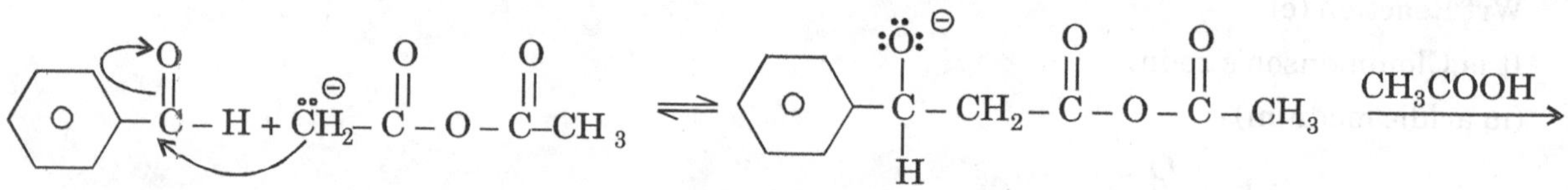

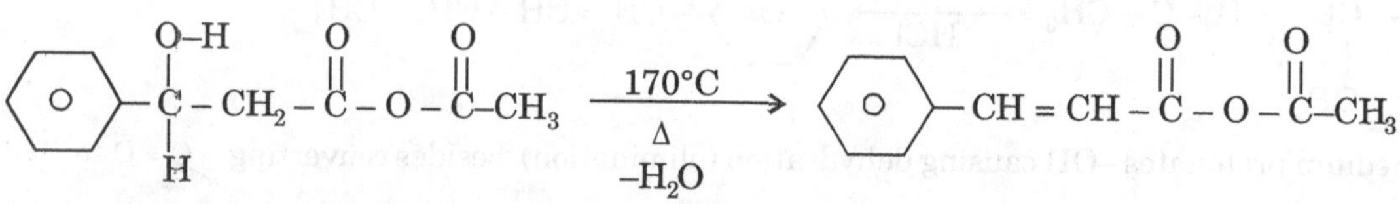

$\xrightarrow{H_2O} C_6H_5 - CH = CH - COOH + CH_3COOH$

111. $>C = O$ bond is highly polar. So attack occurs there firstly.

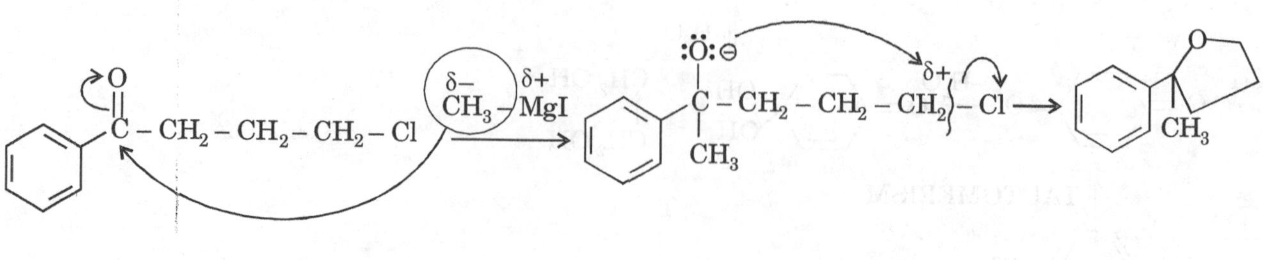

112. Ist step involves acidic hydrolysis of anhydride.

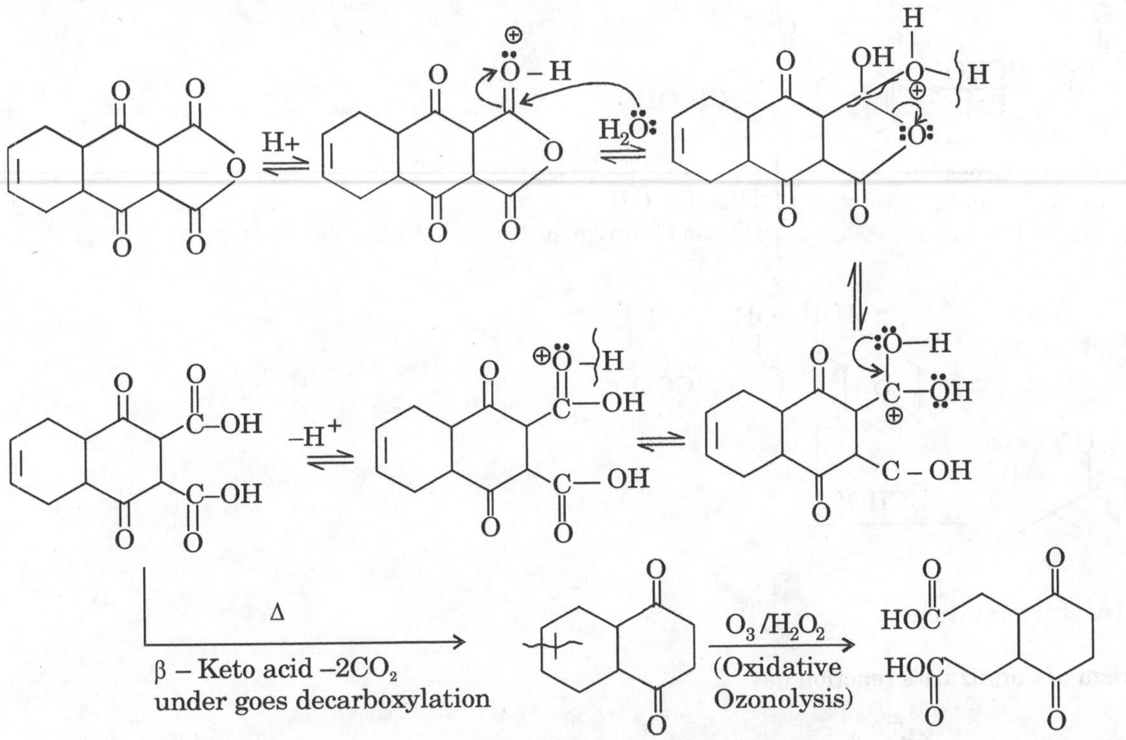

114. Aldehydes (Both aliphatic & aromatic) & α-hydroxy ketones will gives +ve tollen's reagent test.

115. O,O– Dihydroxy benzoic acid is most acidic. After losing H^+ Chelation of two –OH groups occurs with –COO^- group.

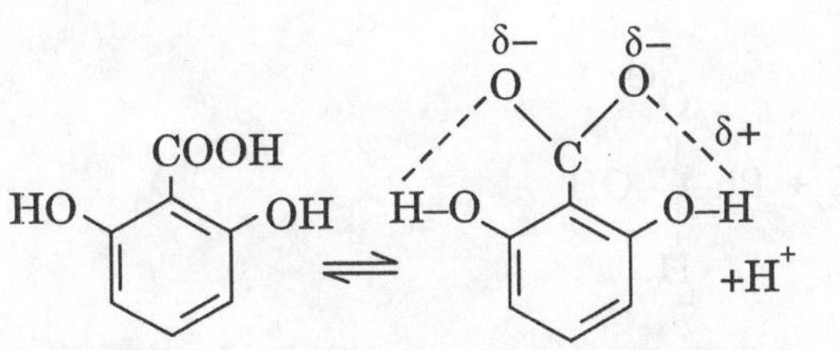

Then, O–hydroxy benzoic acid has its conjugate base stabilised from one end.

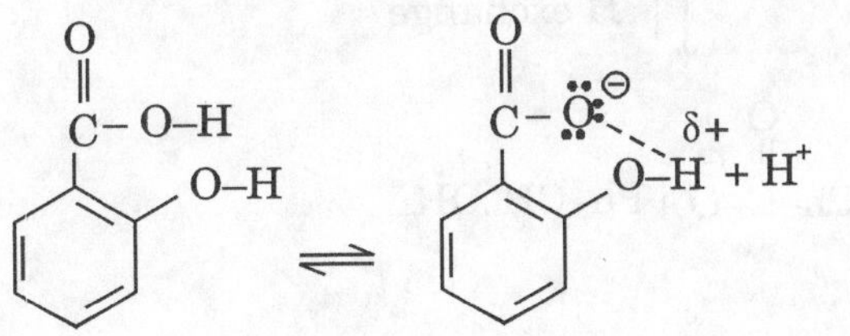

It is followed by meta hydroxy benzoic acid where –I of -OH operates & stabilises the resultant conjugate base.

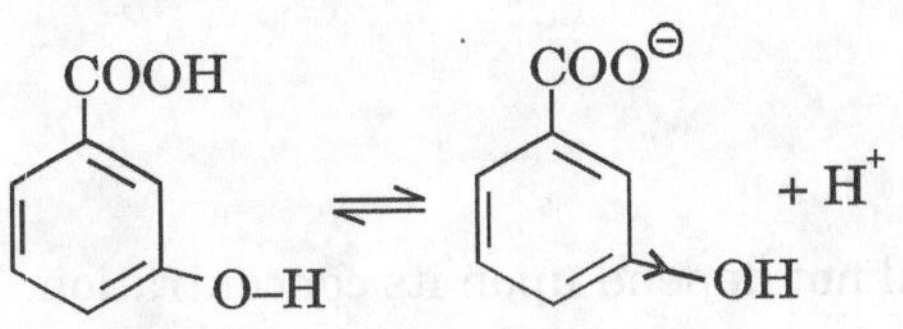

P–Hydroxy Benzoic acid is least acidic because +M effect of – OH at para position decreases its acidic character

116.

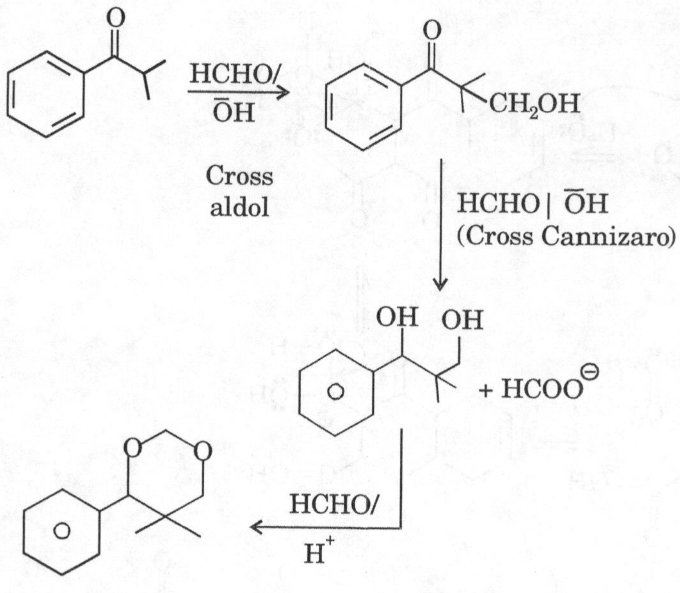

(Acetal formation)

117. Mechanism of Cannizaro's reaction us–

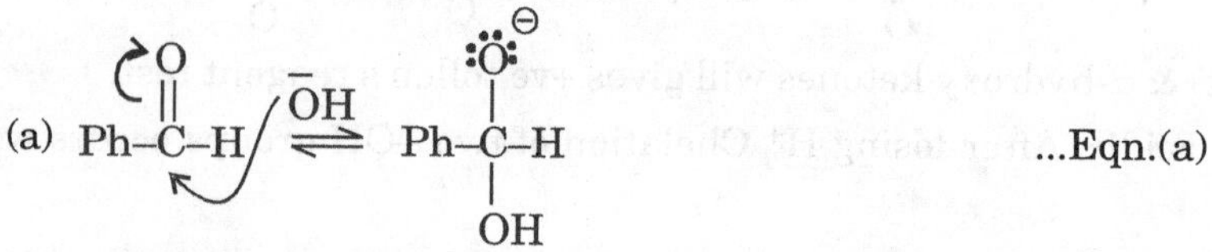

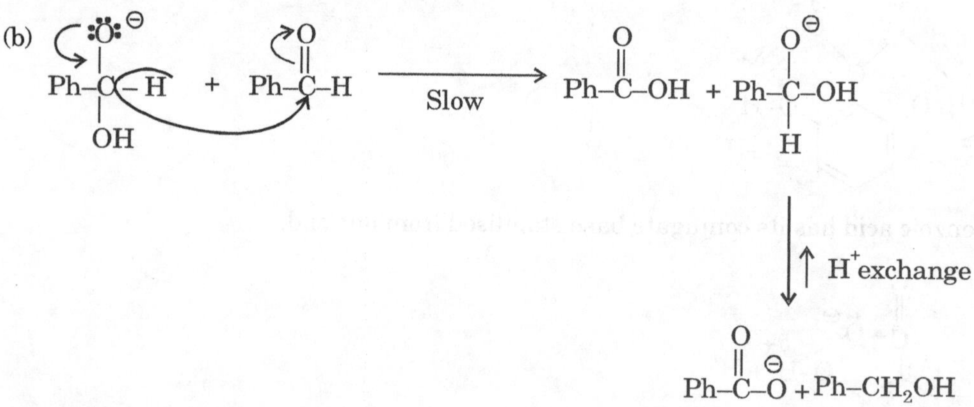

Keeping slow step in mind –

$$\text{Rate of Reaction} = K\,[\text{Ph–C}(O^{\ominus})(OH)\text{–H}]\ [\text{Ph–CHO}] \qquad ...(1)$$

The specie, $\text{Ph–C}(O^{\ominus})(OH)\text{–H}$ is an intermediate, so rate of reaction will not depend upon its concentration. Thus it has to be substituted from rate law.

Now from eqn. (a) –

$$K_{eq.} = \frac{[\text{Ph–C}(\text{O}^{\ominus})(\text{OH})\text{–H}]}{(\text{Ph–CHO})(\bar{\text{O}}\text{H})}$$

$$K_{eq.}(\text{Ph–CHO})(\bar{\text{O}}\text{H}) = [\text{Ph–C}(\text{O}^{\ominus})(\text{OH})\text{–H}]$$

Now, Substituting in eqn. (i)

$$\text{Rate of reaction} = \text{K } K_{eq.}(\text{Ph}-\text{CHO})(\bar{\text{O}}\text{H})(\text{Ph}-\text{CHO})$$

$$\text{Rate of reaction} = \text{K}'(\text{Ph}-\text{CHO})^2(\bar{\text{O}}\text{H})$$

So, it follow 3rd order kinetics

In Presence of high conc. of base –

(a) 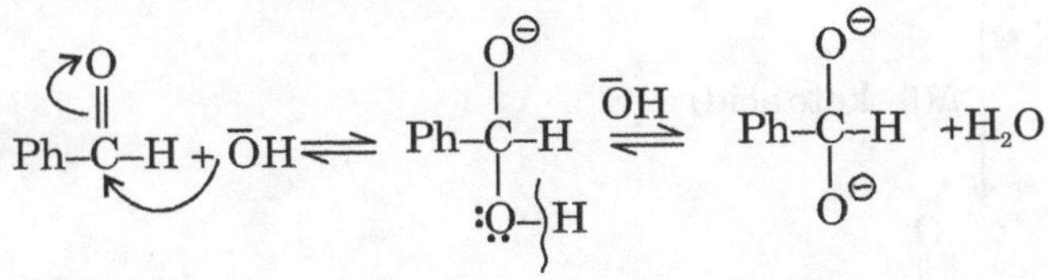

(b) 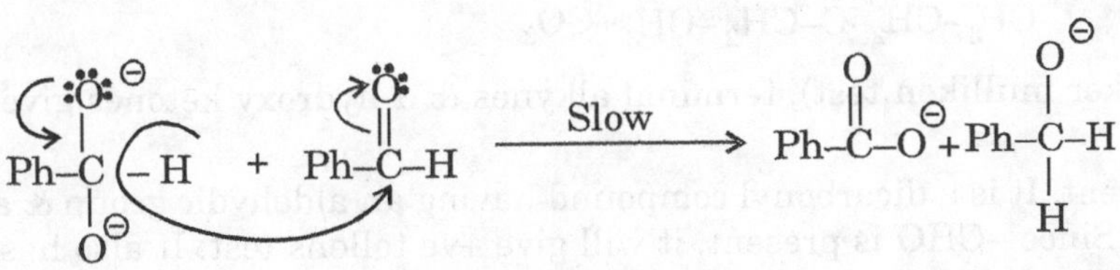

$$\text{Rate of reaction} = \text{K }[\text{Ph–C}(\text{O}^{\ominus})(\text{O}^{\ominus})\text{–H}]\ [\text{Ph–C}(=\text{O})\text{–H}] \quad ...(1)$$

From eqn. (a)

$$K_{eq.} = \frac{[\text{Ph–C}(\text{O}^{\ominus})(\text{O}^{\ominus})\text{–H}]}{(\text{Ph–CHO})(\bar{\text{O}}\text{H})^2}$$

$$K_{eq.}(\text{Ph–CHO})(\bar{\text{O}}\text{H})^2 = [\text{Ph–C}(\text{O}^{\ominus})(\text{O}^{\ominus})\text{–H}]$$

Now, placing the value in eqn.(1)–

$$\text{Rate of reaction} = \text{K } K_{eq}(\text{Ph}-\text{CHO})(\bar{\text{O}}\text{H})^2(\text{Ph}-\text{CHO})$$

$$\text{Rate of reaction} = \text{K}'(\text{Ph}-\text{CHO})^2(\bar{\text{O}}\text{H})^2$$

Now, it follow 4th order Kinetics.

120. In the first step, Claisen ester Condensation Occurs.

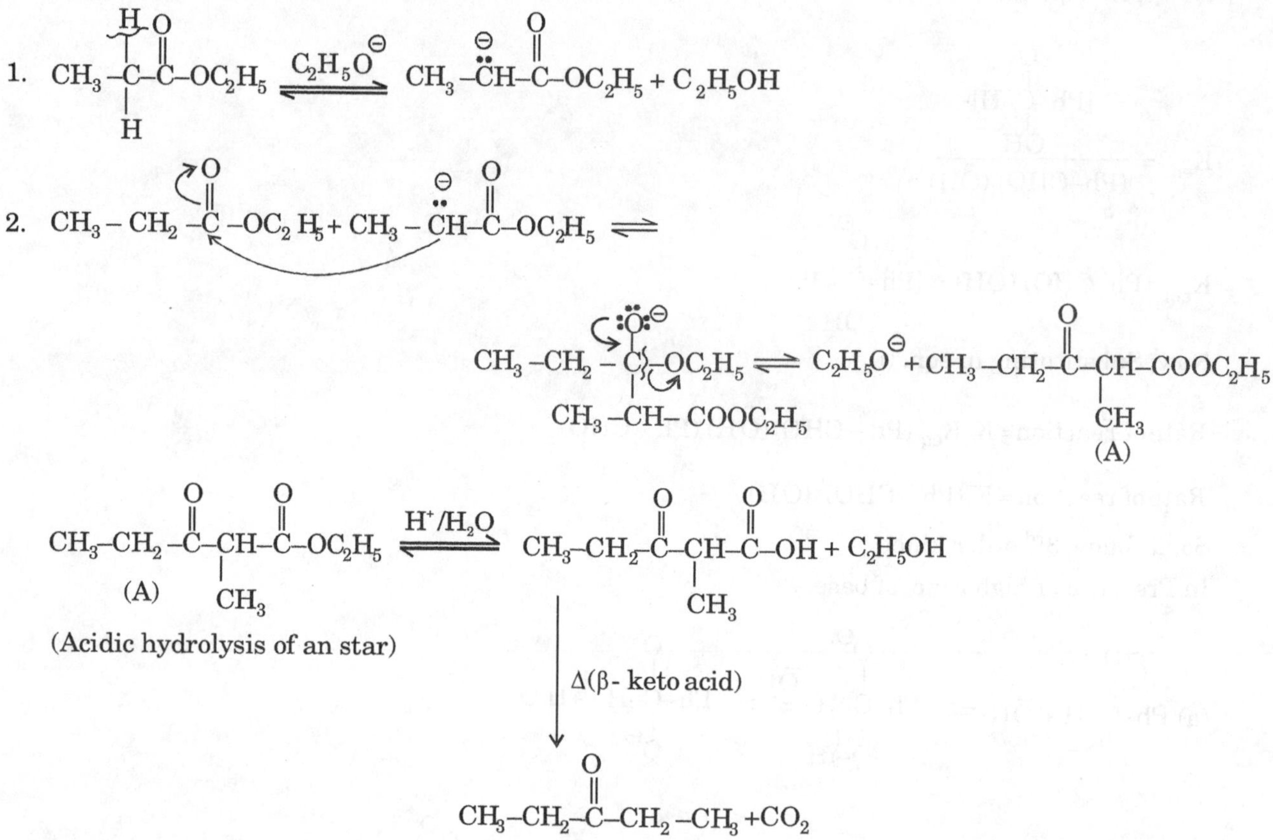

122. Formic acid, hydroxyl amine (Baker mulliken test), terminal alkynes & α-hydroxy ketones give tollen's, reagent test.

123. (b) option fullfils all the requirement. It is a dicarbonyl compound having an aldehydic group & a ketonic group. So, it can form a dioxime. Since –CHO is present, it will give +ve tollens test. It also has CH_3CO group, so it will give + ve iodoform test.

124.

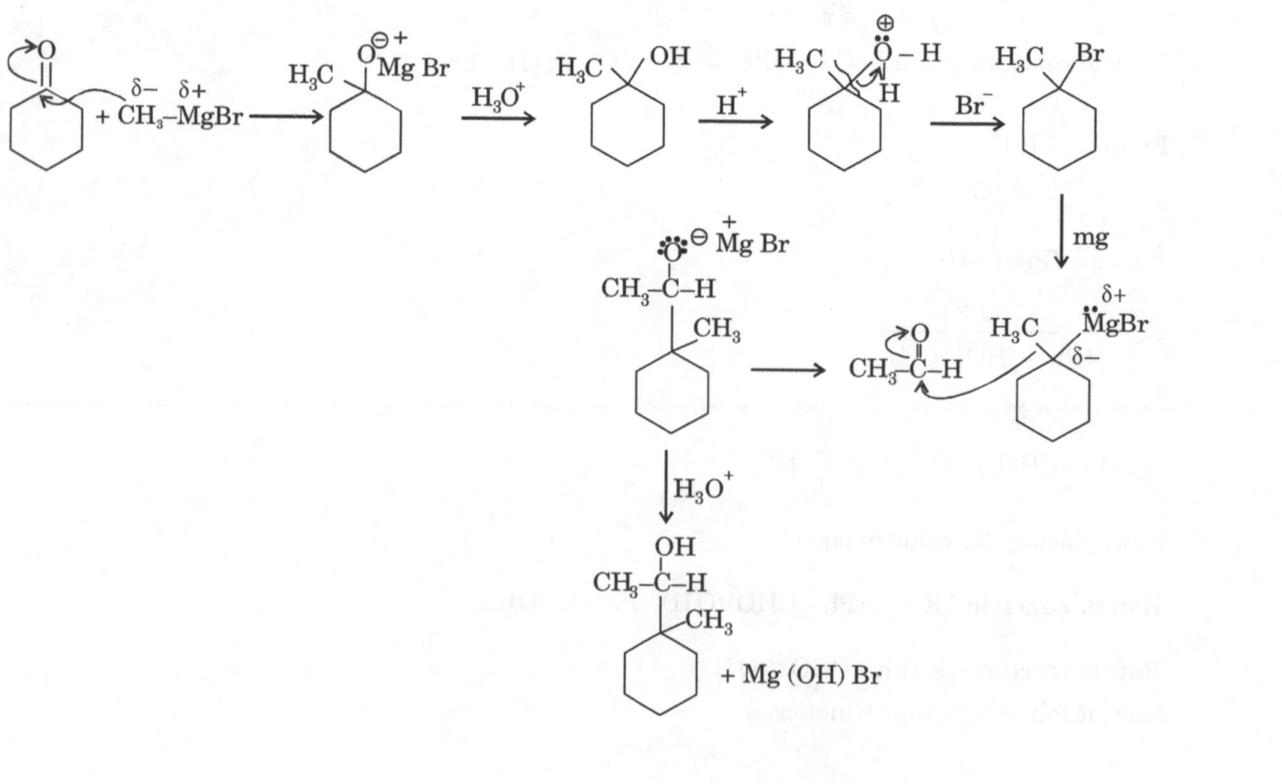

125.

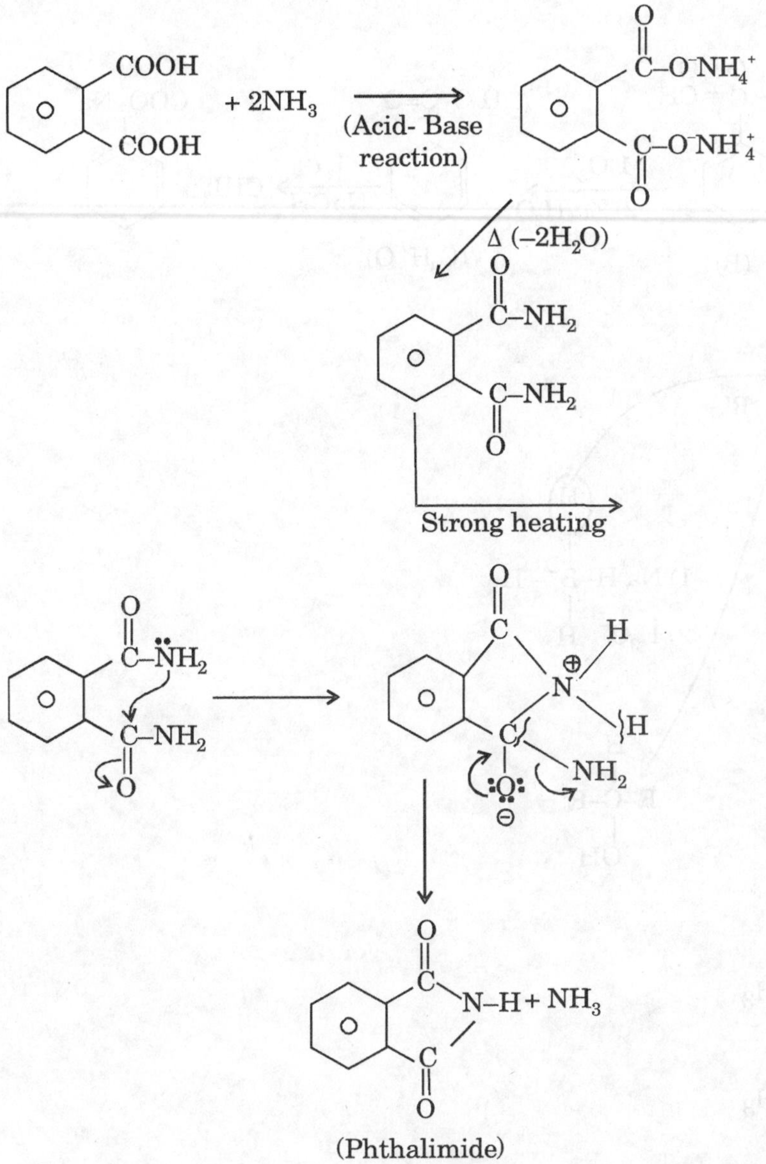
+ 2NH3
(Acid- Base reaction)
Δ (–2H2O)
Strong heating
N–H + NH3
(Phthalimide)

126.

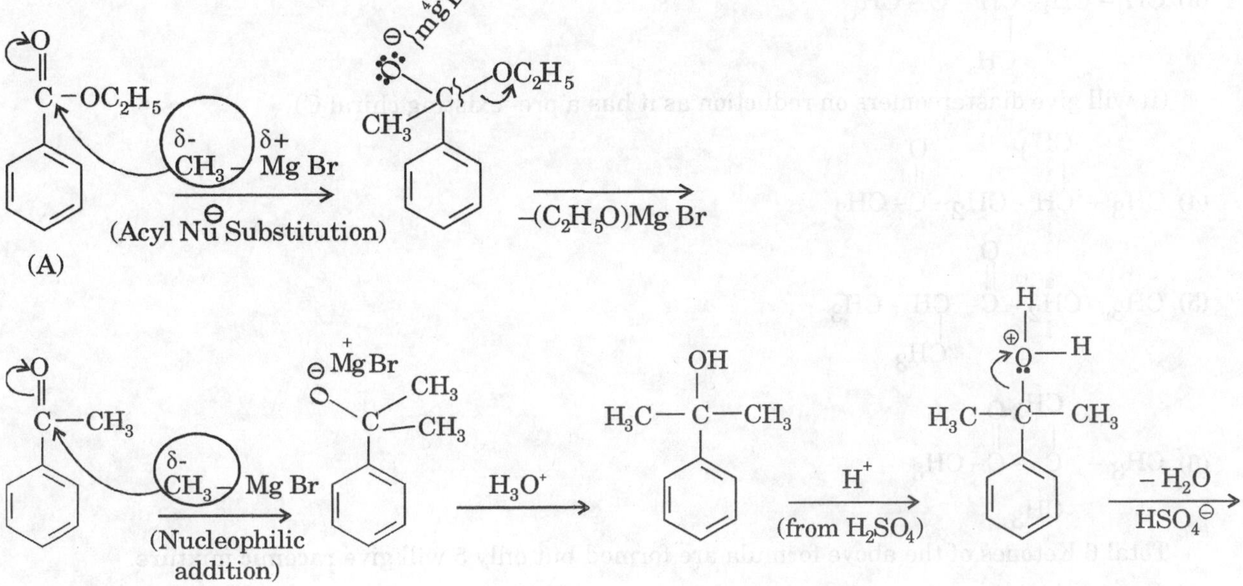
(A)
(Acyl Nu Substitution)
–(C2H5O)Mg Br
(Nucleophilic addition)
H3O+
H+
(from H2SO4)
– H2O
HSO4

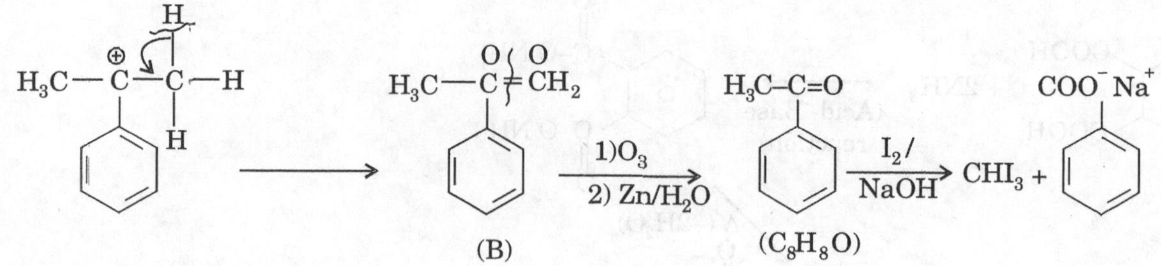

127.

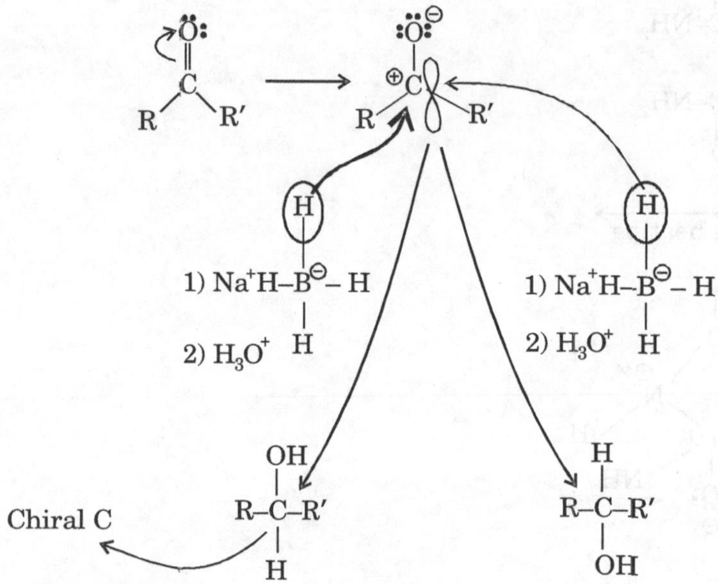

<u>Possible Ketones</u>

(1) $CH_3-CH_2-CH_2-CH_2-\overset{O}{\overset{||}{C}}-CH_3$

(2) $CH_3-CH_2-CH_2-\overset{O}{\overset{||}{C}}-CH_2-CH_3$

(3) $CH_3-CH_2-\overset{*}{C}H(CH_3)-\overset{O}{\overset{||}{C}}-CH_3$

(It will give diastereomers on reduction as it has a pre- existing chiral C)

(4) $CH_3-CH(CH_3)-CH_2-\overset{O}{\overset{||}{C}}-CH_3$

(5) $CH_3-CH_2-\overset{O}{\overset{||}{C}}-CH(CH_3)-CH_3$

(6) $CH_3-C(CH_3)_2-\overset{O}{\overset{||}{C}}-CH_3$

Total 6 Ketones of the above formula are formed but only 5 will give racemic mixture.

128. $CH_3-\overset{\overset{O}{||}}{C}-CH_3 + CH_3-\overset{\overset{O}{||}}{C}-CH_2-CH_3 \xrightarrow[Na^{+}\bar{O}H]{dil.}$

Three self aldol and three cross aldol condensation products are possible, Butan-2-one (unsymmetrical Ketone) can generate nucleophile from 2 sides.

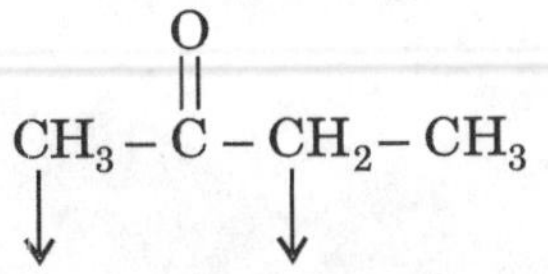

Nucleophile can be generated from these C & can yield different products.

129. 2-Methyl propanal $\left(CH_3-\underset{\underset{CH_3}{|}}{\overset{\overset{H}{|}}{C}}-\overset{\overset{O}{||}}{C}-H\right)$

It has α–H, so can give aldol with dil. NaOH. Also, the α–H is not highly acidic due to the two – CH_3 groups. showing +I. Hence, can also give Cannizaro under suitable conditions.

130. It is the strongest $Nu^{\ominus}$ among these.

131. Option (a) is chloral $\left(Cl_3C-\overset{\overset{O}{||}}{C}-H\right)$. Though it has no α – H but still it will be reluctant to give Cannizaro's reaction. It is because $\overset{\ominus}{C}Cl_3$ is a good leaving group & leaves the molecule readily leading to haloform formation.

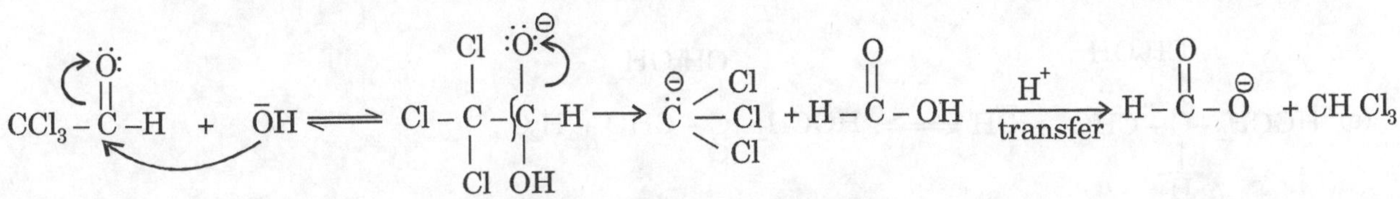

(good leaving group, stabilised by – I of Cl & d-orbital resonance)

In option (b), strong + M of $(CH_3)_2\ddot{N}-$ reduces the electrophilicity of $>C=O$ carbon, hence the attack by $\bar{O}H$ gets hampered.

132. Mechanism

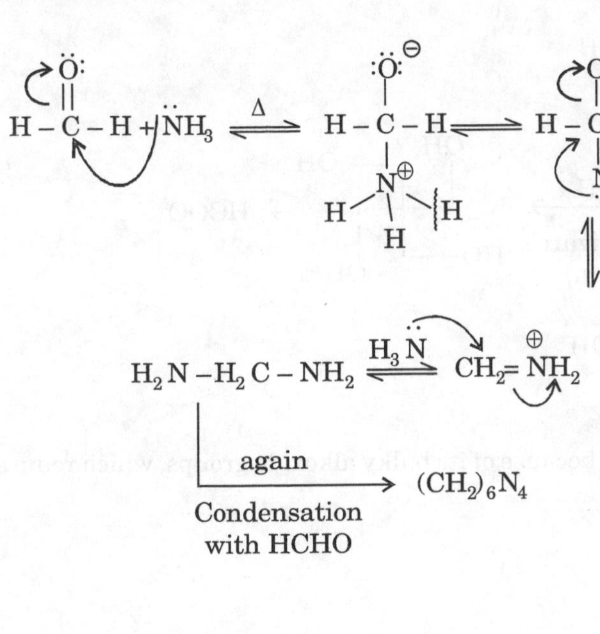

133. 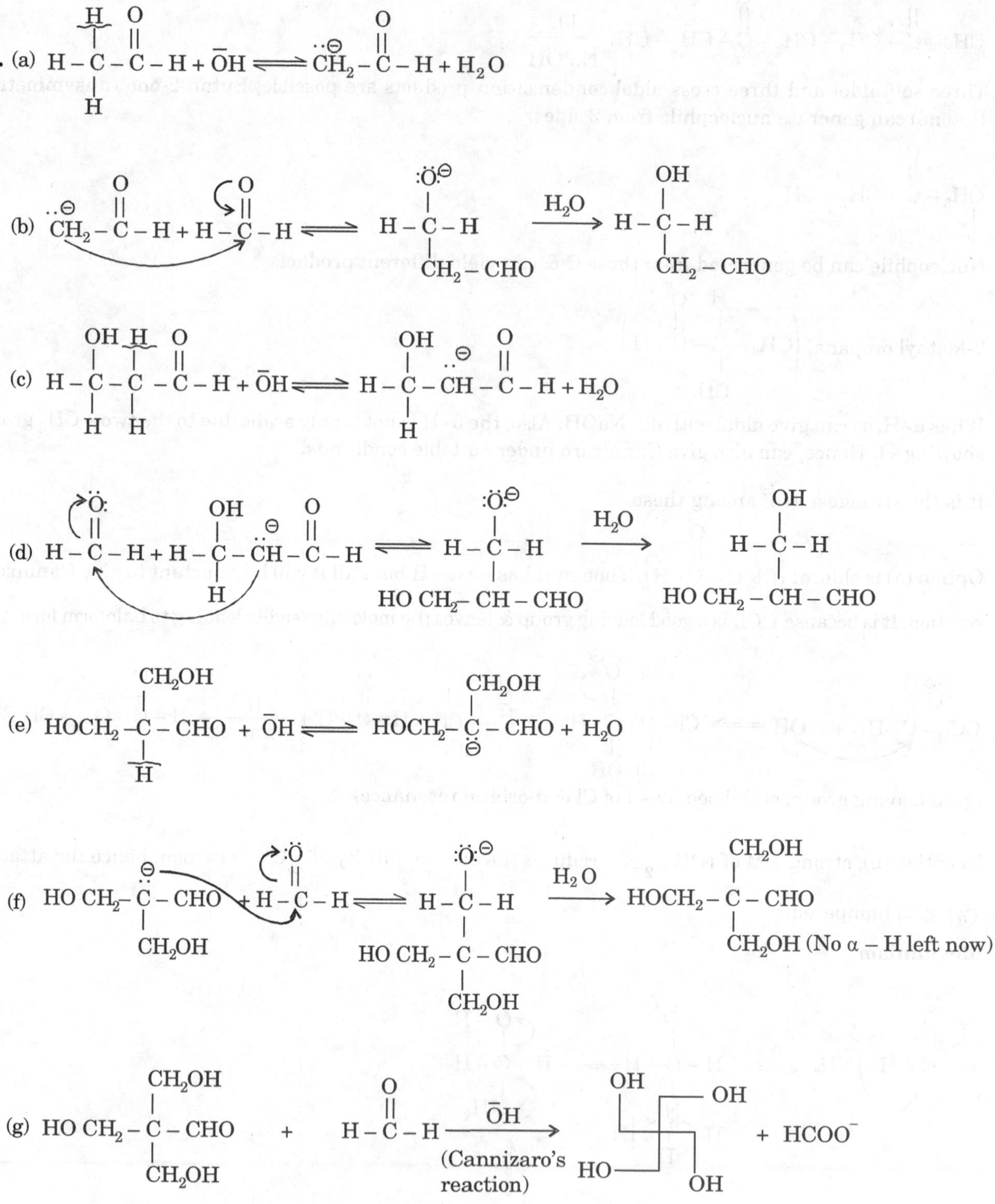

134. (A) is $CH_3-CH(CH_3)-CHO$ & (B) is $CH_3-CH(CH_3)-CH_2OH$

LBAH is a less reactive reducing agent than $LiAlH_4$ because of its bulky alkoxide groups, which reduces its ability to donate H^- ion.

136. Pinacol (Vicinal diol) undergoes rearrangement in acidic medium.

Wrt option (a) –

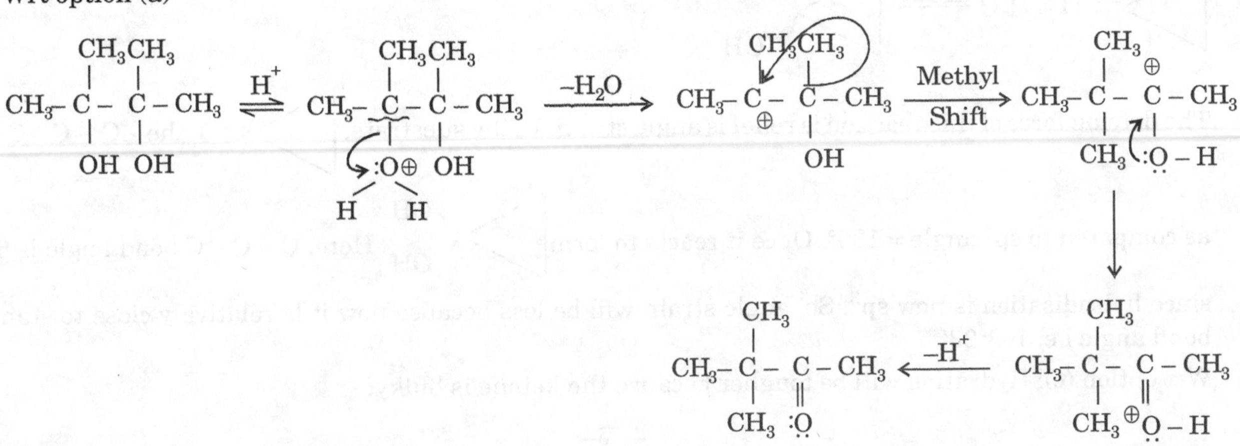

Wrt option (b) –

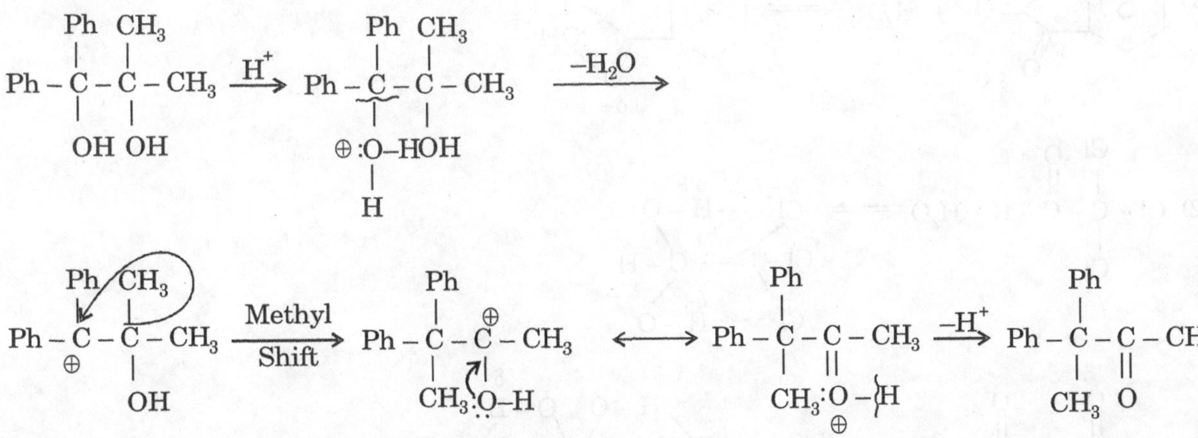

137.

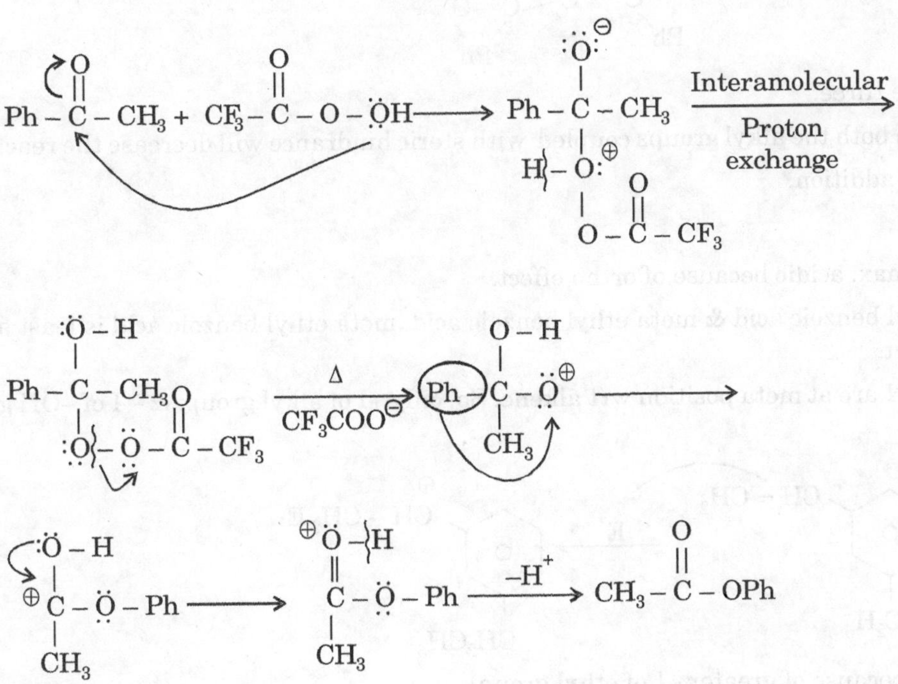

138. Wrt option (a):-

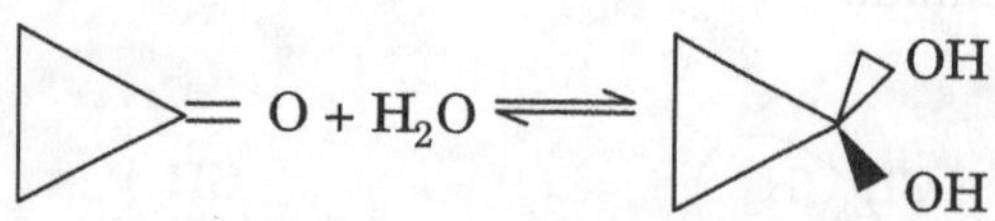

The driving force of this reaction is relief is angle strain. In the substrate, 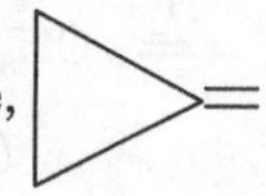, the $\angle C-C-C = 60°$ as compared to sp^2 angle = 120°. Once it reacts to form 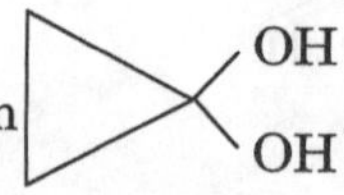. Here, C – C – C bond angle is 60° & since hybridisation is now sp^3. So, angle strain will be less because now it is relatively close to standard bond angle i.e. 109°28′.

Wrt option (c): Hydration will be tougher because the ketone is bulky.

139. (1) 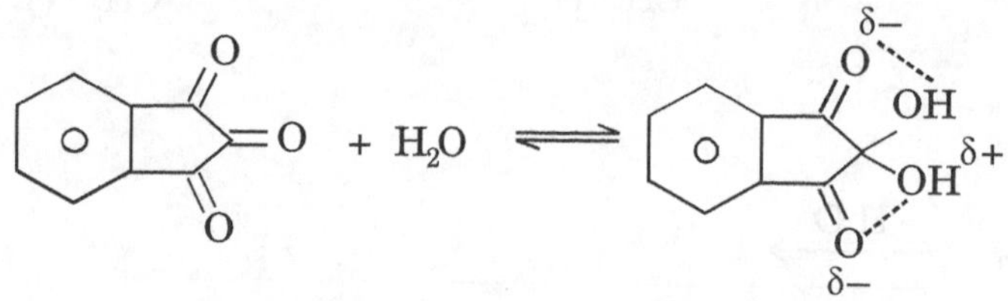

(2) 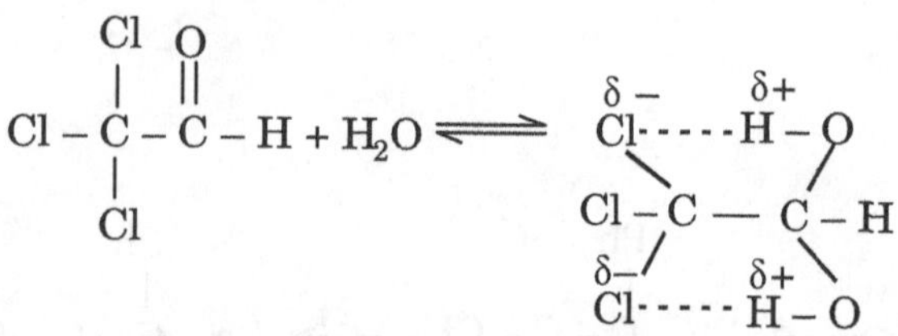

(3) 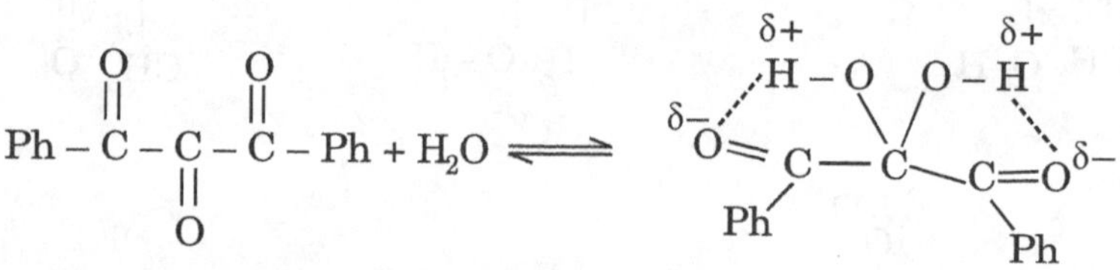

Chelation occurs in all the three.

140. In option (c), +I effect from both the alkyl groups coupled with steric hindrance will decrease the reactivity of molecule towards $Nu^{\ominus}$ addition.

141. wrt option (c),

O-methyl benzoic acid is max. acidic because of ortho effect.

Then, Among meta-methyl benzoic acid & meta ethyl benzoic acid, meta ethyl benzoic acid is least acidic because of greater +I effect.

143. All the alkyl groups & –OH are at meta position wrt alkene. So, only +I of alkyl group. & – I of –OH group is significant.

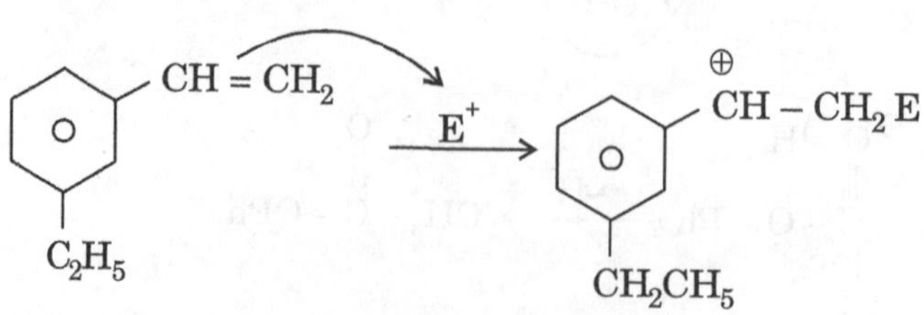

(Carbocation max. stable because of greater +I of ethyl group)

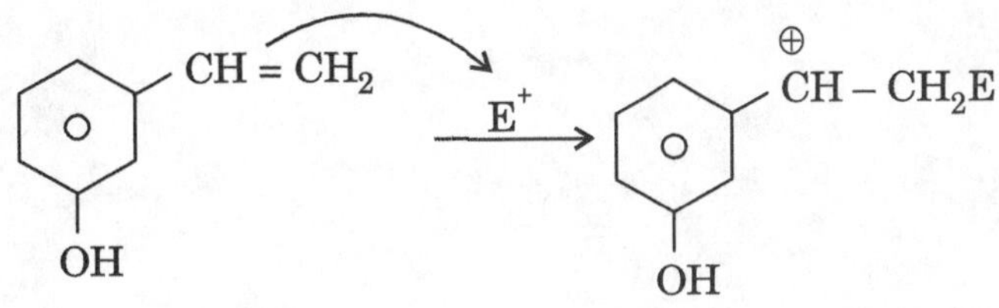

(Carbocation unstable due to –I of –OH group.)

To determine order of reactivity towards electrophillic addition, stability of carbocation should be considered. Greater the stability of carbocation, greater is the reactivity towards electrophillic addition.

wrt option (b).

Actual order of reactivity towards Grignard's reagent is-

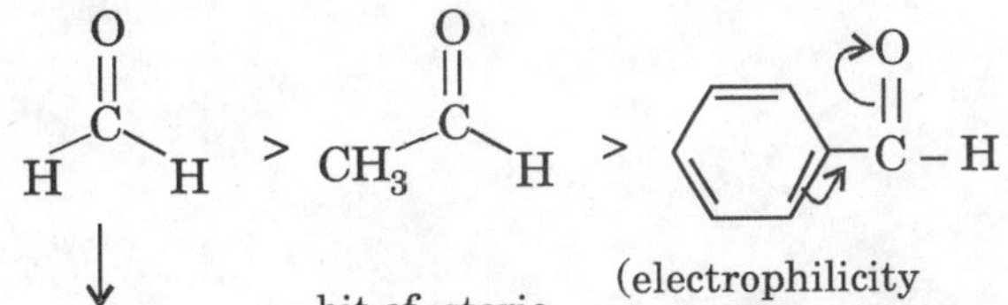

least steric hindrance, least +I

bit of steric hindrance & + I

(electrophilicity of carbonyl compound decreased due to resonance)

wrt option (c),

Actual Reactivity order

R – I > R – Br > R – Cl > R – F.

(because I^- is the best leaving group among halide ions)

wrt option 4,

$F_2 > Cl_2 > Br_2 > I_2$

(order of reactivity of halogens)

144. Both, CH_3CHO & 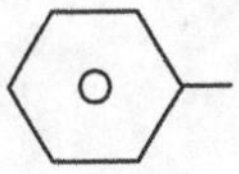 CH_2CHO will give +ve tollens' test.

13 CHAPTER

Organic Compounds Containing Nitrogen

General Introduction & Methods of Preparation of Amines

1. Which one of the following is tertiary amine?

(a) CH_3–CH_2–NH_2

(b) $CH_3 - \underset{NH_2}{\overset{H}{C}} - CH_2CH_3$

(c) $CH_3 - \underset{CH_3}{\overset{CH_3}{C}} - NH_2$

(d) $CH_3 - \underset{CH_3}{N} - CH_2CH_3$

2. Which of the following is optically inactive but non–superimposable on its mirror image?

(a) $(CH_3)_2\ddot{N}C_2H_5$ (b) $H_3C - \underset{C_3H_7}{N} - C_2H_5$

(c) CH_3NH_2 (d) All of these

3. Which of the following will not undergo Hoffmann's Bromamide degradation reaction?

(a) CH_3CONH_2

(b) $CH_3CH_2CONH_2$

(c) $C_6H_5CONH_2$

(d) $CH_3CONHCH_3$

4. Select the incorrect statement (s) about the reaction given below–

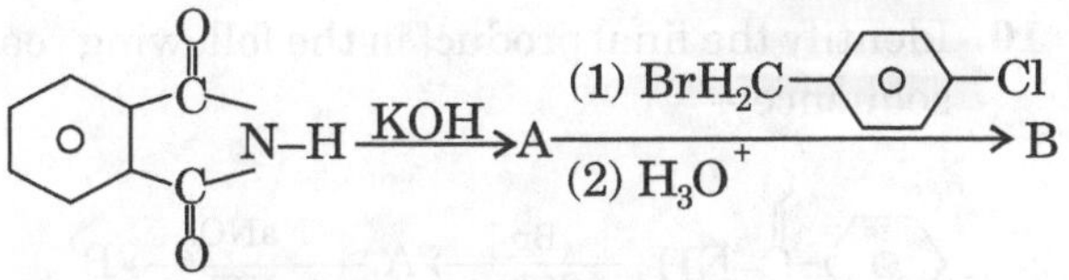

(a) 'A' is formed by acid–base reaction.

(b) Formation of 'B' involves SN^1 reaction followed by hydrolysis.

(c) Formation of 'B' involves SN^2 reaction followed by hydrolysis

(d) Both a & c.

5. Which of the following cannot be prepared by Gabriel phthalamide synthesis?

(a) 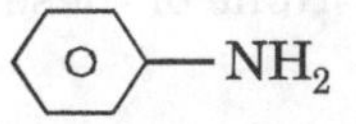 (b) $CH_3 - \underset{CH_3}{\overset{CH_3}{C}} - NH_2$

(c) $CH_3CH_2NH_2$ (d) Both a & b

6. Specie (s) involved in the Hoffmann's bromamide degradation reaction is –

(1) $R - \overset{O}{\overset{||}{C}} - NHBr$ (2) R–N=C=O

(3) $R - \overset{O}{\overset{||}{C}} - \ddot{\underset{\bullet\bullet}{N}}^{\ominus} - Br$

(a) Both 1 & 2 only (b) 2 & 3 only

(c) 1 only (d) All of these

7. Which of the following cannot undergo Hoffmann's ammonolysis?

(a) $CH_3 CH_2 Cl$ (b) $CH_3 CH_2I$

(c) $CH_2 = CH - Cl$ (d) CH_3I

8. Identify 'Y' in the following reaction sequence,

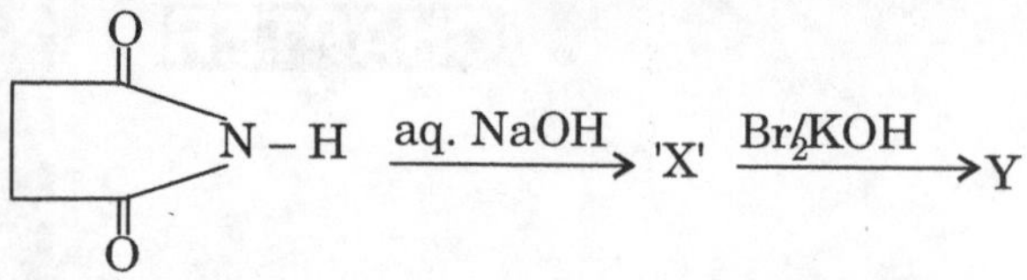

(a) α – alanine (b) β – alanine

(c) γ – alanine (d) γ– amino butyric acid

9. Which of the following will produce an amine ?

(a) $CH_3 - CH_2 - Br + NH_3 \rightarrow$

(b) $CH_3 - CH = N - OH \xrightarrow[C_2H_5OH]{Na}$

(c) $RCONH_2 \xrightarrow[(2) H_3O^+]{(1) LiAlH_4}$

(d) $R - CN \xrightarrow[Hydrolysis]{Complete}$

10. Identify the final product in the following reaction sequence –

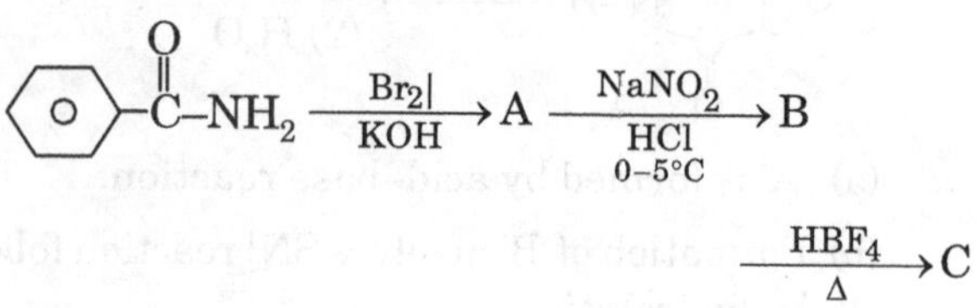

(a) 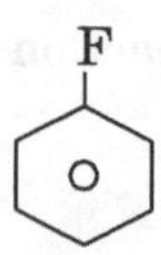 (b) 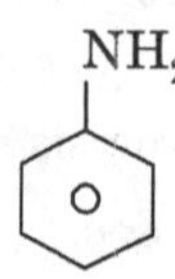

(c) 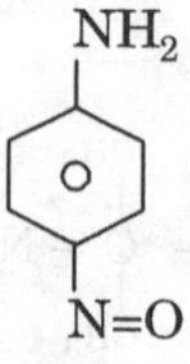 (d) None of these

11. Identify 'X' in the following reaction –

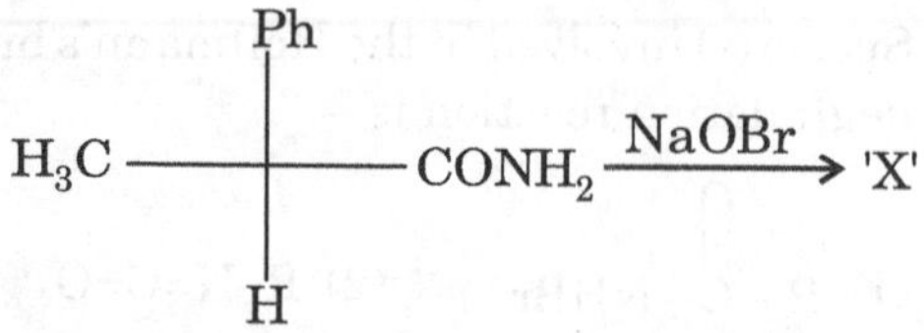

(a) 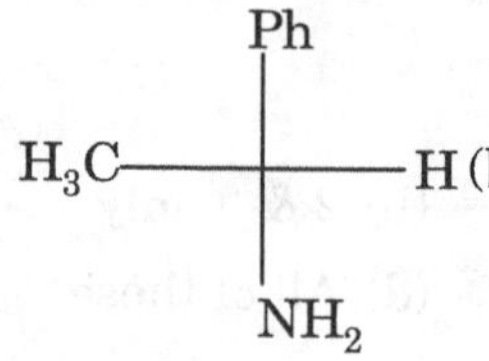 (b) 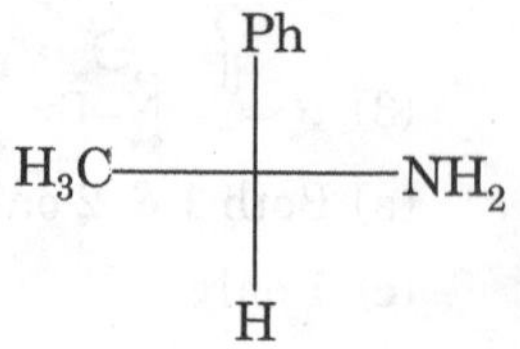

(c) 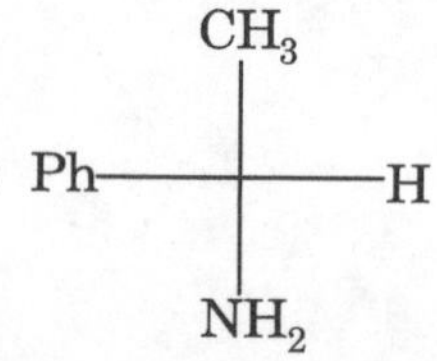 (d) None of these

12. N–alkyl phthalamide can be cleaved better, by –

(a) Acidic Hydrolysis (b) Basic Hydrolysis

(c) Hydrazinolysis (d) None of these

13. Select the correct name reaction

Name reaction	Name
(a) $RCOOH + N_3H \xrightarrow[H_2SO_4]{Conc.} R - NH_2 + N_2 + CO_2$	Schmidt reaction
(b) $R - \overset{O}{\overset{\parallel}{C}} - Cl + NaN_3 \rightarrow R - \overset{O}{\overset{\parallel}{C}} - N_3 \xrightarrow[NaOH]{\Delta} R - NH_2$	Curtius reaction
(c) 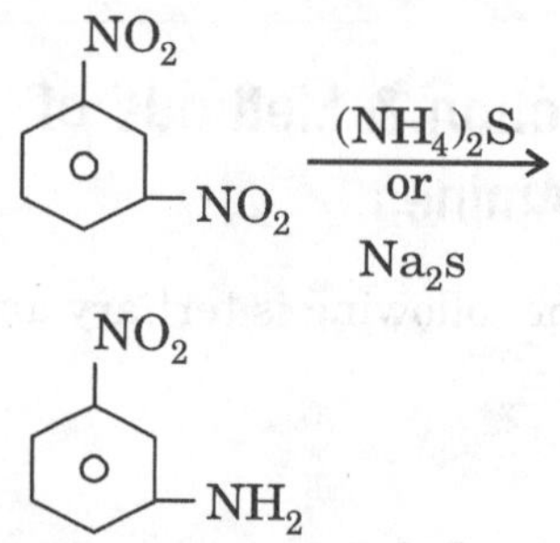	Zinin reduction

(d) All are correct.

14. Which of the following will give a 2° amine?

(a) $R - CHO + NH_3 \xrightarrow{\Delta} A \xrightarrow{H_2/Ni} B$

(b) $R - \overset{O}{\overset{\parallel}{C}} - R + NH_3 \xrightarrow{\Delta} C \xrightarrow{H_2/Ni} D$

(c) $R - \overset{O}{\overset{\parallel}{C}} - R + RNH_2 \xrightarrow{\Delta} E \xrightarrow{H_2/Ni} F$

(d) All of these

Chemical Properties of Amines

15. The Compound which when treated with $CHCl_3$ & NaOH given $R - N \equiv C$ is –

(a) RNH_2

(b) R_2NH

(c) R_3N

(d) $R_4N^+Cl^-$

16. Identify 'A' in the following reaction–

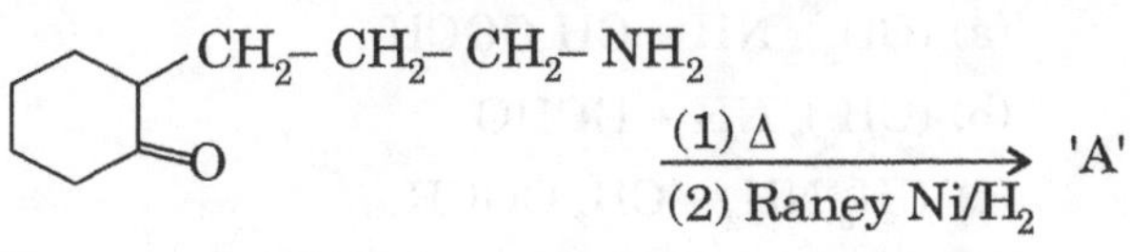

(a) 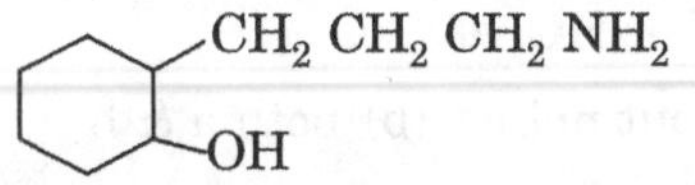

(b) 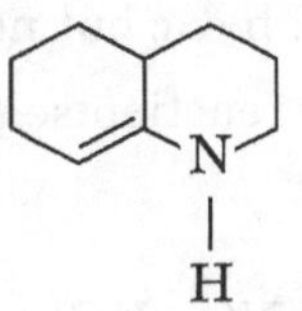

(c) 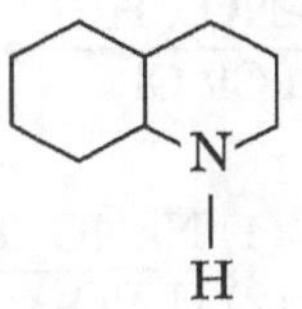

(d) 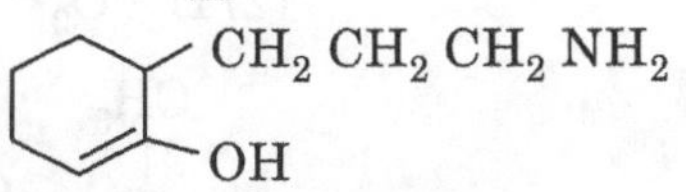

17. Aniline is acetylated, then nitrated & finally hydrolysed to give 'X' as major product. The correct structure of X is–

(a) 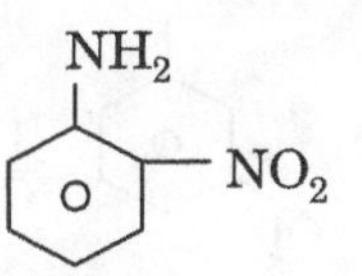

(b) 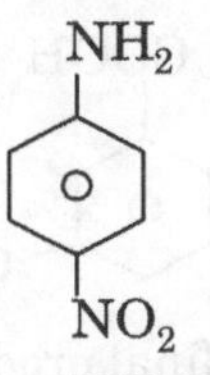

(c) 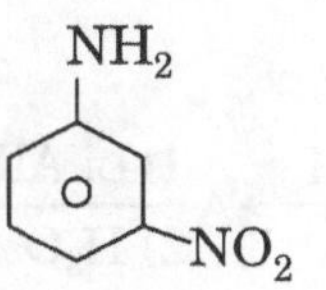

(d) 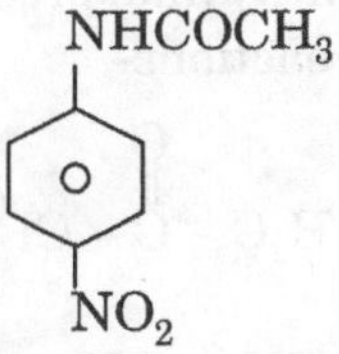

18. Carbylamine test is given by

(a) 1° aliphatic amines only

(b) 1° aliphatic amine & 1° aromatic amines only

(c) 1° Aromatic amines only

(d) Amides Only

19. Arrange the following amides according to their relative reactivity when treated with Br_2/ KOH

P. 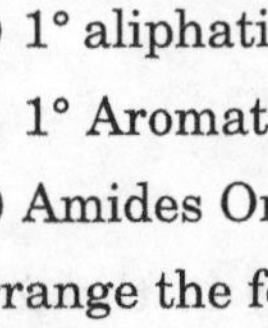

Q. 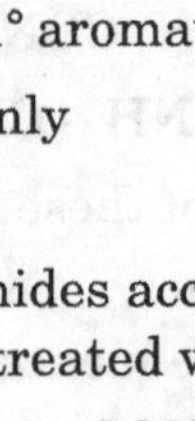

R. 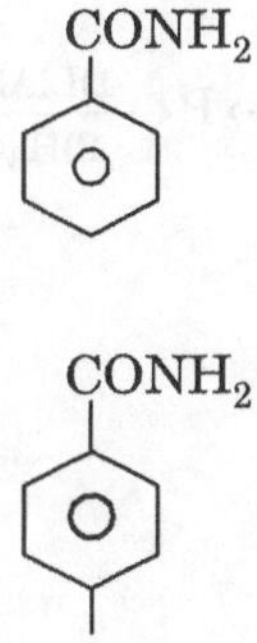

S. 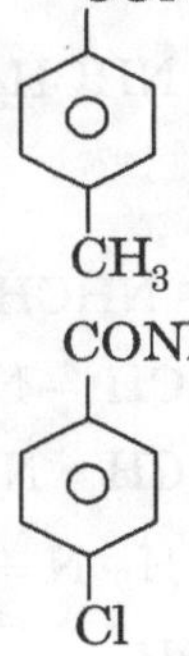

(a) Q > P > S > R (b) P > Q > R > S

(c) R > S > P > Q (d) S > P > Q > R

20. The correct set of reagents for converting benzoic acid to aniline is–

(a) $SOCl_2$, NH_3, Δ (b) $SOCl_2$, NH_3,Br_2/KOH

(c) HCl, NH_3, Br_2/KOH(d)HNO_2, NH_3, Br_2/KOH

21. Consider the following reaction–

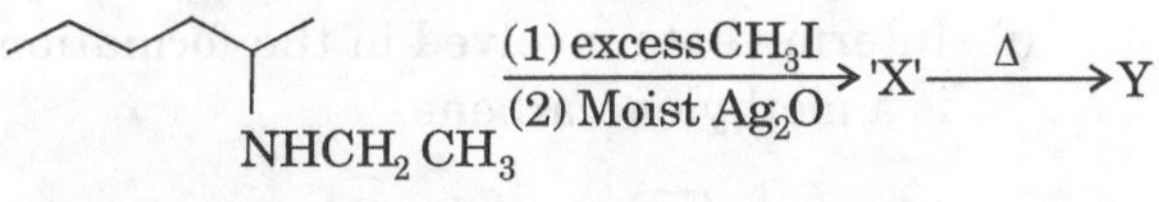

Predict the possible number of alkenes & the major product (alkene) y, in the above reaction.

(a) 2 & $H_3C-CH_2-CH_2-CH=CH-CH_3$

(b) 2 & $CH_3-CH_2-CH_2-CH_2-CH=CH_2$

(c) 3 & $CH_2=CH_2$

(d) 2 & $CH_2=CH_2$

22. Consider the following sequence of reactions –

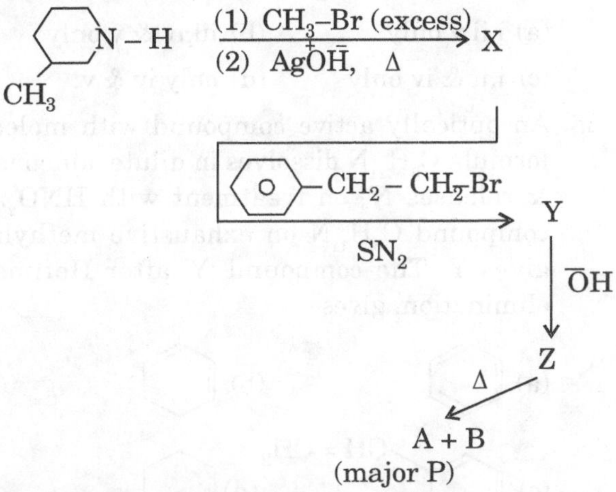

Which of the following is true if 'A' is a nitrogen containing compound?

(a) B is a diene

(b) Y has 2 chiral carbons

(c) X & A are same

(d) X is quarternary ammonium hydroxide

23. An optically inactive amine (A) $C_4H_{11}N$ on treatment with HNO_2 gives an alcohol (B). The compound (B) on heating with conc. H_2SO_4 at 453 K gives an alkene (C). This alkene (C), on treatment with HBr gives an optically active compound (D) having molecular formula C_4H_9Br. Identify A.

(a) $CH_3\ CH_2\ CH\ (NH_2)CH_3$

(b) $CH_3-CH_2-CH_2-CH_2-NH_2$

(c) $CH_3\ NH\ CH_2\ CH_2\ CH_3$

(d) $C_2H_5\ NHC_2H_5$

24. Consider the following sequence of reactions and select the correct statement (s).

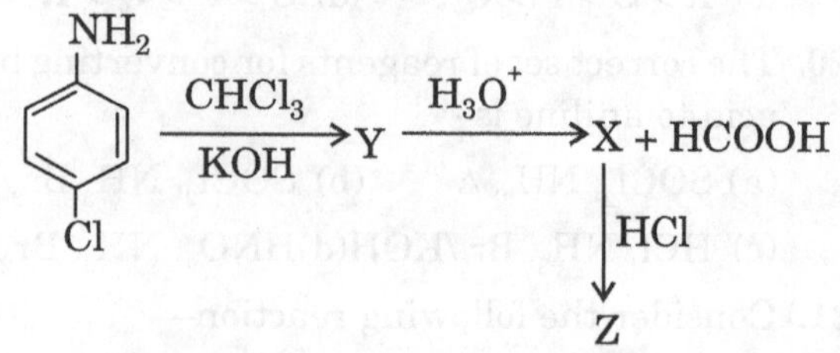

(i) Intermediate involved in the formation of Y is a methylenecarbene.

(ii) X is 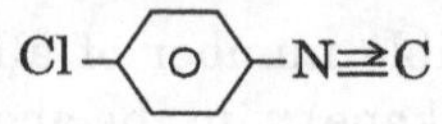

(iii) X & Z can be distinguished with help of $AgNO_3$, Solution

(iv) X is 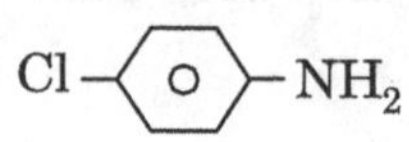

(v) Z on treatment with aq. NaOH followed by $CHCl_3$ / KOH give bad Smelling Compound.

(a) i,ii,v only (b) iii,iv & v only

(c) i,ii & iv only (d) only iv & v.

25. An optically active compound with molecular formula $C_6H_{11}N$ dissolves in dilute aqueous HCl & releases N_2 on treatment with HNO_2. The compound $C_6H_{11}N$ on exhaustive methylation gives Y. The compound 'Y' after Hoffmann's elimination, gives–

(a) 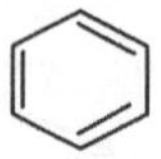 (b) 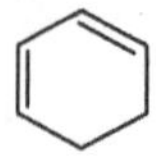

(c) 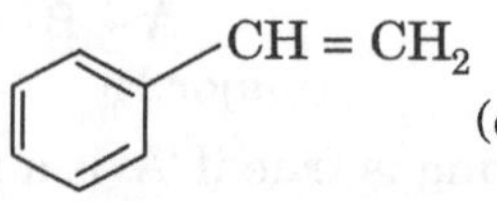 (d) 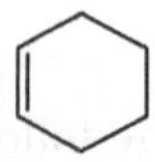

26. Identify 'X' & 'Y' in the following reactions–

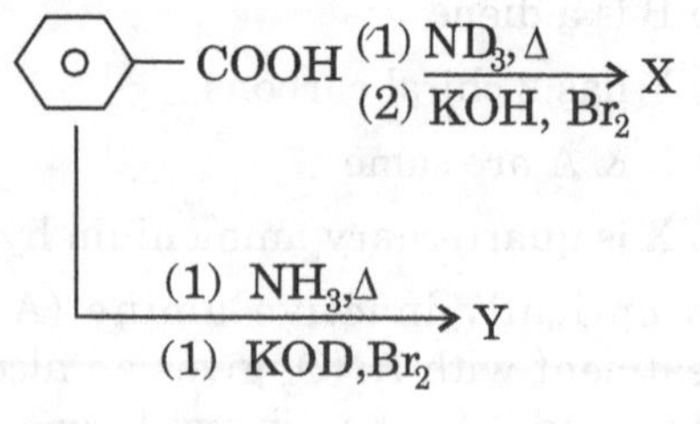

(a) X is 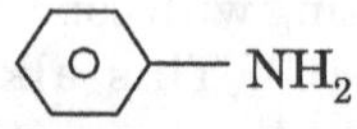 & Y is 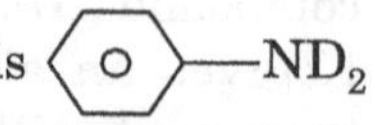

(b) X is 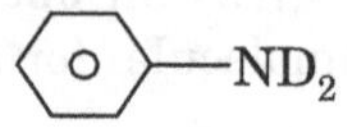 & Y is 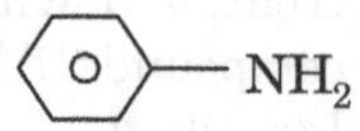

(c) Both are 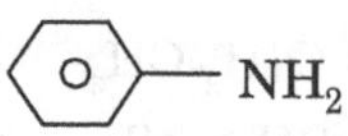

(d) Both are 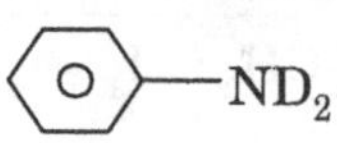

27. Which of the following will give an enamine.

(a) $(CH_3)_2NH + CH_3COCH_3$

(b) $(CH_3)_2NH + HCHO$

(c) $CH_3NH_2 + CH_3COCH_3$

(d) $CH_3NH_2 + HCHO$

(a) a,b & d but not c (b) both a & b

(c) only a (d) a, b & c but not d

28. Identify 'C' in the following reaction sequence–

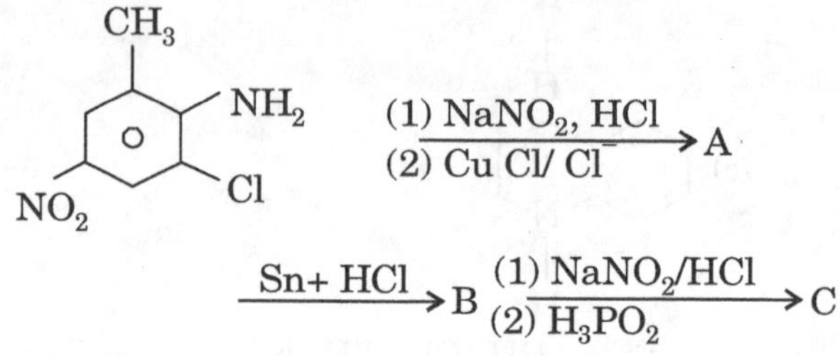

(a) 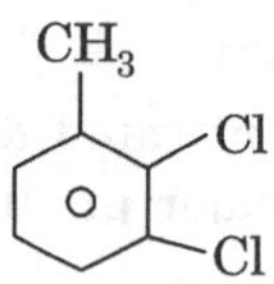 (b) 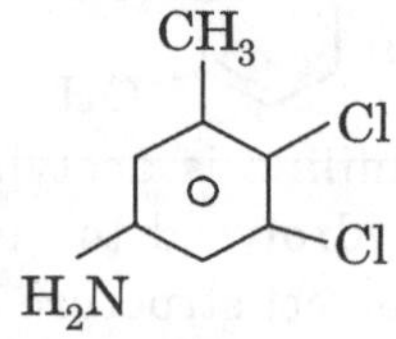

(c) 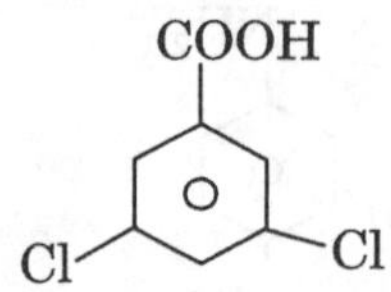 (d) 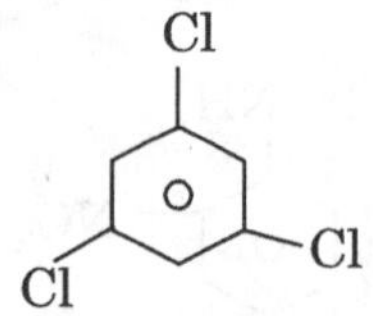

29. Identify final product 'B' in the following sequence of reactions–

$$H_3C-\overset{O}{\overset{||}{C}}-Cl \xrightarrow{(CH_3)_2\ddot{N}H} A \xrightarrow[2)\ H_3O^+]{1)\ LiAlH_4} B$$

(a) $CH_3-CH_2-\underset{CH_3}{\underset{|}{N}}-CH_3$

(b) $CH_3CH_2CONH_2$

(c) $CH_3-NH-CH_2CH_3$

(d) None of these

30. The unknown compound (Q) in the following reaction sequence, cannot be–

$$CH_3-\overset{O}{\overset{||}{C}}-NHCH_3 \xrightarrow[2)H_3O^+]{1)LiAlH_4} P \xleftarrow[2)H_3O^+]{1)LiAlH_4} Q$$

(a) $H-\overset{O}{\overset{||}{C}}-NHCH_2CH_3$

(b) $CH_3-CH_2-N=CH_2$

(c) $CH_3-CH=N-CH_3$

(d) $H-\underset{OH}{\underset{|}{CH}}-N=CH_2$

31. If compound (C) does not reduce Fehling's Solution, then choose the correct option :–

$$\underset{(C_3H_9N)}{(A)} \xrightarrow[-N_2]{HNO_2} (B) \xrightarrow{PCC} (C) \xrightarrow{NH_2OH} \underset{\text{(an oxime)}}{(D)}$$

(a) Both (B) & (C) will give iodoform test.

(b) (D) Can show geometrical isomerism.

(c) (D) on reaction with PCl_5 followed by treatment with H_3O^+ forms 2°amine

(d) Both (B) & (C) will give crystalline adduct with $NaHSO_3$.

32. Identify 'Z' in the following sequence of reactions

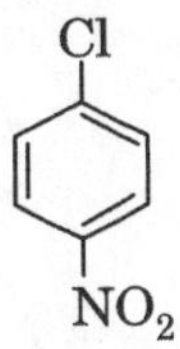

$$CH_2=CH-CH_2-O^{\ominus} \longrightarrow X \xrightarrow{Sn+HCl} Y \xrightarrow[2)H_3PO_2,\Delta]{1)NaNO_2/HCl,\ 0-5°C} Z$$

(a) 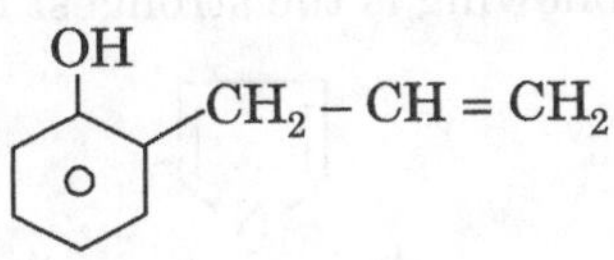

(b) 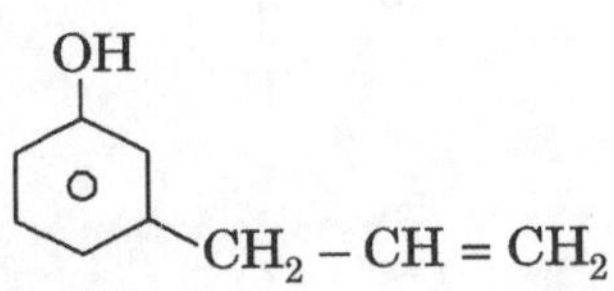

(c) 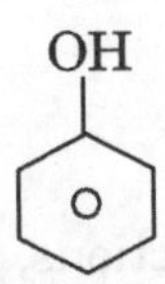

(d) All of these

33. Which of the following will evolve N_2 gas on reaction with HNO_2?

a. acetamide b. isopropylamine

c. ethylmethyl amine d. aniline

e. n-propylamine

(a) a, b & e only (b) c, d & e only

(c) a, c & e only (d) b & c only

34. Which of the following reactions does not involve intramolecular alkyl shift ?

(a) Hoffmann's bromamide degradation

(b) Curtius reaction

(c) Schmidt reaction

(d) Carbylamine reaction

35. Identify 'Y' in the following reaction sequence –

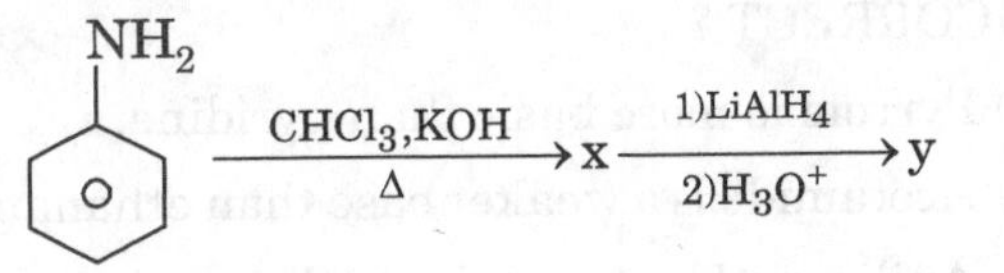

(a) $Ph-\underset{H}{N}-CH_3$ (b) $Ph-CH_2-NH_2$

(c) $Ph-\underset{H}{N}-\overset{O}{\overset{\|}{C}}-H$ (d) $Ph-\overset{\oplus}{N}\equiv C^{\ominus}$

36. The amine that will give off N_2 upon treatment with $NaNO_2/HCl$ at 0°C to 5°C is–

(a) 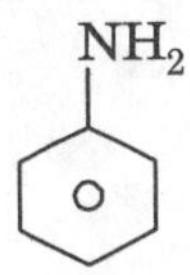 (b) 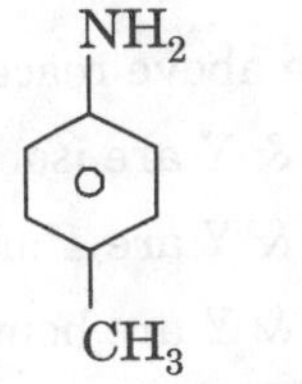

(c) 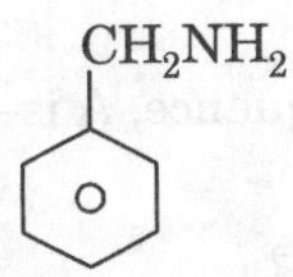 (d) 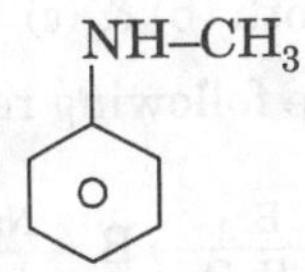

37. Select the correct statement (s) about the reaction given below

$$CH_3-\underset{CH_3}{\overset{CH_3}{\underset{|}{\overset{|}{C}}}}-CH_2-NH_2 \xrightarrow[NaNO_2/HCl]{HNO_2 \text{ or}}$$

(a) $\overset{\oplus}{N}=O$ is the attacking electrophile.

(b) Carbocation undergoes rearrangement here.

(c) N_2 is the leaving group here

(d) All are correct.

38. An amine contains 31.22 % nitrogen by weight. On treatment with nitrous acid (HNO_2), it gives a yellow oily liquid nitrosoamine. Then, the amine is

(a) $(CH_3)_2NH$ (b) $(C_2H_5)_2NH$

(c) $C_2H_5-NHCH_3$ (d) $C_2H_5NH_2$

39. Aniline is treated with Br_2/H_2O to give an organic compound 'X' which when treated with $NaNO_2$/HCl at 0°C gives compound 'Y'. Compound 'Y' on treatment with CuCl & HCl gives a compound–

(a) O–bromo chlorobenzene

(b) p–bromo chlorobenzene

(c) 2,4,6–tribromophenol

(d) 2,4,6–tribromochlorobenzene

40. Which of the following statements is/are INCORRECT ?

(a) Pyrrole is more basic than pyridine.

(b) Acetamide is a weaker base than ethanamine

(c) Aniline is less basic than ethanamine

(d) Ethanamide is more acidic than ethanamine.

41. Consider the following reactions–

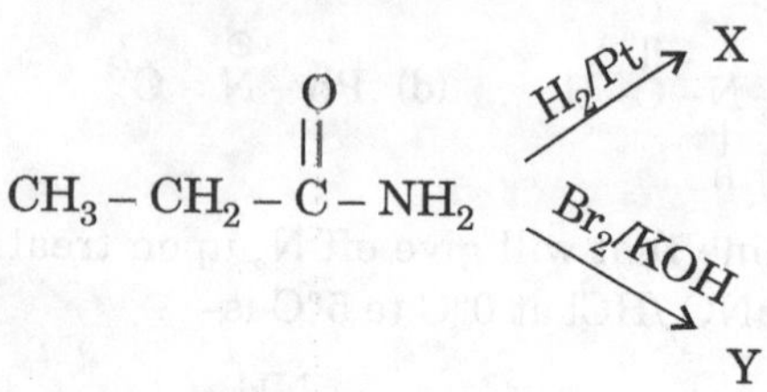

In the above reactions,

(a) X & Y are isomers

(b) X & Y are 1°amines

(c) X & Y are homologues

(d) Both (b) & (c)

42. In the following reaction sequence, A is–

$$A \xrightarrow[H_2O]{Br_2} B \xrightarrow[0-5°C]{NaNO_2-HCl} C \xrightarrow{C_2H_5OH,\Delta} \text{Tribromobenzene}$$

(a) Benzoic acid (b) Salicylic acid

(c) phenol (d) aniline

43. Which of the following will give schiffs base with an aldehyde

(a) $CH_3CH_2NH_2$

(b) $C_6H_5–CH_2–NH_2$

(c) $C_6H_5 – NH_2$

(d) All of these

44. An organic compound (A) having molecular formula $C_9H_{13}N$ dissolves in dil. HCl & releases N_2 with HNO_2 giving an optically active alcohol. Alcohol on oxidation gives dicarboxylic acid which on heating forms an anhydride. The organic compound 'A' is –

(a) 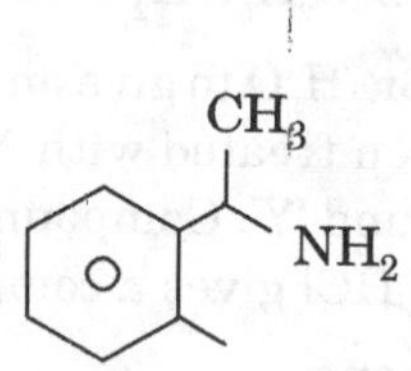 (b) 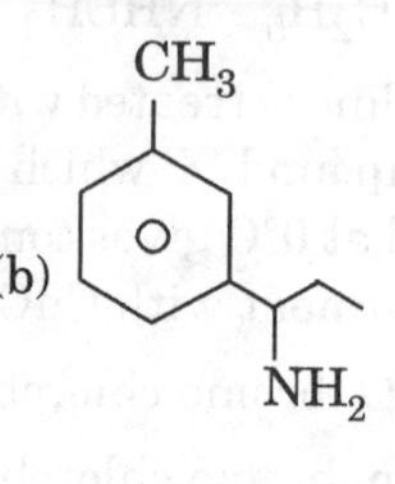

(c) 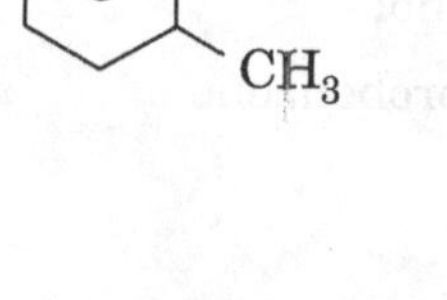 (d) Both (b) & (c)

45. Among the diazonium cations given below, the correct order of decreasing reactivity towards coupling is –

(a) 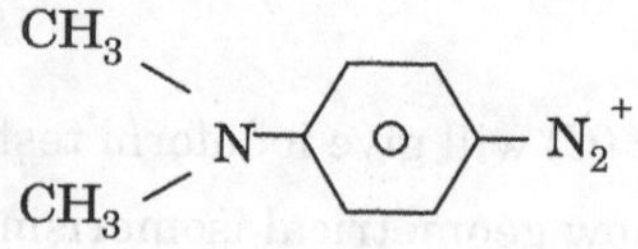

(b) 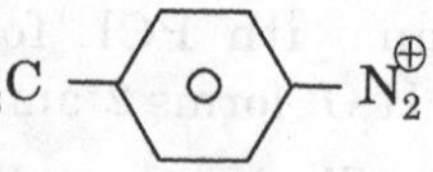

(c) 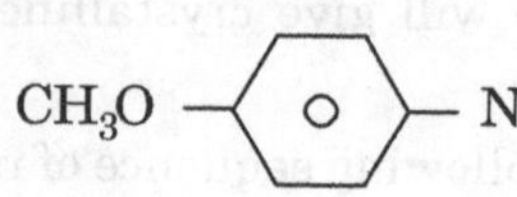

(d) 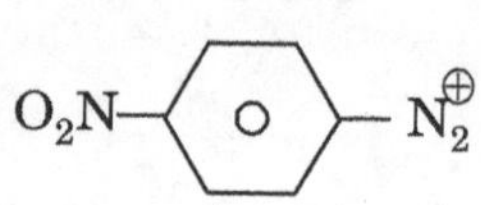

(a) I > II > III > IV

(b) I > III > II > IV

(c) IV > II > III > I

(d) None of these

46. Which of the following is the strongest base?

(a) 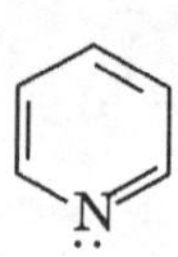 (b) 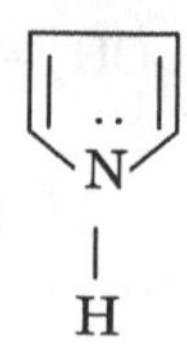

(c) 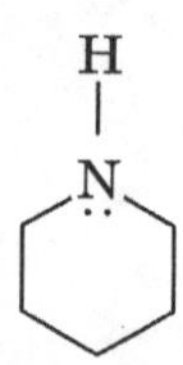 (d) 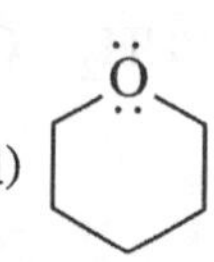

47. In the following sequence of reactions, identify 'C'.

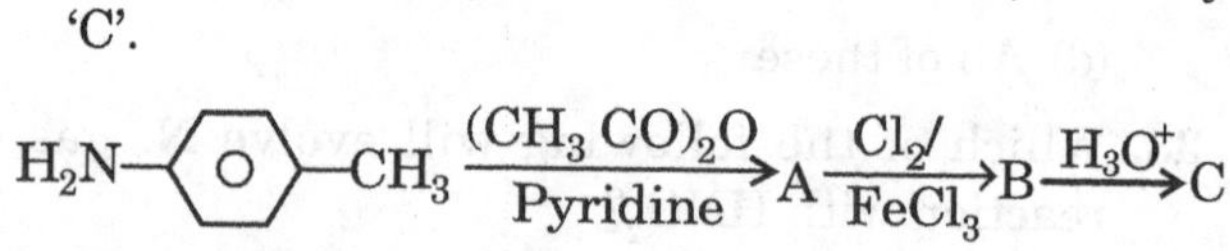

(a) 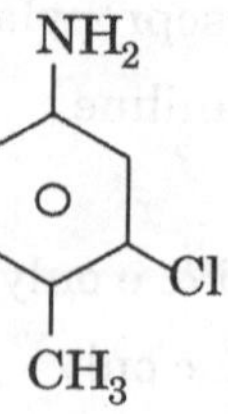 (b) 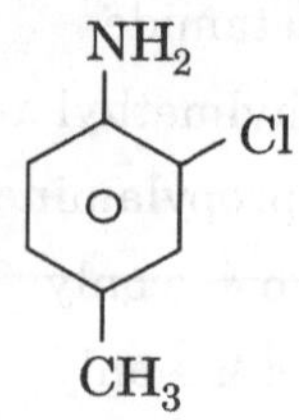

(c) 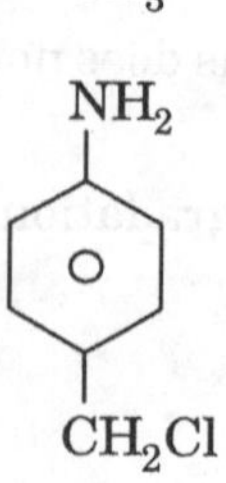 (d) All of these

48. A given nitrogen containing aromatic compound 'A' reacts with Sn/HCl, followed by HNO_2 to give an unstable compound 'B', 'B' on treatment with phenol, forms a beautiful colored compound 'C' with the molecular formula $C_{12}H_{10}N_2O$

The structure of compound 'A' is–

(a) 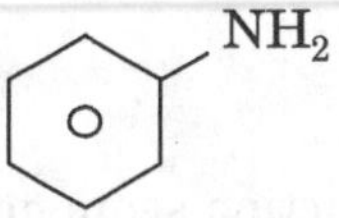

(b) 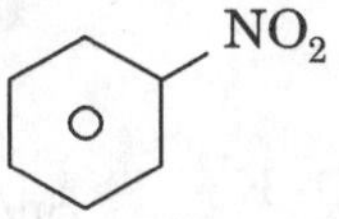

(c) 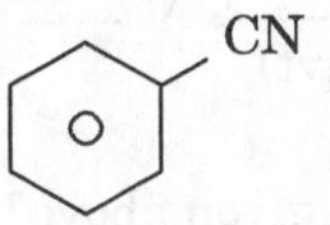

(d) 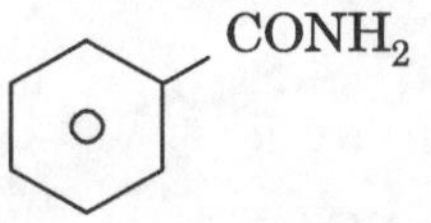

49. Aniline is reacted with Br_2/H_2O & the resulting product is treated with an aqueous solution of $NaNO_2$ in presence of dilute HCl.

The compound so formed is converted into tetrafluoroborate which is subsequently heated dry. The final product is –

(a) p–bromo fluorobenzene

(b) p–bromoaniline

(c) 2,4,6–tribromofluorobenzene

(d) 1,3,5–tribromobenzene

50. The major product of the following reaction is –

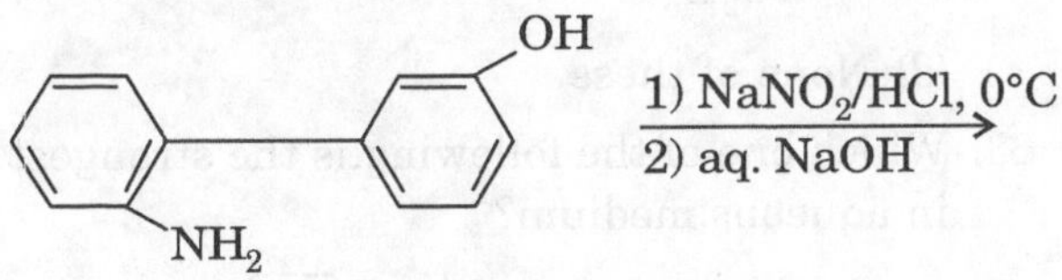

(a) 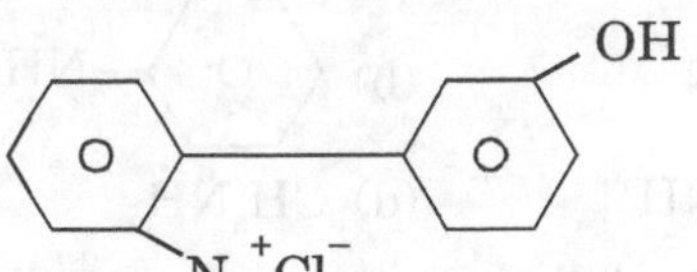

(b) 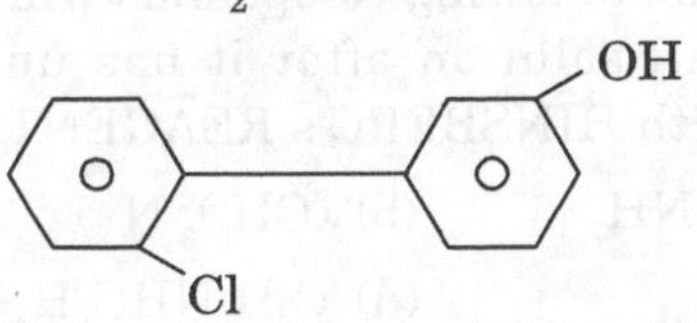

(c) 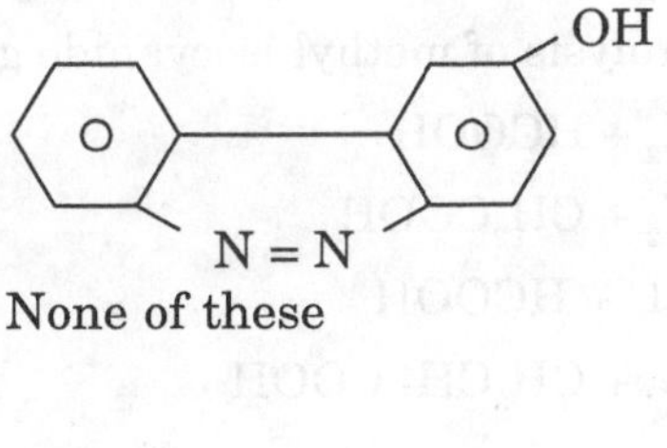

(d) None of these

51. In the diazotisation of arylamine, the use of nitrous acid is that it,

(a) Suppresses hydrolysis of phenol

(b) is a source of nitrosonium ion.

(c) neutralises the base liberated.

(d) All of these

52. 4 – Nitrotoluene is treated with $Br_2/AlCl_3$ to get compound 'P'. 'P' is reduced with Sn/HCl to get compound 'Q', 'Q' is diazotised & the product is treated with phosphinic acid to get compound 'R'. 'R' is oxidised with alkaline $KMnO_4$ to get compound 'S'. The compound 'S' is –

(a) 2 – Bromo – 4 – hydroxybenzoic acid

(b) benzoic acid

(c) 2 – Bromobenzoic acid

(d) 3 – Bromobenzoic acid

53. In the Hoffmann's Bromamide degradation reaction, the number of moles of NaOH & Br_2 used per mole of amine produced, are–

(a) One mole of NaOH & one mole of Br_2.

(b) Four moles of NaOH & two mole of Br_2.

(c) Two moles of NaOH & two moles of Br_2.

(d) Four moles of NaOH & One mole of Br_2

54. The correct order of basic strength of CH_3NH_2 (I), $(CH_3)_2NH$ (II), $(CH_3)_3N$ (III), $C_6H_5CH_2NH_2$ (IV), in gaseous phase is–

(a) I > II > III > IV (b) II > I > III > IV

(c) IV > III > II > I (d) III > II > I > IV

55. An organic compound (C_3H_9N) (A) when treated with HNO_2, gave an alcohol & N_2 gas was evolved. (A) on warming with $CHCl_3$ & Caustic Potash gave (C) which on reduction gave isopropyl methylamine. Predict the structure of 'A'

(a) $CH_3-CH(CH_3)-NH_2$

(b) $CH_3-CH_2-NH-CH_3$

(c) $CH_3-N(CH_3)-CH_3$

(d) $CH_3-CH_2-CH_2-NH_2$

56. The compound which gives an oily nitrosoamine on reaction with HNO_2 at low temperature, is –

(a) CH_3-NH_2 (b) $(CH_3)_2CHNH_2$

(b) $CH_3-NH-CH_3$ (d) $(CH_3)_3N$

57. The order of basicity among the following compounds is –

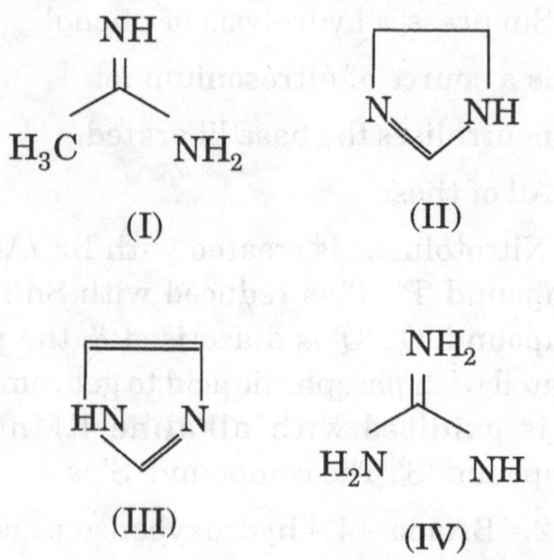

(a) IV > II > III > I (b) II > I > IV > III

(c) IV > I > II > III (d) None of these

58. In the following sequence of reactions, what is D?

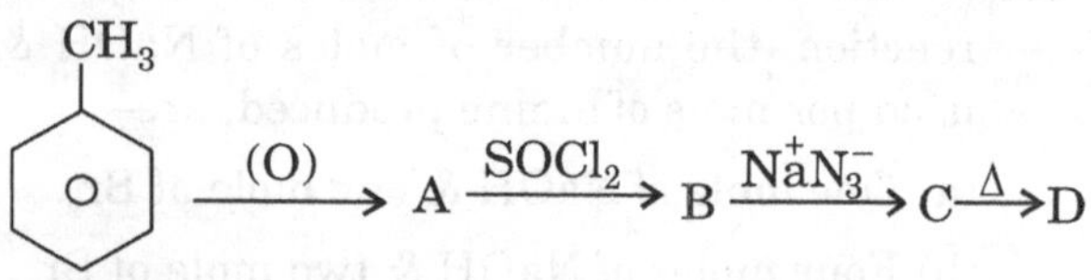

(a) 1° amine

(b) An amide

(c) Phenyl isocyanate

(d) Chain lengthened hydro carbon

59. Among the following, the strongest bronsted base is –

(a) NH_3 (b) 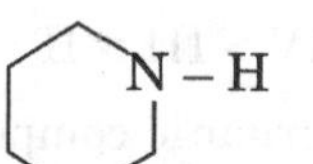

(c) 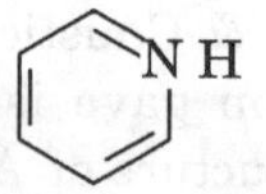

(d) 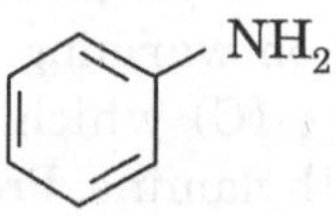

60. The correct sequence of reactions to convert p – nitrophenol into quinol involves –

(a) Reduction, diazotisation & hydrolysis

(b) Hydrolysis, diazotisation & reduction

(c) Hydrolysis, reduction & diazotisation

(d) Diazotisation, reduction & hydrolysis

61. Which one of the following nitro compounds does not react with HNO_2?

(a) $H_3C – CH_2 – CH_2 –NO_2$

(b) $CH_3– \underset{|}{CH}–CH_2NO_2$ (with CH_3 on CH)

(c) $H_3C – C(CH_3)_2 – NO_2$

(d) $H_3C – \overset{O}{\overset{||}{C}} – \underset{CH_3}{CH} – NO_2$

62. Consider the following reaction sequence –

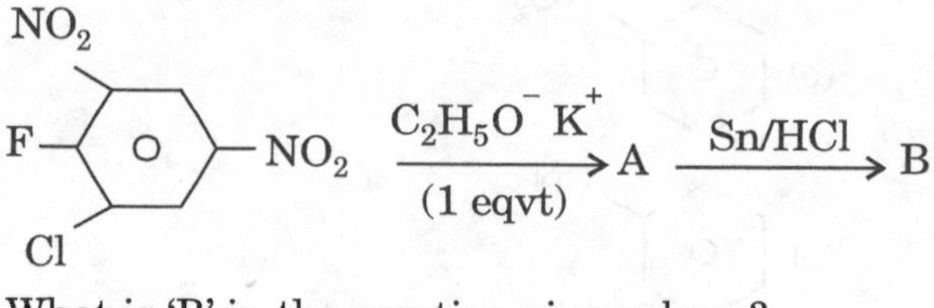

What is 'B' in the reaction given above?

(a) 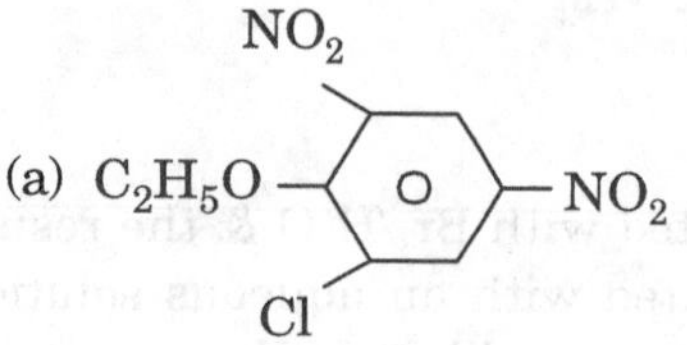

(b) 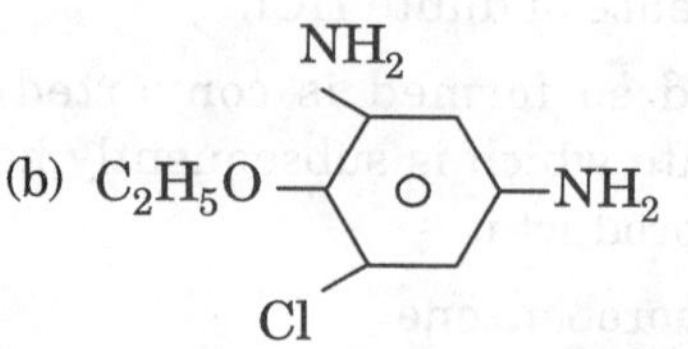

(c) 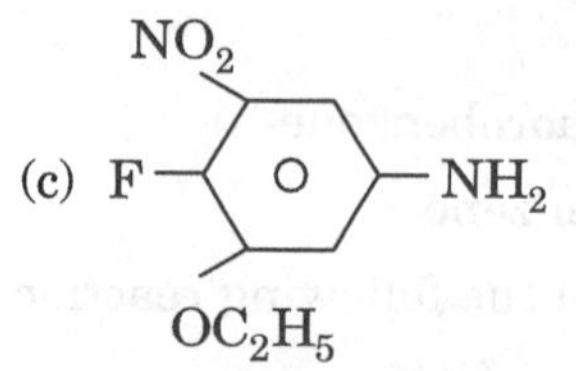

(d) None of these

63. Which one of the following is the strongest base in aqueous medium?

(a) $(CH_3)_3N$ (b) 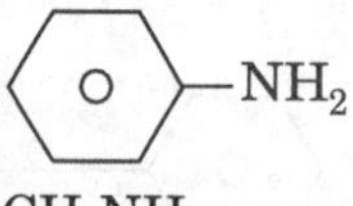

(c) $(CH_3)_2NH$ (d) CH_3NH_2

64. Which of the following compounds will dissolve in an alkali solution after it has undergone reaction with HINSBERG's REAGENT?

(a) $(C_2H_5)_2 NH$ (b) $(CH_3)_3 N$

(d) CH_3NH_2 (d) $C_6H_5NHC_6H_5$

65. Acidic hydrolysis of methyl isocyanide gives –

(a) $CH_3NH_2 + HCOOH$

(b) $CH_3NH_2 + CH_3COOH$

(c) $C_2H_5NH_2 + HCOOH$

(d) $CH_3NH_2 + CH_3CH_2 COOH$

66. Number of Bromine atoms in the final product are –

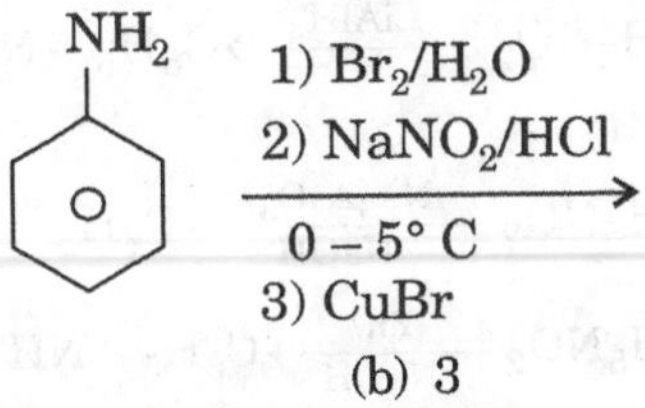

(a) 2 (b) 3

(c) 4 (d) zero

67. Which one of the following is least basic?

(a) p–toluidene (b) m–toluidine

(c) aniline (d) o–toluidine

68. Which of the following will react will $CS_2/HgCl_2$ to give mustard oil like smell ?

(a) RNH_2 (b) R_2NH

(c) R_3N (d) All of these

69. Which of the following is Incorrect?

(a) $R-CH_2-NH_2 \xrightarrow{KMnO_4} R-CH=NH$

(b) $R_2NH \xrightarrow{H_2SO_5} R_2NOH$

(c) $R_2NH \xrightarrow{KMnO_4} R_2N-NR_2$

(d) None of these

70. Select the correct order of basicity

(a) 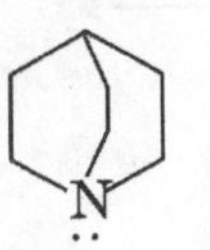 $> Et_3\ddot{N}$

(b) 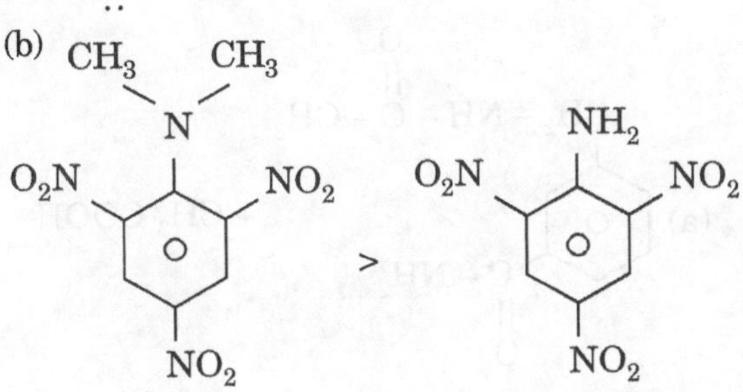

(N, N – Dimethyl picramide)

(c) $(CH_3CH_2)_2NH > (CH_3CH_2)_3N > CH_3CH_2NH_2$ (aq. medium)

(d) All are correct

71. Consider the following sulphonation reaction of Aniline.

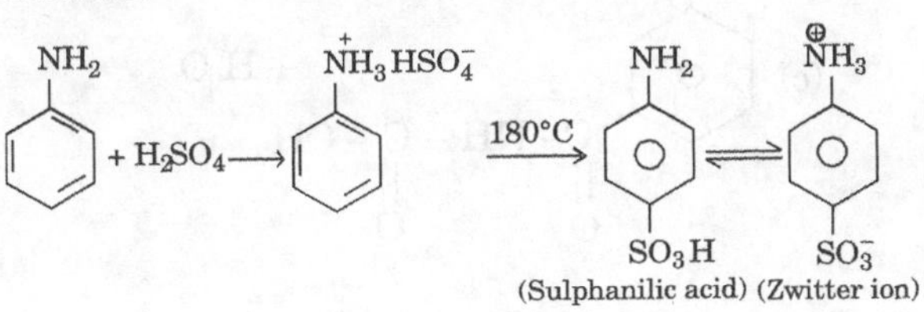

Due to dipolar ionic nature, sulphanilic acid has

(a) High melting point

(b) Insoluble in water due to strong dipole–dipole interaction.

(c) Its solubility in aq. NaOH is because of transfer of H⁺ from $\overset{+}{N}H_3$ to base, $\bar{O}H$ to form 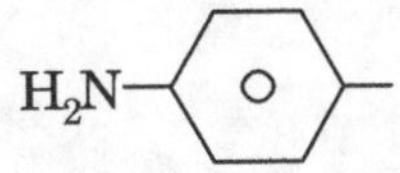 $SO_3^- Na^+$ which is soluble in H_2O

(d) All are correct

72. Which of the following is correct ?

(a) 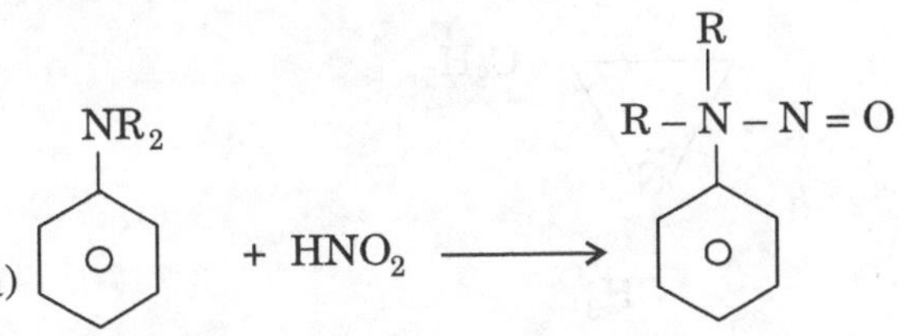

(b) 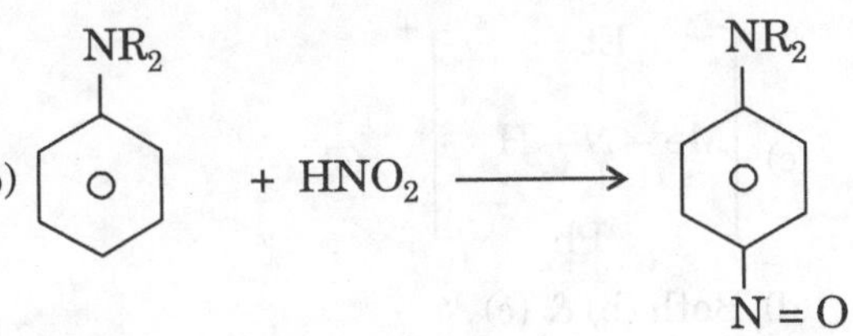

(c) 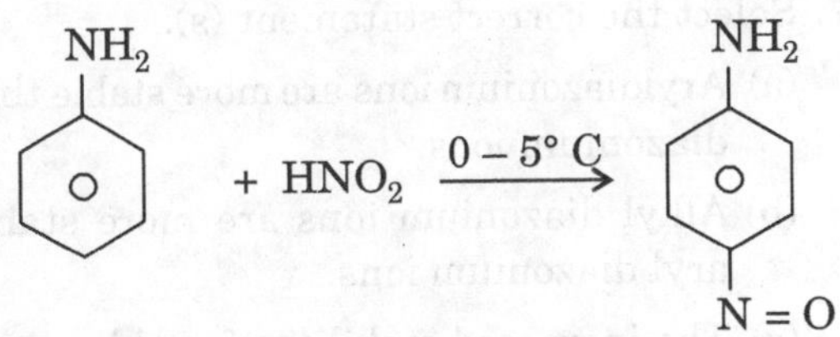

(d) All are correct

73. Amine which cannot undergo benzoylation or acylation is

(a) 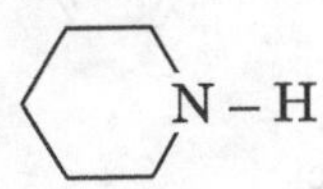 (b) 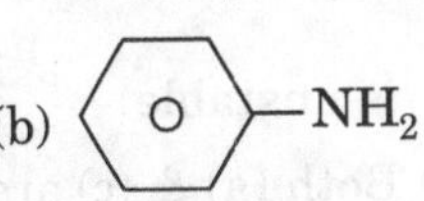

(c) 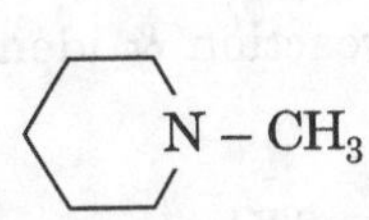 (d) 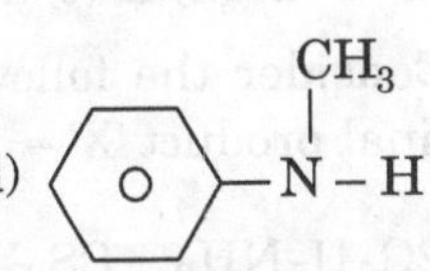

74. The pyramidal inversion from one invertomer of chiral tetrahedral amine to another takes place via –

(a) Carbocationic intermediate

(b) Anionic nitrogen intermediate

(c) Cationic nitrogen intermediate

(d) Planar nitrogen

75. Libermann's nitroso test is used for testing the presence of –

(a) N–methylaniline
(b) Aniline
(c) N, N– dimethylaniline
(d) All of these

76. Which of the following is/are resolvable ?

(a) 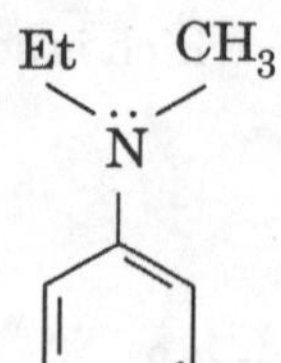

(b) 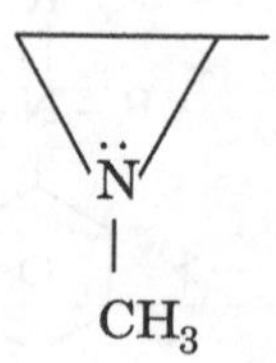

(c) 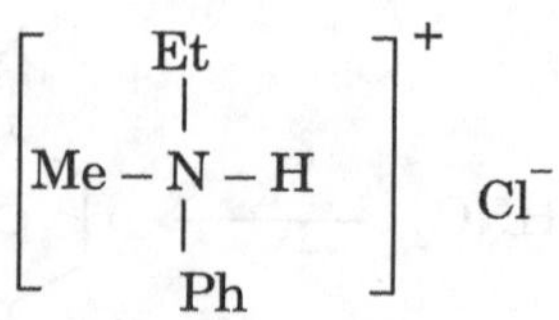

(d) Both (b) & (c)

77. Select the correct statement (s).

(a) Aryldiazonium ions are more stable than alkyl diazonium ions.
(b) Alkyl diazonium ions are more stable than aryl diazonium ions.
(c) The increased stability of aryldiazonium ion is due to resonance stabilisation & also due to great difficulty in forming 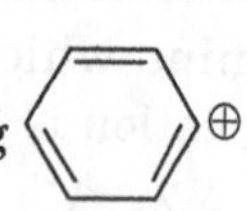 (which is unstable)
(d) Both (a) & (c) are correct

78. Consider the following reaction & identify the final product 'X' –

$$2C_6H_5NH_2 + CS_2 \xrightarrow[KOH]{\Delta} 'X'$$

(a) $C_6H_5N = C = S$
(b) $C_6H_5NH - \overset{\overset{S}{||}}{C} - NHC_6H_5$
(c) $C_6H_5N \equiv C$
(d) Both (b) & (c)

79. Identify the reaction with 'INCORRECT PRODUCTS.'

(a) $2C_6H_5NO_2 \xrightarrow{LiAlH_4} C_6H_5 - N = N - C_6H_5$
(b) $2C_6H_5NO_2 \xrightarrow[NaOH]{Na_3AsO_3/} C_6H_5 - \overset{\overset{O}{\uparrow}}{N} = N - C_6H_5$
(c) $2C_6H_5NO_2 \xrightarrow[NaOH]{Zn/} C_6H_5 - NH - NH - C_6H_5$
(d) None of these

80. During nitration of aniline, with conc. H_2SO_4 and conc. HNO_3, metanitroaniline is also obtained as one of the products, besides ortho & para nitroaniline. It is because–

(a) Aniline is O,P–directing for electrophilic attack.
(b) Aniline gets converted to anilinium ion, which is meta directing for electrophilic attack.
(c) Aniline is meta directing for electrophilic attack
(d) All of these

81. In the reaction shown below, the major product formed is/are –

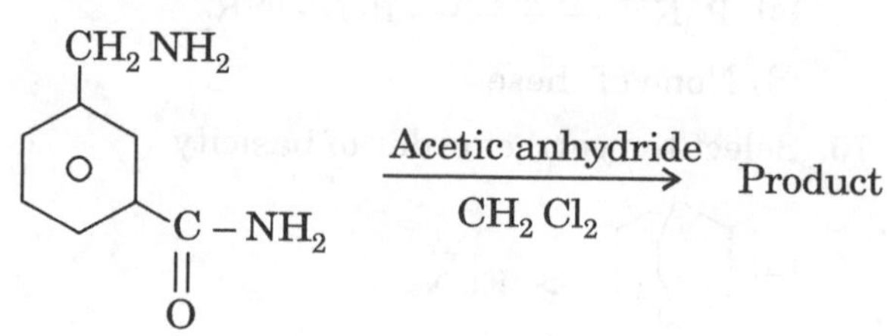

(a) 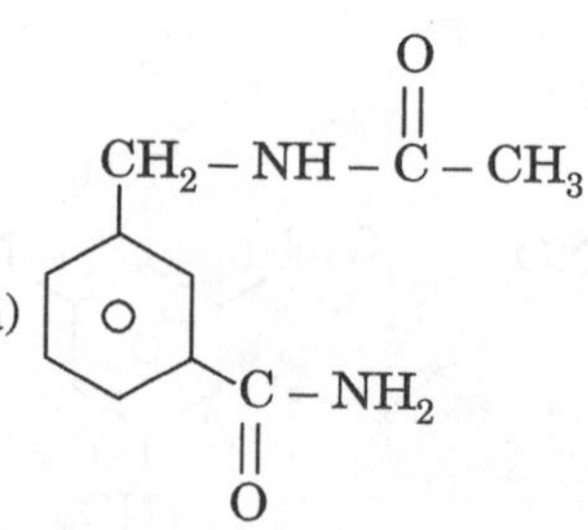 $+ CH_3COOH$

(b) 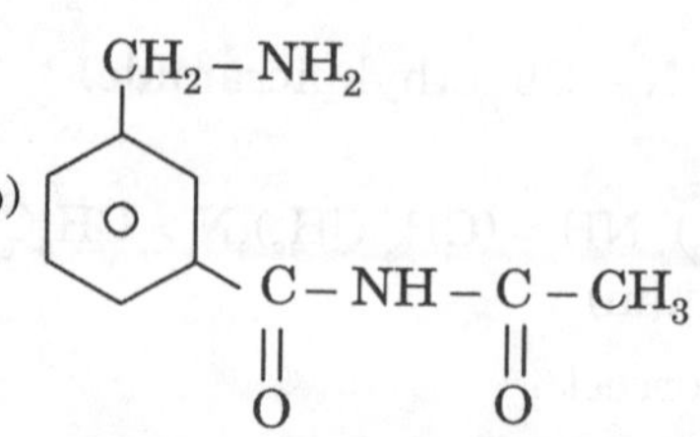 $+ CH_3COOH$

(c) 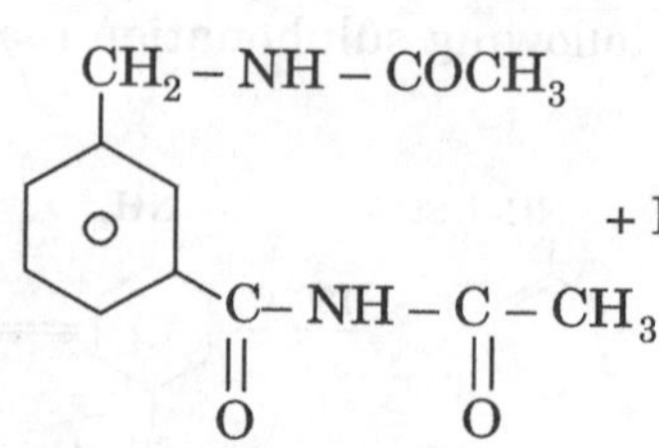 $+ H_2O$

(d) 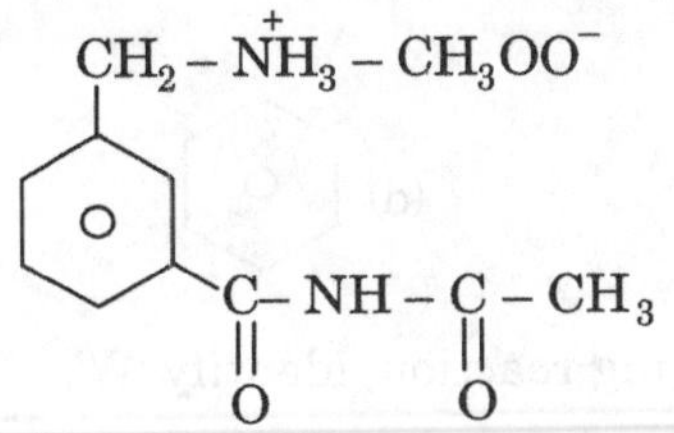

82. The final product formed in the following reaction is –

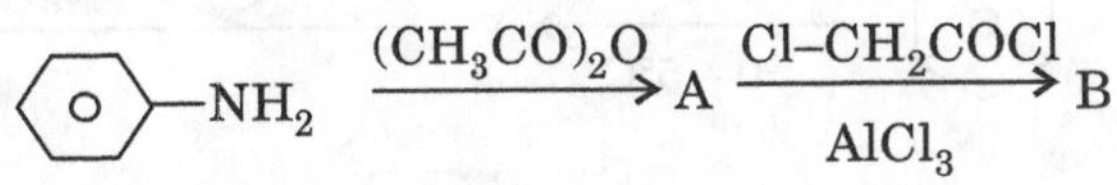

(a) 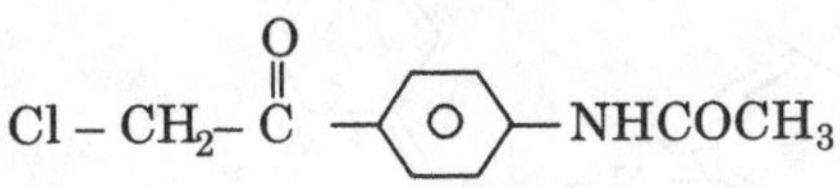

(b) 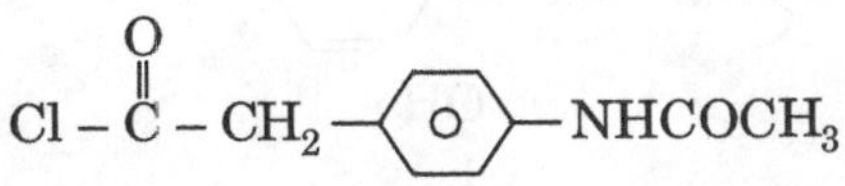

(c) 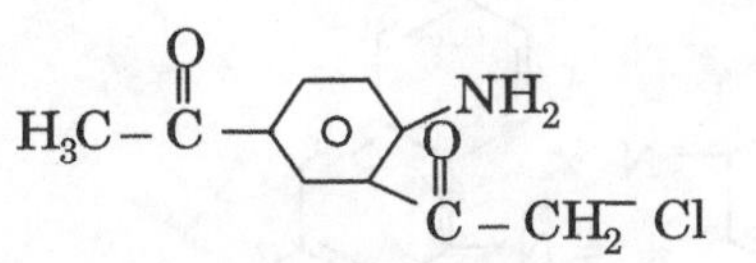

(d) 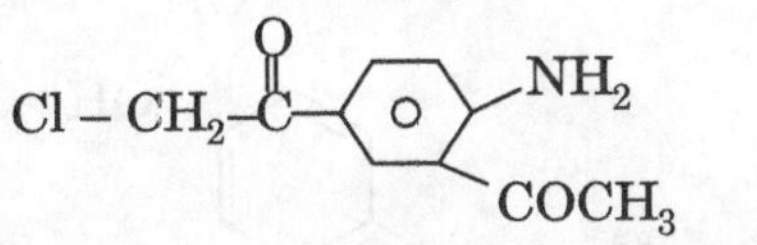

83. A compound with molecular mass 180 is acylated with CH_3COCl to get a compound with molecular mass 390. The number of amino groups present per molecule of the former compound is –

(a) 6

(b) 2

(c) 5

(d) 4

84. The compound that will react most readily with NaOH to form methanol is –

(a) $(CH_3)_4N^+I^-$

(b) CH_3OCH_3

(c) $(CH_3)_4S^+I^-$

(d) $(CH_3)_3CCl$

85. Arrange the following in the decreasing order of their basicities –

$\underset{(I)}{CH_3-CH_2-NH_2}$, $\underset{(II)}{CH_3CONH_2}$ & $\underset{(III)}{C_6H_5CONH_2}$

(a) I > II > III

(b) I > III > II

(c) II > III > I

(d) III > II > I

86. Consider the following reaction sequence

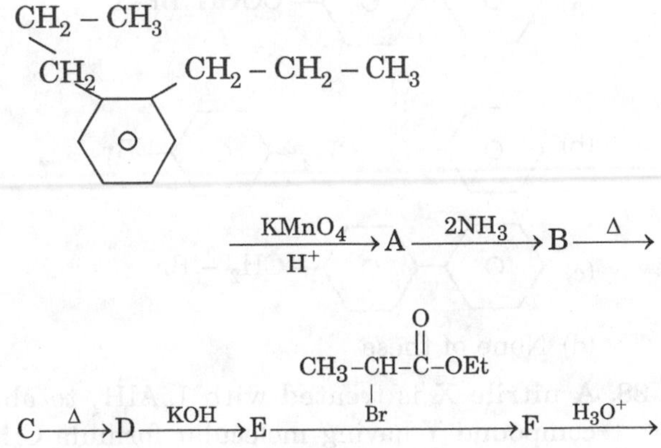

G + H + I

G, H, I in the above reaction, are –

(a) 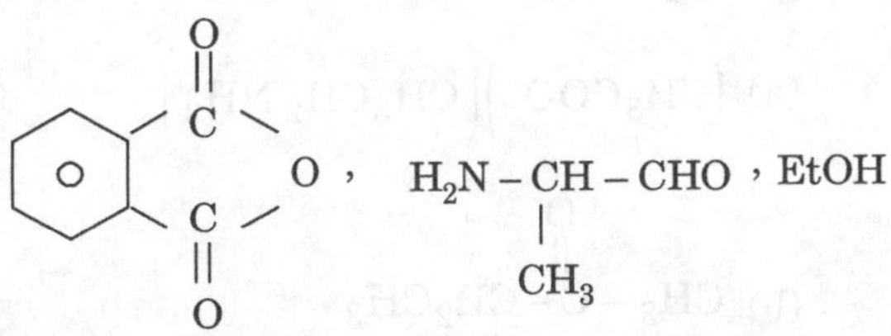

(b) 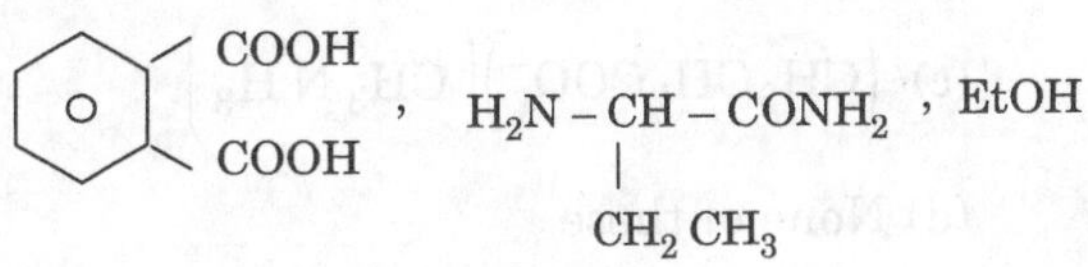

(c) 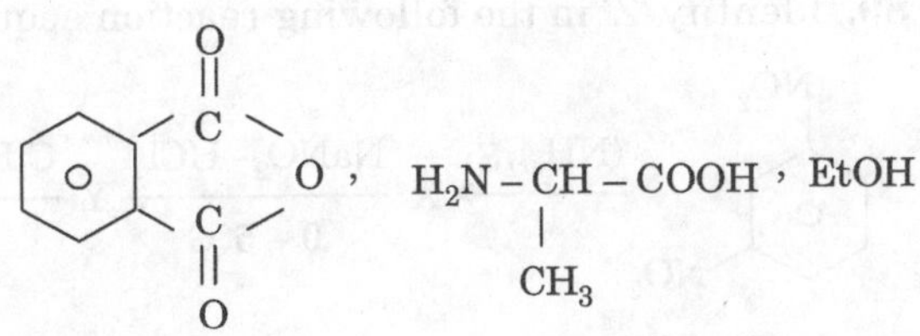

(d) 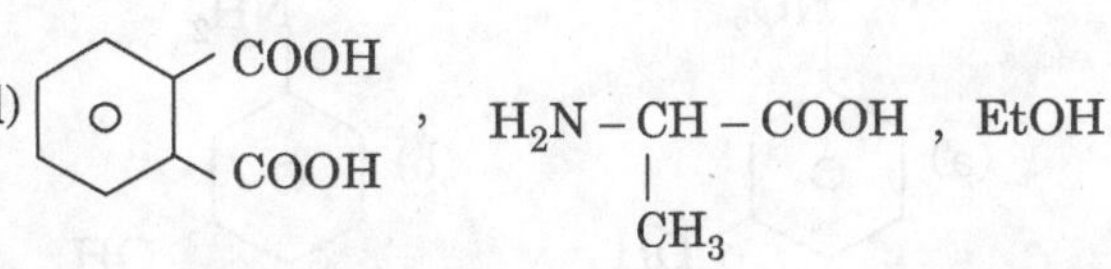

87. Identify the final product 'T' in the following reaction sequence –

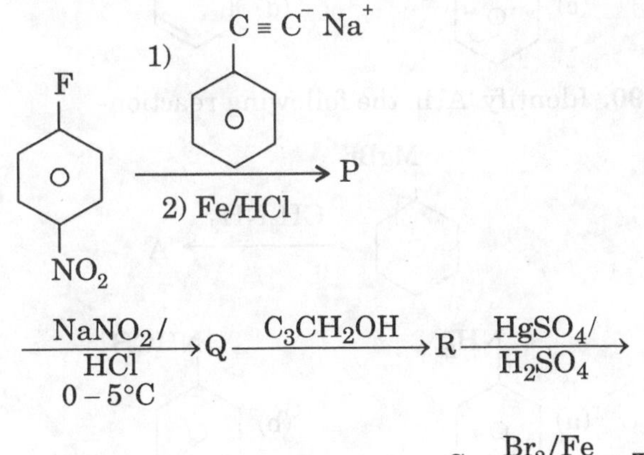

(a) 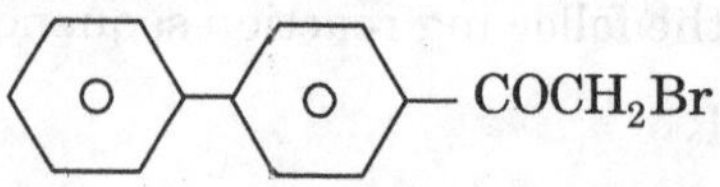

(b) 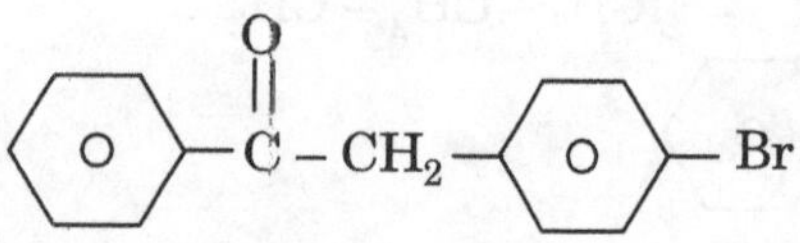

(c) 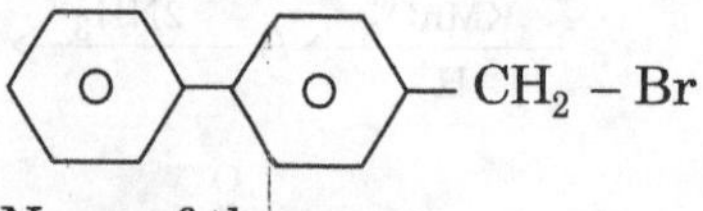

(d) None of these

88. A nitrile X is treated with $LiAlH_4$ to obtain compound Y having molecular formula C_2H_7N. In a separate reaction, X is hydrolysed in acidic medium to obtain Z. The product obtained after mixing Y & Z, will be-

(a) $\left(CH_3COO^-\right)\left(CH_3CH_2\overset{+}{N}H_3\right)$

(b) $CH_3-\overset{O}{\overset{||}{C}}-CH_2CH_3$

(c) $\left(CH_3CH_2COO^-\right)\left(CH_3\overset{+}{N}H_3\right)$

(d) None of these

89. Identify 'Z' in the following reaction sequence-

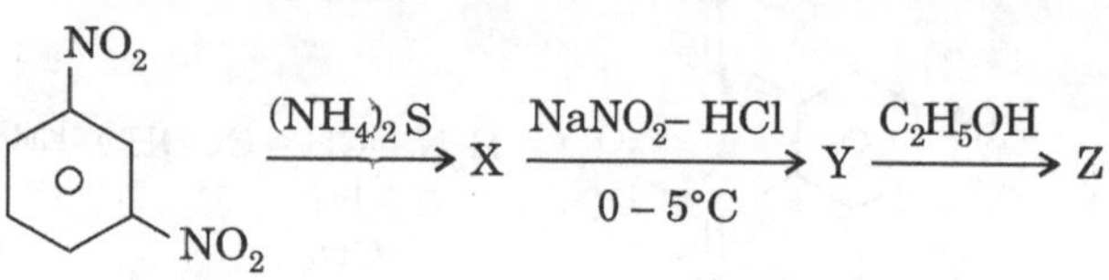

(a) 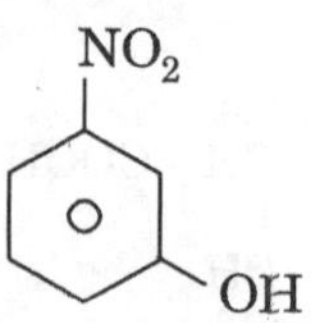

(b) 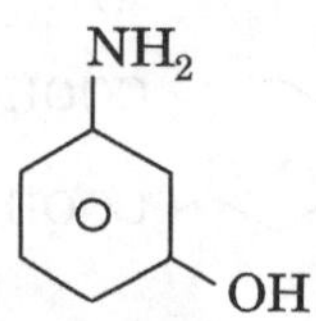

(c) 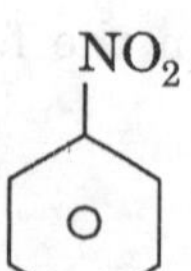

(d) 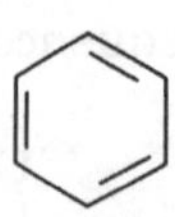

90. Identify 'A' in the following reaction-

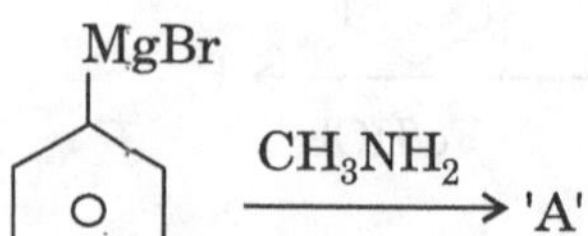

(a) 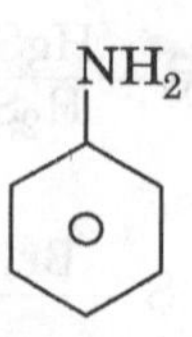

(b) 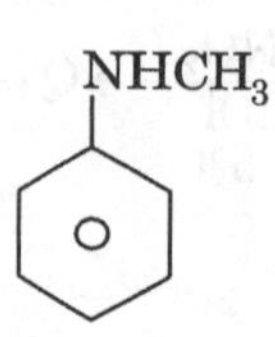

(c) 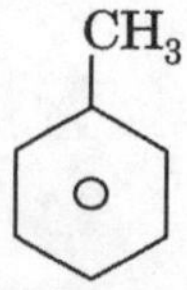

(d) 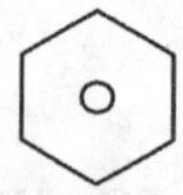

91. In the following reaction, identify 'W'.

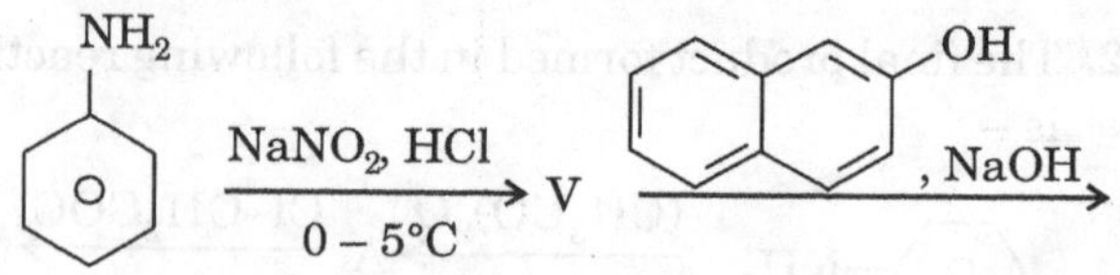

(a) 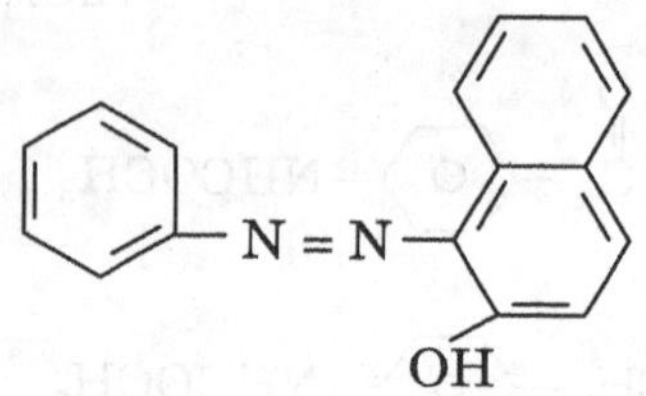

(b) 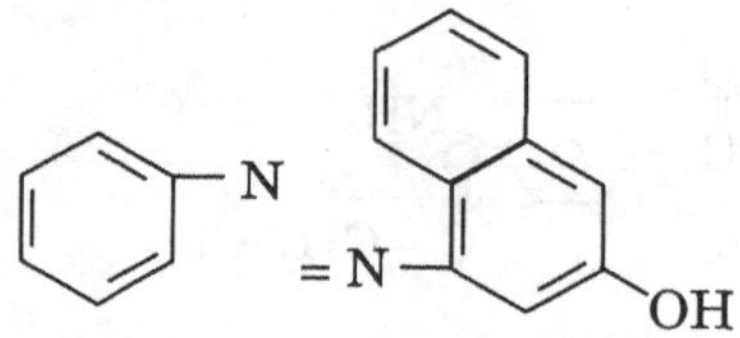

(c) 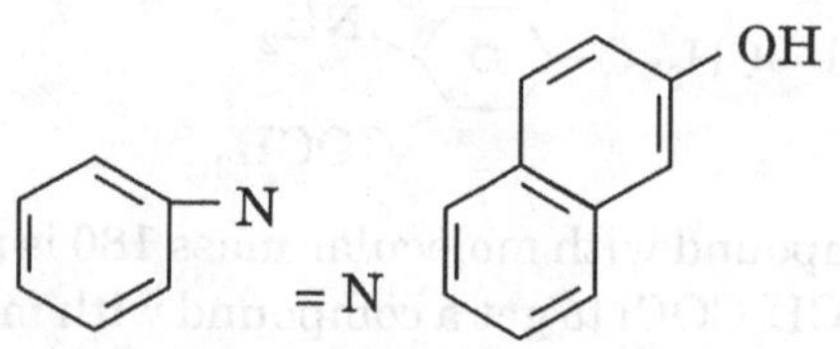

(d) All of these

92. Identify 'A' in the following reaction-

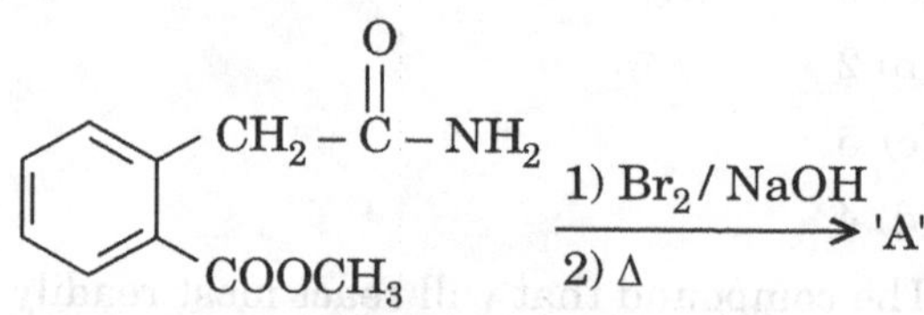

(a) 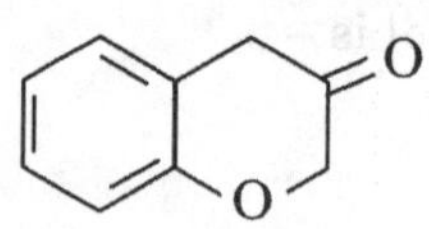

(b) 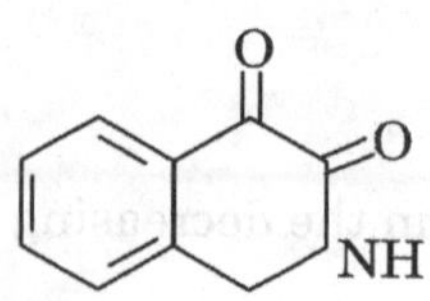

(c) 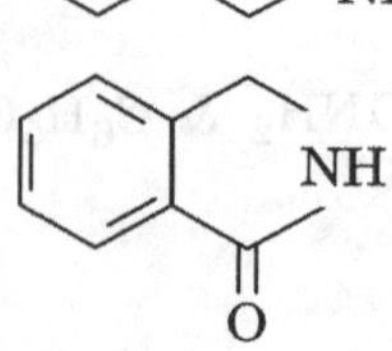

(d) None of these

93. Select the correct structure of 'A' in the following reaction-

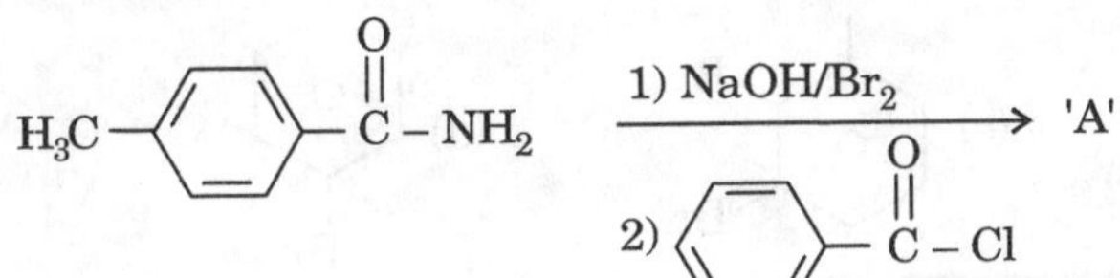

(a) 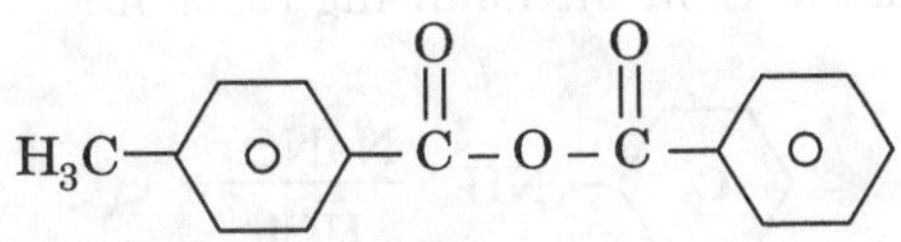

(b) 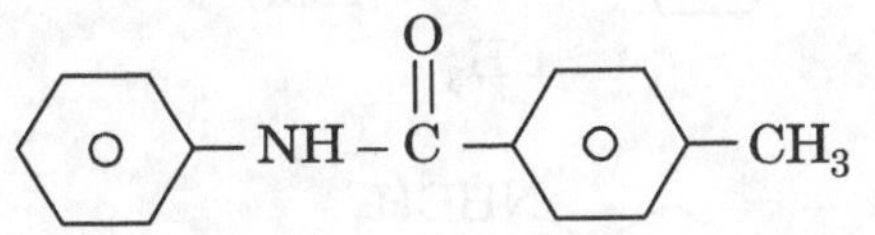

(c) 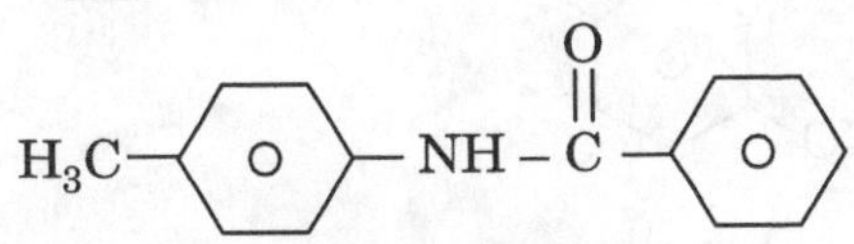

(d) Reaction will not occur.

94. Identify X & Y in the following reaction sequence-

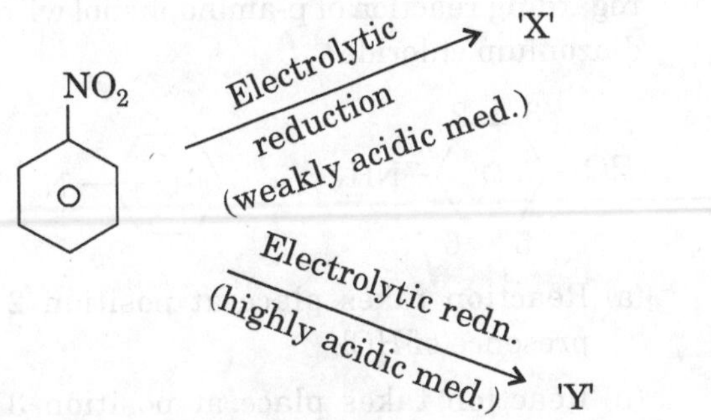

(a) X & Y, both are aniline

(b) X is aniline & Y is p-aminophenol

(c) X is p-aminophenol & Y is aniline

(d) X & Y both are p-aminophenol

95. Identify 'E' in the following sequence of reactions-

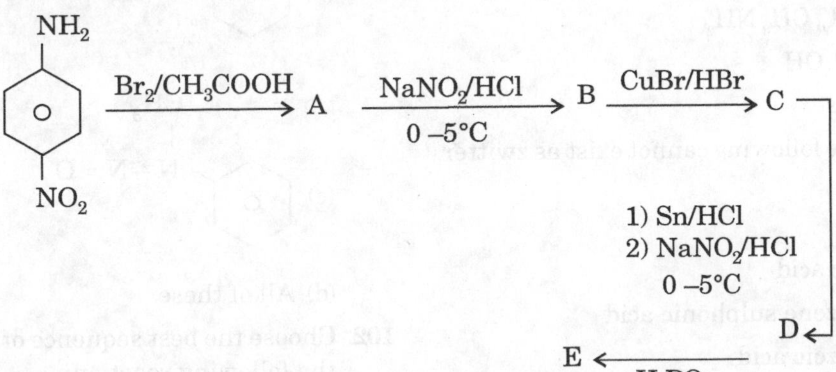

(a) 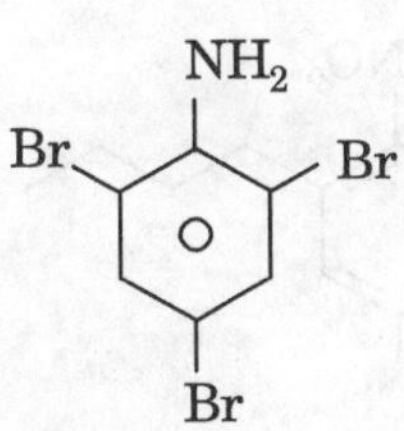

(b) 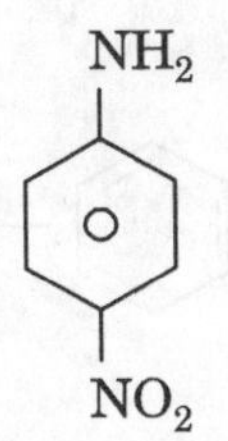

(c) 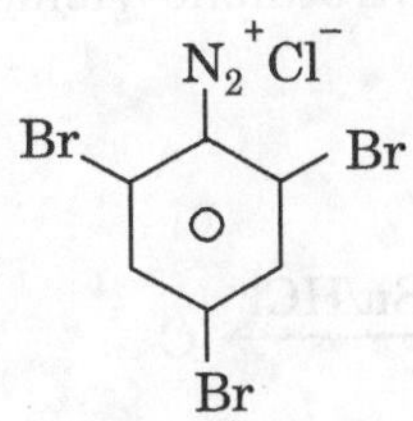

(d) 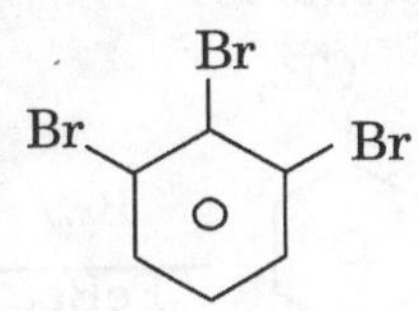

96. What is 'X' in the following sequence of reactions?

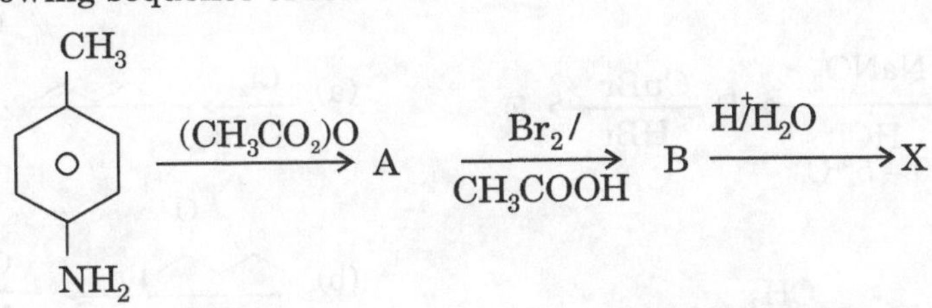

(a) 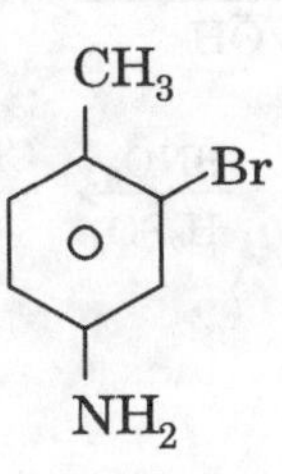

(b) 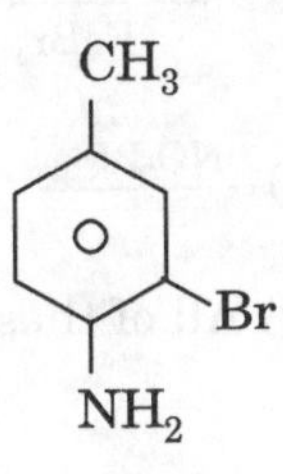

(c) 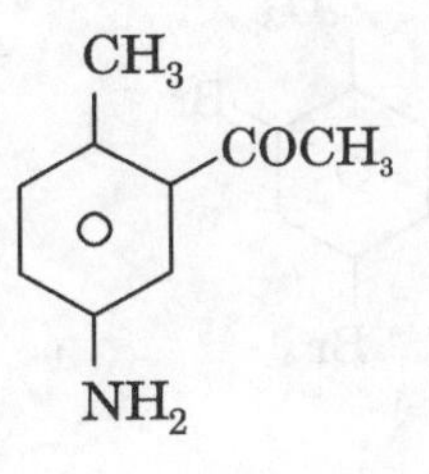

(d) 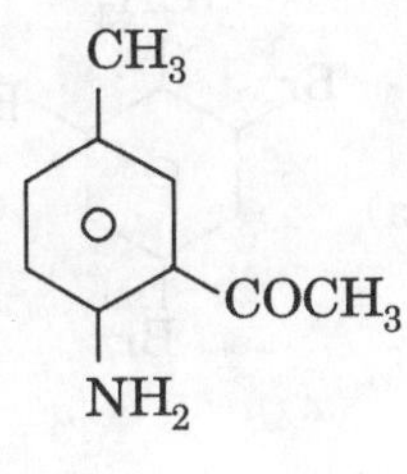

97. Which of the following statement is true regarding reaction of p-aminophenol with arene-diazonium chloride?

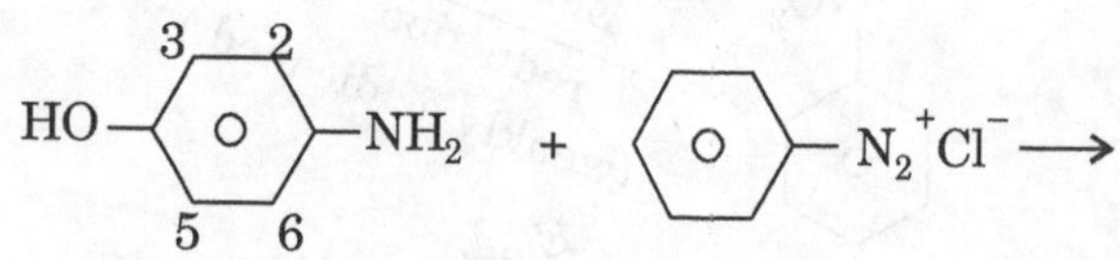

(a) Reaction takes place at position 2 in the presence of HCl.

(b) Reaction takes place at position 3 in the presence of NaOH.

(c) It is an electrophilic substitution reaction

(d) All are true.

98. Identify (C) & (D) in the following series of reactions

$$CH_3NH_2 \xrightarrow[\text{of } CH_3I]{\text{excess}} (A) \xrightarrow{AgOH} (B) \xrightarrow{\Delta} (C) + (D)$$

(a) $(CH_3)_3COH, CH_3NH_2$

(b) $(CH_3)_2C{=}CH_2, CH_3NH_2$

(c) $(CH_3)_3N, CH_3OH$

(d) None of these

99. Which one of the following cannot exist as zwitter ion?

(a) Alanine

(b) Aminoacetic acid

(c) p-aminobenzene sulphonic acid

(d) p-aminobenzoic acid

100. In a set of reactions, p-Nitrotulene yielded a product E-

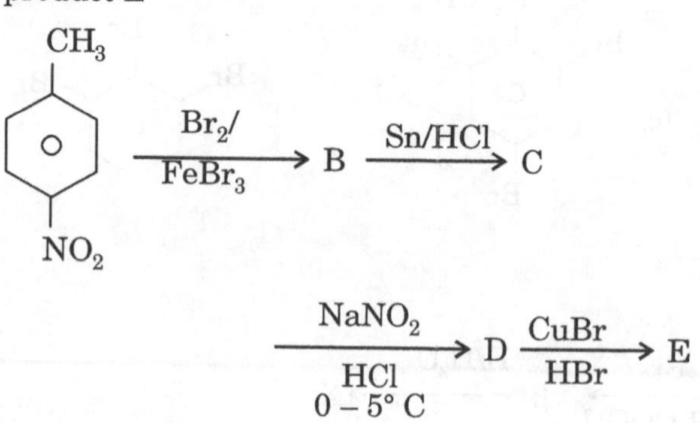

Identify E.

(a) 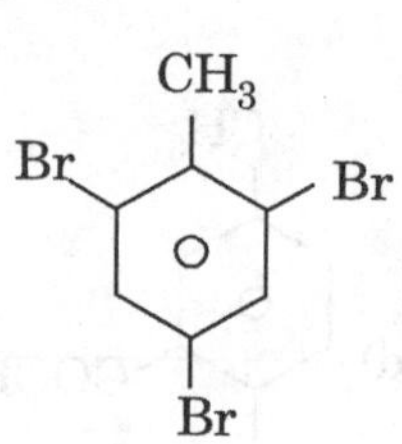

(b) 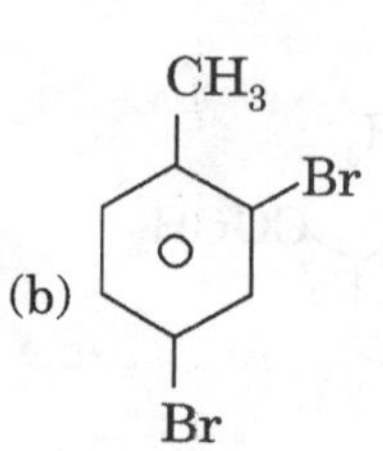

(c) 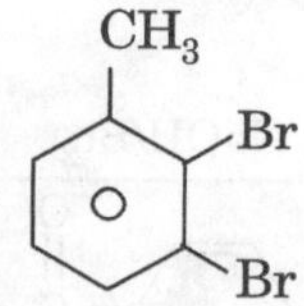

(d) 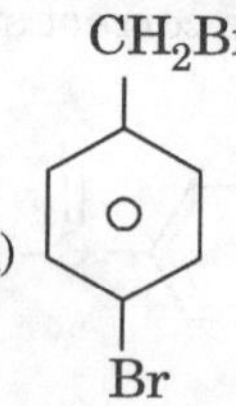

101. What is 'A' in the following reaction?

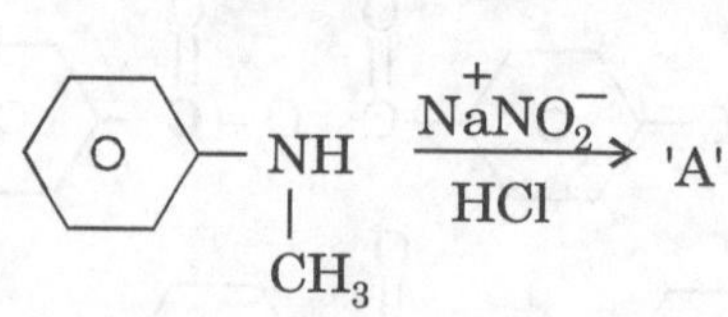

(a) 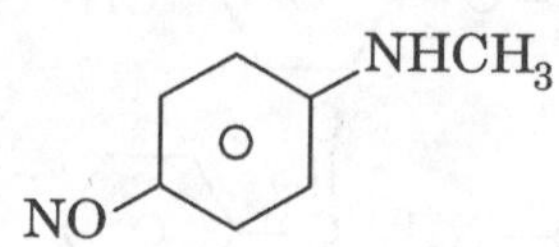

(b) 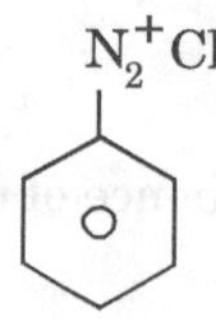

(c) 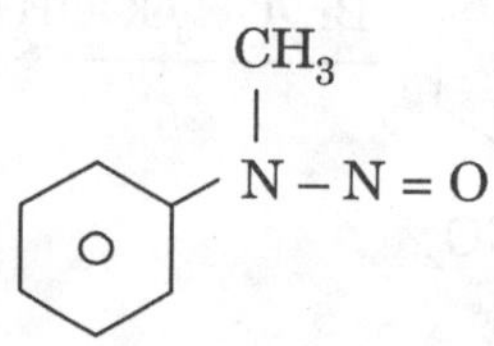

(d) All of these

102. Choose the best sequence of reaction to complete the following reaction:-

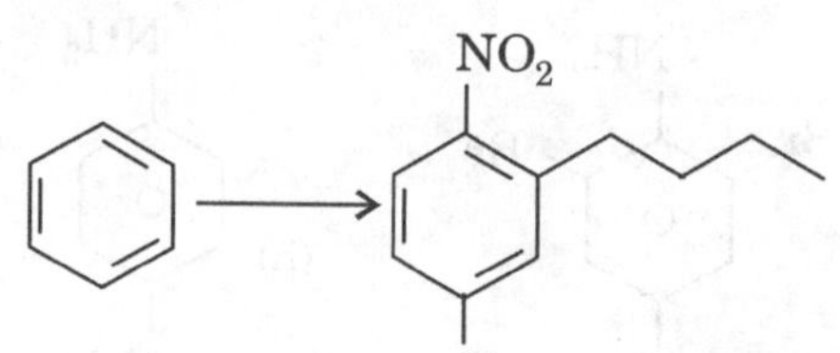

(a) 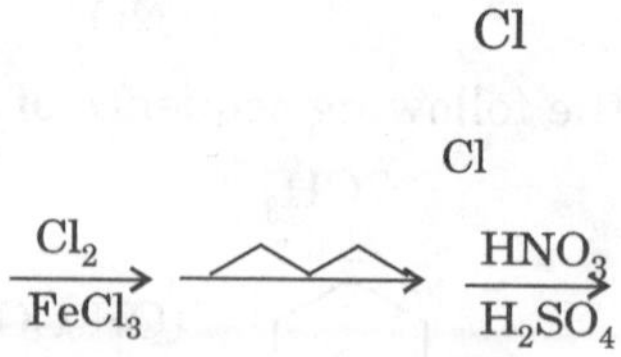

(b) 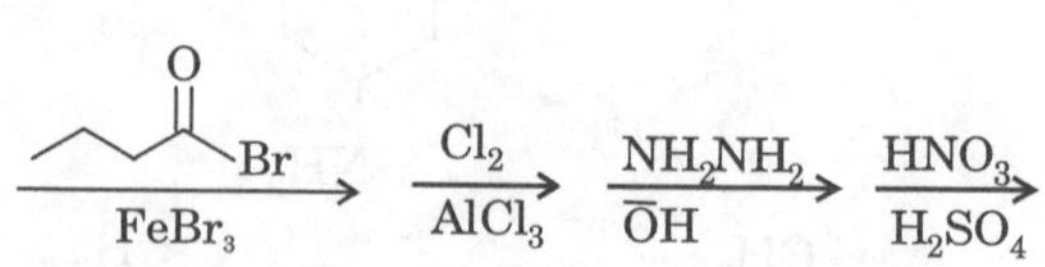

(c) 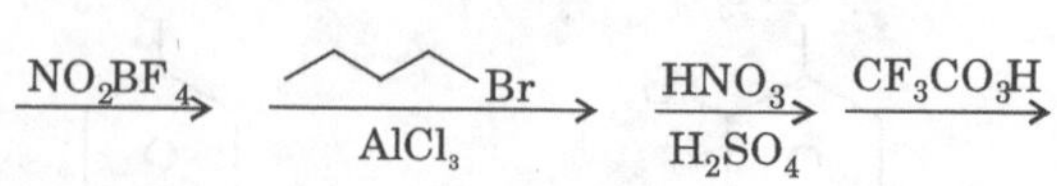

(d) All of these

103. Which one of the following cannot undergo acetylation?

(a) $CH_3 - CH_2 - NH_2$ (b) 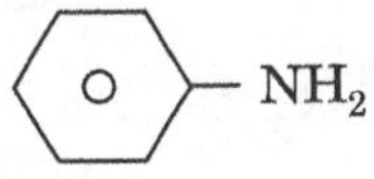

(c) 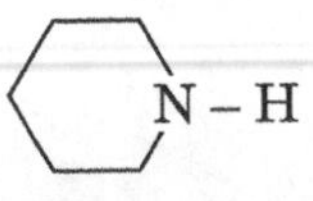 (d) 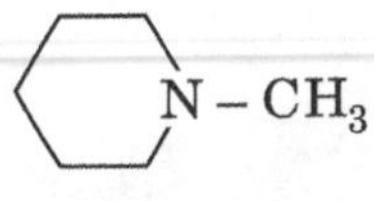

104. Which of the following give(s) Libermann's nitroso reaction?

(a) 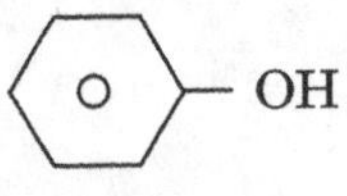 (b) 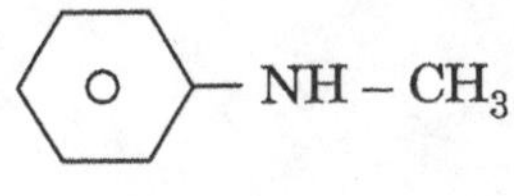

(c) 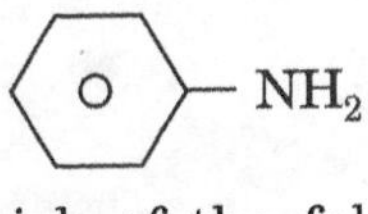 (d) both a & b

105. Which of the following statement(s) is/are incorrect?

(a) Aryldiazonium ions are more stable than alkyldiazonium ions.

(b) Electron release from ortho & para positions of the ring stabilizes the aryl diazonium ions.

(c) The increased stability of aryldiazonium ion is due to great difficulty in forming $Ar^{\oplus}$.

(d) None of these

106. 2° aliphatic amines on oxidation with H_2O_2 give-

(a) Tetra-alkyl hydrazine

(b) Nitro compound

(c) Nitroso compound

(d) N-hydroxyl di alkylamine

Brain Teasers

107. Which of the following is CORRECT regarding basic strength ?

(a) 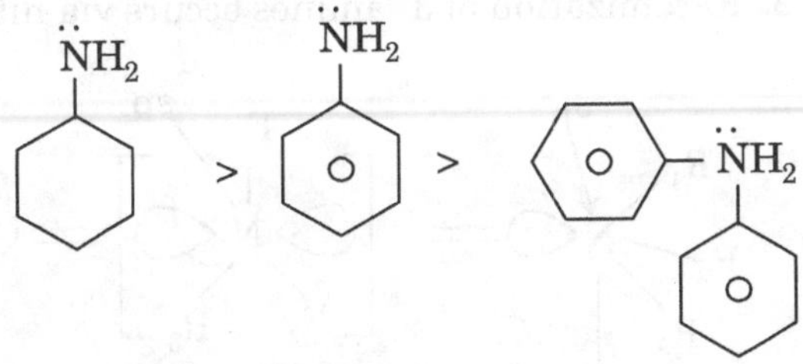

(b) 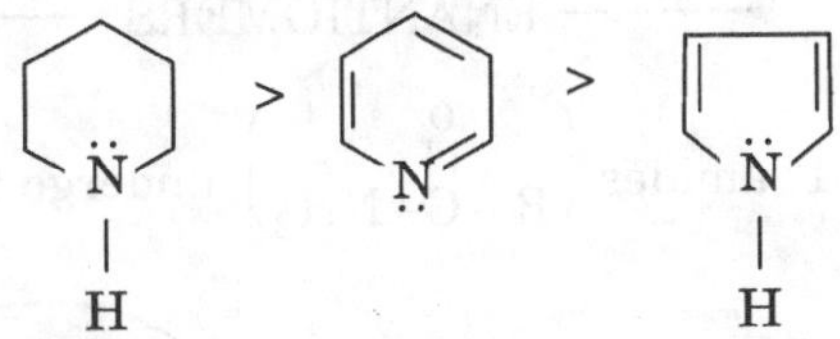

(c) 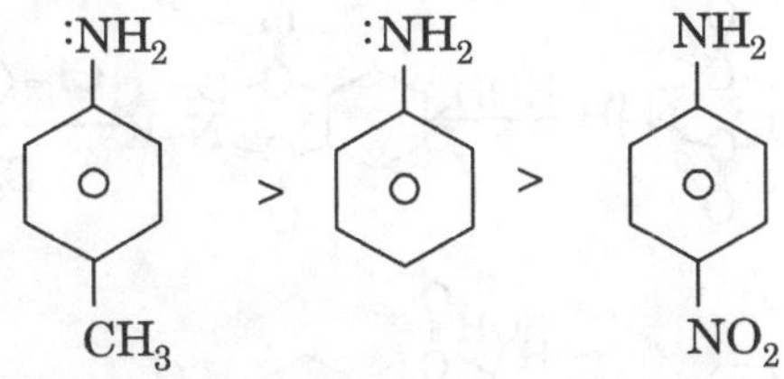

(d) All are correct.

108. Which of the compounds would give nitrogen when treated with HNO_2?

(a) $CH_3CH_2CH_2NH_2$ (b) 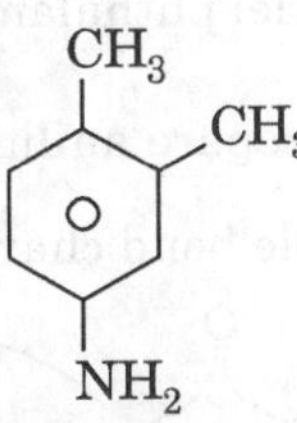

(c) $CH_3CH_2CONHCH_3$ (d) Both a & b

Answers

1. (d)	2. (b)	3. (d)	4. (b)	5. (d)	6. (d)	7. (c)	8. (d)	9. (d)	10. (a)
11. (b)	12. (c)	13. (d)	14. (c)	15. (a)	16. (c)	17. (b)	18. (b)	19. (a)	20. (b)
21. (c)	22. (c)	23. (b)	24. (b)	25. (b)	26. (a)	27. (c)	28. (a)	29. (a)	30. (d)
31. (a)	32. (a)	33. (a)	34. (d)	35. (a)	36. (c)	37. (d)	38. (a)	39. (d)	40. (a)
41. (d)	42. (d)	43. (d)	44. (a)	45. (c)	46. (c)	47. (b)	48. (b)	49. (c)	50. (c)
51. (b)	52. (c)	53. (d)	54. (d)	55. (a)	56. (c)	57. (c)	58. (c)	59. (b)	60. (a)
61. (c)	62. (b)	63. (c)	64. (c)	65. (a)	66. (c)	67. (d)	68. (a)	69. (d)	70. (d)
71. (d)	72. (b)	73. (c)	74. (d)	75. (a)	76. (d)	77. (d)	78. (b)	79. (d)	80. (b)
81. (a)	82. (a)	83. (c)	84. (a)	85. (b)	86. (d)	87. (b)	88. (a)	89. (c)	90. (d)
91. (a)	92. (c)	93. (c)	94. (b)	95. (d)	96. (b)	97. (d)	98. (c)	99. (d)	100. (b)
101. (c)	102. (b)	103. (d)	104. (d)	105. (d)	106. (d)	107. (d)	108. (d)		

Explanations

2. Racemization of 3° amines occurs via nitrogen inversion.

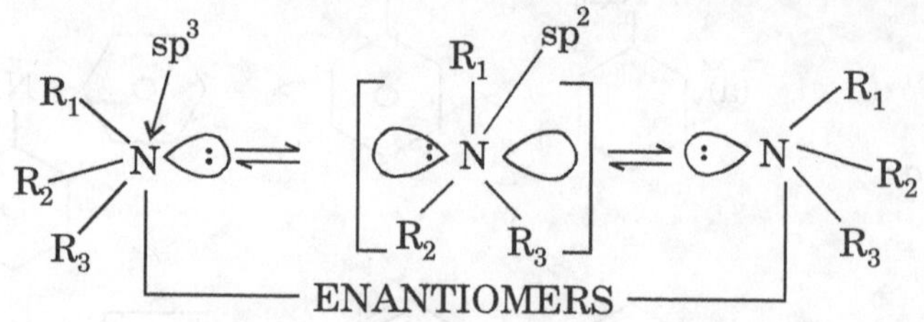

3. Only 1° amides $\left(R-\overset{O}{\overset{||}{C}}-NH_2\right)$ undergo this reaction

4.

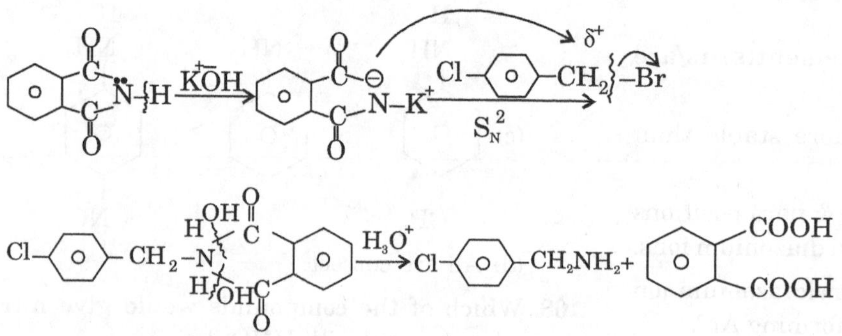

5. Gabriel phthalamide involves SN^2 reaction.

To prepare aniline, C_6H_5–Cl (aryl halide) should undergo SN^2 but it is not possible because of partial double bond character in C-Cl bond.

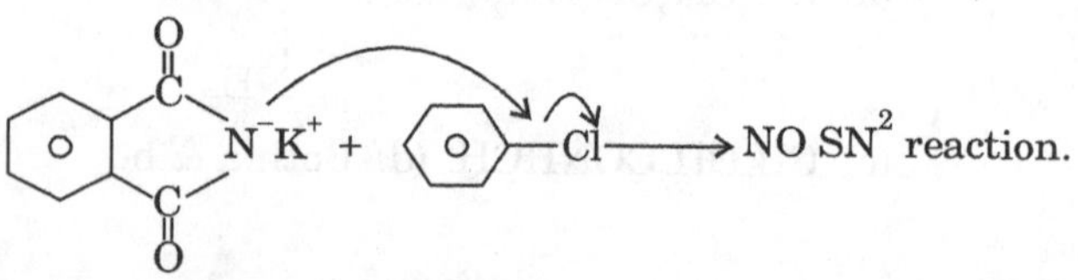

Also, To prepare ter-butyl amine, ter-alkyl halide should participate but it can also NOT undergo S_N^2. Rather, elimination occurs.

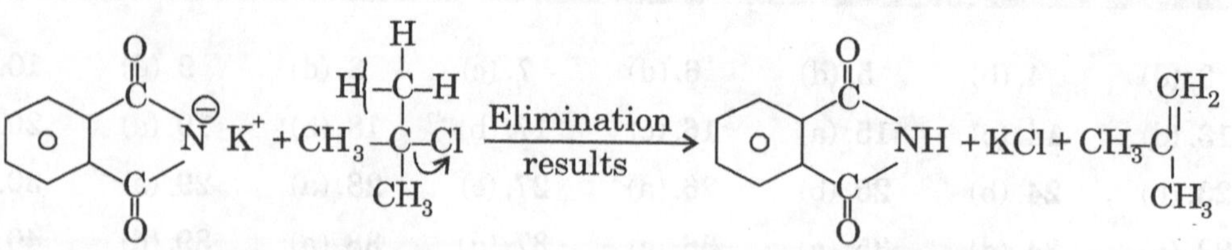

6. Mechanism of Hoffmann's Bromamide degradation is as follows-

(1) $R-\overset{O}{\overset{||}{C}}-\ddot{N}H-H \;\; \bar{O}H \rightleftharpoons R-\overset{O}{\overset{||}{C}}-\ddot{N}\overset{\ominus}{H} + H_2O$

(2) $R-\overset{O}{\overset{||}{C}}-\ddot{N}^{\ominus}-H \;\; + Br-Br \rightarrow R-\overset{O}{\overset{||}{C}}-\ddot{N}(Br)-H \;\; + Br^{\ominus}$

(3) 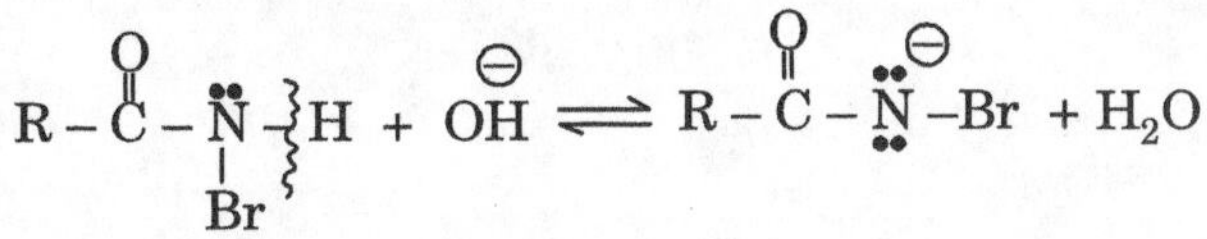

(4) 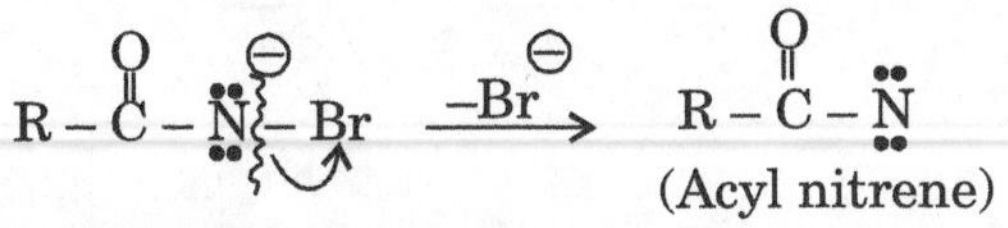

(5) 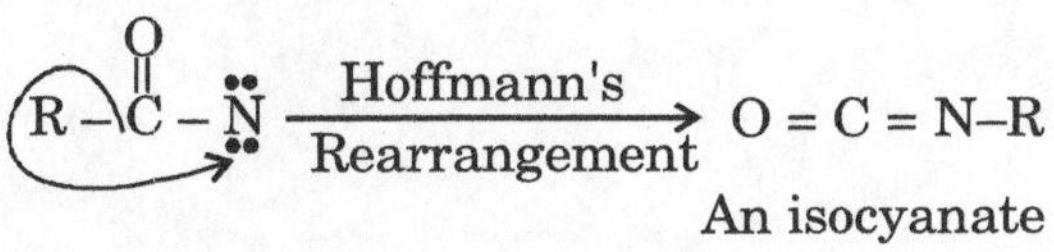

BASIC hydrolysis

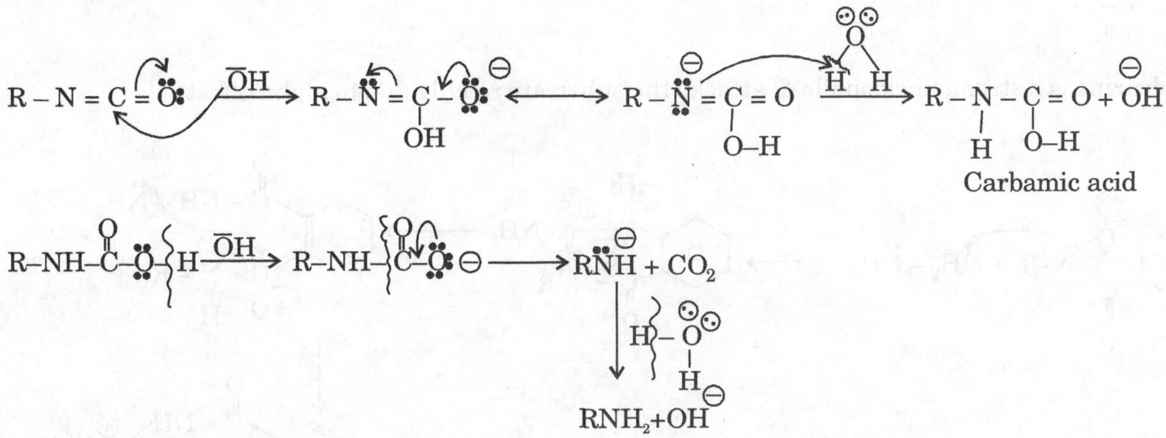

7. 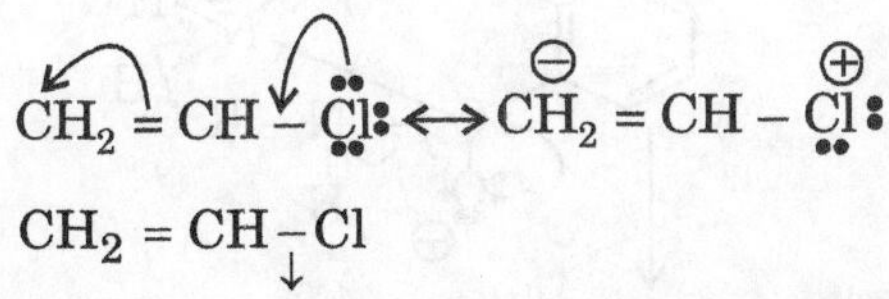

Partial double bond character, SN^2 can't occur.

8. 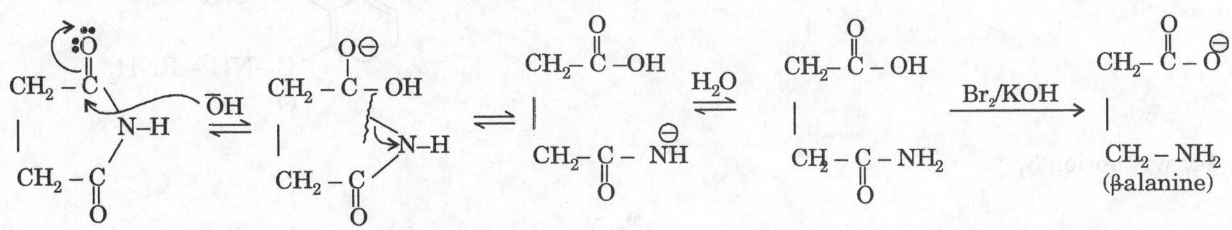

10. 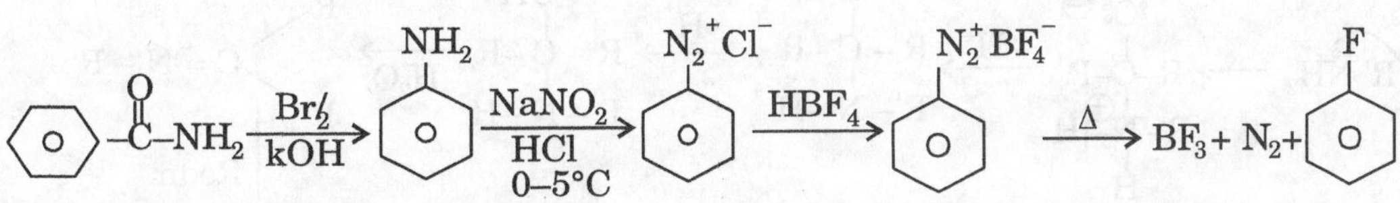

11. Hoffmann's Bromamide degradation proceeds with Retention of Configuration.

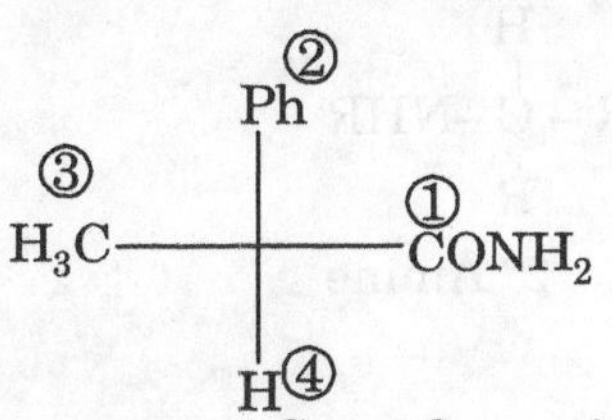

S–configuration

S-Configuration

Option 2 also has S-Configuration.

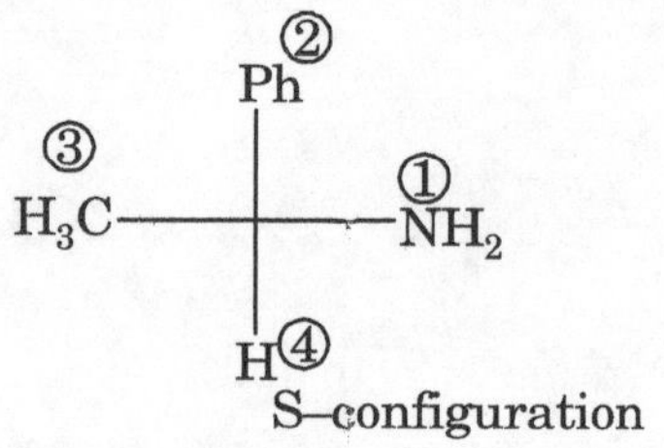

S-Configuration

12. 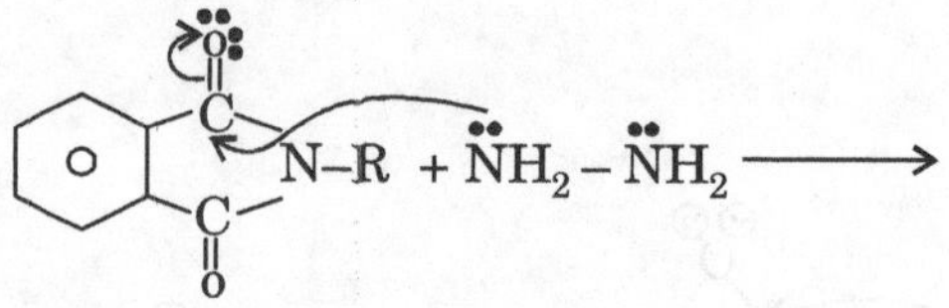

(Hydrazine is a strong nucleophile & attacks the substrate readily due to alpha effect)

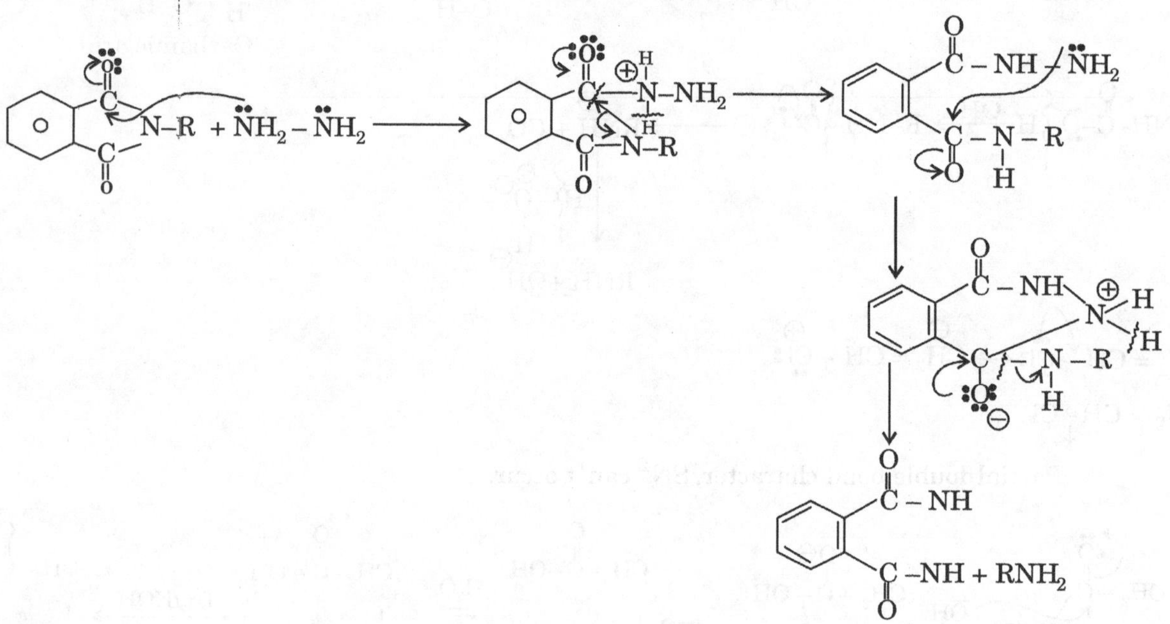

14. wrt option 3,

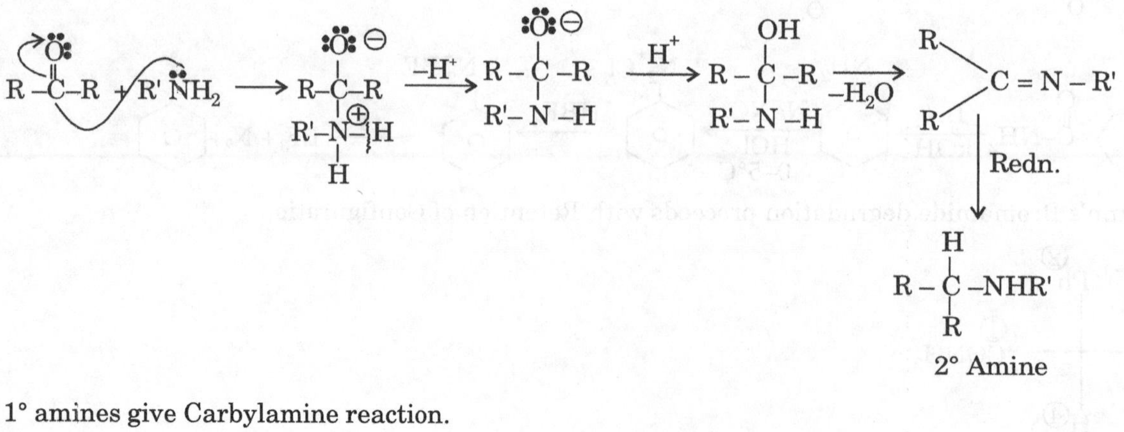

15. 1° amines give Carbylamine reaction.

16. 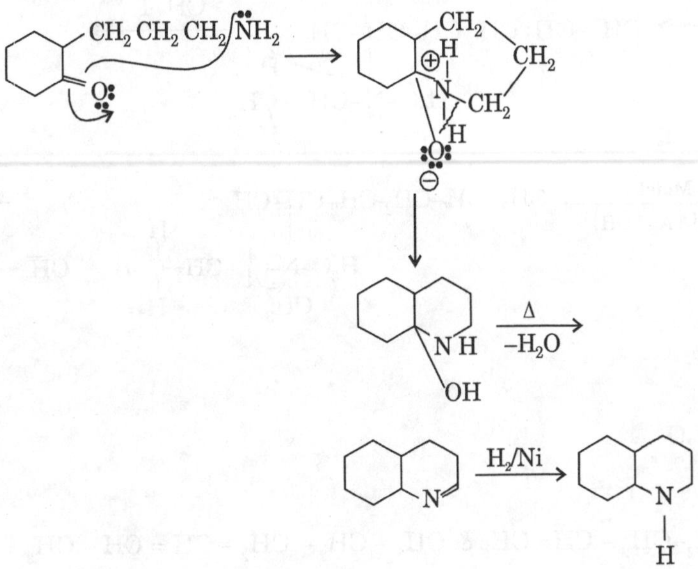

17. 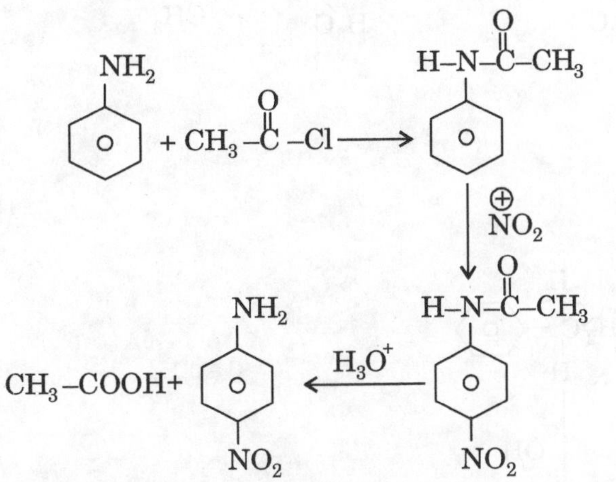

19. It is Hoffmann's bromamide degradation reaction.
Nitrene is formed & it involves Hoffmann's rearrangement i.e. an alkyl shift towards electron deficient N. Electron rich gps/electron rich ring will favour this reaction.

Molecule 'Q' 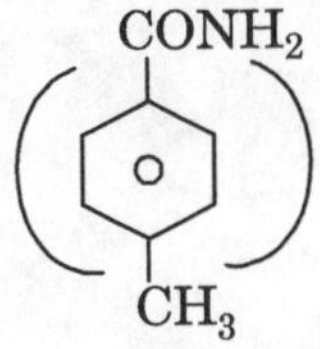

has 'CH_3' at para position which will exert +I & hyperconjugation thus making ring, e⁻ rich.

20. 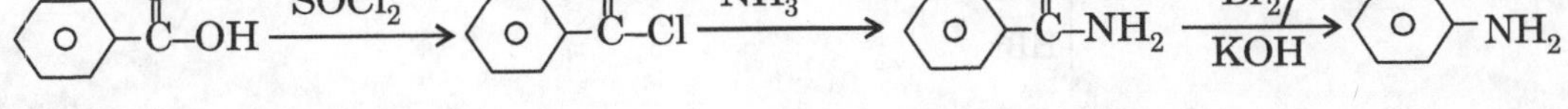

21.

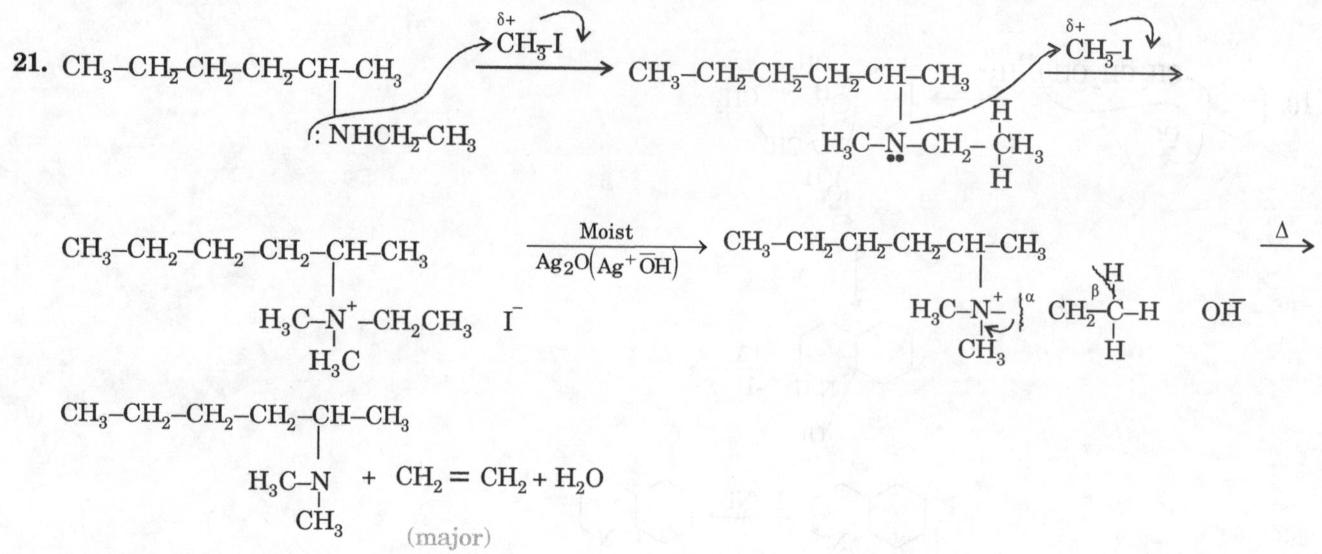

Other possible alkenes are $CH_3-CH_2-CH_2-CH_2-CH=CH_2$ & $CH_3-CH_2-CH_2-CH=CH-CH_3$

22.

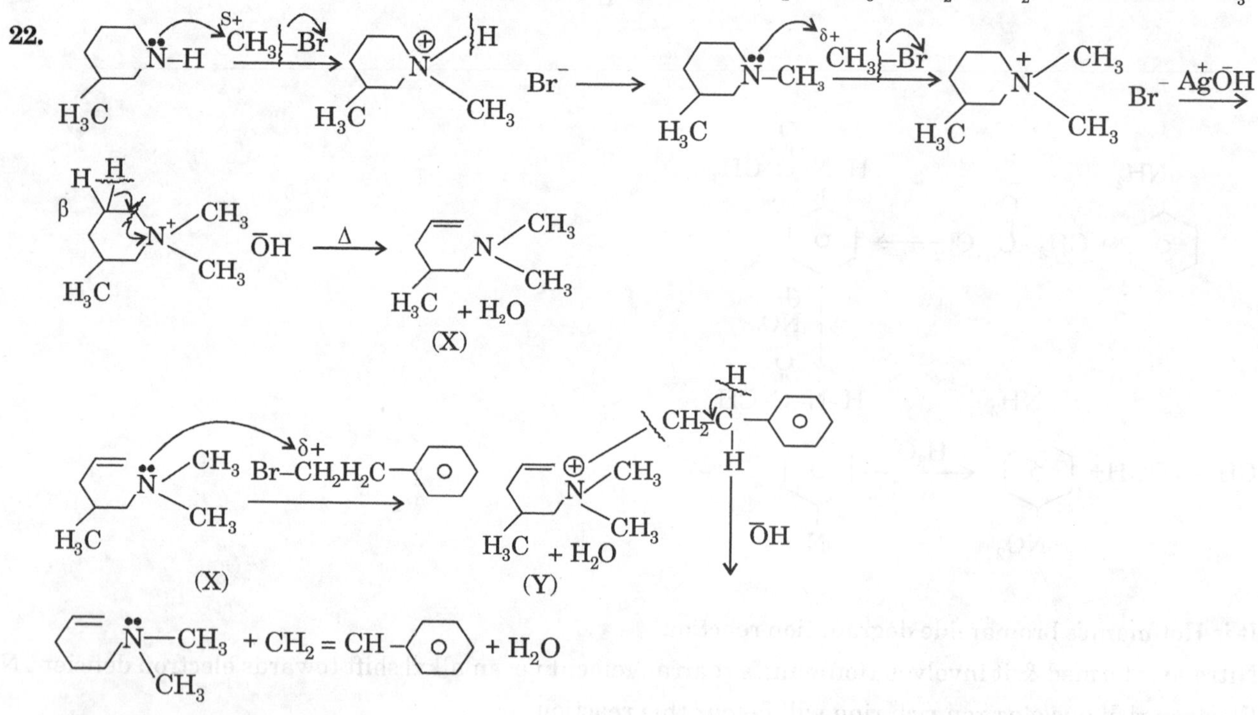

(X) & (A) are same

23.

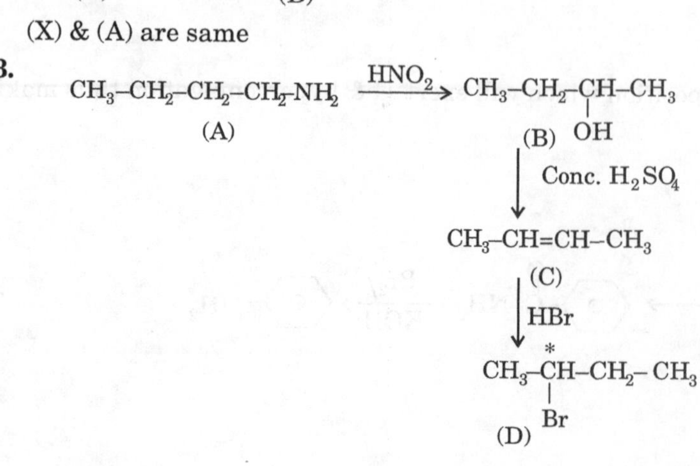

24. Complete mechanism is as follows-

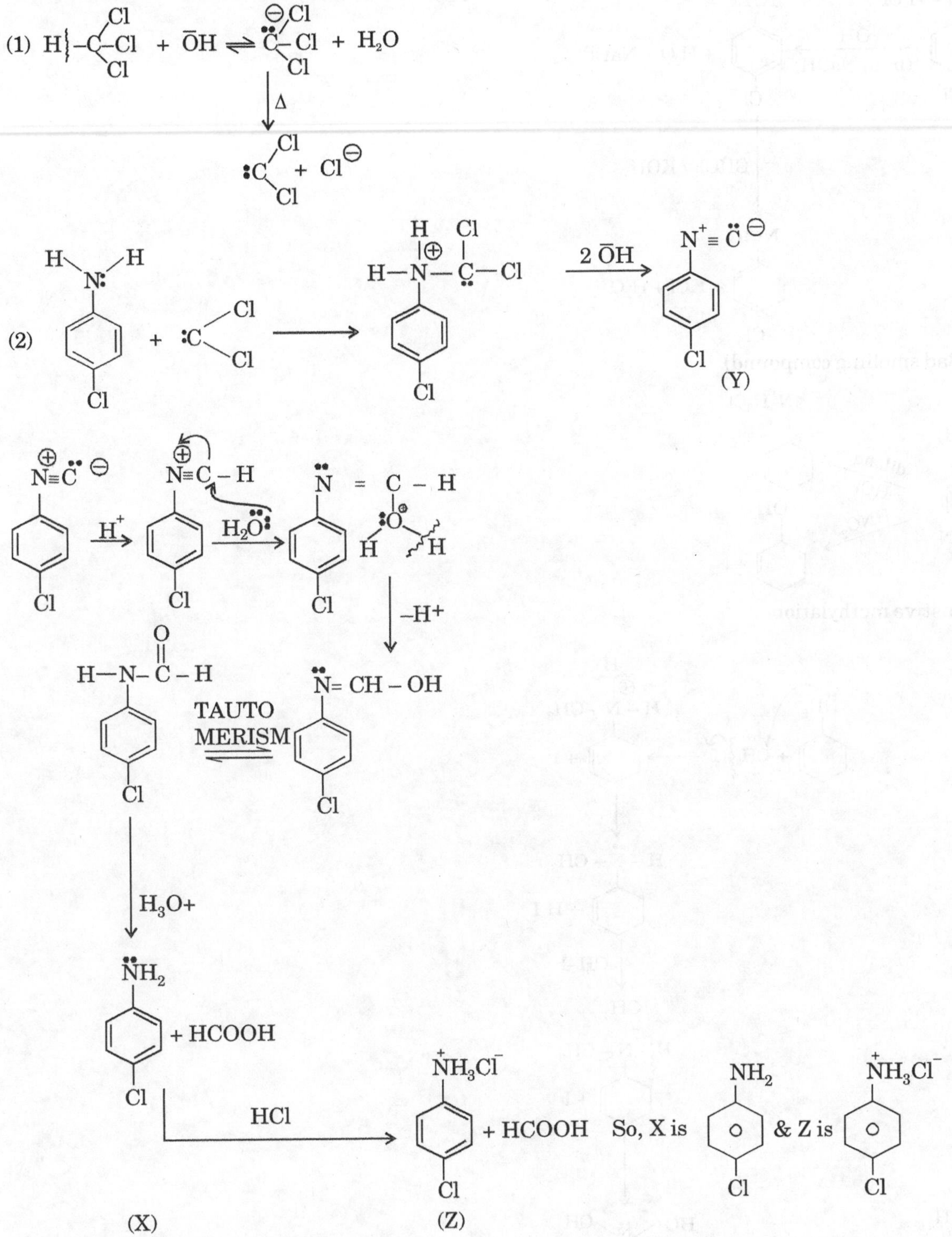

'Z' will be soluble in aq. Ag NO_3 solution.

Also, on treatment with $Na^+\bar{O}H$ & $CHCl_3/KOH$

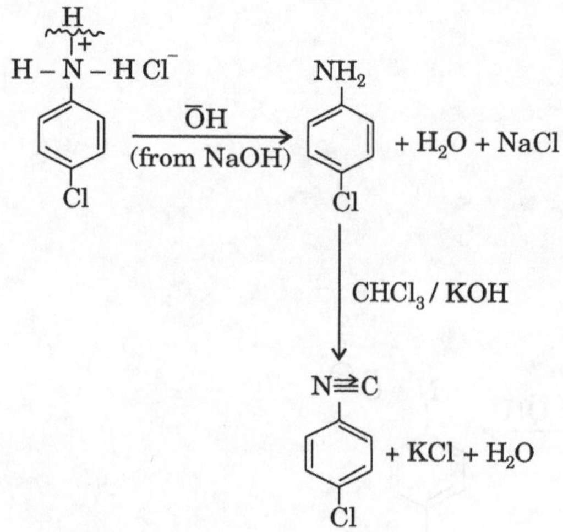

(Bad smelling compound)

25.

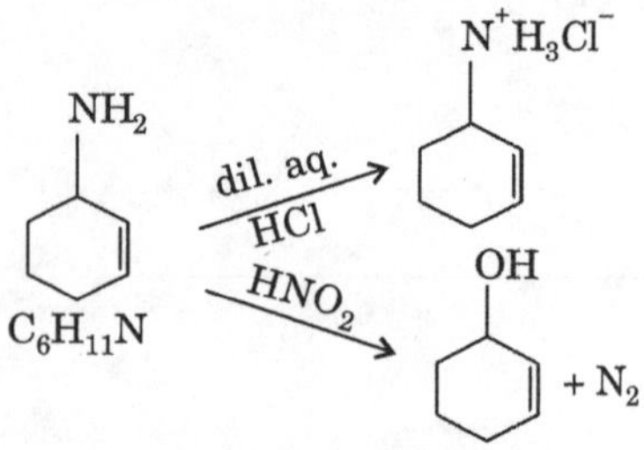

Exhaustive methylation

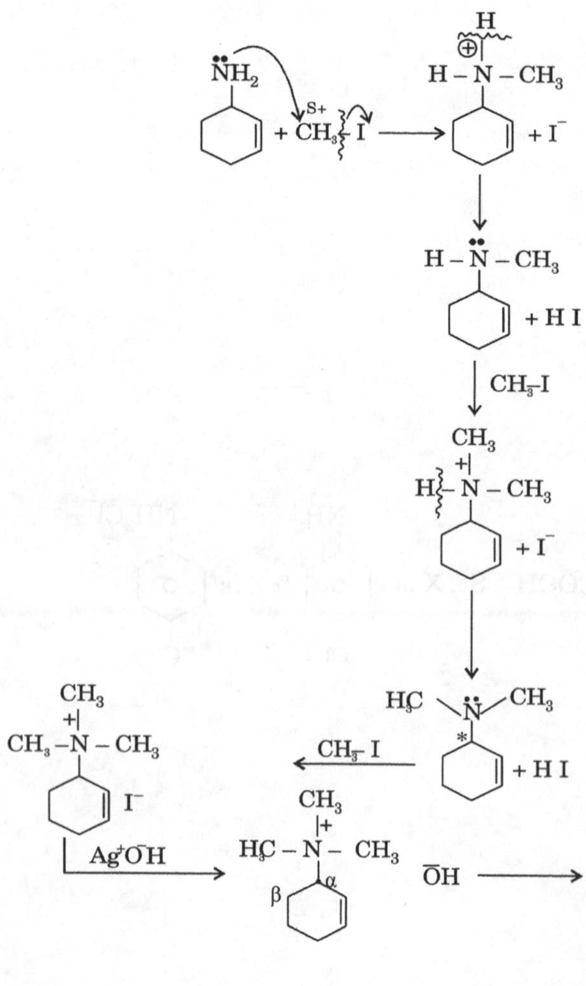

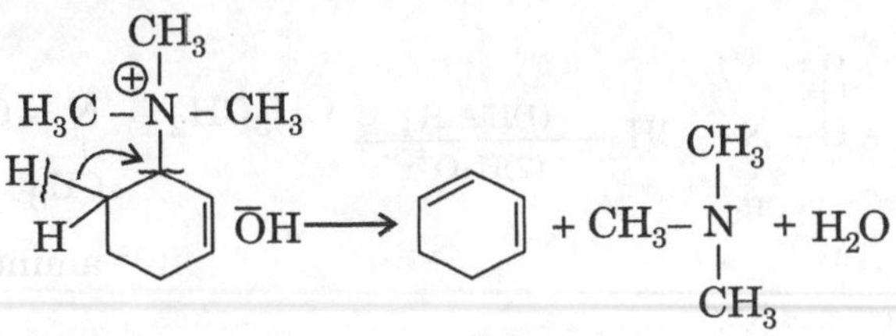

27. 2° Amines react with aldehydes / ketone to give an enamine.

$$(CH_3)_2\ddot{N}H + CH_3-\overset{\overset{O}{||}}{C}-CH_3 \xrightarrow{PTS}$$

Mechanism wrt option a

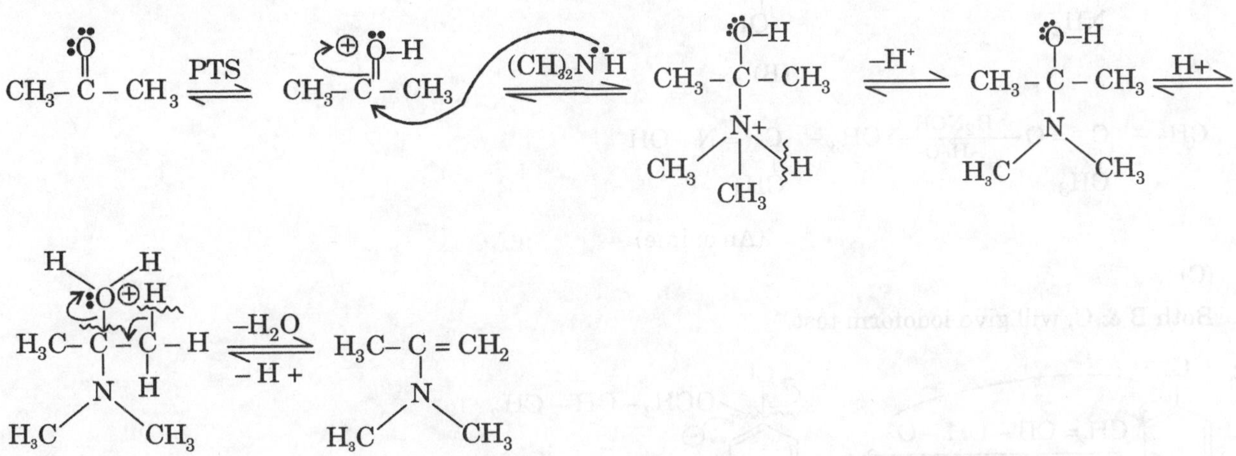

(an enamine)

wrt option b

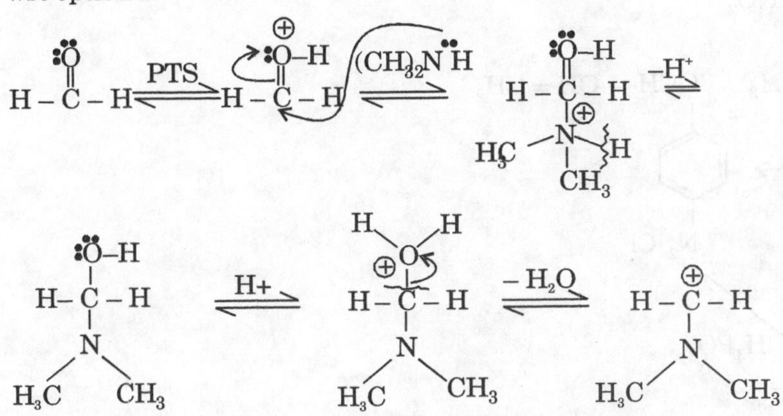

(an enamine CAN'T BE FORMED)

28.

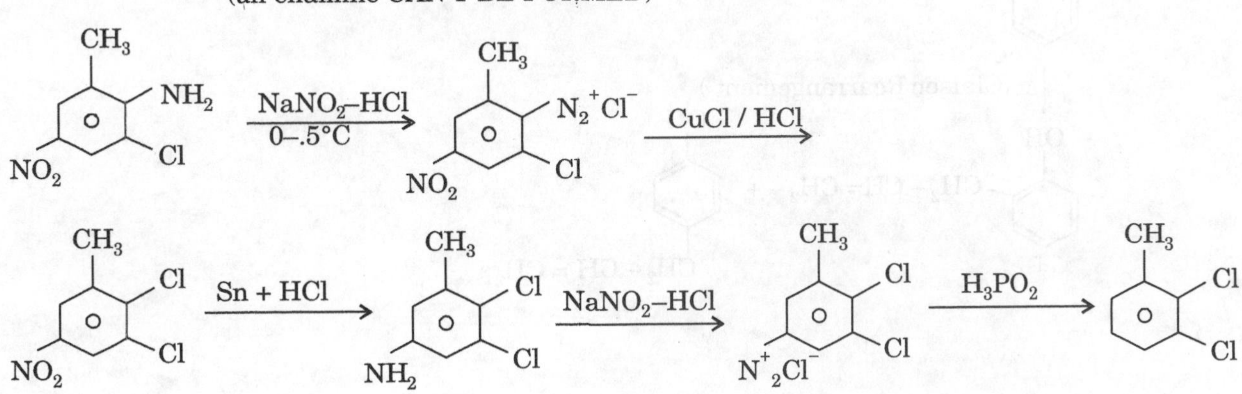

29. 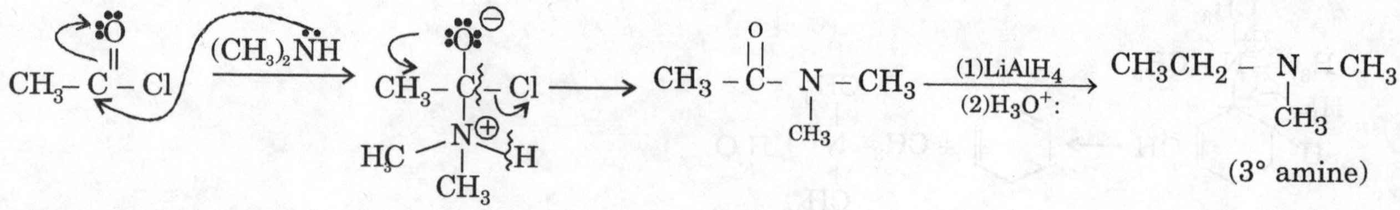

31. If 'C' does not reduce a Fehling's solution, it must be a ketone.

C_3H_9N might be-

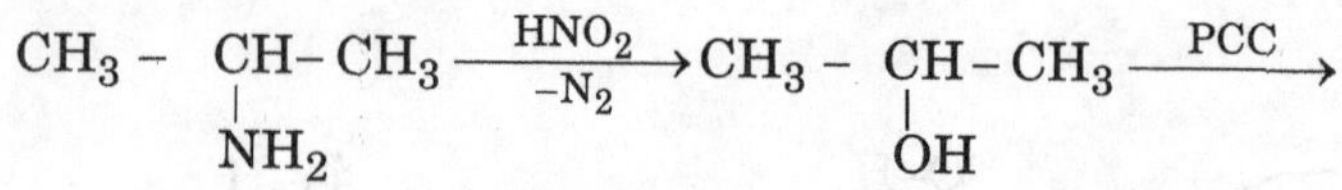

(A) (B)

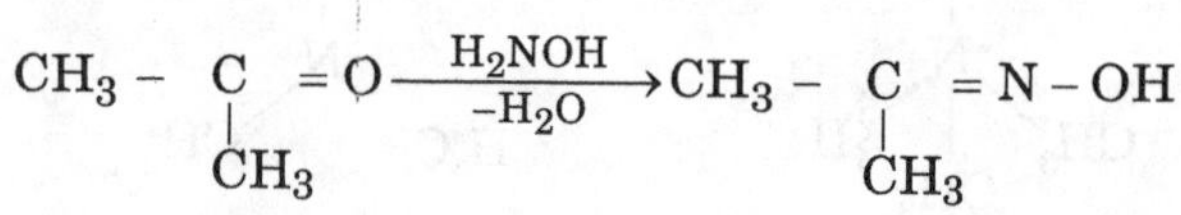

(An oxime)

(C)

Both B & C, will give iodoform test.

32. 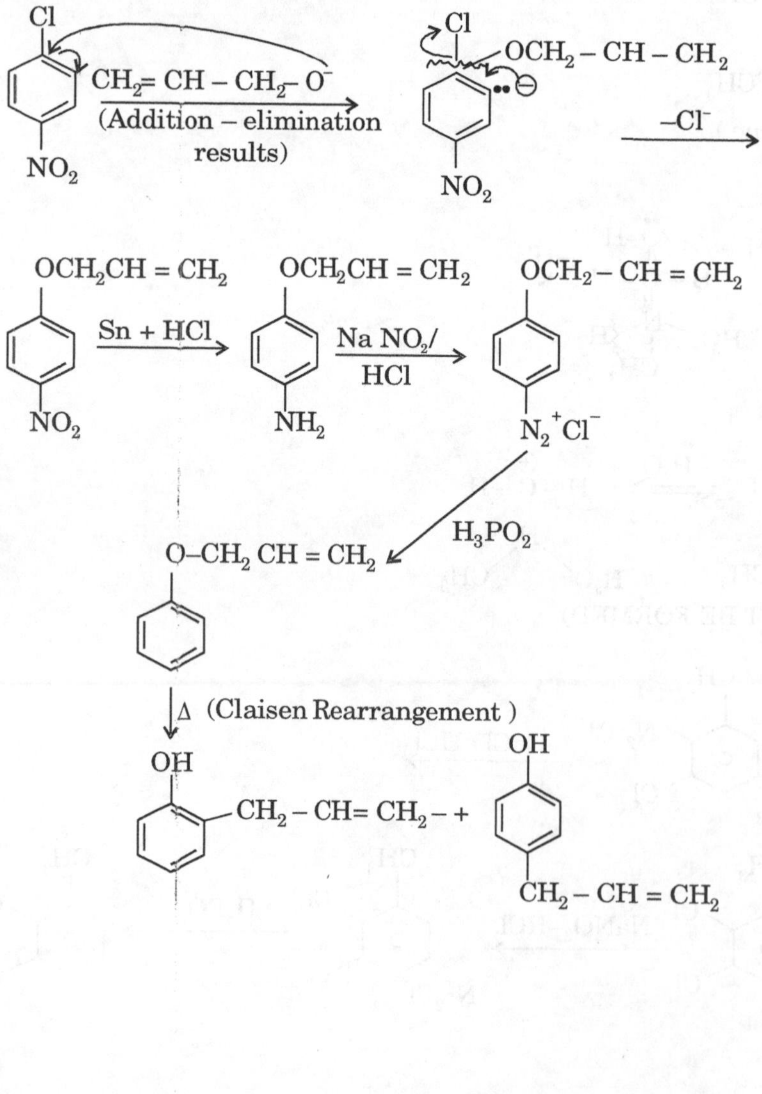

35. 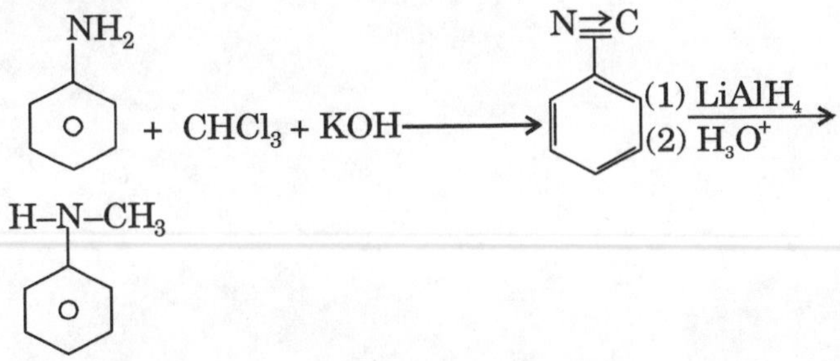

36. Only Aromatic diazonium ions i.e 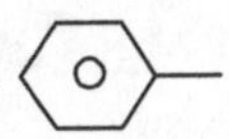 $-\overset{\oplus}{N} \equiv \ddot{N}$, are stable at 0°–5°C.

37. (a) $NaNO_2 + HCl \rightarrow HNO_2 + NaCl$

(b) 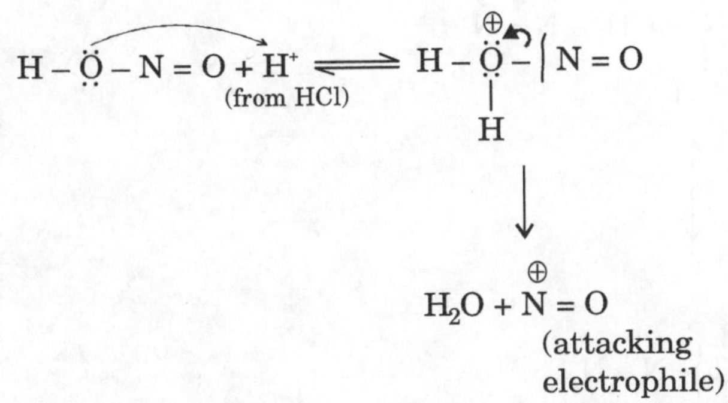

(c) 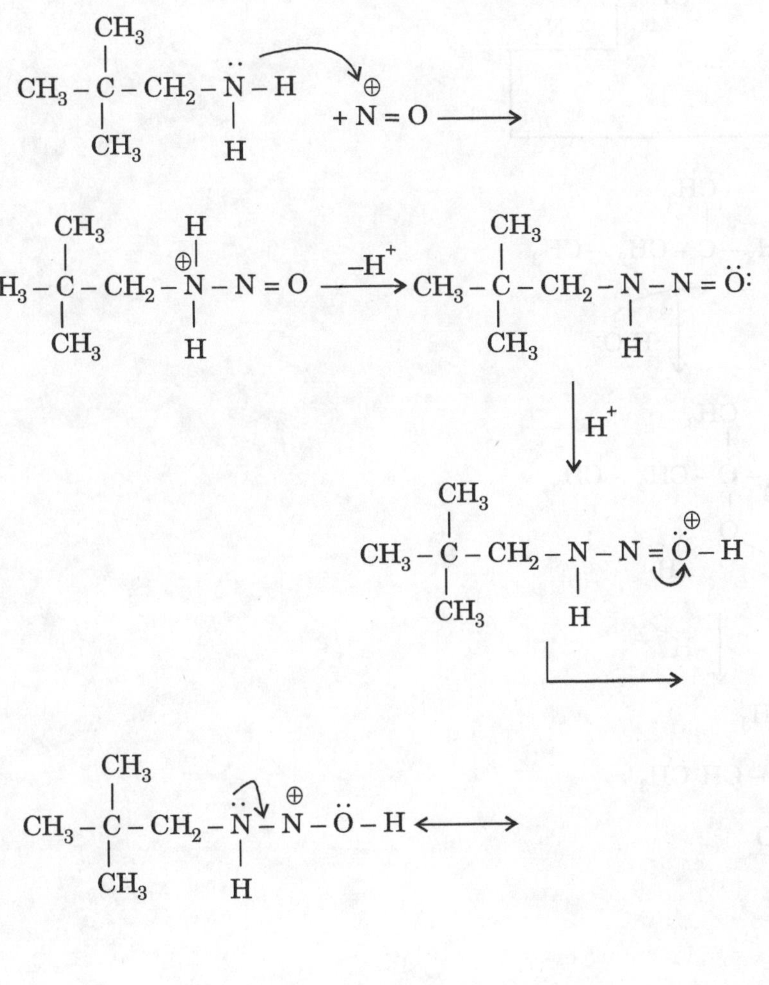

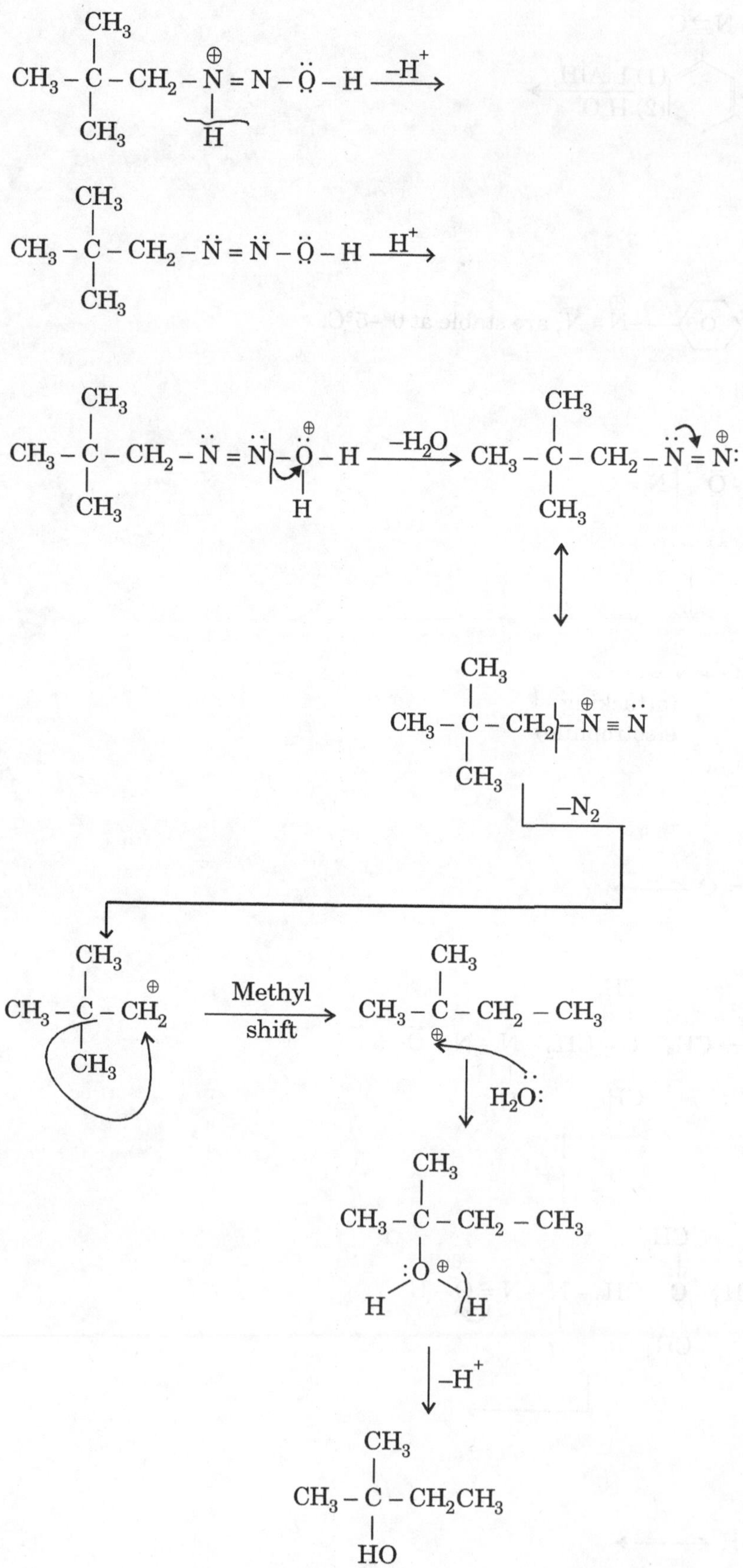
–H⁺
H⁺
–H₂O
–N₂
Methyl shift
H₂O:
–H⁺

39. 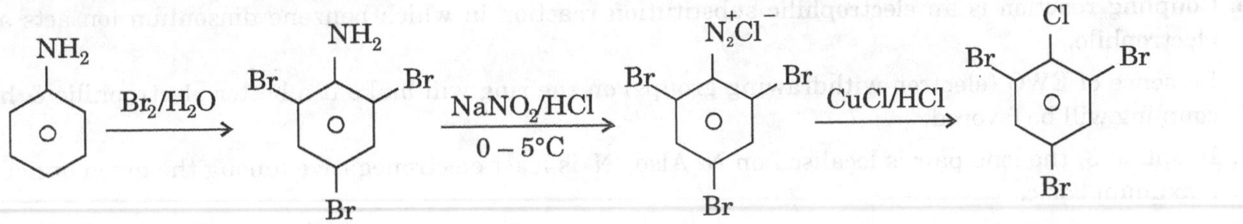

40. 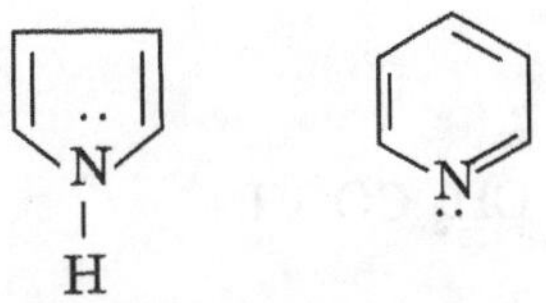

Pyrrole Pyridine

In pyrrole , the lone pair on N is involved in resonance, so it is less basic.

In pyridine, lone pair on N is LOCALISED (not involved in resonance), so it is more basic.

41. 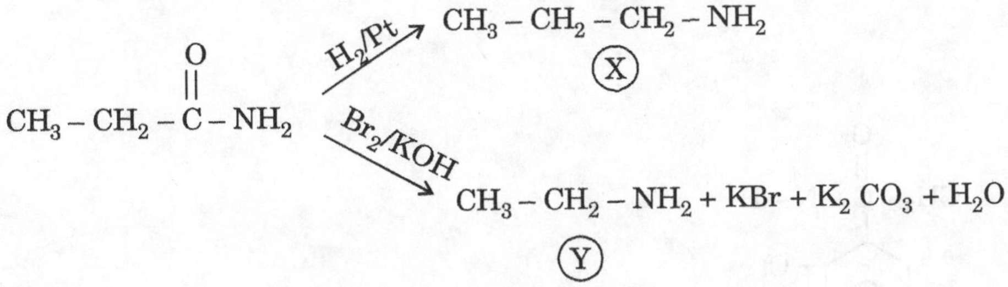

42. 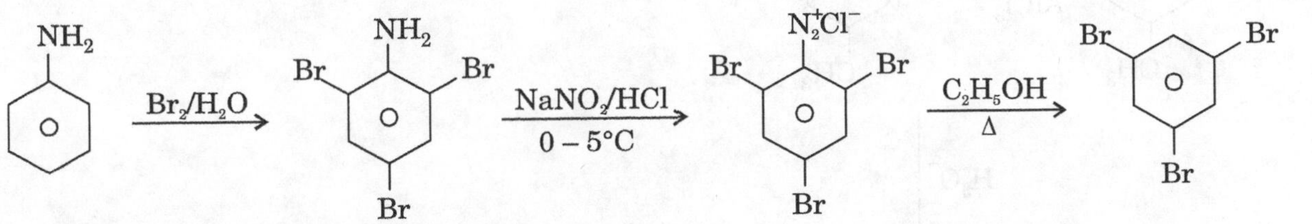

43. 1°Amines react with aldehydes to give schiffs base.

44. 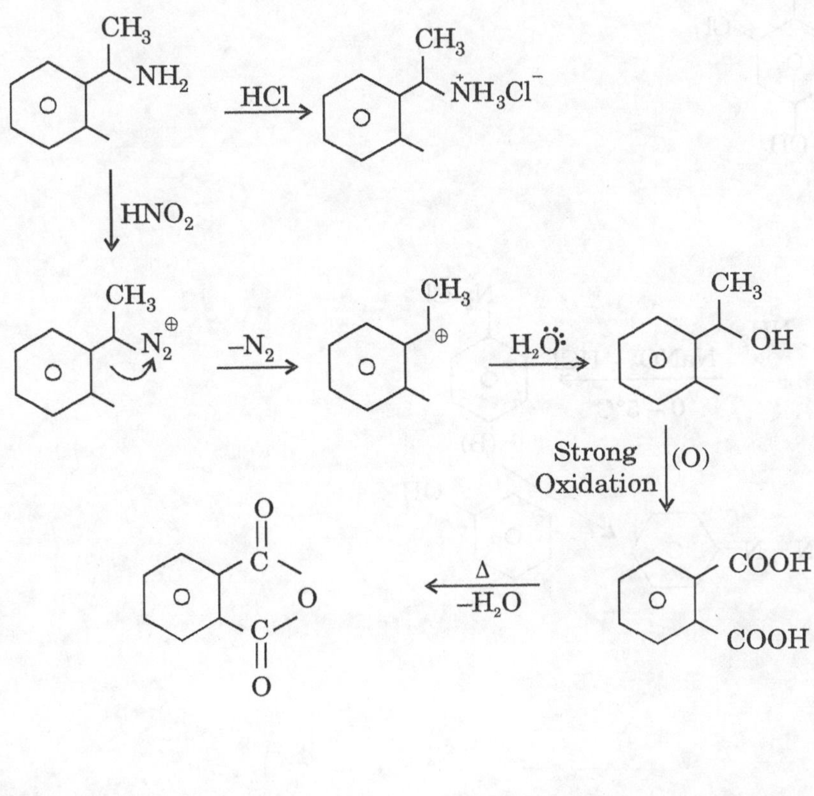

45. Coupling reaction is an electrophilic substitution reaction in which benzene diazonium ion acts as an electrophile.

Presence of EWG (electron withdrawing groups) on the ring will make it a better electrophilie & hence coupling will be favored.

46. In option 3, the lone pair is localised on N. Also, 'N' is least electronegative among the given options, so maximum basic.

47.

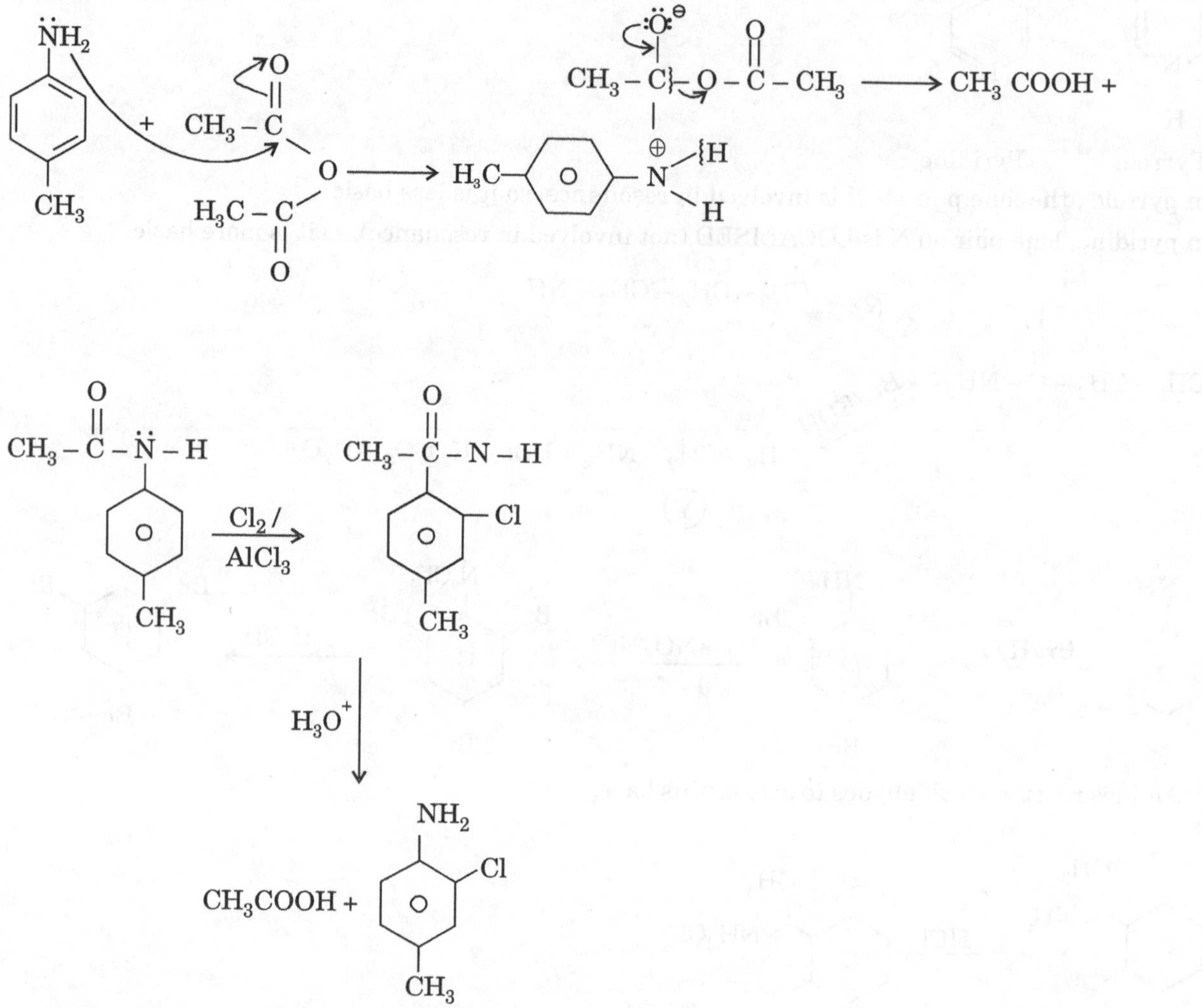

48.

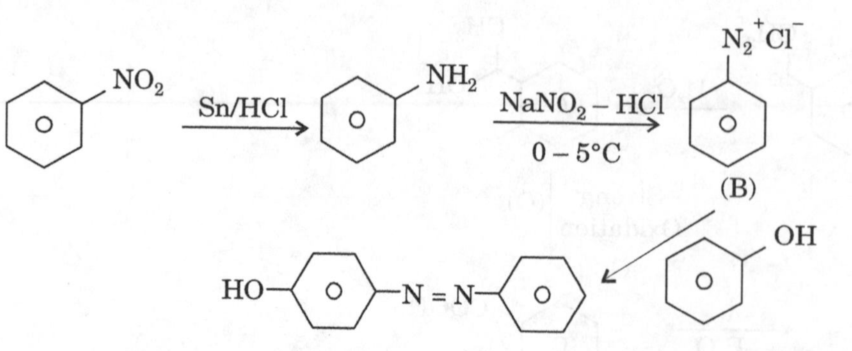

49.

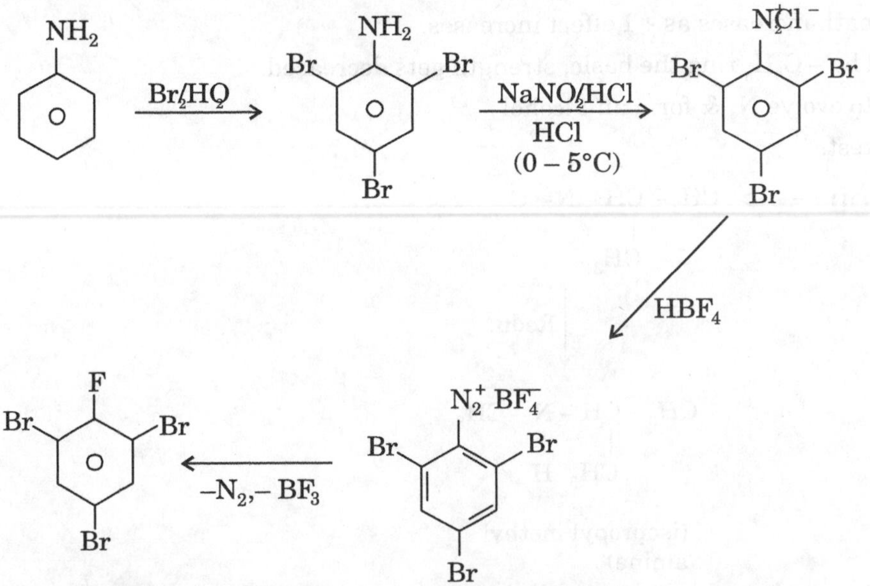

50. It is diazotisation followed by intramolecular coupling.

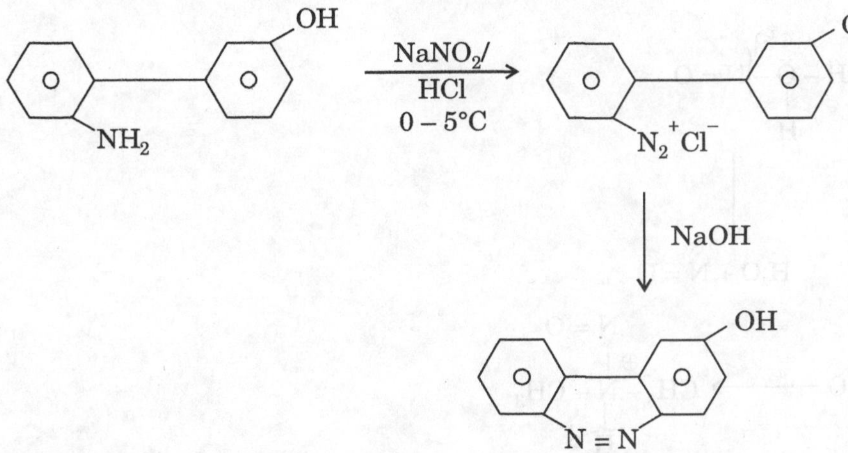

51. (a) $NaNO_2 + HCl \rightarrow HNO_2 + NaCl$

(b) $H-\ddot{O}-N=O + \overset{+}{H} \longrightarrow H-\overset{\overset{\oplus}{}}{\ddot{O}}(H)-N=O \longrightarrow H_2O + \overset{\oplus}{N}=O$

52.

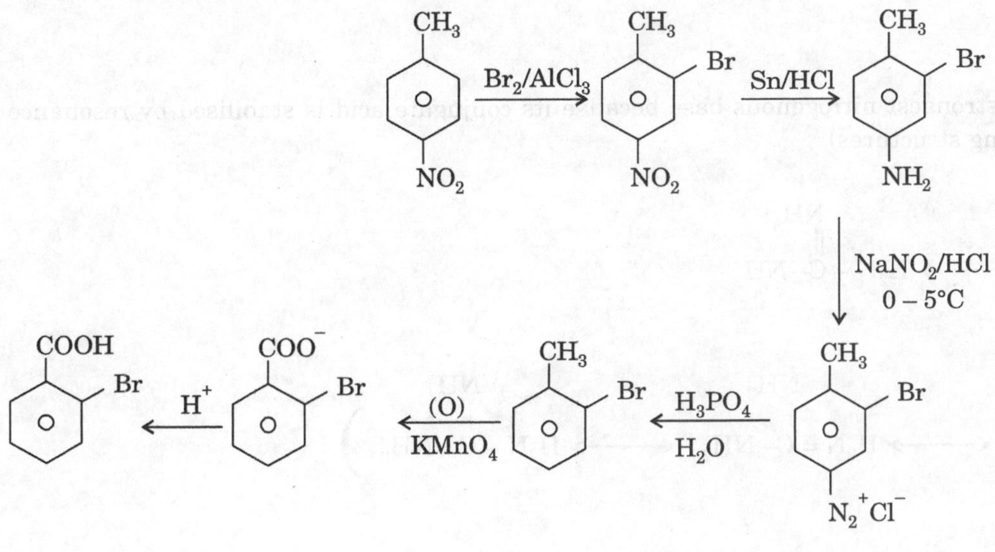

54. In gaseous phase, basic strength increases as + I effect increases.
But due to – I effect exerted by $-C_6H_5$ ring the basic, strength gets decreased.

55. 1° amines react with HNO_2 to evolve N_2 & form an alcohol also, they give carbylamine test.

$$CH_3-\underset{\underset{CH_3}{|}}{CH}-NH_2 + CHCl_3 + KOH \longrightarrow CH_3-\underset{\underset{CH_3}{|}}{CH}-N\equiv C \xrightarrow{\text{Redn.}} CH_3-\underset{\underset{CH_3}{|}}{CH}-\underset{\underset{H}{|}}{N}-CH_3$$

(isopropyl methyl amine)

56. (a) $NaNO_2 + HCl \rightarrow HNO_2 + NaCl$

(b)

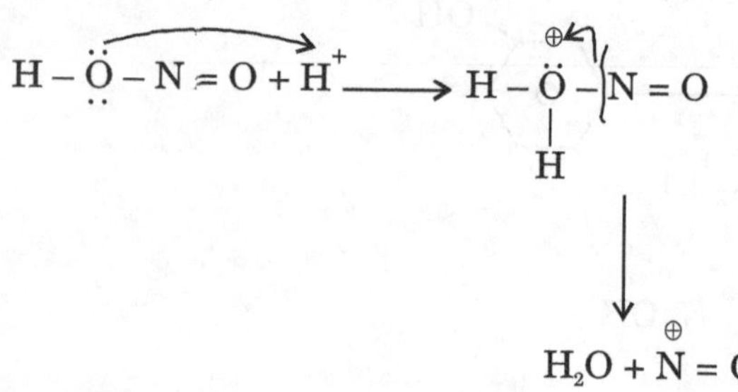

(c)

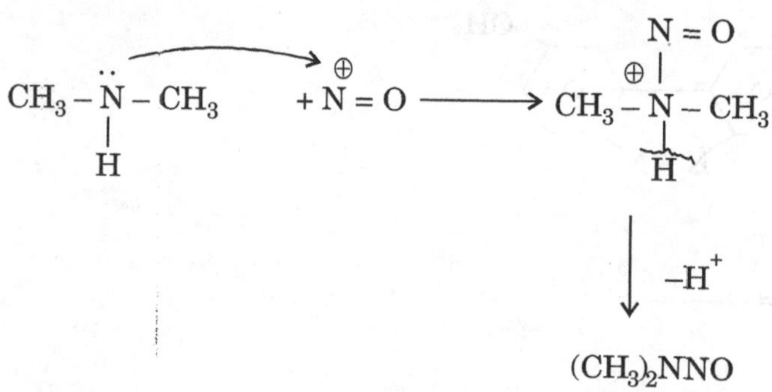

57. $H_2N-\overset{\overset{NH}{||}}{C}-NH_2$

Guanidine is the strongest nitrogenous base because its conjugate acid is stabilised by resonance (two equally contributing structures)

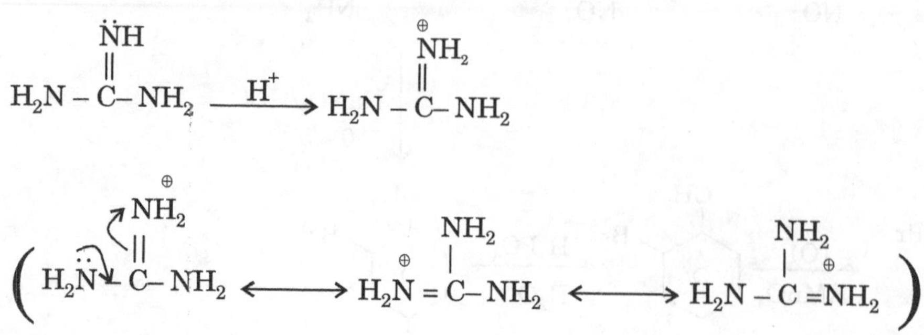

In IVth molecule,

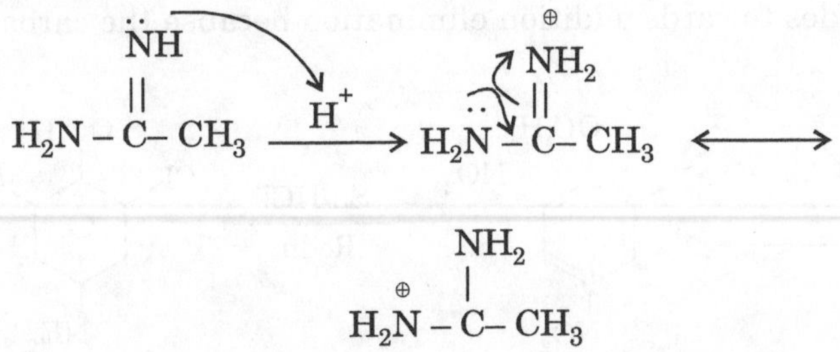

Here, Conjugate acid is stabilised form one end only.

58.

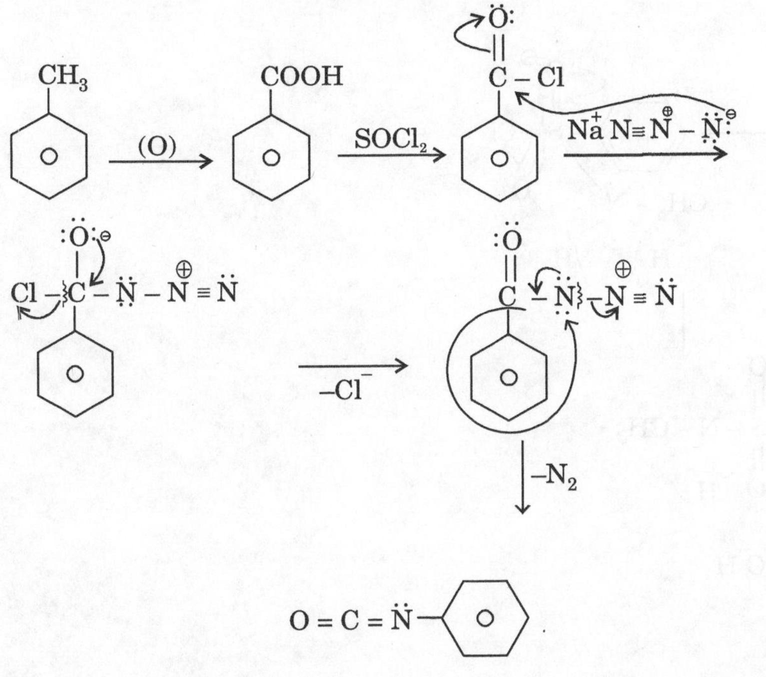

PHENYL ISOCYANATE

59. In, 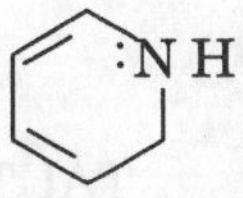 & 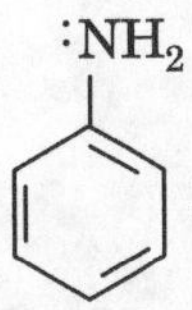, the lone pair is delocalised, option 'b' is a 2° amine & is hence more basic than NH_3

(Also in option 2 l.p. is not delocalised.)

60.

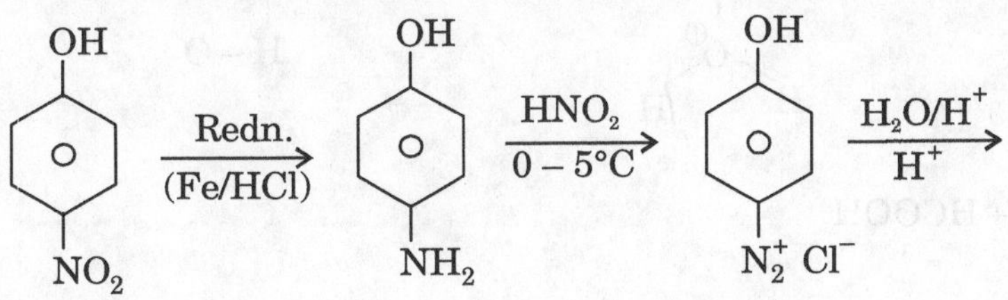

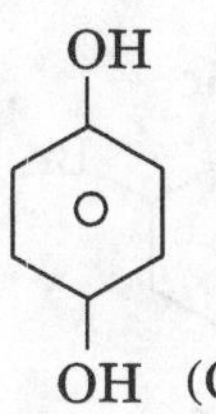

(Quinol)

61. Here, in option (c), 'H' is absent on 'C' to which $-NO_2$ is attached.

62. Aryl fluorides are more reactive then aryl chlorides towards addition elimination because the carbanion formed is more stable in the case of former.

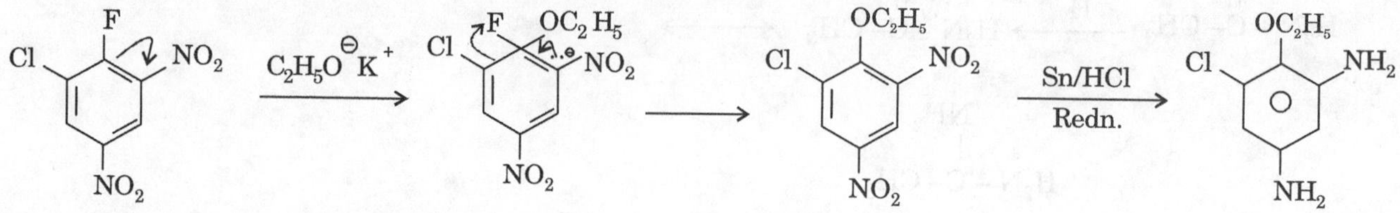

63. 2° amines are maximum basic in aq. medium

64. 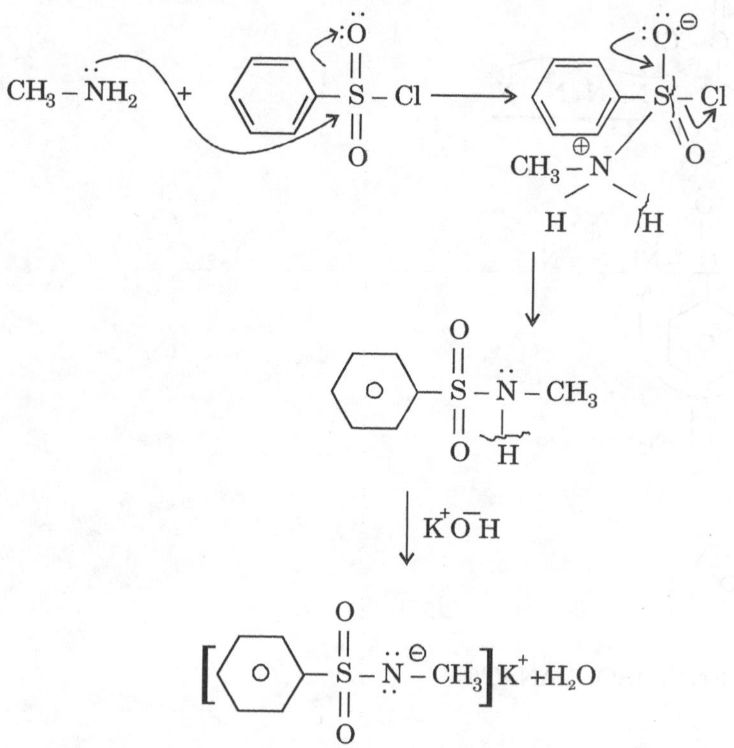

65. 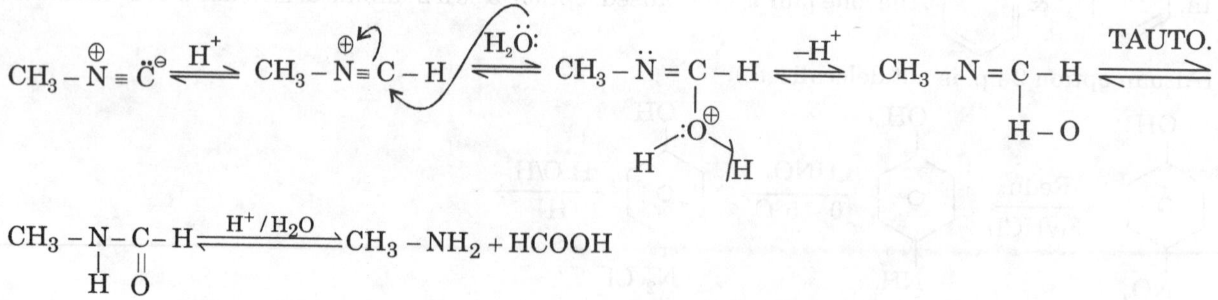

66. 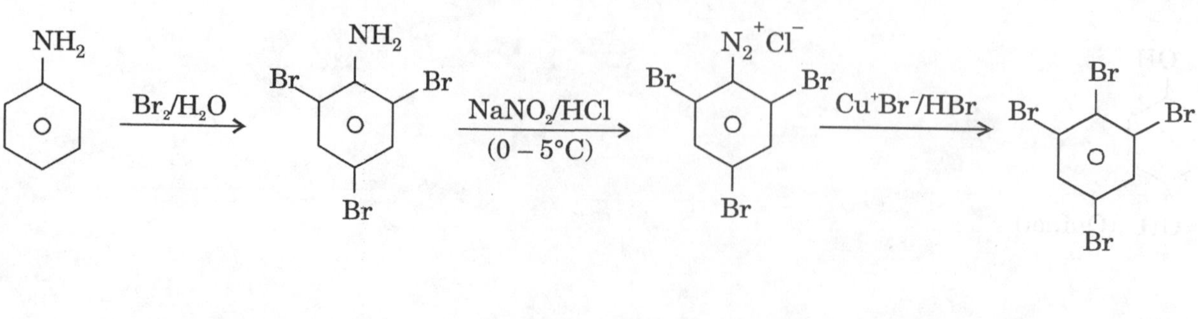

67. O – toluidine is least basic due to ortho effect.

68.

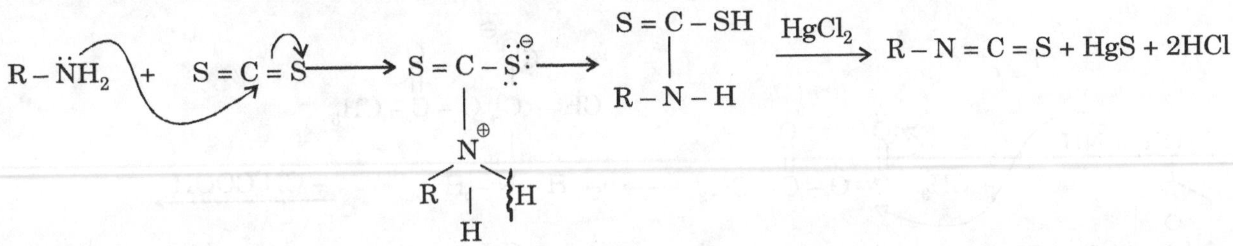

70. In quinuclidine (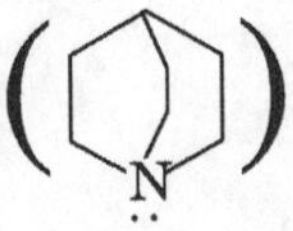), the unshared electron pair is in sp^3 orbital but all the C atoms are tied back to make the lone pair more easily available, so it is slightly more basic then $(C_2H_5)_3N$. Wrt 2 nd option, N, N–dimethyl picramide is a stronger base than picramide.

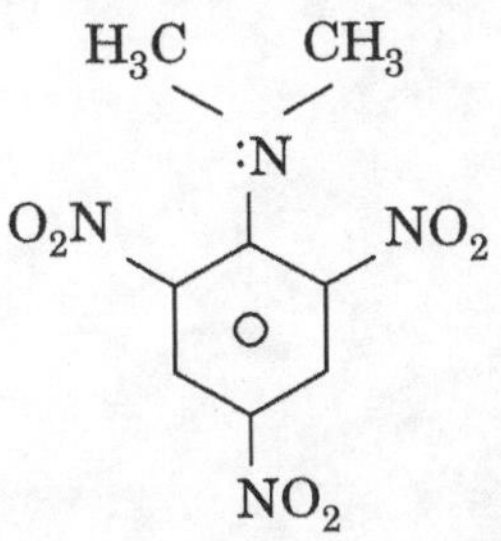

(Here steric Inhibition to Resonance operates and Coplanarity of Ring and dimethyl amino group is lost due to which lone pair of $-\ddot{N}(CH_3)_2$ is not delocalised)

wrt (c) option, order is correct.

72. 3° aromatic amines on reaction with HNO_2 ($\overset{\oplus}{N}=O$ ion is generated), undergo electrophilic substitution at para–position.
1° aromatic amine with HNO_2 (0-5°C) undergoes diazotisation predominantly.

73. Option (c) lacks 'H' attached to 'N'. So, it cannot undergo benzoylation.

75. Used for 2° Amines.

77.

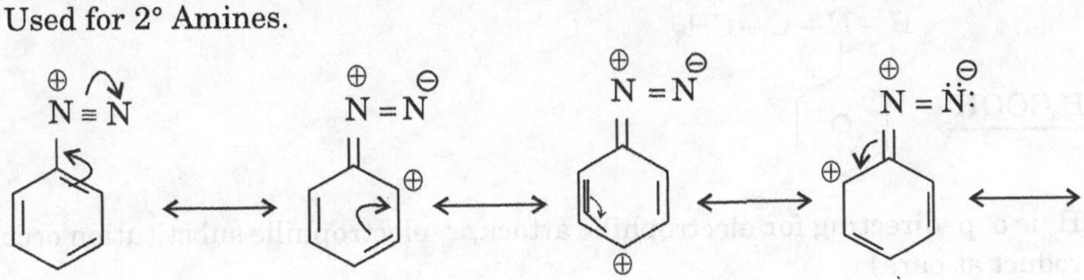

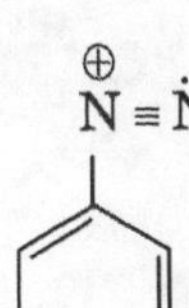

(stabilised by resonance)

$CH_3-CH_2-\overset{\oplus}{N}\equiv\ddot{N}$

↓

(Not stabilised by resonance)

81. An 'amine' is more nucleophilic than an amide ∵ in a amide the lone pair on 'N' is delocalised.

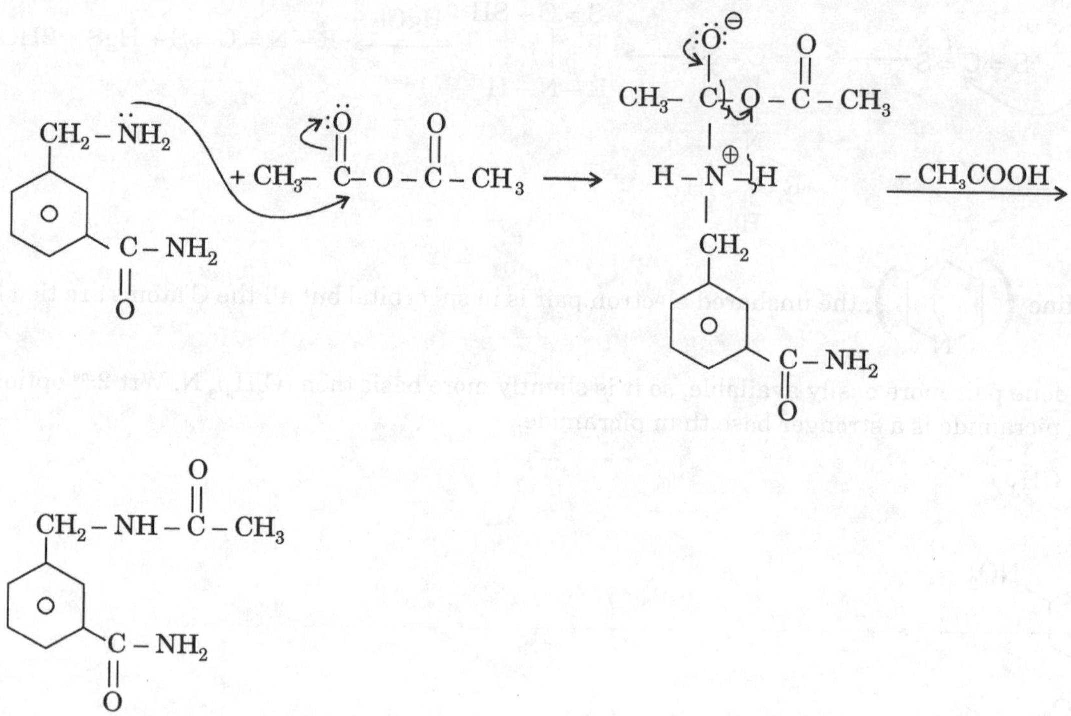

82.

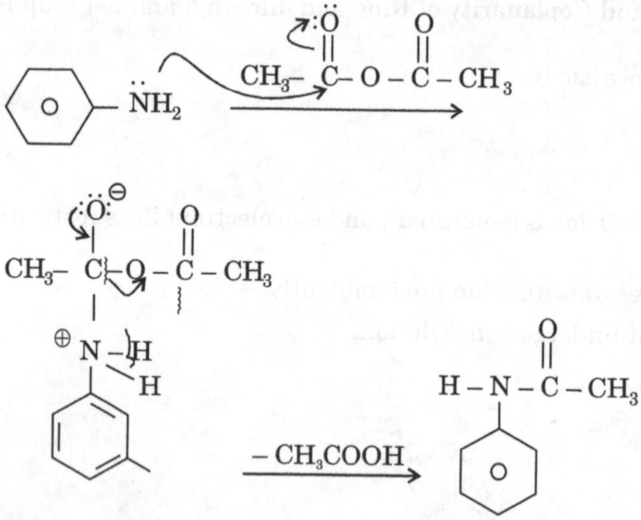

Step 2. Since – NH $COCH_3$ is o, p–directing for electrophilic attack, ∴ electrophilic substitution occurs at O & P locations (major product at para)

1. $Cl-CH_2-\overset{\ddot{O}}{\overset{||}{C}}-Cl + AlCl_3 \longrightarrow \overset{-}{AlCl_4} + Cl-CH_2-\overset{\oplus}{C}=\ddot{O}:$

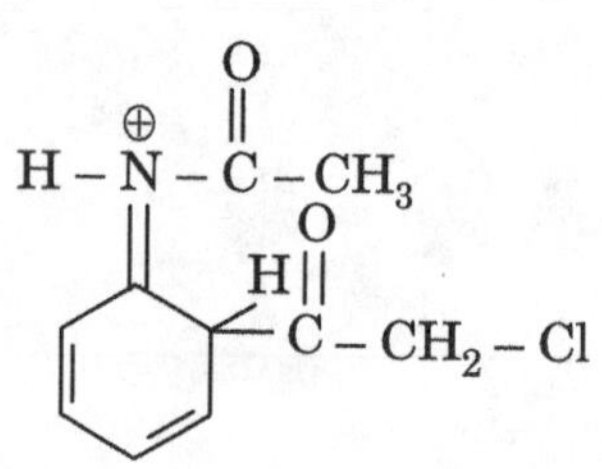

2.
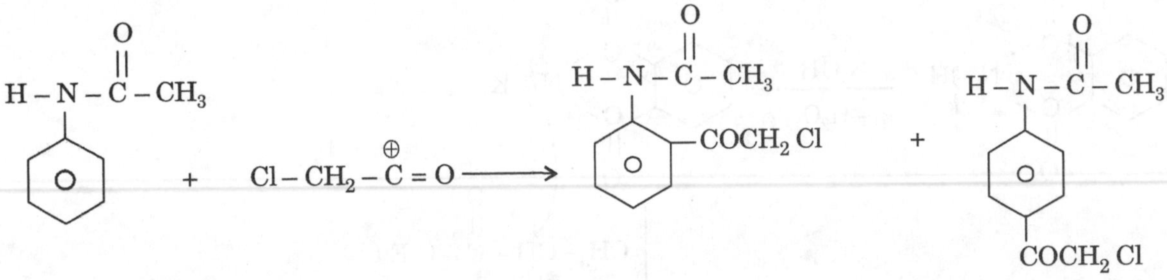

(Major P)

83. During acetylation, one H atom (at. mass = 1 amu) of NH_2 group is replaced by an acetyl group, CH_3CO (mol. mass = 43 amu)

$$-NH_2 + CH_3COCl \longrightarrow -NHCOCH_3 + HCl$$

So, acetylation of each $-NH_2$ group increases the mass by 42 amu (43 – 1).

In this case, increase in mass = 390 – 180 = 210 amu

$$\therefore \text{ No. of } -NH_2 \text{ groups} = \frac{210}{42} = 5$$

84.
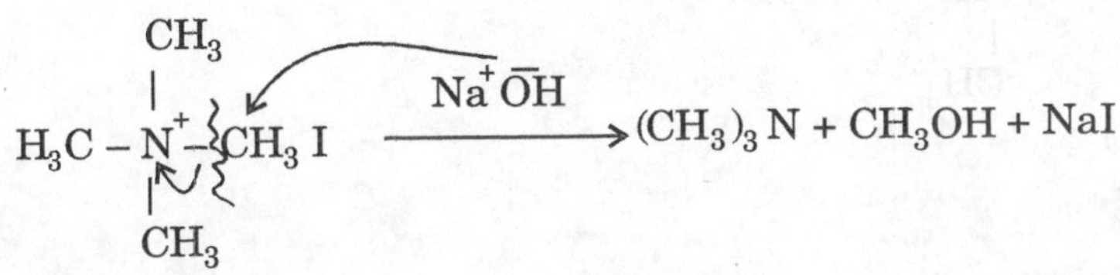

Since 'N' is highly electro –ve and bearing +ve charge have, it will pull maximum electrons towards itself & creating sufficient +ve charge on 'C' & inviting $\overline{O}H$ for attack.

85. Amines are more basic than amides because in amides the lone pair on 'N' is delocalized. So, I is more basic than II & III.

In II, (CH_3CONH_2), the l. p. on 'N' is delocalised with C = O bond

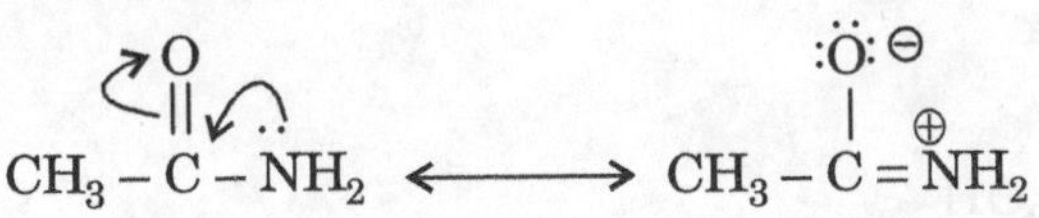

In III, i.e. 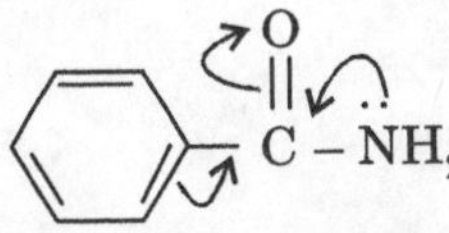, the l. p. on 'N' & the π electrons of ring, both are in conjugation with $-C = O$, so l. p. on N has less probability to participate in resonance. Hence, it is more basic than II.

86.
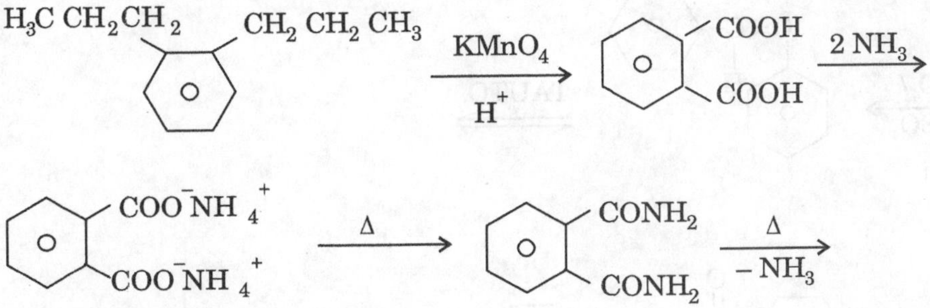

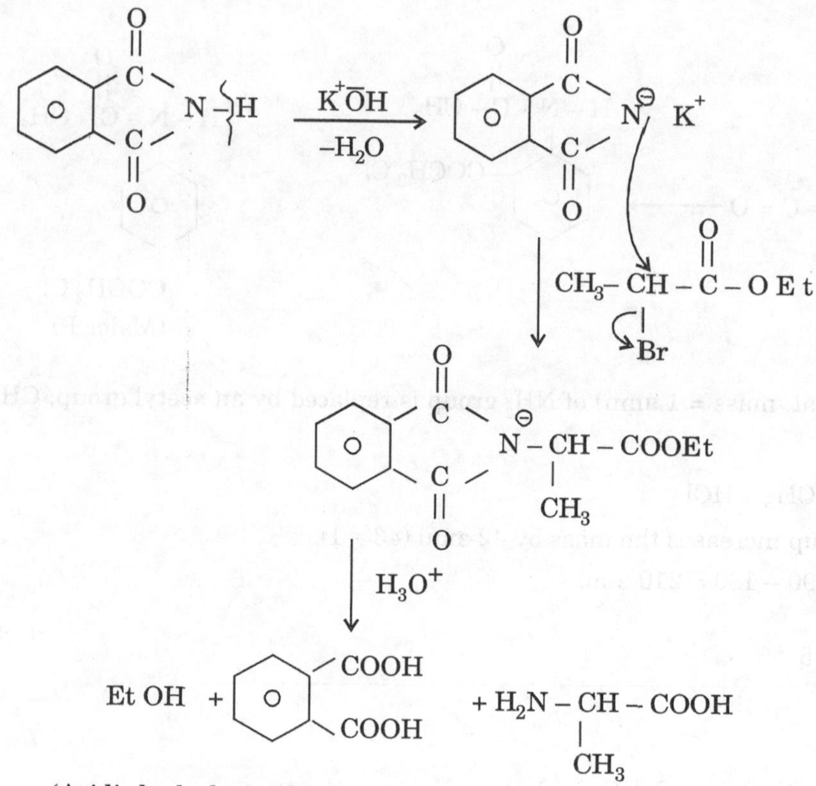

(Acidic hydrolysis of ester also occurs)

87.

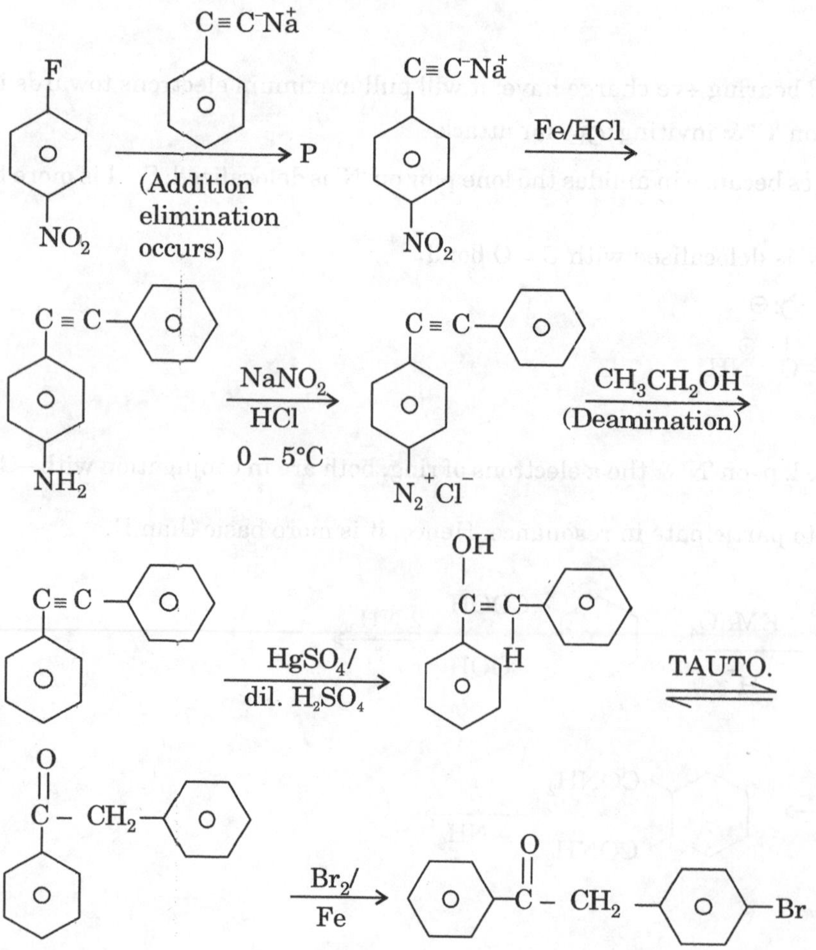

88. $\underset{(X)}{CH_3-C\equiv N} \xrightarrow[2)\ H_3O^+]{1)\ LiAlH_4} \underset{(Y)}{CH_3CH_2NH_2}\ (C_2H_7N)$

$\underset{(X)}{CH_3-C\equiv N} \xrightarrow{H_3O^+} \underset{(Z)}{CH_3COOH}$

Now,

$$\underset{\text{(Acid)}}{CH_3-\overset{\overset{\large O}{||}}{C}-O-H} + \underset{\text{(Base)}}{CH_3CH_2\ddot{N}H_2} \longrightarrow CH_3COO^{\ominus} + CH_3CH_2\overset{+}{N}H_3$$

89. 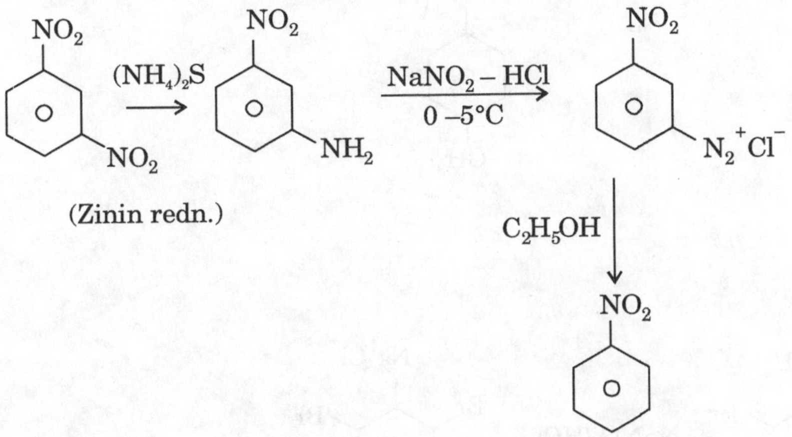

90. 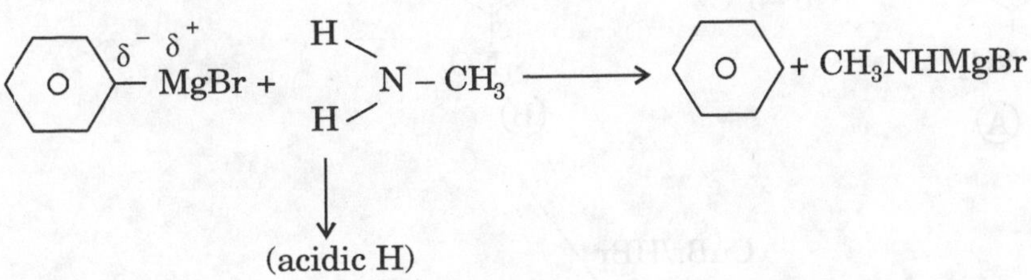

92. 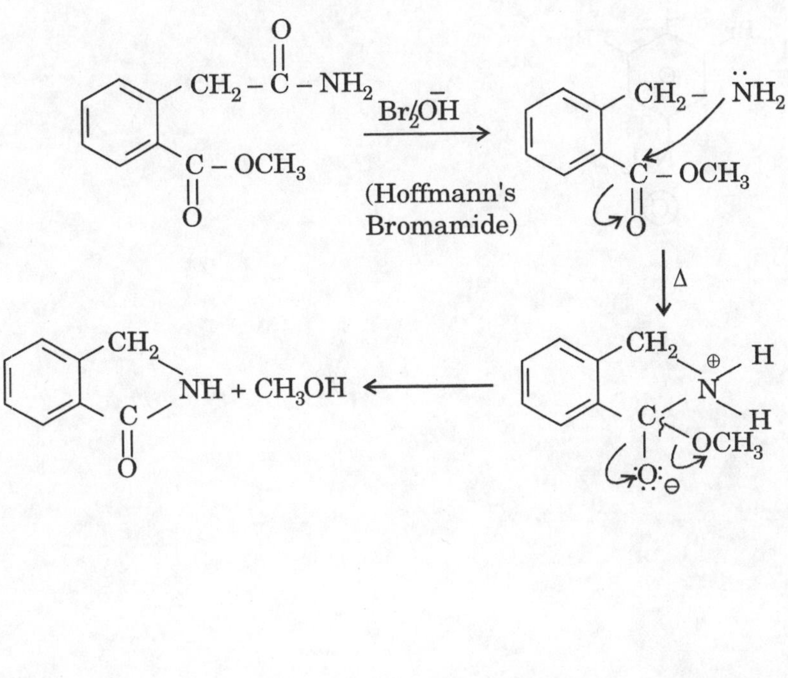

93.

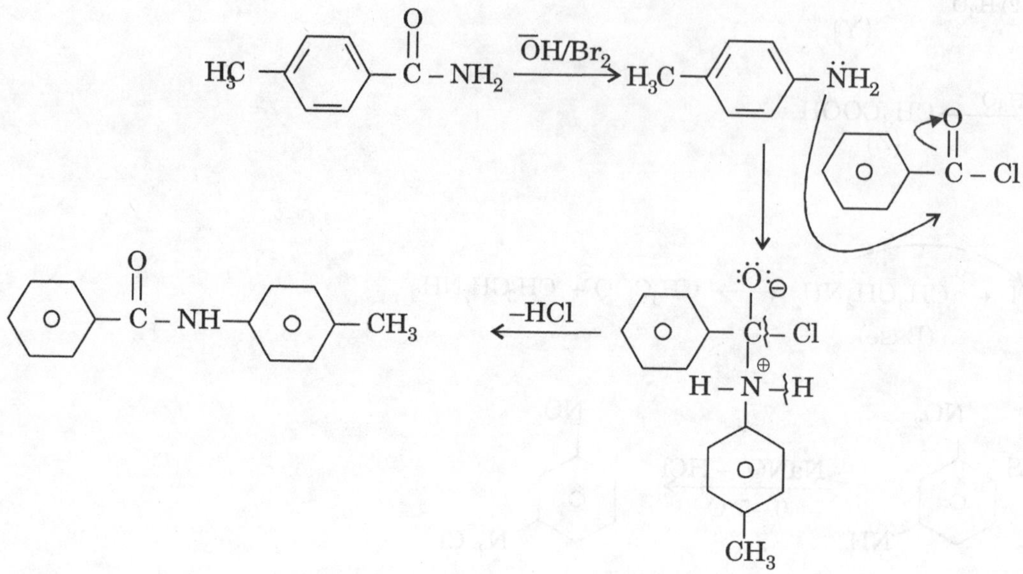
O
H3C
C – NH2
OH/Br2
H3C
NH2
O
C – Cl
O
C – NH
CH3
–HCl
O
C – Cl
H – N – H
CH3

95.

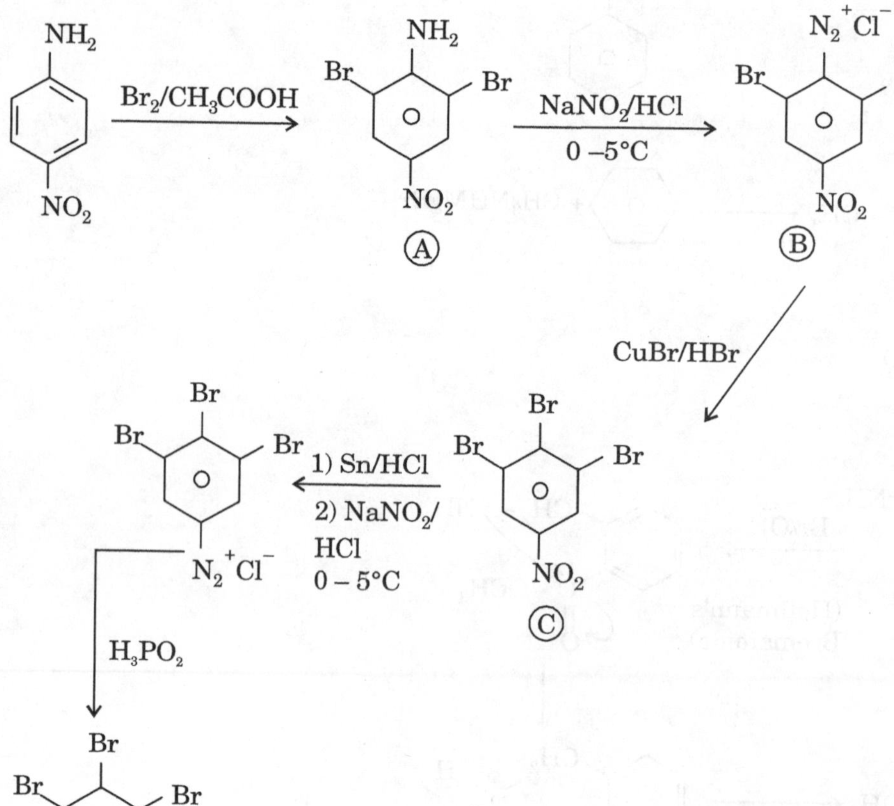
NH2
NO2
Br2/CH3COOH
NH2
Br
Br
NO2
A
NaNO2/HCl
0 –5°C
N2+Cl−
Br
Br
NO2
B
CuBr/HBr
Br
Br
Br
NO2
C
1) Sn/HCl
2) NaNO2/
HCl
0 – 5°C
Br
Br
Br
N2+Cl−
H3PO2
Br
Br
Br

96. 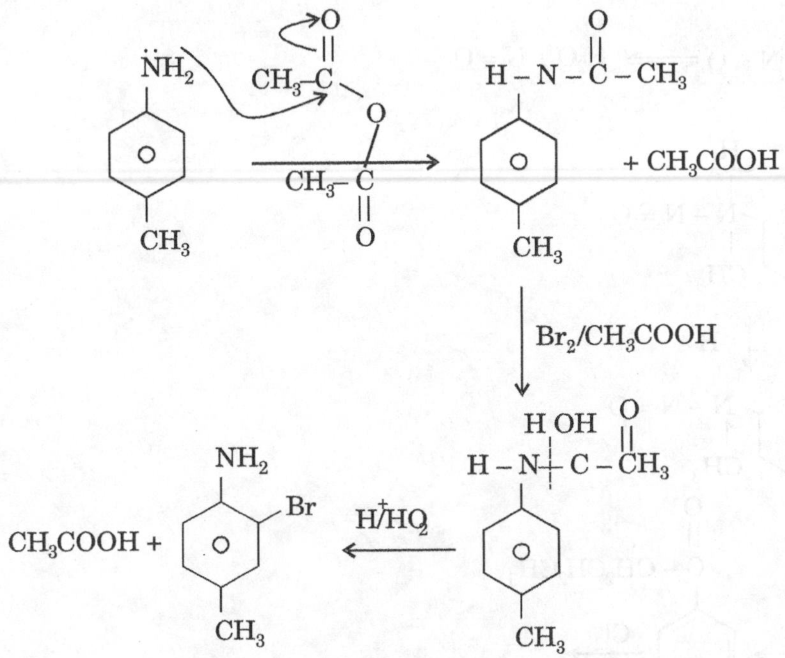

97. Optimum basic medium favours coupling reaction of phenol whereas optimum acidic medium favours coupling reaction of aniline.

98. (1) $CH_3-\ddot{N}H_2 + \overset{\delta+}{CH_3}-I \longrightarrow (CH_3)_2NH + HI$

(2) $(CH_3)_2\ddot{N}H + \overset{\delta+}{CH_3}-I \longrightarrow (CH_3)_3N + HI$

(3) $(CH_3)_3\ddot{N} + \overset{\delta+}{CH_3}-I \longrightarrow CH_3-\overset{+}{N}(CH_3)_2-CH_3\,I^-$

(4) $CH_3-\overset{+}{N}(CH_3)_2-CH_3\,I^- \xrightarrow{AgOH} CH_3-\overset{+}{N}(CH_3)_2-CH_3\,\overline{O}H \xrightarrow{\Delta} (CH_3)_3N + CH_3OH$

99. In P-aminobenzoic acid, –COOH is a relatively weaker acid & hence it cannot transfer H^+ to weakly basic amino group.

100. In p-nitrotoluene, since $-CH_3$ makes the ring activated, so electrophilic attack occurs wrt $-CH_3$ group, which is an o,p – director. Since para is blocked, attack occur at ortho position.

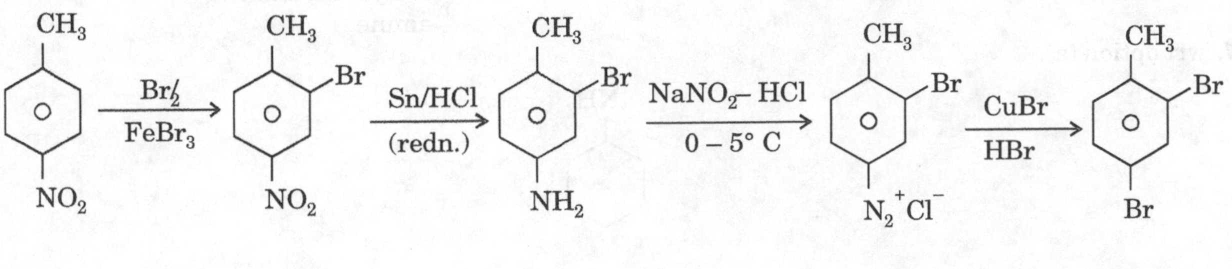

101. $NaNO_2 + HCl \longrightarrow HNO_2 + NaCl$

$$H^+ + H-\ddot{O}-N=O \rightleftharpoons H-\overset{\oplus}{\ddot{O}}(H)-N=O \rightleftharpoons H_2O + \overset{\oplus}{N}=O$$

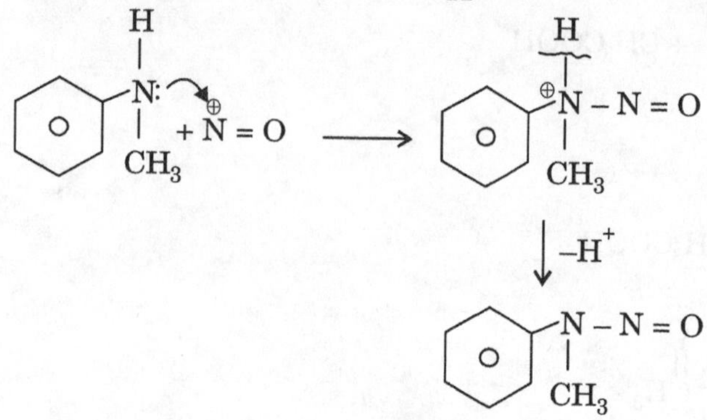

102.

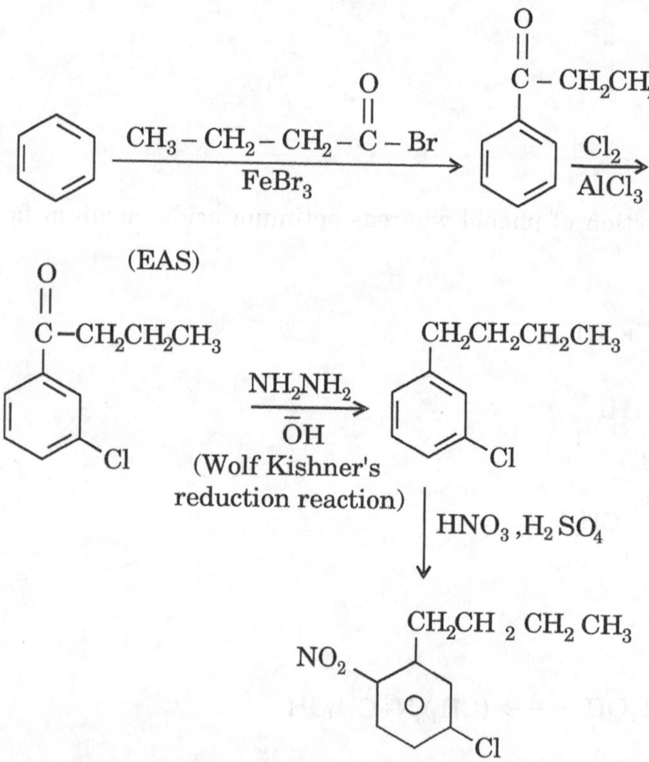

103. 3° amines lack acidic H & hence cannot undergo acetylation.

106.

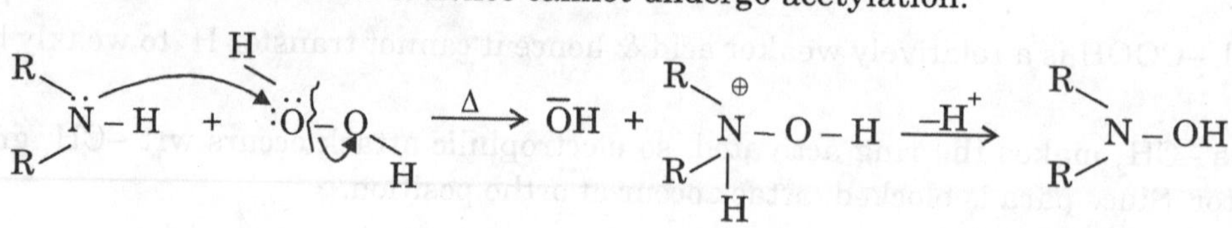

N-hydroxyldialkyl amine

107. wrt option (a).

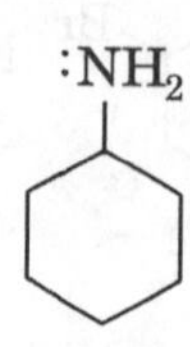

Here lone pair on N is NOT delocalised.

In 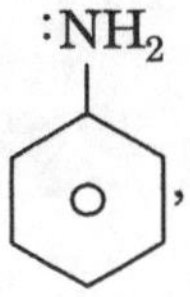, lone pair is delocalised &

in 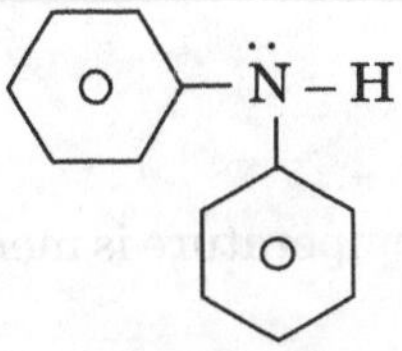, lone pair is delocalised

on two rings, so availability of lone pair is markedly decreased.

Hence, 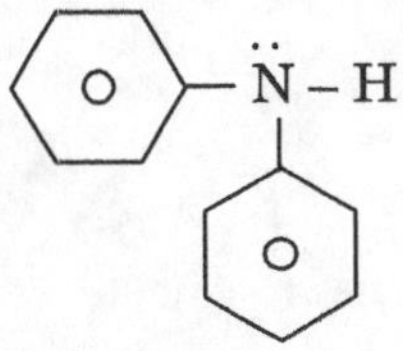 is the weakest base

wrt option (b),

In piperidine,

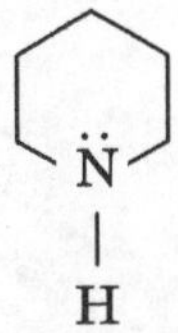

→ lone pair NOT delocalised

→ adjacent C's sp^3 hybridised,

not much eletro –ve.

→ High electron density on N

→ stronger Base.

In pyridine,

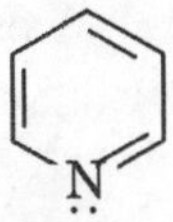

→ lone pair not delocalised

→ adjacent C's sp^2 hybridised. So, electron density on N is relatively less, so less basic.

In pyrrole,

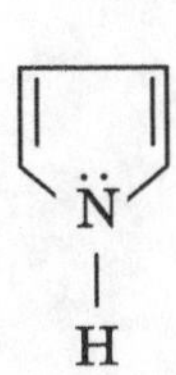

→ lone pair is delocalised.

→ so, it is least basic

wrt option (c),

Presence of EDG (like-CH_3) will increase electron density & increase the basic strength of aniline.

108. $CH_3{-}CH_2{-}CH_2{-}NH_2 + HNO_2 \rightarrow CH_3 - \underset{\displaystyle OH}{\underset{|}{C}} - CH_3 + N_2$

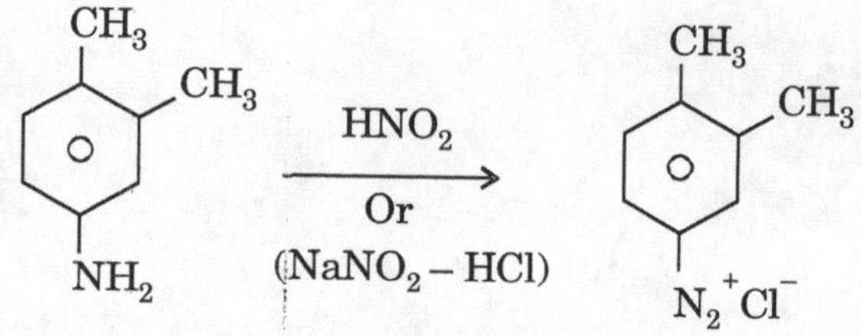

(But here N_2 will be liberated ∵ benzene diazonium is stable at O–5°C & here room temperature is mentioned)

14

CHAPTER

Biomolecules

1. An optically inactive amino acid is –
(a) glycine (b) alanine
(c) proline (d) valine

2. α – D (+) – glucose & β – D (+) – glucose are
(a) enantiomers (b) conformers
(d) epimers (d) anomers

3. Which of the following is / are correct?
(a) D(–) Fructose exists in furanose structure
(b) Maltose is a reducing sugar.
(c) Penta acetate of glucose does not react with NH_2OH.
(d) All are correct.

4. Starch is a mixture of two components, a water soluble component amylose (15–20%) & a water insoluble component amylopectin (80 – 85%). The aqueous solution of amylose gives a blue colour with iodine solution due to the formation of –
(a) amylose iodide
(b) amylose iodate
(c) inclusion complex
(d) amylose tetraiodide complex

5. Select the correct statement (s) about glucose
(a) Glucose give glucaric acid when treated with strong Oxidising agents like HNO_3.
(b) With a mild oxidising agent like bromine water, glucose is oxidised to gluconic acid
(c) glucose on reaction with HI/Red P leads to formation of n–hexane & 2 – iodohexane.
(d) All are correct.

6. Glucose, on treatment with excess of phenyl hydrazine, gives –
(a) Glucose hydroxylamine
(b) Osazone
(c) Glucose phenyl hydrazone
(d) Gluconic acid

7. The rapid interconversion of α – D – glucose & β – D – glucose in aqueous solution is known as –
(a) racemization (b) epimerisation
(c) Mutarotation (d) None of these

8. Glucose & mannose are
(a) enantiomers (b) conformers
(c) epimers (d) anomers

9. Which of the following is a non–reducing sugar ?
(a) Maltose (b) Lactose
(c) Glucose (d) Sucrose

10. Maltose consists of –
(a) One β – D glucopyranose & one α – D – galactopyranose units linked by 1, 2 – glycosidic linkage.
(b) One β – D – glucopyranose & one α – D – galactopyranose units linked by 1, 4 – glycosidic linkage
(c) One β – D – Glucopyranose & one β – D – galactopyranose units linked by 1, 4 – glycosidic linkage.
(d) two α – D – glucopyranose units linked by 1, 4 – glycosidic linkage.

11. Cellulose is soluble in –

(a) Organic solvent

(b) water

(c) ammoniacal Cupric hydroxide solution

(d) None of these

12. Biuret test is not given by –

(a) Urea (b) Carbohydrates

(c) Proteins (d) Polypeptides

13. Lactose consists of –

(a) One β – D – glucopyranose and α – D galactopyranose units linked by 1, 2 – glycosidic linkage.

(b) One β – D – glucopyranose and one α – D – galactopyranose units linked by 1, 4 – glycosidic linkage

(c) One β – D – glucopyranose & one β – D – galactopyranose units linked by 1, 4 glycosidic linkage.

(d) One α – D – glucopyranose & one β – D – galactopyranose units linked by 1, 4 – glycosidic linkage

14. Which of the following will form the same osazone when treated with excess of phenylhydrazine.

(a) D–glucose, D – fructose & D – galactose

(b) D – glucose , D – fructose & D – mannose

(c) D – glucose, D – mannose & D – galactose

(d) Both (a) & (c)

15. A disaccharide consisting of two α – D – glucose units in which C_1 of one glucose is linked to C_4 of another glucose unit is –

(a) Maltose (b) Sucrose

(c) Lactose (d) Cellulose

16. Consider the following structure.

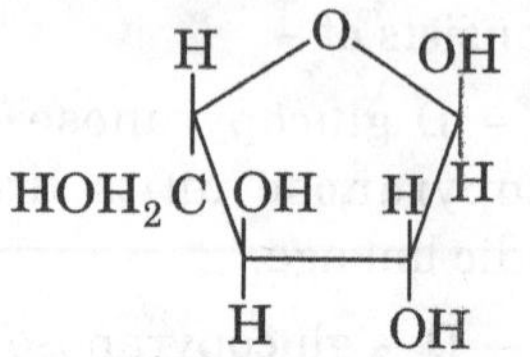

Which set of terms correctly defines the carbohydrate shown ?

(i) Pentose (ii) Hexose

(iii) Aldose (iv) Ketose

(v) Pyranose (vi) Furanose

(a) (i), (iii) & (vi) (b) (i), (iii) & (v)

(c) (ii), (iii) & (v) (d) (i), (iv) & (vi)

17. Amylopectin is water –

(a) Soluble unbranched polymer of α – D – glucose.

(b) Insoluble branched polymer of α – D – glucose.

(c) Soluble branched polymer of α – D – glucose.

(d) Insoluble unbranched polymer of α – D – glucose

18. The corresponding order of names of four aldoses with configuration given below, respectively is –

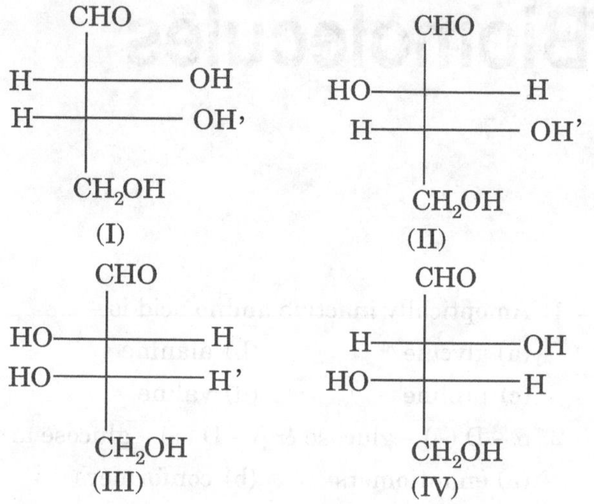

(a) L – erythrose, α – threose, α – erythrose, D – threose

(b) D – threose, L – erythrose, L – threose, D – erythrose

(c) D – erythrose, D – threose, L – erythrose, L –threose

(d) None of these

19. Glucose does not react with–

(a) Br_2 /H_2O

(b) H_2NOH

(c) $CH_3-\overset{\overset{O}{||}}{C}-O-\overset{\overset{O}{||}}{C}-CH_3$

(d) $Na^+HSO_3^-$

20. Fructose reduces tollen's reagent & Fehling's solution, although it does not contain any – CHO group. The rearrangement responsible for this is –

(a) Fries rearrangement

(b) Lossen rearrangement

(c) Curtius rearrangement

(d) Lobry de bruyn van Ekenstein Rearrangement

21. The correct statement about the following disaccharide is –

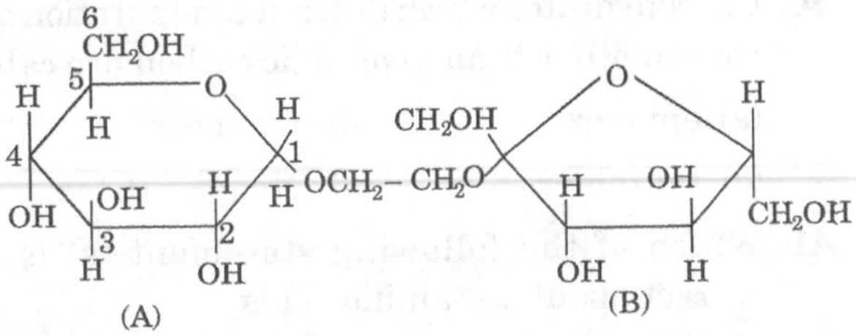

(a) Ring (A) is Pyranose with α – glycosidic linkage

(b) Ring (A) is furanose with α – glycosidic linkage

(c) Ring (B) is furanose with α – glycosidic linkage

(d) Ring (B) is pyranose with α – glycosidic linkage

22. Presence of glucose cannot be tested by –

(a) Silver mirror test

(b) Molisch test

(c) Osazone formation

(d) Ninhydrin solution

23. Same osazone derivative is obtained in case of D-glucose, D–mannose & D–fructose because they–

(a) Have some configuration at C – 5.

(b) Are structural isomers of each other.

(c) Have same configuration at C – 3, C – 4, C – 5 and C – 6 but different functional group and configuration at C – 1 & C – 2

(d) None of these

24. Secondary structure of proteins refers to–

(a) Mainly denaturated proteins and the structure of the prosthetic group

(b) 3 D structure, especially between amino acid residue that are distant from each other in the polypeptide chain.

(c) Linear structure of amino acid residues in the polypeptide chain.

(d) Regular folding patterns of continuos portions of polypeptide chain.

25. Select the wrong statement (s) from the following

(a) Glucose exists in two different crystalline forms, α – D – glucose & β – D – glucose.

(b) α – D – glucose & β – D glucose are enantiomers.

(c) Cellulose is a straight chain polysaccharide made up of only β – D glucose units.

(d) Starch is a mixture of amylase & amylopectin, both contain unbranched chain of α – D – glucose units.

(a) a & b but not c & d

(b) b & c but not a & d

(c) b & d but not a & c

(d) c & d but not a & b

26. Deficiency of vitamin B, causes the disease

(a) sterility (b) Beri – beri

(c) Cheilosis (d) All of these

27. Which of the following bases is NOT present in DNA?

(a) Thymine (b) Cytosine

(c) Quinoline (d) Adenine

28. Which of the following pairs do not give tollen's test ?

(a) Glucose, fructose (b) Glucose, Sucrose

(c) Fructose, Sucrose (d) Both b & c

29. Which of the following monosaccharides are present as five membered cyclic structure ?

(a) Ribose (b) Fructose

(c) Galactose (d) Bothe a & b

30. Hydrolysis of sucrose is called –

(a) Saponification (b) esterification

(c) hydration (d) inversion

31. For an amino acid 'X', isoelectric point is 6.2. Then X is,

(a) acidic amino acid (b) Basic amino acid

(c) neutral amino acid(d) None of these

32. A certain compound gives negative test with ninhydrin & +ve test with Benedict's solution. The compound is –

(a) a protein (b) a mono saccharide

(c) an amino acid (d) both a & c

33. Which of the following is not correct for maltose?

(a) It is a disaccharide

(b) It undergoes mutarotation.

(c) It is reducing sugar

(d) It does not have a hemi–acetal group.

34. Which of the following carbohydrates would be most abundant in the diet of strict vegetarian?

(a) Amylose (b) Glycogen

(c) Cellulose (d) Maltose

35. Consider the given process –

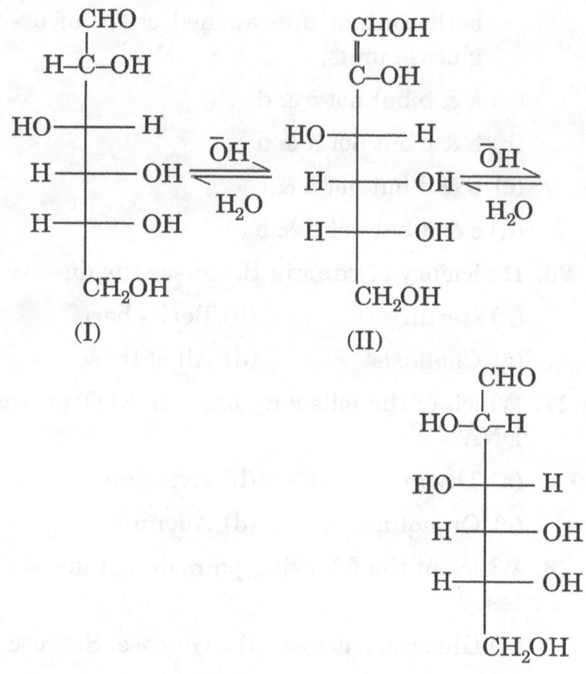

(I) (II) (III)

Identify the correct statement (s)

(a) Configuration at C–2 is lost on enolisation

(b) I & III are epimers.

(d) D – glucose can isomerise to D – fructose through enol intermediate.

(d) All are correct.

36. The pH of the solution containing following zwitter ion species is

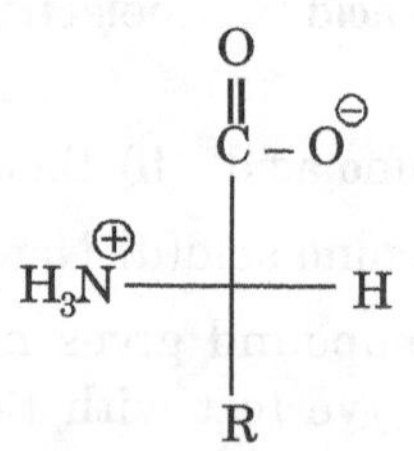

(a) 4 (b) 5

(c) 7 (d) 11

37. A strongly alkaline solution of a monoamino – dicarboxylic acid contains how many basic groups?

(a) 1 (b) 2

(c) 3 (d) 4

38. The total number of stereomers for glucose is are –

(a) 10 (b) 12

(c) 14 (d) 16

39. Select the correct statement.

(a) Maltose forms an osazone.

(b) Galactose is C_4 epimer of glucose

(c) Lactose undergoes mutarotation.

(d) All are correct.

40. Carbohydrates which differ in configuration at any carbon other than glycosidic carbon are called–

(a) epimers (b) anomers

(c) tautomers (d) None of these

41. Which of the following statement (s) is / are correct about α – amino acids

(a) Most naturally occurring amino acids have L – configuration.

(b) Except glycine, all other naturally occurring α – amino acids are optically active.

(c) They are water soluble, high melting solids & behave like salt rather than simple amines & carboxylic acids.

(d) All are true.

42. During denaturation of proteins,

(a) Secondary & tertiary structures are destroyed but primary structure remains intact.

(b) Primary & secondary structures are destroyed but tertiary remains intact.

(c) Primary & tertiary are destroyed but secondary structure remains intact.

(d) None of these occurs.

43. Identify the mismatch

(a) Fibrous protein → Keratin

(b) Globular protein → Haemoglobin

(c) Sucrose $\xrightarrow{\text{Hydrolysis}}$ Glucose + Fructose

(d) None of these

44. Which of the following is correct formula for D – Glyceraldehyde ?

(a) 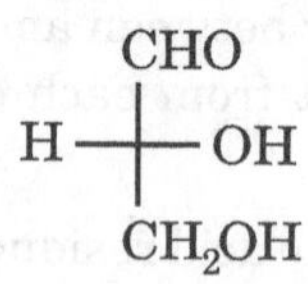 (b) 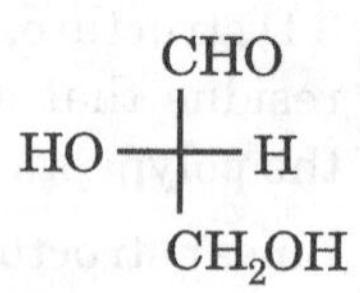

(c) 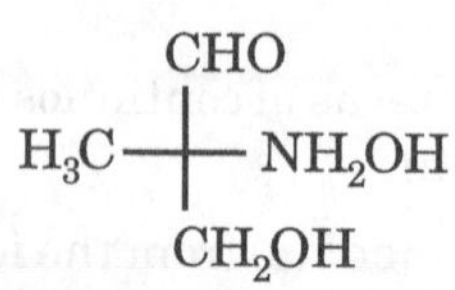 (d) 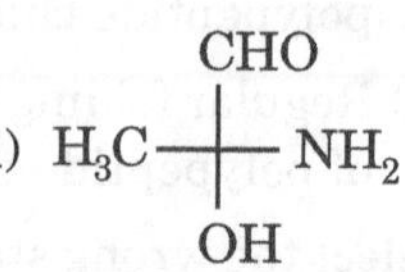

Brain Teasers

45. Sulfa drugs are used as –

(a) Antidiabetics (b) Antibiotic

(c) Anti histamines (d) Analgesic

Answers

1. (a)	**2.** (d)	**3.** (d)	**4.** (c)	**5.** (d)	**6.** (b)	**7.** (c)	**8.** (c)	**9.** (d)	**10.** (d)
11. (c)	**12.** (b)	**13.** (c)	**14.** (b)	**15.** (a)	**16.** (a)	**17.** (b)	**18.** (c)	**19.** (d)	**20.** (d)
21. (a)	**22.** (d)	**23.** (c)	**24.** (d)	**25.** (c)	**26.** (b)	**27.** (c)	**28.** (d)	**29.** (d)	**30.** (d)
31. (c)	**32.** (b)	**33.** (d)	**34.** (c)	**35.** (d)	**36.** (c)	**37.** (c)	**38.** (d)	**39.** (d)	**40.** (a)
41. (d)	**42.** (a)	**43.** (d)	**44.** (a)	**45.** (b)					

Explanations

1. Formula of glycine is NH_2-CH_2-COOH (drawn vertically: NH_2 / CH_2 / COOH)

2.

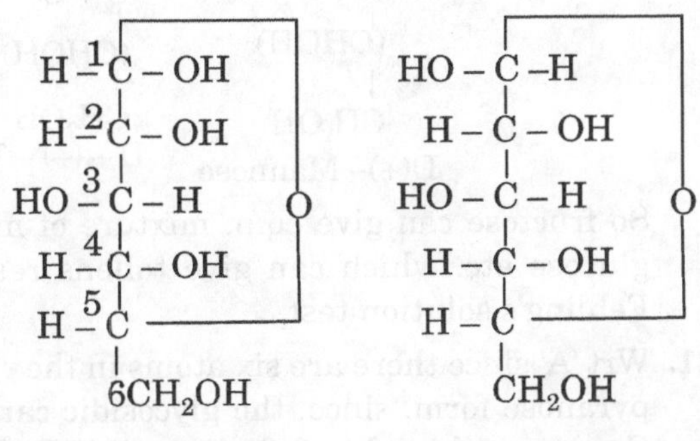

α – D – (+) – Glucose β – D – (+) – Glucose

A pair of stereoisomers which differ in configuration only around C_1 are called anomers & the C_1 carbon is called the anomeric carbon.

5.

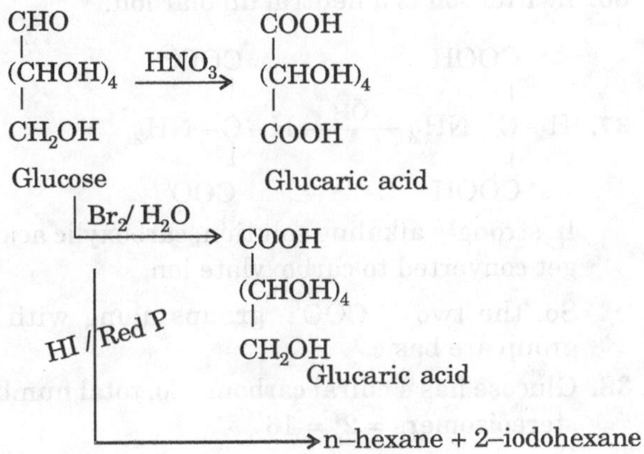

6.

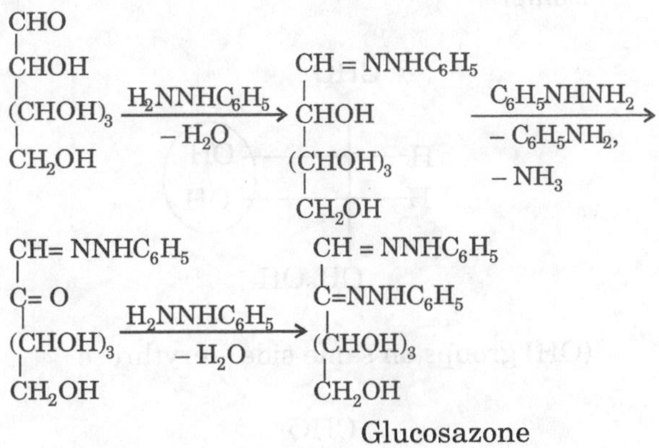

8.

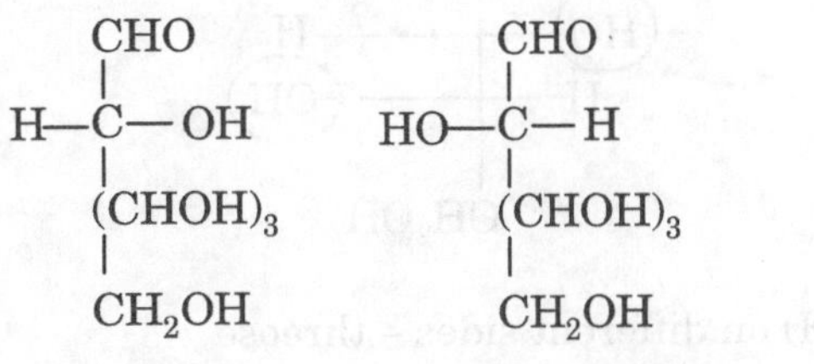

D–(+)–glucose D–(+)–mannose

The stereoisomers which differ in configuration at any carbon except C_1 are called epimers.

10.

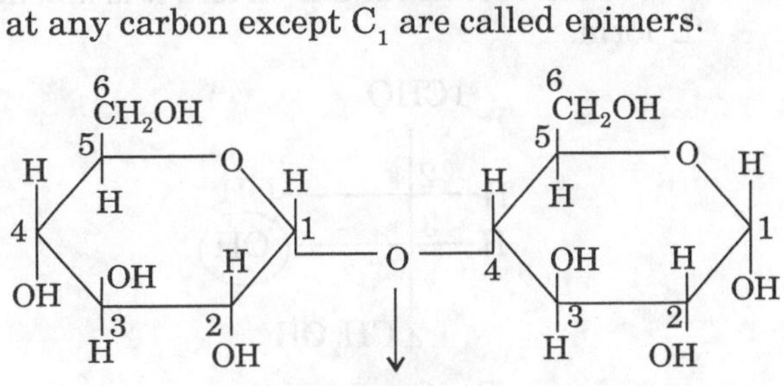

13. In lactose or milk sugar, both glucose & galactose are present in pyranose form. I[st] C of galactose is connected to 4th C of glucose unit, Glucose is reducing half which galactose is not.

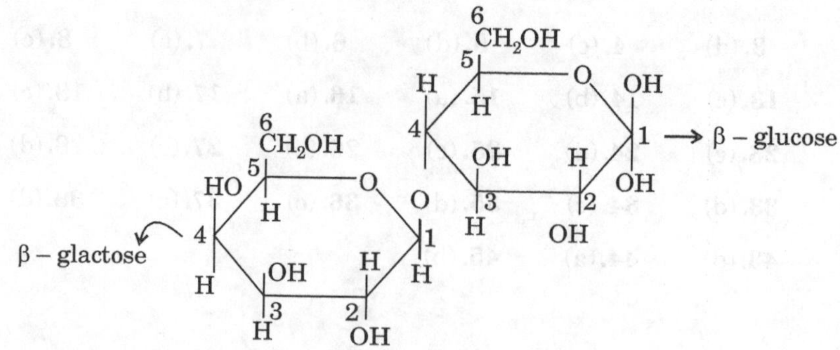

18. The stereoisomers in which the same groups are present on the same side of Fischer projection are called erythro isomers while the stereoisomers in which these groups are present on opposite sides are known as threo isomers

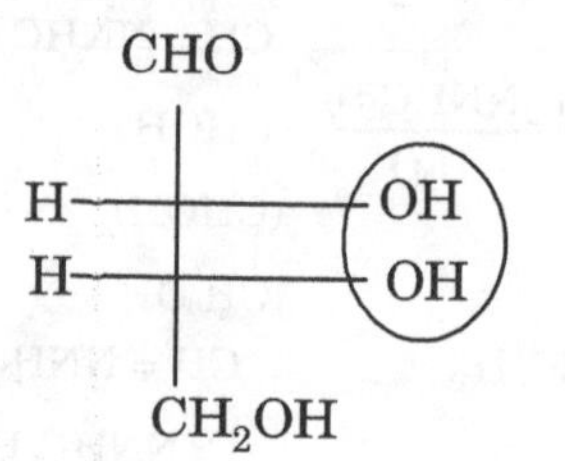

(OH) groups on same side – erythrose

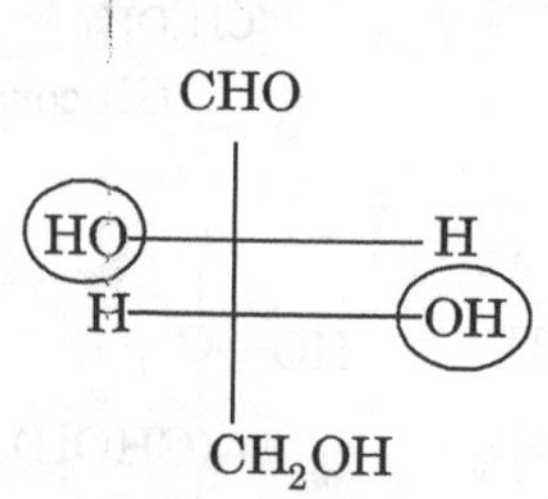

(OH) on different sides – threose

If – OH on the last chiral C is on right side, it is labelled as 'D' form.

If – OH on last chiral C is on left, it is labelled as 'L' form.

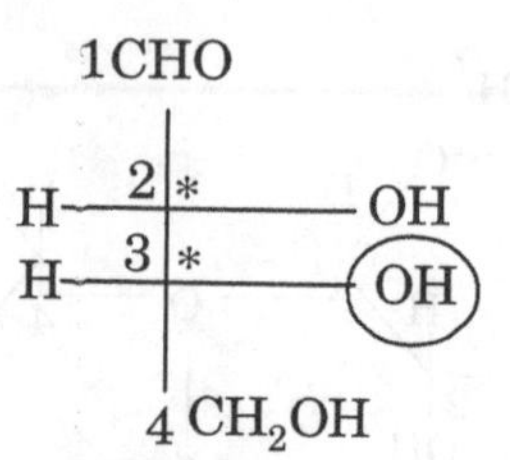

D – Configuration

20. It is as follows –

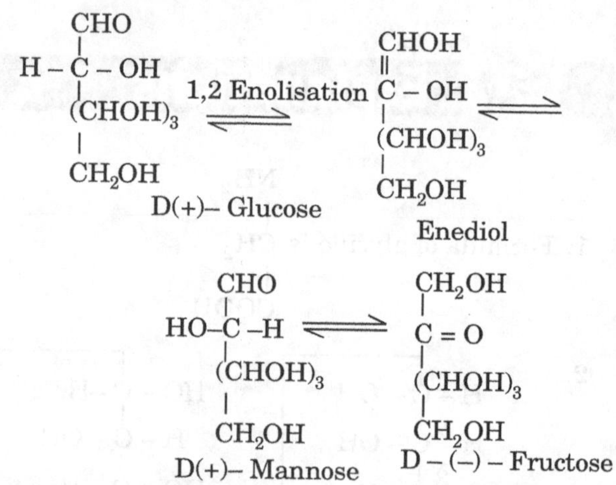

So fructose can give eqm. mixture of mannose, glucose etc. which can give tollens reagent & Fehling's solution test.

21. Wrt 'A' since there are six atoms in the ring, it is pyranose form. since, the glycosidic carbon i.e., C_1 is towards right of 'O' atom, it is D–Series & has OH below the plane in glycosidic carbon. So it is α - glycosidic linkage.

31. At isoelectric point, an amino acid exists as a neutral zwitter ion.

36. Zwitter ion is a neutral dipolar ion.

37. 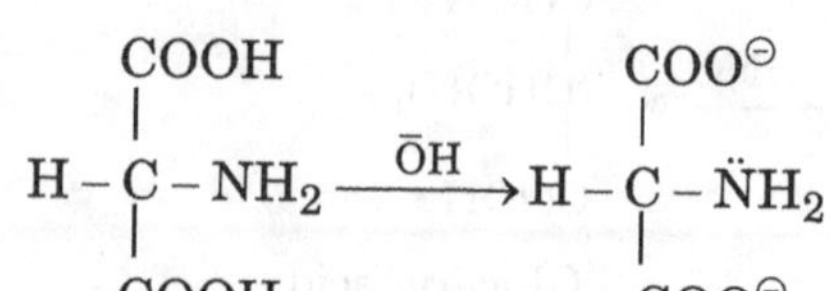

In strongly alkaline solution, carboxylic acid will get converted to carboxylate ion.

So, the two – $COO^{\ominus}$ groups along with $\ddot{N}H_2$ group are basic.

38. Glucose has 4 chiral carbons. So, total number of stereoisomers = $2^4 = 16$

15
CHAPTER

Polymers

1. Which of the following is a condensation polymer?

(a) Polythene (b) PVC

(c) Orlon (d) Terylene

2. Which of the following is NOT an example of Condensation polymer?

(a) Nylon

(b) Bakelite

(c) Urea-formaldehyde resin

(d) Teflon

3. Which of the following is a biodegradable polymer & is a polyester?

(a) Nylon-2-nylon 6

(b) PHBV

(c) Dextron

(d) both (b) & (c)

4. Which one of the following is an example of thermosetting polymer?

(a) $\left(CH_2 - \underset{\underset{Cl}{|}}{C} = CH - CH_2 \right)_n$

(b) $\left(CH_2 - \underset{\underset{Cl}{|}}{CH} \right)_n$

(c) $\left(\overset{\overset{H}{|}}{N} - (CH_2)_6 - \overset{\overset{H}{|}}{N} - \overset{\overset{O}{||}}{C} - (CH_2)_4 - \overset{\overset{O}{||}}{C} \right)_n$

(d)

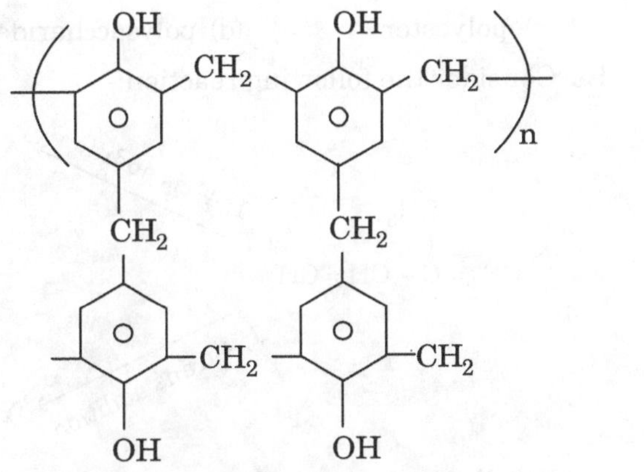

5. BuNa-N synthetic rubber is a copolymer of

(a) $CH_2 = CH - CH = CH_2$ & 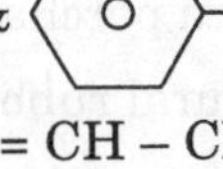 $-CH = CH_2$

(b) $CH_2 = CH - CN$ & $CH_2 = CH - CH = CH_2$

(c) $CH_2 = CH - CN$ & $CH_2 = CH - \underset{\underset{CH_3}{|}}{C} = CH_2$

(d) $CH_2 = CH - \overset{\overset{Cl}{|}}{C} = CH_2$ & $CH_2 = CH - CH = CH_2$

6. A biodegradable polymer which can be produced from glycine & aminocaproic acid is-

(a) buna-N

(b) Nylon-6, 6

(c) nylon -2-nylon-6

(d) PHBV

7. Which of the following monomers has the greatest ability to undergo cationic polymerisation?

(a) 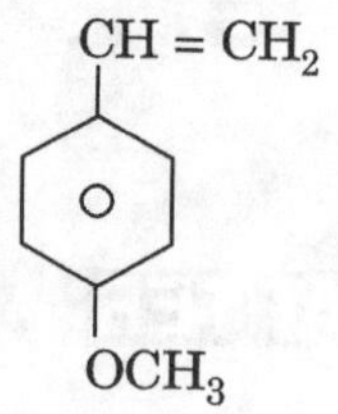

(b) 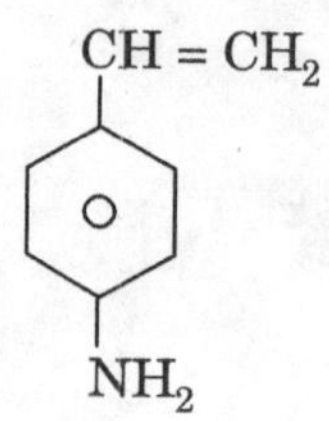

(c) 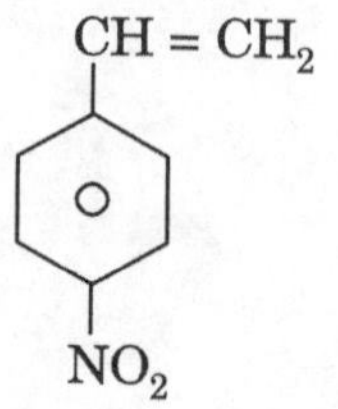

(d) 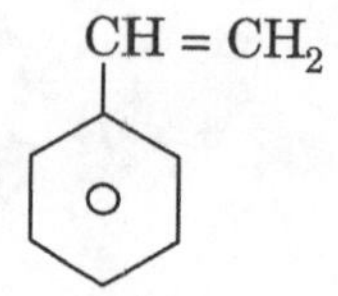

8. Caprolactum is used in the manufacture of-

(a) teflon (b) terylene

(c) nylon-6, 6 (d) nylon-6

9. Nylon is an example of-

(a) polyamide (b) polythene

(c) polyester (d) polysaccharide

10. Consider the following reaction:-

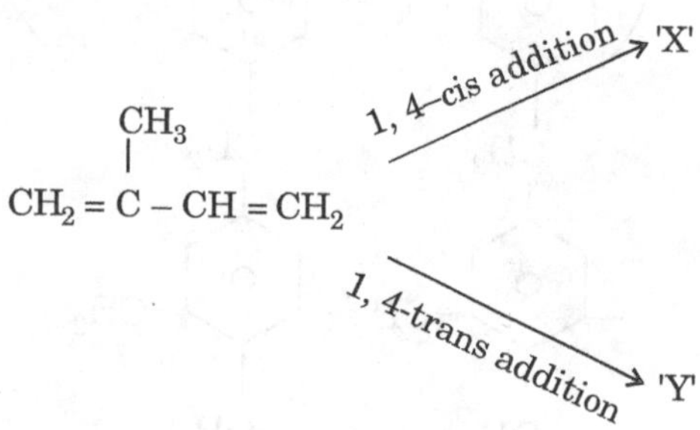

X & Y are, respectively

(a) natural rubber & gutta percha

(b) gutta percha & gutta percha

(c) natural rubber & natural rubber

(d) gutta percha & natural rubber

11. Match the polymer in column A with its main uses in column-B

Column A	**Column B**
A. Polystyrene	i. Paints & lacquers
B. Glyptal	ii. Rain coats
C. Polyvinyl chloride	iii. Manufacture of toys
D. Bakelite	iv. Computer discs

(a) A – ii, B – i, C – iii, D – iv

(b) A – ii, B – iv, C – iii, D – i

(c) A – iii, B – i, C – ii, D – iv

(d) A – iii, B – iv, C – ii, D – i

12. Which of the following sets contain only copolymers?

(a) BuNa-S, Glyptal, Nylon-6, 6

(b) Nylon-6, Neoprene, Bakelite

(c) Polythene, polyester, PVC

(d) Teflon, bakelite, Polythene

13. Plexi glass is commercial name of-

(a) Glyptal (b) Dacron

(c) PMMA (d) Polyacrylonitrile

14. Which of the following is a linear polymer?

(a) Bakelite

(b) Melamine formaldehyde polymer

(c) Nylon

(d) Amylopectin

15. Select the correct statement(s)

(a) Polymers in which the intermolecular forces of attraction between the polymer chains are the weakest are called elastomers.

(b) Examples of elastomers include natural rubber, BuNa-S, BuNa-N

(c) Nylon-6, 6 has H-bonding between the polymeric chains

(d) All are true.

16. Chemical name of melamine is-

(a) 2, 4 diamino-1, 2, 5-triazine

(b) 2-amino – 1, 3, 5-triazine

(c) 3-amino-2, 3, 5,-triazine

(d) 2, 4, 6-Triamino - 1,3,5-Triazine

17. Melamine formaldehyde polymer is also called-

(a) Dacron (b) Glyptal

(c) Melmac (d) PAN

18. Which of the following is not a synthetic polymer?

(a) Polythene (b) BuNa-N

(c) Terylene (d) Cellulose

19. Select the WRONG statement.

(a) Cellulose nitrate & cellulose acetate are semi-synthetic polymers.

(b) Teflon has high thermal stability.

(c) PMMA is used for making lenses.

(d) None of these is wrong.

20. Which of the following is a polymer containing nitrogen?

(a) PVC (b) Bakelite

(c) Nylon-6, 10 (d) Terylene

21. A type of polymer is generally formed from bifunctional & trifunctional monomer & contains very strong covalent bonds between various polymer chains. The polymer may structurally be-

(a) linear polymer

(b) branched chain polymer

(c) cross linked or network polymer

(d) None of these

22. Consider the following polymers-

(i) Polystyrene (ii) Orlon

(ii) Dacron

The above polymers are classified as-

	(i)	(ii)	(iii)
(a)	chain growth	step growth	step growth
(b)	chain growth	chain growth	step growth
(c)	chain growth	step growth	chain growth
(d)	step growth	step growth	step growth

23. Consider the following two reactions-

(a) $CH_3-\underset{|}{\overset{}{CH}}(Cl)-\underset{|}{CH}(Cl)-CH_3 \xrightarrow[\text{(2 moles)}]{\text{alc.KOH}} A$

(b) $H-C\equiv CH + HCN \xrightarrow{Ba(CN)_2} B$

Co-polymerisation of (A) & (B) produces-

(a) BuNa-S

(b) BuNa – N

(c) Neoprene

(d) PAN

24. Identify 'A' in the following reaction sequence-

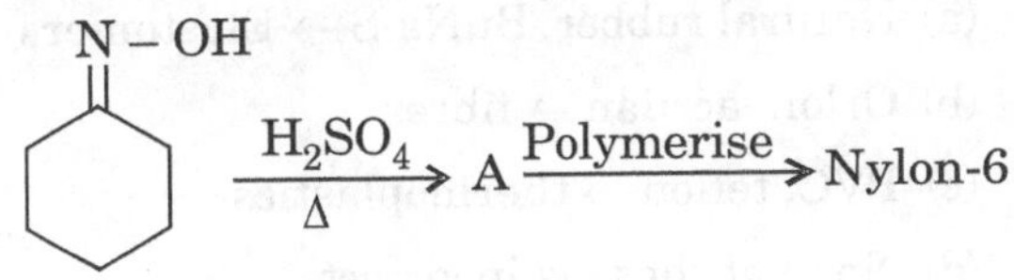

(a) 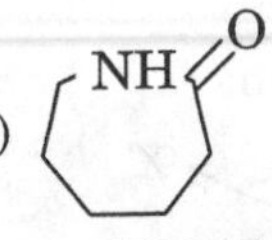 (b) $H_2N-(CH_2)_6-COOH$

(c) 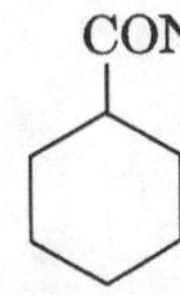 (d) 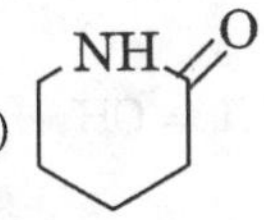

25. Bakelite is a thermosetting polymer formed by condensation of phenol & formaldehyde, by a reaction named-

(a) Lederer - Mannase reaction

(b) Beckmann's Rearrangement

(c) Fries Rearrangement

(d) Curtius reaction

26. Formation of Nylon & polyester is called step growth polymerisation because the-

(a) Polymers are formed by adding a monomer step by step

(b) Polymers are formed by condensation & monomers are joined by loss of simple molecules like water.

(c) Monomers used for condensation are unsaturated molecules.

(d) Polymers are formed by addition of a large number of free radicals formed by monomers.

27. Which of the following is not correctly matched?

	Polymer		Repeating Unit
(a)	Neoprene	→	$\left[CH_2-\underset{\underset{Cl}{|}}{C}=CH-CH_2\right]_n$
(b)	Nylon –6, 6	→	$\left[NH(CH_2)_6NH-\overset{\overset{O}{\|}}{C}-(CH_2)_4-\overset{\overset{O}{\|}}{C}\right]_n$
(c)	Terylene	→	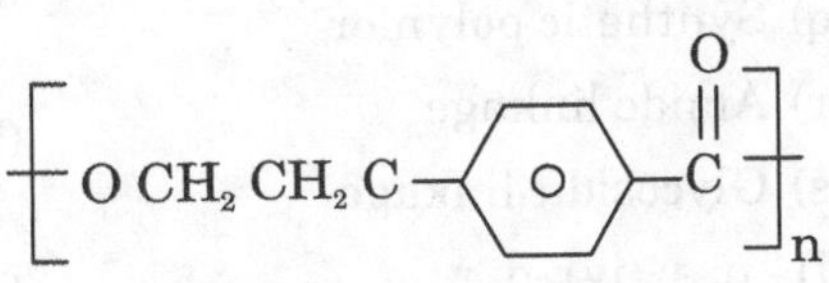
(d)	PMMA	→	$\left[CH_2-\underset{\underset{O=C-OCH_3}{|}}{\overset{\overset{CH_3}{|}}{C}}\right]_n$

28. Select the incorrect match

(a) Natural rubber, BuNa-S → Elastomers

(b) Orlon, acrilan → fibres

(c) PVC, teflon → thermoplastics

(d) None of these is incorrect

29. Consider the following reactions -

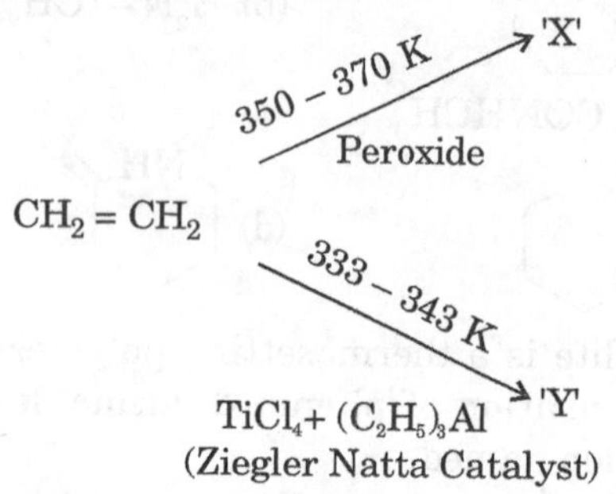

In the above equations,

1. X & Y, both are hard & tough
2. Y has a branched structure & X has a linear structure
3. X is prepared by free radical mechanism & y by co-ordination polymerisation.
4. X is a poor conductor of electricity

(a) Both (1) & (4)

(b) both (2) & (4)

(c) both (3) & (4)

(d) both (1) & (3)

30. Select the correct statement (s).

(a) Crazy glue is a polymer of α-Cyanoacrylate i.e. $CH_2 = C(CN)\ COOCH_3$.

(b) Styrene can undergo anionic polymerisation.

(c) Kevlar is a polyamide & is used to make light weight bullet proof vests.

(d) All are correct.

31. Select the correct match.

Column-I (Polymer)	**Column - II** (Characteristics)
(i) Protein	(p) Natural polymer
(ii) Starch	(q) Synthetic polymer
(iii) Cellulose	(r) Amide linkage
(iv) Nylon-6, 6	(s) Glycosidic linkage

(a) (i) - p, r; (ii) - p, s; (iii) - p, s; (iv) -q, r

(b) (i) - p, s; (ii) - q, p; (iii) - p, r; (iv) -q, s

(c) (i) - q, s; (ii) - q, r; (iii) - p, q; (iv) -r, s

(d) None of these

32. Which of the following statements is/are false?

(a) Natural rubber has trans-configuration at every double bond.

(b) BuNa-S is a Co-polymer of butadiene & styrene.

(c) Natural rubber is a 1,4-polymer of isoprene

(d) All are false.

33. Which one of the bimolecules is not a polymer?

(a) Glycogen

(b) Sucrose

(c) Haemoglobin

(d) DNA

34. Which of the following is not a cross-linked polymer?

(a) Vulcanised rubber

(b) Bakelite

(c) BuNa-S

(d) All of these

35. If 'C' is a polymer & all the products are major products in the following reaction sequences, then correct options is/are-

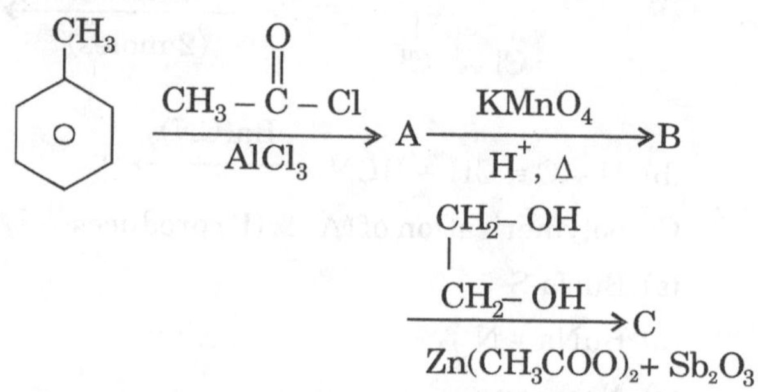

(a) 'B' is soluble in aq. $NaHCO_3$

(b) 'A' will give haloform reaction.

(c) Formation of 'C' is step growth polymerisation.

(d) All are correct

36. The correct functional group 'X' and the reagent/reaction conditions 'Y' in the following scheme are-

$$X-(CH_2)_4-X \xrightarrow[\text{(ii)}HOOC-(CH_2)_4-COOH]{\text{(i)}Y}$$

Condensation polymer

(a) $X = COOCH_3,\ Y = \dfrac{H_2}{Ni/\Delta}$

(b) $X = CONH_2,\ Y = \dfrac{Br_2}{NaOH}$

(c) $X = CN,\ Y = \dfrac{H_2}{Ni/\Delta}$

(d) both (b) & (c)

37. Arrange the following polymers in correct order of their intermolecular forces.

Nylon-6, 6;	BuNa-S;	Polythene
(I)	(II)	(III)

(a) I > III > II (b) I > II > III
(c) III > I > II (d) III > II > I

38. Select the incorrect statement.
(a) Nylon 6 is used to prepare mountaineering ropes.
(b) Glyptal is used to prepare paints & lacquers.
(c) Gutta percha is used in dentistry.
(d) None of these

39. Which of the following can be used as initiator in free radical addition polymerisation?
(a) H_2O_2
(b) Cumyl hydroperoxide

$$\left(C_6H_5-\underset{CH_3}{\overset{CH_3}{\underset{|}{\overset{|}{C}}}}-O-OH\right)$$

(c) Dibenzoyl peroxide
(d) All of these

40. Which of the following alkenes cannot undergo cationic polymerisation?
(a) $CH_2=CH-CH_3$ (b) $C_6H_5-CH=CH_2$
(c) $CH_2=CH-CN$ (d) All of these

41. What is correct about Vulcanisation of rubber?
(a) Vulcanisation leads to formation of sulphur bridges between the chains.
(b) It makes the rubber hard & stiff.
(c) Additives like ZnO are used to increase the rate of Vulcanisation.
(d) All are correct.

42. What is true about PMMA?
(a) Its complete name is Polymethyl methacrylate.
(b) Its alternative name is plexiglass or perspex.
(c) It has excellent light transmission properties, even better than glass.
(d) All are true.

43. Select the correct match.

Polymer		Category
(a) Nylon-6, 6	→	Polyamide
(b) Glyptal	→	Polyester
(c) BuNa-S	→	Polydiene
(d) Polystyrene	→	Polyacrylate

44. Select the WRONG statement.
(a) Bakelite is a cross-linked polymer.
(b) Novolac is a linear polymer.
(c) Nomex is a polyamide formed from benzoic acid & aniline.
(d) All are wrong

45. The initiator most often used in cationic polymerisation is-
(a) BF_3
(b) $AlCl_3$
(c) H_2SO_4
(d) All of these

46. Select the correct statement.
(a) All polymers are macromolecules but all macromolecules are not polymers.
(b) Dacron & Bakelite are copolymers.
(c) Starch is a homopolymer
(d) All are correct.

Brain Teasers

47. Which of the following is NOT TRUE ?
(a) Nylon –2 Nylon – 6 → Biodegradable polymer
(b) Dacron → Polyester
(c) Buna – S → Elastomer
(d) Bakelite → Homopolymer

48. What is the similarity between Buna N & PHBV?
(a) Both are copolymers
(b) Both are biodegradable.
(c) Both have at least one monomeric unit same.
(d) Peroxide is used as catalyst in their preparation

Answers

1. (d)	2. (d)	3. (d)	4. (d)	5. (b)	6. (c)	7. (b)	8. (d)	9. (a)	10. (a)
11. (c)	12. (a)	13. (c)	14. (c)	15. (d)	16. (d)	17. (c)	18. (d)	19. (d)	20. (c)
21. (c)	22. (b)	23. (b)	24. (a)	25. (a)	26. (b)	27. (c)	28. (d)	29. (c)	30. (d)
31. (a)	32. (a)	33. (b)	34. (c)	35. (d)	36. (d)	37. (a)	38. (d)	39. (d)	40. (c)
41. (d)	42. (d)	43. (d)	44. (c)	45. (d)	46. (d)	47. (d)	48. (a)		

Explanations

1. Terylene is a condensation polymer of terephthalic acid & ethylene glycol.

2. Teflon is an addition polymer.

3. PHBV is Poly-β-hydroxybutyrate-co-β-hydroxy valerate. It is formed by condensation of 3-hydroxy butanoic acid & 3-hydroxy pentanoic acid.

The two monomers are connected by ester linkages.

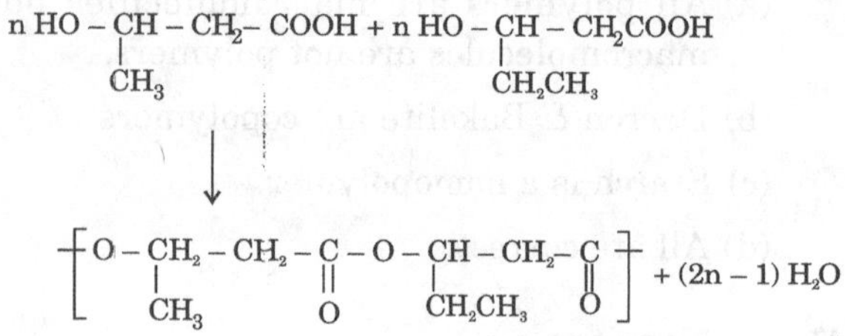

Dextron is Poly (glycollic acid) Poly (lactic acid).

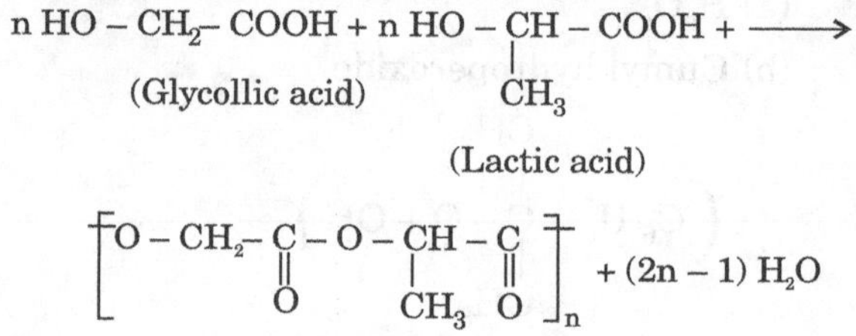

Dextron

4. Option (d) is BAKELITE which is a thermosetting polymer.

7. In cationic polymerisation, carbocation is the reaction intermediate. So, greater the stability of carbocation, greater is the reactivity towards cationic polymerisation.

Out of all the molecules given $-NH_2$ will exert maximum +R & make the carbocation extremely stable.

10.

$$nCH_2=\underset{|}{\overset{CH_3}{C}}-CH=CH_2 \xrightarrow{\text{Polymerisation}} -\!\!(CH_2-\overset{CH_3}{C}=CH-CH_2)\!\!-_n$$

(Polyisoprene)

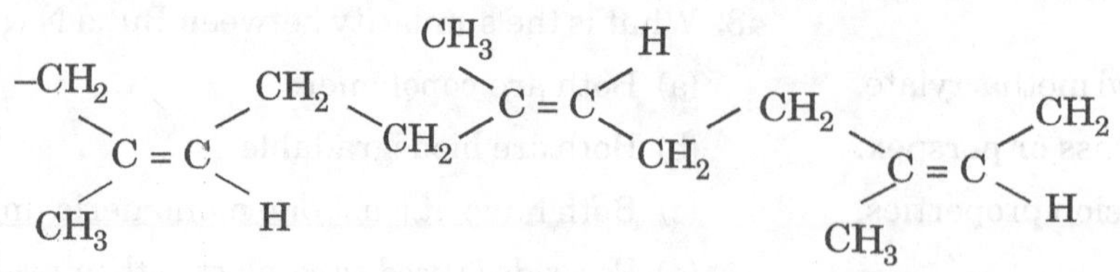

Cis-polyisoprene (Natural rubber)

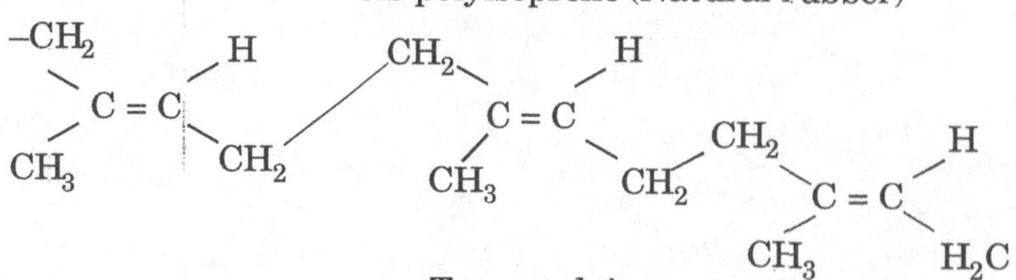

Trans-polyisoprene
(Gutta percha)

12. BuNa-S is made from buta-1, 3-diene & styrene.

Glyptal is made from Ethylene glycol & Phthalic acid.

Nylon-6, 6 is made from hexamethylene diamine & adipic acid.

14. Bakelite & melamine formaldehyde polymer are cross linked polymers.

Amylopectin is branched chain polymer.

Nylon is a linear polymer.

15. Wrt option-c

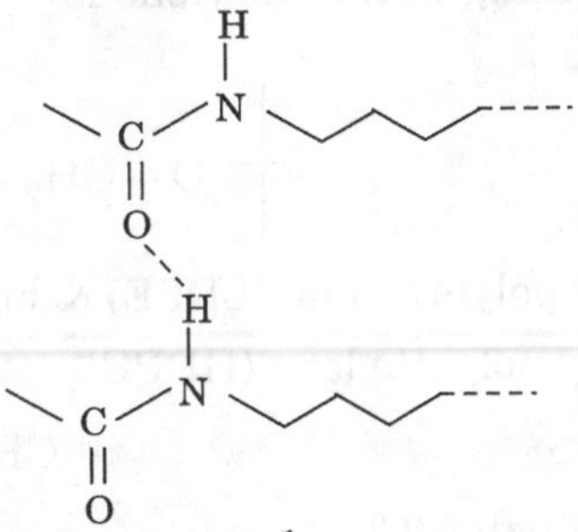

16.

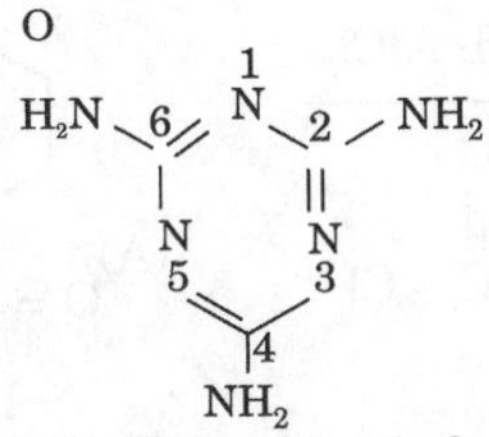

2, 4, 6 - Triamino- 1, 3, 5-triazine

20. $$nH_2N-(CH_2)_6-NH_2 + nHOOC-(CH_2)_8-COOH \xrightarrow{\Delta}$$

Hexamethylenediamine   Sebacic acid

$$\left[NH-(CH_2)_6-NH-\overset{\overset{O}{\|}}{C}-(CH_2)_8-\overset{\overset{O}{\|}}{C} \right]_n + (2n-1)\,H_2O$$

Nylon-6, 10

23. (a) $$CH_3-\underset{\underset{Cl}{|}}{CH}-\underset{\underset{Cl}{|}}{CH}-CH_3 \xrightarrow[\text{(2 moles)}]{\text{alc.KOH}} \underset{(A)}{CH_2=CH-CH=CH_2}$$

(b) $$H-C\equiv C-H + HCN \xrightarrow{Ba(CN)_2} \underset{(B)}{CH_2=CH-CN}$$

Now, co-polymerisation of buta-1, 3-diene & vinyl cyanide will result in formation of BuNa–N.

24.

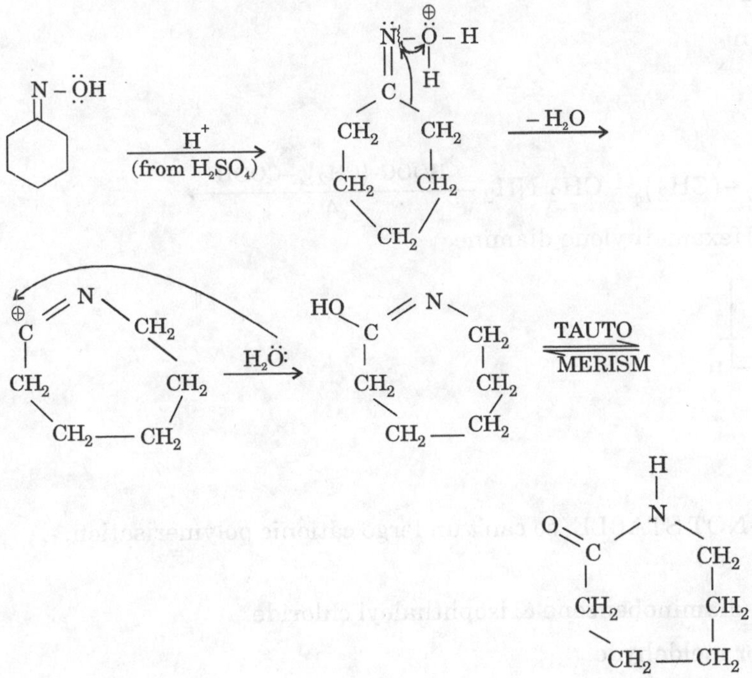

Caprolactum

27. The correct repeating unit of terylene is-

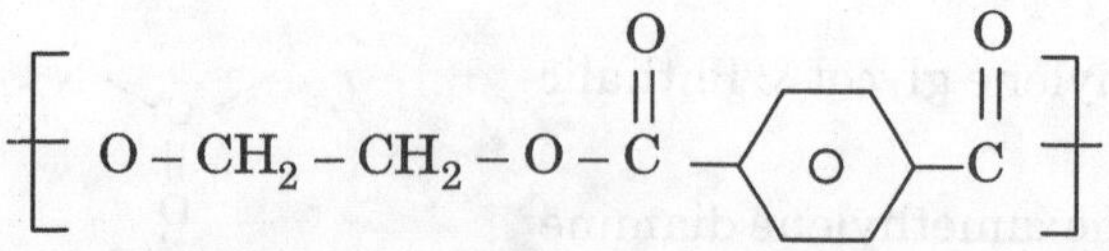

29. 'X' is low density polyethylene (LDPE) & here polymerisation occurs by free radical mechanism.
'Y' is high density polyethylene (HDPE)

35.

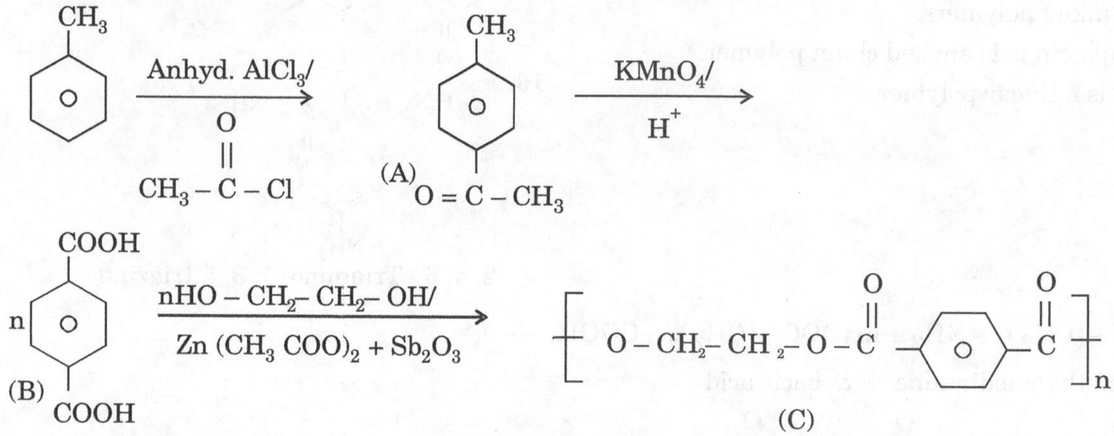

(Terephthalic acid) (Terylene)

36. Wrt option b; if X = $CONH_2$.

$$H_2N-\overset{O}{\overset{\|}{C}}-(CH_2)_4-\overset{O}{\overset{\|}{C}}-NH_2 \xrightarrow[\text{Hoffmann's Bromamide}]{1)\ Br_2/NaOH}$$

$$H_2N-(CH_2)_4-NH_2 \xrightarrow{HOOC-(CH_2)_4-COOH}$$

$$\left[NH-(C_2H_4)-NH-\overset{O}{\overset{\|}{C}}(C_2H_4)-\overset{O}{\overset{\|}{C}} \right]_n$$

Nylon-4, 6

Wrt option c
if X = CN

$$CN-(CH_2)_4-CN \xrightarrow[\Delta]{H_2/Ni} H_2NCH_2-(CH_2)_4-CH_2\,NH_2 \xrightarrow[\Delta]{HOOC-(CH_2)_4-COOH}$$

Hexamethylene diamine

$$\left[NH-(CH_2)_6-NH-\overset{O}{\overset{\|}{C}}-(CH_2)_4-\overset{O}{\overset{\|}{C}} \right]_n$$

Nylon-6, 6

37. Nylon-6, 6 > Polythene > BuNa-S
(Fibres) (Plastic) (elastomer)

40. Carbocation formed in vinyl cyanide is NOT STABLE, so can't undergo cationic polymerisation.

43. Polystyrene is a polyolefin.

44. Nomex is formed by condensation of m-diaminobenzene & isophthaloyl chloride.

47. Bakelite is a Co-polymer of phenol & for meldehyde.

16

CHAPTER

Chemistry in Everyday Life

1. Which of the following is/are antacids?
   (a) Omeprazole
   (b) Lansoprazole
   (c) Ranitidine
   (d) All of these
2. The drugs which are used for the treatment of mental diseases are called-
   (a) Analgesics
   (b) Tranquilizers
   (c) Antibiotics
   (d) Disinfectants
3. Dettol is-
   (a) an analgesic and a mixture of Bithional & boric acid.
   (b) an antiseptic and is a mixture of chloroxylenol & α-terpineol.
   (c) an analgesic and a mixture of chlorhexidine & H_2O_2.
   (d) None of these
4. Which of the following is employed as antihistamine?
   (a) Omeprazole
   (b) Chloramphenicol
   (c) Diphenylhydramine
   (d) Norethindrone
5. Which one of the following is a Tranquilizer?
   (a) Mifepristone
   (b) Promethazine
   (c) Valium
   (d) Naproxen
6. Which of the following is a NARCOTIC ANALGESIC?
   (a) Paracetamol
   (b) Aspirin
   (c) Codeine
   (d) Zantac
7. Bithional, added to soaps is-
   (a) an antiseptic
   (b) a softner
   (c) a drying agent
   (d) a buffering agent
8. Aspirin acts as analgesic because it-
   (a) inhibits the synthesis of prostaglandins which stimulate the inflammation of tissue.
   (b) prevents the release of HCl in the stomach.
   (c) prevents the interaction of histamine with its receptor.
   (d) inhibits activities of enzymes.

9. The sweetest artificial sugar is-

(a) alitame (b) sucrose

(c) sucrolose (d) aspartame

10. Which of the following is/are bacteriostatic antibiotics?

(a) Penicillin (b) Erythromycin

(c) Tetracycline (d) Both b & c

11. Antiseptics & disinfectants either kill or prevent the growth of microorganisms. Then, select the WRONG statement.

(a) Disinfectants harm the living tissues.

(b) A 0.2% solution of phenol is an antiseptic while 1% solution acts a disinfectant.

(c) Chlorine & iodine are strong disinfectants.

(d) Very dilute solutions of Boric acid & H_2O_2 are strong antiseptics.

12. Which one of the following acids have –COOH group?

(a) Picric acid

(b) Barbituric acid

(c) Ascorbic acid

(d) Aspirin

13. Select the correct statement(s).

(a) Sodium 4-(dodecyl) benzene sulphonate is an anionic detergent.

(b) Soaps cannot work in acidic medium as they react with acidic solutions to form insoluble fatty acids.

(c) Promethazine is an antihistamine.

(d) all are correct.

14. Which of the following is/are preservatives?

(a) Sodium benzoate

(b) Sodium metabisulphite ($Na_2S_2O_5$)

(c) Sorbic acid & its salts

(d) All of these

15. Select the WRONG statement.

(a) Soframycin & furacin are antiseptic creams.

(b) Tincture of iodine is a 2-3% solution of iodine in alcohol & water.

(c) Iodoform is an antiseptic

(d) Disinfectants can be applied to the living tissues.

16. Equanil is-

(a) an artificial sweetner

(b) a tranquilizer

(c) an antihistamine

(d) an antifertility drug

17. Which of the following is a narrow spectrum antibiotic?

(a) Rifampicin

(b) Penicillin G

(c) Chloramphenicol

(d) Chloromycetin

18. Select the correct statement (s).

(1) Aspirin and paracetamol are non-narcotic analgesics.

(2) Morphine is a narcotic analgesic.

(3) Iproniazide & phenelzine are tranquilizers.

(4) Chlordiazepoxide & meprobamate are non-hypnotic tranquilizers.

(5) Equanil is used to treat depression & hypertension.

(a) Only 1 & 2 are correct

(b) Only 3, 4 & 5 are correct

(c) Only 3 & 4 are correct

(d) all are correct

19. Select the INCORRECT statement(s).

(a) Broad spectrum antibiotics like Chloramphenicol & vancomycin are effective against different types of gram +ve & gram –ve bacteria.

(b) Narrow spectrum antibiotics like penicillin G are effective mainly against gram +ve or gram –ve bacteria.

(c) Limited spectrum antibiotics like Rifampicin are effective against a single organism.

(d) Sulpha drugs are widely used now-a-days.

20. Choose the incorrect match.

(a) Potassium metabisulphite or SO_2 → used for preservation of colorless food material.

(b) Aspartame → is unstable to heat & therefore, can be used in cold drinks & cold food only.

(c) Sucralose → is stable at cooking temperature.

(d) Aspartame → more stable to heat than alitame.

21. Which of the following is linear alkyl sulphonates?

(a) 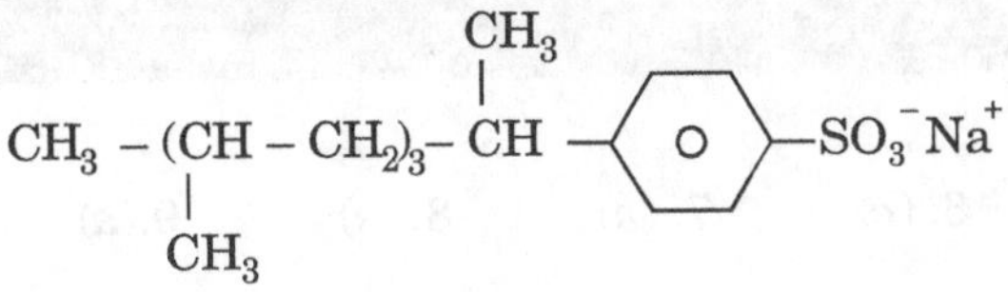

(b) 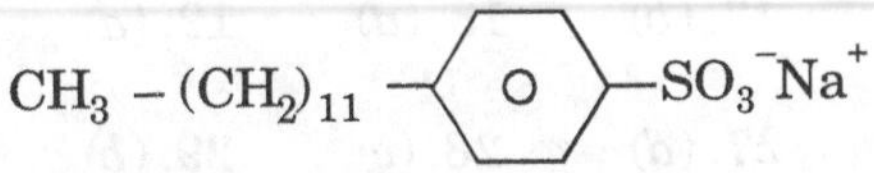

(c) $CH_3(CH_2)_{16}COO(CH_2CH_2O)_n CH_2CH_2OH$

(d) Both (a) & (c)

22. Which of the following statement is correct about Aspirin?

(a) Its alternative name is 2-Acetoxy benzoic acid.

(b) It finds its use in prevention of heart attacks as it has anti blood clotting action.

(c) It should not be taken empty stomach because on hydrolysis it gives salicylic acid which causes bleeding in stomach.

(d) All are correct

23. Soaps cannot be used in hard water since-

(a) it does not interact with Ca^{2+} & Mg^{2+}.

(b) it is soft.

(c) they interact with Ca^{2+} & Mg^{2+} to form scum (white precipitates)

(d) None of these

24. Reserpine, an alkaloid, found in plant Rauwolfia serpentina, is used in treatment of

(a) mental disorder (b) urticaria

(c) hypertension (d) both (a) and (b)

25. An example of antifertility drug is-

(a) Norethindrone (b) Ranitidine

(c) Analgin (d) Phenacitin.

26. The correct structure of 'PARACETAMOL' is-

(a) 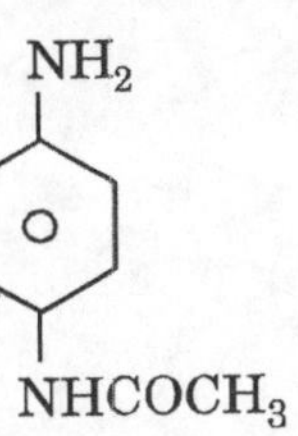

(b) 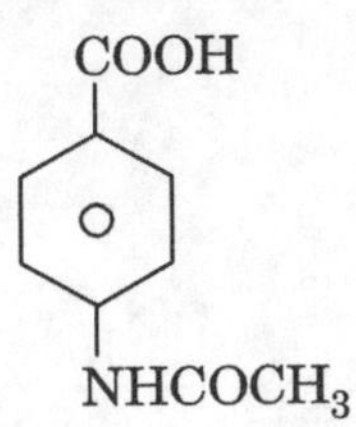

(c) 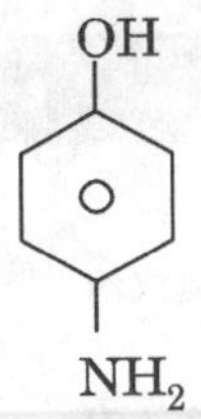

(d) 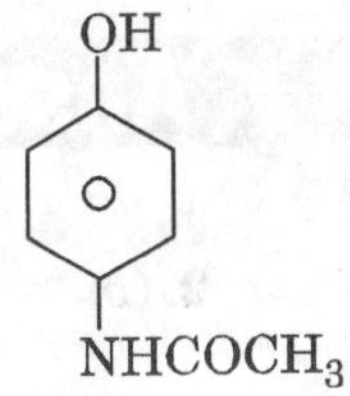

27. Which of the following is correct structure of a sulpha drug?

(a) 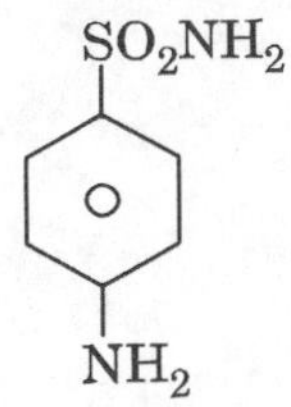

(b) 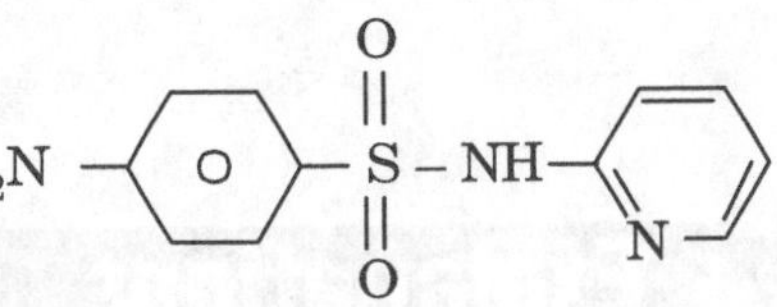

(c) 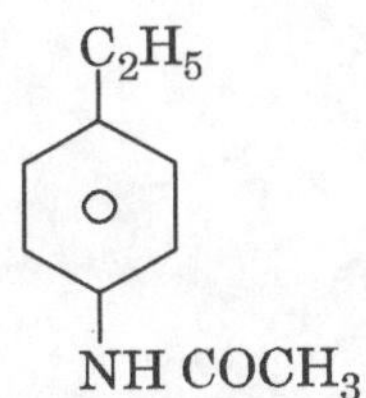

(d) Both (a) & (b)

28. Structure of veronal has-

(a) one methyl group & one ethyl group.

(b) two methyl groups

(c) two ethyl groups

(d) one ethyl & one phenyl group.

29. Drug that binds to receptor site & inhibits its natural function is called-

(a) agonist (b) antagonist

(c) inhibitor (d) All of these

30. Which of the following has maximum sweetness value?

(a) Alitame

(b) Sucralose

(c) Saccharin

(d) Aspartame

Answers

1. (*d*)	2. (*b*)	3. (*b*)	4. (*c*)	5. (*c*)	6. (*c*)	7. (*a*)	8. (*a*)	9. (*a*)	10. (*d*)
11. (*d*)	12. (*d*)	13. (*d*)	14. (*d*)	15. (*d*)	16. (*b*)	17. (*b*)	18. (*d*)	19. (*d*)	20. (*d*)
21. (*b*)	22. (*d*)	23. (*c*)	24. (*c*)	25. (*a*)	26. (*d*)	27. (*d*)	28. (*c*)	29. (*b*)	30. (*a*)

Explanations

12.

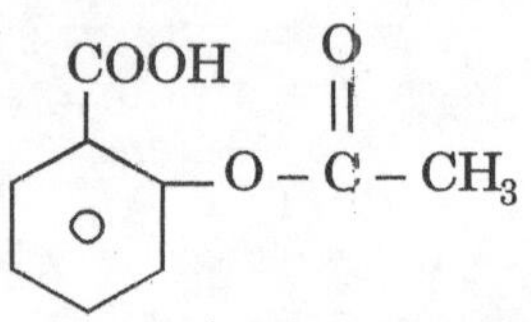

Aspirin

20. Alitame is more stable to heat than aspartame.

28.

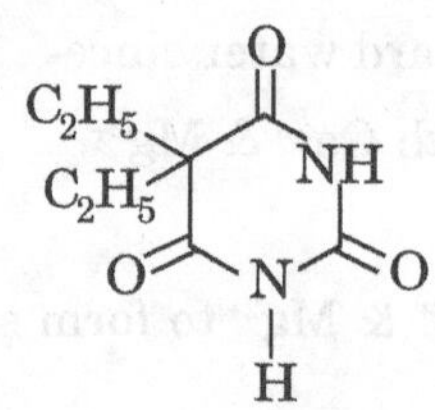

Veronal

Alitame > Sucralose > Saccharin > Aspartame